SAUNDERS

PHARMACEUTICAL WORD BOOK

2002

ELLEN DRAKE, CMT
RANDY DRAKE, BS

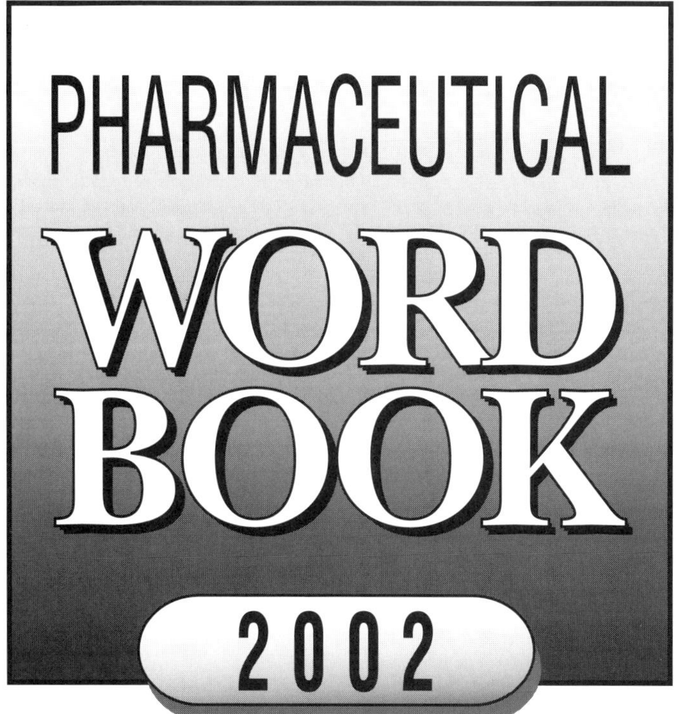

W.B. SAUNDERS COMPANY
Philadelphia London New York St. Louis Sydney Toronto

W.B. SAUNDERS COMPANY

The Curtis Center
Independence Square West
Philadelphia, Pennsylvania 19106

www.wbsaunders.com

NOTICE

We have carefully checked the generic and trade names, approved indications and uses, and dosages of pharmaceuticals appearing in this book. Medicine is an ever-changing field, however, and the information listed here may have changed since its publication. Although we have made every attempt to include as much necessary information as possible, we have by no means tried to provide *prescribing information* as defined by the FDA. The given uses and actions for a particular drug are not all-inclusive, and the indications, contraindications, and side effects are not listed. Physicians should consult the package insert or some other acceptable source for prescribing information.

Herbal and natural remedies are also listed in this book. The indications and uses listed are the historical or traditional uses of the remedy. In most cases, the efficacy of a remedy for a particular indication has been neither proved nor disproved by modern scientific methods. Some of the plants used in herbal remedies are poisonous and may cause illness or death if not properly prepared and used. Therefore, both the authors and the publisher disclaim responsibility for the use or misuse of any information contained herein.

SAUNDERS PHARMACEUTICAL WORD BOOK 2002 ISBN 0–7216–9684–8

ISSN 1072–7779

Printed in the United States of America.

Last digit is the print number: 9 8 7 6 5 4 3 2 1

To the Lord Jesus

Oh, sing to the Lord a new song!
For He has done marvelous things;
His right hand and His holy arm
  have gained Him the victory.
The Lord has made known His salvation;
His righteousness He has revealed
  in the sight of the nations.
He has remembered His mercy
  and His faithfulness
  to the house of Israel;
All the ends of the earth have seen
  the salvation of our God.

Shout joyfully to the Lord, all the earth;
Break forth in song, rejoice, and sing praises.
Sing to the Lord with the harp,
With the harp and the sound of a psalm,
With trumpets and the sound of a horn;
Shout joyfully before the Lord, the King.

— Psalm 98:1–6

Contents

Preface

This edition marks the tenth anniversary of the *Saunders Pharmaceutical Word Book*. Many changes have occurred in this reference over the past decade. It has grown from 18,740 entries on 369 pages in 1993 to 26,498 entries on 693 pages this year. By popular request, dosages were added to brand-name drugs in 1996 and to generic drugs in 1997. Our appendix of sound-alikes, which was unique in the profession in our first edition, was expanded and the appropriate sound-alikes were added to individual entries in 1997. A milestone was achieved in 1998 with the inclusion of over 25,000 entries. Over 1800 medicinal herbs and natural remedies were added in 1999, and the 20th century ended with the introduction of a companion book, *Saunders Pharmaceutical XRef Book*, in 2000.

In January 2001 we launched a new web site—**spwb.saunders.net**—to provide free monthly updates for our readers. In the first ten months, 579 new and updated entries were posted to our web site. (All of those additions and changes and much, much more have been incorporated into this edition.) This year we have added hundreds of Canadian brands to the book, and The Most Prescribed Drugs appendix also includes the drugs most prescribed in Canada. As always, brands available in Canada but not in the United States are designated by the (CAN) symbol.

Through all of the changes, however, some things have remained the same. We are still dedicated to bringing you the most accurate, well-researched drug reference available. We still value and respond to your feedback and suggestions. And yes, we still do all of the work personally—from the annual edition, to the monthly web updates, to answering your letters and e-mails.

We welcome your comments regarding additions, inconsistencies, or inaccuracies in either this book or its companion, *Saunders Pharmaceutical XRef Book*. Please send them to us via e-mail at the address below, or via regular mail to W.B. Saunders Company, The Curtis Center, Independence Square West, Philadelphia, PA 19106-3399.

Authors' e-mail address:
spwb@saunders.net
Authors' web site:
spwb.saunders.net

ELLEN DRAKE, CMT
RANDY DRAKE, BS
Atlanta, Georgia

Notes on Using the Text

The purpose of the *Saunders Pharmaceutical Word Book* is to provide medical transcriptionists (as well as medical records administrators and technicians, coders, nurses, ward clerks, court reporters, legal secretaries, medical assistants, allied health students, physicians, and even pharmacists) with a quick, easy-to-use reference that gives not only the correct spellings and capitalizations of drugs, but the designated uses of those drugs, the cross-referencing of brand names to generics, and the usual methods of administration (e.g., capsule, IV, cream). The indication of the preferred nonproprietary (generic) names and the agencies adopting these names (e.g., USAN, USP) should be particularly useful to those writing for publication. The reader will also find various trademarked or proprietary names (e.g., Spansule, Dosepak) that are not drugs but are closely associated with the packaging or administration of drugs.

There are four different ways to refer to drugs. One of these ways is not by the name of the drug itself but by the class to which it belongs—aminoglycosides, for example. Inexperienced transcriptionists sometimes confuse these classes with the names of drugs. We have included some 200 drug classes in the main list, with a brief description of the therapeutic use and/or method of action common to drugs in the class. Beyond a class description, each drug has three names. The first is the *chemical name*, which describes its chemical composition and how the molecules are arranged. It is often long and complex, sometimes containing numbers, Greek letters, italicized letters, and hyphens between elements. This name is rarely used in dictation except in research hospitals and sometimes in the laboratory section when the blood or urine is examined for traces of the drug. The second name for a drug is the *nonproprietary* or *generic name*. This is a name chosen by the discovering manufacturer or agency and submitted to a nomenclature committee (the United States Adopted Names Council, for example). The name is simpler than the chemical name but often reflects the chemical entity. It is arrived at by using guidelines provided by the nomenclature committee—beta-blockers must end in "olol," for example—and must be unique. There is increasing emphasis on the adoption of the same nonproprietary name by various nomenclature committees worldwide (see the list on page xiii). The third name for a drug is the *trade* or *brand name*. There may be several trade names for the same generic drug, each marketed by a different company. These are the ones that are highly advertised, and sometimes have unusual capitalization. An interesting article on the naming of drugs is "Pharmaceutical Nomenclature: The Lawless Language" in *Perspectives on the Medical Transcription Profession*.[1] *Understanding Pharmacology*[2] also discusses the naming of drugs.

We have included many foreign names of drugs for our Canadian friends, and also because we have so many visitors to the United States from other countries (and they get sick, too). The international and British spellings of generic drugs are cross-referenced to the American spellings, and vice versa. Occasionally there will be three different spellings—one American, one international, and another British—which are all cross-referenced to each other. Other special features that may be useful, especially for students, are the commonly used prescribing abbreviations and the sound-alike lists that are found in the appendices. The Therapeutic Drug Levels and The Most Prescribed Drugs appendices will be useful as well.

This information was compiled using a variety of sources including direct communication with over 500 drug companies. The orphan entries are taken directly from the latest list issued by the FDA. When sources differed, we ranked our sources as to reliability and went with what we thought was the most reliable source. We recognize that there may be several published ways in which to type a single drug, but we have chosen to use only one of those ways. In the instance of internal capitalization (e.g., pHisoHex), it should be recognized that in most instances it is acceptable to type such words with initial capitalization only (Phisohex).

How the Book Is Arranged

Although other pharmaceutical references have separate listings for brand names and generics, or put entries into separate sections by body system or therapeutic use, we have chosen to list all entries in one comprehensive alphabetical listing. Therefore, it is not necessary to know if the term sought is a brand name, a generic, a drug class, a chemotherapy protocol, approved or investigational, or slang; what it is used for; or which body system it affects. If it is given to a patient, it's in "the list." In addition to strict pharmaceuticals, we have included other "consumable" products, such as *in vitro* testing kits, radiographic contrast and other imaging agents, and wound dressings.

All entries are in alphabetical order by word. Initial numbers, chemical prefixes (*N*-, *p*-, L-, D-, etc.), and punctuation (prime, ampersand, etc.) are ignored. For example, L-dopa is alphabetized under "dopa," but levodopa under "levo."

We have indicated brand names with initial capital letters unless an unusual combination of capitals and lowercase has been designated by the manufacturer (e.g., pHisoHex, ALternaGEL). Generic names are rendered in lowercase. Where the same name can be either generic or brand, both have been included.

The general format of a *generic* entry is:

entry	council(s)	*designated use*	[other references]	dosages	sound-alike(s)
#1	#2	#3	#4	#5	#6

1. The name of the drug (in bold).
2. The various agencies that have approved the name, shown in small caps, which may be any or all of the following (listed according to appearance in the book):

USAN	United States Adopted Name Council
USP	United States Pharmacopeial Convention
NF	National Formulary
FDA	U.S. Food and Drug Administration
INN	International Nonproprietary Name (a project of the World Health Organization)
BAN	British Approved Name
JAN	Japanese Accepted Name
DCF	Dénomination Commune Française (French)

3. The indication, sometimes referred to as the drug's "designated use," "approved use," or "therapeutic action." This is provided only for official FDA-approved names or other names for the same substance (e.g., the British name of an official U.S. generic). This entry is always in italic.
4. The entry in brackets is one of four cross-references:

see:	refers the reader to the "official" name(s).
now:	for an older generic name no longer used, refers reader to the current official name(s).
also:	a substance that has two or more different names, each officially recognized by one of the above groups, will cross-reference the other name(s).
q.v.	Latin for quod vide, "which see." Used exclusively for abbreviations, it invites the reader to turn to the reference in parentheses.

   If there is more than one cross-reference, alternate names will follow the order of the above agency list: i.e., U.S. names, then international names, then British, Japanese, and French names. The first cross-reference will always be to the approved U.S. name, unless the entry itself is the U.S. name.
5. Dosage information, including the delivery form(s), is given for medications that may be dispensed generically. No dosage information appears for drugs dispensed only under the brand name, or for those containing multiple ingredients. Some drugs may be available in more than one strength, indicated by a comma in the dosage field:

   erythromycin stearate USP, BAN *macrolide antibiotic* 250, 500 mg oral

   A semicolon in the dosage field separates different delivery forms, such as:

   nitroglycerin USP *coronary vasodilator; antianginal; antihypertensive* [also: glyceryl trinitrate] 2.5, 6.5, 9 mg oral; 5 mg/mL injection; 0.2, 0.4, 0.6 mg/hr. transdermal; 2% topical

   (Note that the oral and transdermal forms come in multiple strengths.)
6. Sound-alike drugs follow the "ear" icon.

The general format for a *brand name* entry is:

Entry (CAN) form(s) ℞/OTC *designated use* [generics] dosages [ear] sound-alike(s)

#1	#2	#3	#4	#5	#6	#7	#8

1. The drug name (in bold), which almost always starts with a capital letter.
2. If a brand is not marketed in the United States, an icon designates the country where it is available. Canadian brands are designated by (CAN).
3. The form of administration, e.g., tablets, capsules, syrup. (Sometimes these words are slurred by the dictator, causing confusion regarding the name.)
4. The prescription (℞) or over-the-counter (OTC) status. A few drugs may be either ℞ or OTC, depending on strength or various state laws.
5. The designated use in italics as for generics. These are more complete or less complete as supplied by the individual drug companies.
6. The brackets that follow contain the generic names of the active ingredients to which the reader may refer for further information.
7. Dosage information follows the generics. For multi-ingredient drugs, a bullet separates the dosages of each ingredient, listed in the same order as the generics. For example, the entry

   Ser-Ap-Es tablets ℞ *antihypertensive; vasodilator; diuretic* [hydrochlorothiazide; reserpine; hydralazine HCl] 15•0.1•25 mg

   shows a three-ingredient product containing 15 mg hydrochlorothiazide, 0.1 mg reserpine, and 25 mg hydralazine HCl.

   Some drugs may have more than one strength, indicated by a comma in the dosage field:

   Norpace capsules ℞ *antiarrhythmic* [disopyramide phosphate] 100, 150 mg

   A semicolon in the dosage field separates either different products listed together, such as:

   Pred Mild; Pred Forte eye drop suspension ℞ *topical ophthalmic corticosteroidal anti-inflammatory* [prednisolone acetate] 0.12%; 1%

   or different delivery forms:

   Phenergan tablets, suppositories, injection ℞ *antihistamine; sedative; antiemetic; motion sickness relief* [promethazine HCl] 12.5, 25, 50 mg; 12.5, 25, 50 mg; 25, 50 mg/mL

   (Note that all three forms of Phenergan come in multiple strengths.)

   Liquid delivery forms show the strength per usual dose where appropriate. Thus, injectables and drops are usually shown per milliliter (mL), whereas oral liquids and syrups are shown per 5 mL or 15 mL.

   The ? symbol indicates that dosage information has not been supplied by the manufacturer for one or more ingredients.

   The * symbol is used when a value *cannot* be given because the generic entry refers to multiple ingredients.
8. Sound-alike drugs follow the "ear" icon.

Experimental, Investigational, and Orphan Drugs

Before a drug can be advertised or sold in the United States, it must first be approved for marketing by the U.S. Food and Drug Administration. With a few exceptions, FDA approval is contingent solely upon the manufacturer's demonstrating that the proposed drug is both safe and effective.

To provide such proof, the manufacturer undertakes a series of tests. Preclinical (before human) research is done through computer simulation, then *in vitro* (L. "in glass," meaning laboratory) tests, then in animals. In most cases neither the public nor the general medical community hears about "experimental drugs" in this stage of testing. Neither are they listed in this reference.

If safety and efficacy are successfully demonstrated during the preclinical stage, an Investigational New Drug (IND) application is filed with the FDA. There are three phases of clinical trials, designated Phase I, Phase II, and Phase III. After each phase, the FDA will review the findings and approve or deny further testing.

Phase I trials involve 20 to 100 patients, primarily to establish safety. Phase II trials may involve several hundred patients for up to two years. The goal in this phase is to determine the drug's effectiveness for the proposed indication. Phase III trials, which routinely last up to four years and involve several thousand patients, determine the optimum effective, but safe, dosage. The manufacturer will then file a New Drug Application (NDA) with the FDA, requesting final marketing approval. Only 20% of drugs entering Phase I trials will ultimately be approved for marketing, at an average cost of $359 million and 8½ years in testing.[3]

An orphan drug is a drug or biological product for the diagnosis, treatment, or prevention of a rare disease or condition. A rare disease is one that affects fewer than 200,000 persons or for which there is no reasonable expectation that the cost of development and testing will be recovered through U.S. sales of the product. Federal subsidies are provided to the manufacturer or sponsor for the development of orphan drugs. Applications for orphan status are made through the FDA, and may be made during drug development or after marketing approval.

A Brief Note on the Transcription of Drug Information

Many references are available describing several acceptable ways to transcribe drug information when dictated. We offer the following only as brief guidelines.

Although some institutions favor capitalizing every drug, others promote not capitalizing any drug, and yet others put drugs in all capital letters, the generally accepted style today for the transcription of medical reports for hospital and doctors' office charts (see the American Medical Association *Manual of Style*[4] for publications) is to capitalize the initial letter of brand name drugs and lowercase generic name drugs. The institution may also designate that brand name drugs with unusual capitalization may be typed with initial capital letter only, or typed using the manufacturer's scheme.

In general, commas are omitted between the drug name, the dosage, and the instructions for purposes of simplification. Items in a series may be separated by either commas (if no internal commas are used) or semicolons. A simple series might be typed thus:

> Procardia, nitroglycerin sublingual, and Tolinase

or

> Procardia 10 mg three times a day, nitroglycerin 1/150 p.r.n., and Tolinase 100 mg twice a day.

or

> Procardia 10 mg t.i.d., nitroglycerin 1/150 p.r.n., and Tolinase 100 mg b.i.d.

A more complex or lengthy list of medications, or a list with internal commas, may require the use of semicolons to separate the items in a series. For example,

> Procardia 10 mg, one t.i.d.; nitroglycerin 1/150 p.r.n., to take one with onset of pain, a second in five minutes, and a third five minutes later, if no relief to go immediately to the ER; Tolinase 100 mg, one b.i.d.; and Coumadin 2.5 mg on Mondays, Wednesdays, and Fridays, and 5 mg on Tuesdays, Thursdays, and Saturdays…

Note that the "one" following Procardia 10 mg and Tolinase 100 mg is not necessary, but many doctors dictate something like this; when they do, it is acceptable to place a comma after the dosage. In addition, when two numbers are adjacent to each other, write out one number and use a numeral for the other.

The typing of chemicals with superscripts or subscripts, italics, small capitals, and Greek letters often presents a problem to the medical transcriptionist. In general, Greek letters are written out (alpha-, beta-, gamma-, etc.). Italics and small capitals are written as standard letters followed by a hyphen (dl-alpha-tocopherol, L-dopa).

When typing nonproprietary (generic) isotope names, element symbols should be included with the name. It may appear to be redundant, but it is the correct form. Therefore, we would type sodium pertechnetate Tc 99m, iodohippurate sodium I 131, or sodium iodide I 125. Occasionally the physician may simply dictate isotopes such as Tc 99m, iodine 131 or I 131, or sodium iodide I 125, and unless he is indicating a trademarked name, it should be typed with a space, no hyphen, and no superscript. This reference indicates proper capitalization, spacing, and hyphenation of isotope entries.

Other combinations of letters and numbers are usually written without spaces or hyphens (OKT1, OKT3, T101, SC1), but this is a complex subject and is dealt with extensively in the AMA *Manual of Style*.

---

[1] Dirckx, John, M.D.: "Pharmaceutical Nomenclature: The Lawless Language," *Perspectives on the Medical Transcription Profession*, Vol. 1, No. 4. Modesto, CA: Health Professions Institute, 1991, p. 9.

[2] Turley, Susan M.: *Understanding Pharmacology for Health Professionals*–2nd ed.. Upper Saddle River, NJ: Prentice-Hall, 1999.

[3] *FDA Consumer*, January, 1995. www.fda.gov/fdac/special/newdrug/ndd_toc.html

[4] American Medical Association: *Manual of Style*, 9th ed. Baltimore: Williams & Wilkins, 1997.

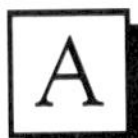

A (vitamin A) [q.v.]

A and D ointment OTC *moisturizer; emollient* [fish liver oil (vitamins A and D); cholecalciferol; lanolin]

A and D Medicated ointment OTC *topical diaper rash treatment* [zinc oxide; vitamins A and D]

A + D (ara-C, daunorubicin) *chemotherapy protocol*

AA (ara-C, Adriamycin) *chemotherapy protocol*

AA-HC Otic ear drops (discontinued 2000) ℞ *topical corticosteroidal anti-inflammatory; antibacterial; antifungal* [hydrocortisone; acetic acid] 1%•2%

abacavir succinate USAN *antiviral nucleoside reverse transcriptase inhibitor for HIV infection*

abacavir sulfate USAN *antiviral nucleoside reverse transcriptase inhibitor for HIV infection*

abacavir sulfate & amprenavir *investigational (Phase III) nucleoside analogue and protease inhibitor combination for HIV and AIDS*

abafilcon A USAN *hydrophilic contact lens material*

abamectin USAN, INN *antiparasitic*

abanoquil INN, BAN

abarelix USAN *investigational (NDA filed) LH-RH antagonist for medical castration (androgen ablation), prostate cancer, uterine fibroids, endometriosis, and precocious puberty*

Abarelix-Depot-M ℞ *investigational (Phase III) antineoplastic for prostate cancer*

abavca & perthon *investigational (Phase I/II) plant derivative combination for HIV and AIDS*

Abbokinase powder for IV or intracoronary artery infusion ℞ *thrombolytic enzymes for pulmonary embolism or coronary artery thrombosis* [urokinase] 250 000 IU/vial

Abbokinase Open-Cath powder for catheter clearance ℞ *thrombolytic enzymes* [urokinase] 5000 IU/mL

Abbo-Pac (trademarked packaging form) *unit dose package*

Abbott TestPack Plus hCG-Urine Plus test kit for professional use *in vitro diagnostic aid; urine pregnancy test* [monoclonal antibody-based enzyme immunoassay]

ABC (Adriamycin, BCNU, cyclophosphamide) *chemotherapy protocol*

ABC to Z tablets OTC *vitamin/mineral/iron supplement* [multiple vitamins & minerals; ferrous fumarate; folic acid; biotin] ≛•18 mg•0.4 mg•30 µg

abciximab USAN, INN *glycoprotein (GP) IIb/IIIa receptor antagonist; antithrombotic monoclonal antibody; antiplatelet agent for PTCA and acute arterial occlusive disorders*

ABCM (Adriamycin, bleomycin, cyclophosphamide, mitomycin) *chemotherapy protocol*

ABD (Adriamycin, bleomycin, DTIC) *chemotherapy protocol*

ABDIC (Adriamycin, bleomycin, DIC, [CCNU, prednisone]) *chemotherapy protocol*

ABDV (Adriamycin, bleomycin, DTIC, vinblastine) *chemotherapy protocol*

ABE (antitoxin botulism equine) [see: botulism equine antitoxin, trivalent]

abecarnil INN *investigational anxiolytic*

Abelcet suspension for IV infusion ℞ *systemic polyene antifungal for aspergillosis and other resistant fungal infections (orphan)* [amphotericin B lipid complex (ABLC)] 100 mg/20 mL

Abelmoschus moschatus *medicinal herb* [see: ambrette]

Abenol (CAN) suppositories OTC *analgesic; antipyretic* [acetaminophen] 120, 325, 650 mg

abetimus sodium USAN *investigational (Phase II/III) oligonucleotide immunosuppressant for systemic lupus erythematosus–associated nephritis*

ABLC [see: TLC ABLC]

ABLC (amphotericin B lipid complex) [q.v.]

ablukast USAN, INN *antiasthmatic; leukotriene antagonist*

ablukast sodium USAN *antiasthmatic; leukotriene antagonist*

Abolic *a veterinary steroid abused as a street drug*

abortifacients *a class of agents that stimulate uterine contractions sufficient to produce uterine evacuation*

ABP (Adriamycin, bleomycin, prednisone) *chemotherapy protocol*

ABPP (aminobromophenylpyrimidinone) [see: bropirimine]

Abreva cream OTC *topical treatment for cold sores and fever blisters* [docosanol] 10%

abrineurin USAN *treatment for amyotrophic lateral sclerosis (ALS)*

Abrus precatorius *medicinal herb* [see: precatory bean]

ABS-205 *investigational (Phase I) treatment for age-related cognitive decline and neurodegeneration*

absinthe; absinthites; absinthium *medicinal herb* [see: wormwood]

absorbable cellulose cotton [see: cellulose, oxidized]

absorbable collagen sponge [see: collagen sponge, absorbable]

absorbable dusting powder [see: dusting powder, absorbable]

absorbable gelatin film [see: gelatin film, absorbable]

absorbable gelatin powder [see: gelatin powder, absorbable]

absorbable gelatin sponge [see: gelatin sponge, absorbable]

absorbable surgical suture [see: suture, absorbable surgical]

Absorbase OTC *ointment base* [water-in-oil emulsion of cholesterolized petrolatum and purified water]

absorbent gauze [see: gauze, absorbent]

Absorbine Antifungal cream, powder (discontinued 1998) OTC *topical antifungal* [tolnaftate] 1%

Absorbine Antifungal Foot aerosol powder OTC *topical antifungal* [miconazole nitrate; alcohol 10%] 2%

Absorbine Arthritis Strength Liquid with Capsaicin OTC *topical analgesic; counterirritant* [menthol; capsaicin] 4%•0.025%

Absorbine Athlete's Foot cream OTC *topical antifungal* [tolnaftate] 1%

Absorbine Athlete's Foot Care liquid (name changed to Absorbine Footcare in 1998)

Absorbine Footcare spray liquid OTC *topical antifungal* [tolnaftate] 1%

Absorbine Jock Itch powder (discontinued 1998) OTC *topical antifungal* [tolnaftate] 1%

Absorbine Jr. liniment OTC *topical analgesic; counterirritant* [menthol] 1.27%, 4%

Absorbine Jr. Antifungal spray liquid (discontinued 1998) OTC *topical antifungal* [tolnaftate] 1%

Absorbine Jr. Extra Strength liquid OTC *topical analgesic; counterirritant* [menthol] 4%

Absorbine Power gel (discontinued 1998) OTC *topical analgesic; counterirritant* [menthol] 4%

ABT-719 *investigational quinolizidine antibiotic*

abunidazole INN

ABV (actimomycin D, bleomycin, vincristine) *chemotherapy protocol*

ABV (Adriamycin, bleomycin, vinblastine) *chemotherapy protocol for Kaposi sarcoma*

ABV (Adriamycin, bleomycin, vincristine) *chemotherapy protocol for Kaposi sarcoma*

ABVD (Adriamycin, bleomycin, vinblastine, dacarbazine) *chemotherapy protocol for Hodgkin lymphoma*

ABVD/MOPP (alternating cycles of ABVD and MOPP) *chemotherapy protocol*

ABX-CBL *investigational (Phase III, orphan) monoclonal antibody for steroid-resistant graft vs. host disease that reverses unwanted immune response* *without general immune system suppression* [also: monoclonal antibody to CD147, murine]

ABX-IL8 *investigational (Phase I/II) for psoriasis*

9-AC (9-aminocamptothecin) [q.v.]

AC (Adriamycin, carmustine) *chemotherapy protocol*

AC (Adriamycin, CCNU) *chemotherapy protocol*

AC (Adriamycin, cisplatin) *chemotherapy protocol for bone sarcoma*

AC; A-C (Adriamycin, cyclophosphamide) *chemotherapy protocol for breast cancer and pediatric neuroblastoma*

AC-2993 *investigational for type 2 diabetes*

acacia NF, JAN *suspending agent; emollient; demulcent*

acacia (*Acacia senegal; A. verek*) gum *medicinal herb for colds, cough, periodontal disease, and wound healing*

acadesine USAN, INN, BAN *platelet aggregation inhibitor*

acamprosate 6473 INN

acamylophenine [see: camylofin]

Acanthopanax senticosus *medicinal herb* [see: Siberian ginseng]

acaprazine INN

acarbose USAN, INN, BAN *α-glucosidase inhibitor for type 2 diabetes*

ACAT (acylCoA transferase) inhibitor *investigational agent to lower serum cholesterol levels*

Accolate film-coated tablets ℞ *leukotriene receptor antagonist (LTRA) for prevention and chronic treatment of asthma* [zafirlukast] 10, 20 mg

Accu-Chek Advantage reagent strips for home use *in vitro diagnostic aid for blood glucose*

AccuNeb solution for inhalation ℞ *sympathomimetic bronchodilator for children 2–12 years* [albuterol sulfate] 0.63, 1.25 mg/3 mL

Accu-Pak (trademarked packaging form) *unit dose blister pack*

Accupep HPF powder OTC *enteral nutritional therapy for GI impairment*

Accupril film-coated tablets ℞ *angiotensin-converting enzyme (ACE) inhibitor; antihypertensive; adjunct to CHF therapy* [quinapril HCl] 5, 10, 20, 40 mg

Accurbron syrup ℞ *antiasthmatic; bronchodilator* [theophylline; alcohol 7.5%] 150 mg/15 mL ⊡ Accutane

Accuretic film-coated tablets ℞ *antihypertensive; angiotensin-converting enzyme (ACE) inhibitor; diuretic* [quinapril HCl; hydrochlorothiazide] 10•12.5, 20•12.5, 20•25 mg

AccuSite injectable gel ℞ *investigational (NDA filed) treatment for genital warts; development discontinued in 1997* [fluorouracil; epinephrine]

Accutane capsules ℞ *internal keratolytic for severe recalcitrant nodular acne* [isotretinoin] 10, 20, 40 mg ⊡ Accurbron

Accuzyme ointment ℞ *topical enzyme for wound debridement; vulnerary* [papain; urea] 1 100 000 IU/g•10%

ACD solution (acid citrate dextrose; anticoagulant citrate dextrose) [see: anticoagulant citrate dextrose solution]

ACD whole blood [see: blood, whole]

ACe (Adriamycin, cyclophosphamide) *chemotherapy protocol for breast cancer*

ACE (Adriamycin, cyclophosphamide, etoposide) *chemotherapy protocol for small cell lung cancer* [also: CAE]

ACE inhibitors (angiotensin-converting enzyme inhibitors) [q.v.]

acebrochol INN, DCF

aceburic acid INN, DCF

acebutolol USAN, INN, BAN *antihypertensive; antiarrhythmic; antiadrenergic (β-blocker)* [also: acebutolol HCl]

acebutolol HCl JAN *antihypertensive; antiarrhythmic; antiadrenergic (β-blocker)* [also: acebutolol] 200, 400 mg oral

acecainide INN *antiarrhythmic* [also: acecainide HCl]

acecainide HCl USAN *antiarrhythmic* [also: acecainide]

acecarbromal INN *CNS depressant; sedative; hypnotic*
aceclidine USAN, INN *cholinergic*
aceclofenac INN, BAN
acedapsone USAN, INN, BAN *antimalarial; antibacterial; leprostatic*
acediasulfone sodium INN, DCF
acedoben INN
acefluranol INN, BAN
acefurtiamine INN
acefylline clofibrol INN
acefylline piperazine INN, DCF [also: acepifylline]
aceglaton JAN [also: aceglatone]
aceglatone INN [also: aceglaton]
aceglutamide INN *antiulcerative* [also: aceglutamide aluminum]
aceglutamide aluminum USAN, JAN *antiulcerative* [also: aceglutamide]
ACEIs (angiotensin-converting enzyme inhibitors) [q.v.]
Acel-Imune IM injection (discontinued 2001) ℞ *active immunizing agent for diphtheria, tetanus, and pertussis* [diphtheria & tetanus toxoids & acellular pertussis (DTaP) vaccine, adsorbed] 7.5 LfU•5 LfU•300 HAU per 0.5 mL
acellular pertussis vaccine [see: diphtheria & tetanus toxoids & acellular pertussis (DTaP) vaccine, adsorbed]
Acel-P (CAN) suspension for IM injection (discontinued 2001) ℞ *active immunization against pertussis* [pertussis vaccine, acellular adsorbed] 300 HAU/0.5 mL
acemannan USAN, INN *investigational (Phase I) antiviral and immunomodulator for AIDS; investigational (NDA filed) hydrogel wound dressing*
acemetacin INN, BAN, JAN
acemethadone [see: methadyl acetate]
aceneuramic acid INN
acenocoumarin [see: acenocoumarol]
acenocoumarol NF, INN [also: nicoumalone]
Aceon tablets ℞ *angiotensin-converting enzyme (ACE) inhibitor for essential hypertension* [perindopril erbumine] 2, 4, 8 mg
aceperone INN
Acephen suppositories OTC *analgesic; antipyretic* [acetaminophen] 120, 325, 650 mg
acephenazine dimaleate [see: acetophenazine maleate]
acepifylline BAN [also: acefylline piperazine]
acepromazine INN, BAN *veterinary sedative* [also: acepromazine maleate]
acepromazine maleate USAN *veterinary sedative* [also: acepromazine]
aceprometazine INN, DCF
acequinoline INN, DCF
acerola *(Malpighia glabra; M. punicifolia)* fruit *natural dietary source of vitamin C*
acesulfame INN, BAN
Aceta tablets, elixir OTC *analgesic; antipyretic* [acetaminophen] 325, 500 mg; 120 mg/5 mL
Aceta with Codeine tablets ℞ *narcotic analgesic* [codeine phosphate; acetaminophen] 30•300 mg
Aceta-Gesic tablets OTC *analgesic; antihistaminic sleep aid* [acetaminophen; phenyltoloxamine citrate] 325•30 mg
***p*-acetamidobenzoic acid** [see: acedoben]
6-acetamidohexanoic acid [see: acexamic acid]
4-acetamidophenyl acetate [see: diacetamate]
acetaminocaproic acid [see: acexamic acid]
acetaminophen USP *analgesic; antipyretic* [also: paracetamol] 80, 325, 500, 650 mg, 100 mg/mL, 120, 160 mg/5 mL, 500/15 mL oral; 120, 300, 325, 650 mg suppository
acetaminophen & butalbital & caffeine *analgesic; barbiturate sedative* 325•50•40 mg oral
acetaminophen & codeine *narcotic analgesic* 300•15, 300•30, 300•60 mg oral; 30•12 mg/5 mL oral

acetaminophen & hydrocodone bitartrate *analgesic; antitussive* 325•10, 500•10, 650•10, 750•7.5 mg oral; 167•2.5 mg/5 mL oral

acetaminophen & pentazocine HCl *narcotic analgesic* 650•25 mg oral

acetaminophenol [see: acetaminophen]

acetaminosalol INN, DCF

acetanilid (or acetanilide) NF

acetannin [see: acetyltannic acid]

acetarsol INN, BAN, DCF [also: acetarsone]

acetarsone NF [also: acetarsol]

acetarsone salt of arecoline [see: drocarbil]

Acetasol ear drops ℞ *antibacterial; antifungal* [acetic acid] 2%

Acetasol HC ear drops ℞ *topical corticosteroidal anti-inflammatory; antibacterial; antifungal* [hydrocortisone; acetic acid] 1%•2%

acetazolamide USP, INN, BAN, JAN *carbonic anhydrase inhibitor; diuretic; anticonvulsant; antiglaucoma; treatment for acute mountain sickness* 125, 250 mg oral; 500 mg injection

acetazolamide sodium USP, JAN *carbonic anhydrase inhibitor; diuretic; anticonvulsant; antiglaucoma; treatment for acute mountain sickness*

acetcarbromal [see: acecarbromal]

acet-dia-mer-sulfonamide (sulfacetamide, sulfadiazine & sulfamerazine) [q.v.]

acetergamine INN

Acetest reagent tablets for professional use *in vitro diagnostic aid for acetone (ketones) in the urine or blood*

acetiamine INN

acetic acid NF, JAN *acidifying agent* 0.25% irrigation

acetic acid, aluminum salt [see: aluminum acetate]

acetic acid, calcium salt [see: calcium acetate]

acetic acid, diluted NF *bladder irrigant*

acetic acid, ethyl ester [see: ethyl acetate]

acetic acid, glacial USP, INN *acidifying agent*

acetic acid, potassium salt [see: potassium acetate]

acetic acid, sodium salt trihydrate [see: sodium acetate]

acetic acid, zinc salt dihydrate [see: zinc acetate]

acetic acid 5-nitrofurfurylidenehydrazide [see: nihydrazone]

aceticyl [see: aspirin]

acetilum acidulatum [see: aspirin]

acetiromate INN

acetohexamide USAN, USP, INN, BAN, JAN *sulfonylurea antidiabetic* 250, 500 mg oral

acetohydroxamic acid (AHA) USAN, USP, INN *urease enzyme inhibitor for chronic urea-splitting urinary infections*

acetol [see: aspirin]

acetomenaphthone BAN

acetomeroctol

acetone NF *solvent; antiseptic*

acetophen [see: aspirin]

acetophenazine INN *antipsychotic* [also: acetophenazine maleate]

acetophenazine maleate USAN, USP *antipsychotic* [also: acetophenazine]

***p*-acetophenetidide** *(withdrawn from market)* [see: phenacetin]

acetophenetidin *(withdrawn from market)* [now: phenacetin]

acetorphan *enkephalinase inhibitor for acute diarrhea*

acetorphine INN, BAN *enkephalinase inhibitor for acute diarrhea; investigational for opioid withdrawal and GERD*

acetosal [see: aspirin]

acetosalic acid [see: aspirin]

acetosalin [see: aspirin]

acetosulfone sodium USAN *antibacterial; leprostatic* [also: sulfadiasulfone sodium]

acetoxyphenylmercury [see: phenylmercuric acetate]

acetoxythymoxamine [see: moxisylyte]

acetphenarsine [see: acetarsone]

acetphenetidin *(withdrawn from market)* [now: phenacetin]

acetphenolisatin [see: oxyphenisatin acetate]

acetrizoate sodium USP [also: sodium acetrizoate]
acetrizoic acid USP
acetryptine INN
acetsalicylamide [see: salacetamide]
acet-theocin sodium [see: theophylline sodium acetate]
aceturate USAN, INN *combining name for radicals or groups*
acetyl adalin [see: acetylcarbromal]
N-acetyl cysteine (NAC) *natural source of cysteine; promotes an increase in the endogenous antioxidant glutathione*
acetyl sulfisoxazole [see: sulfisoxazole acetyl]
***l*-acetyl-α-methadol (LAAM)** [see: levomethadyl acetate]
***p*-acetylaminobenzaldehyde thiosemicarbazone** [see: thioacetazone; thiacetazone]
acetylaminobenzene [see: acetanilid]
N-acetyl-*p*-aminophenol (APAP; NAPA) [see: acetaminophen]
acetylaniline [see: acetanilid]
acetylated polyvinyl alcohol *viscosity-increasing agent*
acetyl-bromo-diethylacetylcarbamide [see: acecarbromal]
acetylcarbromal [see: acecarbromal]
acetylcholine chloride USP, INN, BAN, JAN *cardiac depressant; cholinergic; miotic; peripheral vasodilator*
acetylcholinesterase (AChE) inhibitors *a class of drugs that alter acetylcholine neurotransmitters, used as a cognition adjuvant in Alzheimer dementia* [also called: cholinesterase inhibitors]
acetylcysteine (N-acetylcysteine) USAN, USP, INN, BAN *mucolytic inhaler; treatment for severe acetaminophen overdose (orphan); investigational immunomodulator for AIDS* [also: *N*-acetyl-L-cysteine]
acetylcysteine sodium *mucolytic inhaler* 10%, 20% inhalation
acetyldigitoxin (α-acetyldigitoxin) NF, INN
acetyldihydrocodeinone [see: thebacon]
N-acetyl-DL-leucine [see: acetylleucine]
acetylhydrolase *investigational (Phase II/III) platelet-activating factor*
acetylin [see: aspirin]
acetylkitasamycin JAN *antibacterial* [also: kitasamycin; kitasamycin tartrate]
N-acetyl-L-cysteine JAN *mucolytic inhaler* [also: acetylcysteine]
N-acetyl-L-cysteine salicylate [see: salnacedin]
acetylleucine (*N*-acetyl-DL-leucine) INN
acetylmethadol INN, DCF *narcotic analgesic* [also: methadyl acetate]
acetyloleandomycin [see: troleandomycin]
2-acetyloxybenzoic acid [see: aspirin]
acetylpheneturide JAN [also: pheneturide]
acetylphenylisatin [see: oxyphenisatin acetate]
N-acetyl-procainamide (NAPA) *investigational (orphan) preventative for ventricular arrhythmias in procainamide-induced lupus*
acetylpropylorvinol [see: acetorphine]
acetylresorcinol [see: resorcinol monoacetate]
acetylsal [see: aspirin]
N-acetylsalicylamide [see: salacetamide]
acetylsalicylate aluminum [see: aspirin aluminum]
acetylsalicylic acid (ASA) [now: aspirin]
acetylsalicylic acid, phenacetin & caffeine [see: APC]
acetylspiramycin JAN *macrolide antibiotic* [also: spiramycin]
acetylsulfamethoxazole JAN *broad-spectrum sulfonamide bacteriostatic* [also: sulfamethoxazole; sulphamethoxazole; sulfamethoxazole sodium]
N^1-acetylsulfanilamide [see: sulfacetamide]
acetyltannic acid USP
acetyltannin [see: acetyltannic acid]
acevaltrate INN
acexamic acid INN, DCF

ACFUCY (actinomycin D, fluorouracil, cyclophosphamide) *chemotherapy protocol*

AChE (acetylcholinesterase) inhibitors [q.v.]

Achillea millefolium *medicinal herb* [see: yarrow]

Achromycin V capsules, oral suspension (discontinued 1999) ℞ *broad-spectrum antibiotic* [tetracycline HCl] 250, 500 mg; 125 mg/5 mL

aciclovir INN, JAN *antiviral* [also: acyclovir]

acid acriflavine [see: acriflavine HCl]

acid alpha-glucosidase, human [see: human acid alpha-glucosidase]

acid citrate dextrose (ACD) [see: anticoagulant citrate dextrose solution]

acid histamine phosphate [see: histamine phosphate]

Acid Mantle OTC *cream base*

acid trypaflavine [see: acriflavine HCl]

acidogen [see: glutamic acid HCl]

acidol HCl [see: betaine HCl]

acidophilus *(Lactobacillus acidophilus)* *natural bacteria for replenishment of normal flora in the gastrointestinal tract and vagina; not generally regarded as safe and effective as an antidiarrheal*

acidulated phosphate fluoride (sodium fluoride & hydrofluoric acid) *dental caries prophylactic*

acidum acetylsalicylicum [see: aspirin]

Acid-X tablets OTC *analgesic; antipyretic; antacid* [acetaminophen; calcium carbonate] 500•250 mg

acifran USAN, INN *antihyperlipoproteinemic*

aciglumin [see: glutamic acid HCl]

Aci-jel vaginal jelly OTC *acidity modifier* [acetic acid; oxyquinolone sulfate; ricinoleic acid; glycerin] 0.921%•0.025%•0.7%•5%

acinitrazole BAN *veterinary antibacterial* [also: nithiamide; aminitrozole]

Aciphex enteric-coated delayed-release tablets ℞ *proton pump inhibitor for duodenal ulcers, erosive or ulcerative gastroesophageal reflux disease (GERD), and other gastroesophageal disorders* [rabeprazole sodium] 20 mg ⑨ AcuTect

acipimox INN, BAN

acistrate INN *combining name for radicals or groups*

acitemate INN

acitretin USAN, INN, BAN *systemic antipsoriatic; retinoic acid analogue*

acivicin USAN, INN *antineoplastic*

ackee *(Blighia sapida)* *medicinal herb for colds, fever, edema, and epilepsy; not generally regarded as safe as seeds and unripened fruit are highly toxic*

aclacinomycin A [now: aclarubicin]

aclantate INN

aclarubicin USAN, INN, BAN *antibiotic antineoplastic* [also: aclarubicin HCl]

aclarubicin HCl JAN *antibiotic antineoplastic* [also: aclarubicin]

aclatonium napadisilate INN, BAN, JAN

Aclophen long-acting tablets ℞ *decongestant; antihistamine; analgesic* [phenylephrine HCl; chlorpheniramine maleate; acetaminophen] 40•8•500 mg

Aclovate ointment, cream ℞ *topical corticosteroidal anti-inflammatory* [alclometasone dipropionate] 0.05%

ACM (Adriamycin, cyclophosphamide, methotrexate) *chemotherapy protocol*

A.C.N. tablets OTC *vitamin supplement* [vitamins A, B_3, and C] 25 000 IU•25 mg•250 mg

Acne Lotion 10 OTC *antibacterial and exfoliant for acne* [colloidal sulfur] 10%

Acne-5 lotion, mask OTC *topical keratolytic for acne* [benzoyl peroxide] 5%

Acne-10 lotion OTC *topical keratolytic for acne* [benzoyl peroxide] 10%

Acno lotion OTC *topical acne treatment* [sulfur] 3%

Acno Cleanser liquid OTC *topical cleanser for acne* [isopropyl alcohol] 60%

Acnomel cream OTC *topical acne treatment* [sulfur; resorcinol; alcohol] 8%•2%•11%

Acnotex lotion OTC *topical acne treatment* [sulfur; resorcinol; isopropyl alcohol] 8%•2%•20%

acodazole INN *antineoplastic* [also: acodazole HCl]

acodazole HCl USAN *antineoplastic* [also: acodazole]

aconiazide INN *investigational (orphan) for tuberculosis*

aconite *(Aconitum napellus)* plant and root *medicinal herb for fever, hypertension, and neuralgia; not generally regarded as safe, as it is highly toxic*

aconitine USP

ACOP (Adriamycin, cyclophosphamide, Oncovin, prednisone) *chemotherapy protocol*

ACOPP; A-COPP (Adriamycin, cyclophosphamide, Oncovin, procarbazine, prednisone) *chemotherapy protocol*

acortan [see: corticotropin]

Acorus calamus *medicinal herb* [see: calamus]

Acova IV infusion ℞ *anticoagulant for thrombosis due to heparin-induced thrombocytopenia (HIT); investigational (Phase II) for myocardial infarction* [argatroban] 1 mg/mL

acoxatrine INN

9-acridinamine monohydrochloride [see: aminacrine HCl]

acridinyl anisidide [see: amsacrine]

acridinylamine methanesulfon anisidide (AMSA) [see: amsacrine]

acridorex INN

acrids *a class of agents that have a pungent taste or cause heat and irritation when applied to the skin*

acriflavine NF

acriflavine HCl NF [also: acriflavinium chloride]

acriflavinium chloride INN [also: acriflavine HCl]

acrihellin INN

acrinol JAN [also: ethacridine lactate; ethacridine]

acrisorcin USAN, USP, INN *antifungal*

acrivastine USAN, INN, BAN *antihistamine*

acrocinonide INN, DCF

acronine USAN, INN *antineoplastic*

acrosoxacin BAN *antibacterial* [also: rosoxacin]

AcryDerm Strands wound dressing *high-exudate absorbent dressing for cavitated wounds*

ACT oral rinse OTC *topical dental caries preventative* [sodium fluoride; alcohol 7%] 0.05%

ACT (activated cellular therapy) [q.v.]

Actaea alba; A. pachypoda; A. rubra *medicinal herb* [see: white cohosh]

Actaea racemosa *medicinal herb* [see: black cohosh]

actagardin INN

Actagen tablets, syrup OTC *decongestant; antihistamine* [pseudoephedrine HCl; triprolidine HCl] 60•2.5 mg; 30•1.25 mg/5 mL

Actagen-C Cough syrup ℞ *narcotic antitussive; decongestant; antihistamine* [codeine phosphate; pseudoephedrine HCl; triprolidine HCl] 10•30•2 mg/5 mL

actaplanin USAN, INN, BAN *veterinary growth stimulant*

actarit INN

ACTH powder for IM or subcu injection ℞ *corticosteroid; anti-inflammatory* [corticotropin] 40 U/vial

ACTH (adrenocorticotropic hormone) [see: corticotropin]

ACTH-80 subcu or IM injection ℞ *corticosteroid; anti-inflammatory* [corticotropin repository] 80 U/mL

Acthar powder for IM or subcu injection ℞ *corticosteroid; anti-inflammatory* [corticotropin] 25, 40 U/vial

Acthar Gel [see: H.P. Acthar Gel]

ActHIB powder for injection ℞ *infant (2–18 months) vaccine for Haemophilus influenzae type b (HIB) and invasive diseases (15–18 months) caused by HIB* [Hemophilus b conjugate vaccine; tetanus toxoid] 10•24 μg/ 0.5 mL

ActHIB/Tripedia IM injection ℞ *pediatric vaccine for children younger than 5 months old* [Hemophilus b conjugate vaccine; diphtheria & tetanus toxoids & acellular pertussis (DTaP) vaccine] 10 μg•6.7 LfU•5 LfU•46.8 μg per 0.5 mL

Acthrel IV infusion ℞ *diagnostic aid for adrenocorticotropic hormone (ACTH)-dependent Cushing syndrome (orphan)* [corticorelin ovine triflutate] 100 μg

ActiBath effervescent tablets OTC *moisturizer; emollient* [colloidal oatmeal] 20%

Actical Plus (CAN) tablets OTC *dietary supplement* [calcium citrate; multiple minerals; vitamin D_3] 135 mg•≛•40 IU

Acticin cream ℞ *pediculicide for lice; scabicide* [permethrin] 5%

Acticort 100 lotion ℞ *topical corticosteroidal anti-inflammatory* [hydrocortisone] 1%

Actidose with Sorbitol oral suspension OTC *adsorbent antidote for poisoning; reduces intestinal transit time* [activated charcoal; sorbitol] 25•≟ g/120 mL; 50•≟ g/240 mL

Actidose-Aqua oral suspension OTC *adsorbent antidote for poisoning* [activated charcoal] 25 g/120 mL, 50 g/240 mL

Actifed tablets OTC *decongestant; antihistamine* [pseudoephedrine HCl; triprolidine HCl] 60•2.5 mg ⊡ Actidil

Actifed Allergy daytime caplets + nighttime caplets OTC *decongestant; (antihistamine/sleep aid added at night)* [pseudoephedrine HCl; (diphenhydramine HCl added at night)] 30 mg; 30•25 mg ⊡ Actidil

Actifed Plus caplets, tablets OTC *decongestant; antihistamine; analgesic* [pseudoephedrine HCl; triprolidine HCl; acetaminophen] 30•1.25•500 mg ⊡ Actidil

Actifed Sinus daytime caplets + nighttime caplets OTC *decongestant; analgesic; (antihistamine/sleep aid added at night)* [pseudoephedrine HCl; acetaminophen; (diphenhydramine HCl added at night)] 30•325 mg; 30•500•25 mg ⊡ Actidil

Actifed with Codeine Cough syrup (discontinued 1997) ℞ *narcotic antitussive; decongestant; antihistamine* [codeine phosphate; pseudoephedrine HCl; triprolidine HCl; alcohol 4.3%] 10•30•1.25 mg/5 mL ⊡ Actidil

Actigall capsules ℞ *gallstone dissolving agent; also for primary biliary cirrhosis (orphan)* [ursodiol] 300 mg

Actimmune subcu injection ℞ *immunoregulator for chronic granulomatous disease (orphan) and severe congenital osteopetrosis (orphan); investigational (orphan) for renal cell carcinoma; investigational (Phase III) for multidrug-resistant pulmonary tuberculosis* [interferon gamma-1b] 100 μg (2 million IU) per 0.5 mL

Actinex cream (discontinued 1999) ℞ *antineoplastic for actinic keratoses (AK)* [masoprocol] 10%

actinium *element (Ac)*

actinomycin C BAN *antibiotic antineoplastic* [also: cactinomycin] ⊡ Achromycin; Aureomycin

actinomycin D JAN *antibiotic antineoplastic* [also: dactinomycin] ⊡ Achromycin; Aureomycin

actinoquinol INN *ultraviolet screen* [also: actinoquinol sodium]

actinoquinol sodium USAN *ultraviolet screen* [also: actinoquinol]

actinospectocin [see: spectinomycin]

Actiq "lollipops" ℞ *oral transmucosal narcotic analgesic for breakthrough pain in cancer patients* [fentanyl citrate] 200, 400, 600, 800, 1200, 1600 μg

Actisite periodontal fiber ℞ *oral antibiotic for periodontitis* [tetracycline] 12.7 mg/23 cm

actisomide USAN, INN *antiarrhythmic*

Activase powder for IV infusion ℞ *tissue plasminogen activator (tPA) thrombolytic for acute myocardial infarction, acute ischemic stroke, or pulmonary embolism* [alteplase] 50, 100 mg/vial (29, 58 million IU/vial)

activated attapulgite [see: attapulgite, activated]

activated carbon

activated cellular therapy (ACT) *investigational (Phase II) agent for AIDS*

activated charcoal [see: charcoal, activated]
activated 7-dehydrocholesterol [see: cholecalciferol]
activated ergosterol [see: ergocalciferol]
activated prothrombin complex BAN
Activella film-coated tablets (in packs of 28) ℞ *hormone replacement therapy for postmenopausal symptoms* [estradiol; norethindrone acetate] 1•0.5 mg
actodigin USAN, INN *cardiotonic*
Actonel film-coated tablets ℞ *bisphosphonate bone resorption inhibitor for Paget disease and treatment or prevention of postmenopausal and glucocorticoid-induced osteoporosis* [risedronate sodium] 5, 30 mg
Actos tablets ℞ *thiazolidinedione antidiabetic; increases cellular response to insulin without increasing insulin secretion* [pioglitazone HCl] 15, 30, 45 mg
Act-O-Vial (trademarked packaging form) *vial system*
Actron tablets (discontinued 2000) OTC *analgesic; antiarthritic; nonsteroidal anti-inflammatory drug (NSAID)* [ketoprofen] 12.5 mg
ACU-dyne ointment, perineal wash concentrate, prep solution, skin cleanser, prep swabs, swabsticks OTC *broad-spectrum antimicrobial* [povidone-iodine]
ACU-dyne Douche concentrate OTC *antiseptic/germicidal; vaginal cleanser and deodorizer* [povidone-iodine]
Acular; Acular PF eye drops ℞ *topical ophthalmic nonsteroidal anti-inflammatory drug (NSAID) for allergic conjunctivitis or cataract extraction* [ketorolac tromethamine] 0.5%
AcuTect ℞ *radiopharmaceutical diagnostic aid for acute venous thrombosis* [technetium Tc 99m apcitide] ⑨ Aciphex
Acutrim 16 Hour; Acutrim Late Day; Acutrim II precision-release tablets OTC *diet aid* [phenylpropanolamine HCl] 75 mg
AcuTrim Diet chewing gum OTC *diet aid* [phenylpropanolamine HCl] 75 mg
acycloguanosine [see: acyclovir]
acyclovir USAN, USP, BAN *antiviral* [also: aciclovir] 200, 400, 800 mg oral
acyclovir CD *investigational (Phase I) controlled-delivery antiviral*
acyclovir redox [see: redox-acyclovir]
acyclovir sodium USAN *antiviral* 200 mg oral; 50 mg/mL injection
acylCoA transferase (ACAT) inhibitor *investigational agent to lower serum cholesterol levels*
acylpyrin [see: aspirin]
AD (Adriamycin, dacarbazine) *chemotherapy protocol for soft tissue sarcoma*
AD-32 *investigational (NDA filed) novel anthracycline for treatment of bladder cancer*
AD-439 *investigational (Phase II) antiviral for HIV and AIDS*
AD-519 *investigational (Phase II) antiviral for HIV and AIDS*
ad5CMV-p53 [see: adenoviral p53 gene]
AD7C *investigational urinary test for Alzheimer disease*
ADA (adenosine deaminase) [see: pegademase bovine; pegademase]
Adacel (CAN) IM injection ℞ *active immunizing agent for diphtheria, tetanus, and pertussis* [diphtheria & tetanus toxoids & acellular pertussis (DTaP) vaccine, adsorbed] 2 LfU•5 LfU•2.5 µg per 0.5 mL dose
adafenoxate INN
Adagen IM injection ℞ *adenosine deaminase (ADA) enzyme replacement for severe combined immunodeficiency disease (orphan)* [pegademase bovine] 250 U/mL
Adalat capsules ℞ *antianginal; antihypertensive; calcium channel blocker* [nifedipine] 10, 20 mg
Adalat CC; Adalat Oros sustained-release tablets ℞ *antianginal; antihypertensive; calcium channel blocker* [nifedipine] 30, 60, 90 mg
Adalat XL (CAN) extended-release tablets ℞ *antianginal; antihypertensive; calcium channel blocker* [nifedipine] 20, 30, 60 mg

adamantanamine [see: amantadine]
adamantanamine HCl [see: amantadine HCl]
adamexine INN
adapalene USAN, INN, BAN *synthetic retinoid analogue for topical treatment of acne*
Adapettes solution OTC *rewetting solution for hard contact lenses*
Adapettes Especially for Sensitive Eyes solution OTC *rewetting solution for soft contact lenses*
adaprolol maleate USAN *ophthalmic antihypertensive (β-blocker)*
adatanserin INN *anxiolytic; antidepressant* [also: adatanserin HCl]
adatanserin HCl USAN *anxiolytic; antidepressant* [also: adatanserin]
AdatoSil 5000 intraocular injection ℞ *retinal tamponade for retinal detachment* [polydimethylsiloxane] 10, 15 mL
Adavite tablets OTC *vitamin supplement* [multiple vitamins; folic acid; biotin] ≛ •400•35 μg
Adavite-M tablets OTC *vitamin/mineral/iron supplement* [multiple vitamins & minerals; iron; folic acid; biotin] ≛ •27 mg•0.4 mg•30 μg
ADBC (Adriamycin, DTIC, bleomycin, CCNU) *chemotherapy protocol*
ADC with Fluoride drops ℞ *pediatric vitamin supplement and dental caries preventative* [vitamins A, C, and D; fluoride] 1500 IU•35 mg•400 IU•0.5 mg per mL
Adcon-L gel ℞ *investigational (NDA filed) postsurgical adhesion barrier to inhibit the formation of scars and adhesions following lumbar discectomy and breast augmentation surgery* [carbohydrate polymer gel]
Adcon-P ℞ *investigational (NDA filed) postsurgical adhesion control barrier to inhibit the formation of scars and adhesions in the peritoneal cavity*
Adderall tablets ℞ *CNS stimulant for attention-deficit hyperactivity disorder (ADHD), narcolepsy, and obesity* [amphetamines (equal parts amphetamine aspartate, amphetamine sulfate, dextroamphetamine sulfate, and dextroamphetamine saccharate)] 5, 7.5, 10, 12.5, 15, 20, 30 mg total
Adderall XR extended-release tablets ℞ *once-daily doseform for attention-deficit hyperactivity disorder (ADHD)* [amphetamines (equal parts amphetamine aspartate, amphetamine sulfate, dextroamphetamine sulfate, and dextroamphetamine saccharate)] 5, 30 mg
adder's mouth *medicinal herb* [see: chickweed]
adder's tongue ***(Erythronium americanum)*** bulb and leaves *medicinal herb used as an emetic, antiscrofulous agent, and emollient*
ADD-Vantage (trademarked delivery system) *intravenous drug admixture system*
ADE (ara-C, daunorubicin, etoposide) *chemotherapy protocol*
Adeflor M tablets ℞ *pediatric vitamin deficiency and dental caries prevention* [multiple vitamins; fluoride; calcium; iron] ≛ •1•250•30 mg
adefovir dipivoxil USAN *investigational (NDA filed) oral nucleotide reverse transcriptase inhibitor (NRTI) for advanced HIV and AIDS (clinical trials discontinued 1999); investigational (Phase III) treatment for chronic hepatitis B virus (HBV) infection*
ADEKs chewable tablets OTC *vitamin/mineral supplement* [multiple vitamins & minerals; folic acid; biotin] ≛ •200•50 μg
ADEKs pediatric drops OTC *vitamin/mineral supplement* [multiple vitamins & minerals; biotin] ≛ •15 μg
adelmidrol INN
ademetionine INN
adenazole [see: tocladesine]
adenine USP, JAN *amino acid*
adenine arabinoside (ara-A) [see: vidarabine]
adeno-associated viral-based vector cystic fibrosis gene therapy *investigational (orphan) for cystic fibrosis*

Adenocard IV injection ℞ *antiarrhythmic for paroxysmal supraventricular tachycardia (PSVT)* [adenosine] 3 mg/mL
Adenoscan IV infusion ℞ *cardiac diagnostic aid; cardiac stressor; adjunct to thallium 201 myocardial perfusion scintigraphy* [adenosine] 3 mg/mL
adenosine USAN, BAN *antiarrhythmic for paroxysmal supraventricular tachycardia (PSVT); diagnostic aid*
adenosine deaminase (ADA) [see: pegademase bovine; pegademase]
adenosine monophosphate (AMP) [see: adenosine phosphate]
adenosine phosphate USAN, INN, BAN *nutrient; treatment for varicose veins and herpes infections* 25 mg/mL IM injection
adenosine triphosphate (ATP) disodium JAN
adenoviral p53 gene *investigational (Phase II) gene therapy for cancer* [also: p53 adenoviral gene]
5′-adenylic acid [see: adenosine phosphate]
adepsine oil [see: mineral oil]
adhesive bandage [see: bandage, adhesive]
adhesive tape [see: tape, adhesive]
adibendan INN
A-DIC (Adriamycin, dacarbazine) *chemotherapy protocol*
adicillin INN, BAN
adimolol INN
adinazolam USAN, INN, BAN *antidepressant; sedative*
adinazolam mesylate USAN *antidepressant*
Adipex-P tablets ℞ *anorexiant; CNS stimulant* [phentermine HCl] 37.5 mg
adiphenine INN *smooth muscle relaxant* [also: adiphenine HCl]
adiphenine HCl USAN *smooth muscle relaxant* [also: adiphenine]
adipiodone INN, JAN *parenteral radiopaque contrast medium* [also: iodipamide]
adipiodone meglumine JAN *parenteral radiopaque contrast medium (49.42% iodine)* [also: iodipamide meglumine]
Adipost slow-release capsules ℞ *anorexiant; CNS stimulant* [phendimetrazine tartrate] 105 mg
aditeren INN
aditoprim INN
AdjuVax-100a ℞ *investigational (Phase I/II) liposomal cancer vaccine synergist*
Adlone injection ℞ *corticosteroid; anti-inflammatory* [methylprednisolone acetate] 40, 80 mg/mL
adnephrine [see: epinephrine]
ADOAP (Adriamycin, Oncovin, ara-C, prednisone) *chemotherapy protocol*
Adolph's Salt Substitute OTC *salt substitute* [potassium chloride] 64 mEq/5 g; 35 mEq/5 g
Adolph's Seasoned Salt Substitute (discontinued 1997) OTC *salt substitute* [potassium chloride] 35 mEq/5 g
ADOP (Adriamycin, Oncovin, prednisone) *chemotherapy protocol*
adosopine INN
Adoxa film-coated tablets ℞ *tetracycline antibiotic* [doxycycline monohydrate] 50, 100 mg
adozelesin USAN, INN *antineoplastic*
Adprin-B coated tablets OTC *analgesic; antipyretic; anti-inflammatory; antirheumatic* [aspirin (buffered with calcium carbonate, magnesium oxide, and magnesium carbonate)] 325, 500 mg
ADR (Adriamycin) [see: Adriamycin; doxorubicin HCl]
adrafinil INN
adrenal [see: epinephrine]
adrenal cortical steroids *a class of steroid hormones that stimulate the adrenal cortex*
Adrenalin Chloride nose drops ℞ *nasal decongestant* [epinephrine HCl] 0.1%
Adrenalin Chloride solution for inhalation ℞ *sympathomimetic bronchodilator* [epinephrine HCl] 1:100, 1:1000
Adrenalin Chloride subcu, IV, IM or intracardiac injection ℞ *sympathomimetic bronchodilator for bronchial asthma, bronchospasm, and COPD;*

vasopressor for shock [epinephrine HCl] 1:1000 (1 mg/mL)

adrenaline BAN *vasoconstrictor; sympathomimetic bronchodilator; topical antiglaucoma agent; vasopressor for shock* [also: epinephrine] ⓢ adrenalone

adrenaline bitartrate [see: epinephrine bitartrate]

adrenaline HCl [see: epinephrine HCl]

adrenalone USAN, INN *ophthalmic adrenergic* ⓢ adrenaline

adrenamine [see: epinephrine]

adrenergic agonists *a class of bronchodilators that relax the bronchial muscles, reducing bronchospasm; a class of cardiac agents that increase myocardial contractility, causing a vasopressor effect to counteract shock (inadequate tissue perfusion)* [also called: sympathomimetics]

adrenine [see: epinephrine]

adrenochromazone [see: carbazochrome salicylate]

adrenochrome [see: carbazochrome salicylate]

adrenochrome guanylhydrazone mesilate JAN

adrenochrome monoaminoguanidine sodium methylsulfonate [see: adrenochrome guanylhydrazone mesilate]

adrenochrome monosemicarbazone sodium salicylate [see: carbazochrome salicylate]

adrenocorticotrophin [see: corticotropin]

adrenocorticotropic hormone (ACTH) [see: corticotropin]

adrenone [see: adrenalone]

Adria + BCNU (Adriamycin, BCNU) *chemotherapy protocol*

Adria-L-PAM (Adriamycin, L-phenylalanine mustard) *chemotherapy protocol*

Adriamycin PFS (preservative-free solution) IV injection ℞ *anthracycline antibiotic antineoplastic* [doxorubicin HCl] 2 mg/mL

Adriamycin RDF (rapid dissolution formula) powder for IV injection ℞ *anthracycline antibiotic antineoplastic* [doxorubicin HCl] 10, 20, 50, 150 mg/vial

Adria-Oncoline Chemo-Pin (trademarked delivery system)

adrogolide HCl USAN *dopamine D_1 receptor agonist for Parkinson disease*

Adrucil IV injection ℞ *antimetabolite antineoplastic for colorectal (orphan), breast, stomach, and pancreatic cancers; investigational (orphan) adjuvant to esophageal cancer* [fluorouracil] 50 mg/mL

ADS (azodisal sodium) [now: olsalazine sodium]

adsorbed diphtheria toxoid [see: diphtheria toxoid, adsorbed]

Adsorbocarpine eye drops ℞ *topical antiglaucoma agent; direct-acting miotic* [pilocarpine HCl] 1%, 2%, 4%

Adsorbonac eye drops OTC *corneal edema-reducing agent* [sodium chloride (hypertonic saline solution)] 2%, 5%

Adsorbotear eye drops (discontinued 1998) OTC *ocular moisturizer/lubricant* [hydroxyethylcellulose] 0.4%

ADT (trademarked dosage form) *alternate-day therapy*

Advair Diskus (powder for inhalation) ℞ *bronchodilator and corticosteroidal anti-inflammatory combination for asthma* [salmeterol xinafoate; fluticasone propionate] 50•100, 50•250, 50•500 µg

Advance test stick for home use *in vitro diagnostic aid; urine pregnancy test*

Advanced Care Cholesterol Test kit for home use *in vitro diagnostic aid for cholesterol in the blood*

"Advanced Formula" products [see under product name]

Advantage 24 vaginal gel OTC *spermicidal contraceptive (for use with a diaphragm)* [nonoxynol 9] 3.5%

Advera liquid OTC *enteral nutritional therapy for HIV and AIDS patients* [lactose-free formula] 240 mL

Advicor tablets ℞ *investigational (NDA filed) combination HMG-CoA reductase inhibitor for hypercholesterol-*

emia and hypertriglyceridemia [lovastatin; extended-release niacin]

Advil tablets, Liqui-Gels (soft liquid-filled gelatin capsules) OTC *analgesic; antiarthritic; antipyretic; nonsteroidal anti-inflammatory drug (NSAID)* [ibuprofen] 200 mg ☒ Avail

Advil, Children's chewable tablets, oral suspension OTC *analgesic; antiarthritic; antipyretic; nonsteroidal anti-inflammatory drug (NSAID)* [ibuprofen] 50 mg; 100 mg/5 mL

Advil, Junior Strength chewable tablets OTC *analgesic; antiarthritic; antipyretic; nonsteroidal anti-inflammatory drug (NSAID)* [ibuprofen] 100 mg

Advil Cold & Sinus caplets OTC *decongestant; analgesic; antipyretic* [pseudoephedrine HCl; ibuprofen] 30•200 mg

Advil Migraine liquid-filled capsules OTC *analgesic; antipyretic; nonsteroidal anti-inflammatory drug (NSAID)* [ibuprofen] 200 mg

Advil Pediatric Drops oral suspension OTC *analgesic; antipyretic; nonsteroidal anti-inflammatory drug (NSAID)* [ibuprofen] 100 mg/2.5 mL

AE-941 *investigational (Phase III) shark cartilage–based angiogenesis inhibitor for osteoarthritis, rheumatoid arthritis, and various cancers*

AEDs (anti-epileptic drugs) [see: anticonvulsants]

A-E-R pads OTC *astringent* [hamamelis water] 50%

Aerius (CAN) tablets ℞ *nonsedating antihistamine for allergic rhinitis* [desloratadine] 5 mg

Aeroaid spray OTC *antiseptic; antibacterial; antifungal* [thimerosal; alcohol 72%] 1:1000

AeroBid; AeroBid-M oral inhalation aerosol ℞ *corticosteroidal anti-inflammatory for chronic asthma* [flunisolide] 250 µg/dose

AeroCaine aerosol solution OTC *topical local anesthetic* [benzocaine; benzethonium chloride] 13.6%•0.5%

AeroChamber (trademarked form) *aerosol holding chamber*

Aerodine aerosol OTC *broad-spectrum antimicrobial* [povidone-iodine]

AeroDose (trademarked delivery system) ℞ *investigational (Phase I) inhaler*

Aerofreeze spray OTC *topical vapocoolant anesthetic* [trichloromonofluoromethane; dichlorodifluoromethane] ?•?

Aerolate Sr.; Aerolate Jr.; Aerolate III timed-action capsules ℞ *antiasthmatic; bronchodilator* [theophylline] 260 mg; 130 mg; 65 mg

Aerolizer (trademarked delivery system) *oral inhaler for encapsulated dry powder*

Aeropin ℞ *investigational (orphan) for cystic fibrosis* [heparin, 2-0-desulfated]

Aeroseb-Dex aerosol spray ℞ *topical corticosteroidal anti-inflammatory* [dexamethasone] 0.01%

Aeroseb-HC aerosol spray (discontinued 1997) ℞ *topical corticosteroidal anti-inflammatory; antiseborrheic* [hydrocortisone] 0.5%

aerosol OT [see: docusate sodium]

aerosolized pooled immune globulin [see: globulin, aerosolized pooled immune]

AeroTherm aerosol solution OTC *topical local anesthetic* [benzocaine; benzethonium chloride] 13.6%•0.5%

Aerotrol (trademarked form) *inhalation aerosol*

AeroZoin spray OTC *skin protectant* [benzoin; isopropyl alcohol 44.8%] 30%

AERx ℞ *investigational (Phase II) system that delivers morphine directly to the lungs; investigational (Phase II) insulin inhalation system for diabetes management* [morphine sulfate]

Aesculus hippocastanum; A. californica; A. glabra *medicinal herb* [see: horse chestnut]

Aethusa cynapium *medicinal herb* [see: dog poison]

aethylis chloridum [see: ethyl chloride]

afalanine INN

afloqualone INN, JAN

AFM (Adriamycin, fluorouracil, methotrexate [with leucovorin rescue]) *chemotherapy protocol*

afovirsen INN *antisense antiviral*

afovirsen sodium USAN *antisense antiviral; investigational for genital warts*

African ginger *medicinal herb* [see: ginger]

African pepper; African red pepper *medicinal herb* [see: cayenne]

Afrin extended-release tablets OTC *nasal decongestant* [pseudoephedrine sulfate] 120 mg ⓢ aspirin

Afrin nasal spray, nose drops OTC *nasal decongestant* [oxymetazoline HCl] 0.05% ⓢ aspirin

Afrin Children's Nose Drops OTC *nasal decongestant* [oxymetazoline HCl] 0.025% ⓢ aspirin

Afrin Moisturizing Saline Mist solution OTC *nasal moisturizer* [sodium chloride (saline solution)] 0.64% ⓢ aspirin

Afrin Sinus nasal spray OTC *nasal decongestant* [oxymetazoline HCl] 0.05% ⓢ aspirin

Aftate for Athlete's Foot spray powder, spray liquid OTC *topical antifungal* [tolnaftate] 1%

Aftate for Jock Itch spray powder OTC *topical antifungal* [tolnaftate] 1%

afurolol INN

A/G Pro tablets OTC *dietary supplement* [protein hydrolysate; multiple vitamins & minerals; multiple amino acids] 542•≛ mg

AG-1549 *investigational (Phase II) nonnucleoside reverse transcriptase inhibitor (NNRTI) for HIV and AIDS*

agalsidase alfa USAN *investigational (NDA filed) enzyme replacement therapy for Fabry disease*

agalsidase beta *investigational (NDA filed) enzyme replacement therapy for Fabry disease*

aganodine INN

agar NF, JAN *suspending agent*

agar-agar [see: agar]

Agathosma betulina *medicinal herb* [see: buchu]

agave *(Agave americana)* plant *medicinal herb used as an antiseptic, diuretic, and laxative and for jaundice and liver disease, pulmonary tuberculosis, and syphilis; also used to combat putrefactive bacteria in the stomach and intestines*

age cross-link breakers *a class of investigational antiaging compounds that break age-mediated bonds between proteins*

Agenerase capsules, oral solution ℞ *antiviral protease inhibitor for HIV* [amprenavir] 50, 150 mg; 15 mg/mL

Aggrastat IV infusion ℞ *GP IIb/IIIa platelet aggregation inhibitor for acute coronary syndrome, unstable angina, myocardial infarction, and cardiac surgery* [tirofiban HCl] 50, 250 μg/mL

aggregated albumin [see: albumin, aggregated]

aggregated radio-iodinated I 131 serum albumin [see: albumin, aggregated iodinated I 131 serum]

Aggrenox combination-release capsule ℞ *platelet aggregation inhibitor for stroke* [dipyridamole (extended release); aspirin (immediate release)] 200•25 mg

aglepristone INN

AGN-191024 *investigational (Phase III) agent for glaucoma*

agofollin [see: estradiol]

Agoral oral liquid OTC *stimulant laxative* [sennosides] 25 mg/15 mL ⓢ Argyrol

Agoral Plain emulsion (discontinued 1997) OTC *emollient laxative* [mineral oil] 1.4 g/5 mL

agrimony *(Agrimonia eupatoria)* plant *medicinal herb for diarrhea, gastroenteritis, jaundice, kidney stones, liver disorders, mucous membrane inflammation with discharge; also used topically as an astringent and antiseptic*

agrimony, hemp *medicinal herb* [see: hemp agrimony]

Agropyron repens *medicinal herb* [see: couch grass]

Agrylin capsules ℞ *thrombolytic and antiplatelet agent for essential thrombocytope-*

nia (orphan); investigational (orphan) for thrombocytosis and polycythemia vera [anagrelide HCl] 0.5, 1 mg

ague tree *medicinal herb* [see: sassafras]

agurin [see: theobromine sodium acetate]

AHA (acetohydroxamic acid) [q.v.]

AHA (alpha hydroxy acids) [see: glycolic acid]

AH-chew chewable tablets ℞ *decongestant; antihistamine; anticholinergic* [phenylephrine HCl; chlorpheniramine maleate; methscopolamine nitrate] 10•2•1.25 mg

AH-chew D chewable tablets ℞ *decongestant* [phenylephrine HCl] 10 mg

AHF (antihemophilic factor) [q.v.]

AHG (antihemophilic globulin) [see: antihemophilic factor]

A-Hydrocort IV or IM injection ℞ *corticosteroid; anti-inflammatory* [hydrocortisone sodium succinate] 100, 250, 500, 1000 mg/vial

AIDS vaccine (several different compounds are included in this general category; e.g., gp120, rgp160, rgp160 MN, rp24) *investigational (Phase I–III) antiviral for HIV and AIDS treatment and prophylaxis* [also: gp120; rgp160; rp24]

AIDSVax ℞ *investigational (Phase III) bivalent HIV vaccine* [gp120 antigens]

AIIRAs (angiotensin II receptor antagonists) [q.v.]

air, compressed [see: air, medical]

air, medical USP *medicinal gas*

Airet solution for inhalation ℞ *sympathomimetic bronchodilator* [albuterol sulfate] 0.083%

Airomir (CAN) CFC-free pMDI (pressurized metered-dose inhaler) ℞ *sympathomimetic bronchodilator* [salbutamol sulfate] 100 μg/dose

AI-RSA *investigational (orphan) for autoimmune uveitis*

ajmaline JAN

Akarpine eye drops ℞ *topical antiglaucoma agent; direct-acting miotic* [pilocarpine HCl] 1%, 2%, 4%

AKBeta eye drops ℞ *topical antiglaucoma agent (β-blocker)* [levobunolol HCl] 0.25%, 0.5%

AK-Chlor eye drops, ophthalmic ointment ℞ *topical ophthalmic antibiotic* [chloramphenicol] 5 mg/mL; 10 mg/g

AK-Con eye drops ℞ *topical ophthalmic decongestant and vasoconstrictor* [naphazoline HCl] 0.1%

AK-Dex eye drops ℞ *topical ophthalmic corticosteroidal anti-inflammatory* [dexamethasone sodium phosphate] 0.1%

AK-Dex ophthalmic ointment ℞ *topical ophthalmic corticosteroidal anti-inflammatory* [dexamethasone sodium phosphate] 0.05%

AK-Dilate eye drops ℞ *topical ophthalmic decongestant and vasoconstrictor; mydriatic* [phenylephrine HCl] 2.5%, 10%

AK-Fluor antecubital venous injection ℞ *ophthalmic diagnostic agent* [fluorescein] 10%, 25%

AK-Homatropine eye drops (discontinued 1998) ℞ *mydriatic; cycloplegic* [homatropine hydrobromide] 5%

Akineton IV or IM injection ℞ *anticholinergic; antiparkinsonian* [biperiden lactate] 5 mg/mL

Akineton tablets ℞ *anticholinergic; antiparkinsonian* [biperiden HCl] 2 mg

aklomide USAN, INN, BAN *coccidiostat for poultry*

AK-NaCl eye drops, ophthalmic ointment OTC *corneal edema-reducing agent* [sodium chloride (hypertonic saline solution)] 5%

AK-Nefrin eye drops OTC *topical ophthalmic decongestant* [phenylephrine HCl] 0.12%

Akne-mycin ointment, topical solution ℞ *topical antibiotic for acne* [erythromycin] 2% (S) Ak-Mycin

AK-Neo-Dex eye drops (discontinued 2000) ℞ *topical ophthalmic corticosteroidal anti-inflammatory; antibiotic* [dexamethasone sodium phosphate; neomycin sulfate] 0.1%•0.35%

AK-Pentolate eye drops ℞ *mydriatic; cycloplegic* [cyclopentolate HCl] 1%

AK-Poly-Bac ophthalmic ointment ℞ *topical ophthalmic antibiotic* [polymyxin B sulfate; bacitracin zinc] 10 000•500 U/g

AK-Pred eye drops ℞ *topical ophthalmic corticosteroidal anti-inflammatory* [prednisolone sodium phosphate] 0.125%, 1%

AKPro eye drops ℞ *topical antiglaucoma agent* [dipivefrin HCl] 0.1%

AK-Rinse ophthalmic solution OTC *extraocular irrigating solution* [sterile isotonic solution]

AK-Spore eye drops ℞ *topical ophthalmic antibiotic* [polymyxin B sulfate; neomycin sulfate; gramicidin] 10 000 U•1.75 mg•0.025 mg per mL

AK-Spore ophthalmic ointment ℞ *topical ophthalmic antibiotic* [polymyxin B sulfate; neomycin sulfate; bacitracin zinc] 10 000 U•5 mg•400 U per g

AK-Spore H.C. ear drops, otic suspension ℞ *topical corticosteroidal anti-inflammatory; antibiotic* [hydrocortisone; neomycin sulfate; polymyxin B sulfate] 1%•5 mg•10 000 U per mL

AK-Spore H.C. eye drop suspension (discontinued 2000) ℞ *topical ophthalmic corticosteroidal anti-inflammatory; antibiotic* [hydrocortisone; neomycin sulfate; polymyxin B sulfate] 1%•0.35%•10 000 U per mL

AK-Spore H.C. ophthalmic ointment ℞ *topical ophthalmic corticosteroidal anti-inflammatory; antibiotic* [hydrocortisone; neomycin sulfate; bacitracin zinc; polymyxin B sulfate] 1%•0.35%•400 U/g•10 000 U/g

AK-Sulf eye drops, ophthalmic ointment ℞ *topical ophthalmic antibiotic* [sulfacetamide sodium] 10%

AKTob eye drops ℞ *topical ophthalmic antibiotic* [tobramycin] 0.3%

AK-Tracin ophthalmic ointment ℞ *ophthalmic antibiotic* [bacitracin] 500 U/g

AK-Trol eye drop suspension, ophthalmic ointment ℞ *topical ophthalmic corticosteroidal anti-inflammatory; antibiotic* [dexamethasone; neomycin sulfate; polymyxin B sulfate] 0.1%•0.35%•10 000 U/mL; 0.1%•0.35%•10 000 U/g

Akwa Tears eye drops OTC *ophthalmic moisturizer/lubricant* [polyvinyl alcohol] 1.4%

Akwa Tears ophthalmic ointment OTC *ocular moisturizer/lubricant* [white petrolatum; mineral oil]

AL-721 *investigational (Phase I/II) antiviral for HIV and AIDS*

ALA (alpha lipoic acid) *natural antioxidant* [q.v.]

ALA; 5-ALA HCl [see: aminolevulinic acid HCl]

alacepril INN, JAN

Ala-Cort cream, lotion ℞ *topical corticosteroidal anti-inflammatory* [hydrocortisone] 1%

alafosfalin INN, BAN

Alamag oral suspension OTC *antacid* [aluminum hydroxide; magnesium hydroxide] 225•200 mg/5 mL ⓢ Alma-Mag

Alamag Plus oral suspension OTC *antacid; antiflatulent* [aluminum hydroxide; magnesium hydroxide; simethicone] 225•200•25 mg/5 mL

Alamast eye drops ℞ *mast cell stabilizer for allergic conjunctivitis* [pemirolast potassium] 0.1%

alamecin USAN *antibacterial*

alanine (L-alanine) USAN, USP, INN *nonessential amino acid; symbols: Ala, A*

alanine nitrogen mustard [see: melphalan]

alanosine INN

alaproclate USAN, INN *antidepressant*

Ala-Quin cream ℞ *topical corticosteroidal anti-inflammatory; antifungal; antibacterial* [hydrocortisone; clioquinol] 0.5%•3%

Ala-Scalp lotion ℞ *topical corticosteroidal anti-inflammatory* [hydrocortisone] 2%

AlaSTAT lab test for professional use *test for allergic reaction to latex*

Alasulf vaginal cream ℞ *broad-spectrum antibiotic; antiseptic; vulnerary* [sulfanilamide; aminacrine HCl; allantoin] 15%•0.2%•2%

alatrofloxacin mesylate USAN *broad-spectrum fluoroquinolone antibiotic*

alazanine triclofenate INN

Albalon eye drops ℞ *topical ophthalmic decongestant and vasoconstrictor and lubricant* [naphazoline HCl; polyvinyl alcohol] 0.1%•1.4%

Albamycin capsules ℞ *bacteriostatic antibiotic* [novobiocin sodium] 250 mg

Albay subcu or IM injection ℞ *venom sensitivity testing (subcu); venom desensitization therapy (IM)* [extracts of honeybee, yellow jacket, yellow hornet, white-faced hornet, mixed vespid, and wasp venom]

albendazole USAN, INN, BAN *anthelmintic for neurocysticercosis and hydatid cyst disease (orphan); investigational (Phase III) for AIDS-related microsporidiosis*

albendazole oxide INN, BAN

Albenza Tiltab (film-coated tablets) ℞ *anthelmintic for neurocysticercosis (tapeworm) and cestode-induced hydatid cyst disease (orphan)* [albendazole]

Albright solution (sodium citrate and citric acid) *urine alkalizer; compounding agent*

albucid [see: sulfacetamide]

albumin, aggregated USAN *lung imaging aid (with technetium Tc 99m)*

albumin, aggregated iodinated I 131 serum USAN, USP *radioactive agent*

albumin, chromated Cr 51 serum USAN *radioactive agent*

albumin, human USP *blood volume supporter* 5%, 25% injection

albumin, human (sonicated with chlorofluorocarbons) *ultrasound contrast medium for cardiac imaging; investigational (Phase III) diagnostic aid for infertility due to obstructed fallopian tubes*

albumin, iodinated (^{125}I) human serum INN *radioactive agent; blood volume test* [also: albumin, iodinated I 125 serum]

albumin, iodinated (^{131}I) human serum INN, JAN *radioactive agent; intrathecal imaging agent; blood volume test* [also: albumin, iodinated I 131 serum]

albumin, iodinated I 125 USP *radioactive agent; blood volume test*

albumin, iodinated I 125 serum USAN, USP *radioactive agent; blood volume test* [also: iodinated (^{125}I) human serum albumin]

albumin, iodinated I 131 USP *radioactive agent; intrathecal imaging agent; blood volume test*

albumin, iodinated I 131 serum USAN, USP *radioactive agent; intrathecal imaging agent; blood volume test* [also: iodinated (^{131}I) human serum albumin]

albumin, normal human serum [now: albumin, human]

Albuminar-5; Albuminar-25 IV infusion ℞ *blood volume expander for shock, burns, and hypoproteinemia* [human albumin] 5%; 25%

Albunex injection ℞ *ultrasound heart imaging agent; investigational (Phase III) diagnostic aid for infertility due to obstructed fallopian tubes* [human albumin, sonicated] 5%

Albustix reagent strips for professional use *in vitro diagnostic aid for albumin (protein) in the urine*

Albutein 5%; Albutein 25% IV infusion ℞ *blood volume expander for shock, burns, and hypoproteinemia* [human albumin] 5%; 25%

albuterol USAN, USP *sympathomimetic bronchodilator* [also: salbutamol] 90 µg inhalation

albuterol sulfate USAN, USP *sympathomimetic bronchodilator* [also: salbutamol sulfate] 2, 4 mg oral; 2 mg/5 mL oral; 0.083%, 0.5% inhalation

albutoin USAN, INN *anticonvulsant*

Alcaine Drop-Tainers (eye drops) ℞ *topical ophthalmic anesthetic* [proparacaine HCl] 0.5%

alcanna *medicinal herb* [see: henna (*Alkanna*)]

Alcar ℞ *investigational (Phase III) treatment for Alzheimer disease* [levacecarnine]

Alcare foam OTC *topical antiseptic* [ethyl alcohol] 62%

Alchemilla xanthochlora; A. vulgaris *medicinal herb* [see: lady's mantle]

alclofenac USAN, INN, BAN, JAN *anti-inflammatory*

alclometasone INN, BAN *topical corticosteroidal anti-inflammatory* [also: alclometasone dipropionate]

alclometasone dipropionate USAN, USP, JAN *topical corticosteroidal anti-inflammatory* [also: alclometasone]

alcloxa USAN, INN *astringent; keratolytic* [also: aluminum chlorohydroxy allantoinate]

Alco-Gel OTC *topical antiseptic for instant sanitation of hands* [ethyl alcohol] 60% ⓢ aloe gel

alcohol USP *topical anti-infective/antiseptic; astringent; solvent; a widely abused "legal street drug" used to produce euphoria* [also: ethanol]

alcohol, dehydrated USP *antidote* [also: ethanol, dehydrated]

alcohol, diluted NF *solvent*

alcohol, rubbing USP, INN *rubefacient*

5% Alcohol and 5% Dextrose in Water; 10% Alcohol and 5% Dextrose in Water IV infusion ℞ *for caloric replacement and rehydration* [dextrose; alcohol] 5%•5%; 10%•5%

Alcon Saline Especially for Sensitive Eyes solution OTC *rinsing/storage solution for soft contact lenses* [sodium chloride (preserved saline solution)]

Alconefrin nose drops, nasal spray OTC *nasal decongestant* [phenylephrine HCl] 0.25%, 0.5%

Alconefrin 12 nose drops OTC *nasal decongestant* [phenylephrine HCl] 0.16%

alcuronium chloride USAN, INN, BAN, JAN *skeletal muscle relaxant*

Aldactazide tablets ℞ *antihypertensive; diuretic* [spironolactone; hydrochlorothiazide] 25•25, 50•50 mg ⓢ Aldactone

Aldactone tablets ℞ *antihypertensive; potassium-sparing diuretic* [spironolactone] 25, 50, 100 mg ⓢ Aldactazide

Aldara cream ℞ *immunomodulator for external genital and perianal warts* [imiquimod] 5% in 250 mg single-use packets

alder, spotted *medicinal herb* [see: witch hazel]

alder, striped *medicinal herb* [see: winterberry; witch hazel]

alder buckthorn; European black alder *medicinal herb* [see: buckthorn]

alderlin [see: pronethalol]

aldesleukin USAN, INN, BAN *immunostimulant; biological response modifier; antineoplastic for metastatic melanoma and renal cell carcinoma (orphan); investigational (Phase III, orphan) for immunodeficiency diseases and acute myelogenous leukemia (AML); investigational (Phase II) for Hodgkin lymphoma*

aldesulfone sodium INN, DCF *antibacterial; leprostatic* [also: sulfoxone sodium]

aldioxa USAN, INN, JAN *astringent; keratolytic*

Aldoclor-150; Aldoclor-250 film-coated tablets ℞ *antihypertensive* [chlorothiazide; methyldopa] 150•250 mg; 250•250 mg

aldocorten [see: aldosterone]

Aldomet film-coated tablets, oral suspension ℞ *antihypertensive* [methyldopa] 125, 250, 500 mg; 250 mg/5 mL

Aldomet; Aldomet Ester HCl IV injection ℞ *antihypertensive* [methyldopate HCl] 50 mg/mL

Aldoril 15; Aldoril 25; Aldoril D30; Aldoril D50 film-coated tablets ℞ *antihypertensive; diuretic* [hydrochlorothiazide; methyldopa] 15•250 mg; 25•250 mg; 30•500 mg; 50•500 mg ⓢ Elavil; Eldepryl; Enovil; Equanil; Mellaril

aldosterone INN, BAN, DCF

Aldurazyme ℞ *investigational (Phase III, orphan) enzyme replacement therapy for mucopolysaccharidosis-1 (MPS-1)* [laronidase]

Alec ℞ *investigational (orphan) for neonatal respiratory distress syndrome* [colfosceril palmitate; phosphatidylglycerol]

alefacept USAN *treatment for plaque psoriasis*

alemcinal USAN *motilin agonist to stimulate gastrointestinal peristaltic action*

alemtuzumab *humanized monoclonal antibody (huMAb) immunosuppressant for B-cell chronic lymphocytic leukemia (B-CLL); investigational (Phase II) for non-Hodgkin lymphoma, organ transplants, and multiple sclerosis*

alendronate sodium USAN *bisphosphonate bone resorption inhibitor for Paget disease and corticosteroid-induced or age-related osteoporosis in men and women*

alendronic acid INN, BAN

Alenic Alka chewable tablets OTC *antacid* [aluminum hydroxide; magnesium trisilicate] 80•20 mg

Alenic Alka liquid OTC *antacid* [aluminum hydroxide; magnesium carbonate] 31.7•137.3 mg/5 mL

Alenic Alka, Extra Strength chewable tablets OTC *antacid* [aluminum hydroxide; magnesium carbonate] 160•105 mg

alentemol INN *antipsychotic; dopamine agonist* [also: alentemol hydrobromide]

alentemol hydrobromide USAN *antipsychotic; dopamine agonist* [also: alentemol]

alepride INN

Alertec (CAN) tablets ℞ *analeptic for excessive daytime sleepiness of narcolepsy* [modafinil] 100 mg

Alesse tablets (in packs of 21 or 28) ℞ *monophasic oral contraceptive; emergency postcoital contraceptive* [levonorgestrel; ethinyl estradiol] 100•20 µg

alestramustine INN

aletamine HCl USAN *antidepressant* [also: alfetamine]

Aletris farinosa *medicinal herb* [see: star grass]

Aleurites moluccana; A. cordata *medicinal herb* [see: tung seed]

Aleve tablets, capsules, gelcaps OTC *analgesic; antiarthritic; antipyretic; nonsteroidal anti-inflammatory drug (NSAID)* [naproxen (from naproxen sodium)] 200 (220) mg

alexidine USAN, INN *antibacterial*

alexitol sodium INN, BAN

alexomycin USAN *veterinary growth promoter for poultry and swine*

alfacalcidol (1α-hydroxycholecalciferol; 1α-hydroxyvitamin D_3) INN, BAN, JAN *vitamin D precursor (converted to calcifediol in the body); calcium regulator for treatment of hypocalcemia and osteodystrophy from chronic renal dialysis*

alfadex INN

alfadolone INN, DCF [also: alphadolone]

alfalfa *(Medicago sativa)* leaves and flowers *medicinal herb for anemia, appetite stimulation, arthritis, atherosclerosis, blood cleansing, diabetes, hemorrhages, kidney cleansing, lowering cholesterol levels, nausea, pituitary disorders, and peptic ulcers*

alfaprostol USAN, INN, BAN *veterinary prostaglandin*

alfaxalone INN, JAN, DCF [also: alphaxalone]

Alfenta IV or IM injection ℞ *narcotic analgesic; anesthetic* [alfentanil HCl] 500 µg/mL

alfentanil INN, BAN *narcotic analgesic* [also: alfentanil HCl]

alfentanil HCl USAN *narcotic analgesic* [also: alfentanil]

Alferon LDO (low dose oral) ℞ *investigational (Phase I/II) cytokine for HIV, AIDS, and ARC* [interferon alfa-n3]

Alferon N intralesional injection ℞ *immunomodulator and antiviral for condylomata acuminata; investigational (Phase III) cytokine for HIV, AIDS, ARC, and hepatitis C* [interferon alfa-n3] 5 million IU/mL

alfetamine INN *antidepressant* [also: aletamine HCl]

alfetamine HCl [see: aletamine HCl]
alfuzosin INN, BAN *antihypertensive (α-blocker)* [also: alfuzosin HCl]
alfuzosin HCl USAN *antihypertensive (α-blocker)* [also: alfuzosin]
algeldrate USAN, INN *antacid*
algestone INN *anti-inflammatory* [also: algestone acetonide]
algestone acetonide USAN, BAN *anti-inflammatory* [also: algestone]
algestone acetophenide USAN *progestin*
algin [see: sodium alginate]
alginic acid NF, BAN *tablet binder and emulsifying agent*
alginic acid, sodium salt [see: sodium alginate]
alglucerase USAN, INN, BAN *glucocerebrosidase enzyme replacement for Gaucher disease type I (orphan); investigational (orphan) for types II and III*
alibendol INN, DCF
Alibra ℞ *investigational (NDA filed) treatment for erectile dysfunction*
aliconazole INN
alidine dihydrochloride [see: anileridine]
alidine phosphate [see: anileridine]
alifedrine INN
aliflurane USAN, INN *inhalation anesthetic*
alimadol INN
alimemazine INN *phenothiazine antihistamine; antipruritic* [also: trimeprazine tartrate; trimeprazine; alimemazine tartrate]
alimemazine tartrate JAN *phenothiazine antihistamine; antipruritic* [also: trimeprazine tartrate; alimemazine; trimeprazine]
Alimentum ready-to-use liquid OTC *hypoallergenic infant food* [casein protein formula]
Aliminase ℞ *investigational (Phase III) immunostimulant for ulcerative colitis*
alinidine INN, BAN
alipamide USAN, INN, BAN *diuretic; antihypertensive*
aliphatic alcohol compound *investigational (Phase III) topical antiviral treatment for herpes simplex*
alisactide [see: alsactide]
alisobumal [see: butalbital]
alitame USAN *sweetener*
alitretinoin USAN *retinoic acid for topical treatment of cutaneous lesions of AIDS-related Kaposi sarcoma (orphan); investigational (Phase III, orphan) for acute promyelocytic leukemia*
alitretinoin & interferon *investigational (Phase I/II) combination treatment for AIDS-related Kaposi sarcoma*
alizapride INN
Alka-Mints chewable tablets OTC *antacid* [calcium carbonate] 850 mg
Alkanna tinctoria *medicinal herb* [see: henna]
Alka-Seltzer effervescent tablets OTC *antacid; analgesic* [sodium bicarbonate; citric acid; aspirin; phenylalanine] 1700•1000•325•9 mg
Alka-Seltzer, Extra Strength effervescent tablets OTC *antacid; analgesic* [sodium bicarbonate; citric acid; aspirin] 1985•1000•500 mg
Alka-Seltzer, Gold effervescent tablets OTC *antacid* [sodium bicarbonate; citric acid; potassium bicarbonate] 958•832•312 mg
Alka-Seltzer, Original effervescent tablets OTC *antacid; analgesic* [sodium bicarbonate; citric acid; aspirin] 1916•1000•325 mg
Alka-Seltzer Plus Allergy Liqui-Gels; Alka-Seltzer Plus Cold Liqui-Gels (capsules) OTC *decongestant; antihistamine; analgesic* [pseudoephedrine HCl; chlorpheniramine maleate; acetaminophen] 30•2•250 mg
Alka-Seltzer Plus Children's Cold effervescent tablets OTC *antitussive; decongestant; antihistamine* [dextromethorphan hydrobromide; phenylpropanolamine bitartrate; chlorpheniramine maleate] 5•10•1 mg
Alka-Seltzer Plus Cold & Cough tablets OTC *antitussive; decongestant; antihistamine; analgesic; antipyretic* [dextromethorphan hydrobromide; phenylpropanolamine bitartrate; chlorpheniramine maleate; aspirin] 10•20•2•325 mg

Alka-Seltzer Plus Cold & Cough Liqui-Gels (capsules) OTC *antitussive; decongestant; antihistamine; analgesic* [dextromethorphan hydrobromide; pseudoephedrine HCl; chlorpheniramine maleate; acetaminophen] 10•30•2•250 mg

Alka-Seltzer Plus Cold Medicine; Alka-Seltzer Plus Cold Tablets for oral solution OTC *decongestant; antihistamine; analgesic; antipyretic* [phenylpropanolamine bitartrate; brompheniramine maleate; aspirin] 20•2•325 mg; 24.08•2•325 mg

Alka-Seltzer Plus Cold & Sinus capsules OTC *decongestant; analgesic* [pseudoephedrine HCl; acetaminophen] 30•325 mg

Alka-Seltzer Plus Cold & Sinus effervescent tablets OTC *decongestant; analgesic; antipyretic* [phenylpropanolamine bitartrate; aspirin] 20•325 mg

Alka-Seltzer Plus Flu & Body Aches Non-Drowsy Liqui-Gels (capsules) OTC *antitussive; decongestant; analgesic* [dextromethorphan hydrobromide; pseudoephedrine HCl; acetaminophen] 10•30•250 mg

Alka-Seltzer Plus Night-Time Cold tablets OTC *antitussive; decongestant; antihistamine; analgesic; antipyretic* [dextromethorphan hydrobromide; phenylpropanolamine bitartrate; doxylamine succinate; aspirin] 10•20•6.25•500 mg

Alka-Seltzer Plus Night-Time Cold Liqui-Gels (capsules) OTC *antitussive; decongestant; antihistamine; analgesic* [dextromethorphan hydrobromide; pseudoephedrine HCl; doxylamine succinate; acetaminophen] 10•30•6.25•250 mg

Alka-Seltzer Plus Sinus tablets OTC *decongestant; analgesic; antipyretic* [phenylpropanolamine bitartrate; aspirin] 20•325 mg

Alka-Seltzer with Aspirin effervescent tablets OTC *antacid; analgesic* [sodium bicarbonate; citric acid; aspirin] 1900•1000•325, 1900•1000•500 mg

alkavervir (Veratrum viride alkaloids)

Alkavite extended-release tablets OTC *vitamin/mineral supplement for alcohol-related deficiencies* [multiple vitamins & minerals; calcium carbonate; iron sulfate; folic acid; biotin] ≛•68.5•60•1•0.03 mg

Alkeran tablets, powder for IV infusion ℞ *nitrogen mustard-type alkylating antineoplastic for multiple myeloma (orphan) and ovarian cancer; investigational (orphan) for metastatic melanoma* [melphalan] 2 mg; 50 mg

Alkets chewable tablets OTC *antacid* [calcium carbonate] 500, 750 mg

alkyl aryl sulfonate *surfactant/wetting agent*

alkylamines *a class of antihistamines*

alkylbenzyldimethylammonium chloride [see: benzalkonium chloride]

alkyldimethylbenzylammonium chloride [see: benzalkonium chloride]

alkylpolyaminoethylglycine JAN

alkylpolyaminoethylglycine HCl JAN

allantoin USAN, BAN *topical vulnerary*

Allbee C-800 film-coated tablets OTC *vitamin supplement* [multiple B vitamins; vitamins C and E] ≛•800•45 mg

plus Iron coated tablets OTC *vitamin/iron supplement* [ferrous fumarate; multiple B vitamins; vitamins C and E; folic acid] 27 mg•≛•800 mg•45 IU•0.4 mg

Allbee with C caplets OTC *vitamin supplement* [multiple B vitamins; vitamin C] ≛•300 mg

Allbee-T tablets OTC *vitamin supplement* [multiple B vitamins; vitamin C] ≛•500 mg

Allegra film-coated tablets, capsules ℞ *nonsedating antihistamine for allergic rhinitis and chronic idiopathic urticaria* [fexofenadine HCl] 30, 60, 180 mg; 60 mg

Allegra 24 Hour (CAN) extended-release tablets OTC *nonsedating antihistamine*

for allergic rhinitis [fexofenadine HCl] 120 mg

Allegra-D extended-release film-coated tablets, capsules ℞ *decongestant; nonsedating antihistamine* [pseudoephedrine HCl; fexofenadine HCl] 120•60 mg

Allelix ℞ *investigational (Phase III) agent to increase bone mineral content and density in postmenopausal osteoporosis* [parathyroid hormone (1-84), recombinant human]

Allent sustained-release capsules ℞ *decongestant; antihistamine* [pseudoephedrine HCl; brompheniramine maleate] 120•12 mg

Aller-Chlor tablets, syrup OTC *antihistamine* [chlorpheniramine maleate] 4 mg; 2 mg/5 mL

Allercon tablets OTC *decongestant; antihistamine* [pseudoephedrine HCl; triprolidine HCl] 60•2.5 mg

Allercreme Skin lotion OTC *moisturizer; emollient*

Allercreme Ultra Emollient cream OTC *moisturizer; emollient*

Allerest eye drops OTC *topical ophthalmic decongestant and vasoconstrictor* [naphazoline HCl] 0.012%

Allerest tablets OTC *decongestant; antihistamine* [pseudoephedrine HCl; chlorpheniramine maleate] 30•2 mg

Allerest, Children's chewable tablets OTC *pediatric decongestant and antihistamine* [phenylpropanolamine HCl; chlorpheniramine maleate] 9.4•1 mg

Allerest 12 Hour nasal spray OTC *nasal decongestant* [oxymetazoline HCl] 0.05%

Allerest 12 Hour sustained-release caplets OTC *decongestant; antihistamine* [phenylpropanolamine HCl; chlorpheniramine maleate] 75•12 mg

Allerest Headache; Allerest Sinus Pain Formula tablets OTC *decongestant; antihistamine; analgesic* [pseudoephedrine HCl; chlorpheniramine maleate; acetaminophen] 30•2•325 mg; 30•2•500 mg

Allerest No Drowsiness tablets OTC *decongestant; analgesic* [pseudoephedrine HCl; acetaminophen] 30•325 mg

Allerfrim tablets, syrup OTC *decongestant; antihistamine* [pseudoephedrine HCl; triprolidine HCl] 60•2.5 mg; 30•1.25 mg/5 mL

Allerfrin with Codeine syrup ℞ *narcotic antitussive; decongestant; antihistamine* [codeine phosphate; pseudoephedrine HCl; triprolidine HCl] 10•30•1.25 mg/5 mL

Allergan Enzymatic tablets OTC *enzymatic cleaner for soft contact lenses* [papain] ⑨ allergen; Auralgan

Allergan Hydrocare [see: Hydrocare]

Allergen Ear Drops ℞ *topical local anesthetic; analgesic* [benzocaine; antipyrine] 1.4%•5.4%

allergenic extracts *a class of agents derived from various biological sources containing antigens that possess immunologic activity*

allergenic extracts (aqueous, glycerinated, or alum-precipitated) *over 900 allergens available for diagnosis of and desensitization to specific allergies*

Allergy tablets OTC *antihistamine* [chlorpheniramine maleate] 4 mg

Allergy Drops eye drops OTC *topical ophthalmic decongestant and vasoconstrictor* [naphazoline HCl] 0.012%; 0.03%

AllerMax caplets, oral liquid OTC *antihistamine; sleep aid* [diphenhydramine HCl] 50 mg; 12.5 mg/5 mL

AllerMax liquid (name changed to AllerMax Allergy & Cough Formula in 1997)

AllerMax Allergy & Cough Formula liquid OTC *antihistamine* [diphenhydramine HCl] 6.25 mg/5 mL

Allermed capsules OTC *nasal decongestant* [pseudoephedrine HCl] 60 mg

Allerphed syrup OTC *decongestant; antihistamine* [pseudoephedrine HCl; triprolidine HCl] 30•1.25 mg/5 mL

AlleRx sustained-release tablets (AM and PM) ℞ AM: *decongestant and*

anticholinergic; PM: antihistamine and anticholinergic [AM: pseudoephedrine HCl and methscopolamine nitrate; PM: chlorpheniramine maleate and methscopolamine nitrate] AM: 120•2.5 mg; PM: 8•2.5 mg

alletorphine BAN, INN

all-heal *medicinal herb* [see: mistletoe; valerian]

Allium cepa *medicinal herb* [see: onion]

Allium porrum *medicinal herb* [see: leek]

Allium sativum *medicinal herb* [see: garlic]

All-Nite Cold Formula liquid OTC *antitussive; decongestant; antihistamine; analgesic* [dextromethorphan hydrobromide; pseudoephedrine HCl; doxylamine succinate; acetaminophen; alcohol 25%] 5•10•1.25•167 mg/5 mL

allobarbital USAN, INN *hypnotic*

allobarbitone [see: allobarbital]

alloclamide INN, DCF

allocupreide sodium INN, DCF

AlloDerm *investigational acellular connective tissue skin graft for third-degree burns and plastic surgery* [processed human donor skin]

allomethadione INN, DCF [also: aloxidone]

allopurinol USAN, USP, INN, BAN, JAN *xanthine oxidase inhibitor for gout and hyperuricemia; antineoplastic adjunct for reducing uric acid levels following chemotherapy for leukemia, lymphoma, and solid tumor malignancies (orphan)* 100, 300 mg oral

allopurinol sodium *antineoplastic adjunct for reducing uric acid levels following chemotherapy for leukemia, lymphoma, and solid tumor malignancies (orphan)*

Allovectin-7 ℞ *investigational (Phase II) treatment for head and neck cancer; investigational (Phase II/III, orphan) for invasive and metastatic melanoma*

Allpyral subcu or IM injection ℞ *allergenic sensitivity testing (subcu); allergenic desensitization therapy (IM)* [allergenic extracts, alum-precipitated]

allspice *(Eugenia pimenta; Pimenta dioica; P. officinalis)* unripe fruit and leaves *medicinal herb for diarrhea and gas; also used as a purgative and tonic*

all-*trans*-retinoic acid [see: tretinoin]

allyl isothiocyanate USAN, USP

allylamines *a class of antifungals*

allylbarbituric acid [now: butalbital]

allylestrenol INN, JAN [also: allyloestrenol]

allyl-isobutylbarbituric acid [see: butalbital]

allylisopropylmalonylurea [see: aprobarbital]

4-allyl-2-methoxyphenol [see: eugenol]

N-allylnoretorphine [see: alletorphine]

N-allylnoroxymorphone HCl [see: naloxone HCl]

allyloestrenol BAN [also: allylestrenol]

allylprodine INN, BAN, DCF

5-allyl-5-*sec*-butylbarbituric acid [see: talbutal]

allylthiourea INN

allypropymal [see: aprobarbital]

Almacone chewable tablets, liquid OTC *antacid; antiflatulent* [aluminum hydroxide; magnesium hydroxide; simethicone] 200•200•20 mg; 200•200•20 mg/5 mL

Almacone II liquid OTC *antacid; antiflatulent* [aluminum hydroxide; magnesium hydroxide; simethicone] 400•400•40 mg/5 mL

almadrate sulfate USAN, INN *antacid*

almagate USAN, INN *antacid*

almagodrate INN

almasilate INN, BAN

Almebex Plus B$_{12}$ liquid OTC *vitamin supplement* [multiple B vitamins] ≛

almecillin INN

almestrone INN

alminoprofen INN, JAN

almitrine INN, BAN

almokalant INN *investigational antiarrhythmic*

almond *(Prunus amygdalus)* kernels *medicinal herb used as a demulcent, emollient, and pectoral*

almond oil NF *emollient and perfume; oleaginous vehicle*

Almora tablets OTC *magnesium supplement* [magnesium gluconate] 500 mg

almotriptan USAN, INN *investigational serotonin 5-HT$_{1D}$ agonist for migraine*

almotriptan malate USAN *serotonin 5-HT$_{1B/1D}$ agonist for migraine*

almoxatone INN

alnespirone INN

alniditan dihydrochloride USAN *serotonin 5-HT$_{1D}$ agonist for migraine*

Alnus glutinosa *medicinal herb* [see: black alder]

Alocril eye drops ℞ *mast cell stabilizer for allergic conjunctivitis* [nedocromil sodium] 2%

aloe USP ⑨ Alco-Gel

aloe (*Aloe vera* and over 500 other species) leaves and juice *medicinal herb for burns, hemorrhoids, insect bites, and scalds; also used as a deodorant and to aid digestion and limit scarring; not generally regarded as safe and effective as a cathartic*

Aloe Grande lotion OTC *moisturizer; emollient; skin protectant* [vitamins A and E; aloe] 3333.3•50•≟ U/g

Aloe Vesta Perineal solution OTC *emollient/protectant* [propylene glycol; aloe vera gel]

alofilcon A USAN *hydrophilic contact lens material*

aloin BAN

ALOMAD (Adriamycin, Leukeran, Oncovin, methotrexate, actinomycin D, dacarbazine) *chemotherapy protocol* ⑨ Alomide

Alomide Drop-Tainers (eye drops) ℞ *topical antiallergic for vernal keratoconjunctivitis (orphan)* [lodoxamide tromethamine] 0.1% ⑨ ALOMAD

alonacic INN

alonimid USAN, INN *sedative; hypnotic*

Alophen Pills tablets (discontinued 1998) OTC *stimulant laxative* [phenolphthalein] 60 mg

Aloprim powder for IV infusion ℞ *antineoplastic adjunct for reducing uric acid levels following chemotherapy for leukemia, lymphoma, and solid tumor malignancies (orphan)* [allopurinol sodium] 500 mg

Alor 5/500 tablets ℞ *narcotic analgesic* [hydrocodone bitartrate; aspirin] 5•500 mg

Alora transdermal patch ℞ *estrogen replacement therapy for postmenopausal symptoms* [estradiol] 50, 75, 100 µg/day

aloracetam INN

alosetron INN, BAN *antiemetic; 5-HT$_3$ receptor antagonist for irritable bowel syndrome* [also: alosetron HCl]

alosetron HCl USAN *antiemetic; 5-HT$_3$ receptor antagonist for irritable bowel syndrome* [also: alosetron]

alovudine USAN, INN *antiviral*

aloxidone BAN [also: allomethadione]

aloxiprin INN, BAN, DCF

aloxistatin INN

Aloysiatriphylla **spp.** *medicinal herb* [see: lemon verbena]

alozafone INN

alpertine USAN, INN *antipsychotic*

alpha amylase (α-amylase) USAN *anti-inflammatory*

alpha hydroxy acids (AHA) [see: glycolic acid]

alpha interferon-2A [see: interferon alfa-2A]

alpha interferon-2B [see: interferon alfa-2B]

alpha interferon-N1 [see: interferon alfa-N1]

alpha interferon-N3 [see: interferon alfa-N3]

Alpha Keri Moisturizing Soap bar OTC *therapeutic skin cleanser*

Alpha Keri Spray; Alpha Keri Therapeutic Bath Oil OTC *bath emollient*

alpha lipoic acid (ALA) *natural antioxidant that is both fat- and water-soluble and readily crosses cell membranes; used in the treatment of AIDS, diabetes, liver ailments, oxidative stress injuries, and various cancers*

***d*-alpha tocopherol** *(relative potency: 100%)* [see: vitamin E]

***dl*-alpha tocopherol** *(relative potency: 74%)* [see: vitamin E]

***d*-alpha tocopheryl acetate** *(relative potency: 91%)* [see: vitamin E]

***dl*-alpha tocopheryl acetate** *(relative potency: 67%)* [see: vitamin E]

***d*-alpha tocopheryl acid succinate** *(relative potency: 81%)* [see: vitamin E]

***dl*-alpha tocopheryl acid succinate** *(relative potency: 60%)* [see: vitamin E]

alpha$_1$ PI (alpha$_1$-proteinase inhibitor) [q.v.]

alpha$_1$-antitrypsin (AAT), recombinant *investigational (orphan) for alpha$_1$-antitrypsin deficiency in the ZZ phenotype population; investigational for asthma*

alpha$_1$-antitrypsin, transgenic human *investigational (Phase II, orphan) for cystic fibrosis*

alpha$_1$-proteinase inhibitor (alpha$_1$ PI) *replacement therapy for hereditary alpha$_1$ PI deficiency, which leads to progressive panacinar emphysema (orphan); investigational (Phase II) antiviral for HIV*

alphacemethadone [see: alphacetylmethadol]

alphacetylmethadol BAN, INN, DCF

alpha-chymotrypsin [see: chymotrypsin]

alpha-cypermethrin BAN

alpha-D-galactosidase *digestive enzyme*

alphadolone BAN [also: alfadolone]

alpha-estradiol [see: estradiol]

alpha-estradiol benzoate [see: estradiol benzoate]

alpha-ethyltryptamine (alpha-EtT) *a hallucinogenic street drug chemically related to MDMA* [see also: MDMA; alpha-methyltryptamine]

alphafilcon A USAN *hydrophilic contact lens material*

α-D-galactopyranose [see: galactose]

alpha-galactosidase A *investigational (orphan) enzyme replacement therapy for Fabry disease*

alpha-galactosidase A & ceramide trihexosidase (CTH) *investigational (orphan) enzyme replacement therapy for Fabry disease*

Alphagan; Alphagan P eye drops ℞ *selective α_2 agonist for open-angle glaucoma and ocular hypertension* [brimonidine tartrate] 0.2%; 0.15%

alpha-glucosidase, human acid [see: human acid alpha-glucosidase]

1-alpha-hydroxy vitamin D$_2$ *investigational osteoporosis treatment*

alpha-hypophamine [see: oxytocin]

alpha-L-iduronidase, recombinant [now: laronidase]

alpha-melanocyte stimulating hormone *investigational (orphan) agent for the prevention and treatment of acute renal failure due to ischemia*

alphameprodine INN, BAN, DCF

alphamethadol INN, BAN, DCF

alpha-methyldopa [now: methyldopa]

alpha-methyltryptamine (alpha-MeT) *a hallucinogenic street drug chemically related to MDMA* [see also: MDMA; alpha-ethyltryptamine]

Alphanate powder for IV injection ℞ *antihemophilic; investigational (orphan) for von Willebrand disease* [antihemophilic factor VIII:C, solvent/detergent treated]

AlphaNine IV injection (discontinued 1997; replaced by AlphaNine SD) ℞ *antihemophilic for factor IX deficiency (hemophilia B; Christmas disease) (orphan)* [coagulation factor IX, human]

AlphaNine SD IV injection ℞ *antihemophilic for factor IX deficiency (hemophilia B; Christmas disease) (orphan)* [coagulation factors II, VII, IX, and X, solvent/detergent treated]

alpha-phenoxyethyl penicillin, potassium [see: phenethicillin potassium]

alphaprodine INN, BAN [also: alphaprodine HCl]

alphaprodine HCl USP [also: alphaprodine]

alphasone acetophenide [now: algestone acetonide]

Alphatrex cream, ointment, lotion ℞ *topical corticosteroidal anti-inflammatory* [betamethasone dipropionate] 0.05%

alphaxalone BAN [also: alfaxalone]

alpidem USAN, INN, BAN *anxiolytic*

Alpinia officinarum; A. galanga *medicinal herb* [see: galangal]

Alpinia oxyphylla; A. fructus *medicinal herb* [see: bitter cardamom]

Alpinia speciosa *medicinal herb for edema, fungal infections, hypertension, and thrombosis*

alpiropride INN

alprafenone INN

alprazolam USAN, USP, INN, BAN, JAN *benzodiazepine anxiolytic; sedative; treatment of panic disorders and agoraphobia* 0.25, 0.5, 1, 2 mg, 0.5 mg/5 mL, 1 mg/mL oral

alprenolol INN, BAN *antiadrenergic (β-receptor)* [also: alprenolol HCl]

alprenolol HCl USAN, JAN *antiadrenergic (β-receptor)* [also: alprenolol]

alprenoxime HCl USAN *antiglaucoma agent*

alprostadil USAN, USP, INN, BAN, JAN *vasodilator for erectile dysfunction; platelet aggregation inhibitor; investigational (orphan) for peripheral arterial occlusive disease*

alprostadil, liposomal *investigational (Phase III) for erectile dysfunction; investigational (orphan) for acute respiratory distress and ischemic ulcerations due to peripheral artery disease*

alprostadil alfadex BAN

Alprox-TD cream ℞ *investigational (Phase III) topical therapy for erectile dysfunction* [alprostadil]

Alramucil effervescent powder (discontinued 1999) OTC *bulk laxative* [psyllium hydrophilic mucilloid] 3.6 g/packet

Alredase ℞ *investigational (NDA filed) aldose reductase inhibitor for diabetic neuropathy* [tolrestat]

alrestatin INN *aldose reductase enzyme inhibitor* [also: alrestatin sodium]

alrestatin sodium USAN *aldose reductase enzyme inhibitor* [also: alrestatin]

Alrex eye drop suspension ℞ *corticosteroidal anti-inflammatory* [loteprednol etabonate] 0.2%

alsactide INN

alseroxylon JAN *antihypertensive; rauwolfia derivative*

ALT (autolymphocyte therapy) [q.v.]

ALT-711 *investigational (Phase II) anti-aging compound*

Altace capsules ℞ *angiotensin-converting enzyme (ACE) inhibitor for hypertension, myocardial infarction, and stroke* [ramipril] 1.25, 2.5, 5, 10 mg

altanserin INN *serotonin antagonist* [also: altanserin tartrate]

altanserin tartrate USAN *serotonin antagonist* [also: altanserin]

altapizone INN

alteconazole INN

alteplase USAN, INN, BAN, JAN *tissue plasminogen activator (tPA) for acute myocardial infarction, acute ischemic stroke, or pulmonary embolism*

alteratives *a class of agents that produce gradual beneficial changes in the body, usually by improving nutrition, without having any marked specific effect*

ALternaGEL liquid OTC *antacid* [aluminum hydroxide gel] 600 mg/5 mL

Althaea officinalis *medicinal herb* [see: marsh mallow]

althiazide USAN *antihypertensive* [also: altizide]

Alti-Amiodarone (CAN) tablets ℞ *antiarrhythmic* [amiodarone HCl] 200 mg

Alti-Amoxi Clav (CAN) tablets ℞ *aminopenicillin antibiotic* [amoxicillin; clavulanic acid] 250•125, 500•125 mg

Alti-Clindamycin (CAN) capsules ℞ *lincosamide antibiotic* [clindamycin HCl] 150, 300 mg

Alti-Clobazam (CAN) tablets ℞ *minor tranquilizer and anxiolytic; adjunct to anticonvulsant therapy* [clobazam] 10 mg

Alti-Dexamethasone (CAN) tablets ℞ *corticosteroid; anti-inflammatory* [dexamethasone] 0.5, 0.75, 4 mg

Alti-Doxazosin (CAN) tablets ℞ *antihypertensive (α-blocker)* [doxazosin mesylate] 1, 2, 4 mg

Alti-Famotidine (CAN) film-coated tablets ℞ *histamine H_2 antagonist for gastric and duodenal ulcers* [famotidine] 20, 40 mg

Alti-Flunisolide (CAN) nasal spray ℞ *corticosteroidal anti-inflammatory for chronic asthma and rhinitis* [flunisolide] 0.025% (25 μg/metered dose)

Alti-Fluoxetine (CAN) capsules ℞ *selective serotonin reuptake inhibitor (SSRI) for depression, obsessive-compulsive disorder (OCD), and bulimia nervosa* [fluoxetine HCl] 10, 20 mg

Alti-Ipratropium (CAN) nasal spray, solution for inhalation ℞ *anticholinergic bronchodilator for bronchospasm; antisecretory for rhinorrhea* [ipratropium bromide] 0.03%; 0.0125%, 0.025%

Alti-Metformin HCl (CAN) film-coated tablets ℞ *biguanide antidiabetic* [metformin HCl] 500, 850 mg

Alti-MPA (CAN) tablets ℞ *progestin for secondary amenorrhea, abnormal uterine bleeding, and endometrial hyperplasia* [medroxyprogesterone acetate] 2.5, 5, 10 mg

Altinac cream ℞ *topical keratolytic for acne* [tretinoin] 0.025%, 0.05%, 0.1%

altinicline maleate USAN *investigational (Phase II) nicotinic acetylcholine receptor agonist for Parkinson disease*

Alti-Nortriptylene Hydrochloride (CAN) capsules ℞ *tricyclic antidepressant* [nortriptyline HCl] 10, 25 mg

Alti-Ticlopidine (CAN) film-coated tablets ℞ *platelet aggregation inhibitor for stroke* [ticlopidine HCl] 250 mg

Alti-Timolol (CAN) eye drops ℞ *topical antiglaucoma agent (β-blocker)* [timolol maleate] 0.25%, 0.5%

altizide INN, DCF *antihypertensive* [also: althiazide]

Alti-Zopiclone (CAN) tablets ℞ *sedative; hypnotic* [zopiclone] 7.5 mg

altoqualine INN

Altracin *investigational (orphan) for pseudomembranous enterocolitis* [bacitracin]

altrenogest USAN, INN, BAN *veterinary progestin*

altretamine USAN, INN, BAN *antineoplastic for advanced ovarian adenocarcinoma (orphan)*

Altropane *investigational (Phase III) single photon emission tomography imaging agent for Parkinson disease; investigational (Phase II) radioimaging agent for attention-deficit hyperactivity disorder (ADHD)*

altumomab USAN, INN *radiodiagnostic monoclonal antibody for colorectal carcinoma; anticarcinoembryonic antigen (anti-CEA)* [also: indium In 111 altumomab pentetate]

altumomab pentetate USAN *monoclonal antibody conjugate* [also: indium In 111 altumomab pentetate]

Alu-Cap capsules OTC *antacid* [aluminum hydroxide gel] 400 mg

Aludrox oral suspension OTC *antacid; antiflatulent* [aluminum hydroxide; magnesium hydroxide; simethicone] 307•103•? mg/5 mL

alukalin [see: kaolin]

alum, ammonium USP *topical astringent*

alum, potassium USP *topical astringent* [also: aluminum potassium sulfate]

alum root (*Geranium maculatum*) *medicinal herb used as an astringent, hemostatic, and antiseptic*

Alumadrine tablets ℞ *decongestant; antihistamine; analgesic* [phenylpropanolamine HCl; chlorpheniramine maleate; acetaminophen] 25•4•500 mg

alumina & magnesia USP *antacid*

aluminopara-aminosalicylate calcium (alumino *p*-aminosalicylate calcium) JAN

aluminosilicic acid, magnesium salt hydrate [see: silodrate]

aluminum *element (Al)*

aluminum, micronized *astringent*

aluminum acetate USP *topical astringent; Burow solution*

aluminum aminoacetate [see: dihydroxyaluminum aminoacetate]

aluminum ammonium sulfate dodecahydrate [see: alum, ammonium]

aluminum bismuth oxide [see: bismuth aluminate]
aluminum carbonate, basic USAN, USP *antacid*
aluminum chlorhydroxide [now: aluminum chlorohydrate]
aluminum chlorhydroxide alcohol soluble complex [now: aluminum chlorohydrex]
aluminum chloride USP *topical astringent for hyperhidrosis* 20% topical
aluminum chloride, basic [see: aluminum sesquichlorohydrate]
aluminum chloride hexahydrate [see: aluminum chloride]
aluminum chloride hydroxide hydrate [see: aluminum chlorohydrate]
aluminum chlorohydrate USAN *anhidrotic*
aluminum chlorohydrex USAN *topical astringent*
aluminum chlorohydrol propylene glycol complex [now: aluminum chlorohydrex]
aluminum chlorohydroxy allantoinate JAN *astringent; keratolytic* [also: alcloxa]
aluminum clofibrate INN, BAN, JAN
aluminum dihydroxyaminoacetate [see: dihydroxyaluminum aminoacetate]
aluminum flufenamate JAN
aluminum glycinate, basic [see: dihydroxyaluminum aminoacetate]
aluminum hydroxide gel USP *antacid* 320, 450, 600 mg/5 mL oral
aluminum hydroxide gel, dried USP, JAN *antacid*
aluminum hydroxide glycine [see: dihydroxyaluminum aminoacetate]
aluminum hydroxide hydrate [see: algeldrate]
aluminum hydroxychloride [now: aluminum chlorohydrate]
aluminum magnesium carbonate hydroxide dihydrate [see: almagate]
aluminum magnesium hydroxide carbonate hydrate [see: hydrotalcite]
aluminum magnesium hydroxide oxide sulfate [see: almadrate sulfate]
aluminum magnesium hydroxide oxide sulfate hydrate [see: almadrate sulfate]
aluminum magnesium hydroxide sulfate [see: magaldrate]
aluminum magnesium hydroxide sulfate hydrate [see: magaldrate]
aluminum monostearate NF, JAN
aluminum oxide
Aluminum Paste ointment OTC *occlusive skin protectant* [metallic aluminum] 10%
aluminum phosphate gel USP *antacid (disapproved for use as an antacid in 1989)*
aluminum potassium sulfate JAN *topical astringent* [also: alum, potassium]
aluminum potassium sulfate dodecahydrate [see: alum, potassium]
aluminum sesquichlorohydrate USAN *anhidrotic*
aluminum silicate, natural JAN
aluminum silicate, synthetic JAN
aluminum sodium carbonate hydroxide [see: dihydroxyaluminum sodium carbonate]
aluminum subacetate USP *topical astringent*
aluminum sulfate USP *anhidrotic*
aluminum sulfate hydrate [see: aluminum sulfate]
aluminum zirconium glycine tetrachloro hydrate complex [see: aluminum zirconium tetrachlorohydrex gly]
aluminum zirconium glycine trichloro hydrate complex [see: aluminum zirconium trichlorohydrex gly]
aluminum zirconium octachlorohydrate USP *anhidrotic*
aluminum zirconium octachlorohydrex gly USP *anhidrotic*
aluminum zirconium pentachlorohydrate USP *anhidrotic*
aluminum zirconium pentachlorohydrex gly USP *anhidrotic*
aluminum zirconium tetrachlorohydrate USP *anhidrotic*

aluminum zirconium tetrachlorohydrex gly USAN, USP *anhidrotic*

aluminum zirconium trichlorohydrate USP *anhidrotic*

aluminum zirconium trichlorohydrex gly USAN, USP *anhidrotic*

Alupent tablets (discontinued 1999) ℞ *sympathomimetic bronchodilator* [metaproterenol sulfate] 10, 20 mg

Alupent syrup, inhalation aerosol powder, solution for inhalation ℞ *sympathomimetic bronchodilator* [metaproterenol sulfate] 10 mg/5 mL; 0.65 mg/dose; 0.4%, 0.6%, 5%

Alurate elixir ℞ *sedative; hypnotic* [aprobarbital] 40 mg/5 mL

Alustra cream ℞ *hyperpigmentation bleaching agent* [hydroquinone; tretinoin (in a base containing glycolic acid and vitamins C and E)] 4%•0.1% ⑨ Lustra

alusulf INN

Alu-Tab film-coated tablets OTC *antacid* [aluminum hydroxide gel] 500 mg

ALVAC-120TMG *investigational (Phase II) vaccine for HIV* [also: VCP 205]

ALVAC-HIV 1 ℞ *investigational (Phase I) vaccine for HIV* [also: AIDS vaccine gp160 MN]

alverine INN, BAN *anticholinergic* [also: alverine citrate]

alverine citrate USAN, NF *anticholinergic* [also: alverine]

alvircept sudotox USAN, INN *antiviral; investigational (Phase II) for AIDS*

ALX-0600 *investigational (Phase II, orphan) glucagon analogue for short bowel syndrome*

AM Caps (CAN) OTC *vitamin supplement* [multiple vitamins; folic acid; biotin] ≛•0.2•0.15 mg

amabevan [see: carbarsone]

amacetam HCl [now: pramiracetam HCl]

amacetam sulfate [now: pramiracetam sulfate]

amadinone INN *progestin* [also: amadinone acetate]

amadinone acetate USAN *progestin* [also: amadinone]

amafolone INN, BAN

amalgucin

***Amanita muscaria* mushrooms** *a species that produces muscarine and ibotenic acid, a psychotropic substance ingested as a street drug*

amanozine INN

amantadine INN, BAN *antiviral for influenza A virus; dopaminergic antiparkinsonian* [also: amantadine HCl]

amantadine HCl USAN, USP, JAN *antiviral for influenza A virus; dopaminergic antiparkinsonian* [also: amantadine] 100 mg oral; 50 mg/5 mL oral

amantanium bromide INN

amantocillin INN

Amaphen capsules (discontinued 2000) ℞ *analgesic; barbiturate sedative* [acetaminophen; caffeine; butalbital] 325•40•50 mg

amara; amargo *medicinal herb* [see: quassia]

amaranth (*Amnaranthus* spp.) leaves and flowers *medicinal herb for diarrhea, dysentery, excessive menstruation, and nosebleeds*

amaranth (FD&C Red No. 2) USP

amargo; amara *medicinal herb* [see: quassia]

amarsan [see: acetarsone]

Amaryl tablets ℞ *once-daily sulfonylurea antidiabetic* [glimepiride] 1, 2, 4 mg

ambamustine INN

ambasilide INN *investigational antiarrhythmic*

ambazone INN, BAN, DCF

ambenonium chloride USP, INN, BAN, JAN *anticholinesterase muscle stimulant*

ambenoxan INN, BAN

Ambenyl Cough syrup ℞ *narcotic antitussive; antihistamine* [codeine phosphate; bromodiphenhydramine HCl; alcohol 5%] 10•12.5 mg/5 mL ⑨ Aventyl

Ambenyl-D liquid OTC *antitussive; decongestant; expectorant* [dextromethorphan hydrobromide; pseudoephedrine HCl; guaifenesin; alcohol 9.5%] 10•30•100 mg/5 mL

amber; amber touch-and-heal *medicinal herb* [see: St. John's wort]
Ambi 10 bar OTC *therapeutic skin cleanser*
Ambi 10 cream OTC *topical keratolytic for acne* [benzoyl peroxide] 10%
Ambi Skin Tone cream OTC *hyperpigmentation bleaching agent; sunscreen* [hydroquinone; padimate O]
ambicromil INN, BAN *prophylactic antiallergic* [also: probicromil calcium]
ambicromil calcium [see: probicromil calcium]
Ambien film-coated tablets ℞ *imidazopyridine sedative and hypnotic* [zolpidem tartrate] 5, 10 mg
AmBisome powder for IV infusion ℞ *systemic polyene antifungal for cryptococcal meningitis, visceral leishmaniasis, and histoplasmosis (orphan)* [amphotericin B lipid complex (ABLC)] 50 mg/vial
ambomycin USAN, INN *antineoplastic*
ambrette (*Abelmoschus moschatus*) seeds and oil *medicinal herb for gastric cancer, gonorrhea, hysteria, and respiratory disorders; also used as a fragrance in cosmetics and a flavoring in alcoholic beverages, bitters, and coffees; not generally regarded as safe and effective for medicinal uses*
ambroxol INN [also: ambroxol HCl]
ambroxol HCl JAN [also: ambroxol]
ambruticin USAN, INN *antifungal*
ambucaine INN, DCF
ambucetamide INN, BAN
ambuphylline USAN *diuretic; smooth muscle relaxant* [also: bufylline]
ambuside USAN, INN, BAN *diuretic*
ambuterol [see: mabuterol]
ambutonium bromide BAN
ambutoxate [see: ambucaine]
amcinafal USAN, INN *anti-inflammatory*
amcinafide USAN, INN *anti-inflammatory*
amcinonide USAN, USP, INN, BAN, JAN *topical corticosteroidal anti-inflammatory*
Amcort IM injection ℞ *corticosteroid; anti-inflammatory* [triamcinolone diacetate] 40 mg/mL
AMD-3100 *investigational (Phase II) for HIV infection*
amdinocillin USAN, USP *aminopenicillin antibiotic* [also: mecillinam]
amdinocillin pivoxil USAN *antibacterial* [also: pivmecillinam; pivmecillinam HCl]
Amdray IV infusion, oral solution, capsules ℞ *investigational (Phase III) P-glycoprotein (P-gp) inhibitor for multi-drug–resistant (MDR) cancers, including acute myelogenous leukemia (AML), multiple myeloma, and ovarian cancer* [valspodar]
ameban [see: carbarsone]
amebarsone [see: carbarsone]
amebicides *a class of drugs that kill amoebae*
amebucort INN
amechol [see: methacholine chloride]
amedalin INN *antidepressant* [also: amedalin HCl]
amedalin HCl USAN *antidepressant* [also: amedalin]
Amelorad *investigational agent to reduce chemotherapy side effects (clinical trials discontinued 1998)* [EF-27 (code name—generic name not yet assigned)]
ameltolide USAN, INN, BAN *anticonvulsant*
Amen tablets ℞ *progestin for secondary amenorrhea, abnormal uterine bleeding, and endometrial hyperplasia* [medroxyprogesterone acetate] 10 mg
amenozine [see: amanozine]
Amerge film-coated tablets ℞ *vascular serotonin 5-HT$_1$ receptor agonist for migraine headache* [naratriptan HCl] 1, 2.5 mg
Americaine ointment, anorectal ointment, aerosol spray OTC *topical local anesthetic* [benzocaine] 20%
Americaine Anesthetic Lubricant gel ℞ *anesthetic lubricant for upper GI procedures* [benzocaine] 20%
Americaine First Aid ointment OTC *topical local anesthetic* [benzocaine] 20%

Americaine Otic ear drops ℞ *topical local anesthetic* [benzocaine] 20%
American angelica *medicinal herb* [see: angelica]
American aspen *medicinal herb* [see: poplar]
American centaury *(Sabatia angularis)* plant *medicinal herb used as a bitter tonic, emmenagogue, febrifuge, and vermifuge*
American elder *medicinal herb* [see: elderberry]
American elm *medicinal herb* [see: slippery elm]
American foxglove *medicinal herb* [see: feverweed]
American ginseng *(Panax quinquefolia)* *medicinal herb* [see: ginseng]
American hellebore *(Veratrum viride)* [see: hellebore]
American ivy *(Parthenocissus quinquefolia)* bark and twigs *medicinal herb used as an alterative, astringent, and expectorant*
American nightshade *medicinal herb* [see: pokeweed]
American pepper; American red pepper *medicinal herb* [see: cayenne]
American saffron *medicinal herb* [see: safflower]
American valerian *medicinal herb* [see: lady's slipper]
American vegetable tallow tree; American vegetable wax *medicinal herb* [see: bayberry]
American woodbine *medicinal herb* [see: American ivy]
americium *element (Am)*
Amerigel lotion, ointment OTC *topical diaper rash treatment*
amesergide USAN, INN *serotonin antagonist; investigational antidepressant*
ametantrone INN *antineoplastic* [also: ametantrone acetate]
ametantrone acetate USAN *antineoplastic* [also: ametantrone]
ametazole BAN [also: betazole HCl; betazole]
A-Methapred powder for injection ℞ *corticosteroid; anti-inflammatory; immunosuppressant* [methylprednisolone sodium succinate] 40, 125, 500, 1000 mg/vial
amethocaine BAN *topical anesthetic* [also: tetracaine]
amethocaine HCl BAN *local anesthetic* [also: tetracaine HCl]
amethopterin [now: methotrexate]
Amevive ℞ *investigational (Phase III) for psoriasis*
amezepine INN
amezinium metilsulfate INN, JAN
amfebutamone INN *aminoketone antidepressant; non-nicotine aid to smoking cessation* [also: bupropion HCl; bupropion]
amfebutamone HCl [see: bupropion HCl]
amfecloral INN, BAN *anorectic* [also: amphecloral]
amfenac INN, BAN *anti-inflammatory* [also: amfenac sodium]
amfenac sodium USAN, JAN *anti-inflammatory* [also: amfenac]
amfepentorex INN, DCF
amfepramone INN, DCF *anorexiant* [also: diethylpropion HCl; diethylpropion]
amfepramone HCl *anorexiant* [see: diethylpropion HCl]
amfetamine INN *CNS stimulant* [also: amphetamine sulfate; amphetamine]
amfetaminil INN
amfilcon A USAN *hydrophilic contact lens material*
amflutizole USAN, INN *gout suppressant*
amfodyne [see: imidecyl iodine]
amfomycin INN, DCF *antibacterial* [also: amphomycin]
amfonelic acid USAN, INN, BAN *CNS stimulant*
Amgenal Cough syrup ℞ *narcotic antitussive; antihistamine* [codeine phosphate; bromodiphenhydramine HCl] 10•12.5 mg/5 mL
AMI-7228 *investigational magnetic resonance angiography contrast agent*
amibiarson [see: carbarsone]
Amicar tablets, syrup, IV infusion ℞ *systemic hemostatic to control excessive*

bleeding [aminocaproic acid] 500 mg; 250 mg/mL; 250 mg/mL ⑨ Amikin
amicarbalide INN, BAN
amicibone INN
amicloral USAN *veterinary food additive*
amicycline USAN, INN *antibacterial*
amidantel INN, BAN
amidapsone USAN, INN *antiviral for poultry*
Amidate IV injection ℞ *rapid-acting nonbarbiturate general anesthetic* [etomidate] 2 mg/mL
amidefrine mesilate INN *adrenergic* [also: amidephrine mesylate; amidephrine]
amidephrine BAN *adrenergic* [also: amidephrine mesylate; amidefrine mesilate]
amidephrine mesylate USAN *adrenergic* [also: amidefrine mesilate; amidephrine]
amidofebrin [see: aminopyrine]
amidol [see: dimepheptanol]
amidone HCl [see: methadone HCl]
amidopyrazoline [see: aminopyrine]
amidopyrine [now: aminopyrine]
amidotrizoate sodium [see: diatrizoate sodium]
amidotrizoic acid JAN *radiopaque contrast medium* [also: diatrizoic acid]
amiflamine INN
amifloverine INN, DCF
amifloxacin USAN, INN, BAN *broad-spectrum fluoroquinolone antibiotic*
amifloxacin mesylate USAN *broad-spectrum fluoroquinolone antibiotic*
amifostine USAN, INN, BAN *chemoprotective agent for cisplatin and paclitaxel chemotherapy (orphan); radioprotective agent; treatment for xerostomia following radiation therapy; investigational (orphan) for cyclophosphamide rescue*
Amigesic film-coated tablets, film-coated caplets, capsules ℞ *analgesic; antipyretic; anti-inflammatory; antirheumatic* [salsalate] 500 mg; 750 mg; 500 mg
amikacin USP, INN, BAN *aminoglycoside antibiotic; investigational (Phase II) liposomal formulation for complicated urinary tract infections and AIDS-related Mycobacterial infection*
amikacin sulfate USAN, USP, JAN *aminoglycoside antibiotic* 50, 250 mg/mL injection
amikhelline INN
Amikin IV or IM injection, pediatric injection ℞ *aminoglycoside antibiotic* [amikacin sulfate] 250 mg/mL; 50 mg/mL ⑨ Amicar
amilomer INN
amiloride INN, BAN *antihypertensive; potassium-sparing diuretic* [also: amiloride HCl]
amiloride HCl USAN, USP *antihypertensive; potassium-sparing diuretic; investigational (orphan) inhalant for cystic fibrosis* [also: amiloride]
amiloxate USAN *ultraviolet B sunscreen*
aminacrine BAN *topical anti-infective/antiseptic* [also: aminacrine HCl; aminoacridine]
aminacrine HCl USAN *vaginal antibacterial and antiseptic* [also: aminoacridine; aminacrine]
Amin-Aid Instant Drink powder (discontinued 1997) OTC *enteral nutritional therapy for acute or chronic renal failure* [essential amino acids]
aminarsone [see: carbarsone]
amindocate INN
amine resin [see: polyamine-methylene resin]
amineptine INN
Aminess 5.2% IV infusion ℞ *nutritional therapy for renal failure* [multiple essential amino acids]
aminicotin [see: niacinamide]
aminitrozole INN *veterinary antibacterial* [also: nithiamide; acinitrazole]
2-amino-2-deoxyglucose [see: glucosamine]
aminoacetic acid JAN *nonessential amino acid; urologic irrigant; symbols: Gly, G* [also: glycine]
aminoacridine INN *topical anti-infective/antiseptic* [also: aminacrine HCl; aminacrine]
aminoacridine HCl [see: aminacrine HCl]

9-aminoacridine monohydrochloride [see: aminacrine HCl]
***p*-aminobenzenearsonic acid** [see: arsanilic acid]
***p*-aminobenzenesulfonamide** [see: sulfanilamide]
***p*-aminobenzene-sulfonylacetylimide** [see: sulfacetamide]
aminobenzoate potassium USP *water-soluble vitamin; analgesic; "possibly effective" for scleroderma and other skin diseases and Peyronie disease*
aminobenzoate sodium USP *analgesic*
***p*-aminobenzoic acid** [see: aminobenzoic acid]
aminobenzoic acid (4-aminobenzoic acid) USP *water-soluble vitamin; ultraviolet screen* 100, 1000 mg oral
aminobenzylpenicillin [see: ampicillin]
γ-amino-β-hydroxybutyric acid JAN
aminobromophenylpyrimidinone (ABPP) [see: bropirimine]
γ-aminobutyric acid (GABA) JAN *inhibitory neurotransmitter*
9-aminocamptothecin (9-AC) *topoisomerase I inhibitor; investigational (Phase I/II) anticancer agent; investigational (Phase II) for AIDS-related Kaposi sarcoma*
aminocaproic acid USAN, USP, INN, BAN *systemic hemostatic; investigational (orphan) topical treatment for traumatic hyphema of the eye* [also: ϵ-aminocaproic acid] 250 mg/mL injection
ϵ-aminocaproic acid JAN *systemic hemostatic* [also: aminocaproic acid]
aminocardol [see: aminophylline]
Amino-Cerv pH 5.5 vaginal cream ℞ *emollient; antifungal; anti-inflammatory* [urea; sodium propionate; methionine; cystine; inositol] 8.34%•0.5%•0.83%•0.35%•0.83%
aminodeoxykanamycin [see: bekanamycin]
2-aminoethanethiol [see: cysteamine]
2-aminoethanethiol HCl [see: cysteamine HCl]
2-aminoethanol [see: monoethanolamine]
aminoethyl nitrate (2-aminoethyl nitrate) INN, DCF
amino-ethyl-propanol [see: ambuphylline]
aminoethylsulfonic acid JAN [also: taurine]
aminoform [see: methenamine]
aminoglutethimide USP, INN, BAN *adrenal steroid inhibitor; antisteroidal antineoplastic*
aminoglycosides *a class of bactericidal antibiotics effective against gram-negative organisms*
aminoguanidine monohydrochloride [see: pimagedine HCl]
6-aminohexanoic acid [see: aminocaproic acid]
aminohippurate sodium USP *diagnostic aid for renal function* [also: *p*-aminohippurate sodium] 20% injection
***p*-aminohippurate sodium** JAN *renal function test* [also: aminohippurate sodium]
aminohippuric acid (*p*-aminohippuric acid) USP
aminohydroxypropylidene diphosphonate (APD) [see: pamidronate disodium]
aminoisobutanol [see: ambuphylline]
aminoisometradine [see: methionine]
aminoketones *a class of oral antidepressants*
5-aminolevulinic acid HCl (5-ALA HCl) USAN *photosensitizer for photodynamic therapy of precancerous actinic keratoses of the face and scalp (for use with the BLU-U Blue Light Photodynamic Therapy Illuminator)*
aminometradine INN, BAN
Amino-Min-D capsules OTC *dietary supplement* [calcium carbonate; multiple minerals; vitamin D] 250 mg•≛•100 IU
aminonat [see: protein hydrolysate]
Amino-Opti-C sustained-release tablets OTC *vitamin C supplement with multiple bioflavonoids* [vitamin C; rose hips; lemon bioflavonoids; rutin; hesperidin] 1000•≟•250•≟•≟ mg

Amino-Opti-E capsules (discontinued 1999) OTC *dietary supplement* [vitamin E (as *d*-alpha tocopheryl acid succinate)] 165 mg

aminopenicillins *a subclass of penicillins (q.v.)*

aminopentamide sulfate [see: dimevamide]

aminophenazone INN [also: aminopyrine]

aminophenazone cyclamate INN

***p*-aminophenylarsonic acid** [see: arsanilic acid]

aminophylline USP, INN, BAN, JAN *smooth muscle relaxant; bronchodilator* 100, 200 mg oral; 105 mg/5 mL oral; 250 mg/10 mL injection; 250, 500 suppositories

aminopromazine INN, DCF [also: proquamezine]

aminopterin sodium INN, BAN, DCF *investigational (Phase II) antifolate for breast and ovarian cancer*

4-aminopyridine [see: fampridine]

aminopyrine NF, JAN [also: aminophenazone]

aminoquin naphthoate [see: pamaquine naphthoate]

aminoquinol INN

aminoquinoline [see: aminoquinol]

4-aminoquinoline [see: chloroquine phosphate]

8-aminoquinoline [see: primaquine phosphate]

aminoquinuride INN

aminorex USAN, INN, BAN *anorectic*

aminosalicylate calcium USP [also: calcium para-aminosalicylate]

aminosalicylate potassium USP

aminosalicylate sodium (*p*-aminosalicylate sodium) USP *bacteriostatic; tuberculosis retreatment agent; investigational (orphan) for Crohn disease*

aminosalicylic acid (4-aminosalicylic acid) USP *antibacterial; tuberculostatic (orphan); investigational (orphan) for ulcerative colitis*

5-aminosalicylic acid (5-ASA) [see: mesalamine]

aminosalyle sodium [see: aminosalicylate sodium]

aminosidine *investigational (orphan) for tuberculosis,* Mycobacterium avium *complex, and visceral leishmaniasis*

aminosidine sulfate [see: paromomycin sulfate]

21-aminosteroids *a class of potent antioxidants that can protect against oxygen radical–mediated lipid peroxidation and progressive neuronal degeneration following brain or spinal trauma, subarachnoid hemorrhage, or stroke* [also called: lazaroids]

aminosuccinic acid [see: aspartic acid]

Aminosyn 3.5% (5%, 7%, 8.5%, 10%); Aminosyn (pH6) 10%; Aminosyn II 3.5% (5%, 7%, 8.5%, 10%, 15%); Aminosyn-PF 7% (10%) IV infusion ℞ *total parenteral nutrition (except 3.5%); peripheral parenteral nutrition (all)* [multiple essential and nonessential amino acids]

Aminosyn 3.5% M; Aminosyn II 3.5% M IV infusion ℞ *peripheral parenteral nutrition* [multiple essential and nonessential amino acids; electrolytes]

Aminosyn 7% (8.5%) with Electrolytes; Aminosyn II 7% (8.5%, 10%) with Electrolytes IV infusion ℞ *total parenteral nutrition; peripheral parenteral nutrition* [multiple essential and nonessential amino acids; electrolytes]

Aminosyn II 3.5% in 5% (25%) Dextrose; Aminosyn II 4.25% in 10% (20%, 25%) Dextrose; Aminosyn II 5% in 25% Dextrose IV infusion ℞ *total parenteral nutrition (except 3.5% in 5%); peripheral parenteral nutrition (not 20% and 25%)* [multiple essential and nonessential amino acids; dextrose]

Aminosyn II 3.5% M in 5% Dextrose; Aminosyn II 4.25% M in 10% Dextrose IV infusion ℞ *total parenteral nutrition (4.25% in 10% only); peripheral parenteral nutrition* *(both)* [multiple essential and nonessential amino acids; electrolytes; dextrose]

Aminosyn-HBC 7% IV infusion ℞ *nutritional therapy for high metabolic stress* [multiple branched-chain essential and nonessential amino acids; electrolytes]

Aminosyn-RF 5.2% IV infusion ℞ *nutritional therapy for renal failure* [multiple essential amino acids]

aminothiazole INN

aminotrate phosphate [see: trolnitrate phosphate]

aminoxaphen [see: aminorex]

Aminoxin enteric-coated tablets OTC *vitamin B_6 supplement* [pyridoxal-5′-phosphate] 20 mg

aminoxytriphene INN

aminoxytropine tropate HCl [see: atropine oxide HCl]

Amio-Aqueous ℞ *antiarrhythmic for acute ventricular tachycardia and fibrillation (orphan)* [amiodarone HCl]

amiodarone USAN, INN, BAN *ventricular antiarrhythmic*

amiodarone HCl *ventricular antiarrhythmic for acute ventricular tachycardia and fibrillation (orphan)* 200 mg oral; 50 mg/mL injection (CAN)

Amipaque powder for injection (discontinued 1999) ℞ *radiopaque contrast medium* [metrizamide (48.25% iodine)] 13.5%, 18.75%

amiperone INN

amiphenazole INN, BAN

amipizone INN

amipramidine [see: amiloride HCl]

amiprilose INN *synthetic monosaccharide anti-inflammatory* [also: amiprilose HCl]

amiprilose HCl USAN *investigational (NDA filed) synthetic monosaccharide anti-inflammatory for rheumatoid arthritis* [also: amiprilose]

amiquinsin INN *antihypertensive* [also: amiquinsin HCl]

amiquinsin HCl USAN *antihypertensive* [also: amiquinsin]

amisometradine NF, INN, BAN

amisulpride INN

amiterol INN

Ami-Tex LA long-acting tablets ℞ *decongestant; expectorant* [phenylpropanolamine HCl; guaifenesin] 75•400 mg

amithiozone [see: thioacetazone; thiacetazone]

amitivir INN *investigational influenza vaccine*

Amitone chewable tablets OTC *antacid* [calcium carbonate] 350 mg

amitraz USAN, INN, BAN *scabicide*

amitriptyline (AMT) INN, BAN *tricyclic antidepressant* [also: amitriptyline HCl] (S) nortriptyline

amitriptyline HCl USP, JAN *tricyclic antidepressant* [also: amitriptyline] 10, 25, 50, 75, 100, 150 mg oral

amitriptylinoxide INN

amixetrine INN, DCF

AmLactin cream, lotion OTC *moisturizer; emollient* [ammonium lactate] 12%

amlexanox USAN, INN, JAN *antiallergic; anti-inflammatory; aphthous ulcer treatment*

amlintide USAN *antidiabetic for type 1 diabetes*

amlodipine INN, BAN *antianginal; antihypertensive; calcium channel blocker* [also: amlodipine besylate]

amlodipine besylate USAN *antianginal; antihypertensive; calcium channel blocker* [also: amlodipine]

amlodipine maleate USAN *antianginal; antihypertensive*

ammi *(Ammi majus; A. visnaga)* dried ripe fruits *medicinal herb for angina, bronchial asthma, diabetes, diuresis, kidney and bladder stones, psoriasis, respiratory diseases, and vitiligo*

ammoidin [see: methoxsalen]

[^{13}N]ammonia [see: ammonia N 13]

ammonia [see: ammonia spirit, aromatic]

ammonia N 13 USAN, USP *radioactive diagnostic aid for cardiac and liver imaging*

ammonia solution, strong NF *solvent; source of ammonia* [also: ammonia water]
ammonia spirit, aromatic USP *respiratory stimulant*
ammonia water JAN *solvent; source of ammonia* [also: ammonia solution, strong]
ammoniated mercury [see: mercury, ammoniated]
ammonio methacrylate copolymer NF *coating agent*
ammonium alum [see: alum, ammonium]
ammonium benzoate USP
ammonium biphosphate *urinary acidifier*
ammonium carbonate NF *source of ammonia*
ammonium chloride USP, JAN *urinary acidifier; diuretic; expectorant* 486, 500 mg oral; 5 mEq/mL (26.75%) injection
ammonium 2-hydroxypropanoate [see: ammonium lactate]
ammonium ichthosulfonate [see: ichthammol]
ammonium lactate (lactic acid neutralized with ammonium hydroxide) USAN *antipruritic; emollient for xerosis*
ammonium mandelate USP
ammonium molybdate USP *dietary molybdenum supplement* 25 µg/mL injection
ammonium molybdate tetrahydrate [see: ammonium molybdate]
ammonium phosphate NF *pharmaceutic aid*
ammonium salicylate NF
ammonium tetrathiomolybdate *investigational (orphan) for Wilson disease*
ammonium valerate NF
ammophyllin [see: aminophylline]
Amnaranthus **spp.** *medicinal herb* [see: amaranth]
AMO Endosol; AMO Endosol Extra ophthalmic solution ℞ *intraocular irrigating solution* [sodium chloride (balanced saline solution)]
AMO Vitrax intraocular injection ℞ *viscoelastic agent for ophthalmic surgery* [hyaluronate sodium] 30 mg/mL
amobarbital USP, INN, JAN *sedative; hypnotic; anticonvulsant; also abused as a street drug* [also: amylobarbitone]
amobarbital sodium USP, JAN *hypnotic; sedative; anticonvulsant; also abused as a street drug*
amocaine chloride [see: amolanone HCl]
amocarzine INN
amodiaquine USP, INN, BAN *antiprotozoal*
amodiaquine HCl USP *antimalarial*
Amodopa tablets (discontinued 1998) ℞ *antihypertensive* [methyldopa] 125, 250, 500 mg
amogastrin INN, JAN
amolanone INN
amolanone HCl [see: amolanone]
amonafide INN *investigational antineoplastic*
amoproxan INN, DCF
amopyroquine INN
amorolfine USAN, INN, BAN *antimycotic*
Amorphophallus konjac *medicinal herb* [see: glucomannan]
Amosan powder OTC *oral antibacterial* [sodium peroxyborate monohydrate]
amoscanate INN
amosulalol INN [also: amosulalol HCl]
amosulalol HCl JAN [also: amosulalol]
amotriphene [see: aminoxytriphene]
amoxapine USAN, USP, INN, BAN, JAN *tricyclic antidepressant* 25, 50, 100, 150 mg oral ⊡ amoxicillin; Amoxil
amoxecaine INN
amoxicillin USAN, USP, JAN *aminopenicillin antibiotic* [also: amoxicilline; amoxycillin] 125, 200, 250, 400, 500, 875 mg oral; 125, 250 mg/5 mL oral ⊡ amoxapine
amoxicillin sodium USAN *aminopenicillin antibiotic*
amoxicilline INN *aminopenicillin antibiotic* [also: amoxicillin; amoxycillin]
Amoxil capsules, tablets, chewable tablets, powder for oral suspension, pediatric drops ℞ *aminopenicillin*

antibiotic [amoxicillin] 250, 500 mg; 500, 875 mg; 125, 200, 250, 400 mg; 125, 200, 250, 400 mg/5 mL; 50 mg/mL ⑨ amoxapine

amoxycillin BAN *aminopenicillin antibiotic* [also: amoxicillin; amoxicilline]

amoxydramine camsilate INN [also: amoxydramine camsylate]

amoxydramine camsylate DCF [also: amoxydramine camsilate]

AMP; A_5MP (adenosine monophosphate) [see: adenosine phosphate]

amperozide INN, BAN *investigational antipsychotic for schizophrenia*

amphecloral USAN *anorectic* [also: amfecloral]

amphenidone INN

amphetamine BAN *CNS stimulant; widely abused as a street drug, which causes strong psychic dependence* [also: amphetamine sulfate; amfetamine]

***d*-amphetamine** [see: dextroamphetamine]

(+)-amphetamine [see: dextroamphetamine]

***l*-amphetamine** [see: levamphetamine]

(−)-amphetamine [see: levamphetamine]

amphetamine aspartate *CNS stimulant*

amphetamine complex (resin complex of amphetamine & dextroamphetamine) [q.v.]

amphetamine phosphate, dextro [see: dextroamphetamine phosphate]

amphetamine succinate, levo [see: levamphetamine succinate]

amphetamine sulfate USP *CNS stimulant; widely abused as a street drug, which causes strong psychic dependence* [also: amfetamine; amphetamine] 5, 10 mg oral

amphetamine sulfate, dextro [see: dextroamphetamine sulfate]

amphetamines *a class of CNS stimulants that includes amphetamine, dextroamphetamine, levamphetamine, methamphetamine, and their salts*

Amphocin powder for IV infusion ℞ *systemic polyene antifungal* [amphotericin B deoxycholate] 50 mg/vial

amphocortrin [see: amphomycin]

Amphojel tablets, oral suspension OTC *antacid* [aluminum hydroxide gel] 300, 600 mg; 320 mg/5 mL ⑨ Amphocil

amphomycin USAN, BAN *antibacterial* [also: amfomycin]

amphotalide INN, DCF

Amphotec powder for IV infusion ℞ *systemic polyene antifungal for invasive aspergillosis* [amphotericin B cholesteryl] 50, 100 mg/vial

amphotericin B USP, INN, BAN, JAN *polyene antifungal*

amphotericin B cholesteryl *systemic polyene antifungal for invasive aspergillosis*

amphotericin B deoxycholate *systemic polyene antifungal* 50 mg injection

amphotericin B lipid complex (ABLC) *systemic polyene antifungal for meningitis, leishmaniasis, histoplasmosis, and other invasive infections (orphan)*

ampicillin USAN, USP, INN, BAN, JAN *aminopenicillin antibiotic* 250, 500 mg oral; 125, 250 mg/5 mL oral

ampicillin sodium USAN, USP, JAN *aminopenicillin antibiotic* 125, 250, 500 mg, 1, 2, 10 g injection

ampiroxicam INN, BAN

Amplicor Chlamydia test kit for professional use *in vitro diagnostic aid for Chlamydia trachomatis* [DNA amplification test]

Amplicor HIV-1 Monitor test kit for professional use *in vitro diagnostic aid for HIV-1 in blood* [polymerase chain reaction (PCR) test]

Amplicor MTB test kit for professional use *in vitro diagnostic aid for Mycobacterium tuberculosis* [polymerase chain reaction (PCR) test]

Ampligen ℞ *investigational (Phase III, orphan) RNA synthesis inhibitor and immunomodulator for HIV, renal cell carcinoma, metastatic melanoma, and chronic fatigue syndrome* [poly I: poly C12U]

amprenavir USAN *antiviral protease inhibitor for HIV infection*

amprenavir & abacavir sulfate *investigational (Phase III) protease inhibitor and nucleoside analogue combination for HIV and AIDS*

amprenavir & indinavir sulfate *investigational (Phase II) protease inhibitor combination for AIDS*

amprenavir & lamivudine & zidovudine *investigational (Phase III) second-generation protease inhibitor combination for AIDS*

amprenavir & nelfinavir mesylate *investigational (Phase II) protease inhibitor combination for AIDS*

amprenavir & saquinavir *investigational (Phase II) protease inhibitor combination for AIDS*

amprocidum [see: amprolium]

amprolium USP, INN, BAN *coccidiostat for poultry*

amprotropine phosphate

ampyrimine INN

ampyzine INN *CNS stimulant* [also: ampyzine sulfate]

ampyzine sulfate USAN *CNS stimulant* [also: ampyzine]

amquinate USAN, INN *antimalarial*

amrinone INN, BAN *cardiotonic* [also: inamrinone (USAN changed 2000)]

amrinone lactate [now: inamrinone lactate]

amrubicin INN

AMSA; *m*-AMSA (acridinylamine methanesulfon anisidide) [see: amsacrine]

amsacrine USAN, INN, BAN *investigational (NDA filed) antineoplastic for acute adult leukemias (AML, APL, and ALL) and lymphomas*

Amsidyl ℞ *investigational (NDA filed) antineoplastic for acute adult leukemias (AML, APL, and ALL) and lymphomas* [amsacrine]

amsonate INN, BAN *combining name for radicals or groups*

AMT (amitriptyline HCl) [q.v.]

amtolmetin guacil INN

Amvisc; Amvisc Plus intraocular injection ℞ *viscoelastic agent for ophthalmic surgery* [hyaluronate sodium] 12 mg/mL; 16 mg/mL

amyl alcohol, tertiary [see: amylene hydrate]

amyl nitrite USP, JAN *vasodilator; antianginal; also abused as a euphoric street drug and sexual stimulant* 0.3 mL inhalant

amylase *digestive enzyme* [100 IU/mg in pancrelipase; 25 IU/mg in pancreatin]

amylase [see: alpha amylase]

amylene hydrate NF *solvent*

amylin [see: amlintide]

amylmetacresol INN, BAN

amylobarbitone BAN *sedative; hypnotic; anticonvulsant* [also: amobarbital]

amylocaine BAN

amylopectin sulfate, sodium salt [see: sodium amylosulfate]

amylosulfate sodium [see: sodium amylosulfate]

Amytal Sodium powder for injection ℞ *sedative; hypnotic; anxiolytic; anticonvulsant; also abused as a street drug* [amobarbital sodium]

anabolic steroids *a class of hormones derived from or closely related to testosterone that increase anabolic (tissue-building) and decrease catabolic (tissue-depleting) processes*

Anacin caplets, tablets OTC *analgesic; antipyretic; anti-inflammatory* [aspirin; caffeine] 400•32 mg; 400•32, 500•32 mg ⊠ Unisom; Unasyn

Anacin Aspirin Free tablets, caplets, gelcaps OTC *analgesic; antipyretic* [acetaminophen] 500 mg ⊠ Unisom; Unasyn

Anacin P.M., Aspirin Free film-coated caplets OTC *antihistaminic sleep aid; analgesic* [diphenhydramine HCl; acetaminophen] 25•500 mg ⊠ Unisom; Unasyn

Anadrol-50 tablets ℞ *anabolic steroid for anemias; also abused as a street drug* [oxymetholone] 50 mg

anafebrina [see: aminopyrine]

Anafranil capsules ℞ *tricyclic antidepressant for obsessive-compulsive disorders* [clomipramine HCl] 25, 50, 75 mg ⊡ enalapril

anagestone INN *progestin* [also: anagestone acetate]

anagestone acetate USAN *progestin* [also: anagestone]

anagrelide INN *antithrombotic/antiplatelet drug for essential thrombocythemia (orphan); investigational (orphan) for thrombocytosis and polycythemia vera* [also: anagrelide HCl]

anagrelide HCl USAN *antithrombotic/antiplatelet drug for essential thrombocythemia (orphan); investigational (orphan) for thrombocytosis and polycythemia vera* [also: anagrelide]

Ana-Guard subcu or IM injection ℞ *sympathomimetic bronchodilator for emergency treatment of anaphylaxis; vasopressor for shock* [epinephrine] 1:1000

anakinra USAN, INN *interleukin-1 receptor antagonist (IL-1ra); nonsteroidal anti-inflammatory for inflammatory bowel disease; investigational (NDA filed) for rheumatoid arthritis (RA); investigational (Phase II, orphan) for juvenile rheumatoid arthritis (JRA) and graft vs. host disease (GVHD)*

Ana-Kit ℞ *emergency treatment of anaphylaxis* [epinephrine; chlorpheniramine maleate; alcohol; tourniquet] 1:100 000•2 mg

analeptics *a class of central nervous system stimulants used to maintain or improve alertness*

Analgesia Creme OTC *topical analgesic* [trolamine salicylate] 10%

Analgesic Balm (discontinued 2000) OTC *topical analgesic; counterirritant* [methyl salicylate; menthol]

analgesics *a class of drugs that relieve pain or reduce sensitivity to pain without causing loss of consciousness*

analgesine [see: antipyrine]

Analpram-HC anorectal cream ℞ *topical corticosteroidal anti-inflammatory; local anesthetic* [hydrocortisone acetate; pramoxine] 1%•1%, 2.5%•1% ⊡ Analbalm

Anamine syrup ℞ *decongestant; antihistamine* [pseudoephedrine HCl; chlorpheniramine maleate] 30•2 mg/5 mL

Anamine T.D. sustained-release capsules ℞ *decongestant; antihistamine* [pseudoephedrine HCl; chlorpheniramine maleate] 120•8 mg

Anamirta cocculus; A. paniculata *medicinal herb* [see: levant berry]

ananain *investigational (orphan) proteolytic enzymes for debridement of severe burns*

Ananas comosus *medicinal herb* [see: pineapple]

Anandron (CAN) tablets (also available in Europe and Latin America) ℞ *antiandrogen antineoplastic adjunct to surgical or chemical castration for metastatic prostate cancer* [nilutamide] 50, 100 mg

Anaphalis margaritacea; Gnaphalium polycephalum; G. uliginosum *medicinal herb* [see: everlasting]

anaphrodisiacs *a class of agents that reduce sexual desire or potency*

Anaplex liquid ℞ *decongestant; antihistamine* [pseudoephedrine HCl; chlorpheniramine maleate] 30•2 mg/5 mL

Anaplex DM Cough syrup ℞ *antitussive; decongestant; antihistamine* [dextromethorphan hydrobromide; pseudoephedrine HCl; brompheniramine maleate] 30•60•4 mg/5 mL

Anaplex HD syrup ℞ *narcotic antitussive; decongestant; antihistamine* [hydrocodone bitartrate; pseudoephedrine HCl; brompheniramine maleate] 1.7•30•2 mg/5 mL

Anaprox; Anaprox DS film-coated tablets ℞ *analgesic; antiarthritic; nonsteroidal anti-inflammatory drug (NSAID)* [naproxen (from naproxen sodium)] 250 (275) mg; 500 (550) mg

anarel [see: guanadrel sulfate]

anaritide INN, BAN *antihypertensive; diuretic* [also: anaritide acetate]

anaritide acetate USAN *antihypertensive; diuretic; investigational (orphan)* *for acute renal failure and renal transplants; clinical trials discontinued 1997; orphan status withdrawn 1998*

Anaspaz tablets ℞ *GI/GU antispasmodic; antiparkinsonian; anticholinergic "drying agent" for allergic rhinitis and hyperhidrosis* [hyoscyamine sulfate] 0.125 mg

anastrozole USAN, INN, BAN *aromatase inhibitor; hormone antagonist antineoplastic for advanced breast cancer in postmenopausal women*

Anatrast rectal paste ℞ *radiopaque contrast medium for defecography* [barium sulfate] 100%

Anatrofin *brand name for stenbolone acetate, an anabolic steroid abused as a street drug*

Anatuss film-coated tablets ℞ *antitussive; decongestant; expectorant; analgesic* [dextromethorphan hydrobromide; phenylpropanolamine HCl; guaifenesin; acetaminophen] 15•25•100•325 mg

Anatuss syrup OTC *antitussive; decongestant; expectorant* [dextromethorphan hydrobromide; phenylpropanolamine HCl; guaifenesin] 15•25•100 mg/5 mL

Anatuss DM tablets, syrup OTC *antitussive; decongestant; expectorant* [dextromethorphan hydrobromide; pseudoephedrine HCl; guaifenesin] 20•60•400 mg; 10•30•100 mg/5 mL

Anatuss LA long-acting tablets ℞ *decongestant; expectorant* [pseudoephedrine HCl; guaifenesin] 120•400 mg

Anavar *brand name for oxandrolone, an anabolic steroid abused as a street drug*

anaxirone INN

anayodin [see: chiniofon]

anazocine INN

anazolene sodium USAN, INN *blood volume and cardiac output test* [also: sodium anoxynaphthonate]

Anbesol liquid, gel OTC *topical oral anesthetic; antipruritic/counterirritant; antiseptic* [benzocaine; phenol; alcohol 70%] 6.3%•0.5%

Anbesol, Baby gel OTC *topical oral anesthetic* [benzocaine] 7.5%

Anbesol, Maximum Strength liquid, gel OTC *mucous membrane anesthetic* [benzocaine; alcohol 60%] 20%

ancarolol INN

Ancef powder or frozen premix for IV or IM injection ℞ *cephalosporin antibiotic* [cefazolin sodium] 0.5, 1, 5, 10 g

ancestim USAN *recombinant-methionyl human stem cell factor (r-metHuSCF); hematopoietic growth factor; investigational (orphan) adjunct to myelosuppressive and myeloablative therapy*

Ancet liquid OTC *soap-free therapeutic skin cleanser*

anchusa *medicinal herb* [see: henna (*Alkanna*)]

ancitabine INN [also: ancitabine HCl]

ancitabine HCl JAN [also: ancitabine]

Ancobon capsules ℞ *systemic antifungal* [flucytosine] 250, 500 mg ⊡ Oncovin

ancrod USAN, INN, BAN *anticoagulant enzyme derived from the venom of the Malayan pit viper; investigational (orphan) antithrombotic for heparin-induced thrombocytopenia or thrombosis*

Andehist oral drops ℞ *decongestant; antihistamine* [pseudoephedrine HCl; carbinoxamine maleate] 15•2 mg/mL

Andehist syrup ℞ *decongestant; antihistamine* [pseudoephedrine HCl; brompheniramine maleate] 60•4 mg/5 mL

Andehist DM oral drops ℞ *decongestant; antihistamine; expectorant* [pseudoephedrine HCl; carbinoxamine maleate; dextromethorphan hydrobromide] 15•2•4 mg/mL

Andehist DM syrup ℞ *decongestant; antihistamine; expectorant* [pseudoephedrine HCl; brompheniramine maleate; dextromethorphan hydrobromide] 60•4•15 mg/5 mL

andolast INN

andrachne ***(Andrachne aspera; A. cordifolia; A. phyllanthoides)*** root *medicinal herb for eye inflammation; not generally regarded as safe and effective*

Andro 100; Andro 200 [see: depAndro 100; depAndro 200]

Andro L.A. 200 IM injection (discontinued 2001) ℞ *androgen replacement for delayed puberty or breast cancer* [testosterone enanthate] 200 mg/mL

Androderm transdermal patch (for nonscrotal area) ℞ *hormone replacement therapy for hypogonadism in men; investigational (Phase III) for AIDS-wasting syndrome* [testosterone] 2.5, 5 mg/day (12.2, 24.3 mg total)

AndroGel ℞ *hormone replacement for hypogonadism or testosterone deficiency in men; investigational (orphan) for AIDS-wasting syndrome* [testosterone] 1%

Androgel-DHT ℞ *investigational (Phase III) transdermal testosterone replacement in elderly men; investigational (Phase II, orphan) for AIDS-wasting syndrome* [dihydrotestosterone]

androgens *a class of sex hormones responsible for the development of the male sex organs and secondary sex characteristics*

Androgyn [see: depAndrogyn]

Android capsules ℞ *androgen replacement for hypogonadism or testosterone deficiency in men, delayed puberty in boys, and metastatic breast cancer in women* [methyltestosterone] 10 mg

Android-10; Android-25 tablets (discontinued 2001) ℞ *androgen replacement for hypogonadism or testosterone deficiency in men, delayed puberty in boys, and metastatic breast cancer in women* [methyltestosterone] 10 mg; 25 mg

Androlone-D 200 IM injection (discontinued 2000) ℞ *anabolic steroid for anemia of renal insufficiency* [nandrolone decanoate (in oil)] 200 mg/mL

Andropogon citratus *medicinal herb* [see: lemongrass]

Andropository-200 IM injection (discontinued 2001) ℞ *androgen replacement for delayed puberty or breast cancer* [testosterone enanthate] 200 mg/mL

androstanazole [now: stanozolol]

androstane [see: androstanolone; stanolone]

androstanolone INN *investigational (orphan) for AIDS-wasting syndrome* [also: stanolone]

androtest P [see: testosterone propionate]

Androtest-SL sublingual tablets ℞ *investigational (NDA filed) treatment for hypogonadism; investigational (orphan) for delay of growth and puberty in boys* [testosterone]

Androvite tablets OTC *vitamin/mineral/iron supplement* [multiple vitamins & minerals; iron; folic acid; biotin] ≛ • 3 • 0.06 • ≟ mg

anecortave acetate USAN *angiostatic steroid for neovascularization of the eye*

Anectine IV or IM injection, Flo-Pack (powder for injection) ℞ *muscle relaxant; anesthesia adjunct* [succinylcholine chloride] 20 mg/mL; 500, 1000 mg

Anemagen gelcaps ℞ *hematinic* [ferrous fumarate; cyanocobalamin; ascorbic acid; dessicated stomach substance] 200 mg • 10 µg • 250 mg • 100 mg

Anemone patens *medicinal herb* [see: pasque flower]

Anergan 50 IM injection ℞ *antihistamine; sedative; antiemetic; motion sickness relief* [promethazine HCl] 50 mg/mL

anertan [see: testosterone propionate]

AnervaX *investigational (Phase II) therapeutic peptide vaccine for rheumatoid arthritis*

Anestacon jelly ℞ *mucous membrane anesthetic* [lidocaine HCl] 2%

anesthesin [see: benzocaine]

anesthetics *a class of agents that abolish the sensation of pain*

anesthrone [see: benzocaine]

anethaine [see: tetracaine HCl]

anethole NF *flavoring agent*

anetholtrithion JAN

Anethum foeniculum *medicinal herb* [see: fennel]

Anethum graveolens *medicinal herb* [see: dill]

aneurine HCl [see: thiamine HCl]

Anexsia 5/500; Anexsia 7.5/650; Anexsia 10/660 tablets ℞ *narcotic analgesic* [hydrocodone bitartrate; acetaminophen] 5•500 mg; 7.5•650 mg; 10•660 mg

angelica (Angelica atropurpurea) root *medicinal herb for appetite stimulation, bronchial disorders, colds, colic, cough, exhaustion, gas, heartburn, and rheumatism; also used as a tonic*

Angelica levisticum *medicinal herb* [see: lovage]

Angelica polymorpha; A. sinensis; A. dahurica *medicinal herb* [see: dong quai]

Angio-Conray injection (discontinued 1999) ℞ *radiopaque contrast medium for angiography* [iothalamate sodium (59.9% iodine)] 800 mg/mL (480 mg/mL)

AngioMark injection ℞ *investigational (Phase III) MRI contrast medium for multiple cardiovascular indications* [MS-325 (code name—generic name not yet assigned)]

Angiomax powder for IV injection ℞ *anticoagulant thrombin inhibitor for patients with unstable angina undergoing percutaneous transluminal coronary angioplasty (PTCA)* [bivalirudin] 250 mg/vial

angiotensin II INN

angiotensin II receptor antagonists (AIIRAs) *a class of antihypertensives that reduce the vasoconstricting effects of angiotensin II by blocking the angiotensin II receptor sites in the vascular smooth muscles* [compare to: angiotensin-converting enzyme inhibitors]

angiotensin amide USAN, NF, BAN *vasoconstrictor* [also: angiotensinamide]

angiotensinamide INN *vasoconstrictor* [also: angiotensin amide]

angiotensin-converting enzyme inhibitors (ACEIs) *a class of antihypertensives that reduce the vasoconstricting effects of angiotensin II by blocking the enzyme (kininase II) that converts angiotensin I to angiotensin II* [compare to: angiotensin II receptor antagonists]

Angiovist 282 injection (discontinued 1999) ℞ *radiopaque contrast medium* [diatrizoate meglumine] 60%

Angiovist 292; Angiovist 370 injection (discontinued 1999) ℞ *radiopaque contrast medium* [diatrizoate meglumine; diatrizoate sodium (48.7% total iodine)] 52%•8% (29.3%); 66%•10% (37%)

anhidrotics *a class of agents that reduce or suppress perspiration* [also called: anidrotics; antihydrotics]

anhydrohydroxyprogesterone [now: ethisterone]

anhydrous lanolin [see: lanolin, anhydrous]

anidoxime USAN, INN, BAN *analgesic*

anidrotics *a class of agents that reduce or suppress perspiration* [also called: anhidrotics; antihydrotics]

anidulafungin USAN *antifungal for Candida, Aspergillus, and Pneumocystis infections*

anilamate INN

anileridine USP, INN, BAN *narcotic analgesic*

anileridine HCl USP *narcotic analgesic*

anilopam INN *analgesic* [also: anilopam HCl]

anilopam HCl USAN *analgesic* [also: anilopam]

Animal Shapes chewable tablets OTC *vitamin supplement* [multiple vitamins; folic acid] ≛•0.3 mg

Animal Shapes + Iron chewable tablets OTC *vitamin/iron supplement* [multiple vitamins; iron; folic acid] ≛•15•0.3 mg

anion exchange resin [see: polyamine-methylene resin]

anipamil INN

aniracetam USAN, INN *mental performance enhancer*

anirolac USAN, INN *anti-inflammatory; analgesic*

anisacril INN

anisatil USAN *combining name for radicals or groups*

anise (*Pimpinella anisum*) oil and seeds *medicinal herb for colic, convulsions, cough, gas, intestinal cleansing, iron-deficiency anemia, mucous discharge, promoting expectoration, and psoriasis; also used as an antibacterial, antimicrobial, and antiseptic*

anise oil NF

anise root; sweet anise *medicinal herb* [see: sweet cicely]

anisindione NF, INN, BAN *indandione-derivative anticoagulant*

anisopirol INN

anisopyradamine [see: pyrilamine maleate]

anisotropine methylbromide USAN, JAN *anticholinergic; peptic ulcer adjunct* [also: octatropine methylbromide] 50 mg oral

anisoylated plasminogen streptokinase activator complex (APSAC) [see: anistreplase]

anistreplase USAN, INN, BAN *fibrinolytic; thrombolytic enzyme for acute myocardial infarction*

Anisum officinarum; A. vulgare *medicinal herb* [see: anise]

anitrazafen USAN, INN *topical anti-inflammatory*

anodynes *a class of agents that lessen or relieve pain*

anodynine [see: antipyrine]

anodynon [see: ethyl chloride]

Anogesic ointment ℞ *investigational (Phase III) topical treatment for hemorrhoids and anal fissures* [nitroglycerin]

Anoquan capsules (discontinued 2000) ℞ *analgesic; barbiturate sedative* [acetaminophen; caffeine; butalbital] 325•40•50 mg

anorectics *a class of central nervous system stimulants that suppress the appetite* [also called: anorexiants; anorexigenics]

anorexiants *a class of central nervous system stimulants that suppress the appetite* [also called: anorectics; anorexigenics]

anorexigenics *a class of central nervous system stimulants that suppress the appetite* [also called: anorexiants; anorectics]

anovlar [see: norethindrone & ethinyl estradiol]

anoxomer USAN *antioxidant; food additive*

anoxynaphthonate sodium [see: anazolene sodium]

anpirtoline INN

Ansaid film-coated tablets ℞ *antiarthritic; nonsteroidal anti-inflammatory drug (NSAID)* [flurbiprofen] 50, 100 mg ⊡ NSAID

ansamycin [see: rifabutin]

ansoxetine INN

Answer One-Step; Answer Plus; Answer Quick & Simple test kit for home use *in vitro diagnostic aid; urine pregnancy test*

Answer Ovulation test kit for home use *in vitro diagnostic aid to predict ovulation time*

Antabuse tablets ℞ *deterrent to alcohol consumption* [disulfiram] 250, 500 mg

Antacid chewable tablets OTC *antacid* [calcium carbonate] 500, 750 mg

Antacid oral suspension OTC *antacid* [aluminum hydroxide; magnesium hydroxide] 225•200 mg/5 mL

antacids *a class of drugs that neutralize gastric acid*

antafenite INN

Antagon subcu injection ℞ *gonadotropin-releasing hormone (Gn-RH) antagonist for infertility* [ganirelix acetate] 250 µg/0.5 mL

antastan [see: antazoline HCl]

antazoline INN, BAN [also: antazoline HCl]

antazoline HCl USP [also: antazoline]

antazoline phosphate USP *antihistamine*

antazoline phosphate & naphazoline HCl *topical ocular antihistamine and decongestant* 0.5%•0.05%

antazonite INN
Antegren ℞ *investigational (Phase II) humanized monoclonal antibody for treatment of multiple sclerosis and Crohn disease* [natalizumab]
antelmycin INN *anthelmintic* [also: anthelmycin]
anterior pituitary
anthelmintics *a class of drugs effective against parasitic infections* [also called: vermicides; vermifuges]
anthelmycin USAN *anthelmintic* [also: antelmycin]
Anthemis nobilis *medicinal herb* [see: chamomile]
anthiolimine INN
Anthoxanthum odoratum *medicinal herb* [see: sweet vernal grass]
anthracyclines *a class of antibiotic antineoplastics*
Anthra-Derm ointment ℞ *topical antipsoriatic* [anthralin] 0.1%, 0.25%, 0.5%, 1%
anthralin USP *topical antipsoriatic* [also: dithranol]
anthramycin USAN *antineoplastic* [also: antramycin]
anthraquinone of cascara [see: cascara sagrada]
Anthriscus cerefolium *medicinal herb* [see: chervil]
anti-A blood grouping serum USP *in vitro blood testing*
antiadrenergics *a class of cardiovascular drugs that block the passage of impulses through the sympathetic nervous system* [also called: sympatholytics]
antiandrogens *a class of hormonal antineoplastics*
antib [see: thioacetazone; thiacetazone]
anti-B blood grouping serum USP *in vitro blood testing*
anti-B4-blocked ricin [see: ricin (blocked) ...]
antibason [see: methylthiouracil]
AntibiŌtic ear drops, otic suspension ℞ *topical corticosteroidal anti-inflammatory; antibiotic* [hydrocortisone; neomycin sulfate; polymyxin B sulfate] 1%•5 mg•10 000 U per mL
Antibiotic Ear Solution ℞ *topical corticosteroidal anti-inflammatory; antibiotic* [hydrocortisone; neomycin sulfate; polymyxin B sulfate] 1%•5 mg•10 000 U per mL
Antibiotic Ear Suspension ℞ *topical corticosteroidal anti-inflammatory; antibiotic* [hydrocortisone; neomycin sulfate; polymyxin B sulfate] 1%•5 mg•10 000 U per mL
antibiotics *a class of agents that destroy or arrest the growth of micro-organisms*
antibromics *a class of agents that mask undesirable or offensive odors* [also called: deodorants]
anti-C blood grouping serum [see: blood grouping serum, anti-C]
anti-c blood grouping serum [see: blood grouping serum, anti-c]
anti-CD3 [see: muromonab-CD3]
anti-CD11a monoclonal antibodies [see: HU-1124]
anticholinergics *a class of agents that block parasympathetic nerve impulses, producing antiemetic, antinausea, and antispasmodic effects; also used to dry mucosal secretions*
anticoagulant citrate dextrose (ACD) solution USP *anticoagulant for storage of whole blood and during cardiac surgery*
anticoagulant citrate phosphate dextrose adenine solution USP *anticoagulant for storage of whole blood*
anticoagulant citrate phosphate dextrose solution USP *anticoagulant for storage of whole blood*
anticoagulant heparin solution USP *anticoagulant for storage of whole blood*
anticoagulant sodium citrate solution USP *anticoagulant for plasma and for blood for fractionation*
anticoagulants *a class of therapeutic agents that inhibit or inactivate blood clotting factors*
anticonvulsants *a class of drugs that prevent seizures by suppressing abnormal neuronal discharges in the central nervous system* [also called: anti-epileptic drugs (AEDs)]

Anticort ℞ *investigational anti-aging and anticancer agent; investigational (Phase II) for HIV infection* [procaine HCl]
anti-D antibodies [see: Rh_0(D) immune globulin]
antidopaminergics *a class of antiemetic drugs*
antidotes *a class of drugs that counteract the effects of toxic doses of other drugs or toxic substances*
anti-E blood grouping serum [see: blood grouping serum, anti-E]
anti-e blood grouping serum [see: blood grouping serum, anti-e]
antiemetics *a class of agents that prevent or alleviate nausea and vomiting* [also called: antinauseants]
antiendotoxin MAb E5 [now: edobacomab]
antienite INN
antiepilepsirine [now: ilepcimide]
anti-epileptic drugs (AEDs) *a class of drugs that prevent seizures by suppressing abnormal neuronal discharges in the central nervous system* [also called: anticonvulsants]
antiestrogen [see: tamoxifen citrate]
antiestrogens *a class of hormonal antineoplastics*
antifebriles *a class of agents that relieve or reduce fever* [also called: antipyretics; antithermics; febricides; febrifuges]
antifebrin [see: acetanilide]
antifolic acid [see: methotrexate]
antiformin, dental JAN [also: sodium hypochlorite, diluted]
antihemophilic factor (AHF) USP *antihemophilic; systemic hemostatic; investigational (orphan) for von Willebrand disease*
Antihemophilic Factor (Porcine) Hyate:C powder for IV injection ℞ *antihemophilic to correct coagulation deficiency* [antihemophilic factor VIII:C] 400–700 porcine units/vial
antihemophilic factor, human [now: antihemophilic factor]
antihemophilic factor, recombinant (rFVIII) *antihemophilic for treatment of hemophilia A and presurgical prophylaxis for hemophiliacs (orphan)*
antihemophilic factor A [see: antihemophilic factor]
antihemophilic factor B [see: factor IX complex]
antihemophilic globulin (AHG) [see: antihemophilic factor]
antihemophilic human plasma [now: plasma, antihemophilic human]
antihemophilic plasma, human [now: plasma, antihemophilic human]
antiheparin [see: protamine sulfate]
Antihist-1 tablets OTC *antihistamine* [clemastine fumarate] 1.34 mg
antihistamines *a class of drugs that counteract the effect of histamine*
Antihist-D tablets OTC *decongestant; antihistamine* [phenylpropanolamine HCl (extended release); clemastine fumarate (immediate release)] 75•1.34 mg
anti-human thymocyte immunoglobulin, rabbit *investigational (Phase III) immunosuppressant for kidney transplants*
antihydrotics *a class of agents that reduce or suppress perspiration* [also called: anhidrotics; anidrotics]
antihyperlipidemic agents *a class of drugs that lower serum lipid levels* [also called: antilipemics]
anti-inhibitor coagulant complex *antihemophilic*
antilipemics *a class of drugs that lower serum lipid levels* [also called: antihyperlipidemics]
Antilirium IV or IM injection ℞ *cholinergic to reverse anticholinergic overdose; investigational (orphan) for Friedreich and other inherited ataxias* [physostigmine salicylate] 1 mg/mL
antilithics *a class of agents that prevent the formation of stone or calculus* [see also: litholytics]
antilymphocyte immunoglobulin BAN
Antiminth oral suspension OTC *anthelmintic for ascariasis (roundworm) and*

enterobiasis (pinworm) [pyrantel pamoate] 50 mg/mL

antimony *element (Sb)*

antimony potassium tartrate USP *antischistosomal*

antimony sodium tartrate USP, JAN *antischistosomal*

antimony sodium thioglycollate USP

antimony sulfide [see: antimony trisulfide colloid]

antimony trisulfide colloid USAN *pharmaceutic aid*

antimonyl potassium tartrate [see: antimony potassium tartrate]

antimuscarinics *a class of anticholinergic agents*

anti-MY9-blocked ricin [see: ricin (blocked) ...]

antinauseants *a class of agents that prevent or alleviate nausea and vomiting* [also called: antiemetics]

antineoplastics *a class of chemotherapeutic agents capable of selective action on neoplastic (abnormally proliferating) tissues*

antineoplastons *a class of naturally occurring peptides that suppress cancer oncogenes and stimulate the body's cancer suppressor genes*

Antiox capsules OTC *vitamin supplement* [vitamins C and E; beta carotene] 120 mg•100 IU•25 mg

anti-pellagra vitamin [see: niacin]

antiperiodics *a class of agents that prevent periodic or intermittent recurrence of symptoms, as in malaria*

anti-pernicious anemia principle [see: cyanocobalamin]

antiphlogistics *a class of agents that reduce inflammation and fever*

antipyretics *a class of agents that relieve or reduce fever* [also called: antifebriles; antithermics; febricides; febrifuges]

antipyrine USP, JAN *analgesic; orphan status withdrawn 1996* [also: phenazone]

N-antipyrinylnicotinamide [see: nifenazone]

antirabies serum (ARS) USP *passive immunizing agent*

anti-Rh antibodies [see: $Rh_0(D)$ immune globulin]

anti-Rh typing serums [now: blood grouping serums]

antiscorbutic vitamin [see: ascorbic acid]

antiscorbutics *a class of agents that are sources of vitamin C and are effective in the prevention or relief of scurvy*

antiscrofulous herbs *a class of agents that counteract scrofuloderma (tuberculous cervical lymphadenitis)*

antisense drugs *a class of antiviral drugs that interfere with the replication of viral protein*

antiseptics *a class of agents that inhibit the growth and development of microorganisms, usually on a body surface, without necessarily killing them* [see also: disinfectants; germicides]

Antispas IM injection ℞ *GI antispasmodic* [dicyclomine HCl] 10 mg/mL

Antispasmodic elixir ℞ *GI antispasmodic; anticholinergic; sedative* [atropine sulfate; scopolamine hydrobromide; hyoscyamine sulfate; phenobarbital] 0.0194•0.0065•0.1037•16.2 mg/5 mL

antispasmodics *a class of agents that relieve spasms or cramps, usually of gastrointestinal tract or blood vessels*

antisterility vitamin [see: vitamin E]

anti-tac, humanized; SMART anti-tac [now: daclximab]

antithermics *a class of agents that relieve or reduce fever* [also called: antifebriles; antipyretics; febricides; febrifuges]

antithrombin III (AT-III) INN, BAN *for thrombosis and pulmonary emboli of congenital AT-III deficiency (orphan); investigational (Phase III, orphan) for heparin resistance in patients undergoing coronary artery bypass grafts*

antithrombin III, human [see: antithrombin III]

antithrombin III, recombinant human (rhATIII) [see: antithrombin III]

antithrombin III concentrate IV [see: antithrombin III]

antithymocyte globulin (ATG) *passive immunizing agent to prevent allograft rejection of renal transplants; treatment for aplastic anemia; investigational (orphan) for organ and bone marrow transplants* [also: lymphocyte immune globulin (LIG)]

antithymocyte serum [see: lymphocyte immune globulin, antithymocyte]

anti-TNF (tumor necrosis factor) MAb [now: nerelimomab]

antitoxin botulism equine (ABE) [see: botulism equine antitoxin, trivalent]

antitoxins *a class of drugs used for passive immunization that consist of antibodies which combine with toxins to neutralize them*

α_1-antitrypsin [see: alpha$_1$-antitrypsin]

antituberculous agents *a class of antibiotics, divided into primary and retreatment agents*

Anti-Tuss syrup OTC *expectorant* [guaifenesin; alcohol 3.5%] 100 mg/5 mL

antitussives *a class of drugs that prevent or relieve cough*

antivenin (Crotalidae) polyvalent (equine) USP *passive immunizing agent for pit viper (rattlesnake, copperhead, and cottonmouth moccasin) bites*

antivenin (Crotalidae) polyvalent immune Fab (ovine) *treatment for pit viper (rattlesnake, copperhead, and cottonmouth moccasin) bites (orphan)*

antivenin (Crotalidae) purified (avian) *investigational (orphan) treatment of Crotalidae snake bites*

antivenin (*Latrodectus mactans*) USP *passive immunizing agent for black widow spider bites* 6000 U/vial

antivenin (*Micrurus fulvius*) (equine) USP *passive immunizing agent for coral snake bites*

antivenins *a class of drugs used for passive immunization against or treatment for venomous bites and stings*

Antivert; Antivert/25; Antivert/50 tablets ℞ *anticholinergic; antihistamine; antivertigo agent; motion sickness preventative* [meclizine HCl] 12.5 mg; 25 mg; 50 mg

antivirals *a class of drugs effective against viral infections*

antixerophthalmic vitamin [see: vitamin A]

Antizol IV injection ℞ *alcohol dehydrogenase inhibitor for methanol or ethylene glycol poisoning (orphan)* [fomepizole] 1 g/mL

antler (deer and elk) *natural remedy for aging, energy, hormone balancing, impotence, infertility, and longevity*

antrafenine INN

antramycin INN *antineoplastic* [also: anthramycin]

Antril ℞ *nonsteroidal anti-inflammatory drug (NSAID) for inflammatory bowel disease; investigational (orphan) for juvenile rheumatoid arthritis and graft vs. host disease* [anakinra]

Antrin ℞ *investigational photodynamic therapy for peripheral vascular and cardiovascular atherosclerosis* [motexafin lutetium]

Antrizine tablets ℞ *anticholinergic; antihistamine; antivertigo agent; motion sickness preventative* [meclizine HCl] 12.5 mg

Antrocol elixir ℞ *GI anticholinergic; sedative* [atropine sulfate; phenobarbital] 0.195•16 mg/5 mL

Antrypol (available only from the Centers for Disease Control) ℞ *antiparasitic for African trypanosomiasis and onchocerciasis* [suramin sodium]

antrypol [see: suramin sodium]

Anturane tablets, capsules ℞ *uricosuric for gout* [sulfinpyrazone] 100 mg; 200 mg 🔊 Artane

Anucort HC rectal suppositories ℞ *corticosteroidal anti-inflammatory* [hydrocortisone acetate] 25 mg

Anumed rectal suppositories OTC *temporary relief of hemorrhoidal symptoms* [bismuth subgallate; bismuth resorcin compound; benzyl benzoate; zinc oxide; peruvian balsam] 2.25%•1.75%•1.2%•11%•1.8%

Anumed HC rectal suppositories ℞ *corticosteroidal anti-inflammatory* [hydrocortisone acetate] 10 mg

Anusol anorectal ointment OTC *topical local anesthetic; astringent* [pramoxine HCl; zinc oxide] 1%•12.5% ⓢ Aplisol

Anusol rectal suppositories OTC *emollient* [topical starch] 51%

Anusol-HC anorectal cream ℞ *topical corticosteroidal anti-inflammatory* [hydrocortisone] 2.5%

Anusol-HC rectal suppositories ℞ *corticosteroidal anti-inflammatory* [hydrocortisone acetate] 25 mg

Anusol-HC 1 ointment ℞ *topical corticosteroidal anti-inflammatory* [hydrocortisone acetate] 1%

Anuzinc (CAN) anorectal ointment, suppositories ℞ *topical astringent* [zinc sulfate] 0.5%; 10 mg

Anxanil film-coated tablets (discontinued 1998) ℞ *anxiolytic; minor tranquilizer* [hydroxyzine HCl] 25 mg

Anzemet film-coated tablets, IV injection ℞ *serotonin 5-HT_3 receptor antagonist; antiemetic for nausea following chemotherapy, radiation, or surgery* [dolasetron mesylate] 50, 100 mg; 20 mg/mL

AOD-9604 *investigational (Phase II) antiobesity drug*

AOPA (ara-C, Oncovin, prednisone, asparaginase) *chemotherapy protocol*

AOPE (Adriamycin, Oncovin, prednisone, etoposide) *chemotherapy protocol*

Aosept solution + Aodisc (tablet) OTC *two-step chemical disinfecting system for soft contact lenses* [hydrogen peroxide based] 3%

AP (Adriamycin, Platinol) *chemotherapy protocol for ovarian and endometrial cancer*

AP-1903 *investigational (Phase I, orphan) for graft-versus-host disease*

Apacet chewable tablets, drops OTC *analgesic; antipyretic* [acetaminophen] 80 mg; 100 mg/mL

apafant USAN, INN *platelet activating factor antagonist for allergies, asthma, and acute pancreatitis*

apalcillin sodium USAN, INN *antibacterial*

Apanol ℞ *investigational phospholipase A2 inhibitor* [IPL-576 (code name—generic name not yet assigned)]

APAP (N-acetyl-*p*-aminophenol) [see: acetaminophen]

APAP Plus tablets OTC *analgesic; antipyretic* [acetaminophen; caffeine] 500•65 mg

Apatate chewable tablets, liquid OTC *vitamin supplement* [vitamins B_1, B_6, and B_{12}] 15•0.5•0.025 mg; 15•0.5•0.025 mg/5 mL

Apatate with Fluoride liquid ℞ *pediatric vitamin supplement and dental caries preventative* [vitamins B_1, B_6, and B_{12}; fluoride] 15•0.5•0.025•0.5 mg/5 mL

apaxifylline USAN, INN *selective adenosine A_1 antagonist for cognitive deficits*

apazone USAN *anti-inflammatory* [also: azapropazone]

APC (AMSA, prednisone, chlorambucil) *chemotherapy protocol*

APC (aspirin, phenacetin & caffeine) [q.v.]

APC-366 *investigational (Phase II) tryptase inhibitor for asthma*

APC-2059 *investigational (Phase II) cream for psoriasis (clinical trials discontinued 1999)*

apcitide [see: technetium Tc 99m apcitide]

APD (aminohydroxypropylidene diphosphonate) [see: pamidronate disodium]

APE (Adriamycin, Platinol, etoposide) *chemotherapy protocol*

APE (aminophylline, phenobarbital, ephedrine)

APE (ara-C, Platinol, etoposide) *chemotherapy protocol*

aperients *a class of agents that have a mild purgative or laxative effect* [see also: aperitives]

aperitives *a class of agents that stimulate the appetite or have a mild purgative or laxative effect* [see also: aperients]

Apetil liquid OTC *vitamin/mineral supplement* [multiple B vitamins; multiple minerals] ≛ • ≛

aphrodisiacs *a class of agents that arouse or increase sexual desire or potency*

Aphrodyne tablets ℞ *no FDA-approved uses; sympatholytic; mydriatic; aphrodisiac* [yohimbine HCl] 5.4 mg

Aphthasol oral paste ℞ *anti-inflammatory for aphthous ulcers* [amlexanox] 5%

apicillin [see: ampicillin]

apicycline INN

apiquel fumarate [see: aminorex]

Apium graveolens *medicinal herb* [see: celery]

A.P.L. powder for IM injection ℞ *hormone for prepubertal cryptorchidism and hypogonadism; ovulation stimulant* [chorionic gonadotropin] 500, 1000, 2000 U/mL

APL 400-020 *investigational (orphan) for cutaneous T-cell lymphoma*

Apligraf ℞ *living skin construct for diabetic foot ulcers and pressure sores* [graftskin]

Aplisol intradermal injection *tuberculosis skin test* [tuberculin purified protein derivative] 5 U/0.1 mL ⑨ Anusol; Apresoline

Aplitest single-use intradermal puncture test device *tuberculosis skin test* [tuberculin purified protein derivative] 5 U

aplonidine HCl [see: apraclonidine HCl]

APO (Adriamycin, prednisone, Oncovin) *chemotherapy protocol*

Apo-Acetaminophen (CAN) tablets, film-coated caplets OTC *analgesic; antipyretic* [acetaminophen] 325, 500 mg

Apo-Acyclovir (CAN) tablets ℞ *antiviral for herpes infections* [acyclovir] 200, 400, 800 mg

Apo-Amitriptylene (CAN) film-coated tablets ℞ *tricyclic antidepressant* [amitriptyline HCl] 10, 25, 50, 75 mg

Apo-Amoxi (CAN) capsules, oral suspension ℞ *aminopenicillin antibiotic* [amoxicillin trihydrate] 250, 500 mg; 125, 250 mg/5 mL

Apo-Atenolol (CAN) tablets ℞ *antihypertensive; antianginal; antiadrenergic (β-blocker)* [atenolol] 50, 100 mg

Apo-Beclomethasone (CAN) nasal spray ℞ *corticosteroidal anti-inflammatory for chronic asthma and rhinitis* [beclomethasone dipropionate] 50 μg/spray

Apo-Benzydamine (CAN) oral rinse ℞ *topical analgesic and anti-inflammatory* [benzydamine HCl] 0.15%

Apo-Butorphanol (CAN) nasal spray ℞ *narcotic agonist-antagonist analgesic; antimigraine agent* [butorphanol tartrate] 10 mg/mL

Apo-Cefaclor (CAN) capsules, oral suspension ℞ *cephalosporin antibiotic* [cefaclor] 250, 500 mg; 125, 250, 375 mg/5 mL

Apo-Cefadroxil (CAN) capsules ℞ *cephalosporin antibiotic* [cefadroxil] 500 mg

Apo-Cetirizine (CAN) tablets OTC *antihistamine* [cetirizine HCl] 10 mg

Apo-Chlorhexidine (CAN) oral rinse ℞ *antimicrobial; gingivitis treatment* [chlorhexidine gluconate] 0.12%

Apo-Cimetidine (CAN) film-coated tablets, oral liquid ℞ *histamine H_2 antagonist for gastric and duodenal ulcers and gastric hypersecretory conditions* [cimetidine] 200, 300, 400, 600, 800 mg; 300 mg/5 mL

Apo-Clonazepam (CAN) tablets ℞ *anticonvulsant* [clonazepam] 0.5, 2 mg

Apo-Cromolyn (CAN) nasal spray ℞ *anti-inflammatory/mast cell stabilizer for the prophylaxis of allergic rhinitis* [cromolyn sodium (sodium cromoglycate)] 2% (5.2 mg/dose)

Apo-Cromolyn (CAN) Sterules (solution for nebulization) ℞ *anti-inflammatory/mast cell stabilizer for the prophylaxis of asthma and bronchospasm* [cromolyn sodium (sodium cromoglycate)] 1% (20 mg/2 mL dose)

Apocynum androsaemifolium *medicinal herb* [see: dogbane]

Apo-Desmopressin (CAN) nasal spray ℞ *posterior pituitary hormone; antidiuretic for nocturnal enuresis* [desmopressin acetate] 10 μg/dose

Apo-Diazepam (CAN) tablets ℞ *benzodiazepine sedative; anxiolytic; anticonvulsant; skeletal muscle relaxant* [diazepam] 2, 5, 10 mg

Apo-Diclo Rapide (CAN) tablets ℞ *analgesic; antiarthritic; nonsteroidal anti-inflammatory drug (NSAID)* [diclofenac potassium] 50 mg

Apo-Diltiaz (CAN) IV injection ℞ *calcium channel blocker for atrial fibrillation or paroxysmal supraventricular tachycardia (PSVT)* [diltiazem HCl] 5 mg/mL

Apo-Diltiaz (CAN) tablets ℞ *antianginal; antihypertensive; antiarrhythmic; calcium channel blocker* [diltiazem HCl] 30, 60 mg

Apo-Diltiaz CD (CAN) (once daily) sustained-release capsules ℞ *antihypertensive; antianginal; antiarrhythmic; calcium channel blocker* [diltiazem HCl] 120, 180, 240, 300 mg

Apo-Diltiaz SR (CAN) (twice daily) sustained-release capsules ℞ *antihypertensive; antianginal; antiarrhythmic; calcium channel blocker* [diltiazem HCl] 60, 90, 120 mg

Apo-Dipivefrin (CAN) eye drops ℞ *topical antiglaucoma agent* [dipivefrin HCl] 0.1%

Apo-Divalproex (CAN) enteric-coated tablets ℞ *anticonvulsant* [divalproex sodium] 125, 250, 500 mg

apodol [see: anileridine HCl]

Apo-Domperidone (CAN) film-coated tablets ℞ *antiemetic for diabetic gastroparesis and chronic gastritis* [domperidone maleate] 10 mg

Apo-Doxazosin (CAN) tablets ℞ *antihypertensive (α-blocker); treatment for benign prostatic hyperplasia* [doxazosin mesylate] 1, 2, 4 mg

Apo-Etodolac (CAN) capsules ℞ *nonsteroidal anti-inflammatory drug (NSAID); analgesic; antiarthritic* [etodolac] 200, 300 mg

Apo-Fluconazole (CAN) tablets ℞ *broad-spectrum antifungal* [fluconazole] 50, 100, 150, 200 mg

Apo-Flunisolide (CAN) metered dose nasal spray ℞ *corticosteroidal anti-inflammatory for seasonal or perennial rhinitis* [flunisolide] 25 μg/dose

Apo-Fluphenazine (CAN) tablets ℞ *conventional (typical) antipsychotic* [fluphenazine HCl] 1, 2, 5 mg

Apo-Flutamide (CAN) tablets ℞ *antiandrogen antineoplastic* [flutamide] 250 mg

Apo-Furosemide (CAN) tablets ℞ *antihypertensive; loop diuretic* [furosemide] 20, 40, 80 mg

Apo-Gemfibrozil (CAN) capsules, tablets ℞ *antihyperlipidemic for hypertriglyceridemia and coronary heart disease* [gemfibrozil] 300 mg; 600 mg

Apo-Glyburide (CAN) tablets ℞ *sulfonylurea antidiabetic* [glyburide] 2.5, 5 mg

Apo-Haloperidol LA (CAN) long-acting IM injection ℞ *conventional (typical) antipsychotic* [haloperidol decanoate] 50, 100 mg/mL

Apo-Hydro (CAN) tablets ℞ *antihypertensive; diuretic* [hydrochlorothiazide] 25, 50, 100 mg

Apo-Ipravent (CAN) Sterules (solution for nebulization), solution for inhalation ℞ *anticholinergic bronchodilator for bronchospasm; antisecretory for rhinorrhea* [ipratropium bromide] 250 μg/mL

Apo-Ketoconazole (CAN) tablets ℞ *systemic antifungal* [ketoconazole] 200 mg

Apo-Ketorolac (CAN) tablets ℞ *analgesic; nonsteroidal anti-inflammatory drug (NSAID)* [ketorolac tromethamine] 10 mg

Apokinon injection ℞ *investigational (orphan) treatment for late-stage Parkinson disease* [apomorphine HCl]

Apo-Lactulose (CAN) oral/rectal solution ℞ *hyperosmotic laxative* [lactulose] 10 g/15 mL

Apo-Levobunolol (CAN) eye drops ℞ *topical antiglaucoma agent (β-blocker)* [levobunolol HCl] 0.25%, 0.5%

Apo-Lithium (CAN) capsules ℞ *antipsychotic for manic episodes of a bipolar disorder* [lithium carbonate] 150, 300 mg

Apo-Lorazepam (CAN) tablets ℞ *benzodiazepine anxiolytic* [lorazepam] 0.5, 1, 2 mg

Apo-Loxapine (CAN) film-coated tablets ℞ *conventional (typical) antipsychotic for schizophrenia* [loxapine succinate] 5, 10, 25, 50 mg

Apo-Methoprazine (CAN) tablets ℞ *CNS depressant; neuroleptic* [methotrimeprazine maleate] 2, 5, 25, 50 mg

Apo-Metoprolol (CAN) tablets ℞ *antihypertensive; antianginal; antiadrenergic (β-blocker)* [metoprolol tartrate] 50, 100 mg

Apo-Metoprolol L (CAN) film-coated caplets ℞ *antihypertensive; antianginal; antiadrenergic (β-blocker)* [metoprolol tartrate] 50, 100 mg

Apo-Moclobemide (CAN) film-coated tablets ℞ *antidepressant; MAO inhibitor* [moclobemide] 100, 150 mg

apomorphine BAN *emetic* [also: apomorphine HCl]

apomorphine HCl USP *emetic; investigational (NDA filed) dopamine receptor agonist for erectile dysfunction; investigational (orphan) for late-stage Parkinson disease* [also: apomorphine]

Apo-Nabumetone (CAN) tablets ℞ *antiarthritic; nonsteroidal anti-inflammatory drug (NSAID)* [nabumetone] 500 mg

Apo-Naproxen (CAN) tablets ℞ *analgesic; antiarthritic; nonsteroidal anti-inflammatory drug (NSAID)* [naproxen] 125, 250, 375, 500 mg

Apo-Naproxen SR (CAN) sustained-release tablets ℞ *analgesic; antiarthritic; nonsteroidal anti-inflammatory drug (NSAID)* [naproxen] 750 mg

Apo-Nefazodone (CAN) tablets ℞ *antidepressant* [nefazodone HCl] 50, 100, 150, 200 mg

Apo-Norflox (CAN) tablets ℞ *broad-spectrum fluoroquinolone antibiotic* [norfloxacin] 400 mg

Apo-Oflox (CAN) film-coated tablets ℞ *broad-spectrum fluoroquinolone antibiotic* [ofloxacin] 200, 300, 400 mg

Apo-Orciprenaline (CAN) syrup ℞ *sympathomimetic bronchodilator* [orciprenaline sulfate] 10 mg/5 mL

Apo-Oxazepam (CAN) tablets ℞ *benzodiazepine anxiolytic* [oxazepam] 10, 15, 30 mg

Apo-Pen VK (CAN) tablets, powder for oral solution ℞ *natural penicillin antibiotic* [penicillin V potassium] 300 mg; 125, 300 mg/5 mL

Apo-Perphenazine (CAN) film-coated tablets ℞ *conventional (typical) antipsychotic; antiemetic* [perphenazine] 2, 4, 8, 16 mg

Apo-Pravastatin (CAN) tablets ℞ *HMG-CoA reductase inhibitor for hyperlipidemia and hypertriglyceridemia* [pravastatin sodium] 10, 20, 40 mg

Apo-Prednisone (CAN) tablets ℞ *corticosteroid; anti-inflammatory* [prednisone] 1, 5, 50 mg

Apo-Prochlorazine (CAN) tablets ℞ *conventional (typical) antipsychotic; antiemetic* [prochlorperazine maleate] 5, 10 mg

Apo-Propafenone (CAN) film-coated tablets ℞ *antiarrhythmic* [propafenone HCl] 150, 300 mg

Apo-Ranitidine (CAN) film-coated tablets OTC *histamine H_2 antagonist for episodic heartburn* [ranitidine HCl] 75 mg

Apo-Ranitidine (CAN) film-coated tablets ℞ *histamine H_2 antagonist for gastric and duodenal ulcers* [ranitidine HCl] 150, 300 mg

Apo-Salvent (CAN) inhaler ℞ *sympathomimetic bronchodilator* [salbutamol] 100 μg/dose

Apo-Salvent (CAN) tablets, solution for nebulization ℞ *sympathomimetic bronchodilator* [salbutamol sulfate] 2, 4 mg; 1, 2 mg/mL

Apo-Sertraline (CAN) capsules ℞ *selective serotonin reuptake inhibitor (SSRI) for depression, obsessive-compulsive disorder (OCD), and panic disorder* [sertraline HCl] 25, 50, 100 mg

Apo-Temazepam (CAN) capsules ℞ *benzodiazepine sedative; hypnotic* [temazepam] 15, 30 mg

Apo-Terazosin (CAN) tablets ℞ *antihypertensive (α-blocker); treatment for benign prostatic hyperplasia (BPH)* [terazosin HCl] 1, 2, 5, 10 mg

Apo-Terbinafine (CAN) tablets ℞ *systemic allylamine antifungal* [terbinafine HCl] 250 mg

Apo-Thioridazine (CAN) film-coated tablets ℞ *conventional (typical) antipsychotic* [thioridazine HCl] 10, 25, 50, 100 mg

Apo-Ticlopidine (CAN) film-coated tablets ℞ *platelet aggregation inhibitor for stroke* [ticlopidine HCl] 250 mg

Apo-Trifluoperazine (CAN) film-coated tablets ℞ *conventional (typical) antipsychotic; anxiolytic* [trifluoperazine HCl] 1, 2, 5, 10, 20 mg

Apo-Valproic (CAN) capsules, syrup ℞ *anticonvulsant* [valproic acid] 250 mg; 250 mg/5 mL

apovincamine INN

Apo-Warfarin (CAN) tablets ℞ *coumarin-derivative anticoagulant* [warfarin sodium] 1, 2, 2.5, 4, 5, 10 mg

Appedrine tablets OTC *nonprescription diet aid; vitamin/mineral supplement* [phenylpropanolamine HCl; multiple vitamins & minerals; folic acid] 25•≛•0.4 mg ⓓ aprindine; ephedrine

appetizers *a class of agents that stimulate the appetite* [see also: aperitives]

APPG (aqueous penicillin G procaine) [see: penicillin G procaine]

apple *(Pyrus malus)* fruit *medicinal herb for constipation and diarrhea, dysentery, fever, heart ailments, scurvy, and warts*

apple, ground *medicinal herb* [see: chamomile]

apple, hog; Indian apple; May apple *medicinal herb* [see: mandrake]

Appli-Kit (trademarked form) *ointment and adhesive dosage covers*

Appli-Ruler (trademarked name) OTC *dose-determining pads*

Appli-Tape (trademarked name) OTC *dosage covers*

Apra ℞ *investigational (Phase II) antineoplastic for soft tissue sarcomas* [CT-2584 (code name—generic name not yet assigned)]

apraclonidine INN, BAN *topical adrenergic for glaucoma* [also: apraclonidine HCl]

apraclonidine HCl USAN *topical adrenergic for glaucoma* [also: apraclonidine]

apramycin USAN, INN, BAN *antibacterial*

aprepitant USAN *neurokinin NK_1 antagonist; antidepressant; antiemetic for chemotherapy*

Apresazide 25/25; Apresazide 50/50; Apresazide 100/50 capsules ℞ *antihypertensive; vasodilator; diuretic* [hydralazine HCl; hydrochlorothiazide] 25•25 mg; 50•50 mg; 100•50 mg

Apresoline tablets ℞ *antihypertensive; vasodilator* [hydralazine HCl] 10, 25, 50, 100 mg

Apri tablets (in packs of 21 or 28) ℞ *monophasic oral contraceptive* [desogestrel; ethinyl estradiol] 0.15 mg•30 μg

apricot *(Prunus armeniaca)* fruit, seeds, and kernel oil *medicinal herb for asthma, constipation, cough, eye inflammation, hemorrhage, infertility, spasm, and vaginal infections; not generally regarded as safe, as apricot kernel ingestion causes cyanide poisoning*

apricot kernel water JAN

aprikalim INN *investigational antianginal*

aprindine USAN, INN, BAN *antiarrhythmic* ⓓ Appedrine; ephedrine

aprindine HCl USAN, JAN *antiarrhythmic*

aprobarbital NF, INN, DCF *sedative*

Aprodine tablets, syrup OTC *decongestant; antihistamine* [pseudoephedrine HCl; triprolidine HCl] 60•2.5 mg; 30•1.25 mg/5 mL

Aprodine with Codeine syrup ℞ *narcotic antitussive; decongestant; antihistamine* [codeine phosphate; pseudoephedrine HCl; triprolidine HCl] 10•30•1.25 mg/5 mL

aprofene INN

aprosulate sodium INN

aprotinin USAN, INN, BAN, JAN *systemic hemostatic to reduce blood loss in coronary surgery (orphan); protease inhibitor*

A.P.S. (aspirin, phenacetin & salicylamide) [q.v.]

APSAC (anisoylated plasminogen streptokinase activator complex) [see: anistreplase]

aptazapine INN *antidepressant* [also: aptazapine maleate]

aptazapine maleate USAN *antidepressant* [also: aptazapine]

aptiganel HCl USAN *investigational (Phase III) NMDA ion channel blocker for stroke and traumatic brain injury*

aptocaine INN, BAN, DCF

Aptosyn ℞ *investigational (NDA filed) apoptosis modulator for adenomatous polyposis coli (APC)* [exisulind]

apyron [see: magnesium salicylate]

Aqua-Ban enteric-coated tablets OTC *diuretic* [ammonium chloride; caffeine] 325•100 mg

Aqua-Ban, Maximum Strength tablets OTC *diuretic* [pamabrom] 50 mg

Aqua-Ban Plus enteric-coated tablets OTC *diuretic; iron supplement* [ammonium chloride; caffeine; ferrous sulfate] 650•200•6 mg

Aquabase OTC *ointment base*

Aquacare cream, lotion OTC *moisturizer; emollient; keratolytic* [urea] 10%

Aquachloral Supprettes (suppositories) ℞ *sedative; hypnotic* [chloral hydrate] 324, 648 mg

aquaday [see: menadione]

aquakay [see: menadione]

AquaMEPHYTON IM or subcu injection ℞ *coagulant to correct anticoagulant-induced prothrombin deficiency; vitamin K supplement* [phytonadione] 2 mg/mL

Aquanil lotion OTC *moisturizer; emollient*

Aquanil Cleanser lotion OTC *soap-free therapeutic skin cleanser*

Aquaphilic OTC *ointment base*

Aquaphilic with Carbamide OTC *ointment base* [urea] 10%, 20%

Aquaphor OTC *ointment base*

Aquaphyllin syrup ℞ *antiasthmatic; bronchodilator* [theophylline] 80 mg/15 mL

AquaSite eye drops OTC *ophthalmic moisturizer/lubricant* [polyethylene glycol 400] 0.2%

Aquasol A capsules (discontinued 1999) ℞ *vitamin deficiency therapy* [vitamin A] 25 000, 50 000 IU/mL

Aquasol A IM injection ℞ *vitamin deficiency therapy* [vitamin A] 50 000 IU/mL

Aquasol A drops (discontinued 1999) OTC *vitamin supplement* [vitamin A] 5000 IU/0.1 mL

Aquasol E capsules, drops (discontinued 1999) OTC *vitamin supplement* [vitamin E] 73.5 mg, 400 IU; 50 mg/mL

Aquatab C tablets ℞ *antitussive; decongestant; expectorant* [dextromethorphan hydrobromide; phenylpropanolamine HCl; guaifenesin] 60•75•1200 mg

Aquatab D tablets ℞ *decongestant; expectorant* [phenylpropanolamine HCl; guaifenesin] 75•1200 mg

Aquatab DM tablets ℞ *antitussive; expectorant* [dextromethorphan hydrobromide; guaifenesin] 60•1200 mg

AquaTar gel OTC *topical antipsoriatic; antiseborrheic* [coal tar extract] 2.5%

Aquatensen tablets ℞ *diuretic; antihypertensive* [methyclothiazide] 5 mg

Aquavit-E drops ℞ *vitamin supplement* [vitamin E (as *dl*-alpha tocopheryl acetate)] 15 IU/0.3 mL

aqueous penicillin G procaine (APPG) [see: penicillin G procaine]

Aquest IM injection (discontinued 1998) ℞ *estrogen replacement therapy for postmenopausal symptoms; palliative therapy for inoperable prostatic and breast cancer* [estrone] 2 mg/mL

Aquilegia vulgaris *medicinal herb* [see: columbine]

aquinone [see: menadione]

AR-177 *investigational (Phase I/II) antiviral/oligonucleotide/integrase inhibitor for HIV infection*

ara-A (adenine arabinoside) [see: vidarabine]

ara-AC (azacytosine arabinoside) [see: fazarabine]

arabinofuranosylcytosine [see: cytarabine]

arabinoluranosylcytosine HCl [see: cytarabine HCl]

arabinosyl cytosine [see: cytarabine]

ara-C (cytosine arabinoside) [see: cytarabine] ⑨ ERYC

ara-C + 6-TG (ara-C, thioguanine) *chemotherapy protocol*

ara-C + ADR (ara-C, Adriamycin) *chemotherapy protocol*

ara-C + DNR + PRED + MP (ara-C, daunorubicin, prednisolone, mercaptopurine) *chemotherapy protocol*

ARAC-DNR (ara-C, daunorubicin) *chemotherapy protocol for acute myelocytic leukemia (AML)*

arachis oil [see: peanut oil]

ara-C-HU (ara-C, hydroxyurea) *chemotherapy protocol*

ara-cytidine [see: cytarabine]

Aralen HCl IM injection ℞ *antimalarial; amebicide* [chloroquine HCl] 50 mg/mL ⑨ Arlidin

Aralen Phosphate film-coated tablets ℞ *antimalarial; amebicide* [chloroquine phosphate] 500 mg

Aralia racemosa *medicinal herb* [see: spikenard]

***Aralia* spp.** *medicinal herb* [see: ginseng]

Aramine IV, subcu or IM injection ℞ *vasopressor for acute hypotensive shock, anaphylaxis, or traumatic shock* [metaraminol bitartrate] 10 mg/mL

Aranesp IV or subcu injection ℞ *long-acting epoetin analogue; hematopoietic for anemia of chronic renal failure; investigational (NDA filed) for anemia secondary to cancer chemotherapy* [darbepoetin alfa] 25, 40, 60, 100, 200 µg/mL

aranidipine INN

aranotin USAN, INN *antiviral*

araprofen INN

Arava film-coated tablets ℞ *anti-inflammatory for rheumatoid arthritis (RA)* [leflunomide] 10, 20, 100 mg

ARB (angiotensin II receptor blocker) [see: angiotensin II receptor antagonists]

arbaprostil USAN, INN *gastric antisecretory*

arbekacin INN

arberry *medicinal herb* [see: uva ursi]

arbutamine INN, BAN *cardiac stressor for diagnosis of coronary artery disease* [also: arbutamine HCl]

arbutamine HCl USAN *cardiac stressor for diagnosis of coronary artery disease* [also: arbutamine]

Arbutus uva ursi *medicinal herb* [see: uva ursi]

archangel *medicinal herb* [see: angelica]

arcitumomab USAN *imaging agent for detection of recurrent or metastatic thyroid cancers (orphan)*

arclofenin USAN, INN *hepatic function test*

Arcobee with C caplets OTC *vitamin supplement* [multiple B vitamins; vitamin C] ≛•300 mg

Arco-Lase chewable tablets OTC *digestive enzymes* [amylase; protease; lipase; cellulase] 30•6•25•2 mg

Arco-Lase Plus tablets ℞ *digestive enzymes; GI antispasmodic; sedative* [amylase; protease; lipase; cellulase; hyoscyamine sulfate; atropine sulfate; phenobarbital] 30•6•25•2•0.1•0.02•7.5 mg

Arctium lappa; A. majus; A. minus *medicinal herb* [see: burdock]

Arctostaphylos uva ursi *medicinal herb* [see: uva ursi]

ardacin INN

ardeparin sodium USAN, INN *a low molecular weight heparin–type anticoagulant and antithrombotic for the prevention of deep vein thrombosis (DVT) following knee replacement surgery*

Arduan powder for IV injection ℞ *nondepolarizing neuromuscular* *blocker; adjunct to anesthesia* [pipecuronium bromide] 10 mg/vial

arecoline acetarsone salt [see: drocarbil]

arecoline hydrobromide NF

Aredia powder for IV infusion ℞ *bisphosphonate bone resorption inhibitor for Paget disease, hypercalcemia of malignancy, breast cancer, and multiple myeloma* [pamidronate disodium] 30, 90 mg

Arestin topical microspheres ℞ *bacteriostatic adjunct to scaling and root planing for periodontitis* [minocycline HCl]

arfalasin INN

arfendazam INN

argatroban USAN, INN, JAN *anticoagulant for heparin-induced thrombocytopenia (HIT) and thrombosis; investigational (Phase II) for myocardial infarction*

Argesic cream OTC *topical analgesic; counterirritant* [methyl salicylate; trolamine]

Argesic-SA tablets ℞ *analgesic; anti-inflammatory* [salsalate] 500 mg

argimesna INN

arginine (L-arginine) USP, INN *nonessential amino acid; ammonia detoxicant; diagnostic aid for pituitary function; symbols: Arg, R*

arginine butanoate [see: arginine butyrate]

arginine butyrate (L-arginine butyrate) USAN *investigational (orphan) for beta-hemoglobinopathies, beta-thalassemia, and sickle cell disease*

arginine glutamate (L-arginine L-glutamate) USAN, BAN, JAN *ammonia detoxicant*

arginine HCl USAN, USP, JAN *ammonia detoxicant; pituitary (growth hormone) function diagnostic aid*

L-arginine monohydrochloride [see: arginine HCl]

8-L-arginine vasopressin [see: vasopressin]

8-arginineoxytocin [see: argiprestocin]

8-L-argininevasopressin tannate [see: argipressin tannate]

argipressin INN, BAN *antidiuretic* [also: argipressin tannate]

argipressin tannate USAN *antidiuretic* [also: argipressin]

argiprestocin INN

argon *element (Ar)*

argyn [see: silver protein, mild]

Aricept tablets ℞ *reversible acetylcholinesterase (AChE) inhibitor; cognition adjuvant for Alzheimer dementia* [donepezil HCl] 5, 10 mg ⊡ Erycette

arildone USAN, INN *antiviral*

Arilvax ℞ *investigational (Phase III) single-dose, live attenuated yellow fever vaccine*

Arimidex film-coated tablets ℞ *aromatase inhibitor; hormone antagonist antineoplastic for advanced breast cancer in postmenopausal women* [anastrozole] 1 mg

aripiprazole USAN *antischizophrenic; investigational (Phase III) antipsychotic*

Aristocort ointment, cream ℞ *topical corticosteroidal anti-inflammatory* [triamcinolone acetonide] 0.1%, 0.5%; 0.025%, 0.1%, 0.5%

Aristocort tablets ℞ *corticosteroid; anti-inflammatory* [triamcinolone] 1, 2, 4, 8 mg

Aristocort A ointment, cream ℞ *topical corticosteroidal anti-inflammatory* [triamcinolone acetonide in a water-washable base] 0.1%; 0.025%, 0.1%, 0.5%

Aristocort Forte IM injection ℞ *corticosteroid; anti-inflammatory* [triamcinolone diacetate] 40 mg/mL

Aristocort Intralesional injection ℞ *corticosteroid; anti-inflammatory* [triamcinolone diacetate] 25 mg/mL

Aristolochia clematitis *medicinal herb* [see: birthwort]

Aristospan Intra-articular injection ℞ *corticosteroid; anti-inflammatory* [triamcinolone hexacetonide] 20 mg/mL

Aristospan Intralesional injection ℞ *corticosteroid; anti-inflammatory* [triamcinolone hexacetonide] 5 mg/mL

Arixtra subcu injection ℞ *investigational (NDA filed) factor Xa inhibitor*

for venous thrombosis following orthopedic surgery [fondaparinux sodium]

A.R.M. (Allergy Relief Medicine) caplets OTC *decongestant; antihistamine* [phenylpropanolamine HCl; chlorpheniramine maleate] 25•4 mg

Arm-A-Med (trademarked packaging form) *single-dose plastic vial*

Arm-A-Vial (trademarked packaging form) *single-dose plastic vial*

Armoracia rusticana; A. lapathiofolia *medicinal herb* [see: horseradish]

Armour Thyroid tablets ℞ *natural thyroid replacement for hypothyroidism or thyroid cancer* [thyroid, desiccated] 15, 30, 60, 90, 120, 180, 240, 300 mg

arnica *(Arnica montana; A. cordifolia; A. fulgens)* flowers *medicinal herb used as a topical counterirritant and vulnerary for acne, bruises, rashes, and other dermal lesions; not generally regarded as safe when taken internally, as it is highly toxic*

arnolol INN

arofylline USAN *phosphodiesterase IV inhibitor for asthma*

Aromasin tablets ℞ *aromatase inhibitor; antihormonal antineoplastic for advanced breast cancer in postmenopausal women (orphan)* [exemestane] 25 mg

aromatase inhibitors *a class of antihormonal antineoplastics which block the conversion of androgens to estrogens, effectively depriving hormone-dependent tumors of estrogen in postmenopausal women*

aromatic ammonia spirit [see: ammonia spirit, aromatic]

aromatic cascara fluidextract [see: cascara fluidextract, aromatic]

aromatic cascara sagrada [see: cascara fluidextract, aromatic]

aromatic elixir NF *flavored and sweetened vehicle*

aromatics *a class of agents that have an agreeable odor and stimulating qualities; also, substances with a specific molecular structure in organic chemistry*

aronixil INN

Aroplatin ℞ *investigational (orphan) antineoplastic*

arotinolol INN [also: arotinolol HCl]

arotinolol HCl JAN [also: arotinolol]

arprinocid USAN, INN, BAN *coccidiostat*

arpromidine INN

Arrestin IM injection (discontinued 2000) ℞ *antiemetic; anticholinergic* [trimethobenzamide HCl] 100 mg/mL

arrow wood; Indian arrow wood; Indian arrow *medicinal herb* [see: wahoo]

ARS (antirabies serum) [q.v.]

arsambide [see: carbarsone]

arsanilic acid INN, BAN *investigational (Phase I/II) immunomodulator for AIDS*

arseclor [see: dichlorophenarsine HCl]

arsenic *element (As)*

arsenic acid, sodium salt [see: sodium arsenate]

arsenic trioxide (AsO_3) JAN *antineoplastic for acute promyelocytic leukemia (APL); investigational (NDA filed, orphan) for renal cell carcinoma; investigational (orphan) for multiple myeloma and myelodysplastic syndromes*

arsenobenzene [see: arsphenamine]

arsenobenzol [see: arsphenamine]

arsenphenolamine [see: arsphenamine]

Arsobal (available only from the Centers for Disease Control) ℞ *investigational anti-infective for trypanosomiasis* [melarsoprol]

arsphenamine USP

arsthinenol DCF [also: arsthinol]

arsthinol INN [also: arsthinenol]

Artane tablets, elixir, Sequels (sustained-release capsules) (discontinued 2001) ℞ *anticholinergic; antiparkinsonian* [trihexyphenidyl HCl] 2, 5 mg; 2 mg/5 mL; 5 mg ⑨ Anturane

arteflene USAN, INN *antimalarial*

artegraft USAN *arterial prosthetic aid*

artemether INN

Artemisia absinthium *medicinal herb* [see: wormwood]

Artemisia dracunculus *medicinal herb* [see: tarragon]

Artemisia vulgaris *medicinal herb* [see: mugwort]

artemisinin INN

arterenol [see: norepinephrine bitartrate]

artesunate INN

Artha-G tablets OTC *analgesic; anti-inflammatory* [salsalate] 750 mg

ArthriCare, Double Ice gel OTC *topical analgesic; counterirritant* [menthol; camphor] 4%•3.1%

ArthriCare, Odor Free rub OTC *topical analgesic; counterirritant* [menthol; methyl nicotinate; capsaicin] 1.25%•0.25%•0.025%

ArthriCare Triple Medicated gel OTC *topical analgesic; counterirritant* [methyl salicylate; menthol; methyl nicotinate] 30%•1.5%•0.7%

Arthriten tablets (discontinued 2000) OTC *analgesic; antipyretic* [acetaminophen; magnesium salicylate; caffeine (buffered with magnesium carbonate, magnesium oxide, and calcium carbonate)] 250•250•32.5 mg

"Arthritis Formula"; "Arthritis Strength" products [see under product name]

Arthritis Foundation Ibuprofen tablets (discontinued 1997) OTC *analgesic; antiarthritic; antipyretic; nonsteroidal anti-inflammatory drug (NSAID)* [ibuprofen] 200 mg

Arthritis Foundation Nighttime caplets (discontinued 1997) OTC *antihistaminic sleep aid; analgesic* [diphenhydramine HCl; acetaminophen] 25•500 mg

Arthritis Foundation Pain Reliever tablets (discontinued 1999) OTC *analgesic; antipyretic; anti-inflammatory; antirheumatic* [aspirin] 500 mg

Arthritis Foundation Pain Reliever, Aspirin Free caplets (discontinued 1997) OTC *analgesic; antipyretic* [acetaminophen] 500 mg

Arthritis Hot Creme OTC *topical analgesic; counterirritant* [methyl salicylate; menthol] 15%•10%

Arthritis Pain Formula caplets OTC *analgesic; antipyretic; anti-inflammatory; antirheumatic* [aspirin (buffered with magnesium hydroxide and aluminum hydroxide)] 500 mg

Arthritis Pain Formula Aspirin-Free tablets (discontinued 1997) OTC *analgesic; antipyretic* [acetaminophen] 500 mg

Arthropan IM injection ℞ *analgesic; antipyretic; anti-inflammatory; antirheumatic* [choline salicylate] 870 mg/5 mL

Arthrotec tablets ℞ *antiarthritic NSAID with a coating to protect gastric mucosa* [diclofenac sodium (enteric-coated core); misoprostol (coating)] 50•0.2, 75•0.2 mg

articaine INN *amide local anesthetic for dentistry* [also: articaine HCl; carticaine]

articaine HCl USAN *amide local anesthetic for dentistry* [also: articaine; carticaine]

artichoke (*Cynara scolymus*) flower heads *medicinal herb for albuminuria, bile stimulation, diabetes, diuresis, dyspepsia, jaundice, liver diseases, and postoperative anemia*

Articoat bandages OTC *antimicrobial dressings*

Articulose L.A. IM injection ℞ *corticosteroid; anti-inflammatory* [triamcinolone diacetate] 40 mg/mL

Articulose-50 IM injection (discontinued 1998) ℞ *corticosteroid; anti-inflammatory* [prednisolone acetate] 50 mg/mL

Artificial Tears eye drops OTC *ocular moisturizer/lubricant*

Artificial Tears ophthalmic ointment OTC *ocular moisturizer/lubricant* [white petrolatum; mineral oil; lanolin]

Artificial Tears Plus eye drops OTC *ophthalmic moisturizer/lubricant* [polyvinyl alcohol] 1.4%

artilide INN *antiarrhythmic* [also: artilide fumarate]

artilide fumarate USAN *antiarrhythmic* [also: artilide]

Arvin (available in Canada as Viprinex) ℞ *anticoagulant; orphan status withdrawn 1997* [ancrod]

arzoxifene HCl USAN *selective estrogen receptor modulator (SERM) for breast cancer, uterine fibroids, endometriosis, and dysfunctional uterine bleeding*

AS-013 [see: prostaglandin E_1 enol ester]

^{74}As [see: sodium arsenate As 74]

5-ASA (5-aminosalicylic acid) [see: mesalamine]

ASA (acetylsalicylic acid) [see: aspirin]

Asacol delayed-release tablets ℞ *anti-inflammatory for active ulcerative colitis, proctosigmoiditis and proctitis* [mesalamine] 400 mg

asafetida; asafoetida *(Ferula assafoetida; F. foetida; F. rubricaulis)* gum resin from dried roots and rhizomes *medicinal herb for abdominal tumors, amenorrhea, asthma, colic, convulsions, corns and calluses, edema; also used as an expectorant; not generally regarded as safe for children, as it may induce methemoglobinemia*

asafoetida *medicinal herb* [see: asafetida]

Asarum canadense *medicinal herb* [see: wild ginger]

Asclepias geminata *medicinal herb* [see: gymnema]

Asclepias syriaca *medicinal herb* [see: milkweed]

Asclepias tuberosa *medicinal herb* [see: pleurisy root]

ascorbic acid (L-ascorbic acid; vitamin C) USP, INN, BAN, JAN *water-soluble vitamin; antiscorbutic; urinary acidifier; topical sunscreen* 250, 500, 1000, 1500 mg oral; 240 mg/tsp. oral; 500 mg/5 mL oral; 500 mg/mL injection

L-ascorbic acid, monosodium salt [see: sodium ascorbate]

L-ascorbic acid 6-palmitate [see: ascorbyl palmitate]

Ascorbicap timed-release capsules (discontinued 1999) OTC *vitamin C supplement* [ascorbic acid] 500 mg

ascorbyl palmitate NF *antioxidant*

Ascriptin; Ascriptin A/D coated tablets OTC *analgesic; antipyretic; anti-inflammatory; antirheumatic* [aspirin (buffered with magnesium hydroxide, aluminum hydroxide, and calcium carbonate)] 325, 500 mg; 325 mg

Asendin tablets ℞ *tricyclic antidepressant* [amoxapine] 25, 50, 100, 150 mg

aseptichrome [see: merbromin]

Aseptone 1; Aseptone 2; Aseptone 5; Aseptone QUAT (CAN) solution OTC *antiseptic; disinfectant; germicide*

ash, bitter *medicinal herb* [see: quassia; wahoo]

ash, mountain; American mountain ash; European mountain ash *medicinal herb* [see: mountain ash]

ash, poison *medicinal herb* [see: fringe tree]

ASHAP; A-SHAP (Adriamycin, Solu-Medrol, high-dose ara-C, Platinol) *chemotherapy protocol*

Asimina triloba *medicinal herb* [see: pawpaw]

Asmalix elixir ℞ *antiasthmatic; bronchodilator* [theophylline] 80 mg/15 mL

AsO_3 (arsenic trioxide) [q.v.]

asobamast INN, BAN

asocainol INN

Aspalathus linearis; A. contaminata; Borbonia pinifolia *medicinal herb* [see: red bush tea]

asparaginase (L-asparaginase) USAN, JAN *antineoplastic for acute lymphocytic leukemia* [also: colaspase]

asparagine (L-asparagine) *nonessential amino acid; symbols: Asn, N*

L-asparagine amidohydrolase [see: asparaginase]

asparagus *(Asparagus officinalis)* roots, seeds *medicinal herb for acne, constipation, contraception, edema, neuritis, parasites, rheumatism, stimulating hair growth, and toothache*

aspartame USAN, NF, INN, BAN *sweetener*

L-aspartate potassium JAN

aspartic acid (L-aspartic acid) USAN, INN *nonessential amino acid; symbols: Asp, D*

L-aspartic acid insulin [see: insulin aspart]

aspartocin USAN, INN *antibacterial*

A-Spas S/L sublingual tablets ℞ *GI/GU antispasmodic; anticholinergic* [hyoscyamine sulfate] 0.125 mg

aspen, European *medicinal herb* [see: black poplar]

aspen poplar; American aspen; quaking aspen *medicinal herb* [see: poplar]

Aspercreme cream OTC *topical analgesic* [trolamine salicylate] 10%

Aspercreme Rub lotion OTC *topical analgesic* [trolamine salicylate] 10%

***Aspergillus oryase* proteinase** [see: asperkinase]

Aspergum chewing gum tablets OTC *analgesic; antipyretic; anti-inflammatory; antirheumatic* [aspirin] 227.5 mg

asperkinase

asperlin USAN *antibacterial; antineoplastic*

Asperula odorata *medicinal herb* [see: sweet woodruff]

aspidium *(Dryopteris filix-mas)* plant *medicinal herb for bloody nose, menorrhagia, worm infections including tapeworm and ringworm, and wound healing; not generally regarded as safe for internal use, as it is highly toxic*

aspidosperma USP

aspirin USP, BAN, JAN *analgesic; antipyretic; anti-inflammatory; antirheumatic* 325, 500, 650, 975 mg oral; 120, 200, 300, 600 mg suppositories ⊡ Afrin

aspirin, buffered USP *analgesic; antipyretic; anti-inflammatory; antirheumatic* 325 mg oral

aspirin aluminum NF, JAN

aspirin & butalbital & caffeine *analgesic; barbiturate sedative* 325•50•40 mg oral

aspirin DL-lysine JAN

Aspirin Free Excedrin caplets, geltabs OTC *analgesic; antipyretic* [acetaminophen; caffeine] 500•65 mg

Aspirin with Codeine No. 2, No. 3, and No. 4 tablets ℞ *narcotic analgesic* [codeine phosphate; aspirin] 15•325 mg; 30•325 mg; 60•325 mg

ASPIRINcheck urine test kit for professional use *in vitro diagnostic aid for antiplatelet metabolites of aspirin*

Aspirin-Free Pain Relief tablets, caplets OTC *analgesic; antipyretic* [acetaminophen] 325, 500 mg; 500 mg

Aspirol (trademarked delivery form) *crushable ampule for inhalation*

aspogen [see: dihydroxyaluminum aminoacetate]

aspoxicillin INN, JAN

Asprimox; Asprimox Extra Protection for Arthritis Pain tablets, caplets OTC *analgesic; antipyretic; anti-inflammatory; antirheumatic* [aspirin (buffered with aluminum hydroxide, magnesium hydroxide, and calcium carbonate)] 325 mg

aspro [see: aspirin]

astatine *element (At)*

Astelin nasal spray ℞ *phthalazinone antihistamine and mast cell stabilizer for allergic and vasomotor rhinitis* [azelastine HCl] 137 µg/spray

astemizole USAN, INN, BAN *antiallergic; second-generation piperidine antihistamine*

AsthmaHaler inhalation aerosol OTC *sympathomimetic bronchodilator* [epinephrine bitartrate] 0.35 mg/dose

AsthmaNefrin solution for inhalation OTC *sympathomimetic bronchodilator* [racepinephrine HCl] 2.25%

astifilcon A USAN *hydrophilic contact lens material*

Astracaine; Astracaine Forte (CAN) intraoral injection ℞ *local anesthetic for dentistry* [articaine HCl; epinephrine] 4%•1:200 000; 4%•1:100 000

astragalus *(Astragalus membranaceus)* root *medicinal herb for cancer, chronic fatigue, and Epstein-Barr syndrome; also used to strengthen the immune system, especially after chemotherapy and HIV treatments*

Astramorph PF (preservative free) IV, subcu or IM injection ℞ *narcotic analgesic* [morphine sulfate] 0.5, 1 mg/mL

astringents *a class of agents that contract tissue, reducing secretions or discharges* [see also: hemostatics; styptics]

Astroglide vaginal gel OTC *lubricant* [glycerin; propylene glycol]

astromicin INN *antibacterial* [also: astromicin sulfate]

astromicin sulfate USAN, JAN *antibacterial* [also: astromicin]

AT-III (antithrombin III) [q.v.]

Atacand tablets ℞ *antihypertensive; angiotensin II receptor antagonist* [candesartan cilexetil] 4, 8, 16, 32 mg ⓢ Ativan

Atacand HCT tablets ℞ *antihypertensive; angiotensin II receptor antagonist; diuretic* [candesartan cilexetil; hydrochlorothiazide] 16•12.5, 32•12.5 mg

atamestane INN *investigational aromatase inhibitor for cancer*

ataprost INN

Atarax tablets, syrup ℞ *anxiolytic; minor tranquilizer; antihistamine for allergic pruritus* [hydroxyzine HCl] 10, 25, 50 mg; 10 mg/5 mL ⓢ Marax

Atarax 100 tablets ℞ *anxiolytic; minor tranquilizer; antihistamine for allergic pruritus* [hydroxyzine HCl] 100 mg ⓢ Marax

atarvet [see: acepromazine]

atenolol USAN, INN, BAN, JAN *antihypertensive; antianginal; antiadrenergic (β-blocker)* 25, 50, 100 mg oral ⓢ timolol

atevirdine INN *antiviral* [also: atevirdine mesylate]

atevirdine mesylate USAN *antiviral; investigational (Phase II/III) non-nucleoside reverse transcriptase inhibitor (NNRTI) for HIV and AIDS* [also: atevirdine]

ATG (antithymocyte globulin) [q.v.]

Atgam IV infusion ℞ *immunizing agent to prevent allograft rejection of renal transplants; treatment for aplastic anemia; investigational (orphan) for organ and bone marrow transplants* [lymphocyte immune globulin (antithymocyte globulin), equine] 50 mg/mL

athyromazole [see: carbimazole]

atipamezole USAN, INN, BAN *α_2-receptor antagonist*

atiprimod dihydrochloride USAN *immunomodulator; anti-inflammatory; antiarthritic*

atiprimod dimaleate USAN *immunomodulator; anti-inflammatory; antiarthritic*

atiprosin INN *antihypertensive* [also: atiprosin maleate]

atiprosin maleate USAN *antihypertensive* [also: atiprosin]

Ativan IV or IM injection ℞ *benzodiazepine anxiolytic; anticonvulsive* [lorazepam] 2, 4 mg/mL ⓢ Atacand; Adapin; Avitene

Ativan tablets ℞ *benzodiazepine anxiolytic* [lorazepam] 0.5, 1, 2 mg ⓢ Adapin; Avitene

atlafilcon A USAN *hydrophilic contact lens material*

ATM-027 *investigational (Phase II) monoclonal antibody for multiple sclerosis (clinical trial discontinued 1999)*

ATnativ powder for IV infusion (discontinued 1999) ℞ *for thrombosis and pulmonary emboli of congenital AT-III deficiency (orphan)* [antithrombin III] 500 IU

atolide USAN, INN *anticonvulsant*

Atolone tablets ℞ *corticosteroid; anti-inflammatory* [triamcinolone] 4 mg

atorvastatin calcium USAN *HMG-CoA reductase inhibitor for hypercholesterolemia, dysbetalipoproteinemia, and hypertriglyceridemia*

atosiban USAN, INN *oxytocin antagonist*

atovaquone USAN, INN, BAN *antipneumocystic for Pneumocystis carinii pneumonia (orphan); antimalarial; investigational (orphan) antiprotozoal for Toxoplasma gondii encephalitis*

ATP (adenosine triphosphate) [see: adenosine triphosphate disodium]

ATPase (adenosine triphosphatase) inhibitors *a class of gastric antisecretory agents that inhibit the ATPase "proton pump" within the gastric parietal cell* [also called: proton pump inhibitors; substituted benzimidazoles]

atracurium besilate INN *skeletal muscle relaxant; nondepolarizing neuromuscular blocker; adjunct to anesthesia* [also: atracurium besylate]

atracurium besylate USAN, BAN *skeletal muscle relaxant; nondepolarizing neuromuscular blocker; adjunct to anesthesia* [also: atracurium besilate]

Atragen ℞ *investigational (NDA filed, orphan) antineoplastic for acute promyelocytic leukemia; investigational (orphan) for other leukemias and ophthalmic squamous metaplasia; investigational (Phase II) for relapsed or refractory non-Hodgkin lymphoma and AIDS-related Kaposi sarcoma* [tretinoin]

atrasentan HCl USAN *endothelin* ET_A *receptor antagonist for bone pain due to metastatic prostate cancer*

atreleuton USAN *5-lipoxygenase inhibitor for asthma*

Atretol tablets ℞ *anticonvulsant; analgesic for trigeminal neuralgia; antipsychotic* [carbamazepine] 200 mg

Atridox gel ℞ *subgingival antibiotic for periodontal disease* [doxycycline hyclate] 10%

Atrigel (trademarked delivery system) *sustained-release delivery*

atrimustine INN

atrinositol INN

Atrisone gel ℞ *investigational (Phase II) topical acne treatment*

Atrisorb FreeFlow GTR Barrier ℞ *investigational (NDA filed) guided tissue regeneration (GTR) therapy for severe periodontal disease*

Atrohist Pediatric oral suspension ℞ *pediatric decongestant and antihistamine* [phenylephrine tannate; chlorpheniramine tannate; pyrilamine tannate] 5•2•12.5 mg/5 mL

Atrohist Pediatric sustained-release capsules ℞ *pediatric decongestant and antihistamine* [pseudoephedrine HCl; chlorpheniramine maleate] 60•4 mg

Atrohist Plus sustained-release tablets ℞ *decongestant; antihistamine; anticholinergic* [phenylpropanolamine HCl; phenylephrine HCl; chlorpheniramine maleate; hyoscyamine sulfate; atropine sulfate; scopolamine hydrobromide] 50•25•8•0.19•0.04•0.01 mg

atromepine INN, DCF

Atromid-S capsules ℞ *triglyceride-lowering antihyperlipidemic for primary dysbetalipoproteinemia (type III hyperlipidemia) and hypertriglyceridemia (types IV and V hyperlipidemia)* [clofibrate] 500 mg

Atropa belladonna *medicinal herb* [see: belladonna]

AtroPen auto-injector (automatic IM injection device) ℞ *antidote for organophosphorous or carbamate insecticides* [atropine sulfate]

atropine USP, BAN *anticholinergic*

Atropine Care eye drops ℞ *mydriatic; cycloplegic* [atropine sulfate] 1%

atropine methonitrate INN, BAN *anticholinergic* [also: methylatropine nitrate]

atropine methylnitrate [see: methylatropine nitrate]

atropine oxide INN *anticholinergic* [also: atropine oxide HCl]

atropine oxide HCl USAN *anticholinergic* [also: atropine oxide]

atropine propionate [see: prampine]

atropine sulfate USP, JAN *GI/GU antispasmodic; antiparkinsonian; bronchodilator; cycloplegic; mydriatic; antidote to insecticide poisoning* [also: atropine sulphate] 0.4, 0.6 mg oral; 1%, 2% eye drops; 0.05, 0.1, 0.3, 0.4, 0.5, 0.8, 1 mg/mL injection

atropine sulphate BAN *GI/GU antispasmodic; antiparkinsonian; bronchodilator; cycloplegic; mydriatic* [also: atropine sulfate]

Atropine-1 eye drops ℞ *mydriatic; cycloplegic* [atropine sulfate] 1%

Atropisol Dropperettes (eye drops) ℞ *cycloplegic; mydriatic* [atropine sulfate] 1%

Atrosept sugar-coated tablets ℞ *urinary antibiotic; analgesic; antispasmodic; acidifier* [methenamine; phenyl salicylate; atropine sulfate; methylene blue; hyoscyamine sulfate; benzoic acid] 40.8•18.1•0.03•5.4•0.03•4.5 mg

Atrovent nasal spray, solution for inhalation, inhalation aerosol ℞ *anticholinergic bronchodilator for bronchospasm; antisecretory for rhinorrhea* [ipratropium bromide] 0.03%, 0.06%; 0.02%; 18 μg/dose ⊡ Trovan

A/T/S topical solution, gel ℞ *topical antibiotic for acne* [erythromycin] 2%

Attain liquid OTC *enteral nutritional therapy* [lactose-free formula]

attapulgite, activated USP *suspending agent; GI adsorbent*

Attenuvax powder for subcu injection ℞ *measles vaccine* [measles virus vaccine, live attenuated] 0.5 mL

Atuss DM syrup ℞ *antitussive; decongestant; antihistamine* [dextromethorphan hydrobromide; phenylephrine HCl; chlorpheniramine maleate] 15•5•2 mg/5 mL

Atuss EX syrup ℞ *narcotic antitussive; expectorant* [hydrocodone bitartrate; potassium guaiacolsulfonate] 5•300 mg/5 mL

Atuss G syrup ℞ *narcotic antitussive; decongestant; expectorant* [hydrocodone bitartrate; phenylephrine HCl; guaifenesin] 2•10•100 mg/5 mL

Atuss HD liquid ℞ *narcotic antitussive; decongestant; antihistamine* [hydrocodone bitartrate; phenylephrine HCl; chlorpheniramine maleate] 2.5•5•2 mg/5 mL

"atypical" antipsychotics [see: novel antipsychotics]

^{198}Au [see: gold Au 198]

augmented betamethasone dipropionate *topical corticosteroid*

Augmentin film-coated tablets, chewable tablets, powder for oral suspension ℞ *aminopenicillin antibiotic* [amoxicillin; clavulanate potassium] 250•125, 500•125, 875•125 mg; 125•31.25, 200•28.5, 250•62.5, 400•57 mg; 125•31.25, 200•28.5, 250•62.5, 400•57 mg/5 mL

Augmentin IV injection ℞ *aminopenicillin antibiotic* [amoxicillin sodium; clavulanate potassium]

Augmentin ES powder for oral suspension ℞ *aminopenicillin antibiotic* [amoxicillin; clavulanate potassium] 600•43 mg/5 mL

Auralgan Otic ear drops ℞ *topical local anesthetic; analgesic* [benzocaine; antipyrine] 1.4%•5.4% ⊡ Allergan; allergen

auranofin USAN, INN, BAN, JAN *antirheumatic (29% gold)*

aureoquin [now: quinetolate]

Auriculin *investigational (orphan) for acute renal failure and renal transplants; clinical trials discontinued 1997; orphan status withdrawn 1998* [anaritide acetate]

Auro Ear Drops OTC *agent to emulsify and disperse ear wax* [carbamide peroxide] 6.5%

Auro-Dri ear drops OTC *antibacterial; antifungal* [boric acid] 2.75%

Aurolate IM injection ℞ *antirheumatic* [gold sodium thiomalate] 50 mg/mL

aurolin [see: gold sodium thiosulfate]

auropin [see: gold sodium thiosulfate]

aurosan [see: gold sodium thiosulfate]

aurothioglucose USP *antirheumatic (50% gold)*

aurothioglycanide INN, DCF

aurothiomalate disodium [see: gold sodium thiomalate]

aurothiomalate sodium [see: gold sodium thiomalate]

Auroto Otic ear drops ℞ *topical local anesthetic; analgesic* [antipyrine; benzocaine] 1.4%•5.4%

Australian tea tree *medicinal herb* [see: tea tree oil]

Autohaler (delivery form) *breath-activated metered-dose inhaler*

auto-injector (delivery device) *automatic IM injection device*

autologous cell (AC) vaccine *investigational (Phase III, orphan) therapeutic vaccine for adjuvant treatment of ovarian cancer*

autolymphocyte therapy (ALT) *investigational (orphan) for metastatic renal cell carcinoma (clinical trials discontinued 1998)*

Autoplex T IV injection or drip ℞ *antihemophilic to correct factor VIII deficiency and coagulation deficiency* [anti-inhibitor coagulant complex, heat treated] (each bottle is labeled with dosage)

autoprothrombin I [see: factor VII]

autoprothrombin II [see: factor IX]

autumn crocus *(Colchicum autumnale; C. speciosum; C. vernum)* plant and corm *medicinal herb for edema, gonorrhea, gout, prostate enlargement, and rheumatism; not generally regarded as safe, as it is highly toxic because of its colchicine content*

AV (Adriamycin, vincristine) *chemotherapy protocol*

Avail tablets OTC *vitamin/mineral/iron supplement* [multiple vitamins & minerals; iron; folic acid] ≛•18•0.4 mg Ⓢ Advil

Avakine (name changed to Remicade upon release in 1998)

Avalide tablets ℞ *antihypertensive; angiotensin II receptor antagonist; diuretic* [irbesartan; hydrochlorothiazide] 150•12.5, 300•12.5 mg

Avandia film-coated tablets ℞ *thiazolidinedione antidiabetic; increases cellular response to insulin without increasing insulin secretion* [rosiglitazone maleate] 2, 4, 8 mg

Avapro tablets ℞ *antihypertensive; angiotensin II receptor antagonist* [irbesartan] 75, 150, 300 mg

avasimbe USAN *acylCoA transferase (ACAT) inhibitor for hyperlipidemia and atherosclerosis*

Avaxim; Avaxim Pediatric (CAN) prefilled syringe for IM injection ℞ *immunization against hepatitis A virus (HAV)* [hepatitis A vaccine, inactivated] 0.5 mL

AVC vaginal cream, vaginal inserts (discontinued 2001) ℞ *broad-spectrum antibiotic* [sulfanilamide] 15%; 1.05 g

Aveeno lotion OTC *moisturizer; emollient* [colloidal oatmeal] 1%

Aveeno Anti-Itch cream, lotion OTC *topical poison ivy treatment* [calamine; pramoxine HCl; camphor] 3%•1%•0.3%

Aveeno Cleansing bar OTC *soap-free therapeutic skin cleanser* [colloidal oatmeal] 51%

Aveeno Cleansing for Acne-Prone Skin bar OTC *medicated cleanser for acne* [salicylic acid; colloidal oatmeal]

Aveeno Moisturizing cream OTC *moisturizer; emollient* [colloidal oatmeal] 1%

Aveeno Oilated Bath packets OTC *bath emollient* [colloidal oatmeal; mineral oil] 43%•?̲

Aveeno Regular Bath packets OTC *bath emollient* [colloidal oatmeal] 100%

Aveeno Shave gel OTC *moisturizer; emollient* [oatmeal flour]

Aveeno Shower & Bath oil OTC *bath emollient* [colloidal oatmeal] 5%

Avelox film-coated tablets ℞ *broad-spectrum fluoroquinolone antibiotic* [moxifloxacin HCl] 400 mg

Avena sativa *medicinal herb* [see: oats]

Aventyl HCl Pulvules (capsules), oral solution ℞ *tricyclic antidepressant* [nortriptyline HCl] 10, 25 mg; 10 mg/5 mL Ⓢ Ambenyl; Bentyl

avertin [see: tribromoethanol]

Aviane-28 tablets (in packs of 28) ℞ *monophasic oral contraceptive; emergency postcoital contraceptive* [levonorgestrel; ethinyl estradiol] 100•20 µg

avicatonin INN

Avicidin ℞ *investigational (Phase II) antineoplastic for prostate, colon, and lung cancers*

Avicine ℞ *investigational (Phase III) theraccine for pancreatic cancer; investigational (Phase II) for prostate and advanced colorectal cancers*

avilamycin USAN, INN, BAN *antibacterial*

avinar [see: uredepa]

Avita cream, gel ℞ *topical keratolytic for acne* [tretinoin] 0.025% Ⓢ Evista

Avitene Hemostat nonwoven web ℞ *topical hemostatic aid for surgery* [microfibrillar collagen hemostat] Ⓢ Ativan

avitriptan fumarate USAN *serotonin 5-HT_1 agonist for migraine*
avizafone INN, BAN
avobenzone USAN, INN *sunscreen*
avocado (*Persea americana; P. gratissima*) fruit and seed *medicinal herb for diarrhea, dysentery, inducing menstruation, lowering total cholesterol and improving overall lipid profile, promoting hair growth, and stimulating wound healing; also used as an aphrodisiac*
Avonex powder for IM injection ℞ *immunomodulator for relapsing remitting multiple sclerosis (orphan); investigational (orphan) for non-A, non-B hepatitis, Kaposi sarcoma, brain tumors, and various other cancers* [interferon beta-1a] 33 µg (6.6 million IU)/vial
avoparcin USAN, INN, BAN *glycopeptide antibiotic*
AVP (actinomycin D, vincristine, Platinol) *chemotherapy protocol*
avridine USAN, INN *antiviral*
Award *hydrophilic contact lens material* [hilafilcon A]
axamozide INN
axerophthol [see: vitamin A]
Axert tablets ℞ *selective serotonin agonist for migraine* [almotriptan malate] 6.25, 12.5 mg
axetil USAN, INN *combining name for radicals or groups*
Axid Pulvules (capsules) ℞ *histamine H_2 antagonist for treatment of gastric and duodenal ulcers* [nizatidine] 150, 300 mg ⑨ Biaxin
Axid AR ("acid reducer") tablets OTC *histamine H_2 antagonist for heartburn* [nizatidine] 75 mg
axitirome USAN *antihyperlipidemic*
Axocet capsules ℞ *analgesic; barbiturate sedative* [acetaminophen; butalbital] 650•50 mg
Axokine ℞ *investigational (Phase II) second-generation ciliary neurotrophic factor for obesity; investigational agent for the treatment of obesity associated with type 2 diabetes*
Axotal tablets (discontinued 1997) ℞ *analgesic; sedative* [aspirin; butalbital] 650•50 mg
Aygestin tablets ℞ *progestin for amenorrhea, abnormal uterine bleeding, or endometriosis* [norethindrone acetate] 5 mg
Ayr Saline nasal mist, nose drops, nasal gel OTC *nasal moisturizer* [sodium chloride (saline solution)] 0.65%
5-AZA (5-azacitidine) [see: azacitidine]
azabon USAN, INN *CNS stimulant*
azabuperone INN
azacitidine (5-AZA; 5-AZC) USAN, INN *antineoplastic for acute myelogenous leukemia*
azaclorzine INN *coronary vasodilator* [also: azaclorzine HCl]
azaclorzine HCl USAN *coronary vasodilator* [also: azaclorzine]
azaconazole USAN, INN *antifungal*
azacosterol INN *avian chemosterilant* [also: azacosterol HCl]
azacosterol HCl USAN *avian chemosterilant* [also: azacosterol]
AZA-CR [see: azacitidine]
Azactam powder for IV or IM injection ℞ *monobactam bactericidal antibiotic* [aztreonam] 0.5, 1, 2 g
azacyclonol INN, BAN [also: azacyclonol HCl]
azacyclonol HCl NF [also: azacyclonol]
5-azacytosine arabinoside (ara-AC) [see: fazarabine]
5-aza-2′-deoxycytidine *investigational (orphan) for acute leukemia*
Azadirachta indica *medicinal herb* [see: neem tree]
azaftozine INN
azalanstat dihydrochloride USAN *hypolipidemic*
azalomycin INN, BAN
azaloxan INN *antidepressant* [also: azaloxan fumarate]
azaloxan fumarate USAN *antidepressant* [also: azaloxan]
azamethiphos BAN
azamethonium bromide INN, BAN
azamulin INN
azanator INN *bronchodilator* [also: azanator maleate]

azanator maleate USAN *bronchodilator* [also: azanator]
azanidazole USAN, INN, BAN *antiprotozoal*
azaperone USAN, INN, BAN *antipsychotic*
azapetine BAN
azapetine phosphate [see: azapetine]
azaprocin INN
azapropazone INN, BAN, DCF *anti-inflammatory* [also: apazone]
azaquinzole INN
azaribine USAN, INN, BAN *antipsoriatic*
azarole USAN *immunoregulator*
azaserine USAN, INN *antifungal*
azasetron INN
azaspirium chloride INN
azaspirones *a class of anxiolytics*
azastene
azatadine INN, BAN *piperidine antihistamine* [also: azatadine maleate]
azatadine maleate USAN, USP *piperidine antihistamine for allergic rhinitis and chronic urticaria* [also: azatadine]
azatepa INN *antineoplastic* [also: azetepa]
azathioprine USAN, USP, INN, BAN, JAN *immunosuppressant*
azathioprine sodium USP *immunosuppressant* 100 mg injection
5-AZC (5-azacitidine) [see: azacitidine]
Azdone tablets ℞ *narcotic analgesic* [hydrocodone bitartrate; aspirin] 5•500 mg
azdU (azidouridine) [q.v.]
azelaic acid USAN, INN *topical antimicrobial and keratolytic for inflammatory acne vulgaris*
azelastine INN, BAN *phthalazinone antihistamine; mast cell stabilizer; antiallergic; antiasthmatic* [also: azelastine HCl]
azelastine HCl USAN, JAN *phthalazinone antihistamine; mast cell stabilizer; antiallergic; antiasthmatic* [also: azelastine]
Azelex cream ℞ *antimicrobial and keratolytic for inflammatory acne vulgaris* [azelaic acid] 20%
azelnidipine INN
azepexole INN, BAN
azephine [see: azapetine phosphate]
azepinamide [see: glypinamide]
azepindole USAN, INN *antidepressant*
azetepa USAN, BAN *antineoplastic* [also: azatepa]
azetirelin INN
azidamfenicol INN, BAN, DCF
azidoamphenicol [see: azidamfenicol]
azidocillin INN, BAN
azidothymidine (AZT) [now: zidovudine]
azidouridine (azdU) *investigational (Phase I) antiviral for HIV and AIDS*
azimexon INN
azimilide dihydrochloride USAN *investigational (NDA filed) antiarrhythmic and antifibrillatory*
azintamide INN
azinthiamide [see: azintamide]
azipramine INN *antidepressant* [also: azipramine HCl]
azipramine HCl USAN *antidepressant* [also: azipramine]
aziridinyl benzoquinone [see: diaziquone]
azithromycin USAN, USP, INN, BAN *macrolide antibiotic*
azlocillin USAN, INN, BAN *penicillin antibiotic*
azlocillin sodium USP *penicillin antibiotic*
Azmacort oral inhalation aerosol ℞ *corticosteroidal anti-inflammatory for chronic asthma* [triamcinolone acetonide] 100 µg/dose
Azo Test Strips reagent strips for home use *in vitro diagnostic aid for urinary tract infections*
azoconazole [now: azaconazole]
azodisal sodium (ADS) [now: olsalazine sodium]
"azoles" *a class of fungicides that include all with generic names ending in "azole," such clotrimazole and fluconazole*
azolimine USAN, INN *diuretic* ⑨ Azulfidine
Azopt eye drop suspension ℞ *carbonic anhydrase inhibitor for glaucoma* [brinzolamide] 1%
azosemide USAN, INN, JAN *diuretic*
Azo-Standard tablets OTC *urinary analgesic* [phenazopyridine HCl] 95 mg

Azostix reagent strips for professional use *in vitro diagnostic aid to estimate the amount of BUN in whole blood*

Azo-Sulfisoxazole tablets ℞ *urinary anti-infective; urinary analgesic* [sulfisoxazole; phenazopyridine HCl] 500•50 mg

azotomycin USAN, INN *antibiotic antineoplastic*

azovan blue BAN *blood volume test* [also: Evans blue]

azovan sodium [see: Evans blue]

AZT (azidothymidine) [now: zidovudine]

Aztec controlled release ℞ *investigational (Phase III) antiviral for early HIV and AIDS* [zidovudine]

AZT-P-ddI [see: zidovudine & didanosine]

aztreonam USAN, USP, INN, BAN, JAN *monobactam bactericidal antibiotic*

azulene sulfonate sodium JAN [also: sodium gualenate]

Azulfidine tablets ℞ *broad-spectrum bacteriostatic; anti-inflammatory for ulcerative colitis* [sulfasalazine] 500 mg ⑨ Silvadene

Azulfidine EN-tabs enteric-coated delayed-release tablets ℞ *broad-spectrum bacteriostatic; anti-inflammatory for ulcerative colitis, rheumatoid arthritis (RA), and juvenile rheumatoid arthritis (JRA)* [sulfasalazine] 500 mg

azumolene INN *skeletal muscle relaxant* [also: azumolene sodium]

azumolene sodium USAN *skeletal muscle relaxant* [also: azumolene]

azure A carbacrylic resin [see: azuresin]

azuresin NF, BAN

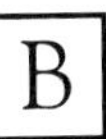

1,4-B (1,4-butanediol) *a precursor to gamma hydroxybutyrate (GHB); a formerly legal alternative to GHB, now also illegal (Schedule I)* [see: gamma hydroxybutyrate (GHB)]

B Complex + C timed-release tablets OTC *vitamin supplement* [multiple B vitamins; vitamin C] ≛•500 mg

B Complex with C and B-12 injection ℞ *parenteral vitamin supplement* [multiple vitamins]

B Complex-50 sustained-release tablets OTC *vitamin supplement* [multiple B vitamins; folic acid; biotin] ≛•400•50 µg

B Complex-150 sustained-release tablets OTC *vitamin supplement* [multiple B vitamins; folic acid; biotin] ≛•400•150 µg

B & O Supprettes No. 15A; B & O Supprettes No. 16A suppositories ℞ *narcotic analgesic* [belladonna extract; opium] 16.2•30 mg; 16.2•60 mg

B vitamins [see: vitamin B]

B_1 (vitamin B_1) [see: thiamine HCl]

B_2 (vitamin B_2) [see: riboflavin]

B_3 (vitamin B_3) [see: niacin; niacinamide]

B_5 (vitamin B_5) [see: calcium pantothenate]

B_6 (vitamin B_6) [see: pyridoxine HCl]

B_8 (vitamin B_8) [see: adenosine phosphate]

B_{12} (vitamin B_{12}) [see: cyanocobalamin]

B_{12a} (vitamin B_{12a}) [see: hydroxocobalamin]

B_{12b} (vitamin B_{12b}) [see: hydroxocobalamin]

B-50 tablets OTC *vitamin supplement* [multiple B vitamins; folic acid; biotin] ≛•100•50 µg

B-100 tablets, timed-release tablets OTC *vitamin supplement* [multiple B vitamins; folic acid; biotin] ≛•100•100 µg; ≛•400•50 µg

B_c (vitamin B_c) [see: folic acid]
B_t (vitamin B_t) [see: carnitine]
Babee Teething lotion OTC *topical oral anesthetic; antiseptic* [benzocaine; cetalkonium chloride] 2.5%•0.02%
baby brain I *chemotherapy protocol for pediatric brain tumors* [see: COPE]
Baby Vitamin drops OTC *vitamin supplement* [multiple vitamins] ≛
Baby Vitamin with Iron drops OTC *vitamin/iron supplement* [multiple vitamins; iron] ≛•10 mg/mL
Babylax [see: Fleet Babylax]
BAC (BCNU, ara-C, cyclophosphamide) *chemotherapy protocol*
BAC (benzalkonium chloride) [q.v.]
bacampicillin INN, BAN *aminopenicillin antibiotic* [also: bacampicillin HCl]
bacampicillin HCl USAN, USP, JAN *aminopenicillin antibiotic* [also: bacampicillin]
bachelor's buttons *medicinal herb* [see: cornflower; feverfew; tansy; buttercup]
Bacid capsules OTC *dietary supplement; fever blister treatment; not generally regarded as safe and effective as an antidiarrheal* [*Lactobacillus acidophilus*] 500 million cultures ⓢ Banacid
Baciguent ointment OTC *topical antibiotic* [bacitracin] 500 U/g
Baci-IM powder for IM injection ℞ *bactericidal antibiotic* [bacitracin] 50 000 U
bacillus Calmette-Guérin (BCG) vaccine [see: BCG vaccine]
bacitracin USP, INN, BAN, JAN *bactericidal antibiotic; investigational (orphan) for pseudomembranous enterocolitis* 500 U/g topical; 50 000 U/vial injection ⓢ Bacitrin; Bactrim
bacitracin zinc USP, BAN *bactericidal antibiotic*
bacitracin zinc & neomycin sulfate & polymyxin B sulfate *topical antibiotic* 400 U•5 mg•10 000 U per g ophthalmic
bacitracin zinc & polymyxin B sulfate *topical antibiotic* 500•10 000 U/g ophthalmic
bacitracins zinc complex [see: bacitracin zinc]
Backache Maximum Strength Relief film-coated caplets OTC *analgesic; antirheumatic* [magnesium salicylate] 467 mg
Back-Pack (trademarked packaging form) *unit-of-use package*
baclofen (L-baclofen) USAN, USP, INN, BAN, JAN *skeletal muscle relaxant for intractable spasticity due to spinal cord injury or disease (orphan); investigational (orphan) for trigeminal neuralgia* 10, 20 mg oral
bacmecillinam INN
Bacmin tablets ℞ *vitamin/mineral/iron supplement* [multiple vitamins & minerals; iron; folic acid; biotin] ≛•27•0.8•0.15 mg
BACOD (bleomycin, Adriamycin, CCNU, Oncovin, dexamethasone) *chemotherapy protocol*
BACON (bleomycin, Adriamycin, CCNU, Oncovin, nitrogen mustard) *chemotherapy protocol*
BACOP (bleomycin, Adriamycin, cyclophosphamide, Oncovin, prednisone) *chemotherapy protocol*
BACT (BCNU, ara-C, cyclophosphamide, thioguanine) *chemotherapy protocol*
bactericidal and permeability-increasing (BPI) protein, recombinant *investigational (Phase III, orphan) treatment for gram-negative sepsis, hemorrhagic shock, and meningococcemia*
bactericidal/permeability-increasing protein [see: rBPI-21]
bacteriostatic sodium chloride [see: sodium chloride]
Bacteriostatic Sodium Chloride Injection ℞ *IV diluent* [sodium chloride (normal saline solution)] 0.9% (normal)
Bacti-Cleanse liquid OTC *soap-free therapeutic skin cleanser* [benzalkonium chloride]
Bactigen B Streptococcus-CS slide test for professional use *in vitro diag-*

nostic aid for Group B streptococcal antigens in vaginal and cervical swabs

Bactigen Meningitis Panel slide test for professional use *in vitro diagnostic aid for H influenzae, N meningitidis, and S pneumoniae in various fluids* [latex agglutination test]

Bactigen N meningitidis slide test for professional use *in vitro diagnostic aid for Neisseria meningitidis* [latex agglutination test]

Bactigen Salmonella-Shigella slide test for professional use *in vitro diagnostic aid for salmonella and shigella* [latex agglutination test]

Bactine Antiseptic Anesthetic liquid, spray OTC *topical local anesthetic; antiseptic* [lidocaine HCl; benzalkonium chloride] 2.5%•0.13%

Bactine First Aid Antibiotic Plus Anesthetic ointment OTC *topical antibiotic; topical local anesthetic* [polymyxin B sulfate; neomycin sulfate; bacitracin; diperodon HCl] 5000 U•3.5 mg•400 U•10 mg per g

Bactine Hydrocortisone; Maximum Strength Bactine cream OTC *topical corticosteroidal anti-inflammatory* [hydrocortisone] 0.5%; 1%

Bactocill capsules (discontinued 1998) ℞ *penicillinase-resistant penicillin antibiotic* [oxacillin sodium] 250, 500 mg ⑨ Pathocil

Bactocill powder for IV or IM injection ℞ *penicillinase-resistant penicillin antibiotic* [oxacillin sodium] 0.5, 1, 2, 4, 10 g ⑨ Pathocil

BactoShield aerosol foam, solution OTC *broad-spectrum antimicrobial; germicidal* [chlorhexidine gluconate; alcohol 4%] 4%

BactoShield 2 solution OTC *broad-spectrum antimicrobial; germicidal* [chlorhexidine gluconate; alcohol 4%] 2%

Bactrim; Bactrim DS tablets ℞ *anti-infective; antibacterial* [trimethoprim; sulfamethoxazole] 80•400 mg; 160•800 mg ⑨ bacitracin

Bactrim IV infusion ℞ *anti-infective; antibacterial* [trimethoprim; sulfamethoxazole] 80•400 mg/5 mL

Bactrim Pediatric oral suspension ℞ *anti-infective; antibacterial* [trimethoprim; sulfamethoxazole] 40•200 mg/5 mL

Bactroban cream ℞ in the U.S.; OTC in Canada *topical antibiotic* [mupirocin calcium] 2%

Bactroban ointment ℞ *topical antibiotic for impetigo* [mupirocin] 2%

Bactroban Nasal ointment in single-use tubes ℞ *antibiotic for iatrogenic methicillin-resistant Staphylococcus aureus (MRSA) infections* [mupirocin calcium] 2%

Bagshawe protocol, modified *chemotherapy protocol* [see: CHAMOCA]

bakeprofen INN

baker's yeast *natural source of protein and B-complex vitamins*

BAL (British antilewisite) [now: dimercaprol]

BAL in Oil deep IM injection ℞ *antidote for arsenic, gold, and mercury poisoning; lead poisoning adjunct* [dimercaprol in peanut oil] 100 mg/mL ⑨ Balneol

balafilcon A USAN *hydrophilic contact lens material*

balipramine BAN [also: depramine]

balm *medicinal herb* [see: lemon balm]

balm, eye; eye root *medicinal herb* [see: goldenseal]

balm, mountain *medicinal herb* [see: yerba santa]

balm, squaw; squaw mint *medicinal herb* [see: pennyroyal]

balm of Gilead *(Populus balsamifera; P. candicans)* buds *medicinal herb used as an antiscorbutic, balsamic, diuretic, stimulant, and vulnerary*

Balmex ointment OTC *astringent; moisturizer; emollient* [zinc oxide] 11.3%

Balmex Baby powder OTC *topical diaper rash treatment* [zinc oxide; peruvian balsam; corn starch]

Balmex Emollient lotion OTC *moisturizer; emollient*

balmony *medicinal herb* [see: turtlebloom]

Balneol Perianal Cleansing lotion OTC *emollient/protectant* [mineral oil; lanolin] ⑨ BAL in Oil

Balnetar bath oil OTC *antipsoriatic; antiseborrheic; antipruritic; emollient* [coal tar] 2.5%

balsalazide INN, BAN *gastrointestinal anti-inflammatory for ulcerative colitis* [also: balsalazide disodium]

balsalazide disodium USAN *gastrointestinal anti-inflammatory for ulcerative colitis* [also: balsalazide]

balsalazide sodium [see: balsalazide disodium]

balsalazine [see: balsalazide disodium; balsalazide]

balsam apple; balsam pear *medicinal herb* [see: bitter melon]

balsam Peru [see: peruvian balsam; balsam tree]

balsam poplar *medicinal herb* [see: balm of Gilead]

balsam tree *medicinal herb* [see: Peruvian balsam]

balsamics; balsams *a class of agents that soothe or heal; balms; also, certain resinous substances of vegetable origin*

Balsamodendron myrrha *medicinal herb* [see: myrrh]

balsan [see: peruvian balsam]

bamaluzole INN

bambermycin INN, BAN *antibacterial antibiotic* [also: bambermycins]

bambermycins USAN *antibacterial antibiotic* [also: bambermycin]

bambuterol INN, BAN

bamethan INN, BAN *vasodilator* [also: bamethan sulfate]

bamethan sulfate USAN, JAN *vasodilator* [also: bamethan]

bamifylline INN, BAN *bronchodilator* [also: bamifylline HCl]

bamifylline HCl USAN *bronchodilator* [also: bamifylline]

bamipine INN, BAN, DCF

bamnidazole USAN, INN *antiprotozoal (Trichomonas)*

BAMON (bleomycin, Adriamycin, methotrexate, Oncovin, nitrogen mustard) *chemotherapy protocol*

Banadyne-3 solution OTC *topical oral anesthetic; analgesic; counterirritant; antiseptic* [lidocaine; menthol; alcohol 45%] 4%•1%

Banalg lotion OTC *topical analgesic; counterirritant* [methyl salicylate; camphor; menthol] 4.9%•2%•1%

Banalg Hospital Strength lotion OTC *topical analgesic; counterirritant* [methyl salicylate; menthol] 14%•3%

Bancap HC capsules ℞ *narcotic analgesic* [hydrocodone bitartrate; acetaminophen] 5•500 mg

bandage, adhesive USP *surgical aid*

bandage, gauze USP *surgical aid*

Banflex IV or IM injection ℞ *skeletal muscle relaxant* [orphenadrine citrate] 30 mg/mL

banocide [see: diethylcarbamazine citrate]

Banophen caplets, capsules OTC *antihistamine* [diphenhydramine HCl] 25 mg

Banophen elixir OTC *antihistamine* [diphenhydramine HCl] 12.5 mg/5 mL

Banophen Allergy oral liquid OTC *antihistamine* [diphenhydramine HCl] 12.5 mg/5 mL

Banophen Decongestant capsules OTC *decongestant; antihistamine* [pseudoephedrine HCl; diphenhydramine HCl] 60•25 mg ⑨ Barophen

Banthīne tablets (discontinued 2001) ℞ *anticholinergic; peptic ulcer treatment adjunct* [methantheline bromide] 50 mg ⑨ Brethine; Vantin

Bantron tablets (discontinued 1999) OTC *smoking deterrent* [lobeline sulfate alkaloids; tribasic calcium phosphate; magnesium carbonate] 2•130•130 mg ⑨ Vantin

Baptisia tinctoria *medicinal herb* [see: wild indigo]

baquiloprim INN, BAN

Barbados aloe *medicinal herb* [see: aloe]

barbenyl [see: phenobarbital]

barberry *(Berberis vulgaris)* bark *medicinal herb for bacteria-associated* *diarrhea, blood cleansing, cough, fever, indigestion, jaundice, liver disorders, sciatica, and sore throat*

barberry, California *medicinal herb* [see: Oregon grape]

barbexaclone INN

Barbidonna; Barbidonna No. 2 tablets ℞ *GI antispasmodic; anticholinergic; sedative* [atropine sulfate; scopolamine hydrobromide; hyoscyamine hydrobromide; phenobarbital] 0.025•0.0074•0.1286•16 mg; 0.025•0.0074•0.1286•32 mg

barbiphenyl [see: phenobarbital]

barbital NF, INN, JAN [also: barbitone]

barbital, soluble [now: barbital sodium]

barbital sodium NF, INN [also: barbitone sodium]

barbitone BAN [also: barbital]

barbitone sodium BAN [also: barbital sodium]

barbiturates *a class of sedatives and hypnotics that produce a wide range of mood alteration; also widely abused as addictive street drugs*

Barc liquid OTC *pediculicide for lice* [pyrethrins; piperonyl butoxide; petroleum distillate] 0.18%•2.2%•5.52%

bardana *medicinal herb* [see: burdock]

Baricon powder for oral suspension ℞ *radiopaque contrast medium for gastrointestinal imaging* [barium sulfate] 98%

Baridium tablets ℞ *urinary analgesic* [phenazopyridine HCl] 100 mg

barium *element (Ba)*

barium hydroxide lime USP *carbon dioxide absorbent*

barium sulfate USP, JAN *oral/rectal radiopaque contrast medium for gastrointestinal imaging*

barley *(Hordeum vulgare)* juice powder *medicinal herb for anemia, arthritis, blood cleansing, boils, bronchitis, cancer, metal poisoning, poor circulation, and reducing total and LDL cholesterol and increasing HDL cholesterol*

barley malt soup extract *bulk laxative*

barmastine USAN, INN *antihistamine*

BarnesHind Saline for Sensitive Eyes solution OTC *rinsing/storage solution for soft contact lenses* [sodium chloride (preserved saline solution)]

barnidipine INN

Barobag rectal suspension ℞ *radiopaque contrast medium for gastrointestinal imaging* [barium sulfate] 97%

Baro-cat oral suspension ℞ *radiopaque contrast medium for gastrointestinal imaging* [barium sulfate] 1.5%

Baroflave powder for oral suspension (discontinued 1999) ℞ *radiopaque contrast medium for gastrointestinal imaging* [barium sulfate]

Baros effervescent granules ℞ *adjunct to gastrointestinal imaging* [sodium bicarbonate; tartaric acid; simethicone] 460•420•≟ mg/g

Barosma betulina; B. cenulata; B. serratifolia *medicinal herb* [see: buchu]

barosmin [see: diosmin]

Barosperse powder for oral suspension ℞ *radiopaque contrast medium for gastrointestinal imaging* [barium sulfate] 95%

Barosperse, Liquid oral/rectal suspension ℞ *radiopaque contrast medium for gastrointestinal imaging* [barium sulfate] 60%

barucainide INN

BAS (benzyl analogue of serotonin) [see: benanserin HCl]

Basaljel tablets, capsules, suspension OTC *antacid* [aluminum carbonate gel, basic] 500 mg; 500 mg; 400 mg/5 mL

Basen ℞ *investigational α-glucosidase inhibitor for diabetes* [voglibose]

basic aluminum acetate [see: aluminum subacetate]

basic aluminum aminoacetate [see: dihydroxyaluminum aminoacetate]

basic aluminum carbonate [see: aluminum carbonate, basic]

basic aluminum chloride [see: aluminum sesquichlorohydrate]

basic aluminum glycinate [see: dihydroxyaluminum aminoacetate]

basic bismuth carbonate [see: bismuth subcarbonate]

basic bismuth gallate [see: bismuth subgallate]

basic bismuth nitrate [see: bismuth subnitrate]

basic bismuth potassium bismuthotartrate [see: bismuth potassium tartrate]

basic bismuth salicylate [see: bismuth subsalicylate]

basic fibroblast growth factor (bFGF) [see: ersofermin]

basic fuchsin [see: fuchsin, basic]

basic zinc acetate [see: zinc acetate, basic]

basifungin USAN, INN *antifungal*

basil *(Ocimum basilicum)* leaves *medicinal herb for colds, headache, indigestion, insect and snake bites, and whooping cough*

basiliximab USAN *immunosuppressant; IL-2 receptor antagonist for the prevention of acute rejection of renal transplants (orphan)*

basswood; bast tree *medicinal herb* [see: linden tree]

bastard hemp *medicinal herb* [see: hemp nettle]

bastard saffron *medicinal herb* [see: safflower]

batanopride INN *antiemetic* [also: batanopride HCl]

batanopride HCl USAN *antiemetic* [also: batanopride]

batebulast INN

batelapine INN *antipsychotic* [also: batelapine HCl]

batelapine maleate USAN *antipsychotic* [also: batelapine]

batilol INN

batimastat USAN, INN *investigational (Phase III) antineoplastic; matrix metalloproteinase (MMP) inhibitor*

batoprazine INN

batroxobin INN, JAN

batyl alcohol [see: batilol]

batylol [see: batilol]

BAVIP (bleomycin, Adriamycin, vinblastine, imidazole carboxamide, prednisone) *chemotherapy protocol*

baxitozine INN

bay; bay laurel; bay tree; Indian bay; sweet bay *medicinal herb* [see: laurel]

bay, holly; red bay; white bay *medicinal herb* [see: magnolia]

bayberry *(Myrica cerifera)* bark, berries, root bark *medicinal herb for cholera, diarrhea, dysentery, glands, goiter, indigestion, jaundice, excessive menstruation, scrofuloderma, and uterine hemorrhage; not generally regarded as safe because of its high tannin content*

Baycol tablets (discontinued 2001 due to safety concerns) ℞ *HMG-CoA reductase inhibitor for hyperlipidemia and hypertriglyceridemia* [cerivastatin sodium] 0.2, 0.3, 0.4, 0.8 mg

Bayer Arthritis Regimen delayed-release enteric-coated tablets OTC *analgesic; antipyretic; anti-inflammatory; antirheumatic* [aspirin] 500 mg

Bayer Aspirin, Genuine; Maximum Bayer Aspirin film-coated tablets, film-coated caplets OTC *analgesic; antipyretic; anti-inflammatory; antirheumatic* [aspirin] 325 mg; 500 mg

Bayer Aspirin Regimen delayed-release enteric-coated tablets and caplets OTC *analgesic; antipyretic; anti-inflammatory; antirheumatic* [aspirin] 81, 325 mg

Bayer Buffered Aspirin tablets OTC *analgesic; antipyretic; anti-inflammatory; antirheumatic* [aspirin, buffered] 325 mg

Bayer Children's Aspirin chewable tablets OTC *analgesic; antipyretic; anti-inflammatory; antirheumatic* [aspirin] 81 mg

Bayer Plus caplets OTC *analgesic; antipyretic; anti-inflammatory; antirheumatic; antacid* [aspirin; calcium carbonate] 500•250 mg

Bayer PM Aspirin Plus Sleep Aid caplet OTC *analgesic; antipyretic; anti-inflammatory; antirheumatic; antihistaminic sleep aid* [aspirin; diphenhydramine HCl] 500•25 mg

Bayer Select Allergy Sinus, Aspirin-Free caplets OTC *decongestant; antihistamine; analgesic; antipyretic*

[pseudoephedrine HCl; chlorpheniramine maleate; acetaminophen] 30•2•500 mg

Bayer Select Backache caplets OTC *analgesic; antipyretic; anti-inflammatory; antirheumatic* [magnesium salicylate] 580 mg

Bayer Select Chest Cold caplets OTC *antitussive; analgesic; antipyretic* [dextromethorphan hydrobromide; acetaminophen] 15•500 mg

Bayer Select Flu Relief caplets OTC *antitussive; decongestant; antihistamine; analgesic; antipyretic* [dextromethorphan hydrobromide; pseudoephedrine HCl; chlorpheniramine maleate; acetaminophen] 15•30•2•500 mg

Bayer Select Head & Chest Cold, Aspirin-Free caplets OTC *antitussive; decongestant; expectorant; analgesic; antipyretic* [dextromethorphan hydrobromide; pseudoephedrine HCl; guaifenesin; acetaminophen] 10•30•100•325 mg

Bayer Select Head Cold; Bayer Select Sinus Pain Relief caplets OTC *decongestant; analgesic; antipyretic* [pseudoephedrine HCl; acetaminophen] 30•500 mg

Bayer Select Headache caplets (discontinued 2000) OTC *analgesic; antipyretic* [acetaminophen; caffeine] 500•65 mg

Bayer Select Menstrual caplets (discontinued 2000) OTC *analgesic; antipyretic; diuretic* [acetaminophen; pamabrom] 500•25 mg

Bayer Select Night Time Cold caplets OTC *antitussive; decongestant; antihistamine; analgesic; antipyretic* [dextromethorphan hydrobromide; pseudoephedrine HCl; triprolidine HCl; acetaminophen] 15•30•1.25•500 mg

Bayer Select Night Time Pain Relief caplets (name changed to Bayer PM Aspirin Plus Sleep Aid in 2000)

Bayer Select Pain Relief Formula caplets (discontinued 2000) OTC *analgesic; antiarthritic; antipyretic; nonsteroidal anti-inflammatory drug (NSAID)* [ibuprofen] 200 mg

Bayer Timed Release, 8-Hour caplets OTC *analgesic; antipyretic; anti-inflammatory; antirheumatic* [aspirin] 650 mg

BayGam IM injection ℞ *immunizing agent for hepatitis A, measles, varicella, and rubella; treatment for immunoglobulin G (IgG) deficiency and acquired agammaglobulinemia* [immune globulin, solvent/detergent treated] 2, 10 mL

BayHep B IM injection ℞ *hepatitis B immunizing agent* [hepatitis B immune globulin, solvent/detergent treated] 0.5, 1, 5 mL

Baypress ℞ *investigational (NDA filed) antihypertensive; calcium channel blocker* [nitrendipine]

BayRab IM injection ℞ *passive immunizing agent for rabies prophylaxis and treatment* [rabies immune globulin, solvent/detergent treated] 150 IU/mL

BayRho-D Full Dose; BayRho-D Mini-Dose IM injection ℞ *obstetric Rh factor immunity suppressant* [Rh_0(D) immune globulin, solvent/detergent treated] 300 µg; 50 µg

BayTet IM injection ℞ *passive immunizing agent for post-exposure tetanus prophylaxis in patients with incomplete or uncertain pre-exposure immunization with tetanus toxoids* [tetanus immune globulin, solvent/detergent treated] 250 U

bazinaprine INN

BB-2893 *investigational disease-modifying oral anti-inflammatory (discontinued 1997)*

BBVP-M (BCNU, bleomycin, VePesid, prednisone, methotrexate) *chemotherapy protocol*

BC powder OTC *analgesic; antipyretic; anti-inflammatory* [aspirin; salicylamide; caffeine] 650•195•33.3 mg/packet

BC tablets (discontinued 2000) OTC *analgesic; antipyretic; anti-inflammatory* [aspirin; salicylamide; caffeine] 325•95•16 mg

B_c (vitamin B_c) [see: folic acid]
BC Arthritis Strength powder OTC *analgesic; antipyretic; anti-inflammatory* [aspirin; salicylamide; caffeine] 742•222•38 mg
BC Cold-Sinus Powder packets OTC *decongestant; analgesic; antipyretic* [phenylpropanolamine HCl; aspirin] 25•650 mg
BC Cold-Sinus-Allergy Powder packets OTC *decongestant; antihistamine; analgesic; antipyretic* [phenylpropanolamine HCl; chlorpheniramine maleate; aspirin] 25•4•650 mg
B-C with Folic Acid tablets ℞ *vitamin supplement* [multiple B vitamins; vitamin C; folic acid] ≛•500•0.5 mg
B-C with Folic Acid Plus tablets ℞ *vitamin/mineral/iron supplement* [multiple vitamins & minerals; ferrous fumarate; folic acid; biotin] ≛•27•0.8•0.15 mg
BCAA (branched-chain amino acids) [see: isoleucine; leucine; valine]
BCAP (BCNU, cyclophosphamide, Adriamycin, prednisone) *chemotherapy protocol*
BCAVe; B-CAVe (bleomycin, CCNU, Adriamycin, Velban) *chemotherapy protocol for Hodgkin lymphoma*
B-C-Bid caplets OTC *vitamin supplement* [multiple B vitamins; vitamin C] ≛•300 mg
BCD (bleomycin, cyclophosphamide, dactinomycin) *chemotherapy protocol*
BCG vaccine (bacillus Calmette-Guérin) USP *active bacterin for tuberculosis prevention; antineoplastic for urinary bladder cancer*
BCH 10652 *investigational (Phase II) reverse transcriptase inhibitor for HIV infection*
B-CHOP (bleomycin, Cytoxin, hydroxydaunomycin, Oncovin, prednisone) *chemotherapy protocol*
BCMF (bleomycin, cyclophosphamide, methotrexate, fluorouracil) *chemotherapy protocol*
BCNU (bis-chloroethyl-nitrosourea) [see: carmustine]
B-Complex elixir OTC *vitamin supplement* [multiple B vitamins] ≛
B-Complex and B-12 tablets OTC *vitamin supplement* [multiple B vitamins; protease] ≛•10 mg
B-Complex with B-12 tablets OTC *vitamin supplement* [multiple B vitamins] ≛
B-Complex/Vitamin C caplets OTC *vitamin supplement* [multiple B vitamins; vitamin C] ≛•300 mg
BCOP (BCNU, cyclophosphamide, Oncovin, prednisone) *chemotherapy protocol*
BCP (BCNU, cyclophosphamide, prednisone) *chemotherapy protocol*
BCVP (BCNU, cyclophosphamide, vincristine, prednisone) *chemotherapy protocol*
BCVPP (BCNU, cyclophosphamide, vinblastine, procarbazine, prednisone) *chemotherapy protocol for Hodgkin lymphoma*
BCX-1470 *investigational (Phase I) agent for use in patients receiving heparin during cardiopulmonary bypass surgery*
B-D glucose chewable tablets OTC *glucose elevating agent* [glucose] 5 g
BDNF (brain-derived neurotrophic factor) [q.v.]
BDO (1,4-butanediol) *a precursor to gamma hydroxybutyrate (GHB); a formerly legal alternative to GHB, now also illegal (Schedule I)* [see: gamma hydroxybutyrate (GHB)]
B-DOPA (bleomycin, DTIC, Oncovin, prednisone, Adriamycin) *chemotherapy protocol*
BDP (beclomethasone dipropionate) [q.v.]
BEAC (BCNU, etoposide, ara-C, cyclophosphamide) *chemotherapy protocol*
BEACOPP (bleomycin, etoposide, Adriamycin, cyclophosphamide, Oncovin, procarbazine, prednisone, [filgrastim]) *chemotherapy protocol for Hodgkin lymphoma*

BEAM (BCNU, etoposide, ara-C, melphalan) *chemotherapy protocol*

bean herb *medicinal herb* [see: summer savory]

bean trefoil *medicinal herb* [see: buckbean]

Beano liquid, tablets OTC *digestive aid* [alpha-D-galactosidase enzyme]

bearberry *medicinal herb* [see: uva ursi]

beard, old man's *medicinal herb* [see: fringe tree; woodbine]

Bear-E-Bag Pediatric rectal suspension ℞ *radiopaque contrast medium for gastrointestinal imaging* [barium sulfate] 95%

Bear-E-Yum CT oral suspension ℞ *radiopaque contrast medium for gastrointestinal imaging* [barium sulfate] 1.5%

Bear-E-Yum GI oral/rectal suspension ℞ *radiopaque contrast medium for gastrointestinal imaging* [barium sulfate] 60%

bear's grape *medicinal herb* [see: uva ursi]

bear's weed *medicinal herb* [see: yerba santa]

bearsfoot *medicinal herb* [see: hellebore]

Beaumont root *medicinal herb* [see: Culver root]

beaver tree *medicinal herb* [see: magnolia]

Bebulin VH powder for injection ℞ *antihemophilic for hemophilia B (orphan)* [factor IX complex, vapor heated]

becanthone HCl USAN *antischistosomal* [also: becantone]

becantone INN *antischistosomal* [also: becanthone HCl]

becantone HCl [see: becanthone HCl]

becaplermin USAN *recombinant platelet-derived growth factor B for chronic diabetic foot ulcers*

Because vaginal foam OTC *spermicidal contraceptive* [nonoxynol 9] 8%

beciparcil INN

beclamide INN, BAN, DCF

becliconazole INN

beclobrate INN, BAN

Becloforte Inhaler (CAN) oral inhalation aerosol (discontinued 2001) ℞ *corticosteroidal anti-inflammatory for chronic asthma* [beclomethasone dipropionate] 250 µg/dose

beclometasone INN *corticosteroidal inhalant for asthma; intranasal steroid* [also: beclomethasone dipropionate; beclomethasone; beclometasone dipropionate]

beclometasone dipropionate JAN *corticosteroidal inhalant for asthma; intranasal steroid* [also: beclomethasone dipropionate; beclomethasone; beclometasone]

beclomethasone BAN *corticosteroidal anti-inflammatory for chronic asthma* [also: beclomethasone dipropionate; beclometasone; beclometasone dipropionate]

beclomethasone dipropionate (BDP) USAN, USP *corticosteroidal anti-inflammatory for chronic asthma and rhinitis; investigational (orphan) oral treatment for intestinal graft vs. host disease* [also: beclometasone; beclomethasone; beclometasone dipropionate]

beclotiamine INN

Beclovent oral inhalation aerosol (discontinued 2001) ℞ *corticosteroidal anti-inflammatory for chronic asthma* [beclomethasone dipropionate] 42 µg/dose

Beclovent Inhaler (CAN) oral inhalation aerosol (discontinued 2001) ℞ *corticosteroidal anti-inflammatory for chronic asthma* [beclomethasone dipropionate] 50 µg/dose

Beconase nasal inhalation aerosol ℞ *corticosteroidal anti-inflammatory for seasonal or perennial rhinitis* [beclomethasone dipropionate] 42 µg/dose

Beconase AQ nasal spray ℞ *corticosteroidal anti-inflammatory for seasonal or perennial rhinitis* [beclomethasone dipropionate] 0.042%

bectumomab USAN *monoclonal antibody; investigational (Phase III, orphan) diagnostic aid for non-Hodgkin lymphoma and AIDS-related lymphoma* [also: technetium Tc 99m bectumomab]

Bedoz (CAN) injection ℞ *hematopoietic; vitamin B_{12}* [cyanocobalamin] 100 µg/mL
bedstraw *(Galium aparine; G. verum)* plant *medicinal herb used as an antispasmodic, aperient, diaphoretic, diuretic, and vulnerary*
bee balm *medicinal herb* [see: lemon balm]
bee pollen *natural remedy for anemia, bodily weakness, cerebral hemorrhage, colitis, constipation, enteritis, and weight loss; also used as an anti-aging agent and prenatal nutritional supplement; not generally regarded as safe and effective because of widespread allergic reactions*
bee venom (derived from *Apis mellifera*) *natural remedy for arthritis and multiple sclerosis, and for hyposensitization of persons highly sensitive to bee stings*
beechwood creosote [see: creosote carbonate]
beef tallow JAN
Beelith tablets OTC *dietary supplement* [vitamin B_6; magnesium oxide] 20•362 mg
Beepen-VK tablets, powder for oral solution ℞ *natural penicillin antibiotic* [penicillin V potassium] 250, 500 mg; 125, 250 mg/5 mL
bee's nest plant *medicinal herb* [see: carrot]
beeswax, white JAN [also: wax, white]
beeswax, yellow JAN [also: wax, yellow]
Bee-Zee tablets OTC *vitamin/zinc supplement* [multiple vitamins; zinc] ≛•22.5 mg
befiperide INN
befloxatone INN
befunolol INN [also: befunolol HCl]
befunolol HCl JAN [also: befunolol]
befuraline INN
behenyl alcohol [see: docosanol]
behepan [see: cyanocobalamin]
bekanamycin INN *antibiotic* [also: bekanamycin sulfate]
bekanamycin sulfate JAN *antibiotic* [also: bekanamycin]
belarizine INN
belfosdil USAN, INN *antihypertensive; calcium channel blocker*
Belganyl (available only from the Centers for Disease Control) ℞ *antiparasitic for African trypanosomiasis and onchocerciasis* [suramin sodium]
Belix elixir (discontinued 1997) OTC *antihistamine* [diphenhydramine HCl] 12.5 mg/5 mL
Bellacane elixir ℞ *GI antispasmodic; anticholinergic; sedative* [atropine sulfate; scopolamine hydrobromide; hyoscyamine sulfate; phenobarbital] 0.0194•0.0065•0.1037•16.2 mg/5 mL
Bellacane tablets ℞ *GI antispasmodic; anticholinergic; sedative* [hyoscyamine sulfate; phenobarbital] 0.125•15 mg
Bellacane SR sustained-release tablets ℞ *GI anticholinergic; sedative; analgesic* [belladonna alkaloids; phenobarbital; ergotamine tartrate] 0.2•40•0.6 mg
belladonna *(Atropa belladonna)* leaves, tops, and berries *medicinal herb used as an antispasmodic, calmative, diaphoretic, diuretic, and narcotic*
belladonna extract USP *GI/GU anticholinergic/antispasmodic; antiparkinsonian* 27–33 mg/100 mL oral
Bellafoline tablets (discontinued 1998) ℞ *GI anticholinergic; antispasmodic; antiparkinsonian agent* [belladonna extract] 0.25 mg
Bell/ans tablets OTC *antacid* [sodium bicarbonate] 520 mg
Bellatal tablets ℞ *long-acting barbiturate sedative, hypnotic, and anticonvulsant* [phenobarbital] 16.2 mg
Bellergal-S tablets ℞ *GI anticholinergic; sedative; analgesic* [belladonna extract; phenobarbital; ergotamine tartrate] 0.2•40•0.6 mg
Bellis perennis *medicinal herb* [see: wild daisy]
bells, May *medicinal herb* [see: lily of the valley]
beloxamide USAN, INN *antihyperlipoproteinemic*

beloxepin USAN *norepinephrine uptake inhibitor for depression*

Bel-Phen-Ergot SR sustained-release tablets ℞ *GI anticholinergic; sedative; analgesic* [belladonna alkaloids; phenobarbital; ergotamine tartrate] 0.2•40•0.6 mg

bemarinone INN *cardiotonic; positive inotropic; vasodilator* [also: bemarinone HCl]

bemarinone HCl USAN *cardiotonic; positive inotropic; vasodilator* [also: bemarinone]

bemegride USP, INN, BAN, JAN

bemesetron USAN, INN *antiemetic*

bemetizide INN, BAN

Beminal 500 tablets OTC *vitamin supplement* [multiple B vitamins; vitamin C] ≛•500 mg ⊡ Benemid

bemitradine USAN, INN *antihypertensive; diuretic*

bemoradan USAN, INN *cardiotonic*

BEMP (bleomycin, Eldisine, mitomycin, Platinol) *chemotherapy protocol*

benactyzine INN, BAN

benactyzine HCl *mild antidepressant; anticholinergic*

Benadryl injection ℞ *antihistamine; motion sickness preventative; sleep aid; antiparkinsonian* [diphenhydramine HCl] 50 mg/mL ⊡ Bentyl; Benylin; Caladryl

Benadryl Kapseals (capsules), tablets (name changed to Benadryl Allergy in 1997)

Benadryl; Benadryl 2% cream, spray OTC *topical antihistamine* [diphenhydramine HCl] 1%; 2% ⊡ Bentyl; Benylin; Caladryl

Benadryl 25 capsules (name changed to Benadryl Allergy Kapseals in 1997)

Benadryl 25 tablets (name changed to Benadryl Allergy Ultratabs in 1997)

Benadryl Allergy Kapseals (sealed capsules), Ultratabs (tablets), chewable tablets OTC *antihistamine* [diphenhydramine HCl] 25 mg; 25 mg; 12.5 mg ⊡ Bentyl; Benylin; Caladryl

Benadryl Allergy liquid ℞ *antihistamine* [diphenhydramine HCl] 6.25 mg/5 mL ⊡ Bentyl; Benylin; Caladryl

Benadryl Allergy Decongestant liquid OTC *pediatric decongestant and antihistamine* [pseudoephedrine HCl; diphenhydramine HCl] 30•12.5 mg/5 mL ⊡ Bentyl; Benylin; Caladryl

Benadryl Allergy/Sinus Headache caplets OTC *decongestant; antihistamine; analgesic* [pseudoephedrine HCl; diphenhydramine HCl; acetaminophen] 30•12.5•500 mg ⊡ Bentyl; Benylin; Caladryl

Benadryl Decongestant Allergy film-coated tablets OTC *decongestant; antihistamine* [pseudoephedrine HCl; diphenhydramine HCl] 60•25 mg ⊡ Bentyl; Benylin; Caladryl

Benadryl Dye-Free Allergy Liqui Gels (soft capsules), liquid OTC *antihistamine* [diphenhydramine HCl] 25 mg; 6.25 mg/5 mL ⊡ Bentyl; Benylin; Caladryl

Benadryl Itch Relief spray, cream, stick OTC *topical antihistamine; astringent* [diphenhydramine HCl; zinc acetate] 2%•0.1% ⊡ Bentyl; Benylin; Caladryl

Benadryl Itch Relief, Children's spray, cream OTC *topical antihistamine; astringent* [diphenhydramine HCl; zinc acetate] 1%•0.1% ⊡ Bentyl; Benylin; Caladryl

Benadryl Itch Stopping Gel; Benadryl Itch Stopping Gel Children's Formula OTC *topical antihistamine; astringent* [diphenhydramine HCl; zinc acetate] 2%•1%; 1%•1% ⊡ Bentyl; Benylin; Caladryl

Benadryl Itch Stopping Spray OTC *topical antihistamine; astringent* [diphenhydramine HCl; zinc acetate] 1%•0.1%, 2%•0.1%

Benadryl Junior (CAN) chewable tablets OTC *antihistamine* [diphenhydramine HCl] 12.5 mg

benafentrine INN

Ben-Allergin-50 injection (discontinued 1997) ℞ *antihistamine; motion*

sickness preventative; sleep aid; antiparkinsonian [diphenhydramine HCl] 50 mg/mL
benanserin HCl
benapen [see: benethamine penicillin]
benaprizine INN *anticholinergic* [also: benapryzine HCl; benapryzine]
benapryzine BAN *anticholinergic* [also: benapryzine HCl; benaprizine]
benapryzine HCl USAN *anticholinergic* [also: benaprizine; benapryzine]
benaxibine INN
benazepril INN, BAN *antihypertensive; angiotensin-converting enzyme (ACE) inhibitor* [also: benazepril HCl]
benazepril HCl USAN *antihypertensive; angiotensin-converting enzyme (ACE) inhibitor* [also: benazepril]
benazeprilat USAN, INN *angiotensin-converting enzyme inhibitor*
bencianol INN
bencisteine INN, DCF
benclonidine INN
bencyclane INN [also: bencyclane fumarate]
bencyclane fumarate JAN [also: bencyclane]
bendacalol mesylate USAN *antihypertensive*
bendamustine INN
bendazac USAN, INN, BAN, JAN *anti-inflammatory*
bendazol INN, DCF
benderizine INN
bendrofluazide BAN *diuretic; antihypertensive* [also: bendroflumethiazide]
bendroflumethiazide USP, INN *diuretic; antihypertensive* [also: bendrofluazide]
BeneFin ℞ *investigational (Phase III) angiogenesis inhibitor for the treatment of solid tumors* [squalamine (shark cartilage powder)]
Benefix powder for IV injection ℞ *antihemophilic for factor IX deficiency (hemophilia B; Christmas disease) (orphan)* [nonacog alfa] 250, 500, 1000 IU
Benemid (CAN) tablets (discontinued 2001; discontinued in U.S. 1996) ℞ *uricosuric for gout* [probenecid] 500 mg ⦻ Beminal
benethamine penicillin INN, BAN
benexate INN
benexate HCl JAN
benfluorex INN, DCF
benfosformin INN, DCF
benfotiamine INN, JAN, DCF
benfurodil hemisuccinate INN, DCF
bengal gelatin [see: agar]
Ben-Gay, Arthritis Formula cream OTC *topical analgesic; counterirritant* [methyl salicylate; menthol] 30%•8%
Ben-Gay Extra Strength cream (name changed to Arthritis Formula Ben-Gay in 1999)
Ben-Gay Original ointment OTC *topical analgesic; counterirritant* [methyl salicylate; menthol] 18.3%•16%
Ben-Gay Regular Strength cream OTC *topical analgesic; counterirritant* [methyl salicylate; menthol] 15%•10%
Ben-Gay SPA cream OTC *topical analgesic; counterirritant* [menthol] 10%
Ben-Gay Ultra Strength cream OTC *topical analgesic; counterirritant* [methyl salicylate; menthol; camphor] 30%•10%•4%
Ben-Gay Vanishing Scent gel OTC *topical analgesic; counterirritant* [menthol; camphor] 3%•?
benhepazone INN
benidipine INN
benmoxin INN, DCF
benolizime INN
Benoquin cream ℞ *depigmenting agent for vitiligo* [monobenzone] 20%
benorilate INN, DCF [also: benorylate]
benorterone USAN, INN *antiandrogen*
benorylate BAN [also: benorilate]
benoxafos INN
benoxaprofen USAN, INN, BAN *anti-inflammatory; analgesic*
benoxinate HCl USP *topical ophthalmic anesthetic* [also: oxybuprocaine; oxybuprocaine HCl]
Benoxyl #5 lotion, mask OTC *topical keratolytic for acne* [benzoyl peroxide] 5% ⦻ PanOxyl

Benoxyl 10 lotion OTC *topical keratolytic for acne* [benzoyl peroxide] 10%
benpenolisin INN
benperidol USAN, INN, BAN *antipsychotic*
benproperine INN [also: benproperine phosphate]
benproperine phosphate JAN [also: benproperine]
benrixate INN, DCF
Bensal HP ointment ℞ *topical antifungal; keratolytic* [benzoic acid; salicylic acid] 6%•3%
bensalan USAN, INN *disinfectant*
benserazide USAN, INN, BAN *decarboxylase inhibitor; antiparkinsonian adjunct* [also: benserazide HCl]
benserazide HCl JAN *decarboxylase inhibitor; antiparkinsonian adjunct* [also: benserazide]
bensuldazic acid INN, BAN
Bensulfoid cream OTC *topical acne treatment* [colloidal sulfur; resorcinol; alcohol] 8%•2%•12%
bensylyte HCl [see: phenoxybenzamine HCl]
bentazepam USAN, INN *sedative*
bentemazole INN
bentiamine INN
bentipimine INN
bentiromide USAN, INN, BAN, JAN *diagnostic aid for pancreas function*
bentonite NF, JAN *suspending agent*
bentoquatam USAN *topical skin protectant for allergic contact dermatitis*
Bentyl capsules, tablets, IM injection, syrup ℞ *GI antispasmodic* [dicyclomine HCl] 10 mg; 20 mg; 10 mg/mL; 10 mg/5 mL ⑨ Aventyl; Benadryl; Bontril
benurestat USAN, INN *urease enzyme inhibitor*
Benuryl (CAN) tablets ℞ *uricosuric for gout* [probenecid] 500 mg
Benylin Adult oral liquid OTC *antitussive* [dextromethorphan hydrobromide; alcohol 5%] 15 mg/5 mL ⑨ Benadryl
Benylin DM syrup OTC *antitussive* [dextromethorphan hydrobromide] 10 mg/5 mL ⑨ Benadryl
Benylin DM 12-Hour; Benylin DM for Children 12-Hour (CAN) controlled-release syrup OTC *antitussive* [dextromethorphan polistirex] 30 mg/5 mL; 15 mg/5 mL ⑨ Benadryl
Benylin DM-D; Benylin DM-D for Children (CAN) syrup OTC *antitussive; decongestant* [dextromethorphan hydrobromide; pseudoephedrine HCl] 15•30 mg/5 mL; 7.5•15 mg/5 mL ⑨ Benadryl
Benylin DM-D-E (CAN) syrup OTC *antitussive; decongestant; expectorant* [dextromethorphan hydrobromide; pseudoephedrine HCl; guaifenesin; alcohol 5%] 15•30•100, 15•30•200 mg/5 mL ⑨ Benadryl
Benylin DM-E (CAN) syrup OTC *antitussive; expectorant* [dextromethorphan hydrobromide; guaifenesin; alcohol 5%] 15•100 mg/5 mL ⑨ Benadryl
Benylin Expectorant liquid OTC *antitussive; expectorant* [dextromethorphan hydrobromide; guaifenesin] 5•100 mg/5 mL ⑨ Benadryl
Benylin First Defense (CAN) lozenges, syrup OTC *herbal remedy for coughs, nasal congestion, and sore throat due to cough or cold* [echinacea; menthol] 65•8 mg; 100•12.5 mg/10 mL
Benylin Multi-Symptom liquid OTC *antitussive; decongestant; expectorant* [dextromethorphan hydrobromide; pseudoephedrine HCl; guaifenesin] 5•15•100 mg/5 mL ⑨ Benadryl
Benylin Pediatric oral liquid OTC *antitussive* [dextromethorphan hydrobromide] 7.5 mg/5 mL ⑨ Benadryl
Benz 42 *hydrophilic contact lens material* [hefilcon A]
Benza solution OTC *topical antiseptic* [benzalkonium chloride] 1:750
Benzac AC 2½; Benzac W 2½; Benzac 5; Benzac AC 5; Benzac W 5; Benzac 10; Benzac AC 10; Benzac W 10 gel ℞ *topical keratolytic for acne* [benzoyl peroxide] 2.5%; 2.5%; 5%; 5%; 5%; 10%; 10%; 10%

Benzac AC Wash 2½; Benzac AC Wash 5; Benzac W Wash 5; Benzac AC Wash 10; Benzac W Wash 10 liquid ℞ *topical keratolytic for acne* [benzoyl peroxide] 2.5%; 5%; 5%; 10%; 10%

Benzaclin gel ℞ *topical antibiotic and keratolytic for acne* [clindamycin phosphate; benzoyl peroxide] 1%•5%

5 Benzagel; 10 Benzagel gel ℞ *topical keratolytic for acne* [benzoyl peroxide] 5%; 10%

Benzagel Wash foamless cleanser ℞ *topical keratolytic for acne* [benzoyl peroxide]

benzaldehyde NF *flavoring agent*

benzalkonium chloride (BAC) NF, INN, BAN, JAN *preservative; bacteriostatic antiseptic; surfactant/wetting agent* 17% topical

Benzamycin gel ℞ *topical antibiotic and keratolytic for acne* [erythromycin; benzoyl peroxide] 30•50 mg/mL

benzaprinoxide INN

benzarone INN, DCF

Benzashave shaving cream ℞ *topical keratolytic for acne* [benzoyl peroxide] 5%, 10%

benzathine benzylpenicillin INN *natural penicillin antibiotic* [also: penicillin G benzathine; benzathine penicillin; benzylpenicillin benzathine]

benzathine penicillin BAN *natural penicillin antibiotic* [also: penicillin G benzathine; benzathine benzylpenicillin; benzylpenicillin benzathine]

benzathine penicillin G [see: penicillin G benzathine]

benzatropine INN *antiparkinsonian; anticholinergic* [also: benztropine mesylate; benztropine]

benzazoline HCl [see: tolazoline HCl]

benzbromaron JAN *uricosuric* [also: benzbromarone]

benzbromarone USAN, INN, BAN *uricosuric* [also: benzbromaron]

benzchinamide [see: benzquinamide]

benzchlorpropamide [see: beclamide]

Benzedrex inhaler ℞ *nasal decongestant* [propylhexedrine] 250 mg

benzene ethanol [see: phenylethyl alcohol]

benzene hexachloride, gamma [now: lindane]

benzeneacetic acid, sodium salt [see: sodium phenylacetate]

benzenebutanoic acid, sodium salt [see: sodium phenylbutyrate]

1,3-benzenediol [see: resorcinol]

benzenemethanol [see: benzyl alcohol]

benzestrofol [see: estradiol benzoate]

benzestrol USP, INN, BAN

benzethacil [see: penicillin G benzathine]

benzethidine INN, BAN, DCF

benzethonium chloride USP, INN, BAN, JAN *topical anti-infective; preservative*

benzetimide INN *anticholinergic* [also: benzetimide HCl]

benzetimide HCl USAN *anticholinergic* [also: benzetimide]

benzfetamine INN *anorexiant; CNS stimulant* [also: benzphetamine HCl; benzphetamine]

benzhexol BAN *anticholinergic; antiparkinsonian* [also: trihexyphenidyl HCl; trihexyphenidyl]

N-benzhydryl-N-methylpiperazine [see: cyclizine HCl]

benzilone bromide [see: benzilonium bromide]

benzilonium bromide USAN, INN, BAN *anticholinergic*

benzimidavir *investigational (Phase II) DNA inhibitor for AIDS-related cytomegalovirus infection*

2-benzimidazolepropionic acid [see: procodazole]

benzimidazoles, substituted *a class of gastric antisecretory agents that inhibit the ATPase "proton pump" within the cell* [also called: proton pump inhibitors; ATPase inhibitors]

benzin, petroleum JAN

benzindamine HCl [see: benzydamine HCl]

benzindopyrine INN *antipsychotic* [also: benzindopyrine HCl]

benzindopyrine HCl USAN *antipsychotic* [also: benzindopyrine]

benzinoform [see: carbon tetrachloride]
benziodarone INN, BAN, DCF
benzisoxazoles *a class of novel (atypical) antipsychotic agents*
benzmalecene INN
benzmethoxazone [see: chlorthenoxazine]
benznidazole INN
benzoaric acid [see: ellagic acid]
benzoate & phenylacetate [see: sodium benzoate & sodium phenylacetate]
benzobarbital INN
benzocaine USP, INN, BAN *topical anesthetic; nonprescription diet aid* [also: ethyl aminobenzoate] 5% topical
benzoclidine INN
benzoctamine INN, BAN *sedative; muscle relaxant* [also: benzoctamine HCl]
benzoctamine HCl USAN, INN *sedative; muscle relaxant* [also: benzoctamine]
Benzodent ointment OTC *topical oral anesthetic* [benzocaine] 20%
benzodepa USAN, INN *antineoplastic*
benzodiazepine HCl [see: medazepam HCl]
benzodiazepines *a class of nonbarbiturate sedatives, hypnotics, and anticonvulsants*
benzododecinium chloride INN
benzogynestryl [see: estradiol benzoate]
benzoic acid USP, JAN *antifungal; urinary acidifier*
benzoic acid, phenylmethyl ester [see: benzyl benzoate]
benzoic acid, potassium salt [see: potassium benzoate]
benzoic acid, sodium salt [see: sodium benzoate]
benzoin USP, JAN *topical protectant*
Benzoin Compound tincture OTC *skin protectant* [benzoin; aloe; alcohol 74–80%]
benzol [see: benzene ...]
benzonatate USP, INN, BAN *antitussive* 100, 200 mg oral
benzophenone
benzopyrrolate [see: benzopyrronium]
benzopyrronium bromide INN
benzoquinone amidoinohydrazone thiosemicarbazone hydrate [see: ambazone]
benzoquinonium chloride
benzorphanol [see: levophenacylmorphan]
benzosulfinide [see: saccharin]
benzosulphinide sodium [see: saccharin sodium]
benzothiazepines *a class of calcium channel blockers*
benzothiozon [see: thioacetazone; thiacetazone]
benzotript INN
Benzox-10 gel ℞ *topical keratolytic for acne* [benzoyl peroxide] 10%
benzoxiquine USAN, INN *antiseptic/disinfectant*
benzoxonium chloride INN
benzoyl *p*-aminosalicylate (B-PAS) [see: benzoylpas calcium]
benzoyl peroxide USAN, USP *keratolytic* 5%, 10% topical
***m*-benzoylhydratropic acid** [see: ketoprofen]
benzoylmethylecgonine [see: cocaine]
benzoylpas calcium USAN, USP *antibacterial; tuberculostatic* [also: calcium benzamidosalicylate]
benzoylsulfanilamide [see: sulfabenzamide]
benzoylthiamindisulfide [see: bisbentiamine]
benzoylthiaminmonophosphate [see: benfotiamine]
benzphetamine BAN *anorexiant; CNS stimulant* [also: benzphetamine HCl; benzfetamine]
benzphetamine chloride [see: benzphetamine HCl]
benzphetamine HCl NF *anorexiant; CNS stimulant* [also: benzfetamine; benzphetamine]
benzpiperylon [see: benzpiperylone]
benzpiperylone INN
benzpyrinium bromide NF, INN
benzquercin INN
benzquinamide USAN, INN, BAN *postanesthesia antinauseant and antiemetic*

benzthiazide USP, INN, BAN *diuretic; antihypertensive*
benztropine BAN *anticholinergic; antiparkinsonian* [also: benztropine mesylate; benzatropine]
benztropine mesylate USP *anticholinergic; antiparkinsonian* [also: benzatropine; benztropine] 0.5, 1, 2 mg oral
benztropine methanesulfonate [see: benztropine mesylate]
benzydamine INN, BAN *analgesic; antipyretic; anti-inflammatory* [also: benzydamine HCl]
benzydamine HCl USAN, JAN *analgesic; antipyretic; anti-inflammatory; investigational (orphan) radioprotectant for oral mucosa* [also: benzydamine]
benzydroflumethiazide [see: bendroflumethiazide]
benzyl alcohol NF, INN, JAN *antimicrobial agent; antiseptic; local anesthetic*
benzyl analogue of serotonin (BAS) [see: benanserin HCl]
benzyl antiserotonin [see: benanserin HCl]
benzyl benzoate USP, JAN
benzyl carbinol [see: phenylethyl alcohol]
***S*-benzyl thiobenzoate** [see: tibenzate]
benzylamide [see: beclamide]
benzylamines *a class of antifungals structurally related to the allylamines*
N-benzylanilinoacetamidoxime [see: cetoxime]
2-benzylbenzimidazole [see: bendazol]
benzyldimethyltetradecylammonium chloride [see: miristalkonium chloride]
benzyldodecyldimethylammonium chloride [see: benzododecinium chloride]
benzylhexadecyldimethylammonium [see: cetalkonium]
benzylhexadecyldimethylammonium chloride [see: cetalkonium chloride]
benzylhydrochlorothiazide JAN
***p*-benzyloxyphenol** [see: monobenzone]
benzylpenicillin INN, BAN *natural penicillin antibiotic; investigational (orphan) for penicillin hypersensitivity assessment*
benzylpenicillin benzathine JAN *natural penicillin antibiotic* [also: penicillin G benzathine; benzathine benzylpenicillin; benzathine penicillin]
benzylpenicillin potassium BAN, JAN *natural penicillin antibiotic* [also: penicillin G potassium]
benzylpenicillin procaine *natural penicillin antibiotic* [see: penicillin G procaine]
benzylpenicillin sodium BAN *natural penicillin antibiotic* [also: penicillin G sodium]
benzylpenicilloic acid [see: benzylpenicillin]
benzylpenicilloyl polylysine USP *diagnostic aid for penicillin sensitivity*
benzylpenilloic acid [see: benzylpenicillin]
benzylsulfamide INN, DCF
benzylsulfanilamide [see: benzylsulfamide]
BEP (bleomycin, etoposide, Platinol) *chemotherapy protocol for testicular cancer and germ cell tumors*
bepafant INN
bepanthen [see: panthenol]
beperidium iodide INN
bephene oxinaphthoate [see: bephenium hydroxynaphthoate]
bephenium embonate [see: bephenium hydroxynaphthoate]
bephenium hydroxynaphthoate USP, INN, BAN
bepiastine INN, DCF
bepridil INN, BAN *vasodilator; antianginal; calcium channel blocker* [also: bepridil HCl]
bepridil HCl USAN *vasodilator; antianginal; calcium channel blocker* [also: bepridil]
beractant USAN *pulmonary surfactant for neonatal respiratory distress syndrome or respiratory failure (orphan)*
beraprost USAN, INN *platelet aggregation inhibitor; peripheral vasodilator;*

investigational (Phase III) prostacyclin analogue for peripheral vascular disease (PVD) and pulmonary arterial hypertension (PAH)

beraprost sodium USAN *platelet aggregation inhibitor; peripheral vasodilator*

berberine chloride JAN

berberine sulfate JAN

berberine tannate JAN

Berberis vulgaris *medicinal herb* [see: barberry]

berculon A [see: thioacetazone; thiacetazone]

berefrine USAN, INN *mydriatic*

bergamot, scarlet *medicinal herb* [see: Oswego tea]

bergamot, wild *medicinal herb* [see: wild bergamot]

bergamot oil *(Citrus aurantium; C. bergamia)* fruit peel *medicinal herb used in conjunction with long-wave UV light therapy for psoriasis and vitiligo; not generally regarded as safe and effective because of its photosensitizing properties*

bergenin JAN

Berinert-P ℞ *investigational (orphan) for acute angioedema* [C1-esterase-inhibitor, human]

berkelium *element (Bk)*

berlafenone INN

bermastine [see: barmastine]

bermoprofen INN

Berocca tablets ℞ *vitamin supplement* [multiple B vitamins; vitamin C; folic acid] ≛•500•0.5 mg

Berocca Parenteral Nutrition injection (discontinued 1997) ℞ *parenteral vitamin supplement* [multiple vitamins; folic acid; biotin] ≛•400•60 µg/mL

Berocca Plus tablets ℞ *vitamin/mineral/iron supplement* [multiple vitamins & minerals; ferrous fumarate; folic acid; biotin] ≛•27•0.8•0.15 mg

Berotec ℞ *investigational (NDA filed) bronchodilator; antiasthmatic* [fenoterol hydrobromide]

Berplex Plus tablets (discontinued 2000) ℞ *vitamin/mineral/iron supplement* [multiple vitamins & minerals; ferrous fumarate; folic acid; biotin] ≛•27•0.8•0.15 mg

bertosamil INN

beryllium *element (Be)*

berythromycin USAN, INN *antiamebic; antibacterial*

besigomsin INN

besilate INN *combining name for radicals or groups* [also: besylate]

besipirdine INN *cognition enhancer for Alzheimer disease* [also: besipiridine HCl]

besipirdine HCl USAN *cognition enhancer for Alzheimer disease* [also: besipiridine]

besulpamide INN

besunide INN

besylate USAN *combining name for radicals or groups* [also: besilate]

beta alethine *investigational (Phase I/II, orphan) antineoplastic and immunostimulant for B-cell lymphoma, multiple myeloma, and metastatic melanoma*

beta blockers (β-blockers) *a class of cardiac agents characterized by their antihypertensive, antiarrhythmic, and antianginal actions; a class of topical antiglaucoma agents* [also called: beta-adrenergic antagonists]

beta carotene USAN, USP *vitamin A precursor* [also: betacarotene] 15 mg (25 000 IU) oral

beta cyclodextrin (β-cyclodextrin) *(previously used NF name)* [now: betadex]

Beta LT ℞ *investigational (Phase I/II, orphan) antineoplastic and immunostimulant for B cell lymphoma, multiple myeloma, and metastatic melanoma* [beta alethine]

Beta-2 solution for inhalation (discontinued 1999) ℞ *sympathomimetic bronchodilator* [isoetharine HCl] 1%

betacarotene INN *vitamin A precursor* [also: beta carotene]

betacetylmethadol INN, BAN

Betachron E-R extended-release capsules (discontinued 2001) ℞ *antiarrhythmic; antihypertensive; antiangi-*

nal; antiadrenergic (β-blocker); migraine prophylaxis [propranolol HCl] 60, 80, 120, 160 mg

betadex USAN, INN *sequestering agent* [previous NF name: beta cyclodextrin]

beta-D-galactosidase *digestive enzyme* [see: tilactase]

Betadine aerosol, gauze pads, lubricating gel, cream, mouthwash, ointment, perineal wash, skin cleanser, foam, solution, swab, swabsticks, surgical scrub OTC *broad-spectrum antimicrobial* [povidone-iodine] 5%; 10%; 5%; 5%; 0.5%; 10%; 10%; 7.5%; 7.5%; 10%; 10%; 10%; 7.5%

Betadine shampoo OTC *broad-spectrum antimicrobial for dandruff* [povidone-iodine] 7.5%

Betadine 5% Sterile Ophthalmic Prep solution ℞ *broad-spectrum antimicrobial for eye surgery* [povidone-iodine] 5%

Betadine First Aid Antibiotics + Moisturizer ointment OTC *topical antibiotic* [polymyxin B sulfate; bacitracin zinc] 10 000•500 IU/g

Betadine Medicated vaginal suppositories, vaginal gel OTC *antiseptic/germicidal; vaginal cleanser and deodorant* [povidone-iodine] 10%

Betadine Medicated Douche; Betadine Medicated Disposable Douche; Betadine Premixed Medicated Disposable Douche solution OTC *antiseptic/germicidal; vaginal cleanser and deodorant* [povidone-iodine] 10%

Betadine Plus First Aid Antibiotics and Pain Reliever ointment OTC *topical antibiotic and anesthetic* [polymyxin B sulfate; bacitracin zinc; pramoxine HCl] 10 000 IU•500 IU•10 mg per g

Betadine PrepStick swab OTC *broad-spectrum antimicrobial* [povidone-iodine] 10%

Betadine PrepStick Plus swab OTC *broad-spectrum antimicrobial* [povidone-iodine; alcohol] 10%•?

beta-estradiol [see: estradiol]

beta-estradiol benzoate [see: estradiol benzoate]

betaeucaine HCl [now: eucaine HCl]

Betafectin ℞ *investigational (Phase III) immunotherapeutic to prevent postsurgical infections in non-colorectal GI surgery patients (clinical trials discontinued 1999)* [PGG glucan]

Betagan Liquifilm eye drops ℞ *topical antiglaucoma agent (β-blocker)* [levobunolol HCl] 0.25%, 0.5% ⓢ Betagen

Betagen ointment, solution, surgical scrub OTC *broad-spectrum antimicrobial* [povidone-iodine] 1%; 10%; 7.5% ⓢ Betagan

beta-glucocerebrosidase [see: alglucerase]

betahistine INN, BAN *vasodilator* [also: betahistine HCl; betahistine mesilate]

betahistine HCl USAN *vasodilator* [also: betahistine; betahistine mesilate]

betahistine mesilate JAN *vasodilator* [also: betahistine HCl; betahistine]

beta-hypophamine [see: vasopressin]

betaine HCl USP *electrolyte replenisher for homocystinuria (orphan)*

Betaject (CAN) injection ℞ *corticosteroidal anti-inflammatory* [betamethasone sodium phosphate; betamethasone acetate] 3•3 mg/mL

beta-lactams *a class of antibiotics*

beta-lactone [see: propiolactone]

betameprodine INN, BAN, DCF

betamethadol INN, BAN, DCF

betamethasone USAN, USP, INN, BAN, JAN *corticosteroid; anti-inflammatory*

betamethasone acetate USP, JAN *corticosteroid; anti-inflammatory*

betamethasone acibutate INN, BAN *corticosteroid; anti-inflammatory*

betamethasone benzoate USAN, USP, BAN *topical corticosteroidal anti-inflammatory*

betamethasone dipropionate USAN, USP, BAN, JAN *topical corticosteroidal anti-inflammatory* 0.05% topical

betamethasone dipropionate, augmented *topical corticosteroidal anti-inflammatory* 0.05% topical

betamethasone dipropionate & clotrimazole *topical corticosteroidal anti-inflammatory and antifungal* 0.05%•1%

betamethasone sodium phosphate USP, BAN, JAN *corticosteroid; anti-inflammatory* 4 mg/mL injection

betamethasone valerate USAN, USP, BAN, JAN *topical corticosteroidal anti-inflammatory; investigational (NDA filed) mousse for scalp psoriasis* 0.1% topical

betamicin INN *antibacterial* [also: betamicin sulfate]

betamicin sulfate USAN *antibacterial* [also: betamicin]

betamipron INN

betanaphthol NF

betanidine INN *antihypertensive* [also: bethanidine sulfate; bethanidine; betanidine sulfate]

betanidine sulfate JAN *antihypertensive* [also: bethanidine sulfate; betanidine; bethanidine]

Betapace caplets ℞ *antiadrenergic (β-blocker); antiarrhythmic for life-threatening ventricular arrhythmias (orphan)* [sotalol HCl] 80, 120, 160, 240 mg

Betapace AF caplets ℞ *antiadrenergic (β-blocker); antiarrhythmic for atrial fibrillation or atrial flutter* [sotalol HCl] 80, 120, 160 mg

Betapen-VK film-coated tablets, powder for oral solution (discontinued 1998) ℞ *natural penicillin antibiotic* [penicillin V potassium] 250, 500 mg; 125, 250 mg/5 mL ⊠ Adapin; Phenaphen

betaprodine INN, BAN, DCF

beta-propiolactone [see: propiolactone]

beta-pyridylcarbinol [see: nicotinyl alcohol]

BetaRx *investigational (orphan) antidiabetic for type 1 patients on immunosuppression* [porcine islet preparation, encapsulated]

Betasept liquid OTC *broad-spectrum antimicrobial; germicidal* [chlorhexidine gluconate; alcohol 4%] 4%

Betaseron powder for subcu injection ℞ *immunomodulator for relapsing-remitting multiple sclerosis (orphan); investigational (Phase II/III) cytokine for AIDS* [interferon beta-1b] 0.3 mg (9.6 mIU)/vial

BetaSite ℞ *investigational (Phase III) agent for glaucoma* [levobunolol]

Betathine *investigational (orphan) for multiple myeloma and metastatic melanoma* [beta alethine]

Beta-Tim (CAN) eye drops (discontinued 1998) ℞ *topical antiglaucoma agent (β-blocker)* [timolol maleate] 0.25%, 0.5%

Betatrex cream, ointment, lotion ℞ *topical corticosteroidal anti-inflammatory* [betamethasone valerate] 0.1%

Beta-Val cream, lotion ℞ *topical corticosteroidal anti-inflammatory* [betamethasone valerate] 0.1%

betaxolol INN, BAN *antihypertensive; antiadrenergic (β-blocker)* [also: betaxolol HCl]

betaxolol HCl USAN, USP *antihypertensive; antiadrenergic (β-blocker); topical antiglaucoma agent* [also: betaxolol] 0.5% eye drops

Betaxon eye drops ℞ *topical antiglaucoma agent (β-blocker)* [levobetaxolol HCl] 0.5%

betazole INN [also: betazole HCl; ametazole]

betazole HCl USP [also: betazole; ametazole]

betazolium chloride [see: betazole HCl]

betel nut *(Areca catechu)* leaves and quids (a mixture of tobacco, powdered or sliced areca nut, and slaked lime wrapped in a *Piper betel* leaf) *medicinal herb used as a digestive aid and mild stimulant; not generally regarded as safe, as it causes leukoplakia and oral cancer*

beth root *medicinal herb* [see: birthroot]

bethanechol chloride USP, BAN, JAN *cholinergic urinary stimulant for postsurgical and postpartum urinary retention* 5, 10, 25, 50 mg oral

bethanidine BAN *antihypertensive* [also: bethanidine sulfate; betanidine; betanidine sulfate]

Bextra

bethanidine sulfate USAN *antihypertensive; orphan status withdrawn 1996* [also: betanidine; bethanidine; betanidine sulfate]

betiatide USAN, INN, BAN *pharmaceutic aid*

Betimol eye drops ℞ *topical antiglaucoma agent (β-blocker)* [timolol hemihydrate] 0.25%, 0.5%

Betonica officinalis *medicinal herb* [now: *Stachys officinalis*] [see: betony]

betony *(Stachys officinalis)* plant *medicinal herb for anxiety, delirium, diarrhea, fever, jaundice, liver and spleen sclerosis, migraine headache, mouth or throat irritation, nervousness, palpitations, and toothache; also used as a purgative and emetic agent*

Betoptic; Betoptic S Drop-Tainer (eye drops) ℞ *topical antiglaucoma agent (β-blocker)* [betaxolol HCl] 0.5%; 0.25%

betoxycaine INN

betoxycaine HCl [see: betoxycaine]

betula oil [see: methyl salicylate]

***Betula* spp.** *medicinal herb* [see: birch]

Betuline lotion OTC *topical analgesic; counterirritant* [methyl salicylate; camphor; menthol; peppermint oil]

bevantolol INN, BAN *antianginal; antihypertensive; antiarrhythmic* [also: bevantolol HCl]

bevantolol HCl USAN *antianginal; antihypertensive; antiarrhythmic* [also: bevantolol]

bevonium methylsulphate BAN [also: bevonium metilsulfate]

bevonium metilsulfate INN [also: bevonium methylsulphate]

bexarotene USAN *synthetic retinoid analogue antineoplastic for cutaneous T-cell lymphoma (CTCL); investigational (Phase II/III) for AIDS-related Kaposi sarcoma (clinical trials discontinued 1999)*

bexlosteride USAN *antineoplastic 5α-reductase inhibitor for prostate cancer*

Bexxar ℞ *investigational (NDA filed, orphan) treatment for low-grade B cell non-Hodgkin lymphoma* [iodine I 131 tositumomab]

bezafibrate USAN, INN, BAN, JAN *antihyperlipidemic*

bezitramide INN, BAN, DCF

bezomil INN *combining name for radicals or groups*

bFGF (basic fibroblast growth factor) [see: ersofermin]

B.F.I. Antiseptic powder OTC *topical antiseptic* [bismuth-formic-iodide] 16%

BGM-24 *investigational for prostatitis*

BHA (butylated hydroxyanisole) [q.v.]

BHAPs (bisheteroarylpiperazines) *a class of antiviral drugs*

BHD (BCNU, hydroxyurea, dacarbazine) *chemotherapy protocol*

BHDV; BHD-V (BCNU, hydroxyurea, dacarbazine, vincristine) *chemotherapy protocol*

BHT (butylated hydroxytoluene) [q.v.]

bialamicol INN, BAN *antiamebic* [also: bialamicol HCl]

bialamicol HCl USAN *antiamebic* [also: bialamicol]

biallylamicol [see: bialamicol]

biantrazole [now: losoxantrone HCl]

biapenem USAN, INN *antibacterial*

Biavax II powder for subcu injection ℞ *mumps and rubella vaccine* [mumps and rubella virus vaccine, live] 1000•20 000 U/0.5 mL

Biaxin Filmtabs (film-coated tablets), granules for oral suspension ℞ *macrolide antibiotic* [clarithromycin] 250, 500 mg; 125, 187.5, 250 mg/5 mL ⊠ Axid

Biaxin XL film-coated extended-release tablets ℞ *once-daily macrolide antibiotic* [clarithromycin] 500 mg

bibapcitide USAN *glycoprotein (GP) IIb/IIIa receptor antagonist; investigational (Phase III) diagnostic imaging aid for deep vein thrombosis*

bibenzonium bromide INN, BAN

bibrocathin [see: bibrocathol]

bibrocathol INN, DCF

bicalutamide USAN, INN, BAN *antiandrogen antineoplastic for prostatic cancer*

Bichloracetic Acid liquid ℞ *cauterant; keratolytic* [dichloroacetic acid] 10 mL ⊡ dichloroacetic acid

bicifadine INN *analgesic* [also: bicifadine HCl]

bicifadine HCl USAN *analgesic* [also: bicifadine]

Bicillin C-R; Bicillin C-R 900/300 deep IM injection, Tubex (cartridge-needle unit) ℞ *natural penicillin antibiotic* [penicillin G benzathine; penicillin G procaine] 150 000•150 000, 300 000•300 000, 600 000•600 000, 1 200 000•1 200 000 U; 900 000•300 000 U ⊡ V-Cillin; Wycillin

Bicillin L-A deep IM injection, Tubex (cartridge-needle units) ℞ *natural penicillin antibiotic* [penicillin G benzathine] 300 000, 600 000, 1 200 000, 2 400 000 U

biciromab USAN, INN, BAN *antifibrin monoclonal antibody*

Bicitra oral solution ℞ *urinary alkalinizing agent* [sodium citrate; citric acid] 500•334 mg/5 mL

biclodil INN *antihypertensive; vasodilator* [also: biclodil HCl]

biclodil HCl USAN *antihypertensive; vasodilator* [also: biclodil]

biclofibrate INN, DCF

biclotymol INN, DCF

BiCNU powder for IV injection ℞ *nitrosourea-type alkylating antineoplastic* [carmustine] 100 mg

bicozamycin INN

Bicozene cream OTC *topical local anesthetic; antifungal* [benzocaine; resorcinol] 6%•1.67%

bicyclomycin [see: bicozamycin]

bidCAP (trademarked dosage form) *twice-daily capsule*

Bidil ℞ *investigational (NDA filed) nitric oxide donor; investigational vasodilator for congestive heart failure* [hydralazine; isosorbide dinitrate]

bidimazium iodide INN, BAN

bidisomide USAN, INN *antiarrhythmic*

Biebrich scarlet red [see: scarlet red]

Biebrich scarlet-picroaniline blue

bietamiverine INN

bietamiverine HCl [see: bietamiverine]

bietaserpine INN, DCF

bifemelane INN [also: bifemelane HCl]

bifemelane HCl JAN [also: bifemelane]

bifepramide INN

bifeprofen INN

bifluranol INN, BAN

bifonazole USAN, INN, BAN, JAN *antifungal*

Big Shot B-12 tablets OTC *vitamin B_{12} supplement* [cyanocobalamin] 5000 µg

Bignonia sempervirens *medicinal herb* [see: gelsemium]

bilberry *(Myrtilli fructus; Vaccinium myrtillus)* fruit *medicinal herb for cold hands and feet, diarrhea, edema, increasing microvascular blood flow, mild gastroenteritis, mucous membrane inflammation, night blindness, and varicose veins*

bile acid sequestrants *a class of antihyperlipidemic agents*

bile acids, oxidized [see: dehydrocholic acid]

bile salts BAN *digestive enzymes; laxative*

BiliCheck breath analyzer device *in vitro diagnostic aid for infant jaundice*

Bili-Labstix reagent strips *in vitro diagnostic aid for multiple urine products*

Bilivist capsules (discontinued 1999) ℞ *radiopaque contrast medium for cholecystography* [ipodate sodium (61.4% iodine)] 500 mg (307 mg)

Bilopaque capsules ℞ *radiopaque contrast medium for cholecystography* [tyropanoate sodium (57.4% iodine)] 750 mg (430.5 mg)

Biltricide film-coated tablets ℞ *anthelmintic for schistosomiasis (flukes)* [praziquantel] 600 mg

bimakalim INN

bimatoprost *topical prostamide analogue for glaucoma and ocular hypertension*

bimazol [see: carbimazole]

bimethadol [see: dimepheptanol]

bimethoxycaine lactate

bimoclomol *investigational (Phase II) agent for microalbuminuria and diabetic neuropathy*

bimosiamose disodium USAN *anti-inflammatory for asthma, psoriasis, and reperfusion injury following transplants or coronary revascularization*

bindarit USAN, INN *antirheumatic; investigational (orphan) for lupus nephritis*

bindazac [see: bendazac]

binedaline INN

binetrakin USAN *immunomodulator for gastrointestinal carcinoma and rheumatoid arthritis*

binfloxacin USAN, INN *veterinary antibacterial*

binifibrate INN

biniramycin USAN, INN *antibacterial antibiotic*

binizolast INN

binodaline [see: binedaline]

binospirone INN *anxiolytic* [also: binospirone mesylate]

binospirone mesylate USAN *anxiolytic* [also: binospirone]

Bio-Acerola C Complex wafers (discontinued 1999) OTC *vitamin C supplement with multiple bioflavonoids* [vitamin C; citrus bioflavonoids; rutin] 500•10•5 mg

bioallethrin BAN *pediculicide*

Biobrane wound dressing *nylon fabric matrix bound to a silicon film*

Biobrane-L light adherence wound dressing *nylon fabric matrix bound to a silicon film*

Biocef capsules, powder for oral suspension ℞ *cephalosporin antibiotic* [cephalexin] 500 mg; 250 mg/5 mL

Bioclate powder for IV injection ℞ *antihemophilic to correct coagulation deficiency* [antihemophilic factor VIII, recombinant] 250, 500, 1000 IU

BioCox intradermal injection ℞ *diagnostic aid for coccidioidomycosis* [coccidioidin] 1:100, 1:10

Biocult-GC culture paddles for professional use *in vitro diagnostic aid for Neisseria gonorrhoeae*

Biodel Implant/BCNU (name changed to Gliadel upon marketing release in 1998)

Biodine Topical solution OTC *broad-spectrum antimicrobial* [povidone-iodine] 1%

bioflavonoids (vitamin P) *a group of more than 4000 natural substances with widespread biological activity, including anthelmintic, antimicrobial, antimalarial, antineoplastic, antioxidant, anti-inflammatory, and antiviral activity; historically named "vitamin P"*

biogastrone [see: carbenoxolone]

Biohist-LA timed-release tablets ℞ *decongestant; antihistamine* [pseudoephedrine HCl; chlorpheniramine maleate] 120•12 mg

Biojector 2000 (trademarked delivery system) ℞ *investigational (Phase I) jet injector for malaria DNA vaccine*

biological indicator for dry-heat sterilization USP *sterilization indicator*

biological indicator for ethylene oxide sterilization USP *sterilization indicator*

biological indicator for steam sterilization USP *sterilization indicator*

Biomox capsules, powder for oral suspension (discontinued 1998) ℞ *aminopenicillin antibiotic* [amoxicillin] 250, 500 mg; 250 mg/5 mL

Bion Tears eye drops OTC *ophthalmic moisturizer/lubricant* [hydroxypropyl methylcellulose] 0.3%

bioral [see: carbenoxolone]

Bio-Rescue ℞ *investigational (orphan) for acute iron poisoning* [dextran; deferoxamine]

bioresmethrin INN

bios I [see: inositol]

bios II [see: biotin]

Biosafe HbA_{1c} (hemoglobin A_{1c}) test kit for home use *in vitro diagnostic aid for glycemic control*

Biosafe PSA (prostate-specific antigen) test kit for home use *in vitro diagnostic aid for prostate function*

Biosafe Total Cholesterol home test kit for serum cholesterol *in vitro diagnostic aid for hypercholesterolemia*

Biosafe Total Cholesterol Panel home test kit for serum cholesterol,

HDL, LDL, and triglycerides *in vitro diagnostic aid for hypercholesterolemia and hypertriglyceridemia*

Biosafe TSH (thyroid-stimulating hormone) test kit for home use *in vitro diagnostic aid for thyroid function*

Biosynject ℞ *investigational (orphan) for newborn hemolytic disease and ABO blood incompatibility of organ or bone marrow transplants* [trisaccharides A and B]

biosynthetic human parathyroid hormone (1-34) [see: teriparatide]

Bio-Tab film-coated tablets ℞ *tetracycline antibiotic* [doxycycline hyclate] 100 mg

Biotel kidney reagent strips *in vitro diagnostic aid for urine hemoglobin, RBCs, and albumin (predictor of kidney diseases)*

biotexin [see: novobiocin]

biotin USP, INN, JAN *B complex vitamin; vitamin H*

Biotin Forte tablets OTC *vitamin supplement* [multiple B vitamins; vitamin C; folic acid; biotin] ≛ •200• 0.8•3 mg, ≛ •100•0.8•5 mg

BioTropin *orphan status withdrawn 1997* [somatropin]

BIP (bleomycin, ifosfamide [with mesna rescue], Platinol) *chemotherapy protocol for cervical cancer*

bipenamol INN *antidepressant* [also: bipenamol HCl]

bipenamol HCl USAN *antidepressant* [also: bipenamol]

biperiden USP, INN, BAN, JAN *anticholinergic; antiparkinsonian*

biperiden HCl USP, BAN, JAN *anticholinergic; antiparkinsonian*

biperiden lactate USP, BAN, JAN *anticholinergic; antiparkinsonian*

biphasic insulin [see: insulin, biphasic]

biphenamine HCl USAN *topical anesthetic; antibacterial; antifungal* [also: xenysalate]

biprofenide [see: bifepramide]

birch (*Betula* spp.) bark and leaves *medicinal herb for bladder problems, blood cleansing, and eczema*

birch oil, sweet [see: methyl salicylate]

bird lime *medicinal herb* [see: mistletoe]

bird pepper *medicinal herb* [see: cayenne]

bird's nest root *medicinal herb* [see: carrot]

biricodar dicitrate USAN *investigational (Phase II) multi-drug–resistance inhibitor for prostate and ovarian cancers*

biriperone INN

birthroot (*Trillium erectum; T. grandiflorum; T. pendulum*) plant *medicinal herb for insect and snake bites, stimulating menses and diaphoresis, and stopping bleeding after childbirth; also used as an antiseptic and astringent*

birthwort (*Aristolochia clematitis*) root and flowering plant *medicinal herb used as a diaphoretic, emmenagogue, febrifuge, oxytocic, and stimulant*

Bisac-Evac enteric-coated tablets, suppositories OTC *stimulant laxative* [bisacodyl] 5 mg; 10 mg

bisacodyl USP, INN, BAN, JAN *stimulant laxative* 5 mg oral; 10 mg suppositories

bisacodyl tannex USAN *stimulant laxative*

bisantrene INN *antineoplastic* [also: bisantrene HCl]

bisantrene HCl USAN *antineoplastic* [also: bisantrene]

bisaramil INN

bisatin [see: oxyphenisatin acetate]

bisbendazole INN

bisbentiamine INN, JAN

bisbutiamine [see: bisbutitiamine]

bisbutitiamine JAN

bis-chloroethyl-nitrosourea (BCNU) [see: carmustine]

Bisco-Lax suppositories (discontinued 1999) OTC *stimulant laxative* [bisacodyl] 10 mg

bisdequalinium diacetate JAN

bisfenazone INN, DCF

bisfentidine INN

bisheteroarylpiperazines (BHAPs) *a class of antiviral drugs*

bishop's wort *medicinal herb* [see: nutmeg; betony]

bishydroxycoumarin [now: dicumarol]

bisibutiamine JAN [also: sulbutiamine]
Bismatrol chewable tablets, liquid OTC *antidiarrheal; antinauseant* [bismuth subsalicylate] 262 mg; 524 mg/5 mL
bismucatebrol [see: bibrocathol]
bismuth *element (Bi)*
bismuth, milk of USP *antacid; astringent*
bismuth aluminate USAN
bismuth betanaphthol USP
bismuth carbonate USAN
bismuth carbonate, basic [see: bismuth subcarbonate]
bismuth citrate USP
bismuth cream [see: bismuth, milk of]
bismuth gallate, basic [see: bismuth subgallate]
bismuth glycollylarsanilate BAN [also: glycobiarsol]
bismuth hydroxide [see: bismuth, milk of]
bismuth hydroxide nitrate oxide [see: bismuth subnitrate]
bismuth magma [now: bismuth, milk of]
bismuth magnesium aluminosilicate JAN
bismuth oxycarbonate [see: bismuth subcarbonate]
bismuth potassium tartrate NF
bismuth sodium triglycollamate USP
bismuth subcarbonate USAN, JAN *antacid; GI adsorbent*
bismuth subgallate USAN, USP *antacid; GI adsorbent*
bismuth subnitrate USP, JAN *skin protectant*
bismuth subsalicylate (BSS) USAN, JAN *antiperistaltic; antacid; GI adsorbent*
bisnafide dimesylate USAN *antineoplastic; DNA and RNA synthesis inhibitor*
bisobrin INN *fibrinolytic* [also: bisobrin lactate]
bisobrin lactate USAN *fibrinolytic* [also: bisobrin]
bisoprolol USAN, INN, BAN *antihypertensive; antiadrenergic (β-blocker)*
bisoprolol fumarate USAN, JAN *antihypertensive; antiadrenergic (β-blocker)* 5, 10 mg oral
bisoprolol fumarate & hydrochlorothiazide *antihypertensive; β-blocker; diuretic* 2.5•6.5, 5•6.5, 10•6.5 mg oral
bisorcic INN
bisoxatin INN, BAN *laxative* [also: bisoxatin acetate]
bisoxatin acetate USAN *laxative* [also: bisoxatin]
Bispan ℞ *investigational agent for rheumatoid arthritis* [IPL-423 (code name—generic name not yet assigned)]
bispecific antibody 520C9x22 *investigational (orphan) for ovarian cancer*
bisphosphonates *a class of calcium-regulating agents that inhibit normal and abnormal bone resorption*
bispyrithione magsulfex USAN *antibacterial; antidandruff; antifungal*
bistort *(Polygonum bistorta)* root *medicinal herb for bleeding, cholera, cuts, diarrhea, dysentery, gum disease (mouthwash), and hemorrhoids*
bis-tropamide [now: tropicamide]
Bite Rx solution OTC *astringent wet dressing (Burow solution) for insect bites* [aluminum acetate] 0.5%
bithionol NF, INN, BAN, JAN *investigational anti-infective for paragonimiasis and fascioliasis*
bithionolate sodium USAN *topical anti-infective* [also: sodium bitionolate]
bithionoloxide INN
Bitin (available only from the Centers for Disease Control) ℞ *investigational anti-infective for paragonimiasis and fascioliasis* [bithionol]
bitipazone INN
bitolterol INN, BAN *sympathomimetic bronchodilator* [also: bitolterol mesylate; bitolterol mesilate]
bitolterol mesilate JAN *sympathomimetic bronchodilator* [also: bitolterol mesylate; bitolterol]
bitolterol mesylate USAN *sympathomimetic bronchodilator* [also: bitolterol; bitolterol mesilate]
bitoscanate INN
bitter ash *medicinal herb* [see: quassia; wahoo]

bitter ash; bitter quassia; bitter wood *medicinal herb* [see: quassia]

bitter buttons *medicinal herb* [see: tansy]

bitter cardamom ***(Alpinia fructus; A. oxyphylla)*** *medicinal herb for dementia, excessive water loss, and gastric lesions*

bitter cucumber *medicinal herb* [see: bitter melon]

bitter dogbane *medicinal herb* [see: dogbane]

bitter grass *medicinal herb* [see: star grass]

bitter herb *medicinal herb* [see: centaury]

bitter melon ***(Momordica charantia)*** fruit, leaves, seeds, oil *medicinal herb used as an antimicrobial and hypoglycemic; also used to reduce fertility in both males and females, and can act as an abortifacient*

bitter quassia; bitter ash; bitter wood *medicinal herb* [see: quassia tree]

bitter tonics; bitters *a class of agents that have a bitter taste, used as tonics, alteratives, or appetizers*

bitter wintergreen *medicinal herb* [see: pipsissewa]

bitter wood; bitter ash; bitter quassia *medicinal herb* [see: quassia tree]

bitterroot; bitterwort *medicinal herb* [see: dogbane; gentian]

bitters; bitter tonics *a class of agents that have a bitter taste, used as tonics, alteratives, or appetizers*

bittersweet herb; bittersweet twigs *medicinal herb* [see: bittersweet nightshade]

bittersweet nightshade ***(Solanum dulcamara)*** *medicinal herb for topical application on abrasions and felons; not generally regarded as safe for internal use, as it is highly toxic*

bitterweed *medicinal herb* [see: fleabane; horseweed]

bitterwort; bitterroot *medicinal herb* [see: gentian]

bivalirudin USAN *anticoagulant thrombin inhibitor for patients with unstable angina undergoing PTCA and to prevent DVT and reocclusion after MI*

bizelesin USAN, INN *antineoplastic*

B-Ject-100 injection ℞ *parenteral vitamin therapy* [multiple B vitamins]

black alder ***(Alnus glutinosa)*** bark and leaves *medicinal herb used as an astringent, demulcent, emetic, hemostatic, and tonic*

black alder dogwood *medicinal herb* [see: buckthorn; cascara sagrada]

black birch *medicinal herb* [see: birch]

black cherry; poison black cherry *medicinal herb* [see: belladonna]

black choke *medicinal herb* [see: wild black cherry]

black cohosh ***(Cimicifuga racemosa)*** root and rhizome *medicinal herb for asthma, bronchitis, dysmenorrhea, dyspepsia, epilepsy, hypertension, hormone imbalance, lung disorders, menopause, rheumatism, snake bite, sore throat, St. Vitus dance, and tuberculosis* 100 mg oral

black currant ***(Ribes nigrum)*** *medicinal herb* [see: currant]

black dogwood *medicinal herb* [see: buckthorn; cascara sagrada]

black elder *medicinal herb* [see: elderberry]

black false hellebore ***(Veratrum niger)*** [see: hellebore]

black ginger *medicinal herb* [see: ginger]

black hellebore ***(Helleborus niger)*** [see: hellebore]

black mulberry ***(Morus nigra)*** *medicinal herb* [see: mulberry]

black oak ***(Quercus tinctoria)*** *medicinal herb* [see: white oak]

black poplar ***(Populus nigra; P. tremula)*** buds *medicinal herb used as a diaphoretic, diuretic, expectorant, and vulnerary*

black root *medicinal herb* [see: Culver root]

black sanicle *medicinal herb* [see: sanicle]

black snakeroot *medicinal herb* [see: black cohosh; sanicle]

black walnut ***(Juglans nigra)*** hulls and leaves *medicinal herb for parasites, ringworm, skin rashes, and stop-*

ping lactation; also used as an external antiseptic

black widow spider antivenin [see: antivenin (Latrodectus mactans)]

black willow *(Salix nigra)* *medicinal herb* [see: willow]

blackberry *(Rubus fructicosus; R. villosus)* berries, leaves, and root bark *medicinal herb for bleeding, cholera, diarrhea in children, dysentery, sinus drainage, and vomiting*

Black-Draught syrup OTC *stimulant laxative* [casanthranol; senna extract; alcohol 5%] 90•? mg/15 mL

Black-Draught tablets, granules OTC *stimulant laxative* [sennosides] 6 mg; 20 mg/5 mL

blackwort *medicinal herb* [see: comfrey]

bladder fucus; bladderwrack *medicinal herb* [see: kelp *(Fucus)*]

bladderpod *medicinal herb* [see: lobelia]

Blairex Lens Lubricant solution OTC *rewetting solution for soft contact lenses*

Blairex Sterile Saline aerosol solution OTC *rinsing/storage solution for soft contact lenses* [sodium chloride (saline solution)]

blastomycin NF

blazing star *medicinal herb* [see: star grass]

blazing star *(Liatris scariosa; L. spicata; L. squarrosa)* root *medicinal herb used as a diuretic*

BlemErase lotion OTC *topical keratolytic for acne* [benzoyl peroxide] 10%

Blenoxane powder for IM, IV, subcu, or intrapleural injection ℞ *antibiotic antineoplastic for lymphomas, testicular and squamous cell carcinomas and malignant pleural effusion (orphan)* [bleomycin sulfate] 15, 30 U

BLEO-COMF (bleomycin, cyclophosphamide, Oncovin, methotrexate, fluorouracil) *chemotherapy protocol*

bleomycin (BLM) INN, BAN *glycopeptide antibiotic antineoplastic* [also: bleomycin sulfate; bleomycin HCl] ⓢ Cleocin

bleomycin HCl JAN *glycopeptide antibiotic antineoplastic* [also: bleomycin sulfate; bleomycin]

bleomycin sulfate USAN, USP, JAN *glycopeptide antibiotic antineoplastic for multiple carcinomas and malignant pleural effusion (orphan)* [also: bleomycin; bleomycin HCl] 15, 30 U injection

Bleph-10 eye drops, ophthalmic ointment ℞ *topical ophthalmic antibiotic* [sulfacetamide sodium] 10%

Blephamide eye drop suspension, ophthalmic ointment ℞ *topical ophthalmic corticosteroidal anti-inflammatory; antibiotic* [prednisolone acetate; sulfacetamide sodium] 0.2%•10%

blessed cardus; holy thistle *medicinal herb* [see: blessed thistle]

blessed thistle *(Cnicus benedictus)* plant *medicinal herb for blood cleansing, digestive disorders, headache, hormonal imbalance, lactation disorders, liver and gallbladder ailments, menstrual disorders, poor circulation, and strengthening heart and lungs*

Blighia sapida *medicinal herb* [see: ackee]

blind nettle *(Lamium album)* plant and flowers *medicinal herb used as an antispasmodic, astringent, expectorant, and styptic*

Blinx ophthalmic solution OTC *extraocular irrigating solution* [sterile isotonic solution]

BlisterGard liquid OTC *skin protectant*

Blistex ointment OTC *topical antipruritic/counterirritant; mild local anesthetic; vulnerary* [camphor; phenol; allantoin] 0.5%•0.5%•1%

Blistik lip balm OTC *antipruritic/counterirritant; mild local anesthetic; skin protectant; sunscreen (SPF 10)* [camphor; phenol; allantoin; dimethicone; padimate O; oxybenzone] 0.5%•0.5%•1%•2%•6.6%•2.5%

Blis-To-Sol liquid OTC *topical antifungal; keratolytic* [tolnaftate] 1%

Blis-To-Sol powder OTC *topical antifungal* [zinc undecylenate] 12%

BLM (bleomycin) [q.v.]

Blocadren tablets ℞ *antihypertensive; antiadrenergic (β-blocker); migraine prophylaxis* [timolol maleate] 5, 10, 20 mg

blocked ricin conjugated murine MAb [see: ricin (blocked) conjugated murine MAb]

blood, whole USP *blood replenisher*

blood, whole human [now: blood, whole]

blood cells, human red [now: blood cells, red]

blood cells, red USP *blood replenisher*

blood group specific substances A, B & AB USP *blood neutralizer*

blood grouping serum, anti-A [see: anti-A blood grouping serum]

blood grouping serum, anti-B [see: anti-B blood grouping serum]

blood grouping serum, anti-C USP *for in vitro blood testing*

blood grouping serum, anti-c USP *for in vitro blood testing*

blood grouping serum, anti-D USP *for in vitro blood testing*

blood grouping serum, anti-E USP *for in vitro blood testing*

blood grouping serum, anti-e USP *for in vitro blood testing*

blood mononuclear cells, allogenic peripheral *investigational (orphan) treatment for pancreatic cancer*

blood staunch *medicinal herb* [see: fleabane; horseweed]

blood volume expanders *a class of therapeutic blood modifiers used to increase the volume of circulating blood* [also called: plasma expanders]

bloodroot *(Sanguinaria canadensis)* root and rhizome *medicinal herb for diuresis, fever, inducing emesis, nasal polyps, rheumatism, sedation, skin cancer, stimulating menstrual flow, and warts; also used in toothpaste and mouthwash; not generally regarded as safe and effective for internal use*

BLP-25 *investigational liposomal formulation of MUC-1, an investigational cancer vaccine*

Bluboro powder packets OTC *astringent wet dressing (modified Burow solution)* [aluminum sulfate; calcium acetate]

blue cohosh *(Caulophyllum thalictroides)* root *medicinal herb for cramps, epilepsy, induction of labor, menstrual flow stimulant, nerves, and chronic uterine problems*

blue curls *medicinal herb* [see: woundwort]

blue flag *(Iris versicolor)* root *medicinal herb used as a cathartic, diuretic, laxative, sialagogue, and vermifuge*

Blue Gel OTC *pediculicide for lice* [pyrethrins; piperonyl butoxide; petroleum distillate] 0.3%•3%•1.2%

Blue Gel Muscular Pain Reliever gel OTC *topical analgesic; counterirritant* [menthol]

blue ginseng *medicinal herb* [see: blue cohosh]

blue gum tree *medicinal herb* [see: eucalyptus]

blue mountain tea *medicinal herb* [see: goldenrod]

blue pimpernel; blue skullcap *medicinal herb* [see: skullcap]

blue vervain *(Verbena hastata)* plant *medicinal herb for asthma, bladder and bowel disorders, bronchitis, colds, convulsions, cough, fever, insomnia, pulmonary tuberculosis, stomach upset, and worms*

blueberry *medicinal herb* [see: bilberry; blue cohosh]

bluebonnet; bluebottle *medicinal herb* [see: cornflower]

blue-green algae (Chloroplast membrane sulfolipids) *nutritional supplement for boosting the immune system*

bluensomycin INN *antibiotic*

BLyS protein *investigational (orphan) natural immunostimulant for common variable immunodeficiency (CVID, CVI), autoimmune diseases, and B-cell tumors*

B-MOPP (bleomycin, nitrogen mustard, Oncovin, procarbazine, prednisone) *chemotherapy protocol*

BMP (BCNU, methotrexate, procarbazine) *chemotherapy protocol*
BMS 232632 *investigational (Phase I) protease azapeptide inhibitor for HIV infection*
BMS 234475 *investigational (Phase II) second-generation protease inhibitor for HIV infection*
BNP-7787 *investigational (Phase I) chemotherapy protective agent*
BOAP (bleomycin, Oncovin, Adriamycin, prednisone) *chemotherapy protocol*
Bo-Cal tablets OTC *dietary supplement* [calcium; vitamin D; magnesium] 250 mg•100 IU•125 mg
boforsin [see: colforsin]
bofumustine INN
bogbean; bog myrtle *medicinal herb* [see: buckbean]
Boil-Ease ointment OTC *topical local anesthetic* [benzocaine] 20%
bolandiol INN *anabolic* [also: bolandiol dipropionate]
bolandiol dipropionate USAN, JAN *anabolic* [also: bolandiol]
bolasterone USAN, INN *anabolic steroid; also abused as a street drug*
bolazine INN
BOLD (bleomycin, Oncovin, lomustine, dacarbazine) *chemotherapy protocol*
Boldea fragrans *medicinal herb* [see: boldo]
boldenone INN, BAN *veterinary anabolic steroid; also abused as a street drug* [also: boldenone undecylenate]
boldenone undecylenate USAN *veterinary anabolic steroid; also abused as a street drug* [also: boldenone]
boldo *(Peumus boldus)* plant and leaves *medicinal herb for bile stimulation, colds, constipation, digestive disorders, earache, edema, gallstones, gonorrhea, gout, liver disease, rheumatism, syphilis, and worms*
Boldu boldus *medicinal herb* [see: boldo]
bolenol USAN, INN *anabolic*
bolmantalate USAN, INN, BAN *anabolic*
bolus alba [see: kaolin]
Bombay aloe *medicinal herb* [see: aloe]
bometolol INN
BOMP (bleomycin, Oncovin, Matulane, prednisone) *chemotherapy protocol*
BOMP; CLD-BOMP (bleomycin, Oncovin, mitomycin, Platinol) *chemotherapy protocol for cervical cancer*
Bonamil Infant Formula with Iron powder, oral liquid OTC *total or supplementary infant feeding* 453 g; 384, 946 mL
Bonamine (CAN) chewable tablets OTC *anticholinergic; antihistamine; antivertigo agent; motion sickness preventative* [meclizine HCl] 25 mg ⚠ Bonine
Bondronat ℞ *bone resorption inhibitor for postmenopausal osteoporosis, metastatic bone disease, hypercalcemia of malignancy, and Paget disease* [ibandronate sodium]
bone ash [see: calcium phosphate, tribasic]
Bone Meal tablets OTC *dietary supplement* [calcium; phosphorus] 236•118 mg
bone powder, purified [see: calcium phosphate, tribasic]
Bonefos (CAN) capsules, IV infusion ℞ *bisphosphonate bone resorption inhibitor for hypercalcemia and osteolysis of malignancy (investigational [orphan] in the U.S.)* [clodronate disodium tetrahydrate] 400 mg; 60 mg/mL
boneset *(Eupatorium perfoliatum)* plant *medicinal herb for chills, colds, constipation, dengue fever, edema, fever, flu, pneumonia, and rheumatism*
Bonine chewable tablets OTC *anticholinergic; antihistamine; antivertigo agent; motion sickness preventative* [meclizine HCl] 25 mg ⚠ Bonamine
Bontril slow-release capsules ℞ *anorexiant; CNS stimulant* [phendimetrazine tartrate] 105 mg ⚠ Bentyl; Vontrol
Bontril PDM tablets ℞ *anorexiant; CNS stimulant* [phendimetrazine tartrate] 35 mg
Bonviva ℞ *bone resorption inhibitor for postmenopausal osteoporosis, meta-*

static bone disease, hypercalcemia of malignancy, and Paget disease [ibandronate sodium]

bookoo *medicinal herb* [see: buchu]

Boost liquid, pudding OTC *enteral nutritional therapy* [milk-based formula] 237 mL

BOP (BCNU, Oncovin, prednisone) *chemotherapy protocol*

BOPAM (bleomycin, Oncovin, prednisone, Adriamycin, mechlorethamine, methotrexate) *chemotherapy protocol*

bopindolol INN

BOPP (BCNU, Oncovin, procarbazine, prednisone) *chemotherapy protocol*

boracic acid [see: boric acid]

borage *(Borago officinalis)* leaves *medicinal herb for bronchitis, colds, eye inflammation, hay fever, strengthening of heart, lactation stimulation, rashes, rheumatism, ringworm; not generally regarded as safe and effective*

borax [see: sodium borate]

Borbonia pinifolia *medicinal herb* [see: red bush tea]

boric acid NF, JAN *acidifying agent; ophthalmic emollient; antiseptic; astringent* 10% topical

2-bornanone [see: camphor]

bornaprine INN, BAN

bornaprolol INN

bornelone USAN, INN *ultraviolet screen*

bornyl acetate USAN

borocaptate sodium B 10 USAN *antineoplastic; radioactive agent* [also: sodium borocaptate (^{10}B)]

Borocell ℞ *investigational (orphan) for boron neutron capture therapy (BNCT) for glioblastoma multiforme* [sodium monomercaptoundecahydro-closo-dodecaborate]

Borofair Otic ear drops ℞ *antibacterial; antifungal; astringent* [acetic acid; aluminum acetate] 2%•?

Borofax Skin Protectant ointment OTC *astringent* [zinc oxide] 15%

boroglycerin NF

boron *element (B); trace mineral for enhancing mental acuity and improving alertness; not generally regarded as safe, as it is highly toxic if taken internally or absorbed through broken skin*

Boropak powder packets OTC *astringent wet dressing (modified Burrow solution)* [aluminum sulfate; calcium acetate]

bosentan USAN, INN *investigational (NDA filed) endothelin receptor antagonist for pulmonary hypertension; investigational for vasospastic diseases*

Boston Advance Cleaner; Boston Cleaner solution OTC *cleaning solution for rigid gas permeable contact lenses*

Boston Advance Comfort Formula solution OTC *disinfecting/wetting/soaking solution for rigid gas permeable contact lenses*

Boston Conditioning Solution OTC *disinfecting/wetting/soaking solution for rigid gas permeable contact lenses*

Boston Rewetting Drops OTC *rewetting solution for rigid gas permeable contact lenses*

Boswellia serrata *medicinal herb* [see: frankincense]

Botanol (CAN) oral liquid OTC *dietary supplement* [potassium; magnesium; iron; iodine; herbal extracts] 779•25.2•2.7•0.045•335 mg per 30 mL

botiacrine INN

Botox powder for injection ℞ *neurotoxin complex for blepharospasm and strabismus of dystonia (orphan) and cervical dystonia (orphan); investigational (orphan) for pediatric cerebral palsy* [botulinum toxin, type A] 100 U/vial

BottomBetter ointment OTC *topical diaper rash treatment*

botulinum toxin, type A *neurotoxin complex derived from Clostridium botulinum, type A; treatment for blepharospasm and strabismus of dystonia (orphan) and cervical dystonia (orphan); investigational (orphan) for pediatric cerebral palsy*

botulinum toxin, type B *neurotoxin complex derived from Clostridium bot-*

ulinum, type B; symptomatic treatment of cervical dystonia (orphan)

botulinum toxin, type F *investigational (orphan) for spasmodic torticollis (cervical dystonia) and essential blepharospasm*

botulinum toxoid, pentavalent (ABCDE) *investigational vaccine (available only from the Centers for Disease Control and Prevention)*

botulism antitoxin USP *passive immunizing agent*

botulism equine antitoxin, trivalent *passive immunizing agent*

botulism immune globulin *investigational (orphan) for infant botulism*

Bounty Bears chewable tablets OTC *vitamin supplement* [multiple vitamins; folic acid] ≛•0.3 mg

Bounty Bears Plus Iron chewable tablets OTC *vitamin/iron supplement* [multiple vitamins; iron; folic acid] ≛•15•0.3 mg

bourbonal [see: ethyl vanillin]

bovactant BAN

bovine colostrum [see: *Cryptosporidium parvum* bovine colostrum IgG concentrate]

bovine fibrin BAN

bovine immunoglobulin concentrate [see: *Cryptosporidium parvum* bovine colostrum IgG concentrate]

bovine myelin *investigational (Phase III) oral treatment for multiple sclerosis*

bovine superoxide dismutase (bSOD) [see: orgotein]

bovine whey protein concentrate [see: *Cryptosporidium parvum* bovine colostrum IgG concentrate]

bower, virgin's *medicinal herb* [see: woodbine]

Bowman's root *medicinal herb* [see: Culver root]

box, mountain *medicinal herb* [see: uva ursi]

boxberry *medicinal herb* [see: wintergreen]

boxidine USAN, INN *antihyperlipoproteinemic*

Boyol salve OTC *topical anti-infective; anesthetic* [ichthammol; benzocaine] 10%•≟ ⓢ boil

B-PAS (benzoyl para-aminosalicylate) [see: benzoylpas calcium]

BPD-MA (benzoporphyrin derivative) [see: verteporfin]

BPI (bactericidal and permeability-increasing) protein [q.v.]

BPI-21 *investigational agent for multiple drug-resistant bacteria, alone or in combination with antibiotics*

B-Plex tablets ℞ *vitamin supplement* [multiple B vitamins; vitamin C; folic acid] ≛•500•0.5 mg

brain-derived neurotrophic factor (BDNF) *investigational (Phase III) treatment for brain and nerve degenerative diseases; clinical trials for ALS discontinued 1997*

brallobarbital INN

bramble *medicinal herb* [see: blackberry]

BranchAmin 4% IV infusion ℞ *nutritional therapy for high metabolic stress* [multiple branched-chain essential amino acids]

branched-chain amino acids (BCAA) *investigational (orphan) for amyotrophic lateral sclerosis* [see: isoleucine; leucine; valine]

brandy mint *medicinal herb* [see: peppermint]

Brasivol cream OTC *abrasive cleanser for acne* [aluminum oxide]

brasofensine maleate USAN *investigational dopamine reuptake inhibitor for Parkinson disease*

Brassica alba *medicinal herb* [see: mustard]

Bravavir ℞ *investigational (NDA filed) antiviral for varicella zoster and herpes zoster in AIDS; orphan status withdrawn 1997* [sorivudine]

brazergoline INN

Breathe Free nasal spray OTC *nasal moisturizer* [sodium chloride (saline solution)] 0.65%

Breezee Mist Aerosol powder OTC *topical antifungal; analgesic; anhidrotic*

[undecylenic acid; menthol; aluminum chlorohydrate]

Breezee Mist Antifungal powder OTC *topical antifungal* [miconazole nitrate] [note: one of two different products with the same name] 2%

Breezee Mist Antifungal powder OTC *topical antifungal* [tolnaftate] [note: one of two different products with the same name] 1%

Breezee Mist Foot Powder OTC *topical anhidrotic* [talc; aluminum chlorohydrate]

brefonalol INN

bremazocine INN

Breonesin capsules OTC *expectorant* [guaifenesin] 200 mg

brequinar INN *antineoplastic* [also: brequinar sodium]

brequinar sodium USAN *antineoplastic* [also: brequinar]

bretazenil USAN, INN *anxiolytic*

Brethaire oral inhalation aerosol (discontinued 2001) ℞ *sympathomimetic bronchodilator* [terbutaline sulfate] 0.2 mg/dose

Brethine tablets, IV or subcu injection ℞ *sympathomimetic bronchodilator* [terbutaline sulfate] 2.5, 5 mg; 1 mg/mL ⑨ Banthine

bretylium tosilate INN *antiadrenergic; antiarrhythmic* [also: bretylium tosylate]

bretylium tosylate USAN, BAN *antiadrenergic; antiarrhythmic* [also: bretylium tosilate] 500, 1000 mg/vial injection

Bretylol IV or IM injection (discontinued 1997) ℞ *antiarrhythmic* [bretylium tosylate] 50 mg/mL ⑨ Brevital

BrevaRex ℞ *investigational (Phase II, orphan) therapeutic vaccine for solid tumors* [monoclonal antibody B43.13]

Brevibloc IV infusion ℞ *antiadrenergic (β-blocker); antiarrhythmic for supraventricular tachycardia* [esmolol HCl] 10, 250 mg/mL

Brevicon tablets (in Wallettes of 21 or 28) ℞ *monophasic oral contraceptive* [norethindrone; ethinyl estradiol] 0.5 mg•35 µg

Brevital Sodium powder for IV injection ℞ *barbiturate general anesthetic* [methohexital sodium] 0.5, 2.5, 5 g ⑨ Bretylol

Brevoxyl gel ℞ *keratolytic for acne* [benzoyl peroxide] 4%, 8%

Brevoxyl Cleansing lotion ℞ *keratolytic for acne* [benzoyl peroxide] 4%, 8%

Brevoxyl Creamy Wash liquid ℞ *keratolytic for acne* [benzoyl peroxide] 4%, 8%

brewer's yeast *natural source of protein and B-complex vitamins*

Brexidol 20 (CAN) tablets ℞ *analgesic; antirheumatic; nonsteroidal anti-inflammatory drug (NSAID)* [piroxicam betadex] 191.2 mg (equivalent to 20 mg of piroxicam)

Brexin-L.A. sustained-release capsules ℞ *decongestant; antihistamine* [pseudoephedrine HCl; chlorpheniramine maleate] 120•8 mg

Bricanyl tablets, IV or subcu injection ℞ *sympathomimetic bronchodilator* [terbutaline sulfate] 2.5, 5 mg; 1 mg/mL

Brietal Sodium (CAN) powder for IV injection (discontinued 2001) ℞ *barbiturate general anesthetic* [methohexital sodium] 10 mg/mL

brifentanil INN *narcotic analgesic* [also: brifentanil HCl]

brifentanil HCl USAN *narcotic analgesic* [also: brifentanil]

Brigham tea; Brigham Young weed *medicinal herb* [see: ephedra]

Brik-Paks (trademarked delivery form) *ready-to-use liquid containers*

brimonidine INN *ophthalmic α_2-adrenergic agonist for open-angle glaucoma and ocular hypertension* [also: brimonidine tartrate]

brimonidine tartrate USAN *ophthalmic α_2-adrenergic agonist for open-angle glaucoma and ocular hypertension* [also: brimonidine]

brinaldix [see: clopamide]

brinase INN [also: brinolase]
brinazarone INN
brindoxime INN
brineurin [now: abrineurin] [USAN changed 2000]
brinolase USAN *fibrinolytic enzyme* [also: brinase]
brinzolamide USAN, INN *carbonic anhydrase inhibitor for glaucoma*
Bristoject (trademarked delivery form) *prefilled disposable syringe*
British antilewisite (BAL) [now: dimercaprol]
British tobacco *medicinal herb* [see: coltsfoot]
brivudine INN
brobactam INN
brobenzoxaldine [see: broxaldine]
broclepride INN
brocresine USAN, INN, BAN *histidine decarboxylase inhibitor*
brocrinat USAN, INN *diuretic*
brodimoprim INN
brofaromine INN *investigational reversible/selective* MAO *inhibitor*
Brofed elixir ℞ *decongestant; antihistamine* [pseudoephedrine HCl; brompheniramine maleate] 30•4 mg/5 mL
brofezil INN, BAN
brofoxine USAN, INN *antipsychotic*
brolaconazole INN
brolamfetamine INN
Brolene eye drops *investigational (orphan) for Acanthamoeba keratitis* [propamidine isethionate] 0.1%
bromacrylide INN
bromadel [see: carbromal]
Bromadine-DM syrup ℞ *antitussive; decongestant; antihistamine* [dextromethorphan hydrobromide; pseudoephedrine HCl; brompheniramine maleate] 10•30•2 mg/5 mL
Bromadine-DX syrup ℞ *antitussive; decongestant; antihistamine* [dextromethorphan hydrobromide; pseudoephedrine HCl; brompheniramine maleate] 10•30•2 mg/5 mL
bromadoline INN *analgesic* [also: bromadoline maleate]
bromadoline maleate USAN *analgesic* [also: bromadoline]
Bromaline elixir OTC *decongestant; antihistamine* [phenylpropanolamine HCl; brompheniramine maleate] 12.5•2 mg/5 mL
bromamid INN
Bromanate elixir OTC *decongestant; antihistamine* [phenylpropanolamine HCl; brompheniramine maleate] 12.5•2 mg/5 mL
Bromanate DC Cough syrup ℞ *narcotic antitussive; decongestant; antihistamine* [codeine phosphate; phenylpropanolamine HCl; brompheniramine maleate; alcohol] 10•12.5•2 mg/5 mL
Bromanyl syrup (discontinued 2000) ℞ *narcotic antitussive; antihistamine* [codeine phosphate; bromodiphenhydramine HCl] 10•12.5 mg/5 mL
bromanylpromide [see: bromamid]
Bromarest DX Cough syrup ℞ *antitussive; decongestant; antihistamine* [dextromethorphan hydrobromide; pseudoephedrine HCl; brompheniramine maleate; alcohol 0.95%] 10•30•2 mg/5 mL
Bromatane DX Cough syrup ℞ *antitussive; decongestant; antihistamine* [dextromethorphan hydrobromide; pseudoephedrine HCl; brompheniramine maleate] 10•30•2 mg/5 mL
Bromatapp extended-release tablets OTC *decongestant; antihistamine* [phenylpropanolamine HCl; brompheniramine maleate] 75•12 mg
bromauric acid NF
bromazepam USAN, INN, BAN, JAN *benzodiazepine anxiolytic; minor tranquilizer*
bromazine INN, DCF *antihistamine* [also: bromodiphenhydramine HCl; bromodiphenhydramine]
bromazine HCl [see: bromodiphenhydramine HCl]
brombenzonium [see: bromhexine HCl]
bromchlorenone USAN, INN *topical anti-infective*
bromebric acid INN, BAN

bromelain JAN *anti-inflammatory; proteolytic enzymes* [also: bromelains]
bromelains USAN, INN, BAN *anti-inflammatory; proteolytic enzymes* [also: bromelain]
bromelin [see: bromelains]
bromerguride INN
brometenamine INN, DCF
bromethol [see: tribromoethanol]
Bromfed syrup OTC *decongestant; antihistamine* [pseudoephedrine HCl; brompheniramine maleate] 30•2 mg/5 mL ⑨ Bromphen
Bromfed tablets, timed-release capsules ℞ *decongestant; antihistamine* [pseudoephedrine HCl; brompheniramine maleate] 60•4 mg; 120•12 mg
Bromfed-DM Cough syrup ℞ *antitussive; decongestant; antihistamine* [dextromethorphan hydrobromide; pseudoephedrine HCl; brompheniramine maleate] 10•30•2 mg/5 mL
Bromfed-PD timed-release capsules ℞ *pediatric decongestant and antihistamine* [pseudoephedrine HCl; brompheniramine maleate] 60•6 mg
bromfenac INN *long-acting nonsteroidal anti-inflammatory drug (NSAID); analgesic; antipyretic* [also: bromfenac sodium]
bromfenac sodium USAN *long-acting nonsteroidal anti-inflammatory drug (NSAID); analgesic; antipyretic* [also: bromfenac]
Bromfenex extended-release capsules ℞ *decongestant; antihistamine* [pseudoephedrine HCl; brompheniramine maleate] 120•12 mg
Bromfenex PD extended-release capsules ℞ *pediatric decongestant and antihistamine* [pseudoephedrine HCl; brompheniramine maleate] 60•6 mg
bromhexine INN, BAN *expectorant; mucolytic; investigational (orphan) for keratoconjunctivitis sicca of Sjögren syndrome* [also: bromhexine HCl]
bromhexine HCl USAN, JAN *expectorant; mucolytic* [also: bromhexine]
bromindione USAN, INN, BAN *anticoagulant*
bromine *element (Br)*
bromisoval INN [also: bromisovalum; bromvalerylurea; bromovaluree]
bromisovalum NF [also: bromisoval; bromvalerylurea; bromovaluree]
2-bromo-α-ergocryptine [see: bromocriptine]
bromocamphor [see: camphor, monobromated]
bromociclen INN [also: bromocyclen]
bromocriptine USAN, INN, BAN *dopamine agonist; prolactin enzyme inhibitor; antiparkinsonian*
bromocriptine mesilate JAN *dopamine agonist; prolactin enzyme inhibitor; antiparkinsonian* [also: bromocriptine mesylate]
bromocriptine mesylate USAN, USP *dopamine agonist; prolactin enzyme inhibitor; antiparkinsonian; investigational (NDA filed) agent for diabetic control of hypoglycemia; investigational (Phase II/III) treatment for obesity* [also: bromocriptine mesilate]
bromocyclen BAN [also: bromociclen]
bromodeoxyuridine [now: broxuridine]
bromodiethylacetylurea [see: carbromal]
bromodiphenhydramine BAN *antihistamine* [also: bromodiphenhydramine HCl; bromazine]
bromodiphenhydramine HCl USP *antihistamine* [also: bromazine; bromodiphenhydramine]
bromofenofos INN
bromoform USP
bromofos INN
1-bromoheptadecafluorooctane [see: perflubron]
bromoisovaleryl urea (BVU) [see: bromisovalum]
Bromophen T.D. sustained-release tablets ℞ *decongestant; antihistamine* [phenylpropanolamine HCl; phenylephrine HCl; brompheniramine maleate] 15•15•12 mg ⑨ Bromphen
bromophenol blue
bromophin [see: apomorphine HCl]
bromophos [see: bromofos]
bromopride INN, DCF

Bromo-Seltzer effervescent granules OTC *antacid; analgesic; antipyretic* [sodium bicarbonate; citric acid; acetaminophen] 2781•2224•325 mg/dose

bromotheophyllinate aminoisobutanol [see: pamabrom]

bromotheophyllinate pyranisamine [see: pyrabrom]

bromotheophyllinate pyrilamine [see: pyrabrom]

8-bromotheophylline [see: pamabrom]

Bromotuss with Codeine syrup ℞ *narcotic antitussive; antihistamine* [codeine phosphate; bromodiphenhydramine HCl] 10•12.5 mg/5 mL

bromovaluree DCF [also: bromisovalum; bromisoval; bromvalerylurea]

11-bromovincamine [see: brovincamine]

bromovinyl arabinosyluracil (BV-araU) [see: sorivudine]

bromoxanide USAN, INN *anthelmintic*

bromperidol USAN, INN, BAN, JAN *antipsychotic*

bromperidol decanoate USAN, BAN *antipsychotic*

Bromphen elixir (discontinued 1997) OTC *antihistamine* [brompheniramine maleate] 2 mg/5 mL ⊡ Bromfed; Bromophen

Bromphen DC with Codeine Cough syrup (discontinued 2000) ℞ *narcotic antitussive; decongestant; antihistamine* [codeine phosphate; phenylpropanolamine HCl; brompheniramine maleate] 10•12.5•2 mg/5 mL

Bromphen DX Cough syrup ℞ *antitussive; decongestant; antihistamine* [dextromethorphan hydrobromide; pseudoephedrine HCl; brompheniramine maleate; alcohol 0.95%] 10•30•2 mg/5 mL

brompheniramine INN, BAN *alkylamine antihistamine* [also: brompheniramine maleate]

Brompheniramine Cough syrup OTC *antitussive; decongestant; antihistamine* [dextromethorphan hydrobromide; pseudoephedrine HCl; brompheniramine maleate; alcohol 0.95%] 10•30•2 mg/5 mL

Brompheniramine DC Cough syrup ℞ *narcotic antitussive; decongestant; antihistamine* [codeine phosphate; phenylpropanolamine HCl; brompheniramine maleate; alcohol 1.15%] 10•12.5•2 mg/5 mL

brompheniramine maleate USP *alkylamine antihistamine* [also: brompheniramine]

brompheniramine maleate & pseudoephedrine HCl & dextromethorphan hydrobromide *antihistamine; nasal decongestant; antitussive* 4•80•15 mg/5 mL oral

Brompton's Cocktail; Brompton's Mixture (refers to any oral narcotic/alcoholic solution containing morphine and either cocaine or a phenothiazine derivative) *prophylaxis for chronic, severe pain*

bromvalerylurea JAN [also: bromisovalum; bromisoval; bromovaluree]

Bronalide (CAN) oral inhalation aerosol (discontinued 2000) ℞ *corticosteroid for bronchial asthma* [flunisolide] 250 µg/dose

Bronchial capsules ℞ *antiasthmatic; bronchodilator; expectorant* [theophylline; guaifenesin] 150•90 mg

Broncho Saline aerosol OTC *diluent for inhalation bronchodilators; solution for tracheal lavage* [sodium chloride (saline solution)] 0.9%

Broncholate softgels, syrup ℞ *decongestant; expectorant* [ephedrine HCl; guaifenesin] 12.5•200 mg; 6.25•100 mg/5 mL ⊡ Brondelate

Brondelate elixir ℞ *antiasthmatic; bronchodilator; expectorant* [theophylline; guaifenesin] 192•150 mg/15 mL ⊡ Broncholate

Bronitin Mist inhalation aerosol (discontinued 1999) OTC *sympathomimetic bronchodilator* [epinephrine bitartrate] 0.3 mg/dose

Bronkaid Dual Action caplets OTC *decongestant; expectorant* [ephedrine sulfate; guaifenesin] 25•400 mg

Bronkaid Mist inhalation aerosol (discontinued 1999) OTC *sympathomimetic bronchodilator* [epinephrine nitrate & epinephrine HCl] 0.5%

Bronkodyl capsules ℞ *antiasthmatic; bronchodilator* [theophylline] 100, 200 mg

Bronkometer inhalation aerosol (discontinued 1999) ℞ *sympathomimetic bronchodilator* [isoetharine mesylate] 0.61% (340 µg/dose)

Bronkosol solution for inhalation (discontinued 1999) ℞ *sympathomimetic bronchodilator* [isoetharine HCl] 1%

Bronkotuss Expectorant liquid ℞ *decongestant; antihistamine; expectorant* [ephedrine sulfate; chlorpheniramine maleate; guaifenesin; hydriodic acid; alcohol 5%] 8.2•4•100•1.67 mg/5 mL

bronopol INN, BAN, JAN

Brontex tablets, liquid ℞ *narcotic antitussive; expectorant* [codeine phosphate; guaifenesin] 10•300 mg; 2.5•75 mg/5 mL

brook bean *medicinal herb* [see: buckbean]

brooklime *(Veronica beccabunga)* plant *medicinal herb used as a diuretic, emmenagogue, and febrifuge*

broom *(Cytisus scoparius)* plant and bloom *medicinal herb for inducing bowel evacuation, diuresis, and emesis; also used as a homeopathic remedy for arrhythmias, diphtheria, and head and throat congestion*

broom, butcher's *medicinal herb* [see: butcher's broom]

broom, dyer's; green broom *medicinal herb* [see: dyer's broom]

broparestrol INN, DCF

broperamole USAN, INN *anti-inflammatory*

bropirimine USAN, INN *antineoplastic; antiviral*

broquinaldol INN

brosotamide INN, DCF

brosuximide INN

brotianide INN, BAN

brotizolam USAN, INN, BAN, JAN *hypnotic*

brovanexine INN

brovavir [see: sorivudine]

brovincamine INN [also: brovincamine fumarate]

brovincamine fumarate JAN [also: brovinacamine]

brown algae *medicinal herb* [see: kelp *(Laminaria)*]

brownwort *medicinal herb* [see: woundwort]

broxaldine INN, DCF

broxaterol INN

Broxine ℞ *investigational (NDA filed, orphan) radiosensitizer for breast and brain tumors* [broxuridine]

broxitalamic acid INN

broxuridine INN *investigational (NDA filed, orphan) radiosensitizer for breast and brain tumors*

broxyquinoline INN, DCF

brucine sulfate NF

bruisewort *medicinal herb* [see: comfrey; soapwort]

bryony *(Bryonia alba; B. dioica)* root *medicinal herb used as a pectoral and purgative; not generally regarded as safe, as the root is poisonous in high doses (ingestion of as few as 40 berries can be fatal in adults, 15 in children)*

B-Salt Forte ophthalmic solution ℞ *intraocular irrigating solution* [sodium chloride (balanced saline solution)]

bSOD (bovine superoxide dismutase) [see: orgotein]

BSS (bismuth subsalicylate) [q.v.]

BSS; BSS Plus ophthalmic solution ℞ *intraocular irrigating solution* [sodium chloride (balanced saline solution)]

BTA Rapid Urine Test test kit for professional use *in vitro diagnostic aid for bladder tumor analytes in the urine*

BTA Stat Test test kit for home use *in vitro diagnostic aid for bladder tumor analytes in the urine* [rapid immunoassay (RIA)]

BTI-322 *investigational (Phase II) monoclonal antibody for graft vs. host disease*

bucainide INN *antiarrhythmic* [also: bucainide maleate]
bucainide maleate USAN *antiarrhythmic* [also: bucainide]
bucco *medicinal herb* [see: buchu]
Bucet capsules ℞ *sedative; barbiturate analgesic* [butalbital; acetaminophen] 50•650 mg
bucetin INN, BAN, JAN
buchu ***(Agathosma betulina; Barosma betulina; B. cenulata; B. serratifolia)*** leaves *medicinal herb for edema, gas, gout, inflammation, kidney and urinary tract infections, and prostatitis; also used as a douche for leukorrhea and vaginal yeast infections*
buciclovir INN
bucillamine INN, JAN
bucindolol INN, BAN *antihypertensive* [also: bucindolol HCl]
bucindolol HCl USAN *antihypertensive* [also: bucindolol]
buckbean ***(Menyanthes trifoliata)*** leaves *medicinal herb used as a tonic, cathartic, diuretic, anthelmintic, and emetic*
buckeye; California buckeye; Ohio buckeye *medicinal herb* [see: horse chestnut]
buckhorn brake ***(Osmunda cinnamomea; O. regalis)*** root *medicinal herb used as a demulcent and tonic*
buckthorn ***(Rhamnus cathartica; R. frangula)*** bark and berries *medicinal herb for bleeding, bowel disorders, chronic constipation, fever, gallstones, lead poisoning, and liver disorders* [also see: cascara sagrada]
bucku *medicinal herb* [see: buchu]
bucladesine INN [also: bucladesine sodium]
bucladesine sodium JAN [also: bucladesine]
buclizine INN, BAN *antinauseant; antiemetic; anticholinergic; motion sickness relief* [also: buclizine HCl]
buclizine HCl USAN *antinauseant; antiemetic; anticholinergic; motion sickness relief* [also: buclizine]
buclosamide INN, BAN, DCF
bucloxic acid INN, DCF
bucolome INN, JAN
bucricaine INN
bucrilate INN *tissue adhesive* [also: bucrylate]
bucromarone USAN, INN *antiarrhythmic*
bucrylate USAN *tissue adhesive* [also: bucrilate]
bucumolol INN [also: bucumolol HCl]
bucumolol HCl JAN [also: bucumolol]
budesonide USAN, INN, BAN, JAN *corticosteroidal anti-inflammatory for chronic asthma, rhinitis, and inflammatory bowel disease*
budipine INN
budotitane INN
budralazine INN, JAN
bufenadine [see: bufenadrine]
bufenadrine INN
bufeniode INN, DCF
bufetolol INN [also: bufetolol HCl]
bufetolol HCl JAN [also: bufetolol]
bufexamac INN, BAN, JAN, DCF
bufezolac INN
buffered aspirin [see: aspirin, buffered]
Bufferin coated tablets, coated caplets OTC *analgesic; antipyretic; anti-inflammatory; antirheumatic* [aspirin (buffered with calcium carbonate, magnesium oxide, and magnesium carbonate)] 325, 500 mg
Bufferin AF Nite Time tablets OTC *antihistaminic sleep aid; analgesic* [diphenhydramine HCl; acetaminophen] 30•500 mg
Buffets II tablets (discontinued 2000) OTC *analgesic; antipyretic; anti-inflammatory; antacid* [acetaminophen; aspirin; caffeine; aluminum hydroxide] 162•227•32.4•50 mg
Buffex tablets OTC *analgesic; antipyretic; anti-inflammatory; antirheumatic* [aspirin (buffered with aluminum glycinate and magnesium carbonate)] 325 mg
bufilcon A USAN *hydrophilic contact lens material*
buflomedil INN, BAN, DCF
bufogenin INN
buformin USAN, INN *antidiabetic*

Buf-Puf Acne Cleansing bar (discontinued 1997) OTC *medicated cleanser for acne* [salicylic acid; vitamin E] 2%•?

bufrolin INN, BAN

bufuralol INN, BAN

bufylline BAN *diuretic; smooth muscle relaxant* [also: ambuphylline]

bugbane *medicinal herb* [see: hellebore; black cohosh]

bugleweed *(Lycopus virginicus)* plant *medicinal herb for cough, excessive menses, nervous indigestion, and other nervous disorders*

bugloss *medicinal herb* [see: borage]

Bugs Bunny Complete chewable tablets OTC *vitamin/mineral/calcium/iron supplement* [multiple vitamins & minerals; calcium; iron; folic acid; biotin] ≛•100•18•0.4•0.04 mg

Bugs Bunny Plus Iron chewable tablets OTC *vitamin/iron supplement* [multiple vitamins; iron; folic acid] ≛•15•0.3 mg

Bugs Bunny with Extra C Children's chewable tablets OTC *vitamin supplement* [multiple vitamins; folic acid] ≛•0.3 mg

bugwort *medicinal herb* [see: black cohosh]

buku *medicinal herb* [see: buchu]

Bulk Forming Fiber Laxative film-coated tablets OTC *bulk laxative; antidiarrheal* [calcium polycarbophil] 625 mg

bulk-producing laxatives *a subclass of laxatives that work by increasing the hydration and volume of stool to stimulate peristalsis; also form an emollient gel to ease the movement of stool through the intestines* [see also: laxatives]

bull's foot *medicinal herb* [see: coltsfoot]

bumadizone INN, DCF

bumecaine INN

bumepidil INN

bumetanide USAN, USP, INN, BAN, JAN *loop diuretic* 0.25 mg/mL injection

bumetrizole USAN, INN *ultraviolet screen*

Bumex tablets, IV or IM injection ℞ *loop diuretic* [bumetanide] 0.5, 1, 2 mg; 0.25 mg/mL

Buminate 5%; Buminate 25% IV infusion ℞ *blood volume expander for shock, burns, and hypoproteinemia* [human albumin] 5%; 25%

bunaftine INN

bunamidine INN, BAN *anthelmintic* [also: bunamidine HCl]

bunamidine HCl USAN *anthelmintic* [also: bunamidine]

bunamiodyl INN [also: buniodyl]

bunamiodyl sodium [see: bunamiodyl; buniodyl]

bunaprolast USAN, INN *antiasthmatic; 5-lipoxygenase inhibitor*

bunapsilate INN *combining name for radicals or groups*

bunazosin INN [also: bunazosin HCl]

bunazosin HCl JAN [also: bunazosin]

bundlin [now: sedecamycin]

buniodyl BAN [also: bunamiodyl]

bunitrolol INN [also: bunitrolol HCl]

bunitrolol HCl JAN [also: bunitrolol]

bunolol INN *antiadrenergic (β-receptor)* [also: bunolol HCl]

bunolol HCl USAN *antiadrenergic (β-receptor)* [also: bunolol]

Bupap caplets ℞ *analgesic; antipyretic; barbiturate sedative* [acetaminophen; butalbital] 650•50 mg

buparvaquone INN, BAN

buphenine INN, BAN *peripheral vasodilator* [also: nylidrin HCl]

Buphenyl tablets, powder for oral solution ℞ *antihyperammonemic for urea cycle disorders (orphan); investigational (orphan) for various sickling disorders* [sodium phenylbutyrate] 500 mg; 3 g/tsp., 8.6 g/tbsp.

bupicomide USAN, INN *antihypertensive*

bupivacaine INN, BAN *injectable local anesthetic* [also: bupivacaine HCl]

bupivacaine HCl USAN, USP, JAN *injectable local anesthetic* [also: bupivacaine] 0.25%, 0.5%, 0.75%

bupranol [see: bupranolol]

bupranolol INN, DCF [also: bupranolol HCl]

bupranolol HCl JAN [also: bupranolol]

Buprenex IV or IM injection ℞ *narcotic agonist-antagonist analgesic* [buprenorphine HCl] 0.324 mg/mL

buprenorphine INN, BAN *narcotic agonist-antagonist analgesic* [also: buprenorphine HCl]

buprenorphine HCl USAN, JAN *narcotic agonist-antagonist analgesic; investigational (orphan) for opiate addictions* [also: buprenorphine]

buprenorphine HCl & naloxone HCl *investigational (orphan) for opiate addictions*

bupropion BAN *aminoketone antidepressant; non-nicotine aid to smoking cessation* [also: bupropion HCl; amfebutamone]

bupropion HCl USAN *aminoketone antidepressant; non-nicotine aid to smoking cessation* [also: amfebutamone; bupropion] 75, 100 mg oral

buquineran INN, BAN

buquinolate USAN, INN *coccidiostat for poultry*

buquiterine INN

buramate USAN, INN *anticonvulsant; antipsychotic*

burdock *(Arctium lappa; A. majus; A. minus)* root *medicinal herb for arthritis, blood cleansing, dandruff, eczema, edema, fever, gout, kidney and lung disorders, rheumatism, skin diseases, and tumors; also used as an antimicrobial and diaphoretic*

burefrine [now: berefrine]

burnet *(Pimpinella magna; P. saxifrage)* root *medicinal herb used as an antispasmodic, astringent, carminative, diaphoretic, diuretic, stimulant, and stomachic*

burning bush *medicinal herb* [see: fraxinella; wahoo]

burodiline INN

Buro-Sol solution OTC *astringent wet dressing (Burow solution)* [aluminum sulfate] 0.23%

Burow solution [see: aluminum acetate]

burr seed; turkey burr seed; clotbur; hareburr; hurr-burr; thorny burr *medicinal herb* [see: burdock]

burrage *medicinal herb* [see: borage]

buserelin INN, BAN *hormonal antineoplastic; gonad-stimulating principle; luteinizing hormone–releasing hormone (LH-RH) analogue* [also: buserelin acetate]

buserelin acetate USAN, JAN *hormonal antineoplastic; gonad-stimulating principle; luteinizing hormone–releasing hormone (LH-RH) analogue* [also: buserelin]

BuSpar tablets ℞ *azaspirone anxiolytic* [buspirone HCl] 5, 10, 15, 30 mg

BuSpar transdermal patch ℞ *investigational (Phase III) delivery form for anxiety and ADHD* [buspirone HCl]

buspirone INN, BAN *azaspirone anxiolytic; minor tranquilizer* [also: buspirone HCl]

buspirone HCl USAN *azaspirone anxiolytic; minor tranquilizer; investigational (Phase III) transdermal delivery form for anxiety and ADHD* [also: buspirone] 5, 10, 15, 30 mg oral

busulfan USP, INN, JAN *alkylating antineoplastic for chronic myelogenous leukemia (CML); pretreatment for bone marrow transplants (orphan)* [also: busulphan]

Busulfex IV infusion ℞ *alkylating antineoplastic for chronic myelogenous leukemia (CML); pretreatment for bone marrow and stem cell transplants (orphan)* [busulfan] 6 mg/mL

busulphan BAN *alkylating antineoplastic* [also: busulfan]

butabarbital USP *sedative; hypnotic* [also: secbutobarbitone] ⑨ butalbital

butabarbital sodium USP *sedative; hypnotic* [also: secbutabarbital sodium] 15, 30 mg oral; 30 mg/5 mL oral

butacaine INN, BAN [also: butacaine sulfate]

butacaine sulfate USP [also: butacaine]

butacetin USAN *analgesic; antidepressant*

butacetoluide [see: butanilicaine]

butaclamol INN *antipsychotic* [also: butaclamol HCl]
butaclamol HCl USAN *antipsychotic* [also: butaclamol]
butadiazamide INN
butafosfan INN, BAN
butalamine INN, BAN
butalbital USAN, USP, INN *barbiturate sedative* ⓢ butabarbital; Butibel
butalbital & acetaminophen & caffeine *analgesic; barbiturate sedative* 50•325•40 mg oral
butalbital & aspirin & caffeine *analgesic; barbiturate sedative* 50•325•40 mg oral
Butalbital Compound tablets, capsules ℞ *analgesic; barbiturate sedative* [aspirin; caffeine; butalbital] 325•40•50 mg
butalgin [see: methadone HCl]
butallylonal NF
butamben USAN, USP *topical anesthetic*
butamben picrate USAN *topical local anesthetic* 1% topical
butamirate INN *antitussive* [also: butamirate citrate; butamyrate]
butamirate citrate USAN *antitussive* [also: butamirate; butamyrate]
butamisole INN *veterinary anthelmintic* [also: butamisole HCl]
butamisole HCl USAN *veterinary anthelmintic* [also: butamisole]
butamiverine [see: butaverine]
butamoxane INN
butamyrate BAN *antitussive* [also: butamirate citrate; butamirate]
butane (*n*-butane) NF *aerosol propellant*
1,4-butanediol (1,4-B; BDO); butane-1,4-diol *a precursor to gamma hydroxybutyrate (GHB); a formerly legal alternative to GHB, now also illegal (Schedule I)* [see: gamma hydroxybutyrate (GHB)]
butanilicaine INN, BAN
butanixin INN
butanserin INN
butantrone INN
butaperazine USAN, INN *antipsychotic*
butaperazine maleate USAN *antipsychotic*
butaprost USAN, INN, BAN *bronchodilator*
butaverine INN, DCF
butaxamine INN *antidiabetic; antihyperlipoproteinemic* [also: butoxamine HCl; butoxamine]
butcher's broom (*Ruscus aculeatus*) rhizomes *medicinal herb for atherosclerosis, circulatory disorders, hemorrhoids, thrombosis, varicose veins, and venous insufficiency; not generally regarded as safe and effective*
butedronate tetrasodium USAN *bone imaging aid*
butedronic acid INN
butelline [see: butacaine sulfate]
butenafine INN *antifungal*
butenafine HCl USAN *topical benzylamine antifungal*
butenemal [see: vinbarbital]
buteprate INN *former combining name for radicals or groups (name rescinded by the USAN)* [now: probutate]
buterizine USAN, INN *peripheral vasodilator*
Butesin Picrate ointment OTC *topical local anesthetic* [butamben picrate] 1%
butetamate INN [also: butethamate]
butethal NF [also: butobarbitone]
butethamate BAN [also: butetamate]
butethamine HCl NF
butethanol [see: tetracaine]
Butex Forte capsules ℞ *analgesic; barbiturate sedative* [acetaminophen; butalbital] 650•50 mg
buthalital sodium INN [also: buthalitone sodium]
buthalitone sodium BAN [also: buthalital sodium]
buthiazide USAN *diuretic; antihypertensive* [also: butizide]
Butibel tablets, elixir ℞ *GI anticholinergic; sedative* [belladonna extract; butabarbital sodium] 15•15 mg; 15•15 mg/5 mL ⓢ butalbital
butibufen INN
butidrine INN, DCF
butikacin USAN, INN, BAN *antibacterial*
butilfenin USAN, INN *hepatic function test*
butinazocine INN
butinoline INN

butirosin INN *antibacterial antibiotic* [also: butirosin sulfate; butirosin sulphate]

butirosin sulfate USAN *antibacterial antibiotic* [also: butirosin; butirosin sulphate]

butirosin sulphate BAN *antibacterial antibiotic* [also: butirosin sulfate; butirosin]

Butisol Sodium tablets, elixir ℞ *sedative; hypnotic* [butabarbital sodium] 15, 30, 50, 100 mg; 30 mg/5 mL ⓢ Butazolidin

butixirate USAN, INN *analgesic; antirheumatic*

butixocort INN

butizide INN *diuretic; antihypertensive* [also: buthiazide]

butobarbitone BAN [also: butethal]

butobendine INN

butoconazole INN, BAN *topical antifungal* [also: butoconazole nitrate]

butoconazole nitrate USAN, USP *topical antifungal* [also: butoconazole]

butocrolol INN

butoctamide INN [also: butoctamide semisuccinate]

butoctamide semisuccinate JAN [also: butoctamide]

butofilolol INN

butonate USAN, INN *anthelmintic*

butopamine USAN, INN *cardiotonic*

butopiprine INN, DCF

butoprozine INN *antiarrhythmic; antianginal* [also: butoprozine HCl]

butoprozine HCl USAN *antiarrhythmic; antianginal* [also: butoprozine]

butopyrammonium iodide INN

butopyronoxyl USP

butorphanol USAN, INN, BAN *analgesic; antitussive*

butorphanol tartrate USAN, USP, BAN, JAN *narcotic agonist-antagonist analgesic; antimigraine* 1, 2 mg injection

butoxamine BAN *antidiabetic; antihyperlipoproteinemic* [also: butoxamine HCl; butaxamine]

butoxamine HCl USAN *antidiabetic; antihyperlipoproteinemic* [also: butaxamine; butoxamine]

2-butoxyethyl nicotinate [see: nicoboxil]

butoxylate INN

butoxyphenylacethydroxamic acid [see: bufexamac]

butriptyline INN, BAN *antidepressant* [also: butriptyline HCl]

butriptyline HCl USAN *antidepressant* [also: butriptyline]

butropium bromide INN, JAN

butterbur *(Petasites hybridus)* leaves and root *medicinal herb used as an analgesic for migraines and as an antispasmodic for asthma, cough, and gastrointestinal and urinary tract disorders; not generally regarded as safe due to organ damage and carcinogenic properties*

buttercup *(Ranunculus acris; R. bulbosus; R. scleratus)* plant *medicinal herb used as an acrid, anodyne, antispasmodic, diaphoretic, and rubefacient*

butterfly weed *medicinal herb* [see: pleurisy root]

butternut *(Juglans cinerea)* bark, leaves, flowers *medicinal herb used as an anthelmintic, antiseptic, cathartic, cholagogue, and nervine*

butterweed *medicinal herb* [see: fleabane; horseweed]

butydrine [see: butidrine]

butyl alcohol NF *solvent*

butyl aminobenzoate (butyl *p*-aminobenzoate) [now: butamben]

butyl *p*-aminobenzoate picrate [see: butamben picrate]

butyl chloride NF

butyl 2-cyanoacrylate [see: enbucrilate]

butyl DNJ (deoxynojirimycin) [see: deoxynojirimycin]

butyl *p*-hydroxybenzoate [see: butylparaben]

butyl methoxydibenzoylmethane [see: avobenzone]

butyl nitrite; isobutyl nitrite *amyl nitrite substitutes, sold as euphoric street drugs, which produce a quick but short-lived "rush"* [see also: amyl nitrite; volatile nitrites]

butyl parahydroxybenzoate JAN *antifungal agent* [also: butylparaben]

***p*-butylaminobenzoyldiethylaminoethyl HCl** JAN

butylated hydroxyanisole (BHA) NF, BAN *antioxidant*

butylated hydroxytoluene (BHT) NF, BAN *antioxidant*

α-butylbenzyl alcohol [see: fenipentol]

1-butylbiguanide [see: buformin]

N-butyl-deoxynojirimycin [see: deoxynojirimycin]

1,4-butylene glycol (1,4-BG) *a precursor to gamma hydroxybutyrate (GHB); a formerly legal alternative to GHB, now also illegal (Schedule I)* [see: gamma hydroxybutyrate (GHB)]

1,5-(butylimino)-1,5-dideoxy-D-glucitol *investigational (orphan) for Fabry disease and Gaucher disease*

butylmesityl oxide [see: butopyronoxyl]

butylparaben NF *antifungal agent* [also: butyl parahydroxybenzoate]

butylphenamide

butylphenylsalicylamide [see: butylphenamide]

butylscopolamine bromide JAN

butynamine INN

butyrate propionate [see: probutate; buteprate]

butyrophenones *a class of dopamine receptor antagonists with conventional (typical) antipsychotic activity* [also called: phenylbutylpiperadines]

butyrylcholesterinase *investigational (orphan) for reduction and clearance of serum cocaine levels and postsurgical apnea*

butyrylperazine [see: butaperazine]

O-butyrylthiamine disulfide [see: bisbutitiamine]

butyvinyl [see: vinylbital]

buzepide metiodide INN, DCF

BVAP (BCNU, vincristine, Adriamycin, prednisone) *chemotherapy protocol*

BV-araU (bromovinyl arabinosyluracil) [see: sorivudine]

BVCPP (BCNU, vinblastine, cyclophosphamide, procarbazine, prednisone) *chemotherapy protocol*

BVDS (bleomycin, Velban, doxorubicin, streptozocin) *chemotherapy protocol*

BVPP (BCNU, vincristine, procarbazine, prednisone) *chemotherapy protocol*

BVU (bromoisovaleryl urea) [see: bromisovalum]

Byclomine capsules, tablets ℞ *GI antispasmodic* [dicyclomine HCl] 10 mg; 20 mg ⊠ Hycomine

Bydramine Cough syrup (discontinued 1997) OTC *antihistamine; antitussive* [diphenhydramine HCl; alcohol 5%] 12.5 mg/5 mL ⊠ Hydramine

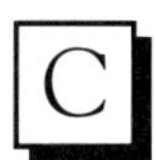

C (vitamin C) [see: ascorbic acid]

C & E softgels OTC *vitamin supplement* [vitamins C and E] 500•400 mg

C Factors "1000" Plus tablets OTC *vitamin C supplement with multiple bioflavonoids* [vitamin C; rose hips; citrus bioflavonoids; rutin; hesperidin] 1000•25•250•50•25 mg

C Speridin sustained-release tablets (discontinued 1999) OTC *vitamin C supplement with multiple bioflavonoids* [ascorbic acid; hesperidin; lemon bioflavonoids] 500•100•100 mg

C vitamin [see: ascorbic acid]

^{14}C urea *diagnostic aid for H. pylori in the stomach* [also: carbon C 14 urea]

C1-esterase-inhibitor, human *investigational (orphan) for acute angioedema*

C242-DM1 *investigational colon cancer therapy*

CA (cyclophosphamide, Adriamycin) *chemotherapy protocol*

CA (cytarabine, asparaginase) *chemotherapy protocol for acute myelocytic leukemia (AML)*

cA2 MAb (chimeric A2 MAb) [see: infliximab]

^{45}Ca [see: calcium chloride Ca 45]

^{47}Ca [see: calcium chloride Ca 47]

cabastine INN

cabbage, cow *medicinal herb* [see: masterwort; white pond lily]

cabbage, meadow; swamp cabbage *medicinal herb* [see: skunk cabbage]

cabbage, water *medicinal herb* [see: white pond lily]

cabergoline USAN, INN *dopamine agonist for hyperprolactinemia; investigational treatment for Parkinson disease and gynecologic disorders*

cabis bromatum [see: bibrocathol]

CABO (cisplatin, Abitrexate, bleomycin, Oncovin) *chemotherapy protocol for head and neck cancer*

CABOP; CA-BOP (Cytoxin, Adriamycin, bleomycin, Oncovin, prednisone) *chemotherapy protocol*

CABS (CCNU, Adriamycin bleomycin, streptozocin) *chemotherapy protocol*

cabufocon A USAN *hydrophobic contact lens material*

cabufocon B USAN *hydrophobic contact lens material*

CAC (cisplatin, ara-C, caffeine) *chemotherapy protocol*

cacao butter JAN

Cachexon ℞ *investigational (orphan) for AIDS-related cachexia* [L-glutathione, reduced]

cactinomycin USAN, INN *antibiotic antineoplastic* [also: actinomycin C]

CAD (cyclophosphamide, Adriamycin, dacarbazine) *chemotherapy protocol*

CAD (cytarabine [and] daunorubicin) *chemotherapy protocol*

cade oil [see: juniper tar]

cadexomer INN

cadexomer iodine USAN, INN, BAN *antiseptic; antiulcerative wound dressing*

cadmium *element (Cd)*

cadralazine INN, BAN, JAN

CAE (cyclophosphamide, Adriamycin, etoposide) *chemotherapy protocol for small cell lung cancer* [also: ACE]

Caelyx (CAN) injection ℞ *antineoplastic for ovarian carcinoma and AIDS-related Kaposi sarcoma* [doxorubicin HCl, liposome-encapsulated] 2 mg/mL

CAF (cyclophosphamide, Adriamycin, fluorouracil) *chemotherapy protocol for breast cancer*

cafaminol INN

Cafatine suppositories ℞ *migraine-specific vasoconstrictor* [ergotamine tartrate; caffeine] 2•200 mg

Cafatine-PB tablets ℞ *migraine treatment; vasoconstrictor; anticholinergic; sedative* [ergotamine tartrate; caffeine; pentobarbital sodium; belladonna extract] 1•100•30•0.125 mg

Cafcit oral solution, IV injection ℞ *analeptic; CNS stimulant for apnea of prematurity (orphan)* [caffeine citrate] 20 mg/mL

cafedrine INN, BAN

Cafergot tablets, suppositories ℞ *migraine treatment; vasoconstrictor* [ergotamine tartrate; caffeine] 1•100 mg; 2•100 mg

Cafetrate suppositories (discontinued 2000) ℞ *migraine-specific vasoconstrictor* [ergotamine tartrate; caffeine] 2•100 mg

Caffedrine tablets OTC *CNS stimulant; analeptic* [caffeine] 200 mg

caffeic acid phenethyl ester (CAPE) *antimicrobial substance found in bee propolis*

caffeine USP, BAN, JAN *CNS stimulant; diuretic; methylxanthine analeptic; investigational (orphan) for apnea of prematurity*

caffeine citrate *methylxanthine analeptic; CNS stimulant for apnea of prematurity (orphan)*

caffeine monohydrate [see: caffeine, citrated]

caffeine nut *medicinal herb* [see: kola nut]

caffeine & sodium benzoate *stimulant for respiratory depression due to an overdose of CNS depressants* 250 mg/mL injection

CAFP (cyclophosphamide, Adriamycin, fluorouracil, prednisone) *chemotherapy protocol*

CAFTH (cyclophosphamide, Adriamycin, fluorouracil, tamoxifen, Halotestin) *chemotherapy protocol*

CAFVP (cyclophosphamide, Adriamycin, fluorouracil, vincristine, prednisone) *chemotherapy protocol*

Cal Carb-HD powder OTC *calcium supplement* [calcium carbonate] 2.5 g/packet

Caladryl cream OTC *topical antihistamine; astringent; antipruritic/anesthetic* [diphenhydramine HCl; calamine] 1%•8% ⓢ Benadryl

Caladryl lotion OTC *topical poison ivy treatment* [calamine; pramoxine HCl; alcohol 2.2%] 8%•1%

Caladryl Clear lotion OTC *topical poison ivy treatment* [pramoxine HCl; zinc acetate; alcohol 2%] 1%•0.1%

Caladryl for Kids cream OTC *topical poison ivy treatment* [calamine; pramoxine HCl] 8%•1%

Cala-gen lotion OTC *topical antihistamine; antipruritic/anesthetic* [diphenhydramine HCl; alcohol 2%] 1%

Calamatum spray OTC *topical poison ivy treatment* [calamine; zinc oxide; menthol; camphor; benzocaine]

calamine USP, JAN *topical protectant; astringent*

calamint *(Calamintha officinalis)* *medicinal herb* [see: summer savory]

Calamintha hortensis *medicinal herb* [see: summer savory]

Calamintha montana *medicinal herb* [see: winter savory]

Calamox ointment OTC *topical poison ivy treatment* [calamine] 17 g/100 g ⓢ Camalox

calamus *(Acorus calamus)* rhizome *medicinal herb for anxiety, bad breath from smoking, colic, digestive disorders, fever, gas, irritated throat, and promoting wound healing; not generally regarded as safe and effective; prohibited in the U.S. as a food additive or supplement*

Calamycin lotion OTC *topical antihistamine; astringent; anesthetic* [pyrilamine maleate; zinc oxide; calamine; benzocaine; chloroxylenol; alcohol 2%]

Calan film-coated tablets ℞ *antianginal; antiarrhythmic; antihypertensive; calcium channel blocker* [verapamil HCl] 40, 80, 120 mg ⓢ kaolin; Kaon

Calan SR film-coated sustained-release tablets ℞ *antihypertensive; antianginal; antiarrhythmic; calcium channel blocker* [verapamil HCl] 120, 180, 240 mg ⓢ kaolin; Kaon

calanolide A *investigational (Phase I/II) non-nucleoside reverse transcriptase inhibitor (NNRTI) for HIV infection*

Calcarb 600 with Vitamin D tablets OTC *antacid* [calcium carbonate] 1.5 g•125 IU

Calcarb 600 with Vitamin D tablets OTC *dietary supplement* [calcium carbonate; vitamin D] 1.5 g•125 IU

Calcet tablets OTC *dietary supplement* [calcium; vitamin D] 152.8 mg•100 IU

Calcet Plus tablets OTC *vitamin/calcium/iron supplement* [multiple vitamins; calcium; iron; folic acid] ≛•152.8•18•0.8 mg

Calcibind powder for oral solution ℞ *antiurolithic to prevent stone formation in absorptive calciuria type I* [cellulose sodium phosphate] 300 g bulk pack

CalciCaps tablets OTC *dietary supplement* [dibasic calcium phosphate; calcium gluconate; calcium carbonate; vitamin D] 125 mg (Ca)•60 mg (P)•67 IU

CalciCaps with Iron tablets OTC *dietary supplement* [dibasic calcium phosphate; calcium gluconate; calcium carbonate; vitamin D; ferrous gluconate] 125 mg (Ca)•60 mg (P)•67 IU•7 mg

Calci-Chew chewable tablets OTC *calcium supplement* [calcium carbonate] 1.25 g

Calciday-667 tablets OTC *calcium supplement* [calcium carbonate] 667 mg

calcidiol [see: calcifediol]

Calcidrine syrup ℞ *narcotic antitussive; expectorant* [codeine phosphate; calcium iodide; alcohol 6%] 8.4•152 mg/5 mL

calcifediol (25-hydroxycholecalciferol; 25-hydroxyvitamin D$_3$) USAN, USP, INN *vitamin D precursor (converted to calcitriol in the body); calcium regulator for treatment of metastatic bone disease or hypocalcemia of chronic renal dialysis*

Calciferol IM injection ℞ *vitamin deficiency therapy for refractory rickets, familial hypophosphatemia, and hypoparathyroidism* [ergocalciferol (vitamin D$_2$)] 500 000 IU/mL

calciferol [now: ergocalciferol]

Calciferol tablets (discontinued 1999) ℞ *vitamin deficiency therapy for refractory rickets, familial hypophosphatemia, and hypoparathyroidism* [ergocalciferol (vitamin D$_2$)] 50 000 IU

Calciferol Drops OTC *vitamin supplement* [ergocalciferol (vitamin D$_2$)] 8000 IU/mL

Calcijex injection ℞ *vitamin D therapy for hypoparathyroidism and hypocalcemia of chronic renal dialysis* [calcitriol] 1 µg/mL

Calcimar subcu or IM injection ℞ *calcium regulator for hypercalcemia, Paget disease, and postmenopausal osteoporosis* [calcitonin (salmon)] 200 IU/mL

Calci-Mix capsules OTC *calcium supplement* [calcium carbonate] 1250 mg

calcipotriene USAN *topical antipsoriatic* [also: calcipotriol]

calcipotriol INN, BAN *topical antipsoriatic* [also: calcipotriene]

calcitonin (human) USAN, INN, BAN, JAN *calcium regulator for symptomatic Paget disease (osteitis deformans) (orphan)* 🔊 calcitriol

calcitonin (salmon) USAN, INN, BAN *calcium regulator for hypercalcemia, postmenopausal osteoporosis, and Paget disease; orphan status withdrawn 1996*

calcitonin salmon (synthesis) JAN *synthetic analogue of calcitonin (salmon); calcium regulator* [also: salcatonin]

calcitonin salmon, recombinant *investigational (Phase III) calcium regulator for hypercalcemia, postmenopausal osteoporosis, and Paget disease*

Cal-Citrate tablets OTC *calcium supplement* [calcium citrate] 250 mg

calcitriol (1,25-hydroxycholecalciferol; 1,25-hydroxyvitamin D$_3$) USAN, INN, BAN, JAN *physiologically active form of vitamin D; calcium regulator for hypoparathyroidism and hypocalcemia due to chronic renal dialysis; decreases the severity of psoriatic lesions* 🔊 calcitonin

calcium *element (Ca)*

Calcium + (CAN) oral liquid OTC *dietary supplement* [calcium; magnesium; vitamin D] 500 mg•200 mg•200 IU per 2 tsp. dose

calcium, oyster shell [see: calcium carbonate]

Calcium 600 tablets OTC *dietary supplement* [calcium carbonate] 600 mg

Calcium 600 + D tablets OTC *dietary supplement* [calcium; vitamin D] 600 mg•125 IU

Calcium 600 with Vitamin D tablets OTC *dietary supplement* [calcium; vitamin D] 600 mg•100 IU

calcium acetate USP, JAN *buffering agent for hyperphosphatemia of end-stage renal disease (orphan)*

calcium alginate fiber *topical local hemostatic*

calcium aminacyl B-PAS (benzoyl para-aminosalicylate) [see: benzoylpas calcium]

calcium 4-aminosalicylate trihydrate [see: aminosalicylate calcium]

calcium amphomycin [see: amphomycin]

calcium antagonists *a class of coronary vasodilators that inhibit cardiac muscle contraction and slow cardiac electrical conduction velocity* [also called: calcium channel blockers; slow channel blockers]

calcium ascorbate (vitamin C) USP *water-soluble vitamin; antiscorbutic* 500 mg oral; 3256 mg/tsp. oral

calcium benzamidosalicylate INN, BAN *antibacterial; tuberculostatic* [also: benzoylpas calcium]

calcium benzoyl *p*-aminosalicylate (B-PAS) [see: benzoylpas calcium]

calcium benzoylpas [see: benzoylpas calcium]

calcium bis-dioctyl sulfosuccinate [see: docusate calcium]

calcium bromide JAN

calcium carbimide INN [also: cyanamide]

calcium carbonate USP *antacid; calcium replenisher; investigational (orphan) for hyperphosphatemia of end-stage renal disease* [also: precipitated calcium carbonate] 500, 600, 650, 1250 mg oral; 1250 mg/5 mL oral

calcium carbonate, precipitated [now: calcium carbonate]

calcium carbophil *bulk laxative*

calcium caseinate *dietary supplement; infant formula modifier*

calcium channel blockers *a class of coronary vasodilators that inhibit cardiac muscle contraction and slow cardiac electrical conduction velocity* [also called: calcium antagonists; slow channel blockers]

calcium chloride USP, JAN *calcium replenisher*

calcium chloride Ca 45 USAN *radioactive agent*

calcium chloride Ca 47 USAN *radioactive agent*

calcium chloride dihydrate [see: calcium chloride]

calcium citrate USP *calcium supplement*

calcium citrate tetrahydrate [see: calcium citrate]

calcium clofibrate INN

calcium cyanamide [see: calcium carbimide]

calcium D-glucarate tetrahydrate [see: calcium saccharate]

calcium D-gluconate lactobionate monohydrate [see: calcium glubionate]

calcium dioctyl sulfosuccinate [see: docusate calcium]

calcium disodium edathamil [see: edetate calcium disodium]

calcium disodium edetate JAN *heavy metal chelating agent* [also: edetate calcium disodium; sodium calcium edetate; sodium calciumedetate]

Calcium Disodium Versenate IM, IV, or subcu injection ℞ *lead chelation therapy; antidote to lead poisoning and lead encephalopathy* [edetate calcium disodium] 200 mg/mL

calcium dobesilate INN

calcium doxybensylate [see: calcium dobesilate]

calcium edetate sodium [see: edetate calcium disodium]

calcium EDTA (ethylene diamine tetraacetic acid) [see: edetate calcium disodium]

calcium folinate INN, BAN, JAN *antianemic; folate replenisher; antidote to folic acid antagonist* [also: leucovorin calcium]

calcium glubionate USAN, INN *calcium replenisher*

calcium gluceptate USP *calcium replenisher* [also: calcium glucoheptonate] 1100 mg/5 mL injection

calcium glucoheptonate INN, DCF *calcium replenisher* [also: calcium gluceptate]

calcium gluconate (calcium D-gluconate) USP *calcium replenisher; investigational (orphan) for hydrofluoric acid burns* 500, 650, 975, 1000 mg oral; 10% injection

calcium glycerinophosphate [see: calcium glycerophosphate]
calcium glycerophosphate NF, JAN
calcium hopantenate JAN
calcium hydroxide USP *astringent*
calcium hydroxide phosphate [see: calcium phosphate, tribasic]
calcium hypophosphite NF
calcium iodide *expectorant*
calcium iododocosanoate [see: iodobehenate calcium]
calcium lactate USP, JAN *calcium replenisher* 325, 650 mg oral
calcium lactate hydrate [see: calcium lactate]
calcium lactate pentahydrate [see: calcium lactate]
calcium lactobionate USP *calcium supplement*
calcium lactobionate dihydrate [see: calcium lactobionate]
calcium lactophosphate NF
calcium L-aspartate JAN
calcium levofolinate [see: levoleucovorin calcium]
calcium levulate [see: calcium levulinate]
calcium levulinate USP *calcium replenisher*
calcium levulinate dihydrate [see: calcium levulinate]
calcium mandelate USP
calcium oxide [see: lime]
calcium pantothenate (calcium D-pantothenate; vitamin B_5) USP, INN, JAN *water-soluble vitamin; enzyme cofactor* [also: pantothenic acid] 100, 218, 545 mg oral
calcium pantothenate, racemic (calcium DL-pantothenate) USP *vitamin; enzyme cofactor*
calcium para-aminosalicylate JAN [also: aminosalicylate calcium]
calcium phosphate, dibasic USP, JAN *calcium replenisher; tablet base*
calcium phosphate, monocalcium [see: calcium phosphate, dibasic]
calcium phosphate, tribasic NF *calcium replenisher* [also: durapatite; hydroxyapatite]
calcium polycarbophil USAN, USP *bulk laxative; antidiarrheal*
calcium polystyrene sulfonate JAN *ion exchange resin for hyperkalemia*
calcium polysulfide & calcium thiosulfate [see: lime, sulfurated]
calcium saccharate USP, INN *stabilizer*
calcium silicate NF *tablet excipient*
calcium sodium ferriclate INN *hematinic* [also: ferriclate calcium sodium]
calcium stearate NF, JAN *tablet and capsule lubricant*
calcium sulfate NF *tablet and capsule diluent*
calcium tetracemine disodium [see: edetate calcium disodium]
calcium trisodium pentetate INN, BAN *plutonium chelating agent* [also: pentetate calcium trisodium]
calcium 10-undecenoate [see: calcium undecylenate]
calcium undecylenate USAN *antifungal*
calciumedetate sodium [see: edetate calcium disodium]
CaldeCort aerosol spray (discontinued 1997) OTC *topical corticosteroidal anti-inflammatory* [hydrocortisone] 0.5%
CaldeCort Anti-Itch; CaldeCort Light with Aloe cream (discontinued 1997) OTC *topical corticosteroidal anti-inflammatory* [hydrocortisone acetate] 0.5%
Calderol capsules ℞ *vitamin D therapy for metastatic bone disease or hypocalcemia of chronic renal dialysis* [calcifediol] 20, 50 µg
Caldesene ointment OTC *moisturizer; emollient; astringent; antiseptic* [cod liver oil (vitamins A and D); zinc oxide; lanolin]
Caldesene powder OTC *topical antifungal* [calcium undecylenate] 10%
caldiamide INN *pharmaceutic aid* [also: caldiamide sodium]
caldiamide sodium USAN, BAN *pharmaceutic aid* [also: caldiamide]
Calel D tablets OTC *dietary supplement* [calcium carbonate; cholecalciferol] 500 mg•200 IU

Calendula officinalis *medicinal herb* [see: marigold]

CALF (cyclophosphamide, Adriamycin, leucovorin [rescue], fluorouracil) *chemotherapy protocol*

calfactant USAN *surface-active extract of saline lavage of calf lungs, used for prevention of respiratory distress syndrome (RDS) in premature infants*

CALF-E (cyclophosphamide, Adriamycin, leucovorin [rescue], fluorouracil, ethinyl estradiol) *chemotherapy protocol*

CAL-G (cyclophosphamide, asparaginase, leurocristine, daunorubicin, prednisone) *chemotherapy protocol for acute lymphocytic leukemia (ALL)*

Calglycine chewable tablets (discontinued 1998) OTC *antacid* [calcium carbonate; glycine] 420•150 mg

Calgonate wash ℞ *investigational (orphan) emergency treatment for hydrofluoric acid burns* [calcium gluconate]

Cal-Guard softgels OTC *calcium supplement* [calcium carbonate] 50 mg

California barberry *medicinal herb* [see: Oregon grape]

California buckthorn *medicinal herb* [see: buckthorn; cascara sagrada]

California false hellebore *(Veratrum californicum)* [see: hellebore]

californium *element (Cf)*

calioben [see: calcium iodobehenate]

Cal-Lac capsules OTC *calcium supplement* [calcium lactate] 500 mg

Calluna vulgaris *medicinal herb* [see: heather]

calmatives *a class of soothing agents that reduce excitement, nervousness, distress, or irritation* [also called: sedatives]

Calmol 4 rectal suppositories OTC *emollient; astringent* [cocoa butter; zinc oxide] 80%•10%

Calm-X tablets OTC *anticholinergic; antiemetic; antivertigo agent; motion sickness preventative* [dimenhydrinate] 50 mg

Calmylin (CAN) oral solution (discontinued 2001) OTC *antitussive; decongestant; expectorant* [dextromethorphan hydrobromide; pseudoephedrine HCl; guaifenesin] 3•6•20 mg/mL

Calmylin #1 (CAN) syrup (discontinued 2001) OTC *antihistamine* [dextromethorphan hydrobromide] 3 mg/mL

Calmylin #2 (CAN) oral solution (discontinued 2001) OTC *antitussive; decongestant* [dextromethorphan hydrobromide; pseudoephedrine HCl] 3•6 mg/mL

Calmylin #4 (CAN) oral solution (discontinued 2001) OTC *antitussive; antihistamine; expectorant* [dextromethorphan hydrobromide; diphenhydramine HCl; ammonium chloride] 2.5•3•25 mg/mL

Calmylin Cough & Cold (CAN) oral solution (discontinued 2001) OTC *antitussive; decongestant; expectorant; analgesic* [dextromethorphan hydrobromide; pseudoephedrine HCl; guaifenesin; acetaminophen] 1•2•6.67•21.67 mg/mL

Calmylin Expectorant (CAN) syrup (discontinued 2001) OTC *expectorant* [guaifenesin] 20 mg/mL

Calmylin Pediatric (CAN) syrup (discontinued 2001) OTC *pediatric antitussive and decongestant* [dextromethorphan hydrobromide; pseudoephedrine HCl] 1.5•3 mg/mL

Calmylin with Codeine (CAN) oral solution ℞ *narcotic antitussive; decongestant; expectorant* [codeine phosphate; pseudoephedrine HCl; guaifenesin] 0.66•6•20 mg/mL

calomel NF

Calphosan IV injection ℞ *calcium replacement* [calcium glycerophosphate; calcium lactate] 50•50 mg/10 mL (0.08 mEq/mL)

Calphron tablets OTC *buffering agent for hyperphosphatemia in end-stage renal failure (orphan)* [calcium acetate] 667 mg

Cal-Plus tablets OTC *calcium supplement* [calcium carbonate] 1.5 g

calteridol INN *pharmaceutic aid* [also: calteridol calcium]

calteridol calcium USAN, BAN *pharmaceutic aid* [also: calteridol]

Caltha palustris *medicinal herb* [see: cowslip]

Caltrate 600 film-coated tablets OTC *calcium supplement* [calcium carbonate] 1.5 g

Caltrate 600 + D tablets OTC *dietary supplement* [calcium carbonate; vitamin D] 600 mg•200 IU

Caltrate 600 + Iron/Vitamin D film-coated tablets OTC *dietary supplement* [calcium carbonate; ferrous fumarate; vitamin D] 600 mg•18 mg•125 IU

Caltrate Jr. chewable tablets OTC *calcium supplement* [calcium carbonate] 750 mg

Caltrate Plus tablets OTC *dietary supplement* [calcium carbonate; vitamin D; multiple minerals] 600 mg•200 IU•≛

Caltro tablets OTC *dietary supplement* [calcium; vitamin D] 250 mg•125 IU

calumba; calumba root; calumbo *medicinal herb* [see: colombo]

calusterone USAN, INN *antineoplastic*

Calypte test kit for professional use *urine test for HIV-1 antibodies*

CAM (cyclophosphamide, Adriamycin, methotrexate) *chemotherapy protocol*

Cama Arthritis Pain Reliever tablets OTC *analgesic; antipyretic; anti-inflammatory; antirheumatic* [aspirin (buffered with magnesium oxide and aluminum hydroxide)] 500 mg

camazepam INN

CAMB (Cytoxin, Adriamycin, methotrexate, bleomycin) *chemotherapy protocol*

cambendazole USAN, INN, BAN *anthelmintic*

CAMELEON (cytosine arabinoside, methotrexate, Leukovorin, Oncovin) *chemotherapy protocol*

camellia oil JAN

Camellia sinensis *medicinal herb* [see: green tea]

CAMEO (cyclophosphamide, Adriamycin, methotrexate, etoposide, Oncovin) *chemotherapy protocol*

Cameo Oil OTC *bath emollient*

CAMF (cyclophosphamide, Adriamycin, methotrexate, folinic acid) *chemotherapy protocol*

camiglibose USAN, INN *antidiabetic*

camiverine INN

camomile *medicinal herb* [see: chamomile]

camonagrel INN

camostat INN [also: camostat mesilate]

camostat mesilate JAN [also: camostat]

cAMP (cyclic adenosine monophosphate) [see: adenosine phosphate]

CAMP (cyclophosphamide, Adriamycin, methotrexate, procarbazine HCl) *chemotherapy protocol for non–small cell lung cancer (NSCLC)*

Campath IV infusion ℞ *immunosuppressant for B-cell chronic lymphocytic leukemia (B-CLL); investigational (Phase II) for non-Hodgkin lymphoma, organ transplants, and multiple sclerosis* [alemtuzumab] 30 mg/3 mL dose

camphetamide [see: camphotamide]

Campho-Phenique liquid, gel OTC *mild anesthetic; anti-infective; counterirritant* [camphor; phenol; eucalyptus oil] 10.8%•4.7%•≟

Campho-Phenique Antibiotic Plus Pain Reliever ointment OTC *topical antibiotic; local anesthetic* [polymyxin B sulfate; neomycin sulfate; bacitracin zinc; lidocaine] 5000 U•3.5 mg•500 U•40 mg per g

camphor (*d*-camphor; *dl*-camphor) USP, JAN *topical antipruritic; mild local anesthetic; counterirritant* [also: *trans*-π-oxocamphor]

camphor, monobromated USP

camphorated opium tincture [now: paregoric]

camphorated parachlorophenol [see: parachlorophenol, camphorated]

camphoric acid USP

camphotamide INN, DCF

Camptosar IV infusion ℞ *topoisomerase I inhibitor; antineoplastic for metastatic colon and rectal cancers* [irinotecan HCl] 20 mg/mL

camptothecin-11 (CPT-11) [see: irinotecan]

Campyvax ℞ *investigational (Phase II/III) Campylobacter vaccine*

camsilate INN *combining name for radicals or groups* [also: camsylate]

camsylate USAN, BAN *combining name for radicals or groups* [also: camsilate]

camylofin INN, DCF

Canada fleabane *medicinal herb* [see: fleabane; horseweed]

Canada pitch tree *medicinal herb* [see: hemlock]

Canada root *medicinal herb* [see: pleurisy root]

Canada tea *medicinal herb* [see: wintergreen]

canaigre *(Rumex hymenosepalus)* *medicinal herb for a variety of disease states and used as a purported substitute for ginseng; not generally regarded as safe because of high tannin content and possible mutagenic effect when used internally*

Canasa suppositories ℞ *anti-inflammatory for active ulcerative colitis, proctosigmoiditis, and proctitis* [mesalamine] 500 mg

canbisol INN

CancerVax ℞ *investigational therapeutic vaccine for melanoma*

Cancidas powder for IV infusion ℞ *systemic antifungal for invasive aspergillosis and other resistant fungal infections* [caspofungin acetate] 50, 70 mg/vial

candesartan USAN, INN *antihypertensive; angiotensin II receptor antagonist*

candesartan cilexetil USAN *antihypertensive; angiotensin II receptor antagonist*

candicidin USAN, USP, INN, BAN *polyene antifungal*

***Candida albicans* skin test antigen** *diagnostic aid for diminished cellular immunity; test for HIV patients to assess TB antigen response*

CandidaSure reagent slides for professional use *in vitro diagnostic aid for Candida albicans in the vagina*

Candin intradermal injection ℞ *diagnostic aid for diminished cellular immunity; test for HIV patients to assess TB antigen response* [Candida albicans skin test antigen] 0.1 mL

candleberry; candleberry myrtle *medicinal herb* [see: bayberry; tung seed]

candocuronium iodide INN

candoxatril USAN, INN, BAN *antihypertensive*

candoxatrilat USAN, INN, BAN *antihypertensive*

Canesten Topical (CAN) cream OTC *topical antifungal* [clotrimazole] 1%

cankerroot *medicinal herb* [see: gold thread]

cannabinol INN, BAN *antiemetic; antinauseant; a nonpsychoactive derivative of the Cannabis sativa plant*

***Cannabis sativa* (marijuana; marihuana; hashish)** *euphoric/hallucinogenic street drug made from the resin or dried leaves and flowering tops of the cannabis plant; medicinal herb for asthma, analgesia, leprosy, and loss of appetite*

canrenoate potassium USAN *aldosterone antagonist* [also: canrenoic acid; potassium canrenoate]

canrenoic acid INN, BAN *aldosterone antagonist* [also: canrenoate potassium; potassium canrenoate]

canrenone USAN, INN *aldosterone antagonist*

cantharides JAN

cantharidin *topical keratolytic*

Cantil tablets ℞ *treatment for peptic ulcer* [mepenzolate bromide] 25 mg

CAO (cyclophosphamide, Adriamycin, Oncovin) *chemotherapy protocol*

CAP (cellulose acetate phthalate) [q.v.]

CAP (cyclophosphamide, Adriamycin, Platinol) *chemotherapy protocol for non–small cell lung cancer (NSCLC)*

CAP (cyclophosphamide, Adriamycin, prednisone) *chemotherapy protocol*

CAP; CAP-I (cyclophosphamide, Adriamycin, Platinol) *chemotherapy protocol*

CAP-II (cyclophosphamide, Adriamycin, high-dose Platinol) *chemotherapy protocol*

Capastat Sulfate powder for IM injection ℞ *tuberculostatic* [capreomycin sulfate] 1 g/10 mL ⊡ Cepastat

CAP-BOP (cyclophosphamide, Adriamycin, procarbazine, bleomycin, Oncovin, prednisone) *chemotherapy protocol*

CAPE (caffeic acid phenethyl ester) *antimicrobial substance found in bee propolis*

Cape aloe *medicinal herb* [see: aloe]

cape gum *medicinal herb* [see: acacia]

capecitabine USAN, INN *oral fluoropyrimidine (5-FU prodrug) antineoplastic for metastatic breast and colorectal cancer*

capers *(Capparis spinosa)* flower buds and leaves *medicinal herb for skin disorders and reducing the effects of enlarged capillaries*

Capex shampoo ℞ *topical corticosteroidal anti-inflammatory; antiseborrheic* [fluocinolone acetonide] 0.01%

capimorelin tartrate [see: capromorelin tartrate]

Capital with Codeine oral suspension ℞ *narcotic analgesic* [codeine phosphate; acetaminophen] 12•120 mg/5 mL

Capitrol shampoo ℞ *antiseborrheic; antibacterial; antifungal* [chloroxine] 2% ⊡ captopril

caplet (dosage form) *capsule-shaped tablet*

capmul 8210 [see: monoctanoin]

capobenate sodium USAN *antiarrhythmic*

capobenic acid USAN, INN *antiarrhythmic*

Capoten tablets ℞ *antihypertensive; angiotensin-converting enzyme (ACE) inhibitor* [captopril] 12.5, 25, 50, 100 mg

Capozide 25/15; Capozide 25/25; Capozide 50/15; Capozide 50/25 tablets ℞ *antihypertensive; angiotensin-converting enzyme (ACE) inhibitor; diuretic* [captopril; hydrochlorothiazide] 25•15 mg; 25•25 mg; 50•15 mg; 50•25 mg

Capparis spinosa *medicinal herb* [see: capers]

CAPPr (cyclophosphamide, Adriamycin, Platinol, prednisone) *chemotherapy protocol*

capreomycin INN, BAN *bactericidal antibiotic; tuberculostatic* [also: capreomycin sulfate]

capreomycin sulfate USAN, USP, JAN *bactericidal antibiotic; tuberculostatic* [also: capreomycin]

Caprogel ℞ *investigational (orphan) topical treatment for traumatic hyphema of the eye* [aminocaproic acid]

capromab INN *monoclonal antibody for diagnosis of prostate cancer* [also: capromab pendetide]

capromab pendetide USAN *monoclonal antibody for diagnosis of prostate cancer* [also: capromab]

capromorelin tartrate USAN *growth hormone secretagogue for anti-aging, congestive heart failure, and catabolic illness* [previous USAN: capimorelin tartrate]

caproxamine INN, BAN

capsaicin *topical analgesic; counterirritant* 0.025%, 0.075% topical

Capsella bursa-pastoris *medicinal herb* [see: shepherd's purse]

Capsicum frutescens; C. annuum *medicinal herb* [see: cayenne]

capsicum oleoresin *topical analgesic; counterirritant*

Capsin lotion OTC *topical analgesic* [capsaicin] 0.025%, 0.075%

Capsulets (trademarked form) *sustained-release caplet*

captab (dosage form) *capsule-shaped tablet*

captamine INN *depigmentor* [also: captamine HCl]

captamine HCl USAN *depigmentor* [also: captamine]

captodiame INN, BAN

captodiame HCl [see: captodiame]

captodiamine HCl [see: captodiame]
captopril USAN, USP, INN, BAN, JAN *antihypertensive; angiotensin-converting enzyme (ACE) inhibitor* 12.5, 25, 50, 100 mg oral ⓢ Capitrol
captopril & hydrochlorothiazide *antihypertensive; angiotensin-converting enzyme (ACE) inhibitor; diuretic* 25•15, 25•25, 50•15, 50•25 mg oral
capuride USAN, INN *hypnotic*
Capzasin-P cream OTC *topical analgesic* [capsaicin] 0.025%
Carac cream ℞ *antimetabolite antineoplastic for actinic keratoses and basal cell carcinomas* [fluorouracil] 0.5%
caracemide USAN, INN *antineoplastic*
Carafate tablets, oral suspension ℞ *treatment for duodenal ulcer* [sucralfate] 1 g; 1 g/10 mL
caramel NF *coloring agent*
caramiphen INN, BAN *antitussive*
caramiphen edisylate *antitussive*
caramiphen HCl [see: caramiphen]
caraway (*Carum carvi*) NF seeds *medicinal herb for acid indigestion, appetite stimulation, colic, gas, gastrointestinal spasms, and uterine cramps*
caraway oil NF
carazolol INN, BAN
carbacephems *a class of bactericidal antibiotics similar to second-generation cephalosporins (q.v.)*
carbachol USP, INN, BAN, JAN *ophthalmic cholinergic; miotic for surgery; antiglaucoma agent* [also: carbacholine chloride]
carbacholine chloride DCF *ophthalmic cholinergic; miotic for surgery; antiglaucoma agent* [also: carbachol]
carbacrylamine resins
carbadipimidine HCl [see: carpipramine dihydrochloride]
carbadox USAN, INN, BAN *antibacterial*
carbaldrate INN
carbamate choline chloride [see: carbachol]
carbamazepine USAN, USP, INN, BAN, JAN *anticonvulsant; analgesic for trigeminal neuralgia; antimanic* 100, 200 mg oral; 100 mg/5 mL oral
carbamide [see: urea]
carbamide peroxide USP *topical dental anti-infective; cerumenolytic to emulsify and disperse ear wax*
N-carbamoylarsanilic acid [see: carbarsone]
carbamoylcholine chloride [see: carbachol]
O-carbamoylsalicylic acid lactam [see: carsalam]
carbamylcholine chloride [see: carbachol]
carbamylglutamic acid *investigational (orphan) treatment for N-acetylglutamate synthetase deficiency*
carbamylmethylcholine chloride [see: bethanechol chloride]
carbantel INN *anthelmintic* [also: carbantel lauryl sulfate]
carbantel lauryl sulfate USAN *anthelmintic* [also: carbantel]
carbaril INN [also: carbaryl]
carbarsone USP, INN
carbaryl BAN [also: carbaril]
carbasalate calcium INN *analgesic* [also: carbaspirin calcium]
carbaspirin calcium USAN *analgesic* [also: carbasalate calcium]
Carbastat solution ℞ *direct-acting miotic for ophthalmic surgery* [carbachol] 0.01%
Carbatrol extended-release capsules ℞ *anticonvulsant; analgesic for trigeminal neuralgia; antipsychotic* [carbamazepine] 200, 300 mg
carbazeran USAN, INN *cardiotonic*
carbazochrome INN, JAN
carbazochrome salicylate INN
carbazochrome sodium sulfonate INN
carbazocine INN
carbenicillin INN, BAN *extended-spectrum penicillin antibiotic* [also: carbenicillin disodium; carbenicillin sodium]
carbenicillin disodium USAN, USP *extended-spectrum penicillin antibiotic* [also: carbenicillin; carbenicillin sodium]

carbenicillin indanyl sodium USAN, USP *extended-spectrum penicillin antibiotic* [also: carindacillin]

carbenicillin phenyl sodium USAN *antibacterial* [also: carfecillin]

carbenicillin potassium USAN *antibacterial*

carbenicillin sodium JAN *antibacterial* [also: carbenicillin disodium; carbenicillin]

carbenoxolone INN, BAN *corticosteroid; anti-inflammatory* [also: carbenoxolone sodium]

carbenoxolone sodium USAN *corticosteroid; anti-inflammatory* [also: carbenoxolone]

carbenzide INN

carbesilate INN *combining name for radicals or groups*

carbetapentane citrate NF *antitussive* [also: pentoxyverine]

carbetapentane tannate *antitussive*

carbetimer USAN, INN *antineoplastic*

carbetocin INN, BAN *uterotonic agent to prevent postpartum hemorrhage following cesarean section*

Carbex tablets ℞ *dopaminergic antiparkinsonian (orphan)* [selegiline HCl] 5 mg

carbidopa USAN, USP, INN, BAN, JAN *decarboxylase inhibitor; antiparkinsonian adjunct*

carbidopa & levodopa *antiparkinsonian* 10•100, 25•100, 25•250, 50•200 mg oral

carbifene INN *analgesic* [also: carbiphene HCl; carbiphene]

carbimazole INN, BAN

carbinoxamine INN, BAN *antihistamine for allergic rhinitis* [also: carbinoxamine maleate]

Carbinoxamine Compound syrup, pediatric drops ℞ *antitussive; decongestant; antihistamine* [dextromethorphan hydrobromide; pseudoephedrine HCl; carbinoxamine maleate] 15•60•4 mg/5 mL; 4•25•2 mg/mL

carbinoxamine maleate USP *antihistamine for allergic rhinitis* [also: carbinoxamine]

carbinoxamine maleate & pseudoephedrine HCl *antihistamine; decongestant* 4•60 mg/5 mL oral; 2•25 mg/mL oral

carbiphene BAN *analgesic* [also: carbiphene HCl; carbifene]

carbiphene HCl USAN *analgesic* [also: carbifene; carbiphene]

Carbiset tablets ℞ *decongestant; antihistamine* [pseudoephedrine HCl; carbinoxamine maleate] 60•4 mg

Carbiset-TR timed-release tablets ℞ *decongestant; antihistamine* [pseudoephedrine HCl; carbinoxamine maleate] 120•8 mg

Carbocaine injection ℞ *injectable local anesthetic* [mepivacaine HCl] 1%, 1.5%, 2%, 3%

Carbocaine with Neo-Cobefrin injection ℞ *injectable local anesthetic* [mepivacaine HCl; levonordefrin] 2%•1:20 000

carbocisteine INN, BAN *mucolytic* [also: carbocysteine]

carbocloral USAN, INN, BAN *hypnotic*

carbocromen INN *coronary vasodilator* [also: chromonar HCl]

carbocysteine USAN *mucolytic* [also: carbocisteine]

Carbodec tablets, syrup ℞ *decongestant; antihistamine* [pseudoephedrine HCl; carbinoxamine maleate] 60•4 mg; 60•4 mg/5 mL

Carbodec DM syrup, pediatric drops ℞ *antitussive; decongestant; antihistamine* [dextromethorphan hydrobromide; pseudoephedrine HCl; carbinoxamine maleate] 15•60•4 mg/5 mL; 4•25•2 mg/mL

Carbodec TR timed-release tablets ℞ *decongestant; antihistamine* [pseudoephedrine HCl; carbinoxamine maleate] 120•8 mg

carbodimid calcium [see: calcium carbimide]

carbofenotion INN [also: carbophenothion]

carbohydrate polymer gel *investigational (NDA filed) postsurgical dressing to inhibit scar formation*

carbol-fuchsin solution (or paint) USP *antifungal*
carbolic acid [see: phenol]
carbolin [see: carbachol]
Carbolith (CAN) capsules ℞ *antipsychotic for manic episodes of a bipolar disorder* [lithium carbonate] 150, 300, 600 mg
carbolonium bromide BAN [also: hexcarbacholine bromide]
carbomer INN, BAN *emulsifying and suspending agent* [also: carbomer 910]
carbomer 1342 NF *emulsifying and suspending agent*
carbomer 910 USAN, NF *emulsifying and suspending agent* [also: carbomer]
carbomer 934 USAN, NF *emulsifying and suspending agent*
carbomer 934P USAN, NF *emulsifying and suspending agent*
carbomer 940 USAN, NF *emulsifying and suspending agent*
carbomer 941 USAN, NF *emulsifying and suspending agent*
carbomycin INN
carbon *element (C)*
carbon, activated
carbon C 13 urea *diagnostic aid for detection of H. pylori in the stomach*
carbon C 14 urea *diagnostic aid for H. pylori in the stomach* [also: ^{14}C urea]
carbon dioxide (CO_2) USP *respiratory stimulant*
carbon tetrachloride NF *solvent*
carbonic acid, calcium salt [see: calcium carbonate]
carbonic acid, dilithium salt [see: lithium carbonate]
carbonic acid, dipotassium salt [see: potassium carbonate]
carbonic acid, disodium salt [see: sodium carbonate]
carbonic acid, magnesium salt [see: magnesium carbonate]
carbonic acid, monoammonium salt [see: ammonium carbonate]
carbonic acid, monopotassium salt [see: potassium bicarbonate]
carbonic acid, monosodium salt [see: sodium bicarbonate]
carbonic anhydrase inhibitors *a class of diuretic agents that reduce the rate of aqueous humor formation, resulting in decreased intraocular pressure; available in both systemic (tablets) and topical (eye drops) forms*
carbonis detergens, liquor (LCD) [see: coal tar]
carbonyl iron *hematinic; iron supplement (100% elemental iron as microparticles)*
carbophenothion BAN [also: carbofenotion]
carboplatin USAN, INN, BAN *alkylating antineoplastic for ovarian and other cancers*
carboplatin & etoposide & paclitaxel *chemotherapy protocol for primary adenocarcinoma and small cell lung cancer*
carboprost USAN, INN, BAN *oxytocic*
carboprost methyl USAN *oxytocic*
carboprost trometanol BAN *oxytocic; prostaglandin-type abortifacient* [also: carboprost tromethamine]
carboprost tromethamine USAN, USP *oxytocic; prostaglandin-type abortifacient* [also: carboprost trometanol]
Carboptic Drop-Tainers (eye drops) ℞ *topical antiglaucoma agent; direct-acting miotic* [carbachol] 3%
carboquone INN
carbose D [see: carboxymethylcellulose sodium]
carbovir *investigational (orphan) for AIDS and symptomatic HIV*
carboxyimamidate [see: carbetimer]
carboxymethylcellulose calcium NF *tablet disintegrant*
carboxymethylcellulose sodium USP *bulk laxative; suspending and viscosity-increasing agent; ophthalmic moisturizer; tablet excipient* [also: carmellose; carmellose sodium]
carboxymethylcellulose sodium 12 NF *suspending and viscosity-increasing agent*
carbromal NF, INN
carbubarb INN
carbubarbital [see: carbubarb]

carburazepam INN
carbutamide INN, BAN
carbuterol INN, BAN *bronchodilator* [also: carbuterol HCl]
carbuterol HCl USAN *bronchodilator* [also: carbuterol]
carcainium chloride INN
carcinoembryonic antigen (CEA)
cardamom seed NF
cardamom [see: bitter cardamom]
Cardec-DM syrup, pediatric syrup, pediatric drops ℞ *antitussive; decongestant; antihistamine* [dextromethorphan hydrobromide; pseudoephedrine HCl; carbinoxamine maleate] 15•60•4 mg/5 mL; 15•60•4 mg/5 mL; 4•25•2 mg/mL
Cardec-S syrup ℞ *decongestant; antihistamine* [pseudoephedrine HCl; carbinoxamine maleate] 60•4 mg/5 mL
Cardene capsules ℞ *antianginal; antihypertensive; calcium channel blocker* [nicardipine HCl] 20, 30 mg ⑨ Cardizem
Cardene I.V. injection ℞ *antihypertensive; calcium channel blocker* [nicardipine HCl] 2.5 mg/mL
Cardene SR sustained-release capsules ℞ *antihypertensive; calcium channel blocker* [nicardipine HCl] 30, 45, 60 mg
cardiac glycosides *a class of cardiovascular drugs that increase the force of cardiac contractions* [also called: digitalis glycosides]
Cardiac T test *in vitro diagnostic aid for troponin T (indicator of cardiac damage) in whole blood*
cardiacs *a class of agents that stimulate or otherwise affect the heart (a term used in folk medicine)*
cardiamid [see: nikethamide]
cardin *medicinal herb* [see: blessed thistle]
Cardio-Green (CG) powder for IV injection ℞ *in vivo diagnostic aid for cardiac output, hepatic function, or ophthalmic angiography* [indocyanine green] 25, 50 mg
Cardiolite injection ℞ *myocardial perfusion agent for cardiac SPECT imaging* [technetium Tc 99m sestamibi] 5 mL
Cardi-Omega 3 capsules OTC *dietary supplement* [omega-3 fatty acids; multiple vitamins & minerals] 1000•≛ mg
cardioplegic solution (calcium chloride, magnesium chloride, potassium chloride, sodium chloride) [q.v.]
cardioprotective agents *a class of potent intracellular chelating agents which protect the heart from the effects of doxorubicin*
Cardioquin tablets ℞ *antiarrhythmic* [quinidine polygalacturonate] 275 mg
Cardizem IV injection, Lyo-Ject (prefilled syringe) ℞ *calcium channel blocker for atrial fibrillation or paroxysmal supraventricular tachycardia (PSVT)* [diltiazem HCl] 5 mg/mL ⑨ Cardene
Cardizem tablets ℞ *antianginal; antihypertensive; antiarrhythmic; calcium channel blocker* [diltiazem HCl] 30, 60, 90, 120 mg
Cardizem CD (once daily) sustained-release capsules ℞ *antihypertensive; antianginal; antiarrhythmic; calcium channel blocker* [diltiazem HCl] 120, 180, 240, 300, 360 mg
Cardizem SR (twice daily) sustained-release capsules ℞ *antihypertensive; antianginal; antiarrhythmic; calcium channel blocker* [diltiazem HCl] 60, 90, 120 mg
Cardizem XL ℞ *investigational (NDA filed) h.s. dosing of Cardizem* [diltiazem HCl]
cardophyllin [see: aminophylline]
Cardura tablets ℞ *antihypertensive (α-blocker); treatment for benign prostatic hyperplasia* [doxazosin mesylate] 1, 2, 4, 8 mg
carebastine INN
carena [see: aminophylline]
carfecillin INN, BAN *antibacterial* [also: carbenicillin phenyl sodium]
carfenazine INN *antipsychotic* [also: carphenazine maleate; carphenazine]

carfentanil INN *narcotic analgesic* [also: carfentanil citrate]
carfentanil citrate USAN *narcotic analgesic* [also: carfentanil]
carfimate INN
cargentos [see: silver protein]
cargutocin INN
Carica papaya *medicinal herb* [see: papaya]
carindacillin INN, BAN *extended-spectrum penicillin antibiotic* [also: carbenicillin indanyl sodium]
Carisolv (CAN) gel ℞ *topical agent for dissolution of dental caries* [sodium hypochlorite] 0.5%
carisoprodol USP, INN, BAN *skeletal muscle relaxant* 350 mg oral
carline thistle *(Carlina acaulis)* root *medicinal herb used as a carminative, diaphoretic, digestive, diuretic, febrifuge, and, in large doses, an emetic and purgative*
carmantadine USAN, INN *antiparkinsonian*
carmellose INN *suspending agent; tablet excipient* [also: carboxymethylcellulose sodium; carmellose sodium]
carmellose sodium BAN *suspending agent; tablet excipient* [also: carboxymethylcellulose sodium; carmellose]
carmetizide INN
carminatives *a class of agents that relieve flatulence*
carminomycin HCl [now: carubicin HCl]
carmofur INN
Carmol 10 lotion OTC *moisturizer; emollient; keratolytic* [urea] 10%
Carmol 20; Carmol 40 cream OTC *moisturizer; emollient; keratolytic* [urea] 20%; 40%
Carmol HC cream ℞ *topical corticosteroidal anti-inflammatory; moisturizer; emollient* [hydrocortisone acetate; urea] 1%•10%
carmoxirole INN
carmustine USAN, INN, BAN *nitrosourea-type alkylating antineoplastic; polymer implant for recurrent malignant glioma (orphan)*
Carnation Follow-Up; Carnation Good Start liquid, powder OTC *total or supplementary infant feeding*
carnauba wax [see: wax, carnauba]
carnidazole USAN, INN, BAN *antiprotozoal*
carnitine INN *vitamin* B_t
L-carnitine [see: levocarnitine]
Carnitor tablets, oral solution, IV injection or infusion ℞ *dietary amino acid for primary and secondary genetic carnitine deficiency (orphan) and end-stage renal disease (orphan); investigational (orphan) for pediatric cardiomyopathy* [levocarnitine] 330 mg; 100 mg/mL; 500 mg/2.5 mL, 1 g/5 mL
carocainide INN
Caroid enteric-coated tablets OTC *stimulant laxative* [bisacodyl] 5 mg
β-carotene [see: beta carotene]
caroverine INN
caroxazone USAN, INN *antidepressant*
carpenter's herb *medicinal herb* [see: woundwort]
carpenter's square *medicinal herb* [see: figwort]
carperidine INN, BAN
carperone INN
carphenazine BAN *antipsychotic* [also: carphenazine maleate; carfenazine]
carphenazine maleate USAN, USP *antipsychotic* [also: carfenazine; carphenazine]
carpindolol INN
carpipramine INN
carpipramine dihydrochloride [see: carpipramine]
carpolene [now: carbomer 934P]
carprazidil INN
carprofen USAN, INN, BAN *nonsteroidal anti-inflammatory drug (NSAID); analgesic; antipyretic*
carpronium chloride INN
Carpuject (trademarked delivery system) *prefilled cartridge-needle unit*
Carpuject Smartpak (trademarked delivery system) *prefilled cartridge-needle unit package*
carrageenan NF *suspending and viscosity-increasing agent*

Carrisyn ℞ *investigational (Phase I) antiviral and immunomodulator for AIDS* [acemannan]

carrot *(Daucus carota)* oil from the dried seed and root *medicinal herb for edema, gas, and worms; also used as a nutritional and vitamin supplement and stimulant; may possibly protect the heart and liver*

carsalam INN, BAN

carsatrin INN *cardiotonic* [also: carsatrin succinate]

carsatrin succinate USAN *cardiotonic* [also: carsatrin]

cartazolate USAN, INN *antidepressant*

carteolol INN, BAN *antihypertensive; antiadrenergic (β-blocker); topical antiglaucoma agent* [also: carteolol HCl]

carteolol HCl USAN *antihypertensive; antiadrenergic (β-blocker); topical antiglaucoma agent* [also: carteolol] 1% eye drops

Carthamus tinctorius *medicinal herb* [see: safflower]

Cartia XT extended-release capsules ℞ *antihypertensive; antianginal; antiarrhythmic; calcium channel blocker* [diltiazem HCl] 120, 180, 240, 300 mg

carticaine BAN *amide local anesthetic for dentistry* [also: articaine]

Carticel ℞ *investigational (NDA filed) process to grow autologous cartilage cells to correct cartilage damage due to acute or chronic trauma* [chondrocytes, cultured autologous]

Cartrix (delivery system) *prefilled syringes*

Cartrol Filmtabs (film-coated tablets) OTC *antihypertensive; antiadrenergic (β-blocker)* [carteolol HCl] 2.5, 5 mg

carubicin INN *antineoplastic* [also: carubicin HCl]

carubicin HCl USAN *antineoplastic* [also: carubicin]

Carum carvi NF *medicinal herb* [see: caraway]

carumonam INN, BAN *antibacterial* [also: carumonam sodium]

carumonam sodium USAN *antibacterial* [also: carumonam]

carvedilol USAN, INN, BAN, JAN *antianginal; antihypertensive; α- and β-blocker for congestive heart failure*

carvotroline HCl USAN *antipsychotic*

Caryophyllus aromaticus *medicinal herb* [see: cloves]

carzelesin USAN *antineoplastic*

carzenide INN

casanthranol USAN, USP *stimulant laxative*

Cascara Aromatic oral liquid OTC *stimulant laxative* [cascara sagrada; alcohol 18%]

cascara fluidextract, aromatic USP *stimulant laxative* 2–6 mL oral

cascara sagrada USP *stimulant laxative* 325 mg oral

cascara sagrada *(Frangula purshiana; Rhamnus purshiana)* bark *medicinal herb for constipation, cough, and gallbladder, intestinal, and liver disorders; chronic use can cause hypokalemia and melanosis coli* [also see: buckthorn]

cascara sagrada fluid extract *investigational (orphan) for oral drug overdose*

cascarin [see: casanthranol]

Casec powder OTC *protein supplement* [calcium caseinate]

Casodex film-coated tablets ℞ *antiandrogen antineoplastic for prostatic cancer* [bicalutamide] 50 mg

caspofungin acetate USAN *systemic echinocandin antifungal for invasive aspergillosis and other resistant fungal infections*

Cassia acutifolia; C. angustifolia; C. senna *medicinal herb* [see: senna]

cassia oil [see: cinnamon oil]

CAST (Color Allergy Screening Test) reagent sticks for professional use *in vitro diagnostic aid for immunoglobulin E in serum*

Castaderm liquid OTC *topical antifungal; astringent; antiseptic* [resorcinol; boric acid; acetone; basic fuchsin; phenol; alcohol 9%]

Castel Minus; Castel Plus liquid OTC *topical antifungal* [resorcinol; acetone; basic fuchsin; alcohol 11.5%]

Castellani paint [see: carbol-fuchsin solution]

Castellani Paint Modified solution ℞ *topical antifungal; antibacterial; keratolytic* [basic fuchsin; phenol; resorcinol]

Castile soap

castor oil USP *stimulant laxative*

CaT (carboplatin, Taxol) *chemotherapy protocol for adenocarcinoma, non–small cell lung cancer (NSCLC), and ovarian cancer*

CAT (cytarabine, Adriamycin, thioguanine) *chemotherapy protocol*

Cataflam tablets ℞ *analgesic; antiarthritic; nonsteroidal anti-inflammatory drug (NSAID) for ankylosing spondylitis* [diclofenac potassium] 50 mg

Catapres tablets ℞ *antihypertensive* [clonidine HCl] 0.1, 0.2, 0.3 mg 🗣 Catarase; Combipres; Ser-Ap-Es

Catapres-TTS-1; Catapres-TTS-2; Catapres-TTS-3 7-day transdermal patch ℞ *antihypertensive* [clonidine HCl] 0.1 mg/day (2.5 mg); 0.2 mg/day (5 mg); 0.3 mg/day (7.5 mg)

Catarase 1:5000 ophthalmic solution (discontinued 1999) ℞ *enzymatic zonulolytic for intracapsular lens extraction* [chymotrypsin] 300 U 🗣 Catapres

Catatrol ℞ *investigational (NDA filed) bicyclic antidepressant* [viloxazine]

catchfly *medicinal herb* [see: dogbane]

catchweed *medicinal herb* [see: bedstraw]

catechol-O-methyltransferase (COMT) [see: COMT inhibitors]

catgut suture [see: absorbable surgical suture]

Catha edulis *the plant from which cathinone, a naturally occurring stimulant, is derived* [see also: cathinone; methcathinone]

Catharanthus roseus *medicinal herb* [see: periwinkle]

cathartics *a class of agents that cause vigorous evacuation of the bowels by increasing bulk, stimulating peristaltic action, etc.* [also called: purgatives]

cathine INN

cathinone INN *an extract of the Catha edulis plant, a naturally occurring stimulant* [see also: *Catha edulis*; methcathinone]

cathomycin sodium [see: novobiocin sodium]

catkins willow *medicinal herb* [see: willow]

catmint *medicinal herb* [see: catnip]

catnip (*Nepeta cataria*) plant *medicinal herb for colds, colic, convulsions, diarrhea, digestion, fever, flu, gas, hives, nervous conditions, and stimulating delayed menses*

Catrix Correction cream OTC *moisturizer; emollient*

catrup *medicinal herb* [see: catnip]

cat's claw (*Uncaria guianensis; U. tomentosa*) inner bark *medicinal herb for cancer, Candida infections, chronic fatigue, contraception, Crohn disease, diverticulitis, hypertension, irritable bowel, lupus, parasites, PMS, ulcers, and viral infections; also used as immune booster*

catswort *medicinal herb* [see: catnip]

Caucasian walnut *medicinal herb* [see: English walnut]

Caulophyllum thalictroides *medicinal herb* [see: blue cohosh]

caustics *a class of escharotic or corrosive agents that destroy living tissue* [also called: cauterants]

cauterants *a class of escharotic or corrosive agents that destroy living tissue* [also called: caustics]

CAV (cyclophosphamide, Adriamycin, vinblastine) *chemotherapy protocol*

CAV (cyclophosphamide, Adriamycin, vincristine) *chemotherapy protocol for small cell lung cancer* [also: VAC]

CAVe; CA-Ve (CCNU, Adriamycin, vinblastine) *chemotherapy protocol*

CAVE (cyclophosphamide, Adriamycin, vincristine, etoposide) *chemotherapy protocol for small cell lung cancer*

Caverject powder for intracavernosal injection, PenInject single-use autoinjector ℞ *vasodilator for erectile dysfunction* [alprostadil] 5, 10, 20 μg/mL

CA-VP16; CAVP16 (cyclophosphamide, Adriamycin, VP-16) *chemotherapy protocol for small cell lung cancer*

cayenne (*Capsicum annuum*; *C. frutescens*) fruit *medicinal herb for arthritis, bleeding, cold feet, diabetes, high blood pressure, kidney disorders, rheumatism, poor circulation, strokes, topical neuritis syndromes, tumors, and ulcers*

CBP-1011 *investigational (Phase III) orally administered steroid for idiopathic thrombocytopenic purpura*

CBV (cyclophosphamide, BCNU, VePesid) *chemotherapy protocol*

CBV (cyclophosphamide, BCNU, VP-16-213) *chemotherapy protocol*

CC (carboplatin, cyclophosphamide) *chemotherapy protocol for ovarian cancer*

CC-Galactosidase ℞ *investigational (orphan) enzyme replacement therapy for Fabry disease* [alpha-galactosidase A]

CCM (cyclophosphamide, CCNU, methotrexate) *chemotherapy protocol*

CCNU (chloroethyl-cyclohexyl-nitrosourea) [see: lomustine]

CCV-AV (CCNU, cyclophosphamide, vincristine [alternates with] Adriamycin, vincristine) *chemotherapy protocol*

CCVPP (CCNU, cyclophosphamide, Velban, procarbazine, prednisone) *chemotherapy protocol*

CD (cytarabine, daunorubicin) *chemotherapy protocol*

CD4, recombinant soluble human (rCD4) *investigational (Phase II, orphan) antiviral for AIDS*

CD4 immunoadhesin [see: CD4 immunoglobulin G, recombinant human]

CD4 immunoglobulin G, recombinant human *investigational (Phase I) antiviral for maternal/fetal transfer of HIV; investigational (orphan) for AIDS*

CD4-IgG [see: CD4 immunoglobulin G, recombinant human]

CD4-PE40 [see: alvircept sudotox]

CD5-T lymphocyte immunotoxin *orphan status withdrawn 1997*

CD19 [see: anti-B4-blocked ricin]

CD20 *investigational for low-grade non-Hodgkin lymphoma*

CD-33 [see: ricin (blocked) conjugated murine MCA myeloid cells]

CD-40 ligand (CD40L) *investigational (Phase II) cytokine for renal cell carcinoma; investigational (Phase I) for rheumatoid arthritis, AIDS, and hyperimmunoglobulin M (HIM) syndrome*

CD-45RB monoclonal antibodies *investigational antirejection antibody*

CdA (2-chloro-2′-deoxyadenosine) [see: cladribine]

CDC (carboplatin, doxorubicin, cyclophosphamide) *chemotherapy protocol*

CDDP; C-DDP (*cis*-diamminedichloroplatinum) [see: cisplatin]

CDDP/VP; CDDP/VP-16 (CDDP, VP-16) *chemotherapy protocol for pediatric brain tumors*

CDE (cyclophosphamide, doxorubicin, etoposide) *chemotherapy protocol*

CDP-571 *investigational (Phase III, orphan) anti-TNFα (tumor necrosis factor alpha) antibody CB-0010 for steroid-dependent Crohn disease; investigational for rheumatoid arthritis*

CDP-cholin [see: citicoline]

CEA (carcinoembryonic antigen)

CEA-Cide ℞ *investigational (orphan) yttrium Y 90–radiolabeled antineoplastic for pancreatic, ovarian, and small cell lung cancer* [monoclonal antibody to CEA, humanized]

CEAker *orphan status withdrawn 1997* [indium In 111 murine anti-CEA MAb, type ZCE 025]

Ceanothus americanus *medicinal herb* [see: New Jersey tea]

CEA-Scan powder for injection ℞ *imaging agent for detection of recurrent or metastatic colorectal cancer* [arcitumomab] 1.25 mg

CEB (carboplatin, etoposide, bleomycin) *chemotherapy protocol*
Cebid Timecelles (sustained-release capsules) (discontinued 1999) OTC *vitamin C supplement* [ascorbic acid] 500 mg
CECA (cisplatin, etoposide, cyclophosphamide, Adriamycin) *chemotherapy protocol*
Ceclor Pulvules (capsules), powder for oral suspension ℞ *cephalosporin antibiotic* [cefaclor] 250, 500 mg; 125, 187, 250, 375 mg/5 mL
Ceclor CD extended-release tablets ℞ *cephalosporin antibiotic* [cefaclor] 375, 500 mg
Ceclor CDpak extended-release tablets in compliance packs of 14 ℞ *cephalosporin antibiotic* [cefaclor] 500 mg
Cecon drops OTC *vitamin C supplement* [ascorbic acid] 100 mg/mL
Cedax capsules, oral suspension ℞ *cephalosporin antibiotic* [ceftibuten] 400 mg; 90, 180 mg/mL
cedefingol USAN *antipsoriatic; antineoplastic adjunct*
cedelizumab USAN *monoclonal antibody; prophylaxis of rejection of solid organ allograft; immunomodulator for autoimmune diseases*
CeeNu capsules, dose pack ℞ *nitrosourea-type alkylating antineoplastic for brain tumors and Hodgkin disease* [lomustine] 10, 40, 100 mg; 2×100 mg + 2×40 mg + 2×10 mg
CEF (cyclophosphamide, epirubicin, fluorouracil, [co-trimoxazole]) *chemotherapy protocol for breast cancer*
cefacetrile INN *antibacterial* [also: cephacetrile sodium]
cefacetrile sodium [see: cephacetrile sodium]
cefaclor USAN, USP, INN, BAN, JAN *second-generation cephalosporin antibiotic* 250, 500 mg oral; 125, 187, 250, 375 mg/5 mL oral
cefadroxil USAN, USP, INN, BAN *first-generation cephalosporin antibiotic* 500, 1000 mg oral
Cefadyl powder for IV or IM injection ℞ *cephalosporin antibiotic* [cephapirin sodium] 1 g ⑨ Cefzil
cefalexin INN, JAN *first-generation cephalosporin antibiotic* [also: cephalexin]
cefaloglycin INN *antibacterial* [also: cephaloglycin]
cefalonium INN [also: cephalonium]
cefaloram INN [also: cephaloram]
cefaloridine INN *antibacterial* [also: cephaloridine]
cefalotin INN *first-generation cephalosporin antibiotic* [also: cephalothin sodium; cephalothin]
cefalotin sodium [see: cephalothin sodium]
cefamandole USAN, INN *second-generation cephalosporin antibiotic* [also: cephamandole]
cefamandole nafate USAN, USP *second-generation cephalosporin antibiotic* [also: cephamandole nafate]
cefamandole sodium USP *second-generation cephalosporin antibiotic*
cefaparole USAN, INN *antibacterial*
cefapirin INN, BAN *first-generation cephalosporin antibiotic* [also: cephapirin sodium]
cefapirin sodium [see: cephapirin sodium]
cefatrizine USAN, INN, BAN *antibacterial*
cefazaflur INN *antibacterial* [also: cefazaflur sodium]
cefazaflur sodium USAN *antibacterial* [also: cefazaflur]
cefazedone INN, BAN
cefazolin USP, INN *first-generation cephalosporin antibiotic* [also: cephazolin] ⑨ cephalothin; Zefazone
cefazolin sodium USAN, USP *first-generation cephalosporin antibiotic* [also: cephazolin sodium] 0.25, 0.5, 1, 5, 10, 20 g injection ⑨ cephalothin; Zefazone
cefbuperazone USAN, INN *antibacterial*
cefcanel INN
cefcanel daloxate INN
cefdinir USAN, INN *third-generation cephalosporin antibiotic*

cefditoren pivoxil *broad-spectrum cephalosporin antibiotic*
cefedrolor INN
cefempidone INN, BAN
cefepime USAN, INN *third-generation cephalosporin antibiotic*
cefepime HCl USAN *third-generation cephalosporin antibiotic*
cefetamet USAN, INN *veterinary antibacterial*
cefetecol USAN, INN, BAN *antibacterial*
cefetrizole INN
cefivitril INN
cefixime USAN, USP, INN, BAN *third-generation cephalosporin antibiotic*
Cefizox powder or frozen premix for IV or IM injection ℞ *cephalosporin antibiotic* [ceftizoxime sodium] 0.5, 1, 2, 10 g
cefmenoxime INN *antibacterial* [also: cefmenoxime HCl]
cefmenoxime HCl USAN, USP *antibacterial* [also: cefmenoxime]
cefmepidium chloride INN
cefmetazole USAN, INN *second-generation cephalosporin antibiotic*
cefmetazole sodium USAN, USP, JAN *second-generation cephalosporin antibiotic*
cefminox INN
Cefobid powder or frozen premix for IV or IM injection ℞ *cephalosporin antibiotic* [cefoperazone sodium] 1, 2, 10 g
cefodizime INN *investigational cephalosporin antibiotic*
Cefol Filmtabs (film-coated tablets) ℞ *vitamin supplement* [multiple vitamins; folic acid] ≛ •0.5 mg
cefonicid INN, BAN *second-generation cephalosporin antibiotic* [also: cefonicid monosodium]
cefonicid monosodium USAN *second-generation cephalosporin antibiotic* [also: cefonicid]
cefonicid sodium USAN, USP *second-generation cephalosporin antibiotic*
cefoperazone INN, BAN *third-generation cephalosporin antibiotic* [also: cefoperazone sodium]
cefoperazone sodium USAN, USP *third-generation cephalosporin antibiotic* [also: cefoperazone]
ceforanide USAN, USP, INN, BAN *bactericidal antibiotic*
Cefotan powder or frozen premix for IV or IM injection ℞ *cephamycin antibiotic* [cefotetan disodium] 1, 2, 10 g
cefotaxime INN, BAN *third-generation cephalosporin antibiotic* [also: cefotaxime sodium] ⁅ cefoxitin
cefotaxime sodium USAN, USP *third-generation cephalosporin antibiotic* [also: cefotaxime]
cefotetan USAN, INN, BAN *cephamycin antibiotic*
cefotetan disodium USAN, USP *cephamycin antibiotic*
cefotiam INN, BAN *antibacterial* [also: cefotiam HCl]
cefotiam HCl USAN *antibacterial* [also: cefotiam]
cefoxazole INN [also: cephoxazole]
cefoxitin USAN, INN, BAN *cephamycin antibiotic* ⁅ cefotaxime
cefoxitin sodium USAN, USP, BAN *cephamycin antibiotic* 1, 2 g/vial injection
cefpimizole USAN, INN *antibacterial*
cefpimizole sodium USAN, JAN *antibacterial*
cefpiramide USAN, USP, INN *antibacterial*
cefpiramide sodium USAN, JAN *antibacterial*
cefpirome INN, BAN *antibacterial* [also: cefpirome sulfate]
cefpirome sulfate USAN, JAN *antibacterial* [also: cefpirome]
cefpodoxime INN, BAN *broad-spectrum third-generation cephalosporin antibiotic* [also: cefpodoxime proxetil]
cefpodoxime proxetil USAN, JAN *broad-spectrum third-generation cephalosporin antibiotic* [also: cefpodoxime]
cefprozil USAN, INN *second-generation cephalosporin antibiotic*
cefprozil monohydrate
cefquinome INN, BAN *veterinary antibacterial*
cefquinome sulfate USAN *veterinary antibacterial*
cefradine INN *first-generation cephalosporin antibiotic* [also: cephradine]

cefrotil INN

cefroxadine USAN, INN *antibacterial*

cefsulodin INN, BAN *antibacterial* [also: cefsulodin sodium]

cefsulodin sodium USAN *antibacterial* [also: cefsulodin]

cefsumide INN

ceftazidime USAN, USP, INN, BAN, JAN *third-generation cephalosporin antibiotic*

cefteram INN

ceftezole INN

ceftibuten USAN, INN, BAN *third-generation cephalosporin antibiotic*

Ceftin film-coated tablets, oral suspension ℞ *cephalosporin antibiotic* [cefuroxime axetil] 125, 250, 500 mg; 125, 250 mg/5 mL

ceftiofur INN, BAN *veterinary antibacterial* [also: ceftiofur HCl]

ceftiofur HCl USAN *veterinary antibacterial* [also: ceftiofur]

ceftiofur sodium USAN *veterinary antibacterial*

ceftiolene INN

ceftioxide INN

ceftizoxime INN, BAN *third-generation cephalosporin antibiotic* [also: ceftizoxime sodium] ⑨ cefuroxime

ceftizoxime sodium USAN, USP *third-generation cephalosporin antibiotic* [also: ceftizoxime]

ceftriaxone INN, BAN *third-generation cephalosporin antibiotic* [also: ceftriaxone sodium]

ceftriaxone sodium USAN, USP *third-generation cephalosporin antibiotic* [also: ceftriaxone]

cefuracetime INN, BAN

cefuroxime USAN, INN, BAN *second-generation cephalosporin antibiotic* ⑨ ceftizoxime

cefuroxime axetil USAN, USP, BAN *second-generation cephalosporin antibiotic*

cefuroxime pivoxetil USAN *second-generation cephalosporin antibiotic*

cefuroxime sodium USP, BAN *second-generation cephalosporin antibiotic* 0.75, 1.5, 7.5 g injection

cefuzonam INN

Cefzil film-coated tablets, powder for oral suspension ℞ *cephalosporin antibiotic* [cefprozil] 250, 500 mg; 125, 250 mg/5 mL ⑨ Cefadyl; Kefzol

Cefzon (foreign name for U.S. product Omnicef)

celandine *(Chelidonium majus)* root and plant *medicinal herb used as an analgesic, antispasmodic, caustic, diaphoretic, diuretic, narcotic, and purgative*

Celebra (name changed to Celebrex upon release in 1999)

Celebrex capsules ℞ *antiarthritic; antipyretic; COX-2 inhibitor; nonsteroidal anti-inflammatory drug (NSAID); reduces polyp proliferation in familial adenomatous polyposis (FAP)* [celecoxib] 100, 200 mg ⑨ Cerebyx

celecoxib USAN *antiarthritic; antipyretic; COX-2 inhibitor; nonsteroidal anti-inflammatory drug (NSAID); reduces polyp proliferation in familial adenomatous polyposis (FAP)*

celery *(Apium graveolens)* root, stem, and seeds *medicinal herb for aiding digestion, arthritis, cancer, diuresis, gas, headache, hysteria, inducing menstruation, lumbago, nervousness, rheumatism, and terminating lactation*

Celestoderm-V; Celestoderm-V/2 (CAN) cream, ointment ℞ *topical corticosteroidal anti-inflammatory* [betamethasone valerate] 0.1%; 0.05%

Celestone tablets, syrup *corticosteroid; anti-inflammatory* [betamethasone] 0.6 mg; 0.6 mg/5 mL

Celestone Phosphate IV, IM injection ℞ *corticosteroid; anti-inflammatory* [betamethasone sodium phosphate] 4 mg/mL

Celestone Soluspan intrabursal, intra-articular, intralesional injection ℞ *corticosteroid; anti-inflammatory* [betamethasone sodium phosphate; betamethasone acetate] 3•3 mg/mL

Celexa film-coated tablets, oral solution ℞ *selective serotonin reuptake inhibitor (SSRI) for depression* [citalopram hydrobromide] 10, 20, 40 mg; 10 mg/5 mL

celgosivir HCl USAN *antiviral; α-glucosidase I inhibitor for HIV*

celiprolol INN, BAN *antiadrenergic (β-receptor)* [also: celiprolol HCl]

celiprolol HCl USAN *antiadrenergic (β-receptor)* [also: celiprolol]

cellacefate INN *tablet-coating agent* [also: cellulose acetate phthalate; cellacephate]

cellacephate BAN *tablet-coating agent* [also: cellulose acetate phthalate; cellacefate]

CellCept capsules, tablets, oral suspension ℞ *immunosuppressant for allogenic heart, liver, and kidney transplants* [mycophenolate mofetil] 250 mg; 500 mg; 200 mg/mL

CellCept powder for IV infusion ℞ *immunosuppressant for allogenic heart, liver, and kidney transplants* [mycophenolate mofetil HCl] 500 mg

Cellufresh eye drops (discontinued 1998) OTC *ophthalmic moisturizer/lubricant* [carboxymethylcellulose] 0.5%

cellulase USAN *digestive enzyme*

cellulolytic enzyme [see: cellulase]

cellulose *bulk laxative*

cellulose, absorbable [see: cellulose, oxidized]

cellulose, ethyl ester [see: ethylcellulose]

cellulose, hydroxypropyl methyl ether [see: hydroxypropyl methylcellulose]

cellulose, microcrystalline NF *tablet and capsule diluent* [also: dispersible cellulose]

cellulose, oxidized USP *topical local hemostatic*

cellulose, oxidized regenerated USP *local hemostatic*

cellulose, sodium carboxymethyl [see: carboxymethylcellulose sodium]

cellulose acetate NF *tablet-coating agent; insoluble polymer membrane*

cellulose acetate butyrate [see: cabufocon A; cabufocon B]

cellulose acetate dibutyrate [see: porofocon A; porofocon B]

cellulose acetate phthalate (CAP) NF *tablet-coating agent* [also: cellacefate; cellacephate]

cellulose carboxymethyl ether, sodium salt [see: carboxymethylcellulose sodium]

cellulose diacetate [see: cellulose acetate]

cellulose dihydrogen phosphate, disodium salt [see: cellulose sodium phosphate]

cellulose disodium phosphate [see: cellulose sodium phosphate]

cellulose ethyl ether [see: ethylcellulose]

cellulose gum, modified [now: croscarmellose sodium]

cellulose methyl ether [see: methylcellulose]

cellulose nitrate [see: pyroxylin]

cellulose sodium phosphate (CSP) USAN, USP *antiurolithic to prevent stone formation in absorptive hypercalciuria Type I*

cellulosic acid [see: cellulose, oxidized]

Celluvisc solution OTC *ophthalmic moisturizer/lubricant* [carboxymethylcellulose] 1%

celmoleukin INN *immunostimulant*

Celontin Kapseals (capsules) ℞ *succinimide anticonvulsant* [methsuximide] 150, 300 mg

celucloral INN, BAN

Cel-U-Jec IV, IM injection ℞ *corticosteroid; anti-inflammatory* [betamethasone sodium phosphate] 4 mg/mL

CEM (cytosine arabinoside, etoposide, methotrexate) *chemotherapy protocol*

Cenafed syrup OTC *nasal decongestant* [pseudoephedrine HCl] 30 mg/5 mL

Cenafed Plus tablets OTC *decongestant; antihistamine* [pseudoephedrine HCl; triprolidine HCl] 60•2.5 mg

Cena-K liquid ℞ *potassium supplement* [potassium chloride] 20, 40 mEq/15 mL

Cenestin film-coated tablets ℞ *estrogen replacement therapy for postmeno-*

pausal symptoms [conjugated estrogens, synthetic] 0.625, 0.9, 1.25 mg

Cenolate IV, IM, or subcu injection ℞ *vitamin C therapy; antiscorbutic* [sodium ascorbate] 562.5 mg/mL

Centara ℞ *investigational treatment for arthritis and multiple sclerosis; transplant rejection preventative* [priliximab]

Centaurea cyanus *medicinal herb* [see: cornflower]

centaury *(Erythraea centaurium)* plant *medicinal herb for aiding digestion, blood cleansing, fever, and promoting menstruation*

Centella asiatica *medicinal herb* [see: gotu kola]

Center-Al subcu or IM injection ℞ *allergenic sensitivity testing (subcu); allergenic desensitization therapy (IM)* [allergenic extracts, alum-precipitated]

Centoxin ℞ *investigational (orphan) for gram-negative bacteremia in endotoxin shock* [nebacumab]

centrazene [see: simtrazene]

centrophenoxine [see: meclofenoxate]

Centrum, Advanced Formula liquid OTC *vitamin/mineral/iron supplement* [multiple vitamins & minerals; ferrous fumarate; biotin; alcohol 6.7%] ≛ •9•0.3 mg/15 mL

Centrum, Advanced Formula tablets OTC *vitamin/mineral/iron supplement* [multiple vitamins & minerals; ferrous fumarate; folic acid; biotin] ≛ •18 mg•0.4 mg•30 µg

Centrum Jr. + Extra C; Centrum Jr. + Extra Calcium chewable tablets OTC *vitamin/mineral/calcium/iron supplement* [multiple vitamins & minerals; calcium; iron; folic acid; biotin] ≛ •108•18•0.4•0.045 mg; ≛ •160•18•0.4•0.045 mg

Centrum Jr. with Iron tablets OTC *vitamin/mineral/iron supplement* [multiple vitamins & minerals; iron; folic acid; biotin] ≛ •18 mg•0.4 mg•45 µg

Centrum Silver tablets OTC *geriatric vitamin/mineral supplement* [multiple vitamins & minerals; folic acid; biotin] ≛ •400•30 µg

Ceo-Two suppository OTC *CO_2-releasing laxative* [sodium bicarbonate; potassium bitartrate]

CEP (CCNU, etoposide, prednimustine) *chemotherapy protocol*

Cēpacol mouthwash/gargle OTC *oral antiseptic* [cetylpyridinium chloride] 0.05%

Cēpacol, Children's oral liquid OTC *pediatric decongestant and analgesic* [pseudoephedrine HCl; acetaminophen] 15•160 mg/5 mL

Cēpacol Anesthetic troches OTC *topical oral anesthetic; antiseptic* [benzocaine; cetylpyridinium chloride] 10 mg•0.07%

Cēpacol Maximum Strength lozenges OTC *topical oral anesthetic* [benzocaine] 10 mg

Cēpacol Throat lozenges OTC *oral antiseptic* [cetylpyridinium chloride] 0.07%

Cēpacol Viractin cream, gel OTC *topical anesthetic for cold sores and fever blisters* [tetracaine HCl] 2%

Cēpastat Sore Throat lozenges OTC *topical antipruritic/counterirritant; mild local anesthetic* [phenol] 14.5, 29 mg 🔊 Capastat

cephacetrile sodium USAN, USP *antibacterial* [also: cefacetrile]

cephalexin USAN, USP, BAN *first-generation cephalosporin antibiotic* [also: cefalexin] 250, 500, 1000 mg oral; 125, 250 mg/5 mL oral 🔊 cefazolin; cephalothin

cephalexin HCl USAN, USP *first-generation cephalosporin antibiotic*

cephaloglycin USAN, USP, BAN *antibacterial* [also: cefaloglycin]

cephalonium BAN [also: cefalonium]

cephaloram BAN [also: cefaloram]

cephaloridine USAN, USP, BAN *antibacterial* [also: cefaloridine]

cephalosporin N [see: adicillin]

cephalosporins *a class of bactericidal antibiotics, divided into first-, second-, and third-generation cephalosporins; higher generations have increasing efficacy against gram-negative and* *decreasing efficacy against gram-positive bacteria*

cephalothin BAN *first-generation cephalosporin antibiotic* [also: cephalothin sodium; cefalotin] ⓢ cefazolin

cephalothin sodium USAN, USP *first-generation cephalosporin antibiotic* [also: cefalotin; cephalothin]

cephamandole BAN *second-generation cephalosporin antibiotic* [also: cefamandole]

cephamandole nafate BAN *second-generation cephalosporin antibiotic* [also: cefamandole nafate]

cephamycins *a class of bactericidal antibiotics similar to second-generation cephalosporins (q.v.)*

cephapirin sodium USAN, USP *first-generation cephalosporin antibiotic* [also: cefapirin] ⓢ cephradine

cephazolin BAN *first-generation cephalosporin antibiotic* [also: cefazolin]

cephazolin sodium BAN *first-generation cephalosporin antibiotic* [also: cefazolin sodium]

cephoxazole BAN [also: cefoxazole]

cephradine USAN, USP, BAN *first-generation cephalosporin antibiotic* [also: cefradine] 250, 500 mg oral; 125, 250 mg/5 mL oral ⓢ cephapirin

Cephulac oral/rectal solution ℞ *synthetic disaccharide used to prevent and treat portal-systemic encephalopathy* [lactulose] 10 g/15 mL

CEPP (cyclophosphamide, etoposide, prednisone) *chemotherapy protocol for non-Hodgkin lymphoma*

CEPPB (cyclophosphamide, etoposide, prednisone, bleomycin) *chemotherapy protocol for non-Hodgkin lymphoma*

Ceprate SC ℞ *investigational (Phase III) stem cell concentration/purification system for multiple myeloma and bone marrow transplants for breast cancer* [monoclonal antibodies]

Ceptaz powder for IV or IM injection ℞ *cephalosporin antibiotic* [ceftazidime pentahydrate] 1, 2, 10 g

ceramide trihexosidase (CTH) & alpha-galactosidase A *investigational (orphan) enzyme replacement therapy for Fabry disease*

CerAxon ℞ *investigational (Phase III) brain tissue protector for ischemic stroke* [citicoline sodium]

Cerebyx IV or IM injection ℞ *hydantoin anticonvulsant for grand mal status epilepticus (orphan)* [fosphenytoin sodium (phenytoin sodium equivalent)] 75 (50) mg/mL ⓢ Celebrex

CereCRIB implant (trials discontinued 1999) ℞ *investigational (Phase II) for severe chronic pain in cancer patients* [encapsulated bovine cell]

Ceredase IV infusion ℞ *glucocerebrosidase enzyme replacement in Gaucher disease type I (orphan); investigational (orphan) for types II and III* [alglucerase] 10, 80 U/mL

cerelose [see: glucose]

Ceresine ℞ *investigational (orphan) pyruvate dehydrogenase activator for acute head trauma and neurologic injury* [sodium dichloroacetate]

Cerestat ℞ *investigational (Phase III) treatment for traumatic brain injury (clinical trials discontinued 1997); investigational (Phase III) treatment for stroke* [aptiganel HCl]

Cerezyme powder for IV infusion ℞ *enzyme replacement therapy for types I, II, and III Gaucher disease (orphan)* [imiglucerase] 40 U/mL

cerium *element (Ce)*

cerium oxalate USP

cerivastatin sodium USAN *HMG-CoA reductase inhibitor for hyperlipidemia and hypertriglyceridemia (discontinued 2001 due to safety concerns)*

Cernevit-12 powder for IV injection ℞ *parenteral vitamin therapy* [multiple vitamins; folic acid; biotin] ≛ •414• 60 μg

ceronapril USAN, INN *antihypertensive*

Cerose-DM liquid OTC *antitussive; decongestant; antihistamine* [dextromethorphan hydrobromide; phenylephrine HCl; chlorpheniramine maleate; alcohol 2.4%] 15•10•4 mg/5 mL

Cerovite; Cerovite Advanced Formula tablets OTC *vitamin/mineral/iron supplement* [multiple vitamins & minerals; ferrous fumarate; folic acid; biotin] ≛•18 mg•0.4 mg•30 µg

Cerovite Jr. tablets OTC *vitamin/mineral/iron supplement* [multiple vitamins & minerals; ferrous fumarate; folic acid; biotin] ≛•18 mg•0.4 mg•45 µg

Cerovite Senior tablets OTC *geriatric vitamin/mineral supplement* [multiple vitamins & minerals; folic acid; biotin] ≛•200•30 µg

Certagen film-coated tablets OTC *vitamin/mineral/iron supplement* [multiple vitamins & minerals; ferrous fumarate; folic acid; biotin] ≛•18 mg•0.4 mg•30 µg

Certagen liquid OTC *vitamin/mineral/iron supplement* [multiple vitamins & minerals; iron; biotin; alcohol 6.6%] ≛•9•0.3 mg

Certagen Senior tablets OTC *geriatric vitamin/mineral supplement* [multiple vitamins & minerals; folic acid; biotin] ≛•200•30 µg

Certa-Vite tablets OTC *vitamin/mineral/iron supplement* [multiple vitamins & minerals; ferrous fumarate; folic acid; biotin] ≛•18 mg•0.4 mg•30 µg

Certa-Vite Golden tablets OTC *geriatric vitamin/mineral supplement* [multiple vitamins & minerals; biotin] ≛•30 µg

Certican ℞ *investigational agent for transplant rejection* [everolimus]

Certiva IM injection ℞ *active immunizing agent for diphtheria, tetanus, and pertussis* [diphtheria & tetanus toxoids & acellular pertussis (DTaP) vaccine, adsorbed] 15 LfU•6 LfU•40 µg per 0.5 mL

Cerubidine powder for IV injection ℞ *antibiotic antineoplastic for multiple nonlymphocytic leukemias* [daunorubicin HCl] 20 mg

ceruletide USAN, INN, BAN *gastric secretory stimulant*

ceruletide diethylamine USAN *gastric secretory stimulant*

Cerumenex ear drops ℞ *cerumenolytic to emulsify and disperse ear wax* [trolamine polypeptide oleate-condensate] 10%

Cervidil vaginal insert ℞ *prostaglandin for cervical ripening at term* [dinoprostone] 10 mg

C.E.S. (CAN) sugar-coated tablets ℞ *estrogen replacement therapy for postmenopausal symptoms* [conjugated estrogens (from plants)] 0.4, 0.625, 0.9, 1.25 mg

cesium *element (Cs)*

cesium (^{131}Cs) chloride INN *radioactive agent* [also: cesium chloride Cs 131]

cesium chloride Cs 131 USAN *radioactive agent* [also: cesium (^{131}Cs) chloride]

Ceta liquid OTC *soap-free therapeutic skin cleanser*

Ceta Plus capsules ℞ *narcotic analgesic* [hydrocodone bitartrate; acetaminophen] 5•500 mg

cetaben INN *antihyperlipoproteinemic* [also: cetaben sodium]

cetaben sodium USAN *antihyperlipoproteinemic* [also: cetaben]

Cetacaine gel, liquid, ointment, aerosol ℞ *topical local anesthetic; antiseptic* [benzocaine; tetracaine HCl; butamben] 14%•2%•2%

Cetacort lotion ℞ *topical corticosteroidal anti-inflammatory* [hydrocortisone] 0.25%, 0.5%

cetalkonium *antiseptic*

cetalkonium chloride USAN, INN, BAN *topical anti-infective*

Cetamide ophthalmic ointment ℞ *topical ophthalmic antibiotic* [sulfacetamide sodium] 10%

cetamolol INN *antiadrenergic (β-receptor)* [also: cetamolol HCl]

cetamolol HCl USAN *antiadrenergic (β-receptor)* [also: cetamolol]

Cetaphil cream, lotion, cleansing bar, cleansing solution OTC *soap-free therapeutic skin cleanser*

Cetapred ophthalmic ointment ℞ *topical ophthalmic corticosteroidal anti-*

inflammatory; antibiotic [prednisolone acetate; sulfacetamide sodium] 0.25%•10%

cethexonium chloride INN

cetiedil INN *peripheral vasodilator* [also: cetiedil citrate]

cetiedil citrate USAN *peripheral vasodilator* [also: cetiedil]

cetirizine INN, BAN *second-generation piperazine antihistamine* [also: cetirizine HCl]

cetirizine HCl USAN *second-generation piperazine antihistamine for allergic rhinitis and chronic idiopathic urticaria* [also: cetirizine]

cetobemidone [see: ketobemidone]

cetocycline INN *antibacterial* [also: cetocycline HCl]

cetocycline HCl USAN *antibacterial* [also: cetocycline]

cetofenicol INN *antibacterial* [also: cetophenicol]

cetohexazine INN

cetomacrogol 1000 INN, BAN

cetophenicol USAN *antibacterial* [also: cetofenicol]

cetophenylbutazone [see: kebuzone]

cetostearyl alcohol NF *emulsifying agent*

cetotetrine HCl [now: cetocycline HCl]

cetotiamine INN

cetoxime INN, BAN

cetoxime HCl [see: cetoxime]

Cetraria islandica *medicinal herb* [see: Iceland moss]

cetraxate INN *GI antiulcerative* [also: cetraxate HCl]

cetraxate HCl USAN *GI antiulcerative* [also: cetraxate]

cetrimide INN, BAN *topical antiseptic*

cetrimonium bromide INN *topical antiseptic* [also: cetrimonium chloride]

cetrimonium chloride BAN *topical antiseptic* [also: cetrimonium bromide]

cetrorelix acetate USAN *gonadotropin-releasing hormone (Gn-RH) antagonist for infertility*

Cetrotide subcu injection ℞ *gonadotropin-releasing hormone (Gn-RH) antagonist for infertility* [cetrorelix acetate] 0.25, 3 mg

cetuximab USAN *antineoplastic for epidermal growth factor (EGF) receptor–expressing cancers; investigational (Phase III) for advanced squamous cell head and neck cancers; investigational (Phase II) for metastatic renal cell carcinoma*

cetyl alcohol NF *emulsifying and stiffening agent*

cetyl esters wax NF *stiffening agent*

cetyldimethylbenzyl ammonium chloride [see: cetalkonium chloride]

cetylpyridinium chloride USP, INN, BAN *topical antiseptic; preservative*

cetyltrimethyl ammonium bromide

CEV (cyclophosphamide, etoposide, vincristine) *chemotherapy protocol for small cell lung cancer*

Cevalin IV, IM, or subcu injection (discontinued 1999) ℞ *vitamin C therapy; antiscorbutic* [ascorbic acid] 500 mg/mL

Cevi-Bid tablets OTC *vitamin C supplement* [ascorbic acid] 500 mg

Cevi-Fer timed-release capsules ℞ *hematinic; iron/vitamin C supplement* [iron (from ferrous fumarate); ascorbic acid; folic acid] 20•300•1 mg

cevimeline HCl USAN *cholinergic and muscarinic receptor agonist for dry mouth due to Sjögren syndrome*

Ce-Vi-Sol drops (discontinued 1999) OTC *vitamin C supplement* [ascorbic acid; alcohol 5%] 35 mg/0.6 mL

cevitamic acid [see: ascorbic acid]

cevitan [see: ascorbic acid]

ceylon gelatin [see: agar]

Cezin-S capsules ℞ *geriatric vitamin/mineral supplement* [multiple vitamins & minerals; folic acid] ≛•0.5 mg

CF (carboplatin, fluorouracil) *chemotherapy protocol for head and neck cancer*

CF (cisplatin, fluorouracil) *chemotherapy protocol for adenocarcinoma and head and neck cancer*

CFL (cisplatin, fluorouracil, leucovorin [rescue]) *chemotherapy protocol*

CFM (cyclophosphamide, fluorouracil, mitoxantrone) *chemotherapy protocol for breast cancer* [also: CNF; FNC]

CFP (cyclophosphamide, fluorouracil, prednisone) *chemotherapy protocol*

CFPT (cyclophosphamide, fluorouracil, prednisone, tamoxifen) *chemotherapy protocol*

CFTR (cystic fibrosis transmembrane conductance regulator) [q.v.]

CG (Cardio-Green) [q.v.]

CG (chorionic gonadotropin) [see: gonadotropin, chorionic]

CGF (Control Gel Formula) dressing [see: DuoDERM CGF]

CGP-61755 *investigational (Phase I) protease inhibitor for HIV infection*

CGP-64128A *investigational (Phase I) antisense anticancer compound*

CGP-69846A *investigational (Phase II) anticancer agent for solid tumors*

CH1VPP; Ch1VPP (chlorambucil, vinblastine, procarbazine, prednisone) *chemotherapy protocol*

CHAD (cyclophosphamide, hexamethylmelamine, Adriamycin, DDP) *chemotherapy protocol*

chalk, precipitated [see: calcium carbonate, precipitated]

Chamaelirium luteum *medicinal herb* [see: false unicorn]

CHAMOCA (cyclophosphamide, hydroxyurea, actinomycin D, methotrexate, Oncovin, calcium folinate, Adriamycin) *chemotherapy protocol for gestational trophoblastic neoplasm*

chamomile *(Anthemis nobilis; Matricaria chamomilla)* flowers *medicinal herb for appetite stimulation, bronchitis, excessive menstruation with cramps, fever, gastrointestinal cramps, hysteria, inflammation, insomnia, nervousness, rheumatic disorders, and parasites*

CHAP (cyclophosphamide, Hexalen, Adriamycin, Platinol) *chemotherapy protocol for ovarian cancer*

CHAP (cyclophosphamide, hexamethylmelamine, Adriamycin, Platinol) *chemotherapy protocol*

Chap Stick Medicated Lip Balm stick, jar, squeezable tube OTC *topical analgesic; counterirritant; moisturizer; protectant; emollient* [camphor; menthol; phenol] 1%•0.6%•0.5%

chaparral *(Larrea divaricata; L. glutinosa; L. tridentata)* leaves and stems *medicinal herb for arthritis, blood cleansing, bronchitis, cancer, chickenpox, colds, leukemia, rheumatic pain, stomach pain, and tumors; not generally regarded as safe because of liver toxicity and stimulation of some tumors*

CharcoAid oral suspension OTC *adsorbent antidote for poisoning* [activated charcoal] 15 g/120 mL, 30 g/150 mL

CharcoAid 2000 oral liquid, granules OTC *adsorbent antidote for poisoning* [activated charcoal] 15 g/120 mL, 50 g/240 mL; 15 g

charcoal *gastric adsorbent/detoxicant; antiflatulent* 260 mg oral

charcoal, activated USP *general purpose antidote/adsorbent* 15, 30, 40, 120, 240 g, 208 mg/mL oral

Charcoal Plus enteric-coated tablets OTC *adsorbent; detoxicant* [activated charcoal] 250 mg

CharcoCaps capsules OTC *adsorbent; detoxicant; antiflatulent* [charcoal] 260 mg

Chardonna-2 tablets ℞ *GI anticholinergic; sedative* [belladonna extract; phenobarbital] 15•15 mg

chaste tree *(Vitex agnus-castus)* dried ripe fruit *medicinal herb for acne, balancing progesterone and estrogen production, increasing lactation, ovarian insufficiency, premenstrual breast pain, regulating menstrual cycle, and uterine bleeding*

chaulmosulfone INN

checkerberry *medicinal herb* [see: squaw vine; wintergreen]

cheese plant; cheeseflower *medicinal herb* [see: mallow]

cheese rennet *medicinal herb* [see: bedstraw]

chelafrin [see: epinephrine]

Chelated Magnesium tablets OTC *magnesium supplement* [magnesium amino acid chelate] 500 mg

Chelated Manganese tablets OTC *manganese supplement* [manganese] 20, 50 mg

chelating agents *a class of agents that prevent bodily absorption of and cause the excretion of substances such as heavy metals*

chelen [see: ethyl chloride]

Chelidonium majus *medicinal herb* [see: celandine]

Chelone glabra *medicinal herb* [see: turtlebloom]

Chemet capsules ℞ *heavy metal chelating agent for lead poisoning (orphan); investigational (orphan) for cystine kidney stones and mercury poisoning* [succimer] 100 mg

Chemo-Pin (trademarked form) *chemical-dispensing pin*

Chemstrip 2 GP; Chemstrip 2 LN; Chemstrip 4 the OB; Chemstrip 6; Chemstrip 7; Chemstrip 8; Chemstrip 9; Chemstrip 10 with SG; Chemstrip uGK reagent strips *in vitro diagnostic aid for multiple urine products*

Chemstrip bG reagent strips for home use *in vitro diagnostic aid for blood glucose*

Chemstrip K reagent strips for professional use *in vitro diagnostic aid for acetone (ketones) in the urine*

Chemstrip Micral reagent strips for professional use *in vitro diagnostic aid for albumin (protein) in the urine*

Chemstrip uG reagent strips for home use *in vitro diagnostic aid for urine glucose*

chenic acid [now: chenodiol]

Chenix tablets ℞ *anticholelithogenic for radiolucent gallstones (orphan)* [chenodiol] 250 mg

chenodeoxycholic acid INN, BAN *anticholelithogenic* [also: chenodiol]

chenodiol USAN *anticholelithogenic for radiolucent gallstones (orphan)* [also: chenodeoxycholic acid]

Cheracol Cough syrup ℞ *narcotic antitussive; expectorant* [codeine phosphate; guaifenesin; alcohol 1.75%] 10•100 mg/5 mL

Cheracol D Cough; Cheracol Plus liquid OTC *antitussive; expectorant* [dextromethorphan hydrobromide; guaifenesin; alcohol 4.75%] 10•100 mg/5 mL

Cheracol Nasal spray (discontinued 2001) OTC *nasal decongestant* [oxymetazoline HCl] 0.05%

Cheracol Sore Throat spray OTC *topical antipruritic/counterirritant; mild local anesthetic* [phenol] 1.4%

cherry, black; choke cherry; rum cherry *medicinal herb* [see: wild black cherry]

cherry, black; poison black cherry *medicinal herb* [see: belladonna]

cherry birch *medicinal herb* [see: birch]

cherry juice NF

chervil *(Anthriscus cerefolium)* flowering plant *medicinal herb used as a digestive, diuretic, expectorant, and stimulant*

chervil, sweet *medicinal herb* [see: sweet cicely]

chestnut *medicinal herb* [see: horse chestnut]

Chewable C chewable tablets (discontinued 1999) OTC *vitamin C supplement* [sodium ascorbate and ascorbic acid] 100, 250, 300, 500 mg

Chewable Multivitamins with Fluoride tablets ℞ *pediatric vitamin supplement and dental caries preventative* [multiple vitamins; fluoride; folic acid] ≛•1•0.3 mg

Chewable Triple Vitamins with Fluoride tablets ℞ *pediatric vitamin supplement and dental caries preventative* [vitamins A, C, and D; fluoride] 2500 IU•60 mg•400 IU•1 mg

Chewable Vitamin C chewable tablets OTC *vitamin C supplement* [ascorbic acid and sodium ascorbate] 250, 500 mg

ChexUP; Chex-Up; CHEX-UP (cyclophosphamide, hexameth-

ylmelamine, fluorouracil, Platinol) *chemotherapy protocol*

CHF (cyclophosphamide, hexamethylmelamine, fluorouracil) *chemotherapy protocol*

Chibroxin Ocumeter (eye drops) ℞ *topical fluoroquinolone antibiotic for bacterial conjunctivitis* [norfloxacin] 0.3%

chicken's toes *medicinal herb* [see: coral root]

chickweed *(Stellaria media)* plant *medicinal herb for appetite suppression, bleeding, blood cleansing, convulsions, obesity, skin rashes, and ulcers; also used as a homeopathic remedy for psoriasis and rheumatic pain*

chicory *(Chicorium intybus)* plant and root *medicinal herb for blood cleansing, cardiac disease, jaundice, liver disorders, promoting expectoration, and removal of calcium deposits*

Chiggerex ointment OTC *topical local anesthetic; analgesic; counterirritant* [benzocaine; camphor; menthol]

Chigger-Tox liquid OTC *topical local anesthetic* [benzocaine]

Chikusetsu ginseng *(Panax pseudoginseng)* *medicinal herb* [see: ginseng]

Children's Formula Cough syrup OTC *pediatric antitussive and expectorant* [dextromethorphan hydrobromide; guaifenesin] 5•50 mg/5 mL

chili pepper; chilies *medicinal herb* [see: cayenne]

chillifolinum [see: quillifoline]

Chimaphila umbellata *medicinal herb* [see: pipsissewa]

chimeric (murine variable, human constant) MAb (C2B8) to CD20 [now: rituximab]

chimeric A2 (human-murine) IgG monoclonal anti-TNF antibody (cA2) [see: infliximab]

chimeric M-T412 (human-murine) IgG monoclonal anti-CD4 *orphan status withdrawn 1997* [now: priliximab]

ChimeriVax ℞ *investigational chimeric flavivirus vaccine*

chinchona *medicinal herb* [see: quinine]

Chinese cucumber *(Trichosanthes kirilowii)* gourd and root *medicinal herb for abscesses, amenorrhea, cough, diabetes, edema, fever, inducing abortion, invasive moles, jaundice, polyuria, and tumors*

Chinese gelatin [see: agar]

Chinese isinglass [see: chiniofon]

Chinese rhubarb *medicinal herb* [see: rhubarb]

chinethazone [see: quinethazone]

chiniofon NF, INN

Chionanthus virginica *medicinal herb* [see: fringe tree]

Chirocaine local or epidural injection ℞ *long-acting local anesthetic* [levobupivacaine HCl] 2.5, 5, 7.5 mg/mL

chitosamine [see: glucosamine]

chitosan *natural cellulose-like biopolymer extracted from marine animal exoskeletons and used as a treatment for hypercholesterolemia, hyperlipidemia, and obesity; also used topically as an antimicrobial and vulnerary*

chittem bark *medicinal herb* [see: buckthorn; cascara sagrada]

CHL + PRED (chlorambucil, prednisone) *chemotherapy protocol*

Chlamydiazyme reagent kit for professional use *in vitro diagnostic aid for Chlamydia trachomatis* [solid phase enzyme immunoassay]

Chlo-Amine chewable tablets OTC *antihistamine* [chlorpheniramine maleate] 2 mg

chlophedianol BAN *antitussive* [also: chlophedianol HCl; clofedanol]

chlophedianol HCl USAN *antitussive* [also: clofedanol; chlophedianol]

chlophenadione [see: clorindione]

chloquinate [see: cloquinate]

Chlor-100 injection (discontinued 1997) ℞ *antihistamine; anaphylaxis* [chlorpheniramine maleate] 100 mg/mL

chloracyzine INN

Chlorafed liquid OTC *decongestant; antihistamine* [pseudoephedrine HCl; chlorpheniramine maleate] 30•2 mg/5 mL

Chlorafed; Chlorafed HS Timecelles (sustained-release capsules) ℞ *decongestant; antihistamine* [pseudoephedrine HCl; chlorpheniramine maleate] 120•8 mg; 60•4 mg

chloral betaine USAN, NF, BAN *sedative* [also: cloral betaine]

chloral hydrate USP, BAN *hypnotic; sedative; also abused as a street drug* 500 mg oral; 250, 500 mg/5 mL oral

chloral hydrate betaine [see: chloral betaine]

chloralformamide USP

chloralodol INN [also: chlorhexadol]

chloralose (α-chloralose) INN

chloralurethane [see: carbocloral]

chlorambucil USP, INN, BAN *nitrogen mustard-type alkylating antineoplastic for multiple leukemias and lymphomas*

chloramidobenzol [see: clofenamide]

chloramine [now: chloramine-T]

chloramine-T NF [also: tosylchloramide sodium]

chloramiphene [see: clomiphene citrate]

chloramphenicol USP, INN, BAN, JAN *bacteriostatic antibiotic; antirickettsial* 250 mg oral; 5 mg/mL eye drops; 10 mg/g topical

chloramphenicol palmitate USP, JAN *antibacterial; antirickettsial* 150 mg/5 mL oral

chloramphenicol pantothenate complex USAN *antibacterial; antirickettsial* [also: cloramfenicol pantotenate complex]

chloramphenicol sodium succinate USP, JAN *antibacterial; antirickettsial* 100 mg/mL injection

chloranautine [see: dimenhydrinate]

ChloraPrep One-Step swabs OTC *topical antiseptic* [chlorhexidine gluconate; isopropyl alcohol] 2%•70%

chlorarsen [see: dichlorophenarsine HCl]

Chloraseptic mouthwash/gargle OTC *topical antipruritic/counterirritant; mild local anesthetic* [phenol] 1.4%

Chloraseptic, Children's lozenges OTC *topical oral anesthetic* [benzocaine] 5 mg

Chloraseptic, Children's throat spray OTC *topical antipruritic/counterirritant; mild local anesthetic* [phenol] 0.5%

Chloraseptic Sore Throat lozenges OTC *topical oral anesthetic; analgesic; counterirritant* [benzocaine; menthol] 6•10 mg

Chlorate tablets (discontinued 1997) OTC *antihistamine* [chlorpheniramine maleate] 4 mg

chlorazanil INN

chlorazanil HCl [see: chlorazanil]

chlorazodin INN [also: chloroazodin]

chlorazone [see: chloramine-T]

chlorbenzoxamine INN

chlorbenzoxamine HCl [see: chlorbenzoxamine]

chlorbetamide INN, BAN

chlorbutanol [see: chlorobutanol]

chlorbutin [see: chlorambucil]

chlorbutol BAN *antimicrobial agent* [also: chlorobutanol]

chlorcinnazine [see: clocinizine]

chlorcyclizine INN, BAN *topical antihistamine* [also: chlorcyclizine HCl]

chlorcyclizine HCl USP *topical antihistamine* [also: chlorcyclizine]

chlordantoin USAN, BAN *antifungal* [also: clodantoin]

chlordiazepoxide USP, INN, BAN, JAN *benzodiazepine anxiolytic; minor tranquilizer; alcohol withdrawal therapy*

chlordiazepoxide HCl USAN, USP, BAN, JAN *benzodiazepine anxiolytic; sedative; sometimes abused as a street drug* 5, 10, 25 mg oral

chlordiazepoxide HCl & clidinium bromide *anxiolytic; GI anticholinergic* 5•2.5 mg

chlordimorine INN

Chlordrine S.R. sustained-release capsules ℞ *decongestant; antihistamine* [pseudoephedrine HCl; chlorpheniramine maleate] 120•8 mg

Chloresium ointment, solution OTC *vulnerary and deodorant for wounds,* *burns, and ulcers* [chlorophyllin copper complex] 0.5%; 0.2%

Chloresium tablets OTC *systemic deodorant for ostomy, breath, and body odors* [chlorophyllin copper complex] 14 mg

chlorethate [see: clorethate]

chlorethyl [see: ethyl chloride]

chlorfenisate [see: clofibrate]

chlorfenvinphos BAN [also: clofenvinfos]

Chlorgest-HD liquid (discontinued 1997) ℞ *narcotic antitussive; decongestant; antihistamine* [hydrocodone bitartrate; phenylephrine HCl; chlorpheniramine maleate] 1.67•5•4 mg/5 mL

chlorguanide HCl [see: chloroguanide HCl]

chlorhexadol BAN [also: chloralodol]

chlorhexidine INN, BAN *antimicrobial* [also: chlorhexidine gluconate]

chlorhexidine gluconate USAN *antimicrobial; investigational (orphan) for oral mucositis in bone marrow transplant patients* [also: chlorhexidine] 0.12%

chlorhexidine HCl USAN, BAN *topical anti-infective*

chlorhexidine phosphanilate USAN *antibacterial*

chlorimiphenin [see: imiclopazine]

chlorimpiphenine [see: imiclopazine]

chlorinated & iodized peanut oil [see: chloriodized oil]

chlorindanol USAN *spermaticide* [also: clorindanol]

chlorine *element (Cl)*

chloriodized oil USP

chlorisondamine chloride INN, BAN

chlorisondamone chloride [see: chlorisondamine chloride]

chlormadinone INN, BAN *progestin* [also: chlormadinone acetate]

chlormadinone acetate USAN, NF *progestin* [also: chlormadinone]

chlormerodrin NF, INN, BAN

chlormerodrin (^{197}Hg) INN *renal function test; radioactive agent* [also: chlormerodrin Hg 197]

chlormerodrin Hg 197 USAN, USP *renal function test; radioactive agent* [also: chlormerodrin (^{197}Hg)]

chlormerodrin Hg 203 USAN, USP *renal function test; radioactive agent*

chlormeroprin [see: chlormerodrin]

chlormethazanone [see: chlormezanone]

chlormethiazole BAN [also: clomethiazole]

chlormethine INN *nitrogen mustard-type alkylating antineoplastic* [also: mechlorethamine HCl; mustine; nitrogen mustard *N*-oxide HCl]

chlormethylencycline [see: clomocycline]

chlormezanone INN, BAN *mild anxiolytic*

chlormidazole INN, BAN

chlornaphazine INN

chloroacetic acid [see: monochloroacetic, dichloroacetic, or trichloroacetic acid]

8-chloroadenosine monophosphate, cyclic (8-Cl cAMP) [see: tocladesine]

chloroazodin USP [also: chlorazodin]

5-chlorobenzoxazolinone [see: chlorzoxazone]

chlorobutanol NF, INN *antimicrobial agent; preservative* [also: chlorbutol]

chlorochine [see: chloroquine]

chlorocresol USAN, NF, INN *antiseptic; disinfectant*

2-chloro-2′-deoxyadenosine (CdA) [now: cladribine]

chlorodeoxylincomycin [see: clindamycin]

chloroethane [see: ethyl chloride]

chloroform NF *solvent*

chloroguanide HCl USP *antimalarial; dihydrofolate reductase inhibitor* [also: proguanil]

chloroguanide triazine pamoate [see: cycloguanil pamoate]

chloro-iodohydroxyquinoline [see: clioquinol]

chlorolincomycin [see: clindamycin]

chloromethapyrilene citrate [see: chlorothen citrate]

Chloromycetin powder for eye drops, ophthalmic ointment ℞ *topical ophthalmic antibiotic* [chloramphenicol] 25 mg/15 mL; 10 mg/g

Chloromycetin Hydrocortisone powder for eye drops (discontinued 2000) ℞ *topical ophthalmic corticosteroidal anti-inflammatory; broad-spectrum antibiotic* [hydrocortisone acetate; chloramphenicol] 0.5%•0.25%

Chloromycetin Otic ear drops ℞ *broad-spectrum antibiotic* [chloramphenicol] 0.5%

Chloromycetin Sodium Succinate powder for IV injection ℞ *broad-spectrum bacteriostatic antibiotic* [chloramphenicol sodium succinate] 100 mg/mL

***p*-chlorophenol** [see: parachlorophenol]

chlorophenothane NF [also: clofenotane; dicophane]

chlorophenoxamide [see: clefamide]

chlorophenylmercury [see: phenylmercuric chloride]

chlorophyll, water soluble [see: chlorophyllin]

chlorophyllin *vulnerary; oral deodorant for ostomy, breath, and body odors; topical deodorant for wounds and ulcers* 20 mg oral

chlorophyllin copper complex USAN *oral deodorant for ostomy, breath, and body odors; topical deodorant for wounds and ulcers*

chloroprednisone INN

chloroprednisone acetate [see: chloroprednisone]

chloroprocaine INN *local anesthetic* [also: chloroprocaine HCl]

chloroprocaine HCl USP *injectable local anesthetic* [also: chloroprocaine]

Chloroptic eye drops ℞ *topical ophthalmic antibiotic* [chloramphenicol] 5 mg/mL

Chloroptic S.O.P. ophthalmic ointment ℞ *topical ophthalmic antibiotic* [chloramphenicol] 10 mg/g

chloropyramine INN [also: halopyramine]

chloropyrilene INN, BAN [also: chlorothen citrate]

chloroquine USP, INN, BAN *amebicide; antimalarial*

chloroquine diphosphate [see: chloroquine phosphate]

chloroquine HCl USP *amebicide; antimalarial* [also: chloroquine]

chloroquine phosphate USP, BAN *amebicide; antimalarial; lupus erythematosus suppressant* 250 mg oral

chloroserpidine INN

N-chlorosuccinimide [see: succinchlorimide]

chlorothen citrate NF [also: chloropyrilene]

chlorothenium citrate [see: chlorothen citrate]

chlorothenylpyramine [see: chlorothen]

chlorothiazide USP, INN, BAN *diuretic; antihypertensive* 250, 500 mg oral

chlorothiazide sodium USAN, USP *diuretic; antihypertensive*

chlorothymol NF

chlorotrianisene USP, INN, BAN *estrogen for hormone replacement therapy or inoperable prostatic cancer*

chloroxine USAN *antiseborrheic*

chloroxylenol USP, INN, BAN *bacteriostatic*

chlorozone [see: chloramine-T]

chlorpenthixol [see: clopenthixol]

Chlorphed-LA nasal spray OTC *nasal decongestant* [oxymetazoline HCl] 0.05%

Chlorphedrine SR sustained-release capsules ℞ *decongestant; antihistamine* [pseudoephedrine HCl; chlorpheniramine maleate] 120•8 mg

chlorphenamine INN *antihistamine* [also: chlorpheniramine maleate; chlorpheniramine]

chlorphenamine maleate [see: chlorpheniramine maleate]

chlorphenecyclane [see: clofenciclan]

chlorphenesin INN, BAN *skeletal muscle relaxant* [also: chlorphenesin carbamate]

chlorphenesin carbamate USAN, JAN *skeletal muscle relaxant* [also: chlorphenesin]
chlorphenindione [see: clorindione]
chlorpheniramine BAN *alkylamine antihistamine* [also: chlorpheniramine maleate; chlorphenamine] ⊠ chlorphentermine
chlorpheniramine maleate USP *alkylamine antihistamine* [also: chlorphenamine; chlorpheniramine] 4, 8, 12 mg oral
chlorpheniramine maleate & phenylpropanolamine HCl *antihistamine; decongestant* 12•75 mg
chlorpheniramine polistirex USAN *alkylamine antihistamine*
chlorpheniramine tannate, pyrilamine tannate, and phenylephrine tannate *alkylamine antihistamine; decongestant* 8•25•25 mg oral
chlorphenoctium amsonate INN, BAN
chlorphenotane [see: chlorophenothane]
chlorphenoxamine INN, BAN [also: chlorphenoxamine HCl]
chlorphenoxamine HCl USP [also: chlorphenoxamine]
chlorphentermine INN, BAN *anorectic* [also: chlorphentermine HCl] ⊠ chlorpheniramine
chlorphentermine HCl USAN *anorectic* [also: chlorphentermine]
chlorphenylindandione [see: clorindione]
chlorphthalidone [see: chlorthalidone]
Chlor-Pro injection (discontinued 1997) ℞ *antihistamine* [chlorpheniramine maleate] 10, 100 mg/mL
chlorprocaine chloride [see: chloroprocaine HCl]
chlorproethazine INN [also: chlorproethazine HCl]
chlorproethazine HCl [also: chlorproethazine]
chlorproguanil INN, BAN
chlorproguanil HCl [see: chlorproguanil]
chlorpromazine USP, INN, BAN *phenothiazine antipsychotic; antiemetic; intractable hiccough relief*
chlorpromazine HCl USP, BAN, JAN *phenothiazine antipsychotic; antiemetic; intractable hiccough relief* 10, 25, 50, 100, 200 mg oral; 30, 100 mg/mL oral; 25 mg/mL injection
chlorpromazine hibenzate JAN *phenothiazine antipsychotic; antiemetic*
chlorpromazine phenolphthalinate JAN *phenothiazine antipsychotic; antiemetic*
chlorpromazine tannate USP, INN, BAN *phenothiazine antipsychotic; antiemetic*
chlorpropamide USP, INN, BAN, JAN *sulfonylurea antidiabetic* 100, 250 mg oral
chlorprophenpyridamine maleate [see: chlorpheniramine maleate]
chlorprothixene USAN, USP, INN, BAN *thioxanthene antipsychotic*
chlorpyrifos BAN
chlorquinaldol INN, BAN
Chlor-Rest tablets OTC *decongestant; antihistamine* [phenylpropanolamine HCl; chlorpheniramine maleate] 18.7•2 mg
Chlorspan-12 timed-release capsules (discontinued 1997) ℞ *antihistamine* [chlorpheniramine maleate] 12 mg
chlortalidone INN *antihypertensive; diuretic* [also: chlorthalidone]
chlortetracycline INN, BAN *antibacterial antibiotic; antiprotozoal* [also: chlortetracycline bisulfate]
chlortetracycline bisulfate USP *antibacterial; antiprotozoal* [also: chlortetracycline]
chlortetracycline calcium
chlortetracycline HCl USP, BAN *antibacterial antibiotic; antiprotozoal*
chlorthalidone USAN, USP, BAN *antihypertensive; diuretic* [also: chlortalidone] 25, 50, 100 mg oral
chlorthenoxazin BAN [also: chlorthenoxazine]
chlorthenoxazine INN [also: chlorthenoxazin]
chlorthiazide [see: chlorothiazide]
chlortrianisestrol [see: chlorotrianisene]

Chlor-Trimeton IV injection (discontinued 1997) ℞ *antihistamine for anaphylaxis* [chlorpheniramine maleate] 10 mg/mL

Chlor-Trimeton syrup (name changed to Chlor-Trimeton Allergy in 1997)

Chlor-Trimeton 4 Hour Relief tablets OTC *decongestant; antihistamine* [pseudoephedrine sulfate; chlorpheniramine maleate] 60•4 mg

Chlor-Trimeton 12 Hour Relief sustained-release tablets OTC *decongestant; antihistamine* [pseudoephedrine sulfate; chlorpheniramine maleate] 120•8 mg

Chlor-Trimeton Allergy 4 Hour syrup (discontinued 2001) OTC *antihistamine* [chlorpheniramine maleate] 2 mg/5 mL

Chlor-Trimeton Allergy 4 Hour tablets OTC *antihistamine* [chlorpheniramine maleate] 4 mg

Chlor-Trimeton Allergy 8 Hour; Chlor-Trimeton Allergy 12 Hour timed-release tablets OTC *antihistamine* [chlorpheniramine maleate] 8 mg; 12 mg

Chlor-Trimeton Allergy-Sinus caplets OTC *decongestant; antihistamine; analgesic* [phenylpropanolamine HCl; chlorpheniramine maleate; acetaminophen] 12.5•2•500 mg

chlorzoxazone USP, INN, BAN, JAN *skeletal muscle relaxant* 250, 500 mg oral

chlosudimeprimylum [see: clopamide]

ChlVPP (chlorambucil, vinblastine, procarbazine, prednisone/prednisolone) *chemotherapy protocol for Hodgkin lymphoma* [note: prednisone is used in the U.S.; prednisolone is used in England]

ChlVPP/EVA (chlorambucil, vinblastine, procarbazine, prednisone/prednisolone, etoposide, vincristine, Adriamycin) *chemotherapy protocol for Hodgkin lymphoma* [note: prednisone is used in the U.S.; prednisolone is used in England]

CHO (cyclophosphamide, hydroxydaunomycin, Oncovin) *chemotherapy protocol*

CHO cells, recombinant [see: CD4, human truncated]

CHOB (cyclophosphamide, hydroxydaunomycin, Oncovin, bleomycin) *chemotherapy protocol*

CHOD (cyclophosphamide, hydroxydaunomycin, Oncovin, dexamethasone) *chemotherapy protocol*

choice dielytra *medicinal herb* [see: turkey corn]

Choice dm oral liquid OTC *enteral nutritional therapy for abnormal glucose tolerance* [lactose-free formula] 240 mL

choke cherry; black choke *medicinal herb* [see: wild black cherry]

Cholac oral/rectal solution ℞ *synthetic disaccharide used to prevent and treat portal-systemic encephalopathy* [lactulose] 10 g/15 mL

cholagogues *a class of agents that stimulate the flow of bile into the duodenum*

cholalic acid [see: dehydrocholic acid]

Cholan-HMB tablets (discontinued 1998) OTC *laxative; hydrocholeretic* [dehydrocholic acid] 250 mg

Cholebrine tablets (discontinued 1999) ℞ *radiopaque contrast medium for cholecystography* [iocetamic acid (62% iodine)] 750 mg

cholecalciferol (vitamin D_3) USP, BAN, JAN *fat-soluble vitamin* [also: colecalciferol] 1000 IU oral

Choledyl SA sustained-action tablets ℞ *antiasthmatic; bronchodilator* [oxtriphylline] 400, 600 mg

cholera vaccine USP *active bacterin for cholera (Vibrio cholerae)* 16 U/mL injection

CholestaGel (name changed to Welchol upon marketing release in 2000)

cholesterin [see: cholesterol]

cholesterol NF *emulsifying agent*

cholestrin [see: cholesterol]

cholestyramine BAN *bile salts ion-exchange resin; antihyperlipoprotein-*

emic [also: cholestyramine resin; colestyramine]

Cholestyramine Light powder for oral suspension ℞ *cholesterol-lowering antihyperlipidemic; also used for biliary obstruction* [cholestyramine resin] 4 g/dose

cholestyramine resin USP *bile salts ion-exchange resin; cholesterol-lowering antihyperlipidemic; also used for biliary obstruction* [also: colestyramine; cholestyramine] 4 g powder for oral solution

cholic acid [see: dehydrocholic acid]

Cholidase tablets OTC *dietary lipotropic with vitamin supplementation* [choline; inositol; vitamins B_6, B_{12}, and E] 185•150•2.5•0.005•7.5 mg

choline *dietary lipotropic supplement* 250, 300, 500, 650 mg oral

choline alfoscerate INN

choline bitartrate NF 250 mg oral

choline bromide hexamethylenedicarbamate [see: hexacarbacholine bromide]

choline chloride INN *investigational (orphan) for choline deficiency of long-term parenteral nutrition*

choline chloride acetate [see: acetylcholine chloride]

choline chloride carbamate [see: carbachol]

choline chloride succinate [see: succinylcholine chloride]

choline dihydrogen citrate NF 650 mg oral

choline gluconate INN

choline glycerophosphate [see: choline alfoscerate]

choline magnesium trisalicylate (choline salicylate + magnesium salicylate) *nonsteroidal anti-inflammatory drug (NSAID)* [q.v.] 500, 750, 1000 mg (293•362, 440•544, 587•725 mg) oral

choline perchlorate, nitrate ester [see: nitricholine perchlorate]

choline salicylate USAN, INN, BAN *analgesic; antipyretic; anti-inflammatory; antirheumatic*

choline theophyllinate INN, BAN *bronchodilator* [also: oxtriphylline]

cholinergic agonists *a class of agents that produce effects similar to those of the parasympathetic nervous system* [also called: parasympathomimetics]

cholinesterase inhibitors *a class of drugs which increase acetylcholine neurotransmitters, used as a cognition adjuvant in Alzheimer dementia* [also called: acetylcholinesterase (AChE) inhibitors]

Cholinoid capsules OTC *dietary lipotropic with vitamin supplementation* [choline; inositol; multiple B vitamins; vitamin C; lemon bioflavonoids] 111•111•≛•100•100 mg

Cholografin Meglumine injection ℞ *radiopaque contrast medium for cholecystography and cholangiography* [iodipamide meglumine (49.2% iodine)] 520 mg/mL (257 mg/mL)

Choloxin tablets (discontinued 1999) ℞ *antihyperlipidemic for primary hypercholesterolemia (types IIa and IIb hyperlipidemia)* [dextrothyroxine sodium] 2, 4 mg

chondodendron tomentosum [see: tubocurarine chloride]

chondrocyte-alginate *investigational (orphan) gel suspension for vesicoureteral reflux in children*

chondroitin 4-sulfate [see: danaparoid sodium]

chondroitin 6-sulfate [see: danaparoid sodium]

chondroitin sulfate *natural remedy for arthritis, blood clots, and extravasation from needle sticks after certain chemotherapy treatments*

chondroitin sulfate sodium JAN

chondroitin sulfuric acid *natural remedy* [see: chondroitin sulfate]

chondroitinase *investigational (orphan) for vitrectomy*

Chondrus crispus *medicinal herb* [see: Irish moss]

chonsurid *natural remedy* [see: chondroitin sulfate]

Chooz chewable tablets OTC *antacid* [calcium carbonate] 500 mg

CHOP (cyclophosphamide, hydroxydaunomycin, Oncovin, prednisone) *chemotherapy protocol for non-Hodgkin lymphoma*

CHOP-BLEO (cyclophosphamide, hydroxydaunomycin, Oncovin, prednisone, bleomycin) *chemotherapy protocol for non-Hodgkin lymphoma*

CHOPE (cyclophosphamide, hydroxydaunomycin, Oncovin, prednisone, etoposide) *chemotherapy protocol*

CHOR (cyclophosphamide, hydroxydaunomycin, Oncovin, radiation therapy) *chemotherapy protocol*

Chorex-5; Chorex-10 powder for IM injection ℞ *hormone for prepubertal cryptorchidism and hypogonadism; ovulation stimulant* [chorionic gonadotropin] 500 U/mL; 1000 U/mL

choriogonadotropin alfa USAN *recombinant human chorionic gonadotropin (rhCG); fertility stimulant for anovulatory women; adjuvant therapy for cryptorchidism*

chorionic gonadotrophin [see: gonadotropin, chorionic]

chorionic gonadotropin (CG) [see: gonadotropin, chorionic]

Choron-10 powder for IM injection ℞ *hormone for prepubertal cryptorchidism and hypogonadism; ovulation stimulant* [chorionic gonadotropin] 1000 U/mL

CHP (chlorhexidine phosphanilate) [q.v.]

Christmas factor [see: factor IX complex]

Chromagen capsules ℞ *hematinic* [ferrous fumarate; cyanocobalamin; ascorbic acid; intrinsic factor concentrate] 66 mg•10 μg•250 mg•100 mg

Chromagen FA; Chromagen Forte capsules OTC *vitamin/iron supplement* [vitamins B_{12} & C; iron; folic acid] 0.01•250•66•1 mg; 0.01•60•151•1 mg

Chromagen OB capsules OTC *prenatal vitamin/mineral/iron supplement* [multiple vitamins & minerals; iron; folic acid] ≛•28•1 mg

Chroma-Pak IV injection ℞ *intravenous nutritional therapy* [chromic chloride hexahydrate] 20.5, 102.5 μg/mL

chromargyre [see: merbromin]

chromated albumin [see: albumin, chromated Cr 51 serum]

Chromelin Complexion Blender OTC *skin darkening agent for vitiligo and hypopigmented areas* [dihydroxyacetone] 5%

chromic acid, disodium salt [see: sodium chromate Cr 51]

chromic chloride USP *dietary chromium supplement* 4, 20 μg/mL injection

chromic chloride Cr 51 USAN *radioactive agent*

chromic chloride hexahydrate [see: chromic chloride]

chromic phosphate Cr 51 USAN *radioactive agent*

chromic phosphate P 32 USAN, USP *antineoplastic; radioactive agent*

chromium *element (Cr); trace mineral important in glucose metabolism*

Chromium Chloride IV injection ℞ *intravenous nutritional therapy* [chromic chloride hexahydrate] 4 μg/mL

chromium chloride [see: chromic chloride; chromic chloride Cr 51]

chromium chloride hexahydrate [see: chromic chloride]

chromium picolinate *trace mineral important in glucose metabolism*

chromium polynicotinate *trace mineral important in glucose metabolism*

chromocarb INN

chromonar HCl USAN *coronary vasodilator* [also: carbocromen]

Chronosule (trademarked dosage form) *sustained-action capsule*

Chronotab (trademarked dosage form) *sustained-action tablet*

Chronovera (CAN) delayed-onset, extended-release tablets ℞ *antihyper-*

tensive; calcium channel blocker [verapamil HCl] 180, 240 mg

Chronulac oral/rectal solution ℞ *hyperosmotic laxative* [lactulose] 10 g/15 mL

Chrysanthemum parthenium *medicinal herb* [see: feverfew]

Chrysanthemum vulgare *medicinal herb* [see: tansy]

chrysazin *(withdrawn from market by FDA)* [see: danthron]

CHVP (cyclophosphamide, hydroxydaunomycin, VM-26, prednisone) *chemotherapy protocol*

Chymex solution (discontinued 1999) ℞ *diagnostic aid for pancreatic function* [bentiromide] 500 mg/7.5 mL

Chymodiactin powder for intradiscal injection ℞ *proteolytic enzyme for herniated nucleus pulposus* [chymopapain] 4 nkat

chymopapain USAN, INN, BAN *proteolytic enzyme for herniated lumbar discs*

chymotrypsin USP, INN, BAN *proteolytic enzyme; zonulolytic for intracapsular lens extraction*

C.I. acid orange 24 monosodium salt (color index) [see: resorcin brown]

C.I. basic violet 3 (color index) [see: gentian violet]

C.I. basic violet 14 monohydrochloride (color index) [see: fuchsin, basic]

C.I. direct blue 53 tetrasodium salt (color index) [see: Evans blue]

C.I. mordant yellow 5, disodium salt (color index) [see: olsalazine sodium]

CI-1012 *investigational (Phase I) antiviral for HIV*

CI-1020 *investigational (Phase I) antiviral for HIV*

ciadox INN

Cialis ℞ *investigational (NDA filed) selective vasodilator for male erectile and female sexual dysfunction* [tadalafil]

ciamexon INN, BAN

cianergoline INN

cianidanol INN

cianidol [see: cianidanol]

cianopramine INN

ciapilome INN

Ciba Vision Cleaner for Sensitive Eyes solution OTC *surfactant cleaning solution for soft contact lenses*

Ciba Vision Saline aerosol solution OTC *rinsing/storage solution for soft contact lenses* [sodium chloride (saline solution)]

Cibacalcin subcu or IM injection ℞ *calcium regulator for Paget disease (osteitis deformans) (orphan)* [calcitonin (human)] 0.5 mg/vial

cibenzoline INN, BAN *antiarrhythmic* [also: cifenline]

cibenzoline succinate JAN *antiarrhythmic* [also: cifenline succinate]

cicaprost INN *prostacyclin analogue*

cicarperone INN

cicely, sweet *medicinal herb* [see: sweet cicely]

Cichorium intybus *medicinal herb* [see: chicory]

ciclacillin INN, BAN *antibacterial* [also: cyclacillin]

ciclactate INN

ciclafrine INN *antihypotensive* [also: ciclafrine HCl]

ciclafrine HCl USAN *antihypotensive* [also: ciclafrine]

ciclazindol USAN, INN, BAN *antidepressant*

cicletanine USAN, INN, BAN *antihypertensive*

ciclindole INN *antidepressant* [also: cyclindole]

cicliomenol INN

ciclobendazole INN, BAN *anthelmintic* [also: cyclobendazole]

ciclofenazine INN *antipsychotic* [also: cyclophenazine HCl]

ciclofenazine HCl [see: cyclophenazine HCl]

cicloheximide INN *antipsoriatic* [also: cycloheximide]

ciclonicate INN

ciclonium bromide INN

ciclopirox USAN, INN, BAN *topical antifungal for onychomycosis*

ciclopirox olamine USAN, USP, JAN *topical antifungal*

ciclopramine INN

cicloprofen USAN, INN, BAN *anti-inflammatory*

cicloprolol INN *antiadrenergic (β-receptor)* [also: cicloprolol HCl; cycloprolol]

cicloprolol HCl USAN *antiadrenergic (β-receptor)* [also: cicloprolol; cycloprolol]

ciclosidomine INN, BAN

ciclosporin INN *immunosuppressive* [also: cyclosporine; cyclosporin]

ciclotate INN *combining name for radicals or groups*

ciclotizolam INN, BAN

ciclotropium bromide INN

cicloxilic acid INN

cicloxolone INN, BAN

cicortonide INN

cicrotoic acid INN

Cidecin injection ℞ *investigational (Phase III) antibiotic for community-acquired pneumonia and complicated urinary tract infections* [daptomycin]

cideferron INN

Cidex; Cidex-7; Cidex Plus 28 solution OTC *broad-spectrum antimicrobial* [glutaral] 2%; 2%; 3.2%

cidofovir USAN, INN *nucleoside antiviral for AIDS-related cytomegalovirus retinitis; investigational (Phase I/II) gel for AIDS-related genital herpes and Kaposi sarcoma*

cidoxepin INN *antidepressant* [also: cidoxepin HCl]

cidoxepin HCl USAN *antidepressant* [also: cidoxepin]

cifenline USAN *antiarrhythmic* [also: cibenzoline]

cifenline succinate USAN *antiarrhythmic* [also: cibenzoline succinate]

cifostodine INN

ciglitazone USAN, INN *antidiabetic*

cignolin [see: anthralin]

ciheptolane INN

ciladopa INN, BAN *antiparkinsonian; dopaminergic agent* [also: ciladopa HCl]

ciladopa HCl USAN *antiparkinsonian; dopaminergic agent* [also: ciladopa]

cilansetron INN *investigational treatment for irritable bowel syndrome*

cilastatin INN, BAN *enzyme inhibitor* [also: cilastatin sodium]

cilastatin sodium USAN, JAN *enzyme inhibitor* [also: cilastatin]

cilazapril USAN, INN, BAN, JAN *antihypertensive; ACE inhibitor*

cilazaprilat INN, BAN

cilexetil USAN *combining name for radicals or groups*

ciliary neurotrophic factor *investigational (orphan) for amyotrophic lateral sclerosis*

cilmostim USAN *hematopoietic; macrophage colony-stimulating factor*

cilobamine INN *antidepressant* [also: cilobamine mesylate]

cilobamine mesylate USAN *antidepressant* [also: cilobamine]

cilofungin USAN, INN *antifungal*

ciloprost [see: iloprost]

cilostamide INN

cilostazol USAN, INN *vasodilator; antithrombotic; phosphodiesterase (PDE) III platelet aggregation inhibitor for intermittent claudication*

Ciloxan Drop-Tainers (eye drops), ointment ℞ *topical ophthalmic antibiotic* [ciprofloxacin HCl] 3.5 mg/mL; 0.3%

ciltoprazine INN

cilutazoline INN

cimaterol USAN, INN *repartitioning agent*

cimemoxin INN

cimepanol INN

cimetidine USAN, USP, INN, BAN, JAN *histamine H_2 antagonist for gastric ulcers* 200, 300, 400, 800 mg oral ⑨ dimethicone

cimetidine HCl USAN *histamine H_2 antagonist for gastric ulcers* 300 mg/5 mL oral; 300 mg/2 mL injection

cimetropium bromide INN

Cimicifuga racemosa *medicinal herb* [see: black cohosh]

cimoxatone INN

cinalukast USAN, INN *antiasthmatic*

cinametic acid INN

cinamolol INN

cinanserin INN *serotonin inhibitor* [also: cinanserin HCl]

cinanserin HCl USAN *serotonin inhibitor* [also: cinanserin]

cinaproxen INN

cincaine chloride [see: dibucaine HCl]
cinchocaine INN, BAN *local anesthetic* [also: dibucaine]
cinchocaine HCl BAN *local anesthetic* [also: dibucaine HCl]
Cinchona succirubra; C. ledgeriana; C. calisaya *medicinal herb* [see: quinine]
cinchonidine sulfate NF
cinchonine sulfate NF
cinchophen NF, INN, BAN
cinecromen INN
cinepaxadil INN
cinepazet INN, BAN *antianginal* [also: cinepazet maleate]
cinepazet maleate USAN *antianginal* [also: cinepazet]
cinepazic acid INN
cinepazide INN, BAN
cinfenine INN
cinfenoac INN, BAN
cinflumide USAN, INN *muscle relaxant*
cingestol USAN, INN *progestin*
cinitapride INN
cinmetacin INN
cinnamaldehyde NF
cinnamaverine INN
cinnamedrine USAN, INN *smooth muscle relaxant*
cinnamedrine HCl *smooth muscle relaxant*
cinnamic aldehyde [now: cinnamaldehyde]
cinnamon NF
cinnamon oil NF
cinnamon *(Cinnamonum zeylanicum)* bark and oil *medicinal herb for diarrhea, dysmenorrhea, gastrointestinal upset, microbial and fungal infections, and gas pain; also used as an aromatic, astringent, and stimulant*
cinnamon wood *medicinal herb* [see: sassafras]
cinnarizine USAN, INN, BAN *antihistamine*
cinnarizine clofibrate INN
cinnofuradione INN
cinnofuron [see: cinnofuradione]
cinnopentazone INN *anti-inflammatory* [also: cintazone]
cinnopropazone [see: apazone]
Cinobac capsules ℞ *urinary antibacterial* [cinoxacin] 250, 500 mg
cinoctramide INN
cinodine HCl USAN *veterinary antibacterial*
cinolazepam INN
cinoquidox INN
cinoxacin USAN, USP, INN, BAN *urinary antibacterial*
cinoxate USAN, USP, INN *ultraviolet screen*
cinoxolone INN, BAN
cinoxopazide INN
cinperene USAN, INN *antipsychotic*
cinprazole INN
cinpropazide INN
cinquefoil *(Potentilla anserina; P. canadensis; P. reptans)* plant *medicinal herb used as an antispasmodic and astringent*
cinromide USAN, INN *anticonvulsant*
cintazone USAN *anti-inflammatory* [also: cinnopentazone]
cintramide INN *antipsychotic* [also: cintriamide]
cintriamide USAN *antipsychotic* [also: cintramide]
cinuperone INN
cioteronel USAN, INN *antiandrogen*
cipamfylline USAN *antiviral agent; tumor necrosis factor alpha inhibitor*
cipemastat USAN *matrix metalloproteinase inhibitor; investigational cartilage protective agent for rheumatoid arthritis*
cipionate INN *combining name for radicals or groups* [also: cypionate]
ciprafamide INN
Cipralan ℞ *investigational antiarrhythmic* [cifenline succinate]
Cipralex ℞ *investigational (NDA filed) selective serotonin reuptake inhibitor (SSRI) for depression* [escitalopram oxalate]
Cipramil (foreign name for U.S. product Celexa)
ciprazafone INN
ciprefadol INN *analgesic* [also: ciprefadol succinate]

ciprefadol succinate USAN *analgesic* [also: ciprefadol]

Cipro Cystitis Pack (6 film-coated tablets) (discontinued 2000) ℞ *broad-spectrum fluoroquinolone antibiotic* [ciprofloxacin] 100 mg ⑨ Septa; Septra

Cipro film-coated tablets, oral suspension, IV infusion ℞ *broad-spectrum fluoroquinolone antibiotic* [ciprofloxacin] 250, 500, 750 mg; 250, 500 mg/5 mL; 200, 400 mg/vial ⑨ Septa; Septra

Cipro HC Otic ear drop suspension ℞ *topical broad-spectrum fluoroquinolone antibiotic; corticosteroidal anti-inflammatory* [ciprofloxacin; hydrocortisone] 0.2%•1% (2•10 mg/mL)

ciprocinonide USAN, INN *adrenocortical steroid*

ciprofibrate USAN, INN, BAN *antihyperlipoproteinemic*

ciprofloxacin USAN, INN, BAN *broad-spectrum fluoroquinolone antibiotic*

ciprofloxacin HCl USAN, USP, JAN *broad-spectrum bactericidal antibiotic*

cipropride INN

ciproquazone INN

ciproquinate INN *coccidiostat for poultry* [also: cyproquinate]

ciprostene INN *platelet antiaggregatory agent* [also: ciprostene calcium]

ciprostene calcium USAN *platelet antiaggregatory agent* [also: ciprostene]

ciproximide INN *antipsychotic; antidepressant* [also: cyproximide]

ciramadol USAN, INN *analgesic*

ciramadol HCl USAN *analgesic*

cirazoline INN

Circavite-T tablets OTC *vitamin/mineral/iron supplement* [multiple vitamins & minerals; iron] ≛•12 mg

cirolemycin USAN, INN *antineoplastic; antibacterial*

cisapride USAN, INN, BAN, JAN *peristaltic stimulant; treatment for nocturnal heartburn due to gastroesophageal reflux disease; (withdrawn from U.S. markets in 2000 due to increased cardiac arrhythmias)*

cisatracurium besylate USAN *nondepolarizing neuromuscular blocker*

CISCA; CisCA (cisplatin, cyclophosphamide, Adriamycin) *chemotherapy protocol for bladder cancer*

$CISCA_{II}/VB_{IV}$ (cisplatin, cyclophosphamide, Adriamycin, vinblastine, bleomycin) *chemotherapy protocol for germ cell tumors*

cisclomiphene [now: enclomiphene]

cisconazole USAN, INN *antifungal*

***cis*-DDP (diamminedichloroplatinum)** [see: cisplatin]

***cis*-diamminedichloroplatinum (DDP)** [see: cisplatin]

cismadinone INN

cisplatin USAN, USP, INN, BAN *alkylating antineoplastic for testicular, ovarian, and bladder cancer* 1 mg/mL injection

cisplatin & docetaxel *chemotherapy protocol for bladder cancer*

cisplatin & epinephrine *investigational (Phase II) injectable gel for inoperable primary liver cancer*

cisplatin & vinorelbine tartrate *chemotherapy protocol for cervical cancer*

***cis*-platinum** [now: cisplatin]

***cis*-platinum II** [now: cisplatin]

9-*cis*-retinoic acid [see: alitretinoin]

13-*cis*-retinoic acid [see: isotretinoin]

cistinexine INN

citalopram INN, BAN *selective serotonin reuptake inhibitor (SSRI) for depression*

citalopram hydrobromide USAN *selective serotonin reuptake inhibitor (SSRI) for depression*

Citanest Forte injection ℞ *injectable local anesthetic for dental procedures* [prilocaine HCl; epinephrine] 4%•1:200 000

Citanest Plain injection ℞ *injectable local anesthetic for dental procedures* [prilocaine HCl] 4%

citatepine INN

citenamide USAN, INN *anticonvulsant*

citenazone INN

citicoline INN, JAN *investigational (Phase III) oral treatment for ischemic stroke and head trauma* [also: citicoline sodium]

citicoline & dizocilpine maleate *investigational (Phase III) neuroprotective treatment for stroke*

citicoline sodium USAN *investigational (Phase III) oral treatment for ischemic stroke and head trauma* [also: citicoline]

citiolone INN, DCF

Citra pH oral solution OTC *antacid* [sodium citrate] 450 mg/5 mL

Citracal tablets OTC *calcium supplement* [calcium citrate] 900 mg ⊡ Citrucel

Citracal Caplets + D OTC *dietary supplement* [calcium citrate; vitamin D] 315 mg•200 IU ⊡ Citrucel

Citracal Liquitab effervescent tablets OTC *calcium supplement* [calcium citrate] 23.76 mg ⊡ Citrucel

Citracal Prenatal tablets ℞ *calcium/iron supplement* [calcium citrate; iron; folic acid; docusate sodium] 125•1•27•50 mg

Citralax effervescent granules OTC *saline laxative* [magnesium citrate; magnesium sulfate]

citrate dextrose [see: ACD solution]

citrate of magnesia [see: magnesium citrate]

citrate phosphate dextrose [see: anticoagulant citrate phosphate dextrose solution]

citrate phosphate dextrose adenine [see: anticoagulant citrate phosphate dextrose adenine solution]

citrated caffeine NF [see: caffeine citrate]

citric acid USP *pH adjusting agent; urinary acidifier*

citric acid, glucono-delta-lactone & magnesium carbonate *irrigant for renal and bladder apatite or struvite calculi (orphan)*

citric acid, magnesium oxide & sodium carbonate [see: Suby solution G]

citrin [see: bioflavonoids]

Citrocarbonate effervescent granules OTC *antacid* [sodium bicarbonate; sodium citrate] 780•1820 mg/dose

Citro-Flav 200 capsules (discontinued 1999) OTC *dietary supplement* [citrus bioflavonoid complex] 200 mg

Citrolith tablets ℞ *urinary alkalinizing agent* [potassium citrate; sodium citrate] 50•950 mg

citronella (*Cymbopogon nardus; C. winterianus*) oil *medicinal herb for gastrointestinal spasms, promoting diuresis, and worms; also used as an antibacterial; not generally regarded as safe for internal use, as it is highly toxic*

Citrotein powder, liquid OTC *enteral nutritional therapy* [lactose-free formula]

citrovorum factor [see: leucovorin calcium]

Citrucel powder OTC *bulk laxative* [methylcellulose] 2 g/tbsp. or scoop ⊡ Citracal

Citrucel Sugar Free powder OTC *bulk laxative* [methylcellulose; phenylalanine] 2 g•52 mg per tbsp. ⊡ Citracal

Citrus bergamia; C. aurantium *medicinal herb* [see: bergamot oil]

citrus bioflavonoids [see: bioflavonoids]

Citrus limon *medicinal herb* [see: lemon]

Citrus paradisi *medicinal herb* [see: grapefruit]

Citrus-flav C 500 tablets (discontinued 1999) OTC *vitamin C supplement with multiple bioflavonoids* [vitamin C; acerola; citrus bioflavonoids; hesperidin; rutin] 200•50•200•40•10 mg

CIVPP (chlorambucil, vinblastine, procarbazine, prednisone) *chemotherapy protocol*

8-Cl cAMP (8-chloroadenosine monophosphate, cyclic) [see: tocladesine]

cladribine *antimetabolite antineoplastic for hairy-cell leukemia (orphan); investigational (orphan) for chronic lymphocytic leukemia, multiple sclerosis, and non-Hodgkin lymphoma* 1 mg/mL injection

Claforan powder or frozen premix for IV or IM injection ℞ *cephalosporin antibiotic* [cefotaxime sodium] 0.5, 1, 2, 10 g

clamidoxic acid INN, BAN

clamoxyquin BAN *antiamebic* [also: clamoxyquin HCl; clamoxyquine]
clamoxyquin HCl USAN *antiamebic* [also: clamoxyquine; clamoxyquin]
clamoxyquine INN *antiamebic* [also: clamoxyquin HCl; clamoxyquin]
clanfenur INN
clanobutin INN
clantifen INN
clara cell 10kDa protein *investigational (orphan) for prevention of bronchopulmonary dysplasia in neonates with respiratory distress syndrome* ▣ Clearasil
claretin-12 [see: cyanocobalamin] ▣ Claritin; Clarityne
clarithromycin USAN, INN, BAN, JAN *macrolide antibiotic* ▣ dirithromycin; erythromycin
Claritin tablets, RediTabs (rapidly disintegrating tablets), syrup ℞ *nonsedating antihistamine for allergic rhinitis and chronic idiopathic urticaria* [loratadine] 10 mg; 10 mg; 5 mg/5 mL ▣ claretin; Clarityne
Claritin-D; Claritin-D 12 Hour; Claritin-D 24 Hour extended-release film-coated tablets ℞ *decongestant; nonsedating antihistamine* [pseudoephedrine sulfate; loratadine] 120•5 mg; 120•5 mg; 240•10 mg
Clarityne (Mexican name for U.S. product Claritin) ▣ claretin; Claritin
Claviceps purpurea *medicinal herb* [see: ergot]
clavulanate potassium USAN, USP *β-lactamase inhibitor; penicillin synergist*
clavulanic acid INN, BAN *β-lactamase inhibitor; penicillin synergist*
claw, scaly dragon's; turkey claw *medicinal herb* [see: coral root]
clay, kaolin *natural material* [see: kaolin]
clazolam USAN, INN *minor tranquilizer*
clazolimine USAN, INN *diuretic*
clazuril USAN, INN, BAN *coccidiostat for pigeons*
CLD-BOMP *chemotherapy protocol for cervical cancer* [see: BOMP]
Clean-N-Soak solution OTC *cleaning/soaking solution for hard contact lenses*
Clear By Design gel OTC *topical keratolytic for acne* [benzoyl peroxide] 2.5%
Clear Eyes eye drops OTC *topical ophthalmic decongestant and vasoconstrictor* [naphazoline HCl] 0.012%
Clear Eyes ACR eye drops OTC *topical ophthalmic decongestant and astringent* [naphazoline HCl; zinc sulfate] 0.012%•0.25%
Clear Total Lice Elimination System kit (shampoo + egg remover enzymes + nit comb) OTC *pediculicide for lice* [pyrethrins; piperonyl butoxide] 0.3%•3%
Clear Tussin 30 liquid OTC *antitussive; expectorant* [dextromethorphan hydrobromide; guaifenesin] 15•100 mg/5 mL
Clearasil cream, lotion OTC *topical keratolytic for acne* [benzoyl peroxide] 10% ▣ clara cell
Clearasil Acne-Fighting Pads OTC *topical keratolytic for acne* [salicylic acid; alcohol ≟%] 2%
Clearasil Adult Care cream OTC *topical acne treatment* [sulfur; resorcinol; alcohol 10%]
Clearasil Antibacterial Soap bar OTC *medicated cleanser for acne* [triclosan]
Clearasil Clearstick liquid OTC *topical keratolytic for acne* [salicylic acid; alcohol 39%] 1.25%, 2%
Clearasil Daily Face Wash liquid OTC *medicated cleanser for acne* [triclosan] 0.3%
Clearasil Double Clear; Clearasil Double Textured medicated pads OTC *topical keratolytic for acne* [salicylic acid; alcohol 40%] 1.25%, 2%; 2%
Clearasil Medicated Deep Cleanser liquid OTC *topical keratolytic cleanser for acne* [salicylic acid; alcohol 42%] 0.5%
Clearblue Easy test stick for home use *in vitro diagnostic aid; urine pregnancy test*
Clearly Cala-gel OTC *topical antihistamine* [diphenhydramine HCl]
Clearplan Easy test kit for home use *in vitro diagnostic aid to predict ovulation time*

Clearview Chlamydia test for professional use *in vitro diagnostic aid for Chlamydia trachomatis* [color-label immunoassay]

cleavers; cleaverwort *medicinal herb* [see: bedstraw]

clebopride USAN, INN *antiemetic*

clefamide INN, BAN

clemastine USAN, BAN *ethanolamine antihistamine*

clemastine fumarate USAN, USP, BAN *ethanolamine antihistamine* 1.34, 2.68 mg oral; 0.5 mg/5 mL

Clematis cirrhosa; C. virginiana *medicinal herb* [see: woodbine]

clemeprol INN, BAN

clemizole INN, BAN

clemizole penicillin INN, BAN

clenbuterol INN, BAN

clenoliximab *investigational (Phase I/II) anti-CD4 antibody for the treatment of rheumatoid arthritis*

clenpirin INN [also: clenpyrin]

clenpyrin BAN [also: clenpirin]

clentiazem INN *calcium channel antagonist* [also: clentiazem maleate]

clentiazem maleate USAN *calcium channel antagonist* [also: clentiazem]

Cleocin capsules ℞ *lincosamide antibiotic; investigational (orphan) for AIDS-related Pneumocystis carinii pneumonia; investigational (NDA filed) vaginal ovules for the 3-day treatment of bacterial vaginosis* [clindamycin HCl] 75, 150, 300 mg ⑨ bleomycin; Lincocin

Cleocin vaginal cream, vaginal ovules (suppositories) ℞ *lincosamide antibiotic for bacterial vaginosis* [clindamycin phosphate] 2%; 100 mg

Cleocin Pediatric granules for oral solution ℞ *lincosamide antibiotic* [clindamycin palmitate HCl] 75 mg/5 mL

Cleocin Phosphate IV infusion, IM injection ℞ *lincosamide antibiotic; investigational (orphan) for AIDS-related Pneumocystis carinii pneumonia* [clindamycin phosphate] 150 mg/mL

Cleocin T gel, topical solution, lotion, pads ℞ *topical antibiotic for acne* [clindamycin phosphate] 10 mg/mL

Clerz 2; Clerz Plus solution OTC *rewetting solution for hard or soft contact lenses*

cletoquine INN, BAN

Clexane (European name for U.S. product Lovenox)

clibucaine INN

clidafidine INN

clidanac INN

clidinium bromide USAN, USP, INN, BAN *GI anticholinergic; peptic ulcer adjunct*

clidinium bromide & chlordiazepoxide HCl *GI anticholinergic; anxiolytic* 2.5•5 mg

Climara transdermal patch ℞ *estrogen replacement therapy for postmenopausal symptoms* [estradiol] 25, 50, 75, 100 µg/day

climazolam INN

climbazole INN, BAN

climiqualine INN

clinafloxacin HCl USAN *quinolone antibacterial*

Clinda-Derm topical solution ℞ *topical antibiotic for acne* [clindamycin phosphate] 10 mg/mL

clindamycin USAN, INN, BAN *lincosamide antibiotic; investigational (orphan) for AIDS-related Pneumocystis carinii pneumonia*

clindamycin HCl USP, BAN *lincosamide antibiotic; investigational (orphan) for AIDS-related Pneumocystis carinii pneumonia; investigational (NDA filed) for bacterial vaginosis* 75, 150 mg oral

clindamycin HCl & primaquine phosphate *investigational (orphan) for AIDS-associated Pneumocystis carinii pneumonia*

clindamycin palmitate HCl USAN, USP *lincosamide antibiotic*

clindamycin phosphate USAN, USP *lincosamide antibiotic* 10 mg/mL topical; 150 mg/mL injection

Clindets pledgets ℞ *topical antibiotic for acne* [clindamycin] 1% (10 mg/mL)
Clindex capsules (discontinued 1998) ℞ *GI anticholinergic; anxiolytic* [clidinium bromide; chlordiazepoxide HCl] 2.5•5 mg
Clinipak (trademarked packaging form) *unit dose package*
Clinistix reagent strips for home use *in vitro diagnostic aid for urine glucose*
Clinitest reagent tablets for home use *in vitro diagnostic aid for urine glucose*
clinocaine HCl [see: procaine HCl]
clinofibrate INN
clinolamide INN
Clinoril tablets ℞ *antiarthritic; nonsteroidal anti-inflammatory drug (NSAID) for ankylosing spondylitis and acute bursitis/tendinitis* [sulindac] 150, 200 mg
clioquinol USP, INN, BAN *topical antibacterial and antifungal* 3% topical
clioxanide USAN, INN, BAN *anthelmintic* ⊡ Clinoxide
clipoxamine [see: cliropamine]
cliprofen USAN, INN *anti-inflammatory*
cliropamine INN
clobamine mesylate [now: cilobamine mesylate]
clobazam USAN, INN, BAN *minor benzodiazepine tranquilizer; anxiolytic*
clobedolum [see: clonitazene]
clobenoside INN
clobenzepam INN
clobenzorex INN
clobenztropine INN
clobetasol INN, BAN *topical corticosteroidal anti-inflammatory* [also: clobetasol propionate]
clobetasol propionate USAN *topical corticosteroidal anti-inflammatory* [also: clobetasol] 0.05% topical
clobetasone INN, BAN *topical corticosteroidal anti-inflammatory* [also: clobetasone butyrate]
clobetasone butyrate USAN *topical corticosteroidal anti-inflammatory* [also: clobetasone]
clobutinol INN
clobuzarit INN, BAN
clocanfamide INN
clocapramine INN
clociguanil INN, BAN
clocinizine INN
clocortolone INN *topical corticosteroid* [also: clocortolone acetate]
clocortolone acetate USAN *topical corticosteroid* [also: clocortolone]
clocortolone pivalate USAN, USP *topical corticosteroid*
clocoumarol INN
Clocream cream OTC *moisturizer; emollient* [cod liver oil (vitamins A and E); cholecalciferol; vitamin A palmitate]
clodacaine INN
clodanolene USAN, INN *skeletal muscle relaxant*
clodantoin INN *antifungal* [also: chlordantoin]
clodazon INN *antidepressant* [also: clodazon HCl]
clodazon HCl USAN *antidepressant* [also: clodazon]
Cloderm cream ℞ *topical corticosteroidal anti-inflammatory* [clocortolone pivalate] 0.1%
clodoxopone INN
clodronate disodium *bisphosphonate bone resorption inhibitor for hypercalcemia of malignancy (investigational (orphan) in the U.S.)* [also: disodium clodronate]
clodronic acid USAN, INN, BAN *calcium regulator*
clofazimine USAN, INN, BAN *bactericidal; tuberculostatic; leprostatic (orphan)*
clofedanol INN *antitussive* [also: chlophedianol HCl; chlophedianol]
clofedanol HCl [see: chlophedianol HCl]
clofenamic acid INN
clofenamide INN
clofenciclan INN
clofenetamine INN
clofenetamine HCl [see: clofenetamine]
clofenotane INN [also: chlorophenothane; dicophane]

clofenoxyde INN
clofenpyride [see: nicofibrate]
clofenvinfos INN [also: chlorfenvinphos]
clofeverine INN
clofexamide INN
clofezone INN
clofibrate USAN, USP, INN, BAN *triglyceride-lowering antihyperlipidemic for primary dysbetalipoproteinemia (type III hyperlipidemia) and hypertriglyceridemia (types IV and V hyperlipidemia)*
clofibric acid INN
clofibride INN
clofilium phosphate USAN, INN *antiarrhythmic*
clofinol [see: nicofibrate]
cloflucarban USAN *disinfectant* [also: halocarban]
clofluperol INN, BAN *antipsychotic* [also: seperidol HCl]
clofluperol HCl [see: seperidol HCl]
clofoctol INN
cloforex INN
clofurac INN
clogestone INN, BAN *progestin* [also: clogestone acetate]
clogestone acetate USAN *progestin* [also: clogestone]
cloguanamil INN, BAN [also: cloguanamile]
cloguanamile BAN [also: cloguanamil]
clomacran INN, BAN *antipsychotic* [also: clomacran phosphate]
clomacran phosphate USAN *antipsychotic* [also: clomacran]
clomegestone INN *progestin* [also: clomegestone acetate]
clomegestone acetate USAN *progestin* [also: clomegestone]
clometacin INN
clometerone INN *antiestrogen* [also: clometherone]
clometherone USAN *antiestrogen* [also: clometerone]
clomethiazole INN [also: chlormethiazole]
clometocillin INN
Clomid tablets ℞ *ovulation stimulant* [clomiphene citrate] 50 mg
clomide [see: aklomide]
clomifene INN *gonad-stimulating principle; ovulation stimulant* [also: clomiphene citrate; clomiphene]
clomifenoxide INN
clominorex USAN, INN *anorectic*
clomiphene BAN *gonad-stimulating principle; ovulation stimulant* [also: clomiphene citrate; clomifene] ⓢ clonidine
clomiphene citrate USAN, USP *gonad-stimulating principle; ovulation stimulant* [also: clomifene; clomiphene] 50 mg oral
clomipramine INN, BAN *tricyclic antidepressant for obsessive-compulsive disorders* [also: clomipramine HCl]
clomipramine HCl USAN *tricyclic antidepressant for obsessive-compulsive disorders* [also: clomipramine] 25, 50, 75 mg oral
clomocycline INN, BAN
clomoxir INN
Clomycin ointment OTC *topical antibiotic; anesthetic* [polymyxin B sulfate; bacitracin; neomycin sulfate; lidocaine] 5000 U•500 U•3.5 mg•40 mg per g
clonazepam USAN, USP, INN, BAN *anticonvulsant; investigational (orphan) for hyperexplexia (startle disease)* 0.5, 1, 2 mg oral
clonazoline INN
clonidine USAN, INN, BAN *centrally acting antiadrenergic antihypertensive; adjunct to epidural opioid analgesics for severe cancer pain (orphan)* ⓢ clomiphene; Klonopin; quinidine
clonidine HCl USAN, USP, BAN *centrally acting antiadrenergic antihypertensive; adjunct to epidural opioid analgesics for severe cancer pain (orphan)* 0.1, 0.2, 0.3 mg oral
clonitazene INN, BAN
clonitrate USAN, INN *coronary vasodilator*
clonixeril USAN, INN *analgesic*
clonixin USAN, INN *analgesic*
clopamide USAN, INN, BAN *antihypertensive; diuretic*

clopenthixol USAN, INN, BAN *antipsychotic*
cloperastine INN
cloperidone INN *sedative* [also: cloperidone HCl]
cloperidone HCl USAN *sedative* [also: cloperidone]
clophenoxate [see: meclofenoxate]
clopidogrel INN, BAN *platelet aggregation inhibitor for stroke, myocardial infarction, and peripheral artery disease*
clopidogrel bisulfate USAN *platelet aggregation inhibitor for stroke, myocardial infarction, and peripheral artery disease*
clopidol USAN, INN, BAN *coccidiostat for poultry*
clopimozide USAN, INN *antipsychotic*
clopipazan INN *antipsychotic* [also: clopipazan mesylate]
clopipazan mesylate USAN *antipsychotic* [also: clopipazan]
clopirac USAN, INN, BAN *anti-inflammatory*
cloponone INN, BAN
clopoxide [see: chlordiazepoxide]
clopoxide chloride [see: chlordiazepoxide HCl]
Clopra tablets ℞ *antidopaminergic; antiemetic for chemotherapy; peristaltic* [metoclopramide HCl] 10 mg
cloprednol USAN, INN, BAN *corticosteroid; anti-inflammatory*
cloprostenol INN, BAN *prostaglandin* [also: cloprostenol sodium]
cloprostenol sodium USAN *prostaglandin* [also: cloprostenol]
cloprothiazole INN
cloquinate INN, BAN
cloquinozine INN
cloracetadol INN
cloral betaine INN *sedative* [also: chloral betaine]
cloramfenicol pantotenate complex INN *antibacterial; antirickettsial* [also: chloramphenicol pantothenate complex]
cloranolol INN
clorarsen [see: dichlorophenarsine HCl]
clorazepate dipotassium USAN, USP *benzodiazepine anxiolytic; minor tranquilizer; anticonvulsant adjunct; alcohol withdrawal aid* [also: dipotassium clorazepate] 3.75, 7.5, 15 mg oral
clorazepate monopotassium USAN *minor tranquilizer*
clorazepic acid BAN
cloretate INN *sedative; hypnotic* [also: clorethate]
clorethate USAN *sedative; hypnotic* [also: cloretate]
clorexolone USAN, INN, BAN *diuretic*
clorgiline INN [also: clorgyline]
clorgyline BAN [also: clorgiline]
cloricromen INN
cloridarol INN
clorindanic acid INN
clorindanol INN *spermaticide* [also: chlorindanol]
clorindione INN, BAN
clormecaine INN
clorofene INN *disinfectant* [also: clorophene]
cloroperone INN *antipsychotic* [also: cloroperone HCl]
cloroperone HCl USAN *antipsychotic* [also: cloroperone]
clorophene USAN *disinfectant* [also: clorofene]
cloroqualone INN
clorotepine INN
Clorpactin WCS-90 powder for solution OTC *topical antimicrobial* [oxychlorosene sodium] 2 g
clorprenaline INN, BAN *adrenergic; bronchodilator* [also: clorprenaline HCl]
clorprenaline HCl USAN *adrenergic; bronchodilator* [also: clorprenaline]
Clorpres tablets ℞ *antihypertensive; diuretic* [clonidine HCl; chlorthalidone] 0.1•15 mg; 0.2•15 mg; 0.3•15 mg
clorquinaldol [see: chlorquinaldol]
clorsulon USAN, INN *antiparasitic; fasciolicide*
clortermine INN *anorectic* [also: clortermine HCl]
clortermine HCl USAN *anorectic* [also: clortermine]

closantel USAN, INN, BAN *anthelmintic*
closilate INN *combining name for radicals or groups* [also: closylate]
closiramine INN *antihistamine* [also: closiramine aceturate]
closiramine aceturate USAN *antihistamine* [also: closiramine]
clostebol INN [also: clostebol acetate]
clostebol acetate BAN [also: clostebol]
clostridial collagenase *investigational (Phase II, orphan) for advanced Dupuytren disease*
***Clostridium botulinum* toxin** [see: botulinum toxin]
closylate USAN, BAN *combining name for radicals or groups* [also: closilate]
clotbur *medicinal herb* [see: burdock]
clothiapine USAN, BAN *antipsychotic* [also: clotiapine]
clothixamide maleate USAN *antipsychotic* [also: clotixamide]
clotiapine INN *antipsychotic* [also: clothiapine]
clotiazepam INN
cloticasone INN, BAN *anti-inflammatory* [also: cloticasone propionate]
cloticasone propionate USAN *anti-inflammatory* [also: cloticasone]
clotioxone INN
clotixamide INN *antipsychotic* [also: clothixamide maleate]
clotixamide maleate [see: clothixamide maleate]
Clotrimaderm (CAN) cream, topical solution, vaginal cream OTC *topical antifungal* [clotrimazole] 1%
clotrimazole (CLT) USAN, USP, INN, BAN, JAN *broad-spectrum antifungal* 1% topical; 1%, 2%, 200 mg vaginal [?] co-trimoxazole
clotrimazole & betamethasone dipropionate *topical antifungal and corticosteroidal anti-inflammatory* 1%• 0.05%
clotrimidazole *investigational (orphan) for sickle cell disease*
cloudberry *medicinal herb* [see: blackberry]
clove oil NF
clover, king's; sweet clover *medicinal herb* [see: melilot]
clover, marsh *medicinal herb* [see: buckbean]
clover, purple; wild clover *medicinal herb* [see: red clover]
clover, winter *medicinal herb* [see: squaw vine]
cloves (*Caryophyllus aromaticus; Eugenia caryophyllata; Syzygium aromaticum*) seed and oil *medicinal herb for bad breath, bronchial secretions, dizziness, earache, fever, nausea, platelet aggregation inhibition, poor circulation, and thrombosis; also used topically as an analgesic and antiseptic*
clovoxamine INN
cloxacepride INN
cloxacillin INN, BAN *penicillinase-resistant penicillin antibiotic* [also: cloxacillin benzathine]
cloxacillin benzathine USP *penicillinase-resistant penicillin antibiotic* [also: cloxacillin]
cloxacillin sodium USAN, USP *penicillinase-resistant penicillin antibiotic* 250, 500 mg oral; 125 mg/5 mL oral
Cloxapen capsules ℞ *penicillinase-resistant penicillin antibiotic* [cloxacillin sodium] 250, 500 mg
cloxazolam INN
cloxestradiol INN
cloxifenol [see: triclosan]
cloximate INN
cloxiquine INN *antibacterial* [also: cloxyquin]
cloxotestosterone INN
cloxphendyl [see: cloxypendyl]
cloxypendyl INN
cloxyquin USAN *antibacterial* [also: cloxiquine]
clozapine USAN, INN, BAN *dibenzodiazepine antipsychotic for severe schizophrenia; sedative* 25, 100 mg oral
Clozaril tablets ℞ *novel (atypical) antipsychotic for severe schizophrenia* [clozapine] 25, 100 mg
CLT (clotrimazole) [q.v.]
club, shepherd's *medicinal herb* [see: mullein]

club moss ***(Lycopodium clavatum)*** spores *medicinal herb used as a hemostatic and vulnerary*

cluster, wax *medicinal herb* [see: wintergreen]

Clysodrast powder for oral solution (discontinued 1999) ℞ *pre-procedure bowel evacuant* [bisacodyl tannex] 2.5 g/packet

C-Max gradual-release tablets OTC *vitamin/mineral supplement* [vitamin C; multiple minerals] 1 • ≟ g

CMC (carboxymethylcellulose) gum [see: carboxymethylcellulose sodium]

CMC (cyclophosphamide, methotrexate, CCNU) *chemotherapy protocol*

CMC-VAP (cyclophosphamide, methotrexate, CCNU, vincristine, Adriamycin, procarbazine) *chemotherapy protocol*

CMF; CMF-IV (cyclophosphamide, methotrexate, fluorouracil) *chemotherapy protocol for breast cancer*

CMF/AV (cyclophosphamide, methotrexate, fluorouracil, Adriamycin, Oncovin) *chemotherapy protocol*

CMFAVP (cyclophosphamide, methotrexate, fluorouracil, Adriamycin, vincristine, prednisone) *chemotherapy protocol*

CMFP; CMF-P (cyclophosphamide, methotrexate, fluorouracil, prednisone) *chemotherapy protocol for breast cancer*

CMFPT (cyclophosphamide, methotrexate, fluorouracil, prednisone, tamoxifen) *chemotherapy protocol*

CMFPTH (cyclophosphamide, methotrexate, fluorouracil, prednisone, tamoxifen, Halotestin) *chemotherapy protocol*

CMFT (cyclophosphamide, methotrexate, fluorouracil, tamoxifen) *chemotherapy protocol*

CMFVAT (cyclophosphamide, methotrexate, fluorouracil, vincristine, Adriamycin, testosterone) *chemotherapy protocol*

CMFVP (cyclophosphamide, methotrexate, fluorouracil, vincristine, prednisone) *chemotherapy protocol for breast cancer* [two dosing protocols: Cooper protocol and SWOG protocol]

CMH (cyclophosphamide, *m*-AMSA, hydroxyurea) *chemotherapy protocol*

C-MOPP (cyclophosphamide, mechlorethamine, Oncovin, procarbazine, prednisone) *chemotherapy protocol*

CMV (cisplatin, methotrexate, vinblastine) *chemotherapy protocol for bladder cancer*

CMV-IGIV (cytomegalovirus immune globulin intravenous) [see: cytomegalovirus immune globulin, human]

CN2 HCl [see: mechlorethamine HCl]

CNF (cyclophosphamide, Novantrone, fluorouracil) *chemotherapy protocol for breast cancer* [also: CFM; FNC]

Cnicus benedictus *medicinal herb* [see: blessed thistle]

CNOP (cyclophosphamide, Novantrone, Oncovin, prednisone) *chemotherapy protocol for non-Hodgkin lymphoma*

CNS-5161 *investigational (Phase I) for neuropathic pain and migraine*

CO Fluoxetine (CAN) capsules ℞ *selective serotonin reuptake inhibitor (SSRI) for depression, obsessive-compulsive disorder (OCD), and bulimia nervosa* [fluoxetine HCl] 10, 20 mg

Co I (coenzyme I) [see: nadide]

CO_2 (carbon dioxide) [q.v.]

^{57}Co [see: cobaltous chloride Co 57]

^{57}Co [see: cyanocobalamin Co 57]

^{58}Co [see: cyanocobalamin (^{58}Co)]

^{60}Co [see: cobaltous chloride Co 60]

^{60}Co [see: cyanocobalamin Co 60]

coachweed *medicinal herb* [see: bedstraw]

Coactinon ℞ *investigational (NDA filed) non-nucleoside reverse transcrip-*

tase inhibitor for naive HIV infection [emivirine]

coagulants *a class of agents that promote or accelerate clotting of the blood*

coagulation factor VIIa [see: factor VIIa, recombinant]

coagulation factor IX (human) [see: factor IX complex]

coakum *medicinal herb* [see: pokeweed]

coal tar USP *topical antieczematic; antiseborrheic*

co-amoxiclav (amoxicillin & potassium clavulanate) [q.v.]

COAP (cyclophosphamide, Oncovin, ara-C, prednisone) *chemotherapy protocol*

Co-Apap tablets OTC *antitussive; decongestant; antihistamine; analgesic* [dextromethorphan hydrobromide; pseudoephedrine HCl; chlorpheniramine maleate; acetaminophen] 15•30•2•325 mg

COAP-BLEO (cyclophosphamide, Oncovin, ara-C, prednisone, bleomycin) *chemotherapy protocol*

Coated Aspirin; Coated Aspirin Extra Strength; Coated Aspirin Arthritis Pain Relief; Coated Aspirin Daily Low Dose (CAN) OTC *analgesic; antipyretic; anti-inflammatory; antirheumatic* [aspirin] 235 mg; 500 mg; 650 mg; 81 mg

COB (cisplatin, Oncovin, bleomycin) *chemotherapy protocol for head and neck cancer*

cobalamin concentrate USP *vitamin* B_{12}*; hematopoietic*

cobalt *element (Co)*

cobalt-labeled vitamin B_{12} [see: cyanocobalamin Co 57 & Co 60]

cobaltous chloride Co 57 USAN *radioactive agent*

cobaltous chloride Co 60 USAN *radioactive agent*

cobamamide INN

cocaine USP, BAN *topical anesthetic for mucous membranes; widely abused as a street drug, derived from coca leaves* 4%, 10% topical

cocaine, crack *street drug made by converting cocaine HCl into a form that can be smoked, which causes a faster, more intense effect*

cocaine HCl USP *topical anesthetic for mucous membranes; widely abused as a street drug, derived from coca leaves* 135 mg oral; 4%, 10% topical

Cocaine Viscous topical solution ℞ *topical mucosal anesthesia* [cocaine] 4%, 10%

cocarboxylase INN [also: co-carboxylase]

co-carboxylase BAN [also: cocarboxylase]

cocashweed *medicinal herb* [see: life root]

coccidioidin USP *dermal coccidioidomycosis test*

cocculin [see: picrotoxin]

Cocculus lacunosus; C. suberosus *medicinal herb* [see: levant berry]

Cocculus palmatus *medicinal herb* [see: colombo]

Cochlearia armoracia *medicinal herb* [see: horseradish]

cocklebur *medicinal herb* [see: agrimony; burdock]

cockspur pepper *medicinal herb* [see: cayenne]

cockspur rye *medicinal herb* [see: ergot]

cocoa NF

cocoa *(Theobromo cacao)* bean *medicinal herb used as a cardiac stimulant, diuretic, and vasodilator*

cocoa butter NF *suppository base; emollient/protectant*

cocowort *medicinal herb* [see: shepherd's purse]

cod liver oil USP, BAN *vitamins A and D source; emollient/protectant*

cod liver oil, nondestearinated NF

codactide INN, BAN

Codamine syrup, pediatric syrup ℞ *narcotic antitussive; decongestant* [hydrocodone bitartrate; phenylpropanolamine HCl] 5•25 mg/5 mL; 2.5•12.5 mg/5 mL

CODE (cisplatin, Oncovin, doxorubicin, etoposide) *chemotherapy protocol for small cell lung cancer*

Codegest Expectorant liquid ℞ *narcotic antitussive; decongestant; expectorant* [codeine phosphate; phenylpropanolamine HCl; guaifenesin] 10•12.5•100 mg/5 mL ⊡ Codehist

Codehist DH elixir ℞ *narcotic antitussive; decongestant; antihistamine* [codeine phosphate; pseudoephedrine HCl; chlorpheniramine maleate; alcohol 5.7%] 10•30•2 mg/5 mL ⊡ Codegest

codehydrogenase I [see: nadide]

codeine USP, BAN *narcotic analgesic used as an antitussive; sometimes abused as a street drug* ⊡ Kaodene

codeine & acetaminophen *narcotic analgesic* 15•300, 30•300, 60•300 mg oral; 12•30 mg/5 mL oral

codeine phosphate USP, BAN *narcotic analgesic used as an antitussive* 15 mg/5 mL oral; 30, 60 mg injection

codeine phosphate & guaifenesin *antitussive; narcotic analgesic; expectorant* 10•300 mg oral; 10•100 mg/5 mL oral

codeine polistirex USAN *narcotic analgesic used as an antitussive*

codeine sulfate USP *narcotic analgesic used as an antitussive* 15, 30, 60 mg oral

codelcortone [see: prednisolone]

co-dergocrine mesylate BAN *cognition adjuvant* [also: ergoloid mesylates]

Codiclear DH syrup ℞ *narcotic antitussive; expectorant* [hydrocodone bitartrate; guaifenesin] 5•100 mg/5 mL

Codimal capsules, film-coated tablets OTC *decongestant; antihistamine; analgesic* [pseudoephedrine HCl; chlorpheniramine maleate; acetaminophen] 30•2•325 mg

Codimal DH syrup ℞ *narcotic antitussive; decongestant; antihistamine* [hydrocodone bitartrate; phenylephrine HCl; pyrilamine maleate] 1.66•5•8.33 mg/5 mL

Codimal DM syrup OTC *antitussive; decongestant; antihistamine* [dextromethorphan hydrobromide; phenylephrine HCl; pyrilamine maleate] 10•5•8.33 mg/5 mL

Codimal PH syrup OTC *narcotic antitussive; decongestant; antihistamine* [codeine phosphate; phenylephrine HCl; pyrilamine maleate] 10•5•8.33 mg/5 mL

Codimal-L.A.; Codimal-L.A. Half extended-release capsules ℞ *decongestant; antihistamine* [pseudoephedrine HCl; chlorpheniramine maleate] 120•8 mg; 60•4 mg

codorphone [now: conorphone HCl]

codoxime USAN, INN *antitussive*

coenzyme Q_{10} *natural enzyme used as a cardiac protectant, free radical scavenger, membrane stabilizer; investigational (Phase I) immune stimulant for AIDS*

COF/COM (cyclophosphamide, Oncovin, fluorouracil + cyclophosphamide, Oncovin, methotrexate) *chemotherapy protocol*

coffeine [see: caffeine]

cofisatin INN

cofisatine [see: cofisatin]

cogazocine INN

Cogentin tablets, IV or IM injection ℞ *anticholinergic; antiparkinsonian* [benztropine mesylate] 0.5, 1, 2 mg; 1 mg/mL

Co-Gesic tablets ℞ *narcotic analgesic* [hydrocodone bitartrate; acetaminophen] 5•500 mg

Cognex capsules ℞ *cognition adjuvant for Alzheimer dementia; reversible cholinesterase inhibitor* [tacrine HCl] 10, 20, 30, 40 mg

Co-Hist tablets OTC *decongestant; antihistamine; analgesic* [pseudoephedrine HCl; chlorpheniramine maleate; acetaminophen] 30•2•325 mg

cohosh *medicinal herb* [see: black cohosh; blue cohosh; white cohosh]

Cola acuminata *medicinal herb* [see: kola nut]

Colace capsules, syrup, oral liquid OTC *laxative; stool softener* [docusate sodium] 50, 100 mg; 60 mg/15 mL; 150 mg/15 mL

Colace suppositories OTC *hyperosmolar laxative* [glycerin]

colaspase BAN *antineoplastic for acute lymphocytic leukemia (ALL)* [also: asparaginase]

Co-Lav powder for oral solution (discontinued 1999) ℞ *pre-procedure bowel evacuant* [polyethylene glycol–electrolyte solution; electrolytes] 60 g/L

Colax tablets (discontinued 1998) OTC *stimulant laxative; stool softener* [phenolphthalein; docusate sodium] 65•100 mg

Colazal capsules ℞ *gastrointestinal anti-inflammatory for ulcerative colitis* [balsalazide disodium] 750 mg

Colazide (European name for U.S. product Colazal)

ColBenemid tablets (discontinued 1997) ℞ *treatment for frequent, recurrent attacks of gouty arthritis* [probenecid; colchicine] 500•0.5 mg

colchamine [see: demecolcine]

colchicine USP, JAN *gout suppressant; orphan status withdrawn 1997* 0.5, 0.6 mg oral; 1 mg injection

colchicine & probenecid *treatment for frequent, recurrent attacks of gouty arthritis* 0.5•500 mg oral

Colchicum autumnale; C. speciosum; C. vernum *medicinal herb* [see: autumn crocus]

Cold & Allergy elixir OTC *decongestant; antihistamine* [phenylpropanolamine HCl; brompheniramine maleate] 12.5•2 mg/5 mL

cold cream USP

Cold Relief tablets OTC *antitussive; decongestant; antihistamine; analgesic* [dextromethorphan hydrobromide; phenylpropanolamine HCl; chlorpheniramine maleate; acetaminophen] 10•12.5•2•325 mg

Cold Symptoms Relief tablets OTC *antitussive; decongestant; antihistamine; analgesic* [dextromethorphan hydrobromide; pseudoephedrine HCl; chlorpheniramine maleate; acetaminophen] 10•30•2•325 mg

Coldec DM syrup ℞ *antitussive; decongestant; antihistamine* [dextromethorphan hydrobromide; pseudoephedrine HCl; brompheniramine maleate] 15•60•4 mg/5 mL

Cold-Gest sustained-release capsules OTC *decongestant; antihistamine* [phenylpropanolamine HCl; chlorpheniramine maleate] 75•8 mg

Coldloc liquid ℞ *decongestant; expectorant* [phenylpropanolamine HCl; phenylephrine HCl; guaifenesin] 20•5•100 mg/5 mL

Coldloc-LA sustained-release caplets ℞ *decongestant; expectorant* [phenylpropanolamine HCl; guaifenesin] 75•600 mg

Coldrine tablets OTC *decongestant; analgesic* [pseudoephedrine HCl; acetaminophen] 30•325 mg

colecalciferol (vitamin D_3) INN *fat-soluble vitamin* [also: cholecalciferol]

colesevelam HCl USAN *bile acid sequestrant; nonabsorbed cholesterol-lowering polymer for hyperlipidemia*

Colestid tablets, granules ℞ *cholesterol-lowering antihyperlipidemic* [colestipol HCl] 1 g; 5 g/dose ▣ colistin

colestipol INN, BAN *bile acid sequestrant; cholesterol-lowering antihyperlipidemic* [also: colestipol HCl] ▣ colistin

colestipol HCl USAN, USP *bile acid sequestrant; cholesterol-lowering antihyperlipidemic* [also: colestipol] ▣ colistin

colestolone USAN, INN *hypolipidemic*

colestyramine INN *bile salt ion-exchange resin; antihyperlipoproteinemic* [also: cholestyramine resin; cholestyramine]

colestyramine resin [see: cholestyramine]

colextran INN

Colfed-A sustained-release capsules ℞ *decongestant; antihistamine* [pseudoephedrine HCl; chlorpheniramine maleate] 120•8 mg

colfenamate INN
colforsin USAN, INN *antiglaucoma agent*
colfosceril palmitate USAN, INN, BAN *pulmonary surfactant for hyaline membrane disease and neonatal respiratory distress syndrome (orphan); investigational (orphan) for adult respiratory distress syndrome (ARDS)*
colfosceril palmitate & phosphatidylglycerol *investigational (orphan) for neonatal respiratory distress syndrome*
colic root *medicinal herb* [see: blazing star; star grass; wild yam]
colimecycline INN
colistimethate sodium USAN, USP, INN *bactericidal antibiotic* [also: colistin sulphomethate]
colistin INN, BAN *bactericidal antibiotic* [also: colistin sulfate] ⊡ Colestid; colestipol
colistin methanesulfonate [see: colistimethate sodium]
colistin sulfate USP *bactericidal antibiotic* [also: colistin]
colistin sulphomethate BAN *bactericidal antibiotic* [also: colistimethate sodium]
collagen *ophthalmic implant to block puncta and retain moisture; urethral injection for stress urinary incontinence*
collagen, purified type II *investigational (Phase III, orphan) oral treatment for juvenile rheumatoid arthritis*
collagen sponge, absorbable *topical local hemostat for surgery*
collagenase *topical proteolytic enzymes for necrotic tissue debridement; investigational (orphan) for Peyronie disease*
collagenase, clostridial [see: clostridial collagenase]
collard *medicinal herb* [see: skunk cabbage]
Collastin Oil Free Moisturizer lotion (discontinued 1998) OTC *moisturizer; emollient* [collagen]
Collinsonia canadensis *medicinal herb* [see: stone root]
collodion USP *topical protectant*
colloidal aluminum hydroxide [see: aluminum hydroxide gel]
colloidal oatmeal *demulcent*
colloidal silicon dioxide [see: silicon dioxide, colloidal]
Colloral *investigational (Phase III, orphan) collagen derivative for treatment of juvenile rheumatoid arthritis* [trinecol (pullus)]
Collyrium for Fresh Eyes ophthalmic solution OTC *extraocular irrigating solution* [sterile isotonic solution]
Collyrium Fresh eye drops OTC *topical ophthalmic decongestant and vasoconstrictor* [tetrahydrozoline HCl] 0.05%
ColoCare test kit for home use *in vitro diagnostic aid for fecal occult blood*
colombo (*Cocculus palmatus*) root *medicinal herb used as an antiemetic and febrifuge*
Colomed enema ℞ *investigational (orphan) for left-sided ulcerative colitis and chronic radiation proctitis* [short chain fatty acids]
colony-stimulating factors *a class of glycoproteins that stimulate the production of granulocytes and macrophages*
Color Allergy Screening Test (CAST) reagent assay tubes *in vitro diagnostic aid for immunoglobulin E in serum*
Color Ovulation Test kit for home use *in vitro diagnostic aid to predict ovulation time*
ColoScreen slide test for professional use *in vitro diagnostic aid for fecal occult blood*
Colovage powder for oral solution (discontinued 1999) ℞ *pre-procedure bowel evacuant* [polyethylene glycol–electrolyte solution (PEG 3350)] 60 g/L
Col-Probenecid tablets (discontinued 1998) ℞ *treatment for frequent, recurrent attacks of gouty arthritis* [probenecid; colchicine] 500•0.5 mg
colterol INN *bronchodilator* [also: colterol mesylate]
colterol mesylate USAN *bronchodilator* [also: colterol]
colt's tail *medicinal herb* [see: fleabane; horseweed]

coltsfoot ***(Tussilago farfara)*** buds, flowers, and leaves *medicinal herb for asthma, bronchitis, dry cough, hay fever, lung disorders, excess mucus, and throat irritation*

columbine ***(Aquilegia vulgaris)*** plant *medicinal herb used as an astringent, diaphoretic, and diuretic*

Coly-Mycin M powder for IV or IM injection ℞ *bactericidal antibiotic* [colistimethate sodium] 150 mg

Coly-Mycin S Otic suspension ℞ *topical corticosteroidal anti-inflammatory; antibiotic* [hydrocortisone acetate; neomycin sulfate; colistin sulfate] 1%•4.71 mg•3 mg per mL

CoLyte powder for oral solution ℞ *pre-procedure bowel evacuant* [polyethylene glycol–electrolyte solution (PEG 3350)] 60 g/L

COM (cyclophosphamide, Oncovin, MeCCNU) *chemotherapy protocol*

COM (cyclophosphamide, Oncovin, methotrexate) *chemotherapy protocol*

COMA-A (cyclophosphamide, Oncovin, methotrexate/citrovorum factor, Adriamycin, ara-C) *chemotherapy protocol*

COMB (cyclophosphamide, Oncovin, MeCCNU, bleomycin) *chemotherapy protocol*

COMB (Cytoxin, Oncovin, methotrexate, bleomycin) *chemotherapy protocol*

Combidex ℞ *investigational (NDA filed) MRI diagnostic aid for lymph node metastases* [ferumoxtran-10]

CombiPatch transdermal patch ℞ *hormone replacement therapy for postmenopausal symptoms* [estradiol; norethindrone acetate] 0.05•0.14, 0.05•0.25 mg/day

Combipres 0.1; Combipres 0.2; Combipres 0.3 tablets ℞ *antihypertensive; diuretic* [clonidine HCl; chlorthalidone] 0.1•15 mg; 0.2•15 mg; 0.3•15 mg ⊠ Catapres

Combistix reagent strips *in vitro diagnostic aid for multiple urine products*

Combivent oral inhalation aerosol ℞ *anticholinergic bronchodilator for chronic bronchospasm with COPD* [ipratropium bromide; albuterol sulfate] 18•103 µg/spray

Combivir film-coated tablets ℞ *nucleoside reverse transcriptase inhibitor combination for HIV* [lamivudine; zidovudine] 150•300 mg

COMe (Cytoxin, Oncovin, methotrexate) *chemotherapy protocol*

COMF (cyclophosphamide, Oncovin, methotrexate, fluorouracil) *chemotherapy protocol*

Comfort eye drops OTC *topical ophthalmic decongestant and vasoconstrictor* [naphazoline HCl] 0.03%

Comfort Tears eye drops OTC *ocular moisturizer/lubricant* [hydroxyethylcellulose]

ComfortCare GP Wetting & Soaking solution OTC *disinfecting/wetting/soaking solution for rigid gas permeable contact lenses*

Comfortine ointment OTC *moisturizer; emollient; astringent; antiseptic* [vitamins A and D; lanolin; zinc oxide]

comfrey ***(Symphytum officinale; S. tuberosum)*** leaves and roots *medicinal herb for anemia, arthritis, blood cleansing, boils and sores, bruises, burns, edema, emphysema, fractures, gastric ulcers, hemorrhoids, and sprains; not generally regarded as safe, as it may be carcinogenic and hepatotoxic*

comfrey, spotted *medicinal herb* [see: lungwort]

Comhist tablets ℞ *decongestant; antihistamine* [phenylephrine HCl; chlorpheniramine maleate; phenyltoloxamine citrate] 10•2•25 mg

Comhist LA long-acting capsules ℞ *decongestant; antihistamine* [phenylephrine HCl; chlorpheniramine maleate; phenyltoloxamine citrate] 20•4•50 mg

COMLA (cyclophosphamide, Oncovin, methotrexate, leucovorin [rescue], ara-C) *chemotherapy protocol for non-Hodgkin lymphoma*

Commiphora abssynica; C. molmol; C. myrrha *medicinal herb* [see: myrrh]
Commiphora mukul *medicinal herb* [see: guggul]
common bugloss *medicinal herb* [see: borage]
common elder *medicinal herb* [see: elderberry]
common flax *medicinal herb* [see: flaxseed]
comosain *investigational (orphan) proteolytic enzymes for debridement of severe burns*
COMP (CCNU, Oncovin, methotrexate, procarbazine) *chemotherapy protocol*
COMP (cyclophosphamide, Oncovin, methotrexate, prednisone) *chemotherapy protocol for pediatric Hodgkin lymphoma*
Compazine suppositories ℞ *conventional (typical) antipsychotic; antiemetic* [prochlorperazine] 2.5, 5, 25 mg
Compazine syrup, IV or IM injection ℞ *conventional (typical) antipsychotic; antiemetic* [prochlorperazine edisylate] 5 mg/5 mL; 5 mg/mL
Compazine tablets, Spansules (sustained-release capsules) ℞ *conventional (typical) antipsychotic; antiemetic* [prochlorperazine maleate] 5, 10 mg; 10, 15 mg
Compete tablets OTC *vitamin/iron supplement* [multiple vitamins; ferrous gluconate; folic acid] ≛•27•0.4 mg
Compleat Modified Formula closed system containers OTC *enteral nutritional therapy* [lactose-free formula]
Compleat Modified Formula ready-to-use liquid OTC *enteral nutritional therapy* [lactose-free formula]
Compleat Regular Formula ready-to-use liquid OTC *enteral nutritional therapy* [milk-based formula]
complement receptor type I, soluble recombinant human *investigational (orphan) for adult respiratory distress syndrome*
Complete solution OTC *rewetting solution for soft contact lenses*
Complete All-in-One solution OTC *cleaning/disinfecting/rinsing/storage solution for soft contact lenses*
Complete Weekly Enzymatic Cleaner effervescent tablets OTC *enzymatic cleaner for soft contact lenses* [subtilisin A]
Complex 15 Face cream OTC *moisturizer; emollient*
Complex 15 Hand & Body cream, lotion OTC *moisturizer; emollient*
Comply liquid OTC *enteral nutritional therapy* [lactose-free formula]
component pertussis vaccine (alternate name for acellular pertussis vacine) [see: diphtheria & tetanus toxoids & acellular pertussis (DTaP) vaccine, adsorbed]
compound 42 [see: warfarin]
compound CB3025 [see: melphalan]
compound E [see: cortisone acetate]
compound F [see: hydrocortisone]
compound orange spirit [see: orange spirit, compound]
compound Q [see: trichosanthin]
compound S [see: zidovudine]
compound solution of sodium chloride INN *fluid and electrolyte replenisher* [also: Ringer injection]
compound solution of sodium lactate INN *electrolyte and fluid replenisher; systemic alkalizer* [also: Ringer injection, lactated]
Compound W liquid, gel OTC *topical keratolytic* [salicylic acid in collodion] 17%
Compound W for Kids pad OTC *topical keratolytic* [salicylic acid] 40%
Compoz gel caps OTC *antihistaminic sleep aid* [diphenhydramine HCl] 25 mg
Compoz Nighttime Sleep Aid tablets OTC *antihistaminic sleep aid* [diphenhydramine HCl] 50 mg
compressible sugar [see: sugar, compressible]
Computer Eye Drops OTC *ophthalmic moisturizer and emollient* [glycerin] 1%
COMT inhibitors (catechol-O-methyltransferase) *a class of antiparkinson agents that stabilize serum*

levodopa levels by inhibiting an enzyme that breaks down the levodopa before it reaches the brain

Comtan film-coated tablets ℞ *COMT inhibitor for Parkinson disease* [entacapone] 200 mg

Comtrex liquid OTC *antitussive; decongestant; antihistamine; analgesic* [dextromethorphan hydrobromide; pseudoephedrine HCl; chlorpheniramine maleate; acetaminophen] 3.3•10•0.67•108.3 mg/5 mL

Comtrex, Cough Formula liquid OTC *antitussive; decongestant; expectorant; analgesic* [dextromethorphan hydrobromide; pseudoephedrine HCl; guaifenesin; acetaminophen; alcohol 20%] 7.5•15•50•125 mg/5 mL

Comtrex Allergy-Sinus caplets, tablets OTC *decongestant; antihistamine; analgesic* [pseudoephedrine HCl; chlorpheniramine maleate; acetaminophen] 30•2•500 mg

Comtrex Liqui-Gels (liquid-filled capsules) OTC *antitussive; decongestant; antihistamine; analgesic* [dextromethorphan hydrobromide; phenylpropanolamine HCl; chlorpheniramine maleate; acetaminophen] 10•12.5•2•325, 15•12.5•2•500 mg

Comtrex Multi-Symptom Cold & Flu Relief tablets, caplets OTC *antitussive; decongestant; antihistamine; analgesic* [dextromethorphan hydrobromide; pseudoephedrine HCl; chlorpheniramine maleate; acetaminophen] 15•30•2•500 mg

Comtrex Multi-Symptom Cold & Flu Relief Liqui-Gels (capsules) OTC *antitussive; decongestant; antihistamine; analgesic* [dextromethorphan hydrobromide; phenylpropanolamine HCl; chlorpheniramine maleate; acetaminophen] 15•12.5•2•500 mg

Comtrex Non-Drowsy caplets OTC *antitussive; decongestant; analgesic* [dextromethorphan hydrobromide; pseudoephedrine HCl; acetaminophen] 15•30•500 mg

Comvax IM injection ℞ *infant (1½–15 months) vaccine for H. influenzae and hepatitis B* [Hemophilus b purified capsular polysaccharide; *Neisseria meningitidis* OMPC; hepatitis B virus vaccine] 7.5•125•5 µg/0.5 mL

Conceive Ovulation Predictor 5-day test kit for professional use *in vitro diagnostic aid to predict ovulation time*

Conceive Pregnancy test kit for home use *in vitro diagnostic aid; urine pregnancy test*

Concentrated Cleaner solution OTC *cleaning solution for rigid gas permeable contact lenses*

Conceptrol Contraceptive Inserts vaginal suppositories OTC *spermicidal contraceptive* [nonoxynol 9] 150 mg

Conceptrol Disposable Contraceptive vaginal gel OTC *spermicidal contraceptive* [nonoxynol 9] 4%

Concerta Oros (extended-release tablets) ℞ *CNS stimulant; once-daily treatment for attention-deficit hyperactivity disorder (ADHD)* [methylphenidate HCl] 18, 36, 54 mg

Condylox solution, gel ℞ *topical antimitotic for external genital and perianal warts* [podofilox] 0.5%

cone flower, purple *medicinal herb* [see: echinacea]

conessine INN

conessine hydrobromide [see: conessine]

Conex syrup OTC *decongestant; expectorant* [phenylpropanolamine HCl; guaifenesin] 12.5•100 mg/5 mL

Conex with Codeine syrup ℞ *narcotic antitussive; decongestant; expectorant* [codeine phosphate; phenylpropanolamine HCl; guaifenesin] 10•12.5•100 mg/5 mL

confectioner's sugar [see: sugar, confectioner's]

Confide test kit for home use *in vitro diagnostic aid for HIV in the blood*

congazone sodium [see: Congo red]

Congess JR capsules ℞ *decongestant; expectorant* [pseudoephedrine HCl; guaifenesin] 60•125 mg

Congess SR sustained-release capsules ℞ *decongestant; expectorant* [pseudoephedrine HCl; guaifenesin] 120•250 mg

Congestac caplets OTC *decongestant; expectorant* [pseudoephedrine HCl; guaifenesin] 60•400 mg

Congestant D tablets OTC *decongestant; antihistamine; analgesic* [phenylpropanolamine HCl; chlorpheniramine maleate; acetaminophen] 12.5•2•325 mg

Congestion Relief tablets (discontinued 2000) OTC *nasal decongestant* [pseudoephedrine HCl] 30, 60 mg

Congestion Relief, Children's liquid OTC *nasal decongestant* [pseudoephedrine HCl] 30 mg/5 mL

Congo red USP

conorfone INN *analgesic* [also: conorphone HCl]

conorfone HCl [see: conorphone HCl]

conorphone HCl USAN *analgesic* [also: conorfone]

CONPADRI; CONPADRI-I (cyclophosphamide, Oncovin, L-phenylalanine mustard, Adriamycin) *chemotherapy protocol*

Conray; Conray 30; Conray 43 injection ℞ *radiopaque contrast medium* [iothalamate meglumine (47% iodine)] 600 mg/mL (282 mg/mL); 300 mg/mL (141 mg/mL); 430 mg/mL (202 mg/mL)

Conray 325 injection (discontinued 1999) ℞ *radiopaque contrast medium* [iothalamate sodium (59.9% iodine)] 543 mg/mL (325 mg/mL)

Conray 400 injection ℞ *radiopaque contrast medium* [iothalamate sodium (59.9% iodine)] 668 mg/mL (400 mg/mL)

Consonar ℞ *investigational reversible/selective MAO inhibitor, type A* [brofaromine]

Constilac oral/rectal solution ℞ *hyperosmotic laxative* [lactulose] 10 g/15 mL

Constulose oral/rectal solution ℞ *hyperosmotic laxative* [lactulose] 10 g/15 mL

consumptive's weed *medicinal herb* [see: yerba santa]

Contac 12 Hour sustained-release capsules, sustained-release caplets OTC *decongestant; antihistamine* [phenylpropanolamine HCl; chlorpheniramine maleate] 75•8 mg; 75•12 mg

Contac Cough & Chest Cold liquid OTC *antitussive; decongestant; expectorant; analgesic* [dextromethorphan hydrobromide; pseudoephedrine HCl; guaifenesin; acetaminophen; alcohol 10%] 5•15•50•125 mg/5 mL

Contac Cough & Sore Throat liquid OTC *antitussive; analgesic* [dextromethorphan hydrobromide; acetaminophen; alcohol 10%] 5•125 mg/5 mL

Contac Day & Night Allergy/Sinus daytime caplets + nighttime caplets OTC *decongestant; analgesic; (antihistamine/sleep aid added nighttime)* [pseudoephedrine HCl; acetaminophen; (diphenhydramine HCl added nighttime)] 60•650 mg daytime; 60•650•50 mg nighttime

Contac Day & Night Cold & Flu daytime caplets + nighttime caplets OTC *decongestant; analgesic; (antitussive added daytime; antihistamine/sleep aid added nighttime)* [pseudoephedrine HCl; acetaminophen; (dextromethorphan hydrobromide added daytime; diphenhydramine HCl added nighttime)] 60•650•30 mg daytime; 60•650•50 mg nighttime

Contac Severe Cold & Flu Nighttime liquid OTC *antitussive; decongestant; antihistamine; analgesic* [dextromethorphan hydrobromide; pseudoephedrine HCl; chlorpheniramine maleate; acetaminophen; alcohol 18.5%] 5•10•0.67•167 mg/5 mL

Contac-C Cold Care Formula caplets (discontinued 1998) OTC *antitussive; decongestant; antihistamine; analgesic* [dextromethorphan hydrobromide; phenylpropanolamine HCl; chlorpheniramine maleate; acetaminophen] 15•12.5•2•500 mg

conteben [see: thioacetazone; thiacetazone]

ConTE-Pak-4 IV injection ℞ *intravenous nutritional therapy* [multiple trace elements (metals)] ≛

Contramid ℞ *investigational (Phase III) controlled-release solid oral form of a racemic albuterol bronchodilator for asthma and COPD* [levalbuterol]

Contrin capsules ℞ *hematinic* [ferrous fumarate; cyanocobalamin; ascorbic acid; intrinsic factor concentrate; folic acid] 110 mg•15 μg•75 mg•240 mg•0.5 mg

Control timed-release capsules OTC *diet aid* [phenylpropanolamine HCl] 75 mg

ControlPak (trademarked packaging form) *tamper-resistant unit-dose package*

Contuss liquid ℞ *decongestant; expectorant* [phenylpropanolamine HCl; phenylephrine HCl; guaifenesin; alcohol 5%] 20•5•100 mg/5 mL

conval lily *medicinal herb* [see: lily of the valley]

Convallaria majalis *medicinal herb* [see: lily of the valley]

conventional (typical) antipsychotics *a class of dopamine receptor antagonists with a higher affinity to the D_2 than D_1 receptors and little affinity to the nondopaminergic receptors; high incidence of extrapyramidal side effects (EPS)* [compare to: novel (atypical) antipsychotics]

Convolvulus sepium *medicinal herb* [see: hedge bindweed]

convulsion root; convulsion weed *medicinal herb* [see: fit root]

ConXn *investigational (Phase II/III) for scleroderma* [relaxin H2, recombinant human]

Conyza canadensis *medicinal herb* [see: horseweed]

cool.click (trademarked device) *needle-free subcutaneous injector*

Cooper regimen *chemotherapy protocol for breast cancer* [see: CMFVP]

COP [see: creatinolfosfate]

COP (cyclophosphamide, Oncovin, prednisone) *chemotherapy protocol for non-Hodgkin lymphoma*

COP 1 (copolymer 1) [see: glatiramer acetate]

COPA (Cytoxin, Oncovin, prednisone, Adriamycin) *chemotherapy protocol*

COPA-BLEO (cyclophosphamide, Oncovin, prednisone, Adriamycin, bleomycin) *chemotherapy protocol*

COPAC (CCNU, Oncovin, prednisone, Adriamycin, cyclophosphamide) *chemotherapy protocol*

Copaxone powder for subcu injection ℞ *immunomodulator for relapsing-remitting multiple sclerosis (orphan)* [glatiramer acetate] 20 mg

COPB (cyclophosphamide, Oncovin, prednisone, bleomycin) *chemotherapy protocol*

COP-BLAM (cyclophosphamide, Oncovin, prednisone, bleomycin, Adriamycin, Matulane) *chemotherapy protocol*

COP-BLEO (cyclophosphamide, Oncovin, prednisone, bleomycin) *chemotherapy protocol*

Cope tablets OTC *analgesic; antipyretic; anti-inflammatory; antacid* [aspirin; caffeine; magnesium hydroxide; aluminum hydroxide] 421•32•50•25 mg

COPE (cyclophosphamide, Oncovin, Platinol, etoposide) *chemotherapy protocol for small cell lung cancer and pediatric brain tumors*

Cophene No. 2 sustained-release capsules ℞ *decongestant; antihistamine* [pseudoephedrine HCl; chlorpheniramine maleate] 120•12 mg

Cophene XP liquid ℞ *narcotic antitussive; decongestant; expectorant* [hydrocodone bitartrate; pseudoephedrine HCl; guaifenesin; alcohol 12.5%] 5•60•200 mg/5 mL

Cophene-B subcu or IM injection (discontinued 1997) ℞ *antihistamine for anaphylaxis* [brompheniramine maleate] 10 mg/mL

Cophene-X capsules ℞ *antitussive; decongestant; expectorant* [carbetapentane citrate; phenylephrine HCl; phenylpropanolamine HCl; potassium guaiacolsulfonate] 20•10•10•45 mg
copolymer 1 (COP 1) [see: glatiramer acetate]
copovithane BAN
COPP (CCNU, Oncovin, procarbazine, prednisone) *chemotherapy protocol*
COPP (cyclophosphamide, Oncovin, procarbazine, prednisone) *chemotherapy protocol for Hodgkin or non-Hodgkin lymphoma*
copper *element (Cu)*
copper chloride dihydrate [see: cupric chloride]
copper gluconate (copper D-gluconate) USP *trace mineral supplement*
copper sulfate pentahydrate [see: cupric sulfate]
copper 10-undecenoate [see: copper undecylenate]
copper undecylenate USAN
copperhead snake antivenin [see: antivenin (Crotalidae) polyvalent]
Coptis trifolia *medicinal herb* [see: gold thread]
Co-Pyronil 2 Pulvules (capsules) OTC *decongestant; antihistamine* [pseudoephedrine HCl; chlorpheniramine maleate] 60•4 mg
Co-Q$_{10}$ (CAN) capsules OTC *dietary supplement* [coenzyme Q$_{10}$ (ubiquinone)] 10, 30, 60 mg
CoQ$_{10}$ [see: coenzyme Q10]
coral (*Goniopora* spp.; *Porite* spp.) *natural material used as a substrate for bone grafts and fractures and in reconstructive surgery*
coral root *(Corallorhiza odontorhiza)* *medicinal herb for diaphoresis, fever, insomnia, and sedation*
coral snake antivenin [see: antivenin (Micrurus fulvius)]
corbadrine INN *adrenergic; vasoconstrictor* [also: levonordefrin]
Cordarone tablets, IV infusion ℞ *antiarrhythmic for acute ventricular tachycardia and fibrillation (orphan)* [amiodarone HCl] 200 mg; 50 mg/mL
Cordase injection ℞ *investigational (Phase II) treatment for Dupuytren disease* [collagenase]
Cordox ℞ *investigational (Phase III) adjunct to coronary artery bypass graft (CABG) surgery; investigational (Phase III, orphan) cytoprotective agent for vaso-occlusive episodes of sickle cell disease; investigational asthma treatment* [fructose-1,6-diphosphate]
Cordran ointment, lotion, tape ℞ *topical corticosteroidal anti-inflammatory* [flurandrenolide] 0.025%, 0.05%; 0.05%; 4 μg/cm^2
Cordran SP cream ℞ *topical corticosteroidal anti-inflammatory* [flurandrenolide] 0.025%, 0.05%
Coreg Tiltab (film-coated tablets) ℞ *antihypertensive; α- and β-blocker for congestive heart failure* [carvedilol] 3.125, 6.25, 12.5, 25 mg
Corgard tablets ℞ *antianginal; antihypertensive; antiadrenergic (β-blocker)* [nadolol] 20, 40, 80, 120, 160 mg
Corgenic ℞ *investigational AC-6 gene therapy for congestive heart failure*
coriander *(Coriandrum sativum)* seed *medicinal herb used as antispasmodic, appetizer, carminative, and stomachic*
coriander oil NF
Coricidin tablets OTC *antihistamine; analgesic* [chlorpheniramine maleate; acetaminophen] 2•325 mg
Coricidin D; Coricidin Sinus Headache tablets OTC *decongestant; antihistamine; analgesic* [phenylpropanolamine HCl; chlorpheniramine maleate; acetaminophen] 12.5•2•325 mg; 12.5•2•500 mg
corkwood tree *(Duboisia myoporoides)* leaves *medicinal herb used as a central nervous system stimulant and in homeopathic therapy for eye disorders; not generally regarded as safe, as it contains scopolamine and related alkaloids, which may be fatal in high doses*
Corlopam IV infusion ℞ *rapid-acting vasodilator for in-hospital management*

of severe hypertension [fenoldopam mesylate] 10 mg/mL

Cormax ointment ℞ *topical corticosteroidal anti-inflammatory* [clobetasol propionate] 0.05%

cormed [see: nikethamide]

cormetasone INN *topical anti-inflammatory* [also: cormethasone acetate]

cormetasone acetate [see: cormethasone acetate]

cormethasone acetate USAN *topical anti-inflammatory* [also: cormetasone]

corn, turkey *medicinal herb* [see: turkey corn]

corn cockle *(Agrostemma githago)* seeds and root *medicinal herb for cancer, edema, exanthema, hemorrhoids, jaundice, and worms; also used as an emmenagogue and expectorant, and in homeopathic remedies for gastritis and paralysis; not generally regarded as safe, as it is extremely poisonous*

Corn Huskers lotion OTC *moisturizer; emollient*

corn oil NF *solvent; caloric replacement*

corn silk (stigmata maidis) *medicinal herb* [see: Indian corn]

cornflower *(Centaurea cyanus)* plant *medicinal herb for conjunctivitis, corneal ulcers and other eye disorders and for nervous disorders and poisonous bites and stings*

corpse plant *medicinal herb* [see: fit root]

corpus luteum extract [see: progesterone]

Corque cream ℞ *topical corticosteroidal anti-inflammatory; antifungal; antibacterial* [hydrocortisone; clioquinol] 1%•3%

Correctol enteric-coated tablets OTC *stimulant laxative* [bisacodyl] 5 mg

Correctol Extra Gentle soft gel capsules (discontinued 1999) OTC *laxative; stool softener* [docusate sodium] 100 mg

CortaGel OTC *topical corticosteroidal anti-inflammatory* [hydrocortisone] 1%

Cortaid cream, ointment OTC *topical corticosteroidal anti-inflammatory* [hydrocortisone acetate] 1%

Cortaid lotion (discontinued 1997) OTC *topical corticosteroidal anti-inflammatory* [hydrocortisone acetate] 1%

Cortaid pump spray OTC *topical corticosteroidal anti-inflammatory* [hydrocortisone] 1%

Cortaid Faststick roll-on stick OTC *topical corticosteroidal anti-inflammatory* [hydrocortisone; alcohol 55%] 1%

Cortaid Intensive Therapy cream OTC *topical corticosteroidal anti-inflammatory* [hydrocortisone] 1%

Cortaid with Aloe cream, ointment OTC *topical corticosteroidal anti-inflammatory* [hydrocortisone acetate] 0.5%

Cortate (CAN) cream, ointment ℞ *topical corticosteroidal anti-inflammatory* [hydrocortisone acetate] 1%

Cortate (CAN) cream, ointment, lotion OTC *topical corticosteroidal anti-inflammatory* [hydrocortisone acetate] 0.5%

Cortatrigen Modified ear drops, otic suspension ℞ *topical corticosteroidal anti-inflammatory; antibiotic* [hydrocortisone; neomycin sulfate; polymyxin B sulfate] 1%•5 mg•10 000 U per mL

Cort-Dome cream ℞ *topical corticosteroidal anti-inflammatory* [hydrocortisone] 0.5%, 1% ⚠ Cortone

Cort-Dome High Potency rectal suppositories ℞ *corticosteroidal anti-inflammatory* [hydrocortisone acetate] 25 mg

Cortef tablets, oral suspension ℞ *corticosteroid; anti-inflammatory* [hydrocortisone] 5, 10, 20 mg; 10 mg/5 mL

Cortef Feminine Itch cream OTC *topical corticosteroidal anti-inflammatory* [hydrocortisone acetate] 0.5%

Cortenema retention enema ℞ *corticosteroid for ulcerative colitis* [hydrocortisone] 100 mg/60 mL ⚠ quart enema

cortenil [see: desoxycorticosterone acetate]

cortexolone [see: cortodoxone]

Cortic ear drops ℞ *topical corticosteroidal anti-inflammatory; topical anesthetic; bacteriostatic* [hydrocortisone;

pramoxine HCl; chloroxylenol] 10•10•1 mg/mL

Corticaine cream OTC *topical corticosteroidal anti-inflammatory* [hydrocortisone acetate] 0.5%

corticorelin ovine triflutate USAN, INN *corticotropin-releasing hormone; diagnostic aid for Cushing syndrome and adrenocortical insufficiency (orphan)*

corticosteroids *a class of anti-inflammatory drugs*

corticotrophin INN, BAN *adrenocorticotropic hormone; corticosteroid; anti-inflammatory; diagnostic aid* [also: corticotropin]

corticotrophin-zinc hydroxide INN *adrenocorticotropic hormone; corticosteroid; anti-inflammatory; diagnostic aid* [also: corticotropin zinc hydroxide]

corticotropin USP *adrenocorticotropic hormone; corticosteroid; anti-inflammatory; diagnostic aid* [also: corticotrophin] 40 U/vial injection

corticotropin, repository USP *adrenocorticotropic hormone; corticosteroid; anti-inflammatory; diagnostic aid*

corticotropin tetracosapeptide [see: cosyntropin]

corticotropin zinc hydroxide USP *adrenocorticotropic hormone; corticosteroid; anti-inflammatory; diagnostic aid* [also: corticotrophin-zinc hydroxide]

corticotropin-releasing factor *investigational (Phase I/II, orphan) agent for peritumoral brain edema*

Cortifoam intrarectal foam aerosol ℞ *corticosteroid for ulcerative proctitis* [hydrocortisone acetate] 90 mg/dose

cortisol [see: hydrocortisone]

cortisol 21-acetate [see: hydrocortisone acetate]

cortisol 21-butyrate [see: hydrocortisone butyrate]

cortisol 21-cyclopentanepropionate [see: hydrocortisone cypionate]

cortisol cyclopentylpropionate [see: hydrocortisone cypionate]

cortisol 21-valerate [see: hydrocortisone valerate]

cortisone INN, BAN *corticosteroid; anti-inflammatory* [also: cortisone acetate] ⓢ Cortizone

cortisone acetate USP *corticosteroid; anti-inflammatory* [also: cortisone] 5, 10, 25 mg oral

Cortisporin cream ℞ *topical corticosteroidal anti-inflammatory; antibiotic* [hydrocortisone acetate; neomycin sulfate; polymyxin B sulfate] 0.5%•0.5%•10 000 U per g

Cortisporin eye drop suspension ℞ *topical ophthalmic corticosteroidal anti-inflammatory; antibiotic* [hydrocortisone; neomycin sulfate; polymyxin B sulfate] 1%•0.35%•10 000 U per mL

Cortisporin ointment ℞ *topical corticosteroidal anti-inflammatory; antibiotic* [hydrocortisone; neomycin sulfate; bacitracin zinc; polymyxin B sulfate] 1%•0.5%•400 U•5000 U per g

Cortisporin ophthalmic ointment ℞ *topical ophthalmic corticosteroidal anti-inflammatory; antibiotic* [hydrocortisone; neomycin sulfate; bacitracin zinc; polymyxin B sulfate] 1%•0.35%•400 U/g•10 000 U/g

Cortisporin Otic ear drops, otic suspension ℞ *topical corticosteroidal anti-inflammatory; antibiotic* [hydrocortisone; neomycin sulfate; polymyxin B sulfate] 1%•5 mg•10 000 U per mL

Cortisporin-TC ear drop suspension ℞ *topical corticosteroidal anti-inflammatory; antibiotic; surface-active synergist* [hydrocortisone acetate; neomycin sulfate; colistin sulfate; thonzonium bromide] 10•3.3•3•0.5 mg/mL

cortisuzol INN

cortivazol USAN, INN *corticosteroid; anti-inflammatory*

Cortizone for Kids cream OTC *topical corticosteroidal anti-inflammatory* [hydrocortisone] 0.5%

Cortizone-5 ointment, cream OTC *topical corticosteroidal anti-inflammatory* [hydrocortisone] 0.5%; 1% ⓢ cortisone

Cortizone-10 ointment OTC *topical corticosteroidal anti-inflammatory* [hydrocortisone] 1%

cortodoxone USAN, INN, BAN *anti-inflammatory*

Cortone Acetate intra-articular or intralesional injection ℞ *corticosteroid; anti-inflammatory* [cortisone acetate] 50 mg/mL ⑨ Cort-Dome

Cortone Acetate tablets (discontinued 1998) ℞ *corticosteroid; anti-inflammatory* [cortisone acetate] 25 mg ⑨ Cort-Dome

Cortrosyn powder for injection ℞ *multiple sclerosis; infantile spasms; diagnostic aid for adrenal function* [cosyntropin] 0.25 mg

Corvert IV infusion ℞ *antiarrhythmic for atrial fibrillation/flutter* [ibutilide fumarate] 0.1 mg/mL

corydalis *(Corydalis cava)* root *medicinal herb used as an antispasmodic, hypnotic, and antiparkinsonian*

Corydalis formosa *medicinal herb* [see: turkey corn]

Corynanthe johimbe *medicinal herb* [see: yohimbe]

Corzide 40/5; Corzide 80/5 tablets ℞ *antihypertensive; β-blocker; diuretic* [nadolol; bendroflumethiazide] 40•5 mg; 80•5 mg

Cosmederm-7 (CAN) (trademarked ingredient) *topical anti-irritant* [strontium chloride]

Cosmegen powder for IV injection ℞ *antibiotic antineoplastic for melanomas, sarcomas, testicular and trophoblastic tumors* [dactinomycin] 0.5 mg

cosmoline [see: petrolatum]

Cosopt eye drops ℞ *topical carbonic anhydrase inhibitor and beta-blocker for glaucoma* [dorzolamide HCl; timolol maleate] 2%•0.5%

cosyntropin USAN *adrenocorticotropic hormone; diagnostic aid for adrenal function* [also: tetracosactide; tetracosactrin]

Cotara ℞ *investigational (Phase II) for glioblastoma multiforme; investigational (Phase I/II) tumor necrosis therapy (TNT) for solid tumors; investigational (Phase I/II) for pancreatic, prostate, and liver cancers* [chimeric monoclonal antibody labeled with iodine-131]

cotarnine chloride NF

cotarnine HCl [see: cotarnine chloride]

Cotazym capsules ℞ *digestive enzymes; antacid* [lipase; protease; amylase; calcium carbonate] 8000 U•30 000 U•30 000 U•25 mg

Cotazym-S capsules containing enteric-coated spheres ℞ *digestive enzymes* [lipase; protease; amylase] 5000•20 000•20 000 U

cotinine INN *antidepressant* [also: cotinine fumarate]

cotinine fumarate USAN *antidepressant* [also: cotinine]

Cotridin (CAN) syrup ℞ *narcotic antitussive; decongestant; antihistamine* [codeine phosphate; pseudoephedrine HCl; triprolidine HCl] 2•6•0.4 mg/mL

Cotridin Expectorant (CAN) oral solution ℞ *narcotic antitussive; decongestant; antihistamine* [codeine phosphate; pseudoephedrine HCl; triprolidine HCl; guaifenesin] 2•6•0.4•20 mg/mL

Cotrim; Cotrim D.S. tablets ℞ *anti-infective; antibacterial* [trimethoprim; sulfamethoxazole] 80•400 mg; 160•800 mg ⑨ Cortin

Cotrim Pediatric oral suspension ℞ *anti-infective; antibacterial* [trimethoprim; sulfamethoxazole] 40•200 mg/5 mL

co-trimoxazole BAN [also: trimethoprim + sulfamethoxazole] ⑨ clotrimazole

cotriptyline INN

cotton, purified USP *surgical aid*

cottonseed oil NF *solvent*

cottonweed *medicinal herb* [see: milkweed]

Co-Tuss V liquid ℞ *narcotic antitussive; expectorant* [hydrocodone bitartrate; guaifenesin] 5•100 mg

couch grass *(Agropyron repens)* rhizomes, roots, and stems *medicinal herb for blood cleansing, cystitis, diabetes, jaundice, kidney problems, upper* *respiratory tract inflammation with mucous discharge, rheumatism, and urinary infections*

Cough syrup OTC *antitussive; decongestant; expectorant* [dextromethorphan hydrobromide; phenylephrine HCl; guaifenesin] 10•5•100 mg/5 mL

Cough Formula liquid OTC *antitussive; antihistamine* [dextromethorphan hydrobromide; chlorpheniramine maleate; alcohol 10%] 15•2 mg/5 mL

Cough Formula with Decongestant liquid OTC *antitussive; decongestant* [dextromethorphan hydrobromide; pseudoephedrine HCl; alcohol 10%] 10•20 mg/5 mL

coughroot *medicinal herb* [see: birthroot]

coughweed *medicinal herb* [see: life root]

coughwort *medicinal herb* [see: coltsfoot]

Cough-X lozenges OTC *antitussive; topical oral anesthetic* [dextromethorphan hydrobromide; benzocaine] 5•2 mg

Coumadin tablets, powder for IV injection ℞ *coumarin-derivative anticoagulant* [warfarin sodium] 1, 2, 2.5, 3, 4, 5, 6, 7.5, 10 mg; 2 mg ⧉ Kemadrin

coumafos INN [also: coumaphos]

coumamycin INN *antibacterial* [also: coumermycin]

coumaphos BAN [also: coumafos]

coumarin NF *anticoagulant; investigational (orphan) for renal cell carcinoma*

coumarins *a class of anticoagulants that interfere with vitamin K-dependent clotting factors*

coumazoline INN

coumermycin USAN *antibacterial* [also: coumamycin]

coumermycin sodium USAN *antibacterial*

coumetarol INN [also: cumetharol]

counterirritants *a class of agents that produce superficial irritation in one part of the body to relieve irritation in another part*

Covangesic tablets OTC *decongestant; antihistamine; analgesic* [phenylpropanolamine HCl; phenylephrine HCl; chlorpheniramine maleate; pyrilamine maleate; acetaminophen] 12.5•7.5•2•12.5•275 mg

covatin HCl [see: captodiame HCl]

Covera-HS extended-release film-coated tablets ℞ *antihypertensive; antianginal; antiarrhythmic; calcium channel blocker* [verapamil HCl] 180, 240 mg ⧉ Provera

Coviracil ℞ *investigational (NDA filed) nucleoside analogue for HIV and AIDS* [emtricitabine]

cow cabbage *medicinal herb* [see: masterwort; white pond lily]

cow parsnip *medicinal herb* [see: masterwort]

cowslip (*Caltha palustris*) plant *medicinal herb used as an analgesic, antispasmodic, diaphoretic, diuretic, expectorant, and rubefacient*

cowslip, Jerusalem *medicinal herb* [see: lungwort]

COX-2 (cyclooxygenase-2) inhibitors *a class of nonsteroidal anti-inflammatory drugs (NSAIDs) for osteoarthritis, rheumatoid arthritis, acute pain, and primary dysmenorrhea; these agents also have antipyretic activity*

Cozaar film-coated tablets ℞ *antihypertensive; angiotensin II receptor antagonist* [losartan potassium] 25, 50, 100 mg

CP (chlorambucil, prednisone) *chemotherapy protocol for chronic lymphocytic leukemia (CLL)*

CP (cyclophosphamide, Platinol) *chemotherapy protocol for ovarian cancer*

CP (cyclophosphamide, prednisone) *chemotherapy protocol*

CPB (cyclophosphamide, Platinol, BCNU) *chemotherapy protocol*

CPB-1011 *investigational (Phase III) treatment for idiopathic thrombocytopenic purpura (ITP)*

CPC (cyclophosphamide, Platinol, carboplatin) *chemotherapy protocol*

CPC-111 *investigational (Phase III) cardioprotective agent used in coronary artery bypass graft surgery; investigational (Phase II) for pain during sickle cell crisis*

CPI-1189 *investigational (Phase II) agent for cognitive impairment in Parkinson disease*

CPM (CCNU, procarbazine, methotrexate) *chemotherapy protocol*

CPOB (cyclophosphamide, prednisone, Oncovin, bleomycin) *chemotherapy protocol*

CPT-11 (camptothecin-11) [see: irinotecan]

CPX *investigational (Phase II) protein repair therapy for cystic fibrosis*

^{51}Cr [see: albumin, chromated Cr 51 serum]

^{51}Cr [see: chromic chloride Cr 51]

^{51}Cr [see: chromic phosphate Cr 51]

^{51}Cr [see: sodium chromate Cr 51]

cramp bark *(Viburnum opulus)* bark and berries *medicinal herb for asthma, convulsions, cramps, heart palpitations, hypertension, hysteria, leg cramps, nervousness, spasm, and urinary disorders*

crampweed *medicinal herb* [see: cinquefoil]

cranberry *(Vaccinium edule; V. erythrocarpum; V. macrocarpon; V. oxycoccos; V. vitis)* fruit *medicinal herb for bladder, kidney, and urinary tract infections; also used to decrease the rate of urine degradation and odor formation in incontinent patients*

cranesbill; spotted cranesbill *medicinal herb* [see: alum root]

Crataegus laevigata; C. monogyna; C. oxyacantha *medicinal herb* [see: hawthorn]

crawley; crawley root *medicinal herb* [see: coral root]

CRDS (curdlan sulfate) [q.v.]

Creamy Tar shampoo OTC *antiseborrheic; antipsoriatic; antipruritic; antibacterial* [coal tar] 7.32%

creatinolfosfate INN

Creon capsules containing enteric-coated microspheres ℞ *digestive enzymes* [pancreatin (lipase; protease; amylase)] 300 mg (8000•13 000•30 000 U)

Creon 5 (CAN) capsules containing enteric-coated microspheres OTC *digestive enzymes* [pancreatin (lipase; protease; amylase)] 75 mg (5000•18 750•16 600 U)

Creon 10 capsules containing enteric-coated microspheres ℞ in the U.S.; OTC in Canada *digestive enzymes* [pancreatin (lipase; amylase; protease)] 150 mg (10 000•33 200•37 500 U)

Creon 20 capsules containing enteric-coated microspheres ℞ in the U.S.; OTC in Canada *digestive enzymes* [pancreatin (lipase; amylase; protease)] 300 mg (20 000•66 400•75 000 U)

Creon 25 (CAN) capsules containing enteric-coated microspheres OTC *digestive enzymes* [pancreatin (lipase; amylase; protease)] 300 mg (25 000•74 700•62 500 U)

creosote carbonate USP

Creo-Terpin liquid OTC *antitussive* [dextromethorphan hydrobromide; alcohol 25%] 10 mg/15 mL

cresol NF *disinfectant*

cresotamide INN

cresoxydiol [see: mephenesin]

crestomycin sulfate [see: paromomycin sulfate]

Crestor ℞ *investigational (NDA filed) HMG-CoA reductase inhibitor for hyperlipidemia* [rosuvastatin calcium]

Cresylate ear drops ℞ *antibacterial; antifungal* [m-cresyl acetate; chlorobutanol; alcohol] 25%•25%•1%

cresylic acid [see: cresol]

crilanomer INN

crilvastatin USAN, INN *antihyperlipidemic*

Crinone vaginal gel ℞ *progestin replacement or supplementation for assisted reproductive technology (ART) treatment* [progesterone] 4%, 8%

crisnatol INN *antineoplastic* [also: crisnatol mesylate]

crisnatol mesylate USAN *antineoplastic* [also: crisnatol]

Criticare HN ready-to-use liquid OTC *enteral nutritional therapy* [lactose-free formula]

Crixivan capsules ℞ *antiviral; HIV protease inhibitor* [indinavir sulfate] 200, 333, 400 mg
crobefate INN *combining name for radicals or groups*
croconazole INN
crocus, autumn *medicinal herb* [see: autumn crocus]
Crocus sativus *medicinal herb* [see: saffron]
CroFab injection ℞ *treatment of pit viper (rattlesnake, copperhead, and cottonmouth moccasin) snake bites (orphan)* [antivenin (Crotalidae) polyvalent immune Fab (ovine)]
crofelemer USAN *investigational (Phase III) treatment for AIDS-related diarrhea; investigational (Phase II) antiviral for AIDS-related genital herpes*
crofilcon A USAN *hydrophilic contact lens material*
Crolom eye drops ℞ *mast cell stabilizer; ocular antiallergic and antiviral for vernal keratoconjunctivitis (orphan)* [cromolyn sodium] 4%
cromacate INN *combining name for radicals or groups*
cromakalim INN, BAN
Cro-Man-Zin tablets OTC *mineral supplement* [chromium; manganese; zinc] 0.2•5•25 mg
cromesilate INN *combining name for radicals or groups*
cromitrile INN *antiasthmatic* [also: cromitrile sodium]
cromitrile sodium USAN *antiasthmatic* [also: cromitrile]
cromoglicic acid INN *prophylactic antiasthmatic* [also: cromolyn sodium; cromoglycic acid]
cromoglycic acid BAN *prophylactic antiasthmatic* [also: cromolyn sodium; cromoglicic acid]
cromolyn sodium USAN, USP *anti-inflammatory; mast cell stabilizer for prophylactic treatment of allergy, asthma, and bronchospasm; treatment for mastocytosis and vernal keratoconjunctivitis (orphan)* [also: cromoglicic acid; cromoglycic acid] 20 mg/2 mL inhalation
cronetal [see: disulfiram]
cronidipine INN
cropropamide INN, BAN
croscarmellose INN *tablet disintegrant* [also: croscarmellose sodium]
croscarmellose sodium USAN, NF *tablet disintegrant* [also: croscarmellose]
crosfumaril [see: hemoglobin crosfumaril]
crospovidone NF *tablet excipient*
cross-linked carboxymethylcellulose sodium [now: croscarmellose sodium]
cross-linked carmellose sodium [see: croscarmellose sodium]
crotaline antivenin [see: antivenin (Crotalidae) polyvalent]
crotamiton USP, INN, BAN *scabicide*
crotetamide INN [also: crotethamide]
crotethamide BAN [also: crotetamide]
crotoniazide INN
crotonylidenisoniazid [see: crotoniazide]
crotoxyfos BAN
crowfoot *medicinal herb* [see: alum root; buttercup]
crowfoot buttercup; acrid crowfoot; cursed crowfoot; marsh crowfoot; meadow crowfoot; tall crowfoot; water crowfoot *medicinal herb* [see: buttercup]
crown, priest's *medicinal herb* [see: dandelion]
crude tuberculin [see: tuberculin, old]
Cruex cream OTC *topical antifungal* [clotrimazole] 1%
Cruex cream, aerosol powder OTC *topical antifungal* [undecylenic acid; zinc undecylenate] 20% total; 19% total
Cruex powder OTC *topical antifungal* [calcium undecylenate] 10%
crufomate USAN, INN, BAN *veterinary anthelmintic*
cryofluorane INN *aerosol propellant* [also: dichlorotetrafluoroethane]
Cryptaz ℞ *investigational (NDA filed, orphan) anti-infective for AIDS-related cryptosporidial diarrhea (NDA withdrawn 1998)* [nitazoxanide]

cryptenamine acetates

Crypto-LA slide test for professional use *in vitro diagnostic aid for Cryptococcus neoformans antigens*

***Cryptosporidium parvum* bovine colostrum IgG concentrate** *investigational (orphan) for Cryptosporidium-induced diarrhea in immunocompromised patients*

crystal violet [see: gentian violet]

crystallized trypsin [see: trypsin, crystallized]

Crystamine IM or subcu injection ℞ *antianemic; vitamin B_{12} supplement* [cyanocobalamin] 1000 μg/mL

Crysti 1000 IM or subcu injection ℞ *antianemic; vitamin B_{12} supplement* [cyanocobalamin] 1000 μg/mL

Crysticillin 300 A.S.; Crysticillin 600 A.S. IM injection (discontinued 1998) ℞ *natural penicillin antibiotic* [penicillin G procaine] 300 000 U/mL; 600 000 U/1.2 mL dose

Crystodigin tablets (discontinued 2000) ℞ *cardiac glycoside to increase cardiac output; antiarrhythmic* [digitoxin] 0.05, 0.1 mg

crystografin [see: meglumine diatriazole]

^{131}Cs [see: cesium chloride Cs 131]

CS-92 *investigational (Phase I/II) nucleoside reverse transcriptase inhibitor (NRTI) for HIV infection*

C-Solve OTC *lotion base*

CSP (cellulose sodium phosphate) [q.v.]

CT (cisplatin, Taxol) *chemotherapy protocol for ovarian cancer*

CT (cytarabine, thioguanine) *chemotherapy protocol*

CT-2584 *investigational (Phase II) antineoplastic for soft tissue sarcomas*

CT-3 *investigational anti-inflammatory*

CTAB (cetyltrimethyl ammonium bromide)

CTCb (cyclophosphamide, thiotepa, carboplatin) *chemotherapy protocol*

CTH (ceramide trihexosidase) [q.v.]

CTLA4-Ig *investigational humanized monoclonal antibody for psoriasis, organ transplant rejection, autoimmune disorders, and graft-versus-host disease*

CTP-37 *investigational theraccine for metastatic colorectal cancer*

C/T/S topical solution ℞ *topical antibiotic for acne* [clindamycin phosphate] 10 mg/mL

CTX (cyclophosphamide) [q.v.]

Ctx-Plat (cyclophosphamide, Platinol) *chemotherapy protocol*

^{64}Cu [see: cupric acetate Cu 64]

cubeb *(Piper cubeba)* unripe berries *medicinal herb used as an antiseptic, antisyphilitic, carminative, diuretic, expectorant, stimulant, and stomachic*

cucurbita *(Cucurbita maxima; C. moschata; C. pepa)* seeds *medicinal herb for prophylaxis, immobilizing, and aiding in the expulsion of intestinal worms and parasites; also used in prostate gland disorders*

Culturette 10 Minute Group A Strep ID slide test for professional use *in vitro diagnostic test for Group A streptococcal antigens in throat swabs* [latex agglutination test]

Culver physic *medicinal herb* [see: Culver root]

Culver root *(Varonicastrum virginicum)* *medicinal herb for blood cleansing, diarrhea, and liver and stomach disorders*

cumetharol BAN [also: coumetarol]

cumin *(Cuminum cyminum; C. odorum)* seeds and oil *medicinal herb for gastric cancer; also used as an antioxidant*

cupric acetate Cu 64 USAN *radioactive agent*

cupric chloride USP *dietary copper supplement*

cupric sulfate USP *antidote to phosphorus; dietary copper supplement* 0.4, 2 mg/mL injection

Cuprimine capsules ℞ *metal chelating agent for rheumatoid arthritis, Wilson disease, and cystinuria* [penicillamine] 125, 250 mg

cuprimyxin USAN, INN *veterinary antibacterial; antifungal*
cuproxoline INN, BAN
Curaçao aloe *medicinal herb* [see: aloe]
curare [see: tubocurarine chloride]
Curcuma domestica; C. longa *medicinal herb* [see: turmeric]
curdlan sulfate (CRDS) *investigational (Phase II) antiviral for HIV*
cure-all *medicinal herb* [see: lemon balm]
curium *element (Cm)*
curled dock; curly dock *medicinal herb* [see: yellow dock]
curled mint *medicinal herb* [see: peppermint]
curls, blue *medicinal herb* [see: woundwort]
Curosurf intratracheal suspension ℞ *porcine lung extract for respiratory distress syndrome (RDS) in premature infants (orphan)* [poractant alfa] 1.5, 3 mL (120, 240 mg phospholipids)
curral [see: diallybarbituric acid]
currant *(Ribes nigrum; R. rubrum)* leaves and fruit *medicinal herb used as a diaphoretic and diuretic*
Curretab tablets ℞ *progestin for secondary amenorrhea, abnormal uterine bleeding, and endometrial hyperplasia* [medroxyprogesterone acetate] 10 mg
custard apple *medicinal herb* [see: pawpaw]
Cūtar Bath Oil Emulsion OTC *antipsoriatic; antiseborrheic; antipruritic; emollient* [coal tar] 7.5%
Cūtemol cream OTC *moisturizer; emollient* [allantoin]
Cuticura Medicated Soap bar OTC *therapeutic skin cleanser* [triclocarban] 1%
Cutivate cream, ointment ℞ *topical corticosteroidal anti-inflammatory* [fluticasone propionate] 0.05%; 0.005%
CV (cisplatin, VePesid) *chemotherapy protocol*
CVA (cyclophosphamide, vincristine, Adriamycin) *chemotherapy protocol*
CVA-BMP; CVA + BMP (cyclophosphamide, vincristine, Adriamycin, BCNU, methotrexate, procarbazine) *chemotherapy protocol*
CVAD; C-VAD (cyclophosphamide, vincristine, Adriamycin, dexamethasone) *chemotherapy protocol*
CVB (CCNU, vinblastine, bleomycin) *chemotherapy protocol*
CVBD (CCNU, bleomycin, vinblastine, dexamethasone) *chemotherapy protocol*
CVD (cisplatin, vinblastine, dacarbazine) *chemotherapy protocol for malignant melanoma*
CVD+IL-2I (cisplatin, vinblastine, dacarbazine, interleukin-2, interferon alfa) *chemotherapy protocol for malignant melanoma*
CVEB (cisplatin, vinblastine, etoposide, bleomycin) *chemotherapy protocol*
CVI (carboplatin, VePesid, ifosfamide [with mesna rescue]) *chemotherapy protocol for non–small cell lung cancer (NSCLC)* [also: VIC]
CVM (cyclophosphamide, vincristine, methotrexate) *chemotherapy protocol*
CVP (cyclophosphamide, vincristine, prednisone) *chemotherapy protocol for non-Hodgkin lymphoma and chronic lymphocytic leukemia (CLL)*
CVPP (CCNU, vinblastine, procarbazine, prednisone) *chemotherapy protocol for Hodgkin lymphoma*
CVPP (cyclophosphamide, Velban, procarbazine, prednisone) *chemotherapy protocol*
CVPP-CCNU (cyclophosphamide, vinblastine, procarbazine, prednisone, CCNU) *chemotherapy protocol*
CVT-124 *investigational (Phase II) for treatment of edema associated with congestive heart failure*
CVT-313 *investigational agent for preventing restenosis*
CVT-510 *investigational (Phase I) selective adenosine A_1 receptor agonist for atrial arrhythmias; investigational (Phase III) for paroxysmal supraventricular tachycardia*

CY-1503 *investigational (Phase III, orphan) adjunct to surgery for congenital heart defects in newborns; investigational (orphan) for postischemic pulmonary reperfusion edema (all clinical trials discontinued 1999)*

CY-1899 *investigational (orphan) for chronic active hepatitis B*

CY-2301 *investigational (Phase I) vaccine for HIV*

cyacetacide INN [also: cyacetazide]

cyacetazide BAN [also: cyacetacide]

CyADIC (cyclophosphamide, Adriamycin, DIC) *chemotherapy protocol*

cyamemazine INN

cyamepromazine [see: cyamemazine]

cyanamide JAN [also: calcium carbimide]

cyani *medicinal herb* [see: cornflower]

Cyanide Antidote Package ℞ *emergency treatment of cyanide poisoning* [sodium nitrite; sodium thiosulfate; amyl nitrite inhalant] 300 mg•12.5 g•0.3 mL

cyanoacetohydrazide [see: cyacetazide]

cyanocobalamin (vitamin B_{12}) USP, INN, BAN, JAN *water-soluble vitamin; hematopoietic* 100, 250, 500, 1000 µg oral; 100, 1000 µg/mL injection

cyanocobalamin (^{57}Co) INN *pernicious anemia test; radioactive agent* [also: cyanocobalamin Co 57]

cyanocobalamin (^{58}Co) INN

cyanocobalamin (^{60}Co) INN *pernicious anemia test; radioactive agent* [also: cyanocobalamin Co 60]

cyanocobalamin Co 57 USAN, USP *pernicious anemia test; radioactive agent* [also: cyanocobalamin (^{57}Co)]

cyanocobalamin Co 60 USAN, USP *pernicious anemia test; radioactive agent* [also: cyanocobalamin (^{60}Co)]

Cyanoject IM or subcu injection ℞ *antianemic; vitamin B_{12} supplement* [cyanocobalamin] 1000 µg/mL

cyclacillin USAN, USP *antibacterial* [also: ciclacillin]

cyclamate calcium NF

cyclamic acid USAN, BAN *non-nutritive sweetener (banned in the U.S.)*

cyclamide [see: glycyclamide]

Cyclan capsules (discontinued 1997) ℞ *peripheral vasodilator; vascular smooth muscle relaxant* [cyclandelate] 200, 400 mg

cyclandelate INN, BAN, JAN *peripheral vasodilator; vascular smooth muscle relaxant*

cyclarbamate INN, BAN

cyclazocine USAN, INN *analgesic*

cyclazodone INN

Cyclessa tablets (in packs of 28) ℞ *triphasic oral contraceptive* [desogestrel; ethinyl estradiol]
Phase 1 (7 days): 100•25 µg;
Phase 2 (7 days): 125•25 µg;
Phase 3 (7 days): 150•25 µg

cyclexanone INN

cyclic adenosine monophosphate (cAMP) [see: adenosine phosphate]

cyclic propylene carbonate [see: propylene carbonate]

cyclindole USAN *antidepressant* [also: ciclindole]

Cyclinex-1 powder OTC *formula for infants with urea cycle disorders or gyrate atrophy*

Cyclinex-2 powder OTC *enteral nutritional therapy for urea cycle disorders or gyrate atrophy* [multiple essential amino acids]

cycliramine INN *antihistamine* [also: cycliramine maleate]

cycliramine maleate USAN *antihistamine* [also: cycliramine]

cyclizine USP, INN, BAN *antihistamine; antiemetic; anticholinergic; motion sickness relief*

cyclizine HCl USP, BAN *antiemetic*

cyclizine lactate USP, BAN *antinauseant*

cyclobarbital NF, INN [also: cyclobarbitone]

cyclobarbital calcium NF

cyclobarbitone BAN [also: cyclobarbital]

cyclobendazole USAN *anthelmintic* [also: ciclobendazole]

cyclobenzaprine INN *skeletal muscle relaxant* [also: cyclobenzaprine HCl]

cyclobenzaprine HCl USAN, USP *skeletal muscle relaxant* [also: cyclobenzaprine] 10 mg oral
cyclobutoic acid INN
cyclobutyrol INN
cyclocarbothiamine [see: cycotiamine]
Cyclocort ointment, cream, lotion ℞ *topical corticosteroidal anti-inflammatory* [amcinonide] 0.1%
cyclocoumarol BAN
cyclocumarol [see: cyclocoumarol]
α-cyclodextrin [see: alfadex]
Cyclofed Pediatric syrup ℞ *pediatric narcotic antitussive, decongestant, and expectorant* [codeine phosphate; pseudoephedrine HCl; guaifenesin; alcohol 6%] 10•30•100 mg/5 mL
cyclofenil INN, BAN
cyclofilcon A USAN *hydrophilic contact lens material*
cycloguanil embonate INN, BAN *antimalarial* [also: cycloguanil pamoate]
cycloguanil pamoate USAN *antimalarial* [also: cycloguanil embonate]
Cyclogyl Drop-Tainers (eye drops) ℞ *cycloplegic; mydriatic* [cyclopentolate HCl] 0.5%, 1%, 2%
cyclohexanehexol [see: inositol]
cyclohexanesulfamate dihydrate [see: sodium cyclamate]
cyclohexanesulfamic acid *(banned in the U.S.)* [see: cyclamic acid]
cycloheximide USAN *antipsoriatic* [also: cicloheximide]
***p*-cyclohexylhydratropic acid** [see: hexaprofen]
N-cyclohexyllinoleamide [see: clinolamide]
4-cyclohexyloxybenzoate [see: cyclomethycaine]
1-cyclohexylpropyl carbamate [see: procymate]
N-cyclohexylsulfamic acid *(banned in the U.S.)* [see: cyclamic acid]
cyclomenol INN
cyclomethicone NF *wetting agent*
cyclomethycaine INN, BAN *local anesthetic* [also: cyclomethycaine sulfate]
cyclomethycaine sulfate USP *local anesthetic* [also: cyclomethycaine]
Cyclomydril Drop-Tainers (eye drops) ℞ *cycloplegic; mydriatic* [cyclopentolate HCl; phenylephrine HCl] 0.2%•1%
cyclonium iodide [see: oxapium iodide]
cyclooxygenase-2 (COX-2) inhibitors *a class of investigational anti-inflammatory drugs*
cyclopentamine INN, BAN [also: cyclopentamine HCl]
cyclopentamine HCl USP [also: cyclopentamine]
cyclopentaphene [see: cyclarbamate]
cyclopenthiazide USAN, INN, BAN *antihypertensive*
cyclopentolate INN, BAN *ophthalmic anticholinergic* [also: cyclopentolate HCl]
cyclopentolate HCl USP *ophthalmic anticholinergic; mydriatic; cycloplegic* [also: cyclopentolate] 1% eye drops
8-cyclopentyl 1,3-dipropylxanthine *investigational (orphan) for cystic fibrosis*
cyclophenazine HCl USAN *antipsychotic* [also: ciclofenazine]
cyclophosphamide USP, INN, BAN, JAN *nitrogen mustard-type alkylating antineoplastic; immunosuppressive*
cycloplegics *a class of drugs that paralyze the ciliary muscles of the eye*
cyclopolydimethylsiloxane [see: cyclomethicone]
cyclopregnol INN
cycloprolol BAN *antiadrenergic (β-receptor)* [also: cicloprolol HCl; cicloprolol]
cyclopropane USP, INN *inhalation general anesthetic*
Cyclo-Prostin ℞ *investigational (orphan) vasodilator for primary pulmonary hypertension* [epoprostenol]
cyclopyrronium bromide INN
cycloserine (L-cycloserine) USP, INN, BAN, JAN *bacteriostatic; tuberculostatic; treatment for acute urinary tract infections; investigational (orphan) for Gaucher disease*
Cyclospasmol capsules (discontinued 1997) ℞ *peripheral vasodilator; vascu-*

lar smooth muscle relaxant [cyclandelate] 200, 400 mg

Cyclospasmol ⓒⓐⓝ film-coated tablets (discontinued 1998) ℞ *peripheral vasodilator; vascular smooth muscle relaxant* [cyclandelate] 200 mg

cyclosporin BAN *immunosuppressant* [also: cyclosporine; ciclosporin]

cyclosporin A [now: cyclosporine]

cyclosporine USAN, USP *immunosuppressant for transplants, rheumatoid arthritis, and psoriasis; investigational (NDA filed, orphan) for Sjögren keratoconjunctivitis sicca; investigational (orphan) for corneal melting syndrome* [also: ciclosporin; cyclosporin] 25, 100 mg oral

CycloTech (trademarked delivery device) *provides premeasured doses of oral liquids and records dosing times*

cyclothiazide USAN, USP, INN, BAN *diuretic; antihypertensive*

cyclovalone INN

cycobemin [see: cyanocobalamin]

Cycofed Pediatric syrup ℞ *narcotic antitussive; decongestant; expectorant* [codeine phosphate; pseudoephedrine HCl; guaifenesin; alcohol 6%] 10•30•100 mg

cycotiamine INN

cycrimine INN, BAN [also: cycrimine HCl]

cycrimine HCl USP [also: cycrimine]

Cycrin tablets ℞ *progestin for secondary amenorrhea, abnormal uterine bleeding, and endometrial hyperplasia* [medroxyprogesterone acetate] 2.5, 5, 10 mg

cyfluthrin BAN

cyhalothrin BAN

cyheptamide USAN, INN *anticonvulsant*

cyheptropine INN

CyHOP (cyclophosphamide, Halotestin, Oncovin, prednisone) *chemotherapy protocol*

Cyklokapron tablets, IV injection ℞ *systemic hemostatic; orphan status withdrawn 1996* [tranexamic acid] 500 mg; 100 mg/mL

Cylert tablets, chewable tablets ℞ *CNS stimulant for attention-deficit hyperactivity disorder (ADHD)* [pemoline] 18.75, 37.5, 75 mg; 37.5 mg

Cylex; Cylex Sugar-Free throat lozenges OTC *topical oral anesthetic; antiseptic* [benzocaine; cetylpyridinium chloride] 15•5 mg

Cylexin ℞ *investigational (Phase III, orphan) adjunct to surgery for congenital heart defects in newborns; investigational (orphan) for postischemic pulmonary reperfusion edema (all clinical trials discontinued 1999)* [CY-1503 (code name—generic name not yet assigned)]

Cymbopogon citratus *medicinal herb* [see: lemongrass]

Cymbopogon nardus; C. winterianus *medicinal herb* [see: citronella]

cymemoxine [see: cimemoxin]

Cymeval (name changed to Valcyte upon marketing release in 2001)

Cymevene (foreign name for U.S. product Cytovene)

Cynara scolymus *medicinal herb* [see: artichoke]

cynarine INN

Cyomin IM or subcu injection ℞ *antianemic; vitamin B_{12} supplement* [cyanocobalamin] 1000 μg/mL

CyPat ℞ *investigational (Phase III) antineoplastic for prostate cancer*

cypenamine INN, BAN *antidepressant* [also: cypenamine HCl]

cypenamine HCl USAN *antidepressant* [also: cypenamine]

cypionate USAN, BAN *combining name for radicals or groups* [also: cipionate]

Cyplex *investigational (Phase II) platelet alternative* [infusible platelet membranes]

cypothrin USAN *veterinary insecticide*

cyprazepam USAN, INN *sedative*

cyprenorphine INN, BAN

cyprenorphine HCl [see: cyprenorphine]

Cypripedium pubescens *medicinal herb* [see: lady's slipper]

cyprodemanol [see: cyprodenate]

cyprodenate INN
cyproheptadine INN, BAN *piperidine antihistamine; antipruritic* [also: cyproheptadine HCl]
cyproheptadine HCl USP, JAN *piperidine antihistamine; antipruritic* [also: cyproheptadine] 4 mg oral; 2 mg/5 mL oral
cyprolidol INN *antidepressant* [also: cyprolidol HCl]
cyprolidol HCl USAN *antidepressant* [also: cyprolidol]
cyproquinate USAN *coccidiostat for poultry* [also: ciproquinate]
cyproterone INN, BAN *antiandrogen* [also: cyproterone acetate]
cyproterone acetate USAN *antiandrogen; orphan status withdrawn 1996* [also: cyproterone]
cyproximide USAN *antipsychotic; antidepressant* [also: ciproximide]
cyren A [see: diethylstilbestrol]
cyren B [see: diethylstilbestrol dipropionate]
cyromazine INN, BAN
Cystadane powder for oral solution ℞ *electrolyte replenisher for homocystinuria (orphan)* [betaine HCl] 1 g
Cystagon capsules ℞ *antiurolithic for nephropathic cystinosis (orphan)* [cysteamine bitartrate] 50, 150 mg
cystamin [see: methenamine]
cysteamine USAN, BAN *antiurolithic for nephropathic cystinosis (orphan)* [also: mercaptamine]
cysteamine bitartrate *antiurolithic for nephropathic cystinosis (orphan)*
cysteamine HCl USAN *antiurolithic; investigational (orphan) for corneal cystine crystal accumulation in cystinosis patients*
cysteine (L-cysteine) INN *nonessential amino acid; symbols: Cys, C; investigational (orphan) for erythropoietic protoporphyria photosensitivity* [also: cysteine HCl]
cysteine HCl (L-cysteine HCl) USP *nonessential amino acid* [also: cysteine] 50 mg/mL injection
L-cysteine HCl monohydrate [see: cysteine HCl]
Cystex tablets ℞ *urinary antibiotic; analgesic; acidifier* [methenamine; sodium salicylate; benzoic acid] 162•162.5•32 mg
cystic fibrosis gene therapy *investigational (orphan) for cystic fibrosis*
cystic fibrosis transmembrane conductance regulator (CFTR) *investigational (orphan) for cystic fibrosis*
cystic fibrosis transmembrane conductance regulator, recombinant adenovirus (AdGV-CFTR) *investigational (orphan) for cystic fibrosis*
cystine (L-cystine) USAN *amino acid*
Cysto-Conray; Cysto-Conray II intracavitary instillation ℞ *radiopaque contrast medium for urological imaging* [iothalamate meglumine (47% iodine)] 430 mg/mL (202 mg/mL); 172 mg/mL (81 mg/mL)
cystogen [see: methenamine]
Cystografin; Cystografin Dilute intracavitary instillation ℞ *radiopaque contrast medium for urological imaging* [diatrizoate meglumine (46.67% iodine)] 300 mg/mL (141 mg/mL); 180 mg/mL (85 mg/mL)
Cystospaz tablets ℞ *GI/GU antispasmodic; antiparkinsonian; anticholinergic "drying agent" for allergic rhinitis and hyperhidrosis* [hyoscyamine sulfate] 0.15 mg
Cystospaz-M timed-release capsules ℞ *GI/GU antispasmodic; antiparkinsonian; anticholinergic "drying agent" for allergic rhinitis and hyperhidrosis* [hyoscyamine sulfate] 0.375 mg
CYT-103-Y-90 *investigational for ovarian cancer; orphan status withdrawn 1998*
CYTABOM (cytarabine, bleomycin, Oncovin, mechlorethamine) *chemotherapy protocol*
Cytadren tablets ℞ *adrenal steroid inhibitor; antisteroidal antineoplastic for corticotropin-producing tumors* [aminoglutethimide] 250 mg
cytarabine USAN, USP, INN, BAN *antimetabolite antineoplastic for various leukemias* 100, 500, 1000, 2000 mg injection ⑨ vidarabine

cytarabine, liposomal *antimetabolite antineoplastic for lymphomatous neoplastic meningitis (orphan)*

cytarabine HCl USAN *antiviral*

Cytisus scoparius *medicinal herb* [see: broom]

CytoGam IV infusion ℞ *adjunct to organ transplants from CMV seropositive donor to CMV seronegative recipient (orphan)* [cytomegalovirus immune globulin, solvent/detergent treated] 50 mg/mL

CytoImplant ℞ *investigational (orphan) for pancreatic cancer* [blood mononuclear cells, allogenic peripheral]

Cytolex cream ℞ *investigational (NDA filed) broad-spectrum antibiotic for impetigo and diabetic foot ulcers* [pexiganan acetate] 1%

cytolin *investigational (Phase I/II) monoclonal antibody for AIDS*

cytomegalovirus immune globulin (CMV-IG), human *prevention of primary cytomegalovirus in organ transplants in immunocompromised patients (orphan)*

cytomegalovirus immune globulin intravenous (CMV-IGIV) & ganciclovir sodium *investigational (orphan) for cytomegalovirus pneumonia in bone marrow transplant patients*

Cytomel tablets ℞ *synthetic thyroid T_3 hormone* [liothyronine sodium] 5, 25, 50 µg

cytoprotective agents *a class of drugs that provide prophylaxis against the side effects of antineoplastic agents*

Cytosar-U powder for subcu, intrathecal or IV injection ℞ *antimetabolite antineoplastic for various leukemias* [cytarabine] 100, 500, 1000, 2000 mg/vial

cytosine arabinoside (ara-C) [see: cytarabine]

cytosine arabinoside HCl [now: cytarabine HCl]

Cytosol liquid ℞ *sterile irrigant* [physiological irrigating solution]

Cyto ℞ *investigational (Phase I) antibody for use in renal transplantation*

Cytotec tablets ℞ *prevents NSAID-induced gastric ulcers* [misoprostol] 100, 200 µg

cytotoxic lymphocyte maturation factor [see: edodekin alfa]

Cytovene capsules ℞ *antiviral for cytomegalovirus (CMV); investigational (Phase I/II) for AIDS prophylaxis* [ganciclovir] 250, 500 mg

Cytovene powder for IV infusion ℞ *antiviral for cytomegalovirus (CMV); investigational (Phase I/II) for AIDS prophylaxis* [ganciclovir sodium] 500 mg/vial

Cytoxan tablets, powder for IV injection ℞ *nitrogen mustard-type alkylating antineoplastic for multiple leukemias, lymphomas, blastomas, sarcomas and organ cancers* [cyclophosphamide] 25, 50 mg; 100 mg

Cytra-2 solution ℞ *urinary alkalizing agent* [sodium citrate; citric acid] 500•334 mg/5 mL

Cytra-3 syrup ℞ *urinary alkalinizing agent* [potassium citrate; sodium citrate; citric acid] 550•500•334 mg/5 mL

Cytra-K oral solution ℞ *urinary alkalizing agent* [potassium citrate; citric acid] 1100•334 mg/5 mL

Cytra-LC solution ℞ *urinary alkalizing agent* [potassium citrate; sodium citrate; citric acid] 550•500•334 mg/5 mL

CY-VA-DACT (Cytoxin, vincristine, Adriamycin, dactinomycin) *chemotherapy protocol*

CYVADIC; CY-VA-DIC; CyVADIC (cyclophosphamide, vincristine, Adriamycin, DIC) *chemotherapy protocol for bone and soft tissue sarcomas*

CYVMAD (cyclophosphamide, vincristine, methotrexate, Adriamycin, DTIC) *chemotherapy protocol*

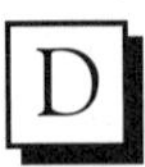

D (vitamin D) [q.v.]

D-2.5-W; D-5-W; D-10-W; D-20-W; D-25-W; D-30-W; D-40-W; D-50-W; D-60-W; D-70-W ℞ *intravenous nutritional therapy* [dextrose]

D_2 (vitamin D_2) [see: ergocalciferol]

D-2163 *investigational (Phase I) anticancer agent*

D_3 (vitamin D_3) [see: cholecalciferol]

d4T [see: stavudine]

D.A. chewable tablets ℞ *decongestant; antihistamine; anticholinergic* [phenylephrine HCl; chlorpheniramine maleate; methscopolamine nitrate] 10•2•1.25 mg

DA (daunorubicin, ara-C) *chemotherapy protocol for acute myelocytic leukemia (AML)*

D.A. II tablets ℞ *decongestant; antihistamine; anticholinergic* [phenylephrine HCl; chlorpheniramine maleate; methscopolamine nitrate] 10•4•1.25 mg

DAA (dihydroxyaluminum aminoacetate) [q.v.]

DAB_{389} IL-2 fusion toxin [now: denileukin diftitox]

dacarbazine USAN, USP, INN, BAN *alkylating antineoplastic for metastatic malignant melanoma and Hodgkin disease* 600 mg/vial injection (CAN) ⑨ Dicarbosil; procarbazine

dacemazine INN

dacisteine INN

dacliximab [see: daclizumab] [USAN changed 2000]

daclizumab USAN, INN, BAN *immunosuppressant monoclonal antibody for organ and bone marrow transplants (orphan)* [also: dacliximab]

Dacplat ℞ *investigational (orphan) alkylating antineoplastic for ovarian and colorectal cancers* [oxaliplatin]

Dacriose ophthalmic solution OTC *extraocular irrigating solution* [sterile isotonic solution]

dactinomycin USAN, USP, BAN *antibiotic antineoplastic* [also: actinomycin D]

dacuronium bromide INN, BAN

DADDS (diacetyl diaminodiphenylsulfone) [see: acedapsone]

dagapamil INN

Daily Care ointment (name changed to Desitin Creamy in 1997)

Daily Vitamins liquid OTC *vitamin supplement* [multiple vitamins] ≛

Daily-Vite with Iron & Minerals tablets OTC *vitamin/mineral/iron supplement* [multiple vitamins & minerals; iron; folic acid; biotin] ≛•18•0.4•?̲ mg

Dairy Ease chewable tablets OTC *digestive aid for lactose intolerance* [lactase enzyme] 3300 U

daisy, wild *medicinal herb* [see: wild daisy]

Dakin solution [see: sodium hypochlorite]

Dakrina eye drops (discontinued 1998) OTC *ophthalmic moisturizer/lubricant* [vitamin A palmitate; polyvinyl alcohol] 350 IU•0.6%

DAL (daunorubicin, ara-C, L-asparaginase) *chemotherapy protocol*

Dalacin (CAN) vaginal cream ℞ *lincosamide antibiotic for bacterial vaginosis* [clindamycin phosphate] 2% (100 mg/5 g dose)

Dalacin C (CAN) capsules ℞ *lincosamide antibiotic* [clindamycin HCl] 150, 300 mg

Dalacin C (CAN) granules for oral solution ℞ *lincosamide antibiotic* [clindamycin palmitate HCl] 75 mg/5 mL

Dalacin C Phosphate (CAN) IV infusion, IM injection ℞ *lincosamide antibiotic; treatment for AIDS-related Pneumocystis carinii pneumonia* [clindamycin phosphate] 150 mg/mL

Dalacin T (CAN) topical solution ℞ *topical antibiotic for acne* [clindamycin phosphate]

Dalalone intra-articular, intralesional, soft tissue, or IM injection ℞ *corticosteroid; anti-inflammatory* [dexamethasone sodium phosphate] 4 mg/mL

Dalalone D.P. intra-articular, soft tissue, or IM injection ℞ *corticosteroid; anti-inflammatory* [dexamethasone acetate] 16 mg/mL

Dalalone L.A. intralesional, intra-articular, soft tissue, or IM injection ℞ *corticosteroid; anti-inflammatory* [dexamethasone acetate] 8 mg/mL

dalanated insulin [see: insulin, dalanated]

dalbraminol INN

daledalin INN *antidepressant* [also: daledalin tosylate]

daledalin tosylate USAN *antidepressant* [also: daledalin]

dalfopristin USAN, INN *streptogramin antibacterial antibiotic for life-threatening infections*

dalfopristin & quinupristin *two streptogramin antibiotics that are synergistically bactericidal to gram-positive infections; investigational (NDA filed) for pneumonia*

Dalgan IV, subcu, or IM injection (discontinued 2000) ℞ *narcotic agonist-antagonist analgesic* [dezocine] 5, 10, 15 mg/mL

Dallergy tablets, sustained-release caplets, syrup ℞ *decongestant; antihistamine; anticholinergic* [phenylephrine HCl; chlorpheniramine maleate; methscopolamine nitrate] 10•4•1.25 mg; 20•8•2.5 mg; 10•2•0.625 mg/5 mL

Dallergy-D syrup OTC *decongestant; antihistamine* [phenylephrine HCl; chlorpheniramine maleate] 5•2 mg/5 mL

Dallergy-JR sustained-release capsules ℞ *pediatric decongestant and antihistamine* [pseudoephedrine HCl; brompheniramine maleate] 60•6 mg

Dalmane capsules ℞ *benzodiazepine sedative; hypnotic; sometimes abused as a street drug* [flurazepam HCl] 15, 30 mg ⊠ Dialume

d'Alpha E 400; d'Alpha E 1000 softgels OTC *vitamin supplement* [vitamin E (as *d*-alpha tocopherol)] 400 IU; 1000 IU

dalteparin sodium USAN, INN, BAN *a low molecular weight heparin–type anticoagulant and antithrombotic for prevention of deep vein thrombosis (DVT), unstable angina, and myocardial infarction*

daltroban USAN, INN *immunosuppressive*

Damason-P tablets ℞ *narcotic analgesic* [hydrocodone bitartrate; aspirin] 5•500 mg

dambose [see: inositol]

dametralast INN

damiana *(Turnera aphrodisiaca; T. diffusa; T. microphylla)* leaves *medicinal herb for bed-wetting, bronchitis, emphysema, headache, hormonal imbalance, hot flashes, menopause, and Parkinson disease; also used as an aphrodisiac*

damotepine INN

D-Amp capsules (discontinued 1997) ℞ *aminopenicillin antibiotic* [ampicillin] 500 mg

danaparoid sodium USAN, BAN *glycosaminoglycan anticoagulant and antithrombotic for prevention of deep vein thrombosis (DVT)*

danazol USAN, USP, INN, BAN *anterior pituitary suppressant; gonadotropin inhibitor for endometriosis, fibrocystic breast disease, and hereditary angioedema* 50, 100, 200 mg oral

dandelion *(Leontodon taraxacum; Taraxacum officinale)* leaves and root *medicinal herb for anemia, analgesia, blisters, blood cleansing, blood glucose regulation, constipation, diaphoresis, dyspepsia, edema, endurance, gallbladder disease, hypertension, and liver disorders*

daniplestim USAN *treatment for chemotherapy-induced bone marrow suppression*

daniquidone BAN

danitamon [see: menadione]

danitracen INN

Danocrine capsules ℞ *gonadotropin inhibitor for endometriosis, fibrocystic breast disease, and hereditary angioedema* [danazol] 50, 100, 200 mg

danofloxacin INN *veterinary antibacterial* [also: danofloxacin mesylate]
danofloxacin mesylate USAN *veterinary antibacterial* [also: danofloxacin]
danosteine INN
danshen *(Salvia miltiorrhiza)* *medicinal herb for abdominal pain, bruises, circulatory problems, insomnia, menstrual irregularity, and stroke; also used as an aid in granulation of wounds*
danthron USP, BAN *(withdrawn from market by FDA)* [also: dantron] ⑨ Dantrium
Dantrium capsules, powder for IV injection ℞ *skeletal muscle relaxant* [dantrolene sodium] 25, 50, 100 mg; 20 mg/vial (0.32 mg/mL) ⑨ danthron
dantrolene USAN, INN, BAN *skeletal muscle relaxant*
dantrolene sodium USAN, BAN *skeletal muscle relaxant*
dantron INN *(withdrawn from market by FDA)* [also: danthron]
Dapa tablets, capsules (discontinued 1997) OTC *analgesic; antipyretic* [acetaminophen] 325 mg; 500 mg
Dapacin Cold capsules OTC *decongestant; antihistamine; analgesic* [phenylpropanolamine HCl; chlorpheniramine maleate; acetaminophen] 12.5•2•325 mg
Daphne mezereum *medicinal herb* [see: mezereon]
dapiprazole INN *α-adrenergic blocker; miotic; neuroleptic* [also: dapiprazole HCl]
dapiprazole HCl USAN *α-adrenergic blocker; miotic; neuroleptic* [also: dapiprazole]
dapsone USAN, USP, BAN *leprostatic; dermatitis herpetiformis treatment; investigational (orphan) for Pneumocystis carinii and toxoplasmosis* 25, 100 mg oral
dapsone & trimethoprim *investigational for Pneumocystis carinii pneumonia; orphan status withdrawn 1998*
daptazole [see: amiphenazole]
daptomycin USAN, INN, BAN *investigational (Phase III) antibiotic*
Daranide tablets ℞ *carbonic anhydrase inhibitor; diuretic* [dichlorphenamide] 50 mg ⑨ Daraprim
Daraprim tablets ℞ *antimalarial; toxoplasmosis treatment adjunct* [pyrimethamine] 25 mg ⑨ Daranide
darbepoetin alfa USAN *novel erythropoiesis stimulating protein (NESP); investigational (NDA filed) epoetin analogue hematopoietic for anemia*
darbufelone mesylate USAN *anti-inflammatory; antiarthritic; cyclo-oxygenase inhibitor; 5-lipoxygenase inhibitor*
darenzepine INN
darglitazone sodium USAN *oral hypoglycemic*
Daricon tablets (discontinued 1997) ℞ *adjunctive therapy for peptic ulcer* [oxyphencyclimine HCl] 10 mg ⑨ Darvon
darifenacin *investigational (Phase III) agent for overactive bladder*
darodipine USAN, INN *antihypertensive; bronchodilator; vasodilator*
Darvocet-N 50; Darvocet-N 100 tablets ℞ *narcotic analgesic* [propoxyphene napsylate; acetaminophen] 50•325 mg; 100•650 mg ⑨ Darvon-N
Darvon Pulvules (capsules) ℞ *narcotic analgesic* [propoxyphene HCl] 65 mg ⑨ Daricon
Darvon Compound-65 Pulvules (capsules) ℞ *narcotic analgesic* [propoxyphene HCl; aspirin; caffeine] 65•389•32.4 mg
Darvon-N film-coated tablets ℞ *narcotic analgesic* [propoxyphene napsylate] 100 mg
DAT (daunorubicin, ara-C, thioguanine) *chemotherapy protocol for acute myelocytic leukemia (AML)* [also: DCT; TAD]
datelliptium chloride INN
Datura stramonium *medicinal herb* [see: jimsonweed]
daturine hydrobromide [see: hyoscyamine hydrobromide]
DATVP (daunorubicin, ara-C, thioguanine, vincristine, prednisone) *chemotherapy protocol*
Daucus carota *medicinal herb* [see: carrot]

daunomycin [see: daunorubicin HCl]
daunorubicin (DNR) INN, BAN *anthracycline antibiotic antineoplastic for various leukemias* [also: daunorubicin HCl] ⓢ doxorubicin
daunorubicin citrate, liposomal *anthracycline antibiotic antineoplastic for advanced HIV-related Kaposi sarcoma (orphan)*
daunorubicin HCl USAN, USP, JAN *anthracycline antibiotic antineoplastic for various leukemias* [also: daunorubicin] 20, 50 mg injection ⓢ doxorubicin
DaunoXome IV infusion ℞ *antibiotic antineoplastic for advanced AIDS-related Kaposi sarcoma (orphan)* [daunorubicin citrate, liposomal] 2 mg/mL
DAV (daunorubicin, ara-C, VePesid) *chemotherapy protocol for acute myelocytic leukemia (AML)*
DAVA (desacetyl vinblastine amide) [see: vindesine]
DAVH (dibromodulcitol, Adriamycin, vincristine, Halotestin) *chemotherapy protocol*
davitamon [see: menadione]
Dayalets Filmtabs (film-coated tablets) OTC *vitamin supplement* [multiple vitamins; folic acid] ≛•0.4 mg
Dayalets + Iron Filmtabs (film-coated tablets) OTC *vitamin/iron supplement* [multiple vitamins; ferrous sulfate; folic acid] ≛•18•0.4 mg
Dayhist-1 tablets OTC *antihistamine* [clemastine fumarate] 1.34 mg
Daypro film-coated caplets ℞ *antiarthritic; nonsteroidal anti-inflammatory drug (NSAID)* [oxaprozin] 600 mg
DayQuil LiquiCaps (soft gel capsules), liquid OTC *antitussive; decongestant; expectorant; analgesic* [dextromethorphan hydrobromide; pseudoephedrine HCl; guaifenesin; acetaminophen] 10•30•100•250 mg; 3.3•10•33.3•108.3 mg/5 mL
DayQuil Allergy Relief 4 Hour tablets OTC *decongestant; antihistamine* [phenylpropanolamine HCl; brompheniramine maleate] 25•4 mg
DayQuil Allergy Relief 12 Hour extended-release tablets OTC *decongestant; antihistamine* [phenylpropanolamine HCl; brompheniramine maleate] 75•12 mg
DayQuil Sinus Pressure & Congestion Relief caplets (discontinued 1997) OTC *decongestant* [phenylpropanolamine HCl; guaifenesin] 25•200 mg
DayQuil Sinus Pressure & Pain Relief caplets OTC *decongestant; analgesic; antipyretic* [pseudoephedrine HCl; acetaminophen] 30•500 mg
Dayto Himbin tablets ℞ *no FDA-approved uses; sympatholytic; mydriatic; aphrodisiac* [yohimbine HCl] 5.4 mg
Dayto Sulf vaginal cream (discontinued 2001) ℞ *broad-spectrum bacteriostatic* [sulfathiazole; sulfacetamide; sulfabenzamide] 3.42%•2.86%•3.7%
dazadrol INN *antidepressant* [also: dazadrol maleate]
dazadrol maleate USAN *antidepressant* [also: dazadrol]
Dazamide tablets ℞ *carbonic anhydrase inhibitor diuretic; treatment for acute mountain sickness* [acetazolamide] 250 mg
dazepinil INN *antidepressant* [also: dazepinil HCl]
dazepinil HCl USAN *antidepressant* [also: dazepinil]
dazidamine INN
dazmegrel USAN, INN, BAN *thromboxane synthetase inhibitor*
dazolicine INN
dazopride INN *peristaltic stimulant* [also: dazopride fumarate]
dazopride fumarate USAN *peristaltic stimulant* [also: dazopride]
dazoquinast INN
dazoxiben INN, BAN *antithrombotic* [also: dazoxiben HCl]
dazoxiben HCl USAN *antithrombotic* [also: dazoxiben]
DBED (dibenzylethylenediamine dipenicillin G) [see: penicillin G benzathine]

DBM (dibromomannitol) [see: mitobronitol]
DC softgels OTC *laxative; stool softener* [docusate calcium] 240 mg
DC (daunorubicin, cytarabine) *chemotherapy protocol*
D&C Brown No. 1 (drugs & cosmetics) [see: resorcin brown]
DCA (desoxycorticosterone acetate) [q.v.]
DCA (dichloroacetate) [see: sodium dichloroacetate]
DCF (2′-deoxycoformycin) [see: pentostatin]
DCL (descarboethoxyloratadine) [q.v.]
DCMP (daunorubicin, cytarabine, mercaptopurine, prednisone) *chemotherapy protocol*
DCPM (daunorubicin, cytarabine, prednisone, mercaptopurine) *chemotherapy protocol*
DCT (daunorubicin, cytarabine, thioguanine) *chemotherapy protocol for acute myelocytic leukemia (AML)* [also: DAT; TAD]
DCV (DTIC, CCNU, vincristine) *chemotherapy protocol*
DDAVP tablets, nasal spray, rhinal tube, subcu or IV injection ℞ *antidiuretic; posterior pituitary hormone for hemophilia A, von Willebrand disease (orphan), central diabetes insipidus, and nocturnal enuresis* [desmopressin acetate] 0.1, 0.2 mg; 10 µg/dose; 0.1 mg/mL; 4 µg/mL
DDAVP (1-deamino-8-D-arginine-vasopressin) [see: desmopressin acetate]
DDC; ddC (dideoxycytidine) [see: zalcitabine]
***o,p′*-DDD** [now: mitotane]
DDI; ddI (dideoxyinosine) [see: didanosine]
DDP; *cis*-DDP (diamminedichloroplatinum) [see: cisplatin]
DDS (diaminodiphenylsulfone) [now: dapsone]
DDT (dichlorodiphenyltrichloroethane) [see: chlorophenothane]
DDVP (dichlorovinyl dimethyl phosphate) [see: dichlorvos]
DEA (diethanolamine) [q.v.]
deacetyllanatoside C [see: deslanoside]
17-deacylnorgestimate [see: norelgestromin]
deadly nightshade *medicinal herb* [see: belladonna]
deadly nightshade leaf [see: belladonna extract]
deal pine *medicinal herb* [see: white pine]
1-deamino-8-D-arginine-vasopressin (DDAVP) [see: desmopressin acetate]
deanil INN *combining name for radicals or groups*
deanol BAN [also: deanol aceglumate]
deanol aceglumate INN [also: deanol]
deanol acetamidobenzoate
deba [see: barbital]
deboxamet INN
Debrisan beads, paste ℞ *debrider and cleanser for wet wounds* [dextranomer]
debrisoquin sulfate USAN *antihypertensive* [also: debrisoquine]
debrisoquine INN, BAN *antihypertensive* [also: debrisoquin sulfate]
Debrox ear drops OTC *agent to emulsify and disperse ear wax* [carbamide peroxide] 6.5%
Decadron tablets, elixir ℞ *corticosteroid; anti-inflammatory* [dexamethasone] 0.5, 0.75, 1.5, 4 mg; 0.5 mg/5 mL ⊡ Decaderm; Percodan
Decadron Phosphate cream (discontinued 1998) ℞ *topical corticosteroidal anti-inflammatory* [dexamethasone sodium phosphate] 0.1%
Decadron Phosphate intra-articular, intralesional, soft tissue or IM injection ℞ *corticosteroid; anti-inflammatory* [dexamethasone sodium phosphate] 4 mg/mL
Decadron Phosphate IV injection ℞ *corticosteroid; anti-inflammatory* [dexamethasone sodium phosphate] 24 mg/mL
Decadron Phosphate Ocumeter (eye drops) ℞ *topical ophthalmic corticosteroidal anti-inflammatory* [dexamethasone sodium phosphate] 0.1%

Decadron Phosphate ophthalmic ointment (discontinued 2000) ℞ *topical ophthalmic corticosteroidal anti-inflammatory* [dexamethasone sodium phosphate] 0.05%

Decadron with Xylocaine soft tissue injection ℞ *corticosteroid; anti-inflammatory* [dexamethasone sodium phosphate; lidocaine HCl] 4•10 mg/mL

Decadron-LA intralesional, intra-articular, soft tissue, or IM injection ℞ *corticosteroid; anti-inflammatory* [dexamethasone acetate] 8 mg/mL

Deca-Durabolin IM injection ℞ *anabolic steroid for anemia of renal insufficiency; sometimes abused as a street drug* [nandrolone decanoate (in oil)] 100, 200 mg/mL

Decagen tablets OTC *vitamin/mineral/iron supplement* [multiple vitamins & minerals; iron; folic acid; biotin] ≛•18 mg•0.4 mg•30 µg

Decaject intra-articular, intralesional, soft tissue, or IM injection ℞ *corticosteroid; anti-inflammatory* [dexamethasone sodium phosphate] 4 mg/mL

Decaject-L.A. intralesional, intra-articular, soft tissue, or IM injection ℞ *corticosteroid; anti-inflammatory* [dexamethasone acetate] 8 mg/mL

DECAL (dexamethasone, etoposide, cisplatin, ara-C, L-asparaginase) *chemotherapy protocol*

decamethonium bromide USP, INN [also: decamethonium iodide]

decamethonium iodide BAN [also: decamethonium bromide]

decapinol [see: delmopinol]

decavitamin USP

Decholin tablets OTC *laxative; hydrocholeretic* [dehydrocholic acid] 250 mg

decicain [see: tetracaine HCl]

decil INN *combining name for radicals or groups*

decimemide INN

decitabine USAN, INN, BAN *antineoplastic*

decitropine INN

declaben [now: lodelaben]

declenperone USAN, INN *veterinary sedative*

Declomycin capsules, film-coated tablets ℞ *broad-spectrum antibiotic* [demeclocycline HCl] 150 mg; 150, 300 mg

decloxizine INN

Decofed syrup OTC *nasal decongestant* [pseudoephedrine HCl] 30 mg/5 mL

Decohistine DH liquid ℞ *narcotic antitussive; decongestant; antihistamine* [codeine phosphate; pseudoephedrine HCl; chlorpheniramine maleate; alcohol 5.8%] 10•30•2 mg/5 mL

decominol INN

Deconamine tablets, syrup ℞ *decongestant; antihistamine* [pseudoephedrine HCl; chlorpheniramine maleate] 60•4 mg; 30•2 mg/5 mL

Deconamine CX tablets, liquid ℞ *narcotic antitussive; decongestant; expectorant* [hydrocodone bitartrate; pseudoephedrine HCl; guaifenesin] 5•30•300 mg; 5•60•200 mg/5 mL

Deconamine SR sustained-release capsules ℞ *decongestant; antihistamine* [pseudoephedrine HCl; chlorpheniramine maleate] 120•8 mg

Decongestabs sustained-release tablets ℞ *decongestant; antihistamine* [phenylpropanolamine HCl; phenylephrine HCl; chlorpheniramine maleate; phenyltoloxamine citrate] 40•10•5•15 mg

Decongestant sustained-release tablets ℞ *decongestant; antihistamine* [phenylpropanolamine HCl; phenylephrine HCl; chlorpheniramine maleate; phenyltoloxamine citrate] 40•10•5•15 mg

Decongestant tablets OTC *decongestant; antihistamine; analgesic* [phenylephrine HCl; chlorpheniramine maleate; acetaminophen] 5•2•325 mg

Decongestant Expectorant liquid (discontinued 2000) ℞ *narcotic antitussive; decongestant; expectorant* [codeine phosphate; pseudoephedrine HCl; guaifenesin; alcohol 7.5%] 10•30•100 mg/5 mL

Deconhist L.A. sustained-release tablets ℞ *decongestant; antihistamine; anticholinergic* [phenylpropanolamine HCl; phenylephrine HCl; chlorpheniramine maleate; hyoscyamine sulfate; atropine sulfate; scopolamine hydrobromide] 50•25•8•0.19•0.04•0.01 mg

Deconomed SR sustained-release capsules ℞ *decongestant; antihistamine* [pseudoephedrine HCl; chlorpheniramine maleate] 120•8 mg

Deconsal II sustained-release tablets ℞ *decongestant; expectorant* [pseudoephedrine HCl; guaifenesin] 60•600 mg ⓢ Deconal

Deconsal Pediatric syrup (discontinued 1998) ℞ *narcotic antitussive; decongestant; expectorant* [codeine phosphate; pseudoephedrine HCl; guaifenesin; alcohol 6%] 10•30•100 mg ⓢ Deconal

Deconsal Sprinkle sustained-release capsules ℞ *decongestant; expectorant* [phenylephrine HCl; guaifenesin] 10•300 mg ⓢ Deconal

decoquinate USAN, INN, BAN *coccidiostat for poultry*

dectaflur USAN, INN *dental caries prophylactic*

Decylenes ointment OTC *topical antifungal* [undecylenic acid; zinc undecylenate]

deditonium bromide INN

Deep-Down Rub OTC *topical analgesic; counterirritant* [methyl salicylate; menthol; camphor] 15%•5%•0.5%

deer musk *(Moschus moschiferus)* *natural remedy in ancient Chinese medicine; reported to have antianginal, antibacterial, antihistaminic, anti-inflammatory, CNS-depressant, and stimulant activity in clinical studies*

deerberry *medicinal herb* [see: holly; squaw vine; wintergreen]

DEET (diethyltoluamide) [q.v.]

DeFed-60 tablets OTC *nasal decongestant* [pseudoephedrine HCl] 60 mg

Defen-LA sustained-release tablets ℞ *decongestant; expectorant* [pseudoephedrine HCl; guaifenesin] 60•600 mg

deferoxamine USAN, INN *iron- and aluminum-chelating agent* [also: desferrioxamine]

deferoxamine & dextran *investigational (orphan) for acute iron poisoning*

deferoxamine HCl USAN

deferoxamine mesylate USAN, USP *antidote to iron poisoning; iron- and aluminum-chelating agent* [also: desferrioxamine mesylate]

defibrotide INN, BAN *investigational (orphan) for thrombotic thrombocytopenic purpura*

Definity suspension for IV injection or infusion ℞ *ultrasound contrast medium for cardiac and gynecologic imaging* [perflutren microspheres]

deflazacort USAN, INN, BAN *anti-inflammatory*

defosfamide INN

defungit sodium salt [see: bensuldazic acid]

Defy eye drops ℞ *topical ophthalmic antibiotic* [tobramycin] 0.3%

Degas chewable tablets OTC *antiflatulent* [simethicone] 80 mg

Degest 2 eye drops OTC *topical ophthalmic decongestant and vasoconstrictor* [naphazoline HCl] 0.012%

Dehist subcu or IM injection (discontinued 1997) ℞ *antihistamine for anaphylaxis* [brompheniramine maleate] 10 mg/mL

Dehistine syrup ℞ *decongestant; antihistamine; anticholinergic* [phenylephrine HCl; chlorpheniramine maleate; methscopolamine nitrate] 10•2•1.25 mg/5 mL

DEHOP (diethylhomospermine) [q.v.]

DEHSPM (diethylhomospermine) [q.v.]

dehydrated alcohol [see: alcohol, dehydrated]

dehydrex *investigational (orphan) for recurrent corneal erosion*

dehydroacetic acid NF *preservative*

dehydroandrosterone [see: prasterone]

dehydrocholate sodium USP [also: sodium dehydrocholate]

7-dehydrocholesterol, activated [now: cholecalciferol]

dehydrocholic acid USP, INN, BAN, JAN *choleretic; laxative* 250 mg oral

dehydrocholin [see: dehydrocholic acid]

dehydroemetine INN, BAN, DCF *investigational anti-infective for amebiasis and amebic dysentery*

dehydroepiandrosterone (DHEA) *natural hormone precursor; investigational (NDA filed, orphan) for systemic lupus erythematosus (SLE)*

dehydroepiandrosterone sulfate (DHEAS) *investigational (Phase II) injectable antiasthmatic*

dehydroepiandrosterone sulfate sodium *investigational (orphan) for re-epithelialization of serious burns and skin graft donor sites*

Del Aqua-5; Del Aqua-10 gel ℞ *topical keratolytic for acne* [benzoyl peroxide] 5%; 10%

delanterone INN

Delaprem (commercially available in several foreign countries) ℞ *investigational (NDA filed) tocolytic and bronchodilator* [hexoprenaline sulfate]

delapril INN *antihypertensive; angiotensin-converting enzyme inhibitor* [also: delapril HCl]

delapril HCl USAN *antihypertensive; angiotensin-converting enzyme inhibitor* [also: delapril]

Delatestryl IM injection ℞ *androgen replacement for testosterone deficiency in men, delayed puberty in boys, and metastatic breast cancer in women; sometimes abused as a street drug* [testosterone enanthate (in oil)] 200 mg/mL

delavirdine INN *antiviral; non-nucleoside reverse transcriptase inhibitor (NNRTI) for HIV and AIDS* [also: delavirdine mesylate]

delavirdine mesylate USAN *antiviral; non-nucleoside reverse transcriptase inhibitor (NNRTI) for HIV-1* [also: delavirdine]

delayed-release aspirin [see: aspirin]

Delcap (trademarked dosage form) *unit dispensing cap*

Delcort cream OTC *topical corticosteroidal anti-inflammatory* [hydrocortisone] 0.5%, 1% ⧉ Dilacor

delequamine INN α_2 *adrenoreceptor antagonist for sexual dysfunction* [also: delequamine HCl]

delequamine HCl USAN α_2 *adrenoreceptor antagonist for sexual dysfunction* [also: delequamine]

delergotrile INN

Delestrogen IM injection ℞ *estrogen replacement therapy for postmenopausal symptoms; antineoplastic for prostatic cancer* [estradiol valerate in oil] 10, 20, 40 mg/mL

delfantrine INN

delfaprazine INN

Delfen Contraceptive vaginal foam OTC *spermicidal contraceptive* [nonoxynol 9] 12.5%

delmadinone INN, BAN *progestin; antiandrogen; antiestrogen* [also: delmadinone acetate]

delmadinone acetate USAN *progestin; antiandrogen; antiestrogen* [also: delmadinone]

delmetacin INN

delmopinol INN

Del-Mycin topical solution ℞ *topical antibiotic for acne* [erythromycin] 2%

delnav [see: dioxathion]

delorazepam INN

deloxolone INN

***m*-delphene** [see: diethyltoluamide]

delprostenate INN, BAN

Delsym sustained-action liquid OTC *antitussive* [dextromethorphan polistirex] 30 mg/5 mL

Delta-Cortef tablets ℞ *corticosteroid; anti-inflammatory* [prednisolone] 5 mg

deltacortone [see: prednisone]

Delta-D tablets OTC *vitamin supplement* [cholecalciferol (vitamin D_3)] 400 IU

deltafilcon A USAN *hydrophilic contact lens material*

deltafilcon B USAN *hydrophilic contact lens material*

delta-1-hydrocortisone [see: prednisolone]

Deltasone tablets ℞ *corticosteroid; anti-inflammatory* [prednisone] 2.5, 5, 10, 20, 50 mg

delta-9-tetrahydrocannabinol (THC) [see: dronabinol]

delta-9-THC (tetrahydrocannabinol) [see: dronabinol]

Delta-Tritex cream, ointment ℞ *topical corticosteroidal anti-inflammatory* [triamcinolone acetonide] 0.1%

Deltavac vaginal cream ℞ *broad-spectrum antibiotic; antiseptic; vulnerary* [sulfanilamide; aminacrine HCl; allantoin] 15%•0.2%•2%

deltibant USAN *bradykinin antagonist for treatment of systemic inflammatory response syndrome*

deltra-stab [see: prednisolone]

Del-Vi-A capsules (discontinued 1999) ℞ *vitamin deficiency therapy* [vitamin A] 50 000 IU

Demadex tablets, IV injection ℞ *antihypertensive; loop diuretic* [torsemide] 5, 10, 20, 100 mg; 10 mg/mL

Demazin Repetabs (repeat-action tablets), syrup OTC *decongestant; antihistamine* [phenylpropanolamine HCl; chlorpheniramine maleate] 25•4 mg; 12.5•2 mg/5 mL

dembrexine INN, BAN

dembroxol [see: dembrexine]

demecarium bromide USP, INN, BAN *antiglaucoma agent; reversible cholinesterase inhibitor miotic*

demeclocycline USP, BAN *tetracycline antibiotic*

demeclocycline HCl USP, BAN *tetracycline antibiotic; antirickettsial*

demecolcine INN, BAN

demecycline USAN, INN *antibacterial*

demegestone INN

demekastigmine bromide [see: demecarium bromide]

demelverine INN

Demerol HCl IV or IM injection (discontinued 1999) ℞ *narcotic analgesic; also abused as a street drug* [meperidine HCl] 50, 100 mg/mL

Demerol HCl tablets, syrup ℞ *narcotic analgesic; also abused as a street drug* [meperidine HCl] 50, 100 mg; 50 mg/5 mL

demetacin [see: delmetacin]

11-demethoxyreserpine [see: deserpidine]

demethylchlortetracycline (DMCT) [now: demeclocycline]

demethylchlortetracycline HCl [see: demeclocycline HCl]

N-demethylcodeine [see: norcodeine]

demexiptiline INN

Demi-Regroton tablets ℞ *antihypertensive; diuretic* [chlorthalidone; reserpine] 25•0.125 mg

democonazole INN

demoxepam USAN, INN *minor tranquilizer*

demoxytocin INN

Demser capsules ℞ *antihypertensive for pheochromocytoma* [metyrosine] 250 mg

demulcents *a class of agents that soothe irritated or abraded tissues, particularly mucous membranes*

Demulen 1/35; Demulen 1/50 tablets (in packs of 21 or 28) ℞ *monophasic oral contraceptive* [ethynodiol diacetate; ethinyl estradiol] 1 mg•35 µg; 1 mg•50 µg ⑨ Demerol; Demolin

denatonium benzoate USAN, NF, INN, BAN *alcohol denaturant; flavoring agent*

denaverine INN

Denavir cream ℞ *nucleoside analogue antiviral for herpes labialis* [penciclovir] 1%

denbufylline INN, BAN

denileukin diftitox USAN, INN *antineoplastic for cutaneous T-cell lymphoma (CTCL) (orphan); investigational (Phase II) agent for non-Hodgkin lymphoma; investigational agent for various malignant diseases and autoimmune disorders* [previously known as DAB_{389} IL-2 fusion toxin]

denipride INN

denofungin USAN *antifungal; antibacterial*

denopamine INN

Denorex shampoo OTC *antiseborrheic; antipsoriatic; antipruritic; antibacterial* [coal tar; menthol; alcohol] 9%•1.5•7.5%; 12.5%•1.5%•10.4%

denpidazone INN

Denquel toothpaste OTC *tooth desensitizer* [potassium nitrate] 5%

dental antiformin [see: antiformin, dental]

dental-type silica [see: silica, dental-type]

Dentipatch transmucosal patch ℞ *mucous membrane anesthetic* [lidocaine HCl] 23, 46.1 mg

Dent's Lotion-Jel lotion/gel OTC *topical oral anesthetic* [benzocaine]

Dent's Toothache Gum; Dent's Toothache Drops OTC *topical oral anesthetic* [benzocaine]

denyl sodium [see: phenytoin sodium]

denzimol INN

deodorants *a class of agents that mask undesirable or offensive odors* [also called: antibromics]

2′-deoxycoformycin (DCF) [see: pentostatin]

deoxycorticosterone acetate [see: desoxycorticosterone acetate]

deoxycorticosterone pivalate [see: desoxycorticosterone pivalate]

deoxycortolone pivalate BAN *salt-regulating adrenocortical steroid* [also: desoxycorticosterone pivalate]

deoxycortone BAN *salt-regulating adrenocortical steroid* [also: desoxycorticosterone acetate; desoxycortone]

2′-deoxycytidine *investigational (orphan) host-protective agent in acute myelogenous leukemia*

deoxyephedrine HCl [see: methamphetamine HCl]

12-deoxyerythromycin [see: berythromycin]

deoxynojirimycin (DNJ) *investigational (Phase II) antiviral for AIDS and ARC*

deoxyribonuclease, recombinant human (rhDNase) [see: dornase alfa]

deoxyribonucleic acid (DNA)

15-deoxyspergualin trihydrochloride [now: gusperimus trihydrochloride]

Depacin capsules OTC *analgesic; antipyretic* [acetaminophen] 325 mg

Depacon IV infusion ℞ *anticonvulsant* [valproate sodium] 100 mg/mL

Depade tablets ℞ *narcotic antagonist for opiate dependence or overdose (orphan) and alcoholism* [naltrexone HCl] 50 mg

Depakene capsules ℞ *anticonvulsant* [valproic acid] 250 mg

Depakene syrup ℞ *anticonvulsant* [valproate sodium] 250 mg/5 mL

Depakote delayed-release tablets ℞ *anticonvulsant; antipsychotic for manic episodes of a bipolar disorder; migraine prophylaxis* [divalproex sodium] 125, 250, 500 mg

Depakote sprinkle capsules ℞ *anticonvulsant* [divalproex sodium] 125 mg

Depakote ER extended-release tablets ℞ *anticonvulsant; antipsychotic for manic episodes of a bipolar disorder; migraine prophylaxis* [divalproex sodium] 500 mg

Depakote ER tablets ℞ *investigational (NDA filed) for the prophylaxis of migraine headaches* [divalproex sodium]

depAndro 100; depAndro 200 IM injection (discontinued 2001) ℞ *androgen replacement for delayed puberty or breast cancer* [testosterone cypionate] 100 mg/mL; 200 mg/mL

depAndrogyn IM injection (discontinued 1999) ℞ *hormone replacement therapy for postmenopausal symptoms* [estradiol cypionate; testosterone cypionate] 2•50 mg/mL

Depen titratable tablets ℞ *metal chelating agent for rheumatoid arthritis, Wilson disease, and cystinuria* [penicillamine] 250 mg

depepsen [see: sodium amylosulfate]

depGynogen IM injection ℞ *estrogen replacement therapy for postmenopausal symptoms* [estradiol cypionate in oil] 5 mg/mL

Depitol tablets (discontinued 1998) ℞ *anticonvulsant; analgesic for trigeminal*

neuralgia; antipsychotic [carbamazepine] 200 mg

depMedalone 40; depMedalone 80 intralesional, soft tissue, and IM injection ℞ *corticosteroid; anti-inflammatory; immunosuppressant* [methylprednisolone acetate] 40 mg/mL; 80 mg/mL

DepoCyt sustained-release intrathecal injection ℞ *antineoplastic for lymphomatous neoplastic meningitis (NM) arising from solid tumors or non-Hodgkin lymphoma (orphan)* [cytarabine, liposomal] 10 mg/mL

Depo-Estradiol Cypionate IM injection ℞ *estrogen replacement therapy for postmenopausal symptoms* [estradiol cypionate in oil] 5 mg/mL

DepoGen IM injection ℞ *estrogen replacement therapy for postmenopausal symptoms* [estradiol cypionate in oil] 5 mg/mL

Depoject intralesional, soft tissue, and IM injection ℞ *corticosteroid; anti-inflammatory; immunosuppressant* [methylprednisolone acetate] 40, 80 mg/mL

Depo-Medrol intralesional, soft tissue, and IM injection ℞ *corticosteroid; anti-inflammatory; immunosuppressant* [methylprednisolone acetate] 20, 40, 80 mg/mL

DepoMorphine ℞ *investigational (Phase II) sustained-release, encapsulated formulation to treat severe post-surgical pain* [morphine sulfate]

Deponit transdermal patch ℞ *antianginal; vasodilator* [nitroglycerin] 16, 32 mg (0.2, 0.4 mg/hr.)

Depopred-40; Depopred-80 intralesional, soft tissue, and IM injection ℞ *corticosteroid; anti-inflammatory; immunosuppressant* [methylprednisolone acetate] 40 mg/mL; 80 mg/mL

Depo-Provera IM injection ℞ *long-term (3 month) injectable contraceptive; hormonal antineoplastic adjunct for metastatic endometrial and renal carcinoma* [medroxyprogesterone acetate] 150, 400 mg/mL

Depotest 100; Depotest 200 IM injection (discontinued 2001) ℞ *androgen replacement for delayed puberty or breast cancer* [testosterone cypionate] 100 mg/mL; 200 mg/mL

Depo-Testadiol IM injection ℞ *hormone replacement therapy for postmenopausal symptoms* [estradiol cypionate; testosterone cypionate] 2•50 mg/mL

Depotestogen IM injection ℞ *hormone replacement therapy for postmenopausal symptoms* [estradiol cypionate; testosterone cypionate] 2•50 mg/mL

Depo-Testosterone IM injection ℞ *androgen replacement for testosterone deficiency in men; sometimes abused as a street drug* [testosterone cypionate (in oil)] 100, 200 mg/mL

depramine INN [also: balipramine]

deprenyl (L-deprenyl) [see: selegiline HCl]

depreotide USAN *radiopharmaceutical imaging agent for lung cancer; investigational (NDA filed) for malignant melanoma and neuroendocrine tumors*

depressants *a class of agents that reduce functional activity and vital energy in general by producing muscular relaxation and diaphoresis*

deprodone INN, BAN

Deproic (CAN) capsules, syrup (discontinued 2001) ℞ *anticonvulsant* [valproic acid] 250, 500 mg; 250 mg/5 mL

Deproist Expectorant with Codeine liquid ℞ *narcotic antitussive; decongestant; expectorant* [codeine phosphate; pseudoephedrine HCl; guaifenesin; alcohol 8.2%] 10•30•100 mg/5 mL

deprostil USAN, INN *gastric antisecretory*

deptropine INN, BAN

deptropine citrate [see: deptropine]

depurants; depuratives *a class of agents that purify or cleanse the system, particularly the blood* [also called: pellants]

dequalinium chloride INN, BAN

Dequasine tablets OTC *dietary supplement* [multiple minerals & amino acids; vitamin C] ≛•200 mg

deracoxib USAN *COX-2 inhibitor anti-inflammatory and analgesic for osteoarthritis and rheumatoid arthritis*

deramciclane *serotonin 5-HT$_2$ receptor antagonist; investigational (Phase III) antidepressant and anxiolytic for generalized anxiety disorder (GAD)*

Derifil tablets OTC *systemic deodorant for ostomy, breath, and body odors* [chlorophyllin] 100 mg

Derma Viva lotion OTC *moisturizer; emollient*

Dermabase OTC *cream base*

Dermabond liquid OTC *topical skin adhesive for closing surgical incisions and traumatic lacerations*

Dermacoat aerosol OTC *topical local anesthetic* [benzocaine] 4.5%

Dermacort cream, lotion ℞ *topical corticosteroidal anti-inflammatory* [hydrocortisone] 1% ⊠ DermiCort

DermaFlex gel OTC *topical local anesthetic* [lidocaine] 2.5%

Dermagraft; Dermagraft-TC (approved for marketing in the UK) ℞ *investigational (NDA filed) fully human skin replacement or temporary wound covering for partial-thickness burns; investigational (NDA filed) for diabetic foot ulcers*

Dermal-Rub balm OTC *counterirritant* [methyl salicylate; camphor; racemic manthol; cajuput oil]

Dermamycin cream, spray OTC *topical antihistamine* [diphenhydramine HCl] 2%

Derma-Pax lotion OTC *topical antihistamine; antiseptic; antipruritic* [pyrilamine maleate; chlorpheniramine maleate; alcohol 35%] 0.44%•0.06%

Dermarest gel OTC *topical antihistamine; antifungal* [diphenhydramine HCl; resorcinol] 2%•2%

Dermarest Dricort Creme OTC *topical corticosteroidal anti-inflammatory* [hydrocortisone acetate] 1%

Dermarest Plus gel, spray OTC *topical antihistamine; analgesic; counterirritant* [diphenhydramine HCl; menthol] 2%•1%

Dermasept Antifungal liquid spray OTC *antifungal; antiseptic; anesthetic; astringent* [tolnaftate; tannic acid; zinc chloride; benzocaine; methylbenzethonium HCl; undecylenic acid; alcohol 58.54%] 1.017%•6.098%•5.081%•2.032%•3.049%•5.081%

Dermasil lotion OTC *bath emollient*

Derma-Smoothe/FS oil ℞ *topical corticosteroidal anti-inflammatory; emollient* [fluocinolone acetonide] 0.01%

dermatan sulfate [see: danaparoid sodium]

dermatol [see: bismuth subgallate]

Dermatop cream ℞ *topical corticosteroidal anti-inflammatory* [prednicarbate] 0.1%

DermaVite tablets OTC *vitamin/mineral/calcium supplement* [multiple vitamins & minerals; calcium; folic acid; biotin] ≛•270•0.4•0.6 mg

Derm-Cleanse liquid OTC *soap-free therapeutic skin cleanser*

Dermol HC anorectal cream, anorectal ointment ℞ *topical corticosteroidal anti-inflammatory* [hydrocortisone] 1%, 2.5%; 1%

Dermolate Anti-Itch cream OTC *topical corticosteroidal anti-inflammatory* [hydrocortisone] 0.5%

Dermolin liniment OTC *topical analgesic; counterirritant; antiseptic* [methyl salicylate; camphor; racemic menthol; mustard oil; alcohol 8%]

Dermoplast aerosol spray, lotion OTC *topical local anesthetic; analgesic* [benzocaine; menthol] 20%•0.5%; 8%•0.5%

Dermovan OTC *cream base*

Dermprotective Factor (DPF) (trademarked ingredient) *aromatic syrup* [eriodictyon]

Dermtex HC with Aloe cream OTC *topical corticosteroidal anti-inflammatory* [hydrocortisone] 0.5%

Dermuspray aerosol spray ℞ *topical enzyme for wound debridement* [trypsin; peruvian balsam] 0.1•72.5 mg/0.82 mL

derpanicate INN

DES (diethylstilbestrol) [q.v.]
desacetyl vinblastine amide (DAVA) [see: vindesine]
desacetyl-lanatoside C [see: deslanoside]
desaglybuzole [see: glybuzole]
desamino-oxytocin [see: demoxytocin]
desaspidin INN
descarboethoxyloratadine (DCL) *investigational antihistamine for allergy*
desciclovir USAN, INN *antiviral*
descinolone INN *corticosteroid; anti-inflammatory* [also: descinolone acetonide]
descinolone acetonide USAN *corticosteroid; anti-inflammatory* [also: descinolone]
Desenex foam, soap OTC *topical antifungal* [undecylenic acid] 10%
Desenex powder, aerosol powder, ointment, cream OTC *topical antifungal* [undecylenic acid; zinc undecylenate] 25% total
Desenex spray liquid (discontinued 1998) OTC *topical antifungal* [tolnaftate] 1%
Desenex, Prescription Strength cream OTC *topical antifungal* [clotrimazole] 1%
Desenex, Prescription Strength spray liquid, spray powder OTC *topical antifungal* [miconazole nitrate] 2%
Desenex Antifungal cream OTC *topical antifungal* [miconazole nitrate] 2%
deserpidine INN, BAN *antihypertensive; peripheral antiadrenergic; rauwolfia derivative* ⑨ desipramine
desert herb; desert tea *medicinal herb* [see: ephedra]
Desert Pure Calcium film-coated tablets OTC *calcium supplement* [calcium carbonate; vitamin D] 500 mg•125 IU
Desferal powder for IM, IV, or subcu injection ℞ *adjunct treatment for iron intoxication or overload* [deferoxamine mesylate] 500 mg ⑨ Disophrol
desferrioxamine BAN *iron- and aluminum-chelating agent* [also: deferoxamine]
desferrioxamine mesylate BAN *antidote to iron poisoning; iron- and aluminum-chelating agent* [also: deferoxamine mesylate] 500 mg/vial injection (CAN)
desflurane USAN, INN *inhalation general anesthetic*
desglugastrin INN
desipramine INN, BAN *tricyclic antidepressant* [also: desipramine HCl] ⑨ deserpidine
desipramine HCl USAN, USP *tricyclic antidepressant* [also: desipramine] 10, 25, 50, 75, 100, 150 mg oral
desirudin USAN *anticoagulant; thrombin inhibitor* [recombinant hirudin]
Desitin ointment OTC *moisturizer; emollient; astringent; antiseptic* [cod liver oil; zinc oxide]
Desitin Creamy ointment OTC *topical diaper rash treatment* [zinc oxide] 10%
Desitin with Zinc Oxide powder OTC *topical diaper rash treatment* [zinc oxide; corn starch] 10%•88.2%
deslanoside USP, INN, BAN *cardiotonic; cardiac glycoside*
desloratadine USAN *investigational (NDA filed) histamine H_1 receptor antagonist for allergic rhinitis (active metabolite of loratadine)*
deslorelin USAN, INN *LH-RH agonist; investigational (orphan) for central precocious puberty*
desmethylmoramide INN
desmophosphamide [see: defosfamide]
desmopressin INN, BAN *posterior pituitary antidiuretic hormone (ADH)* [also: desmopressin acetate]
desmopressin acetate USAN *antidiuretic; posterior pituitary antidiuretic hormone for hemophilia A, von Willebrand disease (orphan), and nocturnal enuresis* [also: desmopressin] 4 µg/mL injection; 10 µg nasal spray
desocriptine INN
Desogen tablets (in packs of 28) ℞ *monophasic oral contraceptive* [desogestrel; ethinyl estradiol] 0.15 mg•30 µg
desogestrel USAN, INN, BAN *progestin*
desolone [see: deprodone]

desomorphine INN, BAN
desonide USAN, INN, BAN *topical corticosteroidal anti-inflammatory* 0.05% topical
DesOwen ointment, cream, lotion ℞ *topical corticosteroidal anti-inflammatory* [desonide] 0.05%
Desoxi (CAN) cream, gel ℞ *topical corticosteroidal anti-inflammatory* [desoximetasone] 0.05%, 0.25%; 0.05%
desoximetasone USAN, USP, INN *topical corticosteroidal anti-inflammatory* [also: desoxymethasone] 0.05%, 0.25% topical ⊠ dexamethasone
desoxycholic acid *increases secretion of bile acids*
desoxycorticosterone acetate (DCA; DOCA) USP *salt-regulating adrenocortical steroid* [also: desoxycortone; deoxycortone]
desoxycorticosterone pivalate USP *salt-regulating adrenocortical steroid* [also: deoxycortolone pivalate]
desoxycorticosterone trimethylacetate USP
desoxycortone INN *salt-regulating adrenocortical steroid* [also: desoxycorticosterone acetate; deoxycortone]
***l*-desoxyephedrine** *nasal decongestant*
desoxyephedrine HCl [see: methamphetamine HCl]
desoxymethasone BAN *topical corticosteroidal anti-inflammatory* [also: desoximetasone]
Desoxyn Gradumets (sustained-release tablets), tablets ℞ *CNS stimulant; sometimes abused as a street drug* [methamphetamine HCl] 5, 10, 15 mg; 5 mg ⊠ digitoxin; digoxin
desoxyribonuclease [see: fibrinolysin & desoxyribonuclease]
Despec liquid ℞ *decongestant; expectorant* [phenylephrine HCl; phenylpropanolamine HCl; guaifenesin] 20•5•100 mg/5 mL
Desquam-E; Desquam-E 5; Desquam-E 10 gel ℞ *topical keratolytic for acne* [benzoyl peroxide] 2.5%; 5%; 10%
Desquam-X 5; Desquam-X 10 gel ℞ *topical keratolytic for acne* [benzoyl peroxide] 5%; 10%
Desquam-X 5 Wash; Desquam-X 10 Wash liquid ℞ *topical keratolytic for acne* [benzoyl peroxide] 5%; 10%
de-Stat 3; de-Stat 4 solution OTC *cleaning/disinfecting/soaking solution for rigid gas permeable contact lenses*
destradiol [see: estradiol]
63-desulfohirudin [see: desirudin]
Desyrel film-coated tablets, Dividose (multiple-scored tablets) ℞ *antidepressant used for panic disorders, aggressive behavior, alcoholism, and cocaine withdrawal* [trazodone HCl] 50, 100 mg; 150, 300 mg
DET (diethyltryptamine) [q.v.]
detajmium bitartrate INN
Detane gel OTC *topical local anesthetic* [benzocaine] 7.5%
detanosal INN
Detect-A-Strep slide tests for professional use *in vitro diagnostic aid for streptococcal antigens in throat swabs*
Detecto-Seal (trademarked packaging form) *tamper-resistant parenteral package*
deterenol INN *ophthalmic adrenergic* [also: deterenol HCl]
deterenol HCl USAN *ophthalmic adrenergic* [also: deterenol]
detergents *a class of agents that cleanse wounds and sores*
detigon HCl [see: chlophedianol HCl]
detirelix INN *luteinizing hormone–releasing hormone (LH-RH) antagonist* [also: detirelix acetate]
detirelix acetate USAN *luteinizing hormone–releasing hormone (LH-RH) antagonist* [also: detirelix]
detomidine INN, BAN *veterinary analgesic; sedative* [also: detomidine HCl]
detomidine HCl USAN *veterinary analgesic; sedative* [also: detomidine]
detorubicin INN
Detox-B ℞ *investigational (Phase III) adjuvant to Theratope-STn for breast cancer*
detralfate INN

Detrol film-coated tablets ℞ *anticholinergic; muscarinic receptor antagonist for urinary frequency, urgency, and incontinence* [tolterodine tartrate] 1, 2 mg

Detrol LA extended-release capsules ℞ *anticholinergic; muscarinic receptor antagonist for urinary frequency, urgency, and incontinence* [tolterodine tartrate] 2, 4 mg

detrothyronine INN

Detrusitol (European name for U.S. product Detrol)

Detussin liquid ℞ *narcotic antitussive; decongestant* [hydrocodone bitartrate; pseudoephedrine HCl; alcohol 5%] 5•60 mg/5 mL

Detussin Expectorant liquid ℞ *narcotic antitussive; decongestant; expectorant* [hydrocodone bitartrate; pseudoephedrine HCl; guaifenesin; alcohol] 5•60•200 mg/5 mL

deuterium oxide USAN *radioactive agent*

devapamil INN

devazepide USAN *cholecystokinin antagonist*

devil's bones *medicinal herb* [see: wild yam]

devil's claw *(Harpagophytum procumbens)* root *medicinal herb for arrhythmias, arteriosclerosis, arthritis, blood cleansing, diabetes, hypertension, liver disease, lowering cholesterol, rheumatism, stomach disorders, and strengthening bladder and kidneys*

devil's club *(Echinopanax horridum; Fatsia horrida; Oplopanax horridus; Panax horridum)* cambium and stem *medicinal herb for arthritis, burns and cuts, colds, cough, fever, inducing vomiting and bowel evacuation, pneumonia, and tuberculosis*

devil's dung *medicinal herb* [see: asafetida]

devil's eye *medicinal herb* [see: henbane]

devil's fuge *medicinal herb* [see: mistletoe]

devil's shrub *medicinal herb* [see: Siberian ginseng]

Devrom chewable tablets OTC *systemic deodorizer for ostomy and incontinence odors* [bismuth subgallate] 200 mg

dewberry *medicinal herb* [see: blackberry]

Dex4 Glucose chewable tablets OTC *glucose elevating agent* [glucose]

dexa [see: dexamethasone]

Dexacidin eye drop suspension, ophthalmic ointment ℞ *topical ophthalmic corticosteroidal anti-inflammatory; antibiotic* [dexamethasone; neomycin sulfate; polymyxin B sulfate] 0.1%•0.35%•10 000 U/mL; 0.1%•0.35%•10 000 U/g

Dexacort Phosphate Respihaler (oral inhalation aerosol) ℞ *corticosteroid for bronchial asthma* [dexamethasone sodium phosphate] 84 µg/dose

Dexacort Phosphate Turbinaire (nasal inhalation aerosol) ℞ *intranasal corticosteroidal anti-inflammatory* [dexamethasone sodium phosphate; alcohol 2%] 84 µg/dose

Dexafed Cough syrup OTC *antitussive; decongestant; expectorant* [dextromethorphan hydrobromide; phenylephrine HCl; guaifenesin] 10•5•100 mg/5 mL

DexAlone gelcaps OTC *antitussive* [dextromethorphan hydrobromide] 30 mg

Dexameth tablets ℞ *corticosteroid; anti-inflammatory* [dexamethasone] 0.5, 0.75, 1.5, 4 mg

dexamethasone USP, INN, BAN *corticosteroidal anti-inflammatory* 0.25, 0.5, 0.75, 1, 1.5, 2, 4, 6 mg oral; 0.5 mg/5 mL oral; 0.5 mg/0.5 mL oral ⑨ desoximetasone

dexamethasone acefurate USAN, INN *corticosteroidal anti-inflammatory*

dexamethasone acetate USAN, USP, BAN *corticosteroidal anti-inflammatory* 8 mg/mL injection

dexamethasone dipropionate USAN *corticosteroidal anti-inflammatory*

dexamethasone & neomycin sulfate & polymyxin B sulfate *topical ophthalmic corticosteroidal anti-inflammatory and antibiotic* 0.1%•0.35%•10 000 U per mL eye drops

dexamethasone sodium phosphate USP, BAN *corticosteroid; anti-inflammatory* 0.05%, 0.1% eye drops; 4, 10 mg/mL injection

dexamfetamine INN *CNS stimulant* [also: dextroamphetamine; dexamphetamine]

dexamisole USAN, INN *antidepressant*

dexamphetamine BAN *CNS stimulant* [also: dextroamphetamine; dexamfetamine]

dexanabinol *investigational treatment for ulcerative colitis, inflammatory bowel disease (IBD), and AIDS-wasting syndrome*

dexanabinol *nonpsychotropic synthetic analogue of marijuana; investigational (Phase II) for severe head trauma*

Dexaphen S.A. sustained-release tablets ℞ *decongestant; antihistamine* [pseudoephedrine sulfate; dexbrompheniramine maleate] 120•6 mg

Dexasone intra-articular, intralesional, soft tissue, or IM injection ℞ *corticosteroid; anti-inflammatory* [dexamethasone sodium phosphate] 4 mg/mL

Dexasone L.A. intralesional, intra-articular, soft tissue, or IM injection ℞ *corticosteroid; anti-inflammatory* [dexamethasone acetate] 8 mg/mL

Dexasporin ophthalmic ointment ℞ *topical ophthalmic corticosteroidal anti-inflammatory; antibiotic* [dexamethasone; neomycin sulfate; polymyxin B sulfate] 0.1%•0.35%•10 000 U/g

Dexatrim extended-release tablets, timed-release capsules OTC *diet aid* [phenylpropanolamine HCl] 75 mg

Dexatrim plus Vitamin C timed-release capsules OTC *diet aid* [phenylpropanolamine HCl; vitamin C] 75•180 mg

Dexatrim Plus Vitamins timed-release caplets (diet aid) + caplets (vitamins) (discontinued 1998) OTC *diet aid + vitamin/mineral/iron supplement* [(phenylpropanolamine HCl; vitamin C) + (multiple vitamins/minerals; iron; folic acid; biotin)] (75•60 mg) + (≛•18•0.4•0.03 mg)

Dexatrim Pre-Meal timed-release capsules OTC *diet aid* [phenylpropanolamine HCl] 25 mg

dexbrompheniramine INN, BAN *antihistamine* [also: dexbrompheniramine maleate]

dexbrompheniramine maleate USP *antihistamine* [also: dexbrompheniramine]

Dexchlor extended-release tablets (discontinued 1997) ℞ *antihistamine* [dexchlorpheniramine maleate] 4, 6 mg

dexchlorpheniramine INN *alkylamine antihistamine* [also: dexchlorpheniramine maleate]

dexchlorpheniramine maleate USP *alkylamine antihistamine* [also: dexchlorpheniramine] 4, 6 mg oral

dexclamol INN *sedative* [also: dexclamol HCl]

dexclamol HCl USAN *sedative* [also: dexclamol]

Dexedrine Spansules (sustained-release capsules), tablets ℞ *amphetamine; CNS stimulant; widely abused as a street drug* [dextroamphetamine sulfate] 5, 10, 15 mg; 5 mg ⑨ dextran

dexetimide USAN, INN, BAN *anticholinergic*

dexetozoline INN

dexfenfluramine INN, BAN *anorexiant; appetite suppressant; serotonin reuptake inhibitor* [also: dexfenfluramine HCl]

dexfenfluramine HCl USAN *anorexiant; appetite suppressant; serotonin reuptake inhibitor* [also: dexfenfluramine]

DexFerrum IV or IM injection ℞ *hematinic* [iron dextran] 50 mg/mL

dexibuprofen USAN, INN *analgesic; cyclooxygenase inhibitor; anti-inflammatory*

dexibuprofen lysine USAN *analgesic; cyclooxygenase inhibitor; anti-inflammatory* [also: dexibuprofen]

deximafen USAN, INN *antidepressant*

dexindoprofen INN

Dexiron (CAN) IM injection ℞ *hematinic* [iron dextran] 50 mg/mL

dexivacaine USAN, INN *anesthetic*

dexlofexidine INN
dexmedetomidine USAN, INN, BAN *sedative*
dexmedetomidine HCl USAN *sedative for intubated and ventilated patients in an intensive care setting; premedication to anesthesia*
dexmethylphenidate HCl *CNS stimulant for attention-deficit hyperactivity disorder (ADHD) and narcolepsy; active isomer of methylphenidate HCl*
dexnorgestrel acetime [now: norgestimate]
Dexone intra-articular, intralesional, soft tissue, or IM injection ℞ *corticosteroid; anti-inflammatory* [dexamethasone sodium phosphate] 4 mg/mL
Dexone tablets ℞ *corticosteroid; anti-inflammatory* [dexamethasone] 0.5, 0.75, 1.5, 4 mg
Dexone LA intralesional, intra-articular, soft tissue, or IM injection ℞ *corticosteroid; anti-inflammatory* [dexamethasone acetate] 8 mg/mL
dexormaplatin USAN, INN *antineoplastic*
dexoxadrol INN *CNS stimulant; analgesic* [also: dexoxadrol HCl]
dexoxadrol HCl USAN *CNS stimulant; analgesic* [also: dexoxadrol]
dexpanthenol USAN, USP, INN, BAN *cholinergic; antipruritic; postoperative prophylaxis for paralytic ileus* 250 mg/mL injection
dexpemedolac USAN *analgesic*
dexpropranolol HCl USAN *antiarrhythmic; antiadrenergic (β-receptor)* [also: dexpropranolol]
dexproxibutene INN
dexrazoxane USAN, INN, BAN *cardioprotectant for doxorubicin-induced cardiomyopathy (orphan); chelates intracellular iron*
dexsecoverine INN
dexsotalol HCl USAN *class III antiarrhythmic*
dextilidine INN
dextran INN, BAN *blood flow adjuvant; plasma volume extender* [also: dextran 40] ⊡ Dexedrine; dextrin
dextran, high molecular weight [see: dextran 70]
dextran, low molecular weight [see: dextran 40]
dextran 1 *monovalent hapten for prevention of dextran-induced anaphylactic reactions*
dextran 40 USAN *blood flow adjuvant; plasma volume extender* [also: dextran] 10% injection
dextran 70 USAN *plasma volume extender; viscosity-increasing agent* 6% injection
dextran 75 USAN *plasma volume extender; viscosity-increasing agent* 6% injection
dextran & deferoxamine *investigational (orphan) for acute iron poisoning*
dextran sulfate *investigational (Phase II) antiviral for HIV and AIDS; investigational (orphan) inhalant for cystic fibrosis*
dextran sulfate, sodium salt, aluminum complex [see: detralfate]
dextran sulfate sodium *investigational (orphan) for AIDS*
dextranomer INN, BAN *wound cleanser and debrider*
dextrates USAN, NF *tablet binder and diluent*
dextriferron NF, INN, BAN
dextrin NF, BAN *suspending agent; tablet binder and diluent* ⊡ dextran
dextroamphetamine USAN *CNS stimulant; widely abused as a street drug, which causes strong psychic dependence* [also: dexamfetamine; dexamphetamine]
dextroamphetamine phosphate USP *CNS stimulant*
dextroamphetamine saccharate *CNS stimulant*
dextroamphetamine sulfate USP *CNS stimulant; widely abused as a street drug, which causes psychic dependence* 5, 10, 15 mg oral
dextrobrompheniramine maleate [see: dexbrompheniramine maleate]
dextrochlorpheniramine maleate [see: dexchlorpheniramine maleate]

dextrofemine INN
dextromethorphan USP, INN, BAN *antitussive*
dextromethorphan hydrobromide USP, BAN *antitussive* 10 mg/5 mL oral
dextromethorphan hydrobromide & brompheniramine maleate & pseudoephedrine HCl *antitussive; antihistamine; nasal decongestant* 15•4•80 mg/5 mL oral
dextromethorphan polistirex USAN *antitussive*
dextromoramide INN, BAN
dextromoramide tartrate [see: dextromoramide]
dextro-pantothenyl alcohol [see: dexpanthenol]
dextropropoxiphene chloride [see: propoxyphene HCl]
dextropropoxyphene INN, BAN *narcotic analgesic* [also: propoxyphene HCl]
dextropropoxyphene HCl BAN [also: propoxyphene HCl]
dextrorphan INN, BAN *adjunct to vasospastic therapy; investigational glutamate receptor antagonist for neurodegenerative disorders* [also: dextrorphan HCl]
dextrorphan HCl USAN *adjunct to vasospastic therapy; investigational glutamate receptor antagonist for neurodegenerative disorders* [also: dextrorphan]
dextrose USP *fluid and nutrient replenisher; parenteral antihypoglycemic*
5% Dextrose and Electrolyte #48; 5% Dextrose and Electrolyte #75; 10% Dextrose and Electrolyte #48 IV infusion ℞ *intravenous nutritional/electrolyte therapy* [combined electrolyte solution; dextrose]
dextrose excipient NF *tablet excipient*
50% Dextrose with Electrolyte Pattern A (or N) IV infusion ℞ *intravenous nutritional/electrolyte therapy* [combined electrolyte solution; dextrose]
Dextrostat tablets ℞ *amphetamine; CNS stimulant* [dextroamphetamine sulfate] 5 mg
Dextrostix reagent strips for home use *in vitro diagnostic aid for blood glucose*
dextrothyronine [see: detrothyronine]
dextrothyroxine BAN *antihyperlipidemic* [also: dextrothyroxine sodium]
dextrothyroxine sodium USAN, USP, INN *antihyperlipidemic* [also: dextrothyroxine]
dexverapamil INN *investigational adjunct to chemotherapy*
Dey-Dose (delivery system) *nebulizer*
Dey-Lute (delivery system) *nebulizer*
Dey-Pak Sodium Chloride 3% & 10% solution ℞ *for inducing sputum production for specimen collection* [sodium chloride] 3%; 10%
dezaguanine USAN, INN *antineoplastic*
dezaguanine mesylate USAN *antineoplastic*
dezinamide USAN, INN *anticonvulsant*
dezocine USAN, INN *narcotic analgesic*
DFMO (difluoromethylornithine) [see: eflornithine]
DFMO (difluoromethylornithine) HCl [see: eflornithine HCl]
DFMO-MGBG (eflornithine, mitoguazone) *chemotherapy protocol* [also see: DFMO; MGBG]
DFP (diisopropyl flurophosphate) [see: isoflurophate]
DFV (DDP, fluorouracil, VePesid) *chemotherapy protocol*
DHA (docosahexaenoic acid) [also: doconexent]
DHAP (dexamethasone, high-dose ara-C, Platinol) *chemotherapy protocol for non-Hodgkin lymphoma*
DHC Plus capsules ℞ *narcotic analgesic* [dihydrocodeine bitartrate; acetaminophen; caffeine] 16•356.4•30 mg
DHE (dihydroergotamine) [see: dihydroergotamine mesylate]
D.H.E. 45 IV or IM injection ℞ *migraine prophylaxis or treatment* [dihydroergotamine mesylate] 1 mg/mL
DHEA (dehydroepiandrosterone) [q.v.]
DHPG (dihydroxy propoxymethyl guanine) [see: ganciclovir]
DHS Tar liquid shampoo, gel shampoo OTC *antiseborrheic; antipsoriatic; antipruritic; antibacterial* [coal tar] 0.5%

DHS Zinc shampoo OTC *antiseborrheic; antibacterial; antifungal* [pyrithione zinc] 2%

DHT tablets, Intensol (concentrated oral solution) ℞ *vitamin D therapy for tetany and hypoparathyroidism* [dihydrotachysterol] 0.125, 0.2, 0.4 mg; 0.2 mg/mL

DHT (dihydrotachysterol) [q.v.]

DHT (dihydrotestosterone) [see: androstanolone; stanolone]

DI (doxorubicin, ifosfamide [with mesna rescue]) *chemotherapy protocol for soft tissue sarcoma*

Diab II ℞ *investigational treatment for type 2 diabetes*

Diaβeta (or DiaBeta) tablets ℞ *sulfonylurea antidiabetic* [glyburide] 1.25, 2.5, 5 mg

Diabetic Tussin liquid OTC *antitussive; decongestant; expectorant* [dextromethorphan hydrobromide; phenylephrine HCl; guaifenesin] 10•5•100 mg/5 mL

Diabetic Tussin DM liquid OTC *antitussive; expectorant* [dextromethorphan hydrobromide; guaifenesin] 10•100 mg/5 mL

Diabetic Tussin EX liquid OTC *expectorant* [guaifenesin] 100 mg/5 mL

Diabinese tablets ℞ *sulfonylurea antidiabetic* [chlorpropamide] 100, 250 mg

diacerein INN

diacetamate INN, BAN

diacetolol INN, BAN *antiadrenergic (β-receptor)* [also: diacetolol HCl]

diacetolol HCl USAN *antiadrenergic (β-receptor)* [also: diacetolol]

diacetoxyphenylisatin [see: oxyphenisatin acetate]

diacetoxyphenyloxindol [see: oxyphenisatin acetate]

diacetrizoate sodium [see: diatrizoate sodium]

diacetyl diaminodiphenylsulfone (DADDS) [see: acedapsone]

diacetylated monoglycerides NF *plasticizer*

diacetylcholine chloride [see: succinylcholine chloride]

diacetyl-dihydroxydiphenylisatin [see: oxyphenisatin acetate]

diacetyldioxphenylisatin [see: oxyphenisatin acetate]

diacetylmorphine HCl USP *(heroin; banned in USA)* [also: diamorphine]

diacetylmorphine salts *(heroin; banned in USA)*

diacetylsalicylic acid [see: dipyrocetyl]

diacetyltannic acid [see: acetyltannic acid]

diacetylthiamine [see: acetiamine]

diagniol [see: sodium acetrizoate]

diallybarbituric acid [see: allobarbital]

diallylbarbituric acid [now: allobarbital]

diallylnortoxiferene dichloride [see: alcuronium chloride]

diallymal [see: allobarbital]

Dialose tablets (discontinued 1999) OTC *stool softener* [docusate sodium] 100 mg

Dialose Plus tablets, capsules (discontinued 1998) OTC *stimulant laxative; stool softener* [yellow phenolphthalein; docusate sodium] 65•100 mg

Dialpak (trademarked packaging form) *reusable patient compliance package for oral contraceptives*

Dialume capsules ℞ *antacid* [aluminum hydroxide gel] 500 mg ⑨ Dalmane

Dialyte Pattern LM solution ℞ *peritoneal dialysis solution* [multiple electrolytes; dextrose] 1.5%•≛, 2.5%•≛, 4.5%•≛

dia-mer-sulfonamides (sulfadiazine & sulfamerazine) [q.v.]

diamethine [see: dimethyltubocurarinium chloride; dimethyltubocurarine]

diamfenetide INN [also: diamphenethide]

Diamine T.D. timed-release tablets (discontinued 1997) ℞ *antihistamine* [brompheniramine maleate] 8, 12 mg

diaminedipenicillin G [see: penicillin G benzathine]

diaminodiphenylsulfone (DDS) [now: dapsone]

3,4-diaminopyridine *investigational (orphan) for Lambert-Eaton myasthenic syndrome*

***cis*-diamminedichloroplatinum (DDP)** [see: cisplatin]
diammonium phosphate [see: ammonium phosphate]
diamocaine INN, BAN *local anesthetic* [also: diamocaine cyclamate]
diamocaine cyclamate USAN *local anesthetic* [also: diamocaine]
diamorphine BAN *(heroin; banned in the U.S.)* [also: diacetylmorphine HCl]
Diamox powder for IV injection ℞ *carbonic anhydrase inhibitor diuretic; antiglaucoma; anticonvulsant; treatment for acute mountain sickness* [acetazolamide sodium] 500 mg
Diamox tablets, Sequels (sustained-release capsules) ℞ *carbonic anhydrase inhibitor diuretic; antiglaucoma; anticonvulsant; treatment for acute mountain sickness* [acetazolamide] 125, 250 mg; 500 mg
diamphenethide BAN [also: diamfenetide]
diampromide INN, BAN
diampron [see: amicarbalide]
diamthazole BAN [also: dimazole]
diamthazole dihydrochloride [see: diamthazole]
Dianabol tablets (discontinued 1982) ℞ *steroid; discontinued for human use, but the veterinary product is still available and sometimes abused as a street drug* [methandrostenolone] 2.5, 5 mg
Diane-35 (CAN) sugar-coated tablets ℞ *antiandrogen/estrogen for severe acne in women* [cyproterone acetate; ethinyl estradiol] 2•0.035 mg
Dianeal Peritoneal Dialysis Solution with 1.1% Amino Acids ℞ *investigational (orphan) nutritional supplement for continuous ambulatory peritoneal dialysis patients*
diapamide USAN *diuretic; antihypertensive* [also: tiamizide]
Diaparene Baby cream OTC *topical diaper rash treatment*
Diaparene Cornstarch Baby powder OTC *topical diaper rash treatment* [corn starch; aloe]
Diaparene Diaper Rash ointment OTC *topical diaper rash treatment* [zinc oxide]
Diaper Guard ointment OTC *topical diaper rash treatment* [dimethicone; vitamins A, D, and E; zinc oxide] 1%•≛•≟
Diaper Rash ointment OTC *topical diaper rash treatment* [zinc oxide]
diaphene [see: dibromsalan]
diaphenylsulfone [see: dapsone]
diaphoretics *a class of agents that promote profuse perspiration* [also called: sudorifics]
Diapid nasal spray (discontinued 2001) ℞ *pituitary antidiuretic hormone for diabetes insipidus* [lypressin] 50 U/mL
Diar-Aid tablets OTC *antidiarrheal; GI adsorbent* [loperamide HCl] 2 mg
diarbarone INN
Diascan reagent strips for home use *in vitro diagnostic aid for blood glucose*
DiaScreen reagent strips for professional use *in vitro diagnostic aid for multiple disease markers in the urine*
Diasorb tablets, liquid OTC *antidiarrheal; GI adsorbent* [activated attapulgite] 750 mg; 750 mg/5 mL
Diastat rectal gel in a disposable applicator ("pediatric" and "adult" refer to the length of the applicator tip) ℞ *benzodiazepine anticonvulsant for acute repetitive seizures (orphan)* [diazepam] 2.5, 5, 10 mg (pediatric); 10, 15, 20 mg (adult)
Diastix reagent strips for home use *in vitro diagnostic aid for urine glucose*
diathymosulfone INN
diatrizoate meglumine USP *oral/parenteral radiopaque contrast medium (46.67% iodine)* [also: meglumine diatrizoate] 76% injection
diatrizoate methylglucamine [see: diatrizoate meglumine]
diatrizoate sodium USP *oral/rectal/parenteral radiopaque contrast medium (59.87% iodine)* [also: sodium amidotrizoate; sodium diatrizoate]
diatrizoate sodium I 125 USAN *radioactive agent*

diatrizoate sodium I 131 USAN *radioactive agent*
diatrizoic acid USAN, USP, BAN *radiopaque contrast medium* [also: amidotrizoic acid]
diaveridine USAN, INN, BAN *antibacterial*
diazacholesterol dihydrochloride [see: azacosterol HCl]
Diazemuls (CAN) emulsified IV injection ℞ *benzodiazepine sedative; anxiolytic; anticonvulsant; skeletal muscle relaxant* [diazepam] 5 mg/mL
diazepam USAN, USP, INN, BAN, JAN *benzodiazepine anxiolytic; anticonvulsant; sedative; skeletal muscle relaxant; investigational (orphan) for acute repetitive seizures; also abused as a street drug* 2, 5, 10 mg oral; 1, 5 mg/mL oral; 5 mg/mL injection
diazinon BAN [also: dimpylate]
diaziquone USAN, INN *antineoplastic*
diazoxide USAN, USP, INN, BAN *emergency antihypertensive; vasodilator; glucose-elevating agent*
dibasic calcium phosphate [see: calcium phosphate, dibasic]
dibasic potassium phosphate [see: potassium phosphate, dibasic]
dibasic sodium phosphate [see: sodium phosphate, dibasic]
dibasol [see: bendazol]
dibazol [see: bendazol]
dibekacin INN, BAN
dibemethine INN
dibencil [see: penicillin G benzathine]
dibencozide [see: cobamamide]
Dibent IM injection ℞ *GI antispasmodic* [dicyclomine HCl] 10 mg/mL
dibenthiamine [see: bentiamine]
dibenzathione [see: sulbentine]
dibenzepin INN, BAN *antidepressant* [also: dibenzepin HCl]
dibenzepin HCl USAN *antidepressant* [also: dibenzepin]
dibenzodiazepines *a class of novel (atypical) antipsychotic agents*
dibenzothiazepines *a class of novel (atypical) antipsychotic agents*
dibenzothiazine [see: phenothiazine]
dibenzothiophene USAN *keratolytic*
dibenzoxazepines *a class of dopamine receptor antagonists with antipsychotic, hypotensive, antiemetic, antispasmodic, and antihistaminic activity*
dibenzoyl peroxide [see: benzoyl peroxide]
dibenzoylthiamin [see: bentiamine]
dibenzthion [see: sulbentine]
dibenzylethylenediamine dipenicillin G (DBED) [see: penicillin G benzathine]
Dibenzyline capsules ℞ *antihypertensive for pheochromocytoma* [phenoxybenzamine HCl] 10 mg
N,N-dibenzylmethylamine [see: dibemethine]
dibromodulcitol [see: mitolactol]
dibromohydroxyquinoline [see: broxyquinoline]
dibromomannitol (DBM) [see: mitobronitol]
dibromopropamidine BAN [also: dibrompropamidine]
dibrompropamidine INN [also: dibromopropamidine]
dibromsalan USAN, INN *disinfectant*
dibrospidium chloride INN
dibucaine USP *topical local anesthetic* [also: cinchocaine] 1% topical
dibucaine HCl USP *local anesthetic* [also: cinchocaine HCl]
dibudinate INN *combining name for radicals or groups*
dibunate INN *combining name for radicals or groups*
dibuprol INN
dibupyrone INN, BAN
dibusadol INN
dibutoline sulfate
DIC (dimethyl imidazole carboxamide) [see: dacarbazine]
Dical CapTabs (capsule-shaped tablets) OTC *dietary supplement* [dibasic calcium phosphate; vitamin D] 117 mg (Ca)•90 mg (P)•133 IU
dicalcium phosphate [see: calcium phosphate, dibasic]
Dical-D tablets, chewable wafers OTC *dietary supplement* [dibasic calcium phosphate; vitamin D] 117 mg

(Ca)•90 mg (P)•133 IU; 232 mg (Ca)•180 mg (P)•200 IU
dicarbine INN
Dicarbosil chewable tablets (discontinued 1998) OTC *antacid* [calcium carbonate] 500 mg ⑨ dacarbazine
dicarfen INN
dichlofenthion BAN
dichloralantipyrine [see: dichloralphenazone]
dichloralphenazone (chloral hydrate & phenazone) BAN *mild sedative*
dichloralpyrine [see: dichloralphenazone]
dichloramine-T NF
dichloranilino imidazolin [see: clonidine HCl]
dichloren [see: mechlorethamine HCl]
dichlorisone INN
dichlorisone acetate [see: dichlorisone]
dichlormethazanone [see: dichlormezanone]
dichlormezanone INN
dichloroacetic acid *strong keratolytic/cauterant* ⑨ Bichloracetic acid
dichlorodifluoromethane NF *aerosol propellant; topical refrigerant anesthetic*
dichlorodiphenyl trichloroethane (DDT) [see: chlorophenothane]
dichlorometaxylenol [see: dichloroxylenol]
dichloromethane [see: methylene chloride]
dichlorophen INN, BAN
dichlorophenarsine INN, BAN [also: dichlorophenarsine HCl]
dichlorophenarsine HCl USP [also: dichlorophenarsine]
dichlorotetrafluoroethane NF *aerosol propellant; topical refrigerant anesthetic* [also: cryofluorane]
dichlorovinyl dimethyl phosphate (DDVP) [see: dichlorvos]
dichloroxylenol INN, BAN
dichlorphenamide USP, BAN *carbonic anhydrase inhibitor; diuretic* [also: diclofenamide]
dichlorvos USAN, INN, BAN *anthelmintic*
dichysterol [see: dihydrotachysterol]
diciferron INN
dicirenone USAN, INN *hypotensive; aldosterone antagonist*
Dick test (scarlet fever streptococcus toxin)
diclazuril USAN, INN, BAN *coccidiostat for poultry; investigational for cryptosporidiosis in AIDS*
diclofenac INN, BAN *analgesic; antiarthritic; nonsteroidal anti-inflammatory drug (NSAID) for ankylosing spondylitis* [also: diclofenac potassium]
diclofenac potassium USAN *analgesic; antiarthritic; nonsteroidal anti-inflammatory drug (NSAID) for ankylosing spondylitis; topical treatment for actinic keratoses* [also: diclofenac] 50 mg oral
diclofenac sodium USAN, JAN *analgesic; antiarthritic; nonsteroidal anti-inflammatory drug (NSAID) for ankylosing spondylitis; ocular treatment for cataract extraction; topical treatment for actinic keratoses (AK)* 25, 50, 75, 100 mg oral; 0.1% eye drops
diclofenamide INN *carbonic anhydrase inhibitor* [also: dichlorphenamide]
diclofensine INN
diclofibrate [see: simfibrate]
diclofurime INN
diclometide INN
diclonixin INN
dicloralurea USAN, INN *veterinary food additive*
Diclotec (CAN) suppositories ℞ *nonsteroidal anti-inflammatory drug (NSAID); antiarthritic; analgesic* [diclofenac sodium] 50, 100 mg
dicloxacillin USAN, INN, BAN *penicillinase-resistant penicillin antibiotic*
dicloxacillin sodium USAN, USP, BAN *penicillinase-resistant penicillin antibiotic* 250, 500 mg oral
dicobalt edetate INN, BAN
dicolinium iodide INN
dicophane BAN [also: chlorophenothane; clofenotane]
dicoumarin [see: dicumarol]
dicoumarol INN *coumarin-derivative anticoagulant* [also: dicumarol]
dicresulene INN

Dictamnus albus *medicinal herb* [see: fraxinella]

dicumarol USAN, USP *coumarin-derivative anticoagulant* [also: dicoumarol] 25 mg oral ⊠ Demerol

dicyclomine BAN *anticholinergic* [also: dicyclomine HCl; dicycloverine]

dicyclomine HCl USP *GI antispasmodic; anticholinergic* [also: dicycloverine; dicyclomine] 10, 20 mg oral; 10 mg/5 mL oral; 10 mg/mL injection

dicycloverine INN *anticholinergic* [also: dicyclomine HCl; dicyclomine]

dicycloverine HCl [see: dicyclomine HCl]

dicysteine [see: cystine]

didanosine USAN, INN, BAN *antiviral nucleoside reverse transcriptase inhibitor (NRTI) for HIV-1 infections*

didanosine & nevirapine & zidovudine *investigational (Phase III) antiviral combination for HIV infection*

didanosine & zidovudine *investigational (Phase II) heterodimer antiviral combination for AIDS*

didehydrodideoxythymidine [see: stavudine]

Di-Delamine gel, spray OTC *topical antihistamine; bacteriostatic* [diphenhydramine HCl; tripelennamine HCl] 1%•0.5%

dideoxycytidine (DDC; ddC) [see: zalcitabine]

dideoxyinosine (DDI; ddI) [see: didanosine]

Didrex tablets ℞ *anorexiant* [benzphetamine HCl] 25, 50 mg

Didrocal (CAN) tablets (in a 90-day therapy pack) ℞ *bisphosphonate bone resorption inhibitor plus calcium supplement for established postmenopausal osteoporosis* [Phase 1 (14 days): etidronate disodium; Phase 2 (76 days): calcium carbonate] 400 mg; 1250 mg

Didro-Kit (Italian name for U.S. product Didronel)

Didronel IV infusion ℞ *bisphosphonate bone resorption inhibitor for hypercalcemia of malignancy (orphan)* [etidronate disodium] 300 mg/ampule

Didronel tablets ℞ *bisphosphonate bone resorption inhibitor for Paget disease and heterotopic ossification* [etidronate disodium] 200, 400 mg

didrovaltrate INN

didroxane [see: dichlorophen]

dieldrin INN, BAN

dielytra; choice dielytra *medicinal herb* [see: turkey corn]

diemal [see: barbital]

dienestrol USP, INN *estrogen* [also: dienoestrol]

dienoestrol BAN *estrogen* [also: dienestrol]

dienogest INN

Diet Ayds candy OTC *decrease taste perception of sweetness* [benzocaine] 6 mg

dietamiphylline [see: etamiphyllin]

dietamiverine HCl [see: bietamiverine HCl]

diethadione INN, BAN

diethanolamine NF *alkalizing agent*

diethazine INN, BAN

diethazine HCl [see: diethazine]

diethyl phthalate NF *plasticizer*

diethylamine *p*-aminobenzenestibonate [see: stibosamine]

3-diethylaminobutyranilide [see: octacaine]

diethylbarbiturate monosodium [see: barbital sodium]

diethylbarbituric acid [see: barbital]

diethylcarbamazine INN, BAN *anthelmintic for Bancroft filariasis, onchocerciasis, tropical eosinophilia, and loiasis* [also: diethylcarbamazine citrate]

diethylcarbamazine citrate USP *anthelmintic for Bancroft filariasis, onchocerciasis, tropical eosinophilia, and loiasis* [also: diethylcarbamazine]

diethylcarbamazine dihydrogen citrate [see: diethylcarbamazine citrate]

diethyldithiocarbamate *investigational (Phase II/III, orphan) immunomodulator for HIV and AIDS*

diethyldixanthogen [see: dixanthogen]

diethylenediamine citrate [see: piperazine citrate]

diethylenetriaminepentaacetic acid (DTPA) [see: pentetic acid]

diethylhomospermine (DEHOP; DEHSPM) *investigational (Phase II) polyamine analogue for AIDS-related non-Hodgkin lymphoma and uncontrolled, refractory diarrhea*

N,N-diethyllysergamide [see: lysergide]

diethylmalonylurea [see: barbital]

diethylmalonylurea sodium [see: barbital sodium]

N,N-diethylnicotinamide [see: nikethamide]

diethylnorspermine *investigational (Phase I) anticancer agent*

diethylpropion BAN *anorexiant; CNS stimulant* [also: diethylpropion HCl; amfepramone] 75 mg oral

diethylpropion HCl USP *anorexiant; CNS stimulant* [also: amfepramone; diethylpropion] 25 mg oral

diethylstilbestrol (DES) USP, INN *hormonal antineoplastic for inoperable prostatic and breast cancer* [also: stilboestrol] 1, 5 mg oral

diethylstilbestrol diphosphate USP *hormonal antineoplastic for palliative therapy of advanced prostatic carcinoma* [also: fosfestrol]

diethylstilbestrol dipropionate NF

***p*-diethylsulfamoylbenzoic acid** [see: etebenecid; ethebenecid]

diethylthiambutene INN, BAN

diethyltoluamide (DEET) USP, BAN *arthropod repellent*

diethyltryptamine (DET) *a hallucinogenic street drug closely related to dimethyltryptamine (DMT), but prepared synthetically*

N,N-diethylvanillamide [see: ethamivan]

dietifen INN

dietroxine [see: diethadione]

Dieutrim T.D. timed-release capsules OTC *diet aid; decrease perception of sweetness* [phenylpropanolamine HCl; benzocaine] 75•9 mg

diexanthogen [see: dixanthogen]

difebarbamate INN

difemerine INN [also: difemerine HCl]

difemerine HCl [also: difemerine]

difemetorex INN

difenamizole INN

difencloxazine INN

difencloxazine HCl [see: difencloxazine]

difenidol INN *antiemetic; antivertigo* [also: diphenidol]

difenoximide INN *antiperistaltic* [also: difenoximide HCl]

difenoximide HCl USAN *antiperistaltic* [also: difenoximide]

difenoxin USAN, INN, BAN *antiperistaltic*

difenoxin HCl *antiperistaltic*

difetarsone INN, BAN

difeterol INN

Differin solution, gel, cream, single-use pledgets ℞ *synthetic retinoid analogue for acne* [adapalene] 0.1%

diflorasone INN, BAN *topical corticosteroidal anti-inflammatory* [also: diflorasone diacetate]

diflorasone diacetate USAN, USP *topical corticosteroidal anti-inflammatory* [also: diflorasone] 0.05% topical

difloxacin INN *anti-infective; DNA gyrase inhibitor* [also: difloxacin HCl]

difloxacin HCl USAN *anti-infective; DNA gyrase inhibitor* [also: difloxacin]

difluanazine INN *CNS stimulant* [also: difluanine HCl]

difluanazine HCl [see: difluanine HCl]

difluanine HCl USAN *CNS stimulant* [also: difluanazine]

Diflucan tablets, powder for oral suspension, IV infusion ℞ *systemic triazole antifungal* [fluconazole] 50, 100, 150, 200 mg; 10, 40 mg/mL; 2 mg/mL

diflucortolone USAN, INN, BAN *corticosteroid; anti-inflammatory*

diflucortolone pivalate USAN *corticosteroid; anti-inflammatory*

diflumidone INN, BAN *anti-inflammatory* [also: diflumidone sodium]

diflumidone sodium USAN *anti-inflammatory* [also: diflumidone]

diflunisal USAN, USP, INN, BAN *anti-inflammatory; analgesic; antipyretic; antiarthritic; antirheumatic* 250, 500 mg oral

difluoromethylornithine (DFMO) [see: eflornithine]

difluoromethylornithine HCl [see: eflornithine HCl]
difluprednate USAN, INN *anti-inflammatory*
difolliculin [see: estradiol benzoate]
diftalone USAN, INN *anti-inflammatory*
digalloyl trioleate USAN
Di-Gel liquid OTC *antacid; antiflatulent* [aluminum hydroxide; magnesium hydroxide; simethicone] 200•200•20 mg/5 mL
Di-Gel, Advanced Formula chewable tablets OTC *antacid; antiflatulent* [magnesium hydroxide; calcium carbonate; simethicone] 128•280•20 mg
Digepepsin dual-coated tablets ℞ *digestive enzymes* [pancreatin; pepsin; bile salts] 300•250•150 mg
digestants; digestives *a class of agents that promote or aid in digestion*
Digestozyme tablets ℞ *digestive enzymes; laxative; choleretic* [pancreatin; pepsin; dehydrocholic acid] 300•250•25 mg
Digibind powder for IV injection ℞ *antidote to digoxin/digitoxin overdose (orphan); investigational (orphan) for other cardiac glycoside intoxication* [digoxin immune Fab (ovine)] 38 mg/vial
Digidote ℞ *antidote to digoxin/digitoxin overdose (orphan); investigational (orphan) for other cardiac glycoside intoxication* [digoxin immune Fab (ovine)]
digitalis USP *cardiotonic*
Digitalis ambigua; D. ferriginea; D. grandiflora; D. lanata; D. lutea; D. purpurea *medicinal herb* [see: foxglove]
digitalis glycosides *a class of cardiovascular drugs that increase the force of cardiac contractions* [also called: cardiac glycosides]
Digitek tablets ℞ *cardiac glycoside to increase cardiac output; antiarrhythmic* [digoxin] 0.125, 0.25 mg
digitoxin USP, INN, BAN *cardiotonic; cardiac glycoside* ⊠ Desoxyn; digoxin
digitoxin, acetyl [see: acetyldigitoxin]
α-digitoxin monoacetate [see: acetyldigitoxin]
digitoxoside [see: digitoxin]
digolil INN *combining name for radicals or groups*
digoxin USP, INN, BAN *cardiotonic; cardiac glycoside antiarrhythmic* 0.125, 0.25 mg oral, 0.05 mg/mL oral, 0.1, 0.25 mg/mL injection ⊠ Desoxyn; digitoxin
digoxin antibody [see: digoxin immune Fab]
digoxin immune Fab (ovine) *antidote to digoxin/digitoxin intoxication (orphan); investigational (orphan) for other cardiac glycoside intoxication*
Digoxin Injection C.S.D. (CAN) ℞ *cardiac glycoside to increase cardiac output; antiarrhythmic* [digoxin] 0.25 mg/mL
Digoxin Pediatric Injection C.S.D. (CAN) ℞ *cardiac glycoside to increase cardiac output; antiarrhythmic* [digoxin] 0.05 mg/mL
dihexyverine INN *anticholinergic* [also: dihexyverine HCl]
dihexyverine HCl USAN *anticholinergic* [also: dihexyverine]
Dihistine DH liquid OTC *narcotic antitussive; decongestant; antihistamine* [codeine phosphate; pseudoephedrine HCl; chlorpheniramine maleate; alcohol] 10•30•2 mg/5 mL
Dihistine Expectorant liquid ℞ *narcotic antitussive; decongestant; expectorant* [codeine phosphate; pseudoephedrine HCl; guaifenesin; alcohol] 10•30•100 mg/5 mL
dihydan soluble [see: phenytoin sodium]
dihydralazine INN, BAN
dihydralazine sulfate [see: dihydralazine]
5,6-dihydro-5-azacytidine *investigational (orphan) for malignant mesothelioma*
dihydrobenzthiazide [see: hydrobentizide]
dihydrocodeine INN, BAN *analgesic* [also: dihydrocodeine bitartrate]

dihydrocodeine bitartrate USP *analgesic* [also: dihydrocodeine]
dihydrocodeinone bitartrate [see: hydrocodone bitartrate]
dihydroergocornine [see: ergoloid mesylates]
dihydroergocristine [see: ergoloid mesylates]
dihydroergocryptine [see: ergoloid mesylates]
dihydroergotamine (DHE) INN, BAN *antiadrenergic; anticoagulant; ergot alkaloid for rapid control of migraines* [also: dihydroergotamine mesylate; dihydroergotamine mesilate]
dihydroergotamine mesilate JAN *antiadrenergic; anticoagulant; ergot alkaloid for rapid control of migraines* [also: dihydroergotamine mesylate; dihydroergotamine]
dihydroergotamine mesylate USAN, USP *antiadrenergic; anticoagulant; ergot alkaloid for rapid control of migraines* [also: dihydroergotamine; dihydroergotamine mesilate]
dihydroergotamine methanesulfonate [see: dihydroergotamine mesylate]
dihydroergotoxine mesylate [now: ergoloid mesylates]
dihydroergotoxine methanesulfonate [now: ergoloid mesylates]
dihydroethaverine [see: drotaverine]
dihydrofollicular hormone [see: estradiol]
dihydrofolliculine [see: estradiol]
dihydrogenated ergot alkaloids [now: ergoloid mesylates]
dihydrohydroxycodeinone [see: oxycodone]
dihydrohydroxycodeinone HCl [see: oxycodone HCl]
6-dihydro-6-iminopurine [see: adenine]
dihydroindolones *a class of dopamine receptor antagonists with conventional (typical) antipsychotic activity* [also called: indolones]
dihydroisoperparine [see: drotaverine]
dihydromorphinone HCl [now: hydromorphone HCl]
dihydroneopine [see: dihydrocodeine bitartrate]
dihydropyridines *a class of calcium channel blockers*
dihydrostreptomycin (DST) INN *antibacterial* [also: dihydrostreptomycin sulfate]
dihydrostreptomycin sulfate USP *antibacterial* [also: dihydrostreptomycin]
dihydrostreptomycin-streptomycin [see: streptoduocin]
dihydrotachysterol (DHT) USP, INN, BAN, JAN *fat-soluble vitamin; synthetic reduction product of a vitamin D isomer; calcium regulator for tetany and hypoparathyroidism* 0.125, 0.2, 0.4 mg oral; 0.2 mg/mL oral
dihydrotestosterone (DHT) *investigational (Phase II, orphan) steroid for AIDS-wasting syndrome* [see: androstanolone; stanolone]
dihydrotheelin [see: estradiol]
dihydroxy(stearato)aluminum [see: aluminum monostearate]
dihydroxy propoxymethyl guanine (DHPG) [see: gancyclovir]
dihydroxyacetone *skin darkener for vitiligo and hypopigmented areas*
dihydroxyaluminum aminoacetate (DAA) USP *antacid*
dihydroxyaluminum sodium carbonate USP *antacid*
dihydroxyanthranol [see: anthralin]
dihydroxyanthraquinone *(withdrawn from market)* [see: danthron]
1,25-dihydroxycholecalciferol [see: calcitriol]
24,25-dihydroxycholecalciferol *investigational (orphan) for uremic osteodystrophy*
dihydroxyestrin [see: estradiol]
dihydroxyfluorane [see: fluorescein]
dihydroxyphenylalanine (DOPA) [see: levodopa]
dihydroxyphenylisatin [see: oxyphenisatin acetate]
dihydroxyphenyloxindol [see: oxyphenisatin acetate]

dihydroxyprogesterone acetophenide [see: algestone acetophenide]
dihydroxypropyl theophylline [see: dyphylline]
diiodobuphenine [see: bufeniode]
diiodohydroxyquin [now: iodoquinol]
diiodohydroxyquinoline INN, BAN *antiamebic* [also: iodoquinol]
diisopromine INN
diisopromine HCl [see: diisopromine]
diisopropanolamine NF *alkalizing agent*
diisopropyl flurophosphate (DFP) [see: isoflurophate]
diisopropyl flurophosphonate [see: isoflurophate]
diisopropyl phosphorofluoridate [see: isoflurophate]
2,6-diisopropylphenol [see: propofol]
Dilacor XR sustained-release capsules ℞ *antihypertensive; antianginal; antiarrhythmic; calcium channel blocker* [diltiazem HCl] 120, 180, 240 mg ⊠ Delcort
Dilantin Infatabs (chewable tablets) ℞ *hydantoin anticonvulsant* [phenytoin] 50 mg ⊠ Milontin; Mylanta; Xalatan
Dilantin Kapseals (capsules) ℞ *hydantoin anticonvulsant* [phenytoin sodium] 30, 100 mg ⊠ Milontin; Mylanta; Xalatan
Dilantin-125 oral suspension ℞ *hydantoin anticonvulsant* [phenytoin] 125 mg/5 mL ⊠ Milontin; Mylanta; Xalatan
Dilatrate-SR sustained-release capsules ℞ *antianginal; vasodilator* [isosorbide dinitrate] 40 mg
Dilaudid tablets, oral liquid, subcu or IM injection, suppositories ℞ *narcotic analgesic; widely abused as a street drug* [hydromorphone HCl] 2, 4, 8 mg; 5 mg/5 mL; 1, 2, 4 mg/mL; 3 mg
Dilaudid Cough syrup ℞ *narcotic antitussive; expectorant* [hydromorphone HCl; guaifenesin; alcohol 5%] 1•100 mg/5 mL
Dilaudid-HP subcu or IM injection ℞ *narcotic analgesic* [hydromorphone HCl] 10 mg/mL (250 mg/vial)
dilazep INN
dilevalol INN, BAN *antihypertensive; antiadrenergic (β-receptor)* [also: dilevalol HCl]
dilevalol HCl USAN, JAN *antihypertensive; antiadrenergic (β-receptor)* [also: dilevalol]
dilithium carbonate [see: lithium carbonate]
dill *(Anethum graveolens)* fruit and seed *medicinal herb used as an aromatic, carminative, diaphoretic, stimulant, and stomachic*
dilmefone INN
Dilocaine injection ℞ *injectable local anesthetic* [lidocaine HCl] 1%, 2%
Dilor tablets, elixir, IM injection ℞ *antiasthmatic; bronchodilator* [dyphylline] 200 mg; 160 mg/15 mL; 250 mg/mL
Dilor 400 tablets ℞ *antiasthmatic; bronchodilator* [dyphylline] 400 mg
Dilor-G tablets, liquid ℞ *antiasthmatic; bronchodilator; expectorant* [dyphylline; guaifenesin] 200•200 mg; 300•300 mg/15 mL
diloxanide INN, BAN, DCF
diloxanide furoate *investigational anti-infective for amebiasis (available only from the Centers for Disease Control and Prevention)*
Diltia XT sustained-release capsules ℞ *antihypertensive; calcium channel blocker* [diltiazem HCl] 120, 180, 240 mg
diltiazem INN, BAN *coronary vasodilator; calcium channel blocker; antianginal; antihypertensive* [also: diltiazem HCl]
diltiazem HCl USAN, USP, JAN *coronary vasodilator; calcium channel blocker; antianginal; antihypertensive; antiarrhythmic* [also: diltiazem] 30, 60, 90, 120, 180, 240 mg oral; 5 mg/mL injection
diltiazem malate USAN *coronary vasodilator; calcium channel blocker; antianginal; antihypertensive; antiarrhythmic*
Dilusol (CAN) OTC *topical solution base* [ethyl alcohol] 38.7%
Dilusol AHA (CAN) OTC *topical solution base* [ethyl alcohol; glycolic acid] 38.7%•8%

diluted acetic acid [see: acetic acid, diluted]
diluted alcohol [see: alcohol, diluted]
diluted hydrochloric acid [see: hydrochloric acid, diluted]
diluted sodium hypochlorite [see: sodium hypochlorite, diluted]
dimabefylline INN
Dimacol caplets OTC *antitussive; decongestant; expectorant* [dextromethorphan hydrobromide; pseudoephedrine HCl; guaifenesin] 10•30•100 mg ⑨ dimercaprol
dimantine INN *anthelmintic* [also: dymanthine HCl]
dimantine HCl INN [also: dymanthine HCl]
Dimaphen tablets, Release-Tabs (timed-release tablets), elixir OTC *decongestant; antihistamine* [phenylpropanolamine HCl; brompheniramine maleate] 25•4 mg; 75•12 mg; 12.5•2 mg/5 mL
dimazole INN [also: diamthazole]
dimazole dihydrochloride [see: dimazole; diamthazole]
dimecamine INN
dimecolonium iodide INN
dimecrotic acid INN
dimedrol [see: diphenhydramine HCl]
dimefadane USAN, INN *analgesic*
dimefilcon A USAN *hydrophilic contact lens material*
dimefline INN, BAN *respiratory stimulant* [also: dimefline HCl]
dimefline HCl USAN *respiratory stimulant* [also: dimefline]
dimefocon A USAN *hydrophobic contact lens material*
dimekolin [see: dimecolonium iodide]
dimelazine INN
dimelin [see: dimecolonium iodide]
dimemorfan INN
dimenhydrinate USP, INN, BAN *antiemetic; anticholinergic; antivertigo; motion sickness prophylaxis* 50 mg oral; 12.5 mg/4 mL oral; 50 mg/mL injection ⑨ diphenhydramine
dimenoxadol INN [also: dimenoxadole]
dimenoxadole BAN [also: dimenoxadol]
dimepheptanol INN, BAN
dimepranol INN *immunomodulator* [also: dimepranol acedoben]
dimepranol acedoben USAN *immunomodulator* [also: dimepranol]
dimepregnen INN, BAN
dimepropion BAN [also: metamfepramone]
dimeprozan INN
dimeprozinum [see: dimeprozan]
dimercaprol USP, INN *antidote to arsenic, gold and mercury poisoning; lead poisoning adjunct; chelating agent* ⑨ Dimacol
dimercaptopropanol [see: dimercaprol]
2,3-dimercaptosuccinic acid (DMSA) [see: succimer]
dimesna INN
dimesone INN, BAN
Dimetabs tablets ℞ *anticholinergic; antiemetic; antivertigo agent; motion sickness preventative* [dimenhydrinate] 50 mg ⑨ Dimetane; Dimetapp
dimetacrine INN
dimetamfetamine INN
Dimetane Extentabs (long-acting tablets) (discontinued 1997) OTC *antihistamine* [brompheniramine maleate] 12 mg ⑨ Dimetabs
Dimetane Decongestant caplets, elixir OTC *decongestant; antihistamine* [phenylephrine HCl; brompheniramine maleate] 10•4 mg; 5•2 mg/5 mL
Dimetane-DC Cough syrup ℞ *narcotic antitussive; decongestant; antihistamine* [codeine phosphate; phenylpropanolamine HCl; brompheniramine maleate; alcohol 0.95%] 10•12.5•2 mg/5 mL
Dimetane-DX Cough syrup ℞ *antitussive; decongestant; antihistamine* [dextromethorphan hydrobromide; pseudoephedrine HCl; brompheniramine maleate; alcohol 0.95%] 10•30•2 mg/5 mL
Dimetapp tablets, Extentabs (long-acting tablets), elixir OTC *decongestant; antihistamine* [phenylpropanolamine HCl; brompheniramine

maleate] 25•4 mg; 75•12 mg; 12.5•2 mg/5 mL ⊠ Dimetabs

Dimetapp 4-Hour Liqui-Gels (liquid-filled capsules) OTC *decongestant; antihistamine* [phenylpropanolamine HCl; brompheniramine maleate] 25•4 mg

Dimetapp Allergy liqui-gels (discontinued 2001) OTC *antihistamine* [brompheniramine maleate] 4 mg

Dimetapp Cold & Allergy chewable tablets, quick-dissolve tablets OTC *pediatric decongestant and antihistamine* [phenylpropanolamine HCl; brompheniramine maleate] 6.25•1 mg

Dimetapp Cold & Flu caplets OTC *decongestant; antihistamine; analgesic* [phenylpropanolamine HCl; brompheniramine maleate; acetaminophen] 12.5•2•500 mg

Dimetapp DM Cold & Cough elixir OTC *antitussive; decongestant; antihistamine* [dextromethorphan hydrobromide; pseudoephedrine HCl; brompheniramine maleate] 5•60•1 mg/5 mL

Dimetapp Sinus caplets OTC *decongestant; analgesic* [pseudoephedrine HCl; ibuprofen] 30•200 mg

dimethadione USAN, INN *anticonvulsant*

dimethazan

dimethazine [see: mebolazine]

dimethicone USAN, NF, BAN *lubricant and hydrophobing agent; soft tissue prosthetic aid* [also: dimeticone] ⊠ cimetidine

dimethicone 350 USAN *soft tissue prosthetic aid*

dimethindene BAN *antihistamine* [also: dimethindene maleate; dimetindene]

dimethindene maleate USP *antihistamine* [also: dimetindene; dimethindene]

dimethiodal sodium INN

dimethisoquin BAN [also: dimethisoquin HCl; quinisocaine]

dimethisoquin HCl USAN [also: quinisocaine; dimethisoquin]

dimethisterone USAN, NF, INN, BAN *progestin*

dimetholizine INN

dimethothiazine BAN *serotonin inhibitor* [also: fonazine mesylate; dimetotiazine]

dimethoxanate INN, BAN

dimethoxanate HCl [see: dimethoxanate]

2,5-dimethoxy-4-methylamphetamine (DOM) *a hallucinogenic street drug derived from amphetamine, popularly called STP*

dimethoxyphenyl penicillin sodium [see: methicillin sodium]

dimethpyridene maleate [see: dimethindene maleate]

dimethyl ketone [see: acetone]

dimethyl phthalate USP

dimethyl polysiloxane [see: dimethicone]

dimethyl sulfoxide (DMSO) USAN, USP, INN *solvent; topical anti-inflammatory for scleroderma; symptomatic relief of interstitial cystitis; investigational (orphan) for traumatic brain coma; investigational (orphan) topical treatment for extravasation of cytotoxic drugs* [also: dimethyl sulphoxide]

dimethyl sulphoxide BAN *topical anti-inflammatory; solvent* [also: dimethyl sulfoxide]

dimethyl triazeno imidazole carboxamide (DIC; DTIC) [see: dacarbazine]

dimethylaminophenazone [see: aminopyrine]

dimethylcysteine [see: penicillamine]

dimethylglycine HCl

dimethylhexestrol [see: methestrol]

1,5-dimethylhexylamine [see: octodrine]

5,5-dimethyl-2,4-oxazolidinedione (DMO) [see: dimethadione]

dimethyloxyquinazine [see: antipyrine]

o,α-dimethylphenethylamine [see: ortetamine]

dimethylsiloxane polymers [see: dimethicone]

dimethylthiambutene INN, BAN

dimethyltryptamine (DMT) *hallucinogenic street drug derived from a plant native to South America and the West Indies*
dimethyltubocurarine BAN [also: dimethyltubocurarinium chloride]
dimethyltubocurarine iodide [see: metocurine iodide]
dimethyltubocurarinium chloride INN [also: dimethyltubocurarine]
dimethylxanthine [see: theophylline]
dimeticone INN *lubricant and hydrophobing agent; soft tissue prosthetic aid* [also: dimethicone]
dimetindene INN *antihistamine* [also: dimethindene maleate; dimethindene]
dimetindene maleate [see: dimethindene maleate]
dimetipirium bromide INN
dimetofrine INN
dimetotiazine INN *serotonin inhibitor* [also: fonazine mesylate; dimethothiazine]
dimetridazole INN, BAN
dimevamide INN
dimevamide sulfate [see: dimevamide]
diminazene INN, BAN
dimoxamine HCl USAN *memory adjuvant*
dimoxaprost INN
dimoxyline INN
dimpylate INN [also: diazinon]
dinaline INN
Dinate IV or IM injection ℞ *anticholinergic; antiemetic; antivertigo agent; motion sickness preventative* [dimenhydrinate] 50 mg/mL
dinazafone INN
diniprofylline INN
dinitolmide INN, BAN
dinitrotoluamide [see: dinitolmide]
dinoprost USAN, INN, BAN *oxytocic; prostaglandin*
dinoprost trometamol BAN *oxytocic; prostaglandin* [also: dinoprost tromethamine]
dinoprost tromethamine USAN *oxytocic; prostaglandin-type abortifacient* [also: dinoprost trometamol]
dinoprostone USAN, INN, BAN *oxytocic for induction of labor; prostaglandin-type abortifacient; cervical ripening agent*
dinsed USAN, INN *coccidiostat for poultry*
Diocto oral liquid, syrup OTC *laxative; stool softener* [docusate sodium] 150 mg/15 mL; 60 mg/15 mL
Diocto-C syrup OTC *stimulant laxative; stool softener* [casanthranol; docusate sodium] 30•60 mg/15 mL
Diocto-K capsules (discontinued 1999) OTC *laxative; stool softener* [docusate potassium] 100 mg
Diocto-K Plus capsules (discontinued 1999) OTC *stimulant laxative; stool softener* [casanthranol; docusate potassium] 30•100 mg
Dioctolose Plus capsules (discontinued 1999) OTC *stimulant laxative; stool softener* [casanthranol; docusate potassium] 30•100 mg
dioctyl calcium sulfosuccinate [now: docusate calcium]
dioctyl potassium sulfosuccinate [now: docusate potassium]
dioctyl sodium sulfosuccinate (DSS) [now: docusate sodium]
Diodex (CAN) eye drops ℞ *topical ophthalmic corticosteroidal anti-inflammatory* [dexamethasone sodium phosphate] 0.1%
diodone INN [also: iodopyracet]
Dioeze capsules (discontinued 1999) OTC *laxative; stool softener* [docusate sodium] 250 mg
diohippuric acid I 125 USAN *radioactive agent*
diohippuric acid I 131 USAN *radioactive agent*
diolamine USAN, INN *combining name for radicals or groups*
diolostene [see: methandriol]
dionin [see: ethylmorphine HCl]
Dionosil Oily suspension for intratracheal use (discontinued 1999) ℞ *radiopaque contrast medium* [propyliodone in peanut oil (56.7% iodine)] 60% (34%)
diophyllin [see: aminophylline]
Dioscorea villosa *medicinal herb* [see: wild yam]

diosmin INN

Diostate D tablets OTC *dietary supplement* [calcium; phosphorus; vitamin D] 114 mg•88 mg•133 IU

diotyrosine I 125 USAN *radioactive agent*

diotyrosine I 131 USAN *radioactive agent*

Dioval XX; Dioval 40 IM injection (discontinued 1998) ℞ *estrogen replacement therapy for postmenopausal symptoms; antineoplastic for prostatic cancer* [estradiol valerate in oil] 20 mg/mL; 40 mg/mL

Diovan capsules ℞ *antihypertensive; angiotensin II receptor antagonist* [valsartan] 80, 160 mg

Diovan HCT tablets ℞ *antihypertensive; angiotensin II receptor antagonist; diuretic* [valsartan; hydrochlorothiazide] 80•12.5, 160•12.5 mg

dioxadilol INN

dioxadrol INN *antidepressant* [also: dioxadrol HCl]

dioxadrol HCl USAN *antidepressant* [also: dioxadrol]

***d*-dioxadrol HCl** [see: dexoxadrol HCl]

dioxamate INN, BAN

dioxaphetyl butyrate INN, BAN

dioxathion BAN [also: dioxation]

dioxation INN [also: dioxathion]

dioxethedrin INN

dioxethedrin HCl [see: dioxethedrin]

dioxifedrine INN

dioxindol [see: oxyphenisatin acetate]

dioxyanthranol [see: anthralin]

dioxyanthraquinone *(withdrawn from market)* [see: danthron]

dioxybenzone USAN, USP, INN *ultraviolet screen*

dipalmitoylphosphatidylcholine (DPPC) [see: colfosceril palmitate]

diparcol HCl [see: diethazine HCl]

dipegyl [see: niacinamide]

dipenicillin G [see: penicillin G benzathine]

dipenine bromide BAN [also: diponium bromide]

Dipentum capsules ℞ *anti-inflammatory for ulcerative colitis* [olsalazine sodium] 250 mg

diperodon USP, INN, BAN *topical anesthetic*

diperodon HCl *topical anesthetic*

diphemanil methylsulfate USP *anticholinergic* [also: diphemanil metilsulfate; diphemanil methylsulphate]

diphemanil methylsulphate BAN *anticholinergic* [also: diphemanil methylsulfate; diphemanil metilsulfate]

diphemanil metilsulfate INN *anticholinergic* [also: diphemanil methylsulfate; diphemanil methylsulphate]

Diphen AF liquid OTC *antihistamine* [diphenhydramine HCl] 6.25 mg/5 mL

Diphen Cough syrup OTC *antihistamine; antitussive* [diphenhydramine HCl; alcohol 5%] 12.5 mg/5 mL

diphenadione USP, INN, BAN

diphenan INN

diphenatil [see: diphemanil methylsulfate]

diphenchloxazine HCl [see: difencloxazine HCl]

diphenesenic acid [see: xenyhexenic acid]

Diphenhist caplets, softgels, liquid OTC *antihistamine* [diphenhydramine HCl] 25 mg; 25 mg; 12.5 mg/5 mL

diphenhydramine INN, BAN *ethanolamine antihistamine; anticholinergic; antiparkinsonian; motion sickness relief* [also: diphenhydramine citrate] ⊡ dimenhydrinate

Diphenhydramine 50 capsules (discontinued 2001) OTC *antihistamine* [diphenhydramine HCl] 50 mg

diphenhydramine citrate USP *ethanolamine antihistamine; anticholinergic; antiparkinsonian; motion sickness relief* [also: diphenhydramine]

diphenhydramine HCl USP, BAN *ethanolamine antihistamine; antitussive; motion sickness preventative; sleep aid* 25, 50 mg oral; 12.5 mg/5 mL oral; 50 mg/mL injection

diphenhydramine theoclate [see: dimenhydrinate]

diphenidol USAN, BAN *antiemetic; antivertigo* [also: difenidol]

diphenidol HCl USAN *antiemetic*
diphenidol pamoate USAN *antiemetic*
diphenmethanil methylsulfate [see: diphemanil methylsulfate]
diphenoxylate INN, BAN *antiperistaltic* [also: diphenoxylate HCl]
diphenoxylate HCl USP *antiperistaltic* [also: diphenoxylate]
diphenylacetylindandione [see: diphenadione]
diphenylalkylamines *a class of calcium channel blockers*
Diphenylan Sodium capsules ℞ *anticonvulsant* [phenytoin sodium] 30, 100 mg ⓢ Diphenylin
diphenylbutazone [see: phenylbutazone]
diphenylbutylpiperidines [see: phenylbutylpiperidines]
diphenylhydantoin [now: phenytoin]
diphenylhydantoin sodium [now: phenytoin sodium]
diphenylisatin [see: oxyphenisatin]
diphenylpyraline INN, BAN *antihistamine* [also: diphenylpyraline HCl]
diphenylpyraline HCl USP *antihistamine* [also: diphenylpyraline]
diphetarsone [see: difetarsone]
diphexamide iodomethylate [see: buzepide metiodide]
diphosphonic acid [see: etidronic acid]
diphosphopyridine nucleotide (DPN) [now: nadide]
diphosphoric acid, tetrasodium salt [see: sodium pyrophosphate]
diphosphothiamin [see: co-carboxylase]
diphoxazide INN
diphtheria antitoxin USP *passive immunizing agent* [also: diphtheria toxoid] 500 U/mL injection
diphtheria CRM_{197} conjugate *carrier protein for hemophilus b and pneumococcal vaccines*
diphtheria equine antitoxin *investigational passive immunizing agent (available only from the Centers for Disease Control and Prevention)*
diphtheria & tetanus toxoids, adsorbed (DT; Td) USP *active immunizing agent* 2•2, 2•5 LfU/0.5 mL injection (adult); 6.7•5 LfU/0.5 mL injection (pediatric)
diphtheria & tetanus toxoids & acellular pertussis (DTaP) vaccine, adsorbed *active immunizing agent*
diphtheria & tetanus toxoids & pertussis vaccine (DTP) USP *active immunizing agent*
diphtheria & tetanus toxoids & whole-cell pertussis vaccine (DTwP) *active immunizing agent*
diphtheria toxin, diagnostic [now: diphtheria toxin for Schick test]
diphtheria toxin, inactivated diagnostic [now: Schick test control]
diphtheria toxin for Schick test USP *dermal diphtheria immunity test*
diphtheria toxoid USP *active immunizing agent* [also: diphtheria antitoxin]
diphtheria toxoid, adsorbed USP *active immunizing agent* 15 LfU/0.5 mL injection
dipipanone INN, BAN
dipipanone HCl [see: dipipanone]
dipiproverine INN
dipiproverine HCl [see: dipiproverine]
dipivalyl epinephrine (DPE) [now: dipivefrin]
dipivefrin USAN *ophthalmic adrenergic* [also: dipivefrine]
dipivefrin HCl USP *topical antiglaucoma agent* 0.1% eye drops
dipivefrine INN, BAN *ophthalmic adrenergic* [also: dipivefrin]
diponium bromide INN [also: dipenine bromide]
dipotassium carbonate [see: potassium carbonate]
dipotassium clorazepate INN *benzodiazepine anxiolytic; minor tranquilizer; anticonvulsant adjunct; alcohol withdrawal aid* [also: clorazepate dipotassium]
dipotassium hydrogen phosphate [see: potassium phosphate, dibasic]
dipotassium phosphate [see: potassium phosphate, dibasic]
dipotassium pyrosulfite [see: potassium metabisulfite]
diprafenone INN

diprenorphine INN, BAN

Diprivan emulsion for IV ℞ *general anesthetic* [propofol] 10 mg/mL

diprobutine INN, BAN

diprofene INN

diprogulic acid INN

diproleandomycin INN

Diprolene ointment, gel, lotion ℞ *topical corticosteroidal anti-inflammatory* [betamethasone dipropionate, augmented] 0.05%

Diprolene AF cream ℞ *topical corticosteroidal anti-inflammatory* [betamethasone dipropionate, augmented] 0.05%

diprophylline INN, BAN *bronchodilator* [also: dyphylline]

dipropylacetic acid [see: valproic acid]

2-dipropylaminoethyl diphenylthioacetate [see: diprofene]

1,1-dipropylbutylamine [see: diprobutine]

diproqualone INN

Diprosone ointment, cream, lotion, aerosol ℞ *topical corticosteroidal anti-inflammatory* [betamethasone dipropionate] 0.05%; 0.05%; 0.05%; 0.1%

diproteverine INN, BAN

diprothazine [see: dimelazine]

diprotrizoate sodium USP [also: sodium diprotrizoate]

diproxadol INN

Dipteryx odorata; D. oppositifolia *medicinal herb* [see: tonka bean]

dipyridamole USAN, USP, INN, BAN *coronary vasodilator; platelet aggregation inhibitor; diagnostic aid for coronary artery function* 25, 50, 75 mg oral

dipyrithione USAN, INN *antibacterial; antifungal*

dipyrocetyl INN

dipyrone USAN, BAN *analgesic; antipyretic* [also: metamizole sodium]

Dirame ℞ *investigational (Phase III) narcotic agonist-antagonist analgesic for moderate to severe pain* [propiram fumarate]

dirithromycin USAN, INN, BAN *macrolide antibiotic* ⑨ clarithromycin; erythromycin

disaccharide tripeptide glycerol dipalmitoyl *investigational (orphan) for pulmonary and hepatic metastases of colorectal adenocarcinoma and osteosarcoma; investigational (Phase II, orphan) for Ewing sarcoma*

Disalcid film-coated tablets, capsules ℞ *analgesic; antipyretic; anti-inflammatory; antirheumatic* [salsalate] 500, 750 mg; 500 mg

disalicylic acid [see: salsalate]

Disanthrol capsules (discontinued 1999) OTC *stimulant laxative; stool softener* [casanthranol; docusate sodium] 30•100 mg

Dis-Co Pack (trademarked packaging form) *unit-dose package*

discutients *a class of agents that cause a dispersal or disappearance of a pathological condition, such as a tumor*

disinfectants *a class of agents that inhibit the growth and development of microorganisms, usually on an inanimate surface, without necessarily killing them* [see also: antiseptics; germicides]

Disinfecting Solution OTC *chemical disinfecting solution for soft contact lenses*

Disipal (CAN) film-coated tablets (discontinued 2001) ℞ *anticholinergic; antiparkinsonian* [orphenadrine HCl] 50 mg

disiquonium chloride USAN, INN *antiseptic*

Disket (trademarked dosage form) *dispersible tablet*

Diskhaler (trademarked device) *inhalation powder dispenser* [used with a Rotadisk]

Diskus (trademarked device) *breath-activated inhalation powder dispenser*

Disobrom sustained-release tablets ℞ *decongestant; antihistamine* [pseudoephedrine sulfate; dexbrompheniramine maleate] 120•6 mg

disobutamide USAN, INN *antiarrhythmic*

disodium carbenicillin [see: carbenicillin disodium]

disodium carbonate [see: sodium carbonate]

disodium cefotetan [see: cefotetan disodium]

disodium chromate [see: sodium chromate]

disodium clodronate [see: clodronate disodium]

disodium clodronate tetrahydrate *investigational (orphan) for increased bone resorption due to malignancy*

disodium cromoglycate (DSC; DSCG) [see: cromolyn sodium]

disodium dihydrogen methylenediphosphonate [see: medronate disodium]

disodium edathamil [see: edathamil disodium]

disodium edetate BAN *metal-chelating agent* [also: edetate disodium]

disodium ethylenediamine tetraacetate [see: edetate disodium]

disodium hydrogen phosphate [see: sodium phosphate]

disodium hydrogen phosphate heptahydrate [see: sodium phosphate, dibasic]

disodium hydrogen phosphate hydrate [see: sodium phosphate, dibasic]

(disodium) methylene diphosphonate (MDP) [now: medronate disodium]

disodium phosphate [see: sodium phosphate, dibasic]

disodium phosphate heptahydrate [see: sodium phosphate]

disodium phosphonoacetate monohydrate [see: fosfonet sodium]

disodium phosphorofluoridate [see: sodium monofluorophosphate]

disodium pyrosulfite [see: sodium metabisulfite]

disodium silibinin dihemisuccinate *orphan status withdrawn 1997*

disodium sulfate decahydrate [see: sodium sulfate]

disodium thiosulfate pentahydrate [see: sodium thiosulfate]

disofenin USAN, INN, BAN *carrier agent in diagnostic tests*

disogluside INN

Disolan capsules (discontinued 1998) OTC *stimulant laxative; stool softener* [phenolphthalein; docusate sodium] 65•100 mg

Disolan Forte capsules (discontinued 1999) OTC *stimulant laxative; bulk laxative; stool softener* [casanthranol; carboxymethylcellulose sodium; docusate sodium] 30•400•100 mg

Disonate capsules, syrup, liquid (discontinued 1999) OTC *laxative; stool softener* [docusate sodium] 100, 240 mg; 60 mg/15 mL; 150 mg/15 mL

Disophrol tablets, Chronotabs (sustained-action tablets) OTC *decongestant; antihistamine* [pseudoephedrine sulfate; dexbrompheniramine maleate] 60•2 mg; 120•6 mg ⊡ Desferal; disoprofol; Stilphostrol

Disoplex capsules (discontinued 1999) OTC *bulk laxative; stool softener* [carboxymethylcellulose sodium; docusate sodium] 400•100 mg

disoprofol [see: propofol] ⊡ Disophrol

disopromine HCl [see: diisopromine HCl]

disoproxil *combining name for radicals or groups* [also: soproxil]

disopyramide USAN, INN, BAN *antiarrhythmic*

disopyramide phosphate USAN, USP, BAN *antiarrhythmic* 100, 150 mg oral

Disotate IV infusion (discontinued 2000) ℞ *chelating agent for hypercalcemia and ventricular arrhythmias due to digitalis toxicity* [edetate disodium] 150 mg/mL

disoxaril USAN, INN *antiviral*

Di-Spaz capsules, IM injection ℞ *GI antispasmodic* [dicyclomine HCl] 10 mg; 10 mg/mL

Dispenserpak (trademarked packaging form) *unit-of-use package*

dispersible cellulose BAN *tablet and capsule diluent* [also: cellulose, microcrystalline]

Dispertab (trademarked dosage form) *delayed-release tablet*

Dispette (trademarked delivery system) *disposable pipette*

Dispos-a-Med (trademarked delivery form) *solution for inhalation*

distaquaine [see: penicillin V]
distigmine bromide INN, BAN
disulergine INN
disulfamide INN [also: disulphamide]
disulfiram USP, INN, BAN *deterrent to alcohol consumption* 250, 500 mg oral
disulfurous acid, dipotassium salt [see: potassium metabisulfite]
disulfurous acid, disodium salt [see: sodium metabisulfite]
disulphamide BAN [also: disulfamide]
disuprazole INN
Dital slow-release capsules ℞ *anorexiant; CNS stimulant* [phendimetrazine tartrate] 105 mg
ditazole INN
ditekiren USAN *antihypertensive; renin inhibitor*
ditercalinium chloride INN
dithiazanine BAN [also: dithiazanine iodide]
dithiazanine iodide USP, INN [also: dithiazanine]
dithranol INN, BAN *topical antipsoriatic* [also: anthralin]
D.I.T.I.-2 vaginal cream ℞ *broad-spectrum antibiotic; antiseptic; vulnerary* [sulfanilamide; aminacrine HCl; allantoin] 15%•0.2%•2%
ditiocarb sodium INN
ditiomustine INN
ditolamide INN
ditophal INN, BAN
Ditropan tablets, syrup ℞ *urinary antispasmodic* [oxybutynin chloride] 5 mg; 5 mg/5 mL ⓢ Intropin
Ditropan XL extended-release tablets ℞ *anticholinergic and urinary antispasmodic for urge urinary incontinence and frequency* [oxybutynin chloride] 5, 10, 15 mg
Diucardin tablets ℞ *diuretic; antihypertensive* [hydroflumethiazide] 50 mg
Diurese tablets ℞ *diuretic; antihypertensive* [trichlormethiazide] 4 mg
diuretics *a class of agents that stimulate increased excretion of urine*
Diurigen tablets ℞ *diuretic* [chlorothiazide] 500 mg
Diuril tablets, oral suspension ℞ *diuretic* [chlorothiazide] 250, 500 mg; 250 mg/5 mL
Diutensen-R tablets ℞ *antihypertensive* [methyclothiazide; reserpine] 2.5•0.1 mg ⓢ Salutensin
divabuterol INN
divalproex sodium USAN *anticonvulsant; antipsychotic for manic episodes; migraine prophylaxis* [also: valproate semisodium; semisodium valproate]
divanilliden cyclohexanone [see: cyclovalone]
divaplon INN
Divide-Tab (trademarked dosage form) *scored tablet*
Dividose (trademarked dosage form) *multiple-scored tablets*
diviminol [see: viminol]
divinyl ether [see: vinyl ether]
divinyl oxide [see: vinyl ether]
dixamone bromide [see: methantheline bromide]
dixanthogen INN
dixarit [see: clonidine]
Dizac emulsified IV injection (discontinued 1999) ℞ *benzodiazepine sedative; anxiolytic; anticonvulsant; skeletal muscle relaxant* [diazepam] 5 mg/mL
dizatrifone INN
Dizmiss chewable tablets (discontinued 2000) OTC *anticholinergic; antivertigo agent; motion sickness preventative* [meclizine HCl] 25 mg
dizocilpine INN *neuroprotective; NMDA (N-methyl-D-aspartate) antagonist* [also: dizocilpine maleate]
dizocilpine maleate USAN *neuroprotective; NMDA (N-methyl-D-aspartate) antagonist* [also: dizocilpine]
dizocilpine maleate & citicoline *investigational (Phase III) neuroprotective treatment for stroke*
D-Lay (trademarked dosage form) *timed-release tablet*
DMC (dactinomycin, methotrexate, cyclophosphamide) *chemotherapy protocol*
DMCT (demethylchlortetracycline) [see: demeclocycline]

DML lotion OTC *moisturizer; emollient*
DML Forte cream OTC *moisturizer; emollient*
DMO (dimethyl oxazolidinedione) [see: dimethadione]
DMP 450 *investigational (Phase I/II) second-generation protease inhibitor for HIV infection*
DMP 504 *investigational (Phase III) hydrogel bile acid sequestrant (BAS) for lowering serum cholesterol*
DMP 777 *investigational (orphan) for management of cystic fibrosis lung disease*
d-MPH (d-methylphenidate HCl) [q.v.]
DMSA (dimercaptosuccinic acid) [see: succimer]
DMSO (dimethyl sulfoxide) [q.v.]
DMT (dimethyltryptamine) *street drug* [q.v.]
DNA (deoxyribonucleic acid)
DNA polymerase [see: reverse transcriptase inhibitors; non-nucleoside reverse transcriptase inhibitors]
DNase (recombinant human deoxyribonuclease I) [see: dornase alfa]
DNJ (deoxynojirimycin) [q.v.]
DNR (daunorubicin) [q.v.]
Doak Tar bath oil, lotion, shampoo OTC *topical antipsoriatic; antiseborrheic; antiseptic* [coal tar] 0.8%; 2%; 1.2%, 3%
Doak Tar Distillate liquid OTC *topical antipsoriatic; antiseborrheic; antiseptic* [coal tar] 40%
Doak Tar Oil liquid OTC *topical antipsoriatic; antiseborrheic; antiseptic* [coal tar] 2%
Doan's Pills caplets OTC *analgesic; antirheumatic* [magnesium salicylate] 325, 500 mg
Doan's P.M. caplets OTC *analgesic; antirheumatic; antihistaminic sleep aid* [magnesium salicylate; diphenhydramine HCl] 500•25 mg
DOAP (daunorubicin, Oncovin, ara-C, prednisone) *chemotherapy protocol*
dobupride INN
dobutamine USAN, INN, BAN *cardiotonic; vasopressor for shock* ⑨ dopamine
dobutamine HCl USAN, USP, BAN *cardiotonic; vasopressor for shock* 12.5 mg/mL injection
dobutamine lactobionate USAN *cardiotonic*
dobutamine tartrate USAN *cardiotonic*
Dobutrex IV infusion ℞ *vasopressor for cardiac shock* [dobutamine HCl] 12.5 mg/mL
DOCA (desoxycorticosterone acetate) [q.v.]
docarpamine INN
docebenone USAN, INN *5-lipoxygenase inhibitor*
docetaxel USAN, INN *antineoplastic for advanced or metastatic breast cancer and non–small cell lung cancer (NSCLC); analogue to paclitaxel*
docetaxel & cisplatin *chemotherapy protocol for bladder cancer*
dock, curled; curly dock; narrow dock; sour dock *medicinal herb* [see: yellow dock]
dock, patience; sweet dock *medicinal herb* [see: bistort]
doconazole USAN, INN *antifungal*
doconexent INN *omega-3 marine triglyceride* [also: docosahexaenoic acid (DHA)]
docosahexaenoic acid (DHA) [also: doconexent]
docosanol (*n*-docosanol) USAN *antiviral for herpes simplex labialis; topical treatment of oral herpes simplex type 1; investigational (Phase II) for HIV infection and AIDS-related Kaposi sarcoma*
docosil INN *combining name for radicals or groups*
Doctar shampoo OTC *antiseborrheic; antipsoriatic; antipruritic; antibacterial* [coal tar] 0.5%
Docu oral liquid; syrup OTC *laxative; stool softener* [docusate sodium] 150 mg/15 mL; 20 mg/5 mL
Docucal-P softgels (discontinued 1998) OTC *stimulant laxative; stool softener* [phenolphthalein; docusate calcium] 65•60 mg

docusate calcium USAN, USP *laxative; stool softener* 240 mg oral

docusate potassium USAN, USP *laxative; stool softener*

docusate sodium USAN, USP, BAN *stool softener; surfactant/wetting agent* [also: sodium dioctyl sulfosuccinate] 50, 100, 250 mg oral; 50 mg/15 mL oral

Docusate with Casanthranol capsules OTC *stool softener; stimulant laxative* [docusate sodium; casanthranol] 100•30 mg

dodecafluoropentane [see: perflenapent]

dodeclonium bromide INN

2-dodecylisoquinolinium bromide [see: lauryl isoquinolinium bromide]

dofamium chloride INN, BAN

dofetilide USAN, INN, BAN *antiarrhythmic for atrial fibrillation/atrial flutter (AF/AFl); potassium channel blocker*

dofosfate INN *combining name for radicals or groups*

dog grass *medicinal herb* [see: couch grass]

dog poison *(Aethusa cynapium)* plant *medicinal herb used as an antispasmodic and emetic in homeopathic remedies; not generally regarded as safe, as ingestion may be fatal*

dogbane *(Apocynum androsaemifolium)* root *medicinal herb used as a cathartic, diuretic, emetic, expectorant, stimulant, and sudorific*

dogwood, black; black alder dogwood *medicinal herb* [see: buckthorn; cascara sagrada]

DOK capsules, syrup, liquid (discontinued 1999) OTC *laxative; stool softener* [docusate sodium] 100, 250 mg; 60 mg/15 mL; 150 mg/15 mL

DOK-Plus syrup OTC *stimulant laxative; stool softener* [casanthranol; docusate sodium; alcohol 10%] 30•60 mg/15 mL

Dolacet capsules ℞ *narcotic analgesic* [hydrocodone bitartrate; acetaminophen] 5•500 mg

Dolanex elixir (discontinued 1997) OTC *analgesic; antipyretic* [acetaminophen] 325 mg/5 mL

dolantal [see: meperidine HCl]

dolantin [see: meperidine HCl]

dolasetron INN *serotonin 5-HT_3 receptor antagonist; antiemetic for nausea following chemotherapy, radiation, or surgery* [also: dolasetron mesylate]

dolasetron mesylate USAN *serotonin 5-HT_3 receptor antagonist; antiemetic for nausea following chemotherapy, radiation, or surgery* [also: dolasetron]

Dolene capsules (discontinued 1999) ℞ *narcotic analgesic* [propoxyphene HCl; acetaminophen] 65 mg

Dolgic caplets ℞ *analgesic; antipyretic; barbiturate sedative* [acetaminophen; butalbital] 650•50 mg

doliracetam INN

Dolobid film-coated tablets ℞ *analgesic; antiarthritic; antirheumatic; anti-inflammatory; antipyretic* [diflunisal] 250, 500 mg

dolomite *nutritional supplement; source of calcium and magnesium*

Dolomite tablets OTC *mineral supplement* [calcium; magnesium] 130•78 mg

Dolono elixir OTC *analgesic; antipyretic* [acetaminophen] 160 mg/5 mL

Dolophine HCl tablets, subcu or IM injection ℞ *narcotic analgesic; treatment for opioid dependence; often abused as a street drug* [methadone HCl] 5, 10 mg; 10 mg/mL

Dolorac cream OTC *topical analgesic* [capsaicin] 0.025%

dolosal [see: meperidine HCl]

Dolsed sugar-coated tablets ℞ *urinary antibiotic; analgesic; antispasmodic; acidifier* [methenamine; phenyl salicylate; atropine sulfate; methylene blue; hyoscyamine sulfate; benzoic acid] 40.8•18.1•0.03•5.4•0.03•4.5 mg

dolvanol [see: meperidine HCl]

DOM (2,5-dimethoxy-4-methylamphetamine) *a hallucinogenic street drug derived from amphetamine, popularly called STP*

domazoline INN *anticholinergic* [also: domazoline fumarate]
domazoline fumarate USAN *anticholinergic* [also: domazoline]
Domeboro powder packets, effervescent tablets OTC *astringent wet dressing (modified Burow solution)* [aluminum sulfate; calcium acetate]
Domeboro Otic [see: Otic Domeboro]
Dome-Paste medicated gauze bandage OTC *protection and support of extremities* [zinc oxide; calamine; gelatin]
domestrol [see: diethylstilbestrol]
domibrom [see: domiphen bromide]
domiodol USAN, INN *mucolytic*
domiphen bromide USAN, BAN *topical anti-infective*
domipizone INN
Domol Bath and Shower Oil OTC *bath emollient*
domoprednate INN
domoxin INN
domperidone USAN, INN, BAN, JAN *antiemetic for diabetic gastroparesis and chronic gastritis*
Donatussin drops ℞ *pediatric decongestant, antihistamine, and expectorant* [phenylephrine HCl; chlorpheniramine maleate; guaifenesin] 2•1•20 mg/mL
Donatussin syrup ℞ *antitussive; decongestant; antihistamine; expectorant* [dextromethorphan hydrobromide; phenylephrine HCl; chlorpheniramine maleate; guaifenesin] 7.5•10•2•100 mg/5 mL
Donatussin DC syrup ℞ *narcotic antitussive; decongestant; expectorant* [hydrocodone bitartrate; phenylephrine HCl; guaifenesin] 2.5•7.5•50 mg/5 mL
donepezil HCl USAN *reversible acetylcholinesterase (AChE) inhibitor; cognition adjuvant for Alzheimer dementia*
donetidine USAN, INN, BAN *antagonist to histamine H_2 receptors*
dong quai (*Angelica polymorpha; A. sinensis; A. dahurica*) root *medicinal herb for allergies, anemia, blood cleansing, constipation, female hormonal problems, hypertension, internal bleeding, menopausal symptoms, nourishing brain, and ulcers; not generally regarded as safe, as it contains safrole and coumarins*
Donnagel chewable tablets, liquid OTC *antidiarrheal; GI adsorbent* [attapulgite] 600 mg; 600 mg/15 mL ⊡ Donnatal
Donnamar tablets ℞ *GI/GU antispasmodic; antiparkinsonian; anticholinergic "drying agent" for allergic rhinitis and hyperhidrosis* [hyoscyamine sulfate] 0.125 mg
Donna-Sed elixir ℞ *GI antispasmodic; anticholinergic; sedative* [atropine sulfate; scopolamine hydrobromide; hyoscyamine hydrobromide; phenobarbital] 0.0194•0.0065•0.1037•16.2 mg/5 mL
Donnatal capsules & tablets, elixir, Extentabs (extended-release tablets) ℞ *GI antispasmodic; anticholinergic; sedative* [atropine sulfate; scopolamine hydrobromide; hyoscyamine sulfate; phenobarbital] 0.0194•0.0065•0.1037•16.2 mg; 0.0194•0.0065•0.1037•16.2 mg/5 mL; 0.0582•0.0195•0.3111•48.6 mg ⊡ Donnagel
Donnatal No. 2 tablets ℞ *GI antispasmodic; anticholinergic; sedative* [atropine sulfate; scopolamine hydrobromide; hyoscyamine sulfate; phenobarbital] 0.0194•0.0065•0.1037•32.4 mg
Donnazyme tablets ℞ *digestive enzymes* [pancreatin; lipase; protease; amylase] 500 mg•1000 U•12 500 U•12 500 U ⊡ Entozyme
DOPA (dihydroxyphenylalanine) [see: levodopa]
L-dopa [see: levodopa]
dopamantine USAN, INN *antiparkinsonian*
dopamine INN, BAN *adrenergic; vasopressor for shock* [also: dopamine HCl] ⊡ dobutamine; Dopram

dopamine HCl USAN, USP *adrenergic; vasopressor for shock* [also: dopamine] 40, 80, 160 mg/mL injection

dopamine HCl in 5% dextrose *adrenergic; vasopressor for shock* 80, 160, 320 mg/100 mL injection

dopaminergics *a class of antiparkinsonian agents that affect the dopamine neurotransmitters in the brain*

Dopar capsules ℞ *dopamine precursor; antiparkinsonian* [levodopa] 100, 250, 500 mg ⊠ Dopram

Dopascan injection *investigational (Phase III) diagnostic imaging aid for dopamine and serotonin transporter sites* [iometopane I 123]

dopexamine USAN, INN, BAN *cardiovascular agent*

dopexamine HCl USAN, BAN *cardiovascular agent*

Dopram IV injection or infusion ℞ *CNS stimulant; analeptic; adjunct to postanesthesia "stir-up"* [doxapram HCl] 20 mg/mL ⊠ dopamine; Dopar

dopropidil INN

doqualast INN

Doral tablets ℞ *sedative; hypnotic* [quazepam] 7.5, 15 mg

dorastine INN *antihistamine* [also: dorastine HCl]

dorastine HCl USAN *antihistamine* [also: dorastine]

Dorcol Children's Cold Formula liquid OTC *pediatric decongestant and antihistamine* [pseudoephedrine HCl; chlorpheniramine maleate] 15•1 mg/5 mL

Dorcol Children's Cough syrup OTC *pediatric antitussive, decongestant, and expectorant* [dextromethorphan hydrobromide; pseudoephedrine HCl; guaifenesin] 5•15•50 mg/5 mL

Dorcol Children's Decongestant liquid OTC *nasal decongestant* [pseudoephedrine HCl] 15 mg/5 mL

Dorcol Children's Fever & Pain Reducer liquid (discontinued 1997) OTC *analgesic; antipyretic* [acetaminophen] 160 mg/5 mL

doreptide INN

doretinel USAN, INN *antikeratinizing agent*

Dormarex 2 tablets OTC *antihistaminic sleep aid; motion sickness preventative* [diphenhydramine HCl] 50 mg

dormethan [see: dextromethorphan hydrobromide]

Dormin caplets, capsules OTC *antihistaminic sleep aid* [diphenhydramine HCl] 25 mg

dormiral [see: phenobarbital]

dormonal [see: barbital]

dornase alfa USAN, INN *reduces respiratory viscoelasticity of sputum in cystic fibrosis (orphan)*

Doryx capsules ℞ *tetracycline antibiotic* [doxycycline hyclate] 100 mg

dorzolamide HCl USAN *topical carbonic anhydrase inhibitor for glaucoma*

D.O.S. softgels OTC *laxative; stool softener* [docusate sodium] 100, 250 mg

Dosalax syrup (discontinued 1999) OTC *stimulant laxative* [senna concentrate; alcohol 7%]

Dosa-Trol Pack (trademarked dosage form) *unit-of-use package*

Dosepak (trademarked dosage form) *unit-of-use package*

dosergoside INN

Dosette (trademarked dosage form) *injectable unit-of-use system (vials, ampules, syringes, etc.)*

Dospan (trademarked form) *controlled-release tablets*

Dostinex tablets ℞ *dopamine agonist for hyperprolactinemia; investigational treatment for Parkinson disease and gynecologic disorders* [cabergoline] 0.5 mg

dosulepin INN *antidepressant* [also: dothiepin HCl; dothiepin; dosulepin HCl]

dosulepin HCl JAN *antidepressant* [also: dothiepin HCl; dosulepin; dothiepin]

dotarizine INN

dotefonium bromide INN

dothiepin BAN *antidepressant* [also: dothiepin HCl; dosulepin; dosulepin HCl]

dothiepin HCl USAN *antidepressant* [also: dosulepin; dothiepin; dosulepin HCl]

Double Ice ArthriCare [see: ArthriCare, Double Ice]

Double-Action Toothache Kit tablets + liquid OTC *analgesic; topical oral anesthetic* [(acetaminophen) + (benzocaine; alcohol 74%)] (325 mg) + (?)

Dovonex cream, ointment, scalp solution ℞ *topical antipsoriatic* [calcipotriene] 0.005%

doxacurium chloride USAN, INN, BAN *nondepolarizing neuromuscular blocker; muscle relaxant; adjunct to anesthesia*

doxaminol INN

doxapram INN, BAN *respiratory stimulant* [also: doxapram HCl]

doxapram HCl USAN, USP *respiratory stimulant; analeptic* [also: doxapram]

doxaprost USAN, INN *bronchodilator*

doxate [see: docusate sodium]

doxazosin INN, BAN *antihypertensive; α_1-adrenergic blocker; treatment for benign prostatic hyperplasia* [also: doxazosin mesylate]

doxazosin mesylate USAN *antihypertensive; α_1-adrenergic blocker; treatment for benign prostatic hyperplasia* [also: doxazosin] 1, 2, 4, 8 mg oral

doxefazepam INN

doxenitoin INN

doxepin INN, BAN *tricyclic antidepressant; anxiolytic; topical antihistamine* [also: doxepin HCl] ⊠ Doxidan; Loxitane

doxepin HCl USAN, USP *tricyclic antidepressant; anxiolytic; topical antihistamine* [also: doxepin] 10, 25, 50, 75, 100, 150 mg oral; 10 mg/mL oral

doxercalciferol USAN *synthetic vitamin D analogue; serum calcium regulator for hyperparathyroidism of chronic renal dialysis*

doxibetasol INN [also: doxybetasol]

Doxidan capsules OTC *stimulant laxative; stool softener* [casanthranol; docusate sodium] 30•100 mg

Doxidan capsules (discontinued 1998) OTC *stimulant laxative; stool softener* [phenolphthalein; docusate calcium] 65•60 mg ⊠ doxepin

doxifluridine INN, JAN *investigational antineoplastic*

Doxil IV injection ℞ *anthracycline antibiotic antineoplastic for Kaposi sarcoma and ovarian cancer; investigational (NDA filed) for prostate cancer* [doxorubicin HCl, liposome-encapsulated] 20 mg/vial

doxofylline USAN, INN *bronchodilator*

doxorubicin USAN, INN, BAN *anthracycline antibiotic antineoplastic* ⊠ daunorubicin

doxorubicin HCl USP *anthracycline antibiotic antineoplastic* 10, 20, 50 mg, 2 mg/mL injection

doxorubicin HCl, liposome-encapsulated (LED) *anthracycline antibiotic antineoplastic for Kaposi sarcoma and ovarian cancer; investigational (NDA filed) for prostate cancer*

Doxovir ℞ *investigational (Phase II) prophylaxis for genital herpes* [CTC-96 (code name—generic name not yet assigned)]

doxpicodin HCl [now: doxpicomine HCl]

doxpicomine INN *analgesic* [also: doxpicomine HCl]

doxpicomine HCl USAN *analgesic* [also: doxpicomine]

Doxy 100; Doxy 200 powder for IV injection ℞ *tetracycline antibiotic* [doxycycline hyclate] 100 mg; 200 mg

Doxy Caps capsules ℞ *tetracycline antibiotic* [doxycycline hyclate] 100 mg

doxybetasol BAN [also: doxibetasol]

Doxychel Hyclate capsules, tablets, powder for IV injection ℞ *tetracycline antibiotic* [doxycycline hyclate] 50, 100 mg; 50, 100 mg; 100, 200 mg

doxycycline USAN, USP, INN, BAN *antibiotic; antirickettsial; malaria prophylaxis*

doxycycline calcium USP *antibiotic; antiprotozoal*

doxycycline fosfatex USAN, BAN *antibiotic*

doxycycline hyclate USP *antibiotic* 50, 100 mg oral; 100, 200 mg/vial injection

doxycycline monohydrate *antibiotic*

doxylamine INN, BAN *antihistamine; sleep aid* [also: doxylamine succinate]

doxylamine succinate USP *antihistamine; sleep aid* [also: doxylamine]

DPE (dipivalyl epinephrine) [now: dipivefrin]

DPF [see: Dermprotective Factor]

DPN (diphosphopyridine nucleotide) [now: nadide]

DPPC (dipalmitoylphosphatidylcholine) [see: colfosceril palmitate]

DPPE (diethyl-phenylmethyl-phenoxy ethenamine) HCl [see: tesmilifene HCl]

Dr. Brown's Home Drug Testing System *in vitro diagnostic aid for detection of multiple illicit drugs in the urine*

Dr. Caldwell Senna Laxative oral liquid (discontinued 1999) OTC *stimulant laxative* [senna concentrate] 33.3 mg/mL

Dr. Dermi-Heal ointment OTC *vulnerary; antipruritic; astringent* [allantoin; zinc oxide; peruvian balsam] 1%•?•?

Dr. Scholl's Advanced Pain Relief Corn Removers; Dr. Scholl's Callus Removers; Dr Scholl's Clear Away; Dr. Scholl's Corn Removers medicated discs OTC *topical keratolytic* [salicylic acid in a rubber-based vehicle] 40%

Dr. Scholl's Athlete's Foot powder, spray powder, spray liquid OTC *topical antifungal* [tolnaftate] 1%

Dr. Scholl's Clear Away OneStep; Dr. Scholl's OneStep Corn Removers medicated strips OTC *topical keratolytic* [salicylic acid in a rubber-based vehicle] 40%

Dr. Scholl's Corn/Callus Remover liquid OTC *topical keratolytic* [salicylic acid in flexible collodion] 17%

Dr. Scholl's Cracked Heel Relief cream OTC *topical local anesthetic; antiseptic* [lidocaine HCl; benzalkonium chloride] 2%•0.13%

Dr. Scholl's Moisturizing Corn Remover Kit medicated discs + cushions + moisturizing cream OTC *topical keratolytic* [salicylic acid in a rubber-based vehicle] 40%

Dr. Scholl's Tritin powder, spray powder OTC *topical antifungal* [tolnaftate] 1%

Dr. Scholl's Wart Remover Kit liquid + adhesive pads OTC *topical keratolytic* [salicylic acid in flexible collodion] 17%

draflazine USAN *cardioprotectant*

dragée (French for "sugar plum") *a sugar-coated pill or medicated confection* [pronounced "drah zhá"]

dragon's claw, scaly *medicinal herb* [see: coral root]

dragonwort *medicinal herb* [see: bistort]

Dramamine liquid ℞ *antinauseant; antiemetic; antivertigo agent; motion sickness preventative* [dimenhydrinate] 15.62 mg/5 mL

Dramamine tablets, chewable tablets, liquid OTC *antinauseant; antiemetic; antivertigo agent; motion sickness preventative* [dimenhydrinate] 50 mg; 50 mg; 12.5 mg/4 mL

Dramamine, Children's liquid OTC *antinauseant; antiemetic; antivertigo agent; motion sickness preventative* [dimenhydrinate; alcohol 5%] 12.5 mg/5 mL

Dramamine II tablets (name changed to Dramamine Less Drowsy Formula in 2000)

Dramamine Less Drowsy Formula tablets OTC *anticholinergic; antihistamine; antivertigo agent; motion sickness preventative* [meclizine HCl] 25 mg

Dramanate IV or IM injection ℞ *antinauseant; antiemetic; antivertigo agent; motion sickness preventative* [dimenhydrinate] 50 mg/mL 🅓 Dommanate

dramarin [see: dimenhydrate]

dramedilol INN

Dramilin IV or IM injection ℞ *antinauseant; antiemetic; antivertigo agent;*

motion sickness preventative [dimenhydrinate] 50 mg/mL

dramyl [see: dimenhydrate]

draquinolol INN

drazidox INN

Drepanol ℞ *investigational (orphan) for prophylactic treatment of sickle cell disease* [OM 401 (code name—generic name not yet assigned)]

dribendazole USAN, INN *anthelmintic*

dricol [see: amidephrine]

Dri/Ear ear drops OTC *antibacterial; antifungal* [boric acid] 2.75%

dried aluminum hydroxide gel [see: aluminum hydroxide gel, dried]

dried basic aluminum carbonate [see: aluminum carbonate, basic]

dried ferrous sulfate [see: ferrous sulfate, dried]

dried yeast [see: yeast, dried]

drinidene USAN, INN *analgesic*

Drisdol capsules ℞ *vitamin deficiency therapy for refractory rickets, familial hypophosphatemia, and hypoparathyroidism* [ergocalciferol (vitamin D_2)] 50 000 IU

Drisdol Drops OTC *vitamin supplement* [ergocalciferol (vitamin D_2)] 8000 IU/mL

Dristan nasal spray OTC *nasal decongestant; antihistamine* [phenylephrine HCl; pheniramine maleate] 0.5%•0.2%

Dristan 12-Hr. nasal spray OTC *nasal decongestant* [oxymetazoline HCl] 0.05%

Dristan Cold caplets OTC *decongestant; analgesic; antipyretic* [pseudoephedrine HCl; acetaminophen] 30•500 mg

Dristan Cold, Maximum Strength caplets OTC *decongestant; antihistamine; analgesic* [pseudoephedrine HCl; brompheniramine maleate; acetaminophen] 30•2•500 mg

Dristan Cold Multi-Symptom Formula tablets OTC *decongestant; antihistamine; analgesic* [phenylephrine HCl; chlorpheniramine maleate; acetaminophen] 5•2•325 mg

Dristan Saline Spray OTC *nasal moisturizer* [sodium chloride (saline solution)]

Dristan Sinus caplets OTC *decongestant; analgesic* [pseudoephedrine HCl; ibuprofen] 30•200 mg

Drithocreme; Drithocreme HP 1%; Dritho-Scalp cream ℞ *topical antipsoriatic* [anthralin] 0.1%, 0.25%, 0.5%; 1%; 0.5%

Drixomed sustained-release tablets ℞ *decongestant; antihistamine* [pseudoephedrine sulfate; dexbrompheniramine maleate] 120•6 mg

Drixoral syrup OTC *decongestant; antihistamine* [pseudoephedrine sulfate; brompheniramine maleate] 30•2 mg/5 mL

Drixoral Cold & Allergy sustained-action tablets OTC *decongestant; antihistamine* [pseudoephedrine sulfate; dexbrompheniramine maleate] 120•6 mg

Drixoral Cold & Flu; Drixoral Plus extended-release tablets OTC *decongestant; antihistamine; analgesic* [pseudoephedrine sulfate; dexbrompheniramine maleate; acetaminophen] 60•3•500 mg

Drixoral Cough & Congestion Liquid Caps (capsules) OTC *antitussive; decongestant* [dextromethorphan hydrobromide; pseudoephedrine HCl] 30•60 mg

Drixoral Cough Liquid Caps (liquid-filled capsules) (discontinued 1998) OTC *antitussive* [dextromethorphan hydrobromide] 30 mg

Drixoral Cough & Sore Throat Liquid Caps (liquid-filled capsules) OTC *antitussive; analgesic* [dextromethorphan hydrobromide; acetaminophen] 15•325 mg

Drixoral Day; Drixoral N.D. (CAN) sustained-action tablets OTC *nasal decongestant* [pseudoephedrine sulfate] 120 mg

Drixoral Night (CAN) tablets OTC *decongestant; antihistamine* [pseudoephedrine sulfate; dexbrompheniramine maleate] 60•2 mg

Drixoral Non-Drowsy Formula extended-release tablets OTC *nasal decongestant* [pseudoephedrine sulfate] 120 mg

Drize sustained-release capsules ℞ *decongestant; antihistamine* [phenylpropanolamine HCl; chlorpheniramine maleate] 75•12 mg

drobuline USAN, INN *antiarrhythmic*

drocarbil NF

drocinonide USAN, INN *anti-inflammatory*

droclidinium bromide INN

drocode [see: dihydrocodeine]

drofenine INN

droloxifene INN *investigational (Phase III) antineoplastic for breast cancer; investigational (Phase III) antiestrogen for postmenopausal osteoporosis*

droloxifene citrate USAN *antineoplastic; antiestrogen*

drometrizole USAN, INN *ultraviolet screen*

dromostanolone propionate USAN, USP *antineoplastic* [also: drostanolone]

dronabinol USAN, USP, INN *antiemetic for nausea following chemotherapy; appetite stimulant for AIDS patients (orphan)*

drop chalk [see: calcium carbonate]

dropberry *medicinal herb* [see: Solomon's seal]

Drop-Dose (trademarked delivery system) *prefilled eye drop dispenser*

dropempine INN

droperidol USAN, USP, INN, BAN *general anesthetic; antiemetic* 2.5 mg/mL injection

Dropperettes (delivery system) *prefilled droppers*

droprenilamine USAN, INN *coronary vasodilator*

dropropizine INN, BAN

Drop-Tainers (trademarked dosage form) *prefilled eye drop dispenser*

drospirenone USAN *progestin; spironolactone analogue; aldosterone antagonist*

drostanolone INN, BAN *antineoplastic* [also: dromostanolone propionate]

drotaverine INN

drotebanol INN, BAN

Drotic ear drops ℞ *topical corticosteroidal anti-inflammatory; antibiotic* [hydrocortisone; neomycin sulfate; polymyxin B sulfate] 1%•5 mg•10 000 U per mL

drotrecogin alfa *investigational (NDA filed) recombinant human activated protein C (rhAPC) for severe sepsis*

droxacin INN *antibacterial* [also: droxacin sodium]

droxacin sodium USAN *antibacterial* [also: droxacin]

Droxia capsules ℞ *sickle cell anemia treatment (orphan)* [hydroxyurea] 200, 300, 400 mg

droxicainide INN

droxicam INN

droxidopa INN

droxifilcon A USAN *hydrophilic contact lens material*

droxinavir HCl USAN *antiviral; HIV-1 protease inhibitor*

droxypropine INN, BAN

Dry E 400 tablets OTC *vitamin supplement* [vitamin E (as *d*-alpha tocopheryl acid succinate)] 400 IU

Dry Eye Therapy eye drops (discontinued 1998) OTC *ophthalmic moisturizer/lubricant* [glycerin] 0.3%

Dry Eyes eye drops OTC *ophthalmic moisturizer/lubricant* [polyvinyl alcohol] 1.4%

Dry Eyes ophthalmic ointment OTC *ocular moisturizer/lubricant* [white petrolatum; mineral oil]

Dryopteris filix-mas *medicinal herb* [see: aspidium]

Dryox 2.5; Dryox 5; Dryox 10; Dryox 20 gel OTC *topical keratolytic for acne* [benzoyl peroxide] 2.5%; 5%; 10%; 20%

Dryox 10S 5; Dryox 20S 10 gel OTC *topical keratolytic for acne* [benzoyl peroxide; sulfur] 10%•5%; 20%•10%

Dryox Wash 5; Dryox Wash 10 liquid OTC *topical keratolytic for acne* [benzoyl peroxide] 5%; 10%

Drysol solution ℞ *astringent for hyperhidrosis* [aluminum chloride] 20%

Drytergent liquid OTC *soap-free therapeutic skin cleanser*

Drytex lotion OTC *topical keratolytic cleanser for acne* [salicylic acid; acetone; isopropyl alcohol] ≟•10%•40%

DSC; DSCG (disodium cromoglycate) [see: cromolyn sodium]

DSMC Plus capsules (discontinued 1999) OTC *stimulant laxative; stool softener* [casanthranol; docusate potassium] 30•100 mg

D-S-S capsules OTC *laxative; stool softener* [docusate sodium] 100 mg

DSS (dioctyl sodium sulfosuccinate) [now: docusate sodium]

DSS 100 Plus capsules OTC *stimulant laxative; stool softener* [casanthranol; docusate sodium] 30•100 mg

D-S-S Plus capsules (discontinued 1997) OTC *stimulant laxative; stool softener* [casanthranol; docusate sodium] 30•100 mg

DST (dihydrostreptomycin) [q.v.]

DT; Td (diphtheria & tetanus [toxoids]) *the designation DT (or TD) denotes the pediatric vaccine; Td denotes the adult vaccine* [see: diphtheria & tetanus toxoids, adsorbed]

DTaP (diphtheria & tetanus [toxoids] & acellular pertussis [vaccine]) [q.v.]

DTI-015 *investigational (orphan) antineoplastic for glioblastoma multiforme*

DTIC (dimethyl triazeno imidazole carboxamide) [see: dacarbazine]

DTIC & tamoxifen citrate *chemotherapy protocol for malignant melanoma*

DTIC-ACTD; DTIC-ACT-D (DTIC, actinomycin D) *chemotherapy protocol*

DTIC-Dome IV injection ℞ *antineoplastic for metastatic malignant melanoma and Hodgkin disease* [dacarbazine] 10 mg/mL

DTP (diphtheria & tetanus [toxoids] & pertussis [vaccine]) [q.v.]

DTPA (diethylenetriaminepentaacetic acid) [see: pentetic acid]

DTPA (diethylenetriaminepentaacetic acid) technetium (^{99m}Tc), human serum albumin [see: technetium Tc 99m pentetate]

DTwP (diphtheria & tetanus [toxoids] & whole-cell pertussis [vaccine]) [q.v.]

Duadacin capsules OTC *decongestant; antihistamine; analgesic* [phenylpropanolamine HCl; chlorpheniramine maleate; acetaminophen] 12.5•2•325 mg

duazomycin USAN, INN *antineoplastic*

duazomycin A [see: duazomycin]

duazomycin B [see: azotomycin]

duazomycin C [see: ambomycin]

Duboisia myoporoides *medicinal herb* [see: corkwood]

duck's foot *medicinal herb* [see: mandrake]

ducodal [see: oxycodone]

Dulcagen enteric-coated tablets, suppositories (discontinued 1999) OTC *stimulant laxative* [bisacodyl] 5 mg; 10 mg

Dulcet (trademarked dosage form) *chewable tablet*

Dulcolax enteric-coated tablets, suppositories OTC *stimulant laxative* [bisacodyl] 5 mg; 10 mg

Dulcolax Bowel Prep Kit 4 enteric-coated tablets + 1 suppository (discontinued 1999) OTC *pre-procedure bowel evacuant* [bisacodyl] 5 mg; 10 mg

Dull-C powder OTC *vitamin C supplement* [ascorbic acid] 4.24 g/tsp.

dulofibrate INN

duloxetine INN *investigational (Phase III) serotonin and norepinephrine uptake inhibitor for depression; investigational (Phase II) for urinary incontinence* [also: duloxetine HCl]

duloxetine HCl USAN *antidepressant* [also: duloxetine]

dulozafone INN

dumorelin INN

duneryl [see: phenobarbital]

Duocet tablets ℞ *narcotic analgesic* [hydrocodone bitartrate; acetaminophen] 5•500 mg

Duo-Cyp IM injection ℞ *hormone replacement therapy for postmenopau-*

sal symptoms [estradiol cypionate; testosterone cypionate] 2•50 mg/mL

DuoDerm CGF; DuoDerm Extra Thin; DuoDerm Hydroactive adhesive dressings OTC *occlusive wound dressing* [hydrocolloid gel]

DuoDerm Hydroactive paste, granules OTC *wound dressing* [hydrocolloid gel] 30 g; 5 g

DuoFilm liquid OTC *topical keratolytic* [salicylic acid in flexible collodion] 17%

DuoFilm transdermal patch OTC *topical keratolytic* [salicylic acid in a rubber-based vehicle] 40%

DuoFilm Gel for Kids (CAN) OTC *topical keratolytic* [salicylic acid in flexible collodion] 11%

Duo-Medihaler inhalation aerosol (discontinued 1997) ℞ *bronchodilator* [isoproterenol HCl; phenylephrine bitartrate] 0.16•0.24 mg/dose

duometacin INN

duomycin [see: chlortetracycline HCl]

DuoNeb solution for nebulization ℞ *anticholinergic bronchodilator for chronic bronchospasm with COPD* [ipratropium bromide; albuterol sulfate] 0.5•2.5 mg/3 mL dose

duoperone INN *neuroleptic* [also: duoperone fumarate]

duoperone fumarate USAN *neuroleptic* [also: duoperone]

DuoPlant gel ℞ *topical keratolytic* [salicylic acid in flexible collodion] 17%

duotal [see: guaiacol carbonate]

Duo-Trach Kit pre-filled syringe with cannula ℞ *injectable local anesthetic* [lidocaine HCl] 4%

Duphalac oral/rectal solution ℞ *hyperosmotic laxative* [lactulose] 10 g/15 mL

Duplex liquid OTC *soap-free therapeutic skin cleanser* [sodium lauryl sulfate] 15%

Duplex T shampoo OTC *antiseborrheic; antipsoriatic; antipruritic; antibacterial* [coal tar] 10%

duponol [see: sodium lauryl sulfate]

dupracetam INN

Durabolin IM injection (discontinued 2000) ℞ *anabolic steroid for metastatic breast cancer in women; also abused as a street drug* [nandrolone phenpropionate (in oil)] 25, 50 mg/mL

Duracaps (dosage form) *sustained-release capsules*

DURAcare II solution OTC *surfactant cleaning solution for soft contact lenses*

Duraclon continuous epidural infusion ℞ *central analgesic; adjunct to opioid analgesics for severe cancer pain (orphan)* [clonidine HCl] 500 µg/mL

Duract capsules (discontinued 1998) ℞ *long-acting nonsteroidal anti-inflammatory drug (NSAID); analgesic; antipyretic* [bromfenac sodium] 25 mg

Duradrin capsules ℞ *vasoconstrictor; sedative; analgesic (for migraine)* [isometheptene mucate; dichloralphenazone; acetaminophen] 65•100•325 mg

DuraGen ℞ *resorbable graft matrix to repair the dura mater following brain surgery or traumatic injury*

Duragesic-25; Duragesic-50; Duragesic-75; Duragesic-100 transdermal patch ℞ *narcotic analgesic* [fentanyl] 25 µg/hr.; 50 µg/hr.; 75 µg/hr.; 100 µg/hr.

Dura-Gest capsules ℞ *decongestant; expectorant* [phenylephrine HCl; phenylpropanolamine HCl; guaifenesin] 45•5•200 mg

Duralex sustained-release capsules ℞ *decongestant; antihistamine* [pseudoephedrine HCl; chlorpheniramine maleate] 120•8 mg

Duralith (CAN) sustained-release tablets ℞ *antipsychotic for manic episodes of a bipolar disorder* [lithium carbonate] 300 mg

Duralone-40; Duralone-80 intralesional, soft tissue, and IM injection ℞ *corticosteroid; anti-inflammatory; immunosuppressant* [methylprednisolone acetate] 40 mg/mL; 80 mg/mL

Duramist Plus nasal spray OTC *nasal decongestant* [oxymetazoline HCl] 0.05%

Duramorph IV, subcu or IM injection ℞ *narcotic analgesic* [morphine sulfate] 0.5, 1 mg/mL

duramycin *investigational (orphan) for cystic fibrosis*

Duranest; Duranest MPF injection ℞ *injectable local anesthetic* [etidocaine HCl] [note: one of two different products with the same name] 1% ⊡ Duratest

Duranest; Duranest MPF injection ℞ *injectable local anesthetic* [etidocaine; epinephrine] [note: one of two different products with the same name] 1%•1:200 000, 1.5%•1:200 000 ⊡ Duratest

durapatite USAN *prosthetic aid* [also: calcium phosphate, tribasic; hydroxyapatite]

DuraSite (delivery system) *polymer-based eye drops*

DuraSolv (trademarked delivery system) *orally disintegrating tablets*

Durasphere injection ℞ *tissue-bulking agent for female stress urinary incontinence* [carbon-coated beads]

Dura-Tabs (trademarked dosage form) *sustained-release tablets*

Dura-Tap/PD prolonged-action capsule ℞ *pediatric decongestant and antihistamine* [pseudoephedrine HCl; chlorpheniramine maleate] 60•4 mg

Duratears Naturale ophthalmic ointment OTC *ocular moisturizer/lubricant* [white petrolatum; mineral oil; lanolin]

Duratest 100; Duratest 200 IM injection (discontinued 2001) ℞ *androgen replacement for delayed puberty or breast cancer* [testosterone cypionate] 100 mg/mL; 200 mg/mL ⊡ Duranest; Duratuss

Duratestrin IM injection (discontinued 1999) ℞ *hormone replacement therapy for postmenopausal symptoms* [estradiol cypionate; testosterone cypionate] 2•50 mg/mL

Durathate-200 IM injection (discontinued 2001) ℞ *androgen replacement for delayed puberty or breast cancer* [testosterone enanthate] 200 mg/mL

Duration nasal spray OTC *nasal decongestant* [oxymetazoline HCl] 0.05%

Duratocin (CAN) IV injection ℞ *uterotonic agent to prevent postpartum hemorrhage following cesarean section* [carbetocin] 100 µg/mL

Duratuss; Duratuss-GP long-acting film-coated tablets ℞ *decongestant; expectorant* [pseudoephedrine HCl; guaifenesin] 120•600 mg; 120•1200 mg ⊡ Duratest

Duratuss DM elixir ℞ *antitussive; expectorant* [dextromethorphan hydrobromide; guaifenesin] 20•200 mg/5 mL

Duratuss-G film-coated tablets ℞ *expectorant* [guaifenesin] 1.2 g

Dura-Vent long-acting tablets ℞ *decongestant; expectorant* [phenylpropanolamine HCl; guaifenesin] 75•600 mg

Dura-Vent/A continuous-release capsule ℞ *decongestant; antihistamine* [phenylpropanolamine HCl; chlorpheniramine maleate] 75•10 mg

Dura-Vent/DA sustained-release tablets ℞ *decongestant; antihistamine; anticholinergic* [phenylephrine HCl; chlorpheniramine maleate; methscopolamine nitrate] 20•8•2.5 mg

Duricef capsules, tablets, powder for oral suspension ℞ *cephalosporin antibiotic* [cefadroxil] 500 mg; 1000 mg; 125, 250, 500 mg/5 mL

DUROS (trademarked delivery system) *investigational (NDA filed) osmotically driven implantable therapeutic system, currently used for Viadur (leuprolide)*

dusting powder, absorbable USP *surgical glove lubricant*

dutasteride USAN *5α-reductase inhibitor for benign prostatic hyperplasia*

Dutonin (British name for U.S. product Serzone)

Duvoid tablets (discontinued 2001) ℞ *cholinergic urinary stimulant for postsurgical and postpartum urinary retention* [bethanechol chloride] 10, 25, 50 mg

DVB (DDP, vindesine, bleomycin) *chemotherapy protocol*

DVP (daunorubicin, vincristine, prednisone) *chemotherapy protocol for acute lymphocytic leukemia (ALL)*

DVPL-ASP (daunorubicin, vincristine, prednisone, L-asparaginase) *chemotherapy protocol*

dwarf ginseng *(Panax trifolius)* *medicinal herb* [see: ginseng]

dwarf palm; dwarf palmetto *medicinal herb* [see: saw palmetto]

dwarf sumach *medicinal herb* [see: sumach]

Dwelle eye drops (discontinued 1998) OTC *ocular moisturizer/lubricant*

Dyazide capsules ℞ *antihypertensive; diuretic* [triamterene; hydrochlorothiazide] 37.5•25 mg ⊠ thiazides; Tiazac

Dycill capsules ℞ *penicillinase-resistant penicillin antibiotic* [dicloxacillin sodium] 250, 500 mg

dyclocaine BAN *topical anesthetic* [also: dyclonine HCl; dyclonine]

Dyclone solution ℞ *anesthetic prior to upper GI and respiratory endoscopies* [dyclonine HCl] 0.5%, 1%

dyclonine INN *topical anesthetic* [also: dyclonine HCl; dyclocaine]

dyclonine HCl USP *topical anesthetic* [also: dyclonine; dyclocaine]

dydrogesterone USAN, USP, INN, BAN *progestin*

dyer's broom *(Genista tinctoria)* flowering twigs *medicinal herb used as an aperient, diuretic, stimulant, and vasoconstrictor*

dyer's bugloss *medicinal herb* [see: henna *(Alkanna)*]

dyer's saffron *medicinal herb* [see: safflower]

dyer's weed *medicinal herb* [see: goldenrod]

Dyflex-G tablets ℞ *antiasthmatic; bronchodilator; expectorant* [dyphylline; guaifenesin] 200•200 mg

dyflos BAN *antiglaucoma agent; irreversible cholinesterase inhibitor miotic* [also: isoflurophate]

Dy-G oral liquid ℞ *antiasthmatic; bronchodilator; expectorant* [dyphylline; guaifenesin] 100•100 mg/5 mL

dylate [see: clonitrate]

Dyline-GG tablets, liquid ℞ *antiasthmatic; bronchodilator; expectorant* [dyphylline; guaifenesin] 200•200 mg; 300•300 mg/15 mL

dymanthine HCl USAN *anthelmintic* [also: dimantine HCl]

Dymelor tablets ℞ *sulfonylurea antidiabetic* [acetohexamide] 250, 500 mg ⊠ Demerol; Pamelor

Dymenate IV or IM injection ℞ *antinauseant; antiemetic; antivertigo; motion sickness preventative* [dimenhydrinate] 50 mg/mL

Dynabac enteric-coated tablets ℞ *once-daily macrolide antibiotic for respiratory and dermatological infections* [dirithromycin] 250 mg

Dynacin capsules ℞ *tetracycline antibiotic* [minocycline HCl] 50, 75, 100 mg

DynaCirc capsules ℞ *antihypertensive; dihydropyridine calcium channel blocker* [isradipine] 2.5, 5 mg

DynaCirc CR controlled-release tablets ℞ *once-daily antihypertensive; dihydropyridine calcium channel blocker* [isradipine] 5, 10 mg

dynacoryl [see: nikethamide]

Dynafed; Dynafed Plus tablets OTC *decongestant; analgesic; antipyretic* [pseudoephedrine HCl; acetaminophen] 30•500 mg

Dynafed Asthma Relief tablets OTC *decongestant; expectorant* [ephedrine HCl; guaifenesin] 25•200 mg

Dynafed E.X. tablets OTC *analgesic; antipyretic* [acetaminophen] 500 mg

Dynafed IB tablets (discontinued 2000) OTC *analgesic; antiarthritic; nonsteroidal anti-inflammatory drug (NSAID)* [ibuprofen] 200 mg

Dynafed Jr., Children's chewable tablets OTC *analgesic; antipyretic* [acetaminophen] 80 mg

Dynafed Pseudo tablets (discontinued 2000) OTC *nasal decongestant* [pseudoephedrine HCl] 60 mg

Dyna-Hex Skin Cleanser; Dyna-Hex 2 Skin Cleanser liquid OTC *broad-spectrum antimicrobial; germicidal* [chlorhexidine gluconate; alcohol 4%] 4%; 2%

dynamine *investigational (orphan) for Lambert-Eaton myasthenic syndrome and Charcot-Marie-Tooth disease*

Dynapen capsules, powder for oral suspension ℞ *penicillinase-resistant penicillin antibiotic* [dicloxacillin sodium] 125, 250, 500 mg; 62.5 mg/5 mL

dynarsan [see: acetarsone]

Dynepo ℞ *investigational (NDA filed) gene therapy for anemia of renal failure* [erythropoietin, gene-activated]

dyphylline USP *antiasthmatic; bronchodilator* [also: diprophylline] 200, 400 mg oral

dyphylline & guaifenesin *antiasthmatic; bronchodilator; expectorant* 200•200 mg

Dyphylline-GG elixir OTC *antiasthmatic; bronchodilator; expectorant* [dyphylline; guaifenesin] 100•100 mg/15 mL

Dyprotex pads OTC *topical diaper rash treatment* [zinc oxide; dimethicone] 40%•2.5%

Dyrenium capsules ℞ *antihypertensive; potassium-sparing diuretic* [triamterene] 50, 100 mg ⑨ Pyridium

Dyrexan-OD sustained-release capsules ℞ *anorexiant; CNS stimulant* [phendimetrazine tartrate] 105 mg

Dysport ℞ *blepharospasm and strabismus of dystonia (orphan); investigational (orphan) for pediatric cerebral palsy and cervical dystonia* [botulinum toxin, type A]

dysprosium *element (Dy)*

DZAPO (daunorubicin, azacitidine, ara-C, prednisone, Oncovin) *chemotherapy protocol*

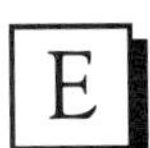

E2II transdermal patch ℞ *investigational (NDA filed) estrogen replacement therapy* [estradiol]

E2III transdermal patch ℞ *investigational (NDA filed) 7-day patch for estrogen replacement therapy* [estrogen]

E_2C (estradiol cypionate) [q.v.]

E5 MAb [now: edobacomab]

E-200; E-400; E-1000 softgels (discontinued 1999) OTC *vitamin supplement* [vitamin E] 147 mg; 400 IU; 1000 IU

E25 (rhuMAb-E25) [now: omalizumab]

EACA (epsilon-aminocaproic acid) [see: aminocaproic acid]

EAP (etoposide, Adriamycin, Platinol) *chemotherapy protocol for gastric and small bowel cancer*

ear, lion's *medicinal herb* [see: motherwort]

Ear-Dry ear drops OTC *antibacterial; antifungal* [boric acid] 2.75%

Ear-Eze ear drops ℞ *topical corticosteroidal anti-inflammatory; antibiotic* [hydrocortisone; neomycin sulfate; polymyxin B sulfate] 1%•5 mg•10 000 U per mL

EarSol ear drops OTC *antiseptic* [alcohol] 44%

EarSol-HC ear drops OTC *topical corticosteroidal anti-inflammatory; antiseptic* [hydrocortisone; alcohol 44%] 1%

earthnut oil [see: peanut oil]

Easprin delayed-release enteric-coated tablets ℞ *analgesic; antipyretic; anti-inflammatory; antirheumatic* [aspirin] 975 mg

Easter giant *medicinal herb* [see: bistort]

Easy A1C fingerstick test kit for home use *in vitro diagnostic aid for glycosylated hemoglobin levels*

EasyInjector (trademarked device) *self-injector*

E-Base delayed-release enteric-coated caplets and tablets ℞ *macrolide antibiotic* [erythromycin] 333, 500 mg
ebastine USAN, INN *antihistamine*
ebiratide INN
ebrotidine INN
ebselen INN
EC (etoposide, carboplatin) *chemotherapy protocol for lung cancer*
ecadotril USAN, INN *antihypertensive*
ecamsule USAN *UVA sunscreen*
ecarazine [see: todralazine]
EC-ASA (enteric-coated aspirin) [see: aspirin]
ecastolol INN
Ecee Plus tablets OTC *vitamin/mineral supplement* [vitamins C and E; zinc sulfate; magnesium sulfate] 100•165•80•70 mg
echinacea *(Echinacea angustifolia; E. purpurea; E. pallida)* root *medicinal herb for anemia, blood diseases, blood poisoning, boils, dizziness, immune system stimulation, lymph disorders, promoting wound healing, prostate disorders, skin infections, and snake bites*
echinocandins *a class of antifungals* [also: glucan synthesis inhibitors]
Echinopanax horridum *medicinal herb* [see: devil's club]
ECHO (etoposide, cyclophosphamide, hydroxydaunomycin, Oncovin) *chemotherapy protocol*
EchoGen emulsion ℞ *investigational (NDA filed) ultrasound contrast agent for stress cardiography and transrectal prostate imaging* [perflenapent; perflisopent] 85%•15%
echothiophate iodide USP *antiglaucoma agent; irreversible cholinesterase inhibitor miotic* [also: ecothiopate iodide]
Echovist (CAN) intrauterine suspension ℞ *ultrasound contrast medium for gynecological imaging* [galactose]
ecipramidil INN
eclanamine INN *antidepressant* [also: eclanamine maleate]
eclanamine maleate USAN *antidepressant* [also: eclanamine]
eclazolast USAN, INN *antiallergic; mediator release inhibitor*
EC-Naprosyn enteric-coated delayed-release tablets ℞ *antiarthritic; nonsteroidal anti-inflammatory drug (NSAID)* [naproxen] 375, 500 mg
ecogramostim BAN
E-Complex-600 capsules (discontinued 1999) OTC *dietary supplement* [vitamin E] 600 IU
ecomustine INN
econazole USAN, INN, BAN *topical antifungal*
econazole nitrate USAN, USP, BAN *topical antifungal*
Econo B & C caplets OTC *vitamin supplement* [multiple B vitamins; vitamin C] ≛•300 mg
Econopred; Econopred Plus Drop-Tainers (eye drop suspension) ℞ *topical ophthalmic corticosteroidal anti-inflammatory* [prednisolone acetate] 0.125%; 1%
ecopipam HCl USAN *selective dopamine receptor antagonist for addiction*
ecostigmine iodide [see: echothiophate iodide]
ecothiopate iodide INN, BAN *antiglaucoma agent; irreversible cholinesterase inhibitor miotic* [also: echothiophate iodide]
Ecotrin enteric-coated tablets, enteric-coated caplets OTC *analgesic; antipyretic; anti-inflammatory; antiarthritic* [aspirin] 325, 500 mg ⑨ Edecrin
Ecotrin Adult Low Strength enteric-coated tablets OTC *analgesic; antipyretic; anti-inflammatory; antiarthritic* [aspirin] 81 mg
ectylurea BAN
Ed A-Hist long-acting capsules, liquid ℞ *decongestant; antihistamine* [phenylephrine HCl; chlorpheniramine maleate] 20•8 mg; 10•4 mg/5 mL
edamine [see: ethylenediamine]
EDAP (etoposide, dexamethasone, ara-C, Platinol) *chemotherapy protocol*
edathamil [now: edetate calcium disodium]

edathamil calcium disodium [now: edetate calcium disodium]
edathamil disodium [now: edetate disodium]
edatrexate USAN, INN *antineoplastic; methotrexate analogue*
Edecrin tablets ℞ *antihypertensive; loop diuretic* [ethacrynic acid] 25, 50 mg ⓢ Ecotrin; Ethaquin
Edecrin Sodium powder for IV injection ℞ *antihypertensive; loop diuretic* [ethacrynate sodium] 50 mg
edelfosine INN
edetate calcium disodium USAN, USP *heavy metal chelating agent for lead poisoning* [also: sodium calcium edetate; sodium calciumedetate; calcium disodium edetate]
edetate dipotassium USAN *chelating agent*
edetate disodium USP *chelating agent; preservative; antioxidant* [also: disodium edetate] 150 mg/mL injection
edetate sodium USAN *chelating agent*
edetate trisodium USAN *chelating agent*
edetic acid NF, INN, BAN *chelating agent*
edetol USAN, INN *alkalizing agent*
Edex injection, pre-filled cartridges ℞ *vasodilator for erectile dysfunction* [alprostadil] 5, 10, 20, 40 μg/mL; 10, 20, 40 μg/mL
edifolone INN *antiarrhythmic* [also: edifolone acetate]
edifolone acetate USAN *antiarrhythmic* [also: edifolone]
Ed-In-Sol drops OTC *hematinic* [ferrous sulfate (source of iron)] 75 mg/0.6 mL (15 mg/0.6 mL)
edisilate INN *combining name for radicals or groups* [also: edisylate]
edisylate USAN, BAN *combining name for radicals or groups* [also: edisilate]
edithamil [see: edetate ...]
edobacomab USAN *antiendotoxin monoclonal antibody for gram-negative sepsis; clinical trials discontinued 1997*
edodekin alfa USAN *antiasthmatic; investigational (Phase I/II) immunomodulator for AIDS-related Kaposi sarcoma; investigational (orphan) for renal cell carcinoma* [previously: interleukin 12 (IL-12)]
edogestrone INN, BAN
edoxudine USAN, INN *antiviral*
edrecolomab USAN *monoclonal antibody; antineoplastic adjuvant*
edrofuradene [see: nifurdazil]
Edronax (commercially available in England) ℞ *investigational (NDA filed) fast-acting selective norepinephrine reuptake inhibitor for depression* [reboxetine mesylate]
edrophone chloride [see: edrophonium chloride]
edrophonium chloride USP, INN, BAN *cholinergic/anticholinesterase muscle stimulant; antidote to curare; myasthenia gravis diagnostic aid*
Ed-Spaz tablets ℞ *GI/GU antispasmodic; antiparkinsonian; anticholinergic "drying agent" for allergic rhinitis and hyperhidrosis* [hyoscyamine sulfate] 0.125 mg
EDTA (ethylenediaminetetraacetic acid) [see: edetate disodium]
EDTA calcium [see: edetate calcium disodium]
ED-TLC; ED Tuss HC liquid ℞ *narcotic antitussive; decongestant; antihistamine* [hydrocodone bitartrate; phenylephrine HCl; chlorpheniramine maleate] 1.67•5•2 mg/5 mL; 2.5•10•4 mg/5 mL
E.E.S. granules for oral suspension ℞ *macrolide antibiotic* [erythromycin ethylsuccinate] 200 mg/5 mL
EES (erythromycin ethylsuccinate) [q.v.]
E.E.S. 200 oral suspension ℞ *macrolide antibiotic* [erythromycin ethylsuccinate] 200 mg/5 mL
E.E.S. 400 film-coated tablets, oral suspension ℞ *macrolide antibiotic* [erythromycin ethylsuccinate] 400 mg; 400 mg/5 mL
EF-27 *investigational agent to reduce chemotherapy side effects (clinical trials discontinued 1998)*
efaroxan INN, BAN

efavirenz *antiviral non-nucleoside reverse transcriptase inhibitor (NNRTI) for HIV infection*

efavirenz & lamivudine & zidovudine *investigational (Phase III) antiviral combination for HIV and AIDS*

efegatran sulfate USAN *antithrombotic*

efetozole INN

Effer-K effervescent tablets ℞ *potassium supplement* [potassium bicarbonate; potassium citrate] 25 mEq

Effervescent Potassium effervescent tablets ℞ *potassium supplement* [potassium bicarbonate; potassium citrate] 25 mEq

Effexor tablets ℞ *antidepressant* [venlafaxine HCl] 25, 37.5, 50, 75, 100 mg

Effexor XR extended-release capsules ℞ *once-daily antidepressant and anxiolytic* [venlafaxine HCl] 37.5, 75, 150 mg

Efidac/24 extended-release tablets OTC *nasal decongestant* [pseudoephedrine HCl] 240 mg

Efidac/24 Chlorpheniramine extended-release tablets OTC *antihistamine* [chlorpheniramine maleate] 16 mg

Eflone eye drop suspension ℞ *topical ophthalmic corticosteroidal anti-inflammatory* [fluorometholone acetate] 0.1%

eflornithine INN, BAN *antineoplastic; antiprotozoal; topical hair growth inhibitor* [also: eflornithine HCl]

eflornithine HCl USAN *antiprotozoal for Trypanosoma brucei gambiense (sleeping sickness) infection (orphan); topical hair growth inhibitor; investigational (Phase III) antineoplastic for bladder cancer* [also: eflornithine]

efloxate INN

eflumast INN

Efodine ointment OTC *broad-spectrum antimicrobial* [povidone-iodine] 1%

eformoterol fumarate BAN *bronchodilator for asthma, COPD, and emphysema* [also: formoterol; formoterol fumarate]

EFP (etoposide, fluorouracil, Platinol) *chemotherapy protocol for gastric and small bowel cancer*

efrotomycin USAN, INN, BAN *veterinary growth stimulant*

Efudex cream, topical solution ℞ *antimetabolite antineoplastic for actinic keratoses and basal cell carcinomas* [fluorouracil] 5%; 2%, 5%

EGF-Genistein *investigational antineoplastic for breast cancer* [genistein]

egtazic acid USAN, INN *pharmaceutic aid*

Egyptian privet *medicinal herb* [see: henna *(Lawsonia)*]

Egyptian thorn *medicinal herb* [see: acacia]

EHDP (ethane hydroxydiphosphonate) [see: etidronate disodium]

Ehrlich 594 [see: acetarsone]

Ehrlich 606 [see: arsphenamine]

eicosapentaenoic acid (EPA) [also: icosapent]

8 in 1 (methylprednisolone, vincristine, lomustine, procarbazine, hydroxyurea, cisplatin, cytarabine, cyclophosphamide) *chemotherapy protocol*

8 in 1 (methylprednisolone, vincristine, lomustine, procarbazine, hydroxyurea, cisplatin, cytarabine, dacarbazine) *chemotherapy protocol for pediatric brain tumors*

8-MOP capsules ℞ *systemic psoralens for repigmentation of idiopathic vitiligo; used to increase tolerance to sunlight and enhance pigmentation* [methoxsalen] 10 mg

einsteinium *element (Es)*

eIPV (enhanced, inactivated polio vaccine) [see: poliovirus vaccine, enhanced inactivated]

elacridar HCl USAN *chemotherapy potentiator; multi–drug-resistance inhibitor*

ELA-Max cream OTC *topical local anesthetic* [lidocaine] 4%

elantrine USAN, INN *anticholinergic*

elanzepine INN

Elase powder, ointment (discontinued 1999) ℞ *topical enzyme for biochemical* *debridement* [fibrinolysin; desoxyribonuclease] 25•15 000 U; 1•666.6 U/g

Elase-Chloromycetin ointment (discontinued 1999) ℞ *topical enzyme for biochemical debridement; antibiotic* [fibrinolysin; desoxyribonuclease; chloramphenicol] 1 U•666.6 U•10 mg per g

elastofilcon A USAN *hydrophilic contact lens material*

Elavil film-coated tablets, IM injection ℞ *tricyclic antidepressant* [amitriptyline HCl] 10, 25, 50, 75, 100, 150 mg; 10 mg/mL ⊡ Aldoril; Eldepryl; Enovil; Equanil; Mellaril

elbanizine INN

elcatonin INN, JAN *investigational (orphan) intrathecal treatment of intractable pain*

eldacimibe USAN *antihyperlipidemic; antiatherosclerotic; AcylCoA transferase (ACAT) inhibitor*

Eldepryl capsules ℞ *dopaminergic antiparkinsonian (orphan)* [selegiline HCl] 5 mg ⊡ Aldoril; Elavil; Enovil; Equanil; Mellaril

elder flower; elderberry *(Sambucus canadensis; S. ebulus; S. nigra; S. racemosa)* berries and flowers *medicinal herb for allergies, asthma, bronchitis, colds, constipation, edema, fever, hay fever, pneumonia, and sinus congestion; also used topically as an astringent*

Eldercaps capsules ℞ *vitamin/mineral supplement* [multiple vitamins & minerals; folic acid] ≛•1 mg

Eldertonic liquid OTC *vitamin/mineral supplement* [multiple B vitamins & minerals; alcohol 13.5%]

eldexomer INN

Eldisine ℞ *investigational (NDA filed) antineoplastic for leukemia, melanoma, breast and lung cancers* [vindesine sulfate]

Eldopaque; Eldopaque-Forte cream OTC *hyperpigmentation bleaching agent; sunscreen* [hydroquinone in a sunblock base] 2%; 4%

Eldoquin; Eldoquin-Forte Sunbleaching cream OTC *hyperpigmentation bleaching agent* [hydroquinone] 2%; 4%

elecampane *(Inula helenium)* root *medicinal herb for chronic bronchitis and cough*

electrocortin [see: aldosterone]

eledoisin INN

eletriptan hydrobromide USAN *investigational (NDA filed) serotonin 5-*HT_{1D}*-receptor agonist for migraine*

Eleutherococcus senticosus *medicinal herb* [see: Siberian ginseng]

ELF (etoposide, leucovorin [rescue], fluorouracil) *chemotherapy protocol for gastric cancer*

elfazepam USAN, INN *veterinary appetite stimulant*

elfdock; elfwort *medicinal herb* [see: elecampane]

elgodipine INN

Elimite cream ℞ *pediculicide for lice; scabicide* [permethrin] 5%

eliprodil INN *investigational treatment for ischemic stroke*

Elixomin elixir ℞ *antiasthmatic; bronchodilator* [theophylline] 80 mg/15 mL

Elixophyllin capsules, elixir ℞ *antiasthmatic; bronchodilator* [theophylline] 100, 200 mg; 80 mg/15 mL

Elixophyllin GG liquid ℞ *antiasthmatic; bronchodilator; expectorant* [theophylline; guaifenesin] 100•100 mg/15 mL

Elixophyllin-KI elixir ℞ *antiasthmatic; bronchodilator; expectorant* [theophylline; potassium iodide] 80•130 mg/15 mL

ellagic acid INN

Ellence IV infusion ℞ *anthracycline antibiotic antineoplastic for breast cancer* [epirubicin HCl] 2 mg/mL

Elliott's B solution *investigational (orphan) intrathecal chemotherapy diluent*

elliptinium acetate INN, BAN

elm, American; Indian elm; moose elm; red elm; rock elm; sweet elm; winged elm *medicinal herb* [see: slippery elm]

Elmiron capsules ℞ *urinary tract anti-inflammatory and analgesic for intersti-*

tial cystitis (orphan) [pentosan polysulfate sodium] 100 mg

elmustine INN

elnadipine INN

Elocom (CAN) ointment, cream, lotion ℞ *topical corticosteroidal anti-inflammatory* [mometasone furoate] 0.1%

Elocon ointment, cream, lotion ℞ *topical corticosteroidal anti-inflammatory* [mometasone furoate] 0.1%

Eloxatin ℞ *investigational (orphan) alkylating antineoplastic for ovarian and colorectal cancers* [oxaliplatin]

elsamitrucin USAN, INN *antineoplastic*

Elspar powder for IV or IM injection ℞ *antineoplastic adjunct for acute lymphocytic leukemia* [asparaginase] 10 000 IU

eltanolone INN *investigational IV anesthetic*

eltenac INN

eltoprazine INN

Eltroxin tablets ℞ *synthetic thyroid T_4 hormone* [levothyroxine sodium] 50, 75, 100, 125, 150, 200, 300 µg

elucaine USAN, INN *gastric anticholinergic*

Elymus repens *medicinal herb* [see: couch grass]

elziverine INN

EMA (estramustine L-alanine) [q.v.]

EMA 86 (etoposide, mitoxantrone, ara-C) *chemotherapy protocol for acute myelocytic leukemia (AML)*

EMACO (etoposide, methotrexate, actinomycin D, cyclophosphamide, Oncovin) *chemotherapy protocol*

Emadine eye drops ℞ *topical antihistamine for allergic conjunctivitis* [emedastine difumarate] 0.05%

embinal [see: barbital sodium]

embonate INN, BAN *combining name for radicals or groups* [also: pamoate]

embramine INN, BAN

embramine HCl [see: embramine]

embutramide USAN, INN, BAN *veterinary anesthetic; veterinary euthanasia*

Emcyt capsules ℞ *nitrogen mustard-type alkylating antineoplastic for palliative treatment of progressive or metastatic prostate cancer* [estramustine phosphate sodium] 140 mg

Emdogain ℞ *investigational (NDA filed) freeze-dried enamel matrix protein for wound healing*

Emecheck liquid (discontinued 1998) OTC *antinauseant; antiemetic* [phosphorated carbohydrate solution (glucose, fructose, and phosphoric acid)]

emedastine INN *ophthalmic antihistamine* [also: emedastine difumarate]

emedastine difumarate USAN, JAN *ophthalmic antihistamine* [also: emedastine]

emepronium bromide INN, BAN

emepronium carrageenate BAN

Emergent-Ez Kit *carry-kit for medical personnel* [multiple drugs and devices for emergencies]

Emersal emulsion ℞ *topical antipsoriatic; antiseborrheic* [ammoniated mercury; salicylic acid] 5%•2.5%

emetic herb; emetic weed *medicinal herb* [see: lobelia]

emetics *a class of agents that induce vomiting*

emetine BAN *antiamebic* [also: emetine HCl] ⑨ Emetrol

emetine bismuth iodide [see: emetine HCl]

emetine HCl USP *amebicide* [also: emetine]

Emetrol oral solution OTC *antiemetic for nausea associated with influenza, morning sickness, motion sickness, inhalation anesthesia, or food and drink indiscretions* [phosphorated carbohydrate solution (fructose, dextrose, and phosphoric acid)] 1.87 g•1.87 g•21.5 mg ⑨ emetine

Emgel gel ℞ *topical antibiotic for acne* [erythromycin] 2%

emiglitate INN, BAN

emilium tosilate INN *antiarrhythmic* [also: emilium tosylate]

emilium tosylate USAN *antiarrhythmic* [also: emilium tosilate]

Eminase powder for IV injection ℞ *thrombolytic enzyme for acute myocardial infarction* [anistreplase] 30 U/vial

Emitasol intranasal ℞ *investigational antiemetic for chemotherapy* [metoclopramide HCl]

emitefur USAN *antineoplastic for stomach, colorectal, breast, pancreatic, and non–small cell lung cancers (NSCLC)*

emivirine *investigational (NDA filed) non-nucleoside reverse transcriptase inhibitor for naive HIV infection*

Emko; Emko Pre-Fil vaginal foam OTC *spermicidal contraceptive* [nonoxynol 9] 8%

EMLA cream, adhesive disc ℞ *topical local anesthetic* [lidocaine; prilocaine] 2.5%•2.5%

emmenagogues *a class of agents that induce or increase menstruation*

Emollia lotion OTC *moisturizer; emollient*

emollient laxatives *a subclass of laxatives that work by retarding colonic absorption of fecal water to soften the stool and ease its movement through the intestines* [see also: laxatives]

emollients *a class of dermatological agents that soften and soothe the skin*

emonapride INN

emopamil INN

emorfazone INN

Empirin tablets OTC *analgesic; antipyretic; anti-inflammatory; antirheumatic* [aspirin] 325 mg

Empirin with Codeine No. 3 & No. 4 tablets ℞ *narcotic analgesic; sometimes abused as a street drug* [codeine phosphate; aspirin] 30•325 mg; 60•325 mg

emtricitabine USAN *investigational (NDA filed) nucleoside analogue antiviral for HIV and AIDS; investigational (Phase I/II) for hepatitis B*

emtryl [see: dimetridazole]

emu oil *natural remedy for arthritis pain, hair loss prevention, and chronic skin disorders*

emulsifying wax [see: wax, emulsifying]

Emulsoil oral emulsion OTC *stimulant laxative* [castor oil] 95%

E-Mycin enteric-coated tablets ℞ *macrolide antibiotic* [erythromycin] 250, 333 mg

emylcamate INN, BAN

Enable ℞ *investigational (NDA filed) anti-inflammatory for rheumatoid arthritis and osteoarthritis* [tenidap]

enadoline INN *analgesic* [also: enadoline HCl]

enadoline HCl USAN *analgesic; investigational (orphan) for severe head injury* [also: enadoline]

enalapril INN, BAN *antihypertensive; angiotensin-converting enzyme (ACE) inhibitor* [also: enalapril maleate]

enalapril maleate USAN, USP *antihypertensive; angiotensin-converting enzyme (ACE) inhibitor* [also: enalapril] 2.5, 5, 10, 20 mg oral; 1.25 mg/mL injection

enalapril maleate & hydrochlorothiazide *antihypertensive; angiotensin-converting enzyme (ACE) inhibitor; diuretic* 5•12.5, 10•25 mg oral

enalaprilat USAN, USP, INN, BAN *antihypertensive; angiotensin-converting enzyme (ACE) inhibitor* 1.25 mg/mL injection

enalkiren USAN, INN *antihypertensive; renin inhibitor*

enallynymal sodium [see: methohexital sodium]

enantate INN *combining name for radicals or groups* [also: enanthate]

enanthate USAN, USP, BAN *combining name for radicals or groups* [also: enantate]

Enbrel powder for subcu injection ℞ *soluble tumor necrosis factor receptor (sTNFR) inhibitor for rheumatoid arthritis (RA) and juvenile rheumatoid arthritis (JRA); investigational (NDA filed) for congestive heart failure* [etanercept] 25 mg ⑨ Incel

enbucrilate INN, BAN

encainide INN, BAN *antiarrhythmic* [also: encainide HCl]

encainide HCl USAN *antiarrhythmic* [also: encainide]

Encare vaginal suppositories OTC *spermicidal contraceptive* [nonoxynol 9] 2.27%

enciprazine INN, BAN *minor tranquilizer* [also: enciprazine HCl]
enciprazine HCl USAN *minor tranquilizer* [also: enciprazine]
enclomifene INN [also: enclomiphene]
enclomiphene USAN [also: enclomifene]
encyprate USAN, INN *antidepressant*
End Lice liquid OTC *pediculicide for lice* [pyrethrins; piperonyl butoxide] 0.3%•3%
Endafed sustained-release capsules ℞ *decongestant; antihistamine* [pseudoephedrine HCl; brompheniramine maleate] 120•12 mg
Endagen-HD liquid ℞ *narcotic antitussive; decongestant; antihistamine* [hydrocodone bitartrate; phenylephrine HCl; chlorpheniramine maleate] 1.67•5•2 mg/5 mL
Endal timed-release tablets ℞ *decongestant; expectorant* [phenylephrine HCl; guaifenesin] 20•300 mg ⊡ Intal
Endal Expectorant syrup ℞ *narcotic antitussive; decongestant; expectorant* [codeine phosphate; phenylpropanolamine HCl; guaifenesin; alcohol 5%] 10•12.5•100 mg/5 mL
Endal-HD; Endal-HD Plus liquid ℞ *narcotic antitussive; decongestant; antihistamine* [hydrocodone bitartrate; phenylephrine HCl; chlorpheniramine maleate] 1.7•5•2 mg/5 mL; 2.5•5•2 mg/5 mL
endiemal [see: metharbital]
endive *medicinal herb* [see: chicory]
endive, white; wild endive *medicinal herb* [see: dandelion]
endixaprine INN
endobenzyline bromide
endocaine [see: pyrrocaine]
Endocet tablets ℞ *narcotic analgesic* [oxycodone HCl; acetaminophen] 5•325 mg
Endocodone tablets ℞ *narcotic analgesic* [oxycodone HCl] 5 mg
endolate [see: meperidine HCl]
Endolor capsules (discontinued 2000) ℞ *analgesic; barbiturate sedative* [acetaminophen; caffeine; butalbital] 325•40•50 mg
endomide INN
endomycin
Endospray (CAN) metered-dose spray OTC *topical anesthetic for oropharyngeal and endotracheal areas* [benzocaine; tetracaine] 18•2 mg/spray
endothelin-1 receptor antagonists *a class of antihypertensives that block the action of endothelin-1, a vascular vasoconstrictor more potent than angiotensin II*
endralazine INN, BAN *antihypertensive* [also: endralazine mesylate]
endralazine mesylate USAN *antihypertensive* [also: endralazine]
Endrate IV infusion ℞ *chelating agent for hypercalcemia and ventricular arrhythmias due to digitalis toxicity* [edetate disodium] 150 mg/mL
endrisone INN *topical ophthalmic anti-inflammatory* [also: endrysone]
endrysone USAN *topical ophthalmic anti-inflammatory* [also: endrisone]
Enduret (trademarked dosage form) *prolonged-action tablet*
Enduron tablets ℞ *diuretic; antihypertensive* [methyclothiazide] 5 mg ⊡ Imuran; Inderal
Enduronyl; Enduronyl Forte tablets ℞ *antihypertensive* [methyclothiazide; deserpidine] 5•0.25 mg; 5•0.5 mg ⊡ Inderal
Enecat concentrated rectal suspension ℞ *radiopaque contrast medium for gastrointestinal imaging* [barium sulfate] 5%
enefexine INN
Ener-B nasal gel (discontinued 1999) OTC *vitamin B_{12} supplement* [cyanocobalamin] 400 µg
Enerjets lozenges OTC *CNS stimulant; analeptic* [caffeine] 75 mg
enestebol INN
Enfalac AR (CAN) powder OTC *total or supplementary infant feeding; thickened formula* [cow's milk–based formula]
Enfalac Iron Fortified (CAN) liquid, powder OTC *total or supplementary infant feeding* [milk-based formula]

Enfalac ProSobee Soy (CAN) liquid, powder OTC *hypoallergenic infant food* [soy protein formula]
Enfalac Regular (CAN) liquid, powder OTC *total or supplementary infant feeding* [milk-based formula]
Enfamil liquid, powder OTC *total or supplementary infant feeding*
Enfamil Human Milk Fortifier powder OTC *supplement to breast milk*
Enfamil LactoFree liquid, liquid concentrate, powder OTC *hypoallergenic infant formula* [milk-based formula, lactose free] 946 mL; 384 mL; 397 g
Enfamil Natalins Rx tablets ℞ *vitamin/mineral/calcium/iron supplement* [multiple vitamins & minerals; calcium; iron; folic acid; biotin] ≛•100•27•0.5 mg•15 μg
Enfamil Next Step liquid, powder OTC *total or supplementary infant feeding*
Enfamil Premature Formula liquid OTC *total or supplementary infant feeding*
Enfamil with Iron liquid, powder OTC *total or supplementary infant feeding*
enfenamic acid INN
enflurane USAN, USP, INN, BAN *inhalation general anesthetic* 125, 250 mL
Engerix-B adult IM injection, pediatric IM injection ℞ *active immunizing agent for hepatitis B and D* [hepatitis B virus vaccine, recombinant] 20 μg/mL, 10 μg/0.5 mL
English elm *(Ulmus campestris)* *medicinal herb* [see: slippery elm]
English hawthorn *medicinal herb* [see: hawthorn]
English ivy *(Hedera helix)* leaves *medicinal herb used as an antispasmodic and antiexanthematous agent*
English oak *(Quercus robur)* *medicinal herb* [see: white oak]
English valerian *medicinal herb* [see: valerian]
English walnut *(Juglans regia)* leaves *medicinal herb used as an astringent*
englitazone INN *antidiabetic* [also: englitazone sodium]
englitazone sodium USAN *antidiabetic* [also: englitazone]
enhanced, inactivated polio vaccine (eIPV) [see: poliovirus vaccine, enhanced inactivated]
Enhancer oral suspension ℞ *radiopaque contrast medium for gastrointestinal imaging* [barium sulfate] 98%
enhexymal [see: hexobarbital]
eniclobrate INN
enilconazole USAN, INN, BAN *antifungal*
enilospirone INN
eniluracil USAN *antineoplastic potentiator for fluorouracil; uracil reductase inhibitor*
enisoprost USAN, INN *antiulcerative; orphan status withdrawn 1996*
Enisyl tablets OTC *dietary amino acid supplement* [L-lysine] 334, 500 mg
Enlon IV or IM injection ℞ *myasthenia gravis treatment; antidote to curare overdose* [edrophonium chloride] 10 mg/mL
Enlon Plus IV or IM injection ℞ *muscle stimulant; neuromuscular blocker antagonist* [edrophonium chloride; atropine sulfate] 10•0.14 mg
enloplatin USAN, INN *antineoplastic*
enocitabine INN
enofelast USAN, INN *antiasthmatic*
enolicam INN *anti-inflammatory; antirheumatic* [also: enolicam sodium]
enolicam sodium USAN *anti-inflammatory; antirheumatic* [also: enolicam]
Enomine capsules ℞ *decongestant; expectorant* [phenylpropanolamine HCl; phenylephrine HCl; guaifenesin] 45•5•200 mg
Enovid tablets (discontinued 1997) ℞ *estrogen/progestin combination for hypermenorrhea or endometriosis* [mestranol; norethynodrel] 75 μg•5 mg; 150 μg•9.85 mg
enoxacin USAN, INN, BAN, JAN *broad-spectrum fluoroquinolone antibiotic*
enoxamast INN
enoxaparin BAN *a low molecular weight heparin–type anticoagulant and antithrombotic for the prevention of deep vein thrombosis (DVT), unstable angina, and myocardial infarction* [also: enoxaparin sodium]

enoxaparin sodium USAN, INN *a low molecular weight heparin–type anticoagulant and antithrombotic for the prevention of deep vein thrombosis (DVT), unstable angina, and myocardial infarction* [also: enoxaparin]

enoximone USAN, INN, BAN *cardiotonic*

enoxolone INN, BAN

enphenemal [see: mephobarbital]

enpiprazole INN, BAN

enpiroline INN *antimalarial* [also: enpiroline phosphate]

enpiroline phosphate USAN *antimalarial* [also: enpiroline]

enprazepine INN

Enpresse tablets ℞ *triphasic oral contraceptive; emergency postcoital contraceptive* [levonorgestrel; ethinyl estradiol] Phase 1 (6 days): 50•30 µg; Phase 2 (5 days): 75•40 µg; Phase 3 (10 days): 125•30 µg

enprofen [now: furaprofen]

enprofylline USAN, INN *bronchodilator*

enpromate USAN, INN *antineoplastic*

enprostil USAN, INN, BAN *investigational antisecretory and antiulcerative for acute peptic ulcers*

enramycin INN

enrofloxacin USAN, INN, BAN *veterinary antibacterial*

Enseal (trademarked dosage form) *enteric-coated tablet*

Ensure liquid, powder OTC *enteral nutritional therapy* [lactose-free formula]

Ensure pudding OTC *enteral nutritional therapy* [milk-based formula] 150 g

Ensure Glucerna beverage, bars OTC *diabetic nutritional supplements/snacks*

Ensure High Calcium ready-to-use liquid OTC *enteral nutritional therapy for postmenopausal women*

Ensure High Protein ready-to-use liquid OTC *enteral nutritional therapy* [lactose-free formula] 237 mL

Ensure HN; Ensure with Fiber ready-to-use liquid OTC *enteral nutritional therapy* [lactose-free formula]

Ensure Plus; Ensure Plus HN liquid OTC *enteral nutritional therapy* [lactose-free formula]

E.N.T. sustained-release tablets (discontinued 1997) ℞ *decongestant; antihistamine* [phenylpropanolamine HCl; brompheniramine maleate] 75•12 mg

EN-tab (trademarked dosage form) *enteric-coated tablet*

entacapone USAN *catechol-O-methyltransferase (COMT) inhibitor for Parkinson disease*

entecavir USAN *antiviral for hepatitis B infection*

enteramine [see: serotonin]

Entero-Test; Entero-Test Pediatric string capsules for professional use *in vitro diagnostic aid for GI disorders*

Entertainer's Secret Throat Relief spray OTC *saliva substitute* [carboxymethylcellulose sodium]

Entex capsules, liquid ℞ *decongestant; expectorant* [phenylephrine HCl; phenylpropanolamine HCl; guaifenesin] 5•45•200 mg; 5•20•100 mg/5 mL

Entex LA long-acting tablets ℞ *decongestant; expectorant* [phenylpropanolamine HCl; guaifenesin] 75•400 mg

Entex PSE prolonged-action tablets ℞ *decongestant; expectorant* [pseudoephedrine HCl; guaifenesin] 60•120 mg

Entocort (CAN) oral capsules for ileal release, retention enema ℞ *steroidal anti-inflammatory for Crohn disease* [budesonide] 3 mg; 2 mg

Entri-Pak (dosage form) *liquid-filled pouch*

Entrition 0.5 liquid OTC *enteral nutritional therapy* [lactose-free formula]

Entrition HN Entri-Pak (liquid-filled pouch) OTC *enteral nutritional therapy* [lactose-free formula]

Entrobar oral suspension (with Entrocel diluent) ℞ *radiopaque contrast medium for gastrointestinal imaging* [barium sulfate; (methylcellulose diluent)] 50% (500 mL)

Entrophen (CAN) enteric-coated tablets, enteric-coated caplets OTC *analgesic; antipyretic; anti-inflammatory; anti-*

rheumatic [aspirin] 325, 500, 650 mg; 325, 650 mg

entsufon INN *detergent* [also: entsufon sodium]

entsufon sodium USAN *detergent* [also: entsufon]

Entuss Expectorant liquid ℞ *narcotic antitussive; expectorant* [hydrocodone bitartrate; potassium guaiacolsulfonate] 5•300 mg/5 mL

Entuss Expectorant tablets ℞ *narcotic antitussive; expectorant* [hydrocodone bitartrate; guaifenesin] 5•300 mg

Entuss-D liquid ℞ *narcotic antitussive; decongestant* [hydrocodone bitartrate; pseudoephedrine HCl] 5•30 mg/5 mL

Entuss-D tablets ℞ *narcotic antitussive; decongestant; expectorant* [hydrocodone bitartrate; pseudoephedrine HCl; guaifenesin] 5•30•300 mg

Entuss-D Jr. liquid ℞ *pediatric narcotic antitussive, decongestant, and expectorant* [hydrocodone bitartrate; pseudoephedrine HCl; guaifenesin; alcohol 5%] 2.5•30•100 mg/5 mL

Enuclene eye drops OTC *cleaning, wetting and lubricating agent for artificial eyes* [tyloxapol] 0.25%

Enulose oral/rectal solution ℞ *synthetic disaccharide used to prevent and treat portal-systemic encephalopathy* [lactulose] 10 g/15 mL

enviomycin INN

enviradene USAN, INN *antiviral*

Enviro-Stress slow-release tablets OTC *vitamin/mineral supplement* [multiple vitamins & minerals; folic acid] ≛ • 0.4 mg

enviroxime USAN, INN *antiviral*

enzacamene USAN *ultraviolet sunscreen*

Enzone cream ℞ *topical corticosteroidal anti-inflammatory; local anesthetic* [hydrocortisone acetate; pramoxine HCl] 1%•1%

Enzymatic Cleaner for Extended Wear tablets OTC *enzymatic cleaner for soft contact lenses* [pork pancreatin]

Enzyme chewable tablets OTC *digestive enzymes* [amylase; protease; lipase; cellulase] 30•6•2•25 mg

EP (etoposide, Platinol) *chemotherapy protocol for adenocarcinoma and lung and testicular cancer*

EPA capsules OTC *dietary supplement* [omega-3 fatty acids] 1000 mg

EPA (eicosapentaenoic acid) [also: icosapent]

epalrestat INN *investigational treatment for diabetic neuropathy*

epanolol INN, BAN

Epaxal Berna (CAN) suspension for IM injection OTC *active immunizing agent for hepatitis* A [hepatitis A vaccine, inactivated] 0.5 mL

eperezolid USAN *antibacterial*

eperisone INN

epervudine INN

ephedra (*Ephedra* spp.) plant *medicinal herb for asthma, blood cleansing, bronchitis, bursitis, chills, colds, edema, fever, flu, headache, kidney disorders, nasal congestion, and venereal disease*

ephedrine USP, BAN *sympathomimetic bronchodilator; nasal decongestant; vasopressor for shock* ⓢ Appedrine; aprindine

ephedrine HCl USP, BAN *sympathomimetic bronchodilator; nasal decongestant; vasopressor for shock* ⓢ Appedrine; aprindine

ephedrine sulfate USP *sympathomimetic bronchodilator; nasal decongestant; vasopressor for acute hypotensive shock* [also: ephedrine sulphate] 25 mg oral; 50 mg/mL injection ⓢ Appedrine; aprindine

ephedrine sulphate BAN *sympathomimetic bronchodilator; nasal decongestant* [also: ephedrine sulfate] ⓢ Appedrine; aprindine

ephedrine tannate *sympathomimetic bronchodilator; nasal decongestant* ⓢ Appedrine; aprindine

EPI-2010 *investigational for asthma*

Epi-C concentrated oral suspension ℞ *radiopaque contrast medium for gastrointestinal imaging* [barium sulfate] 150%

epicainide INN

epicillin USAN, INN, BAN *antibacterial*

epicriptine INN

epidermal growth factor, human *investigational (orphan) for acceleration of corneal regeneration*

epiestriol INN [also: epioestriol]

Epifoam aerosol foam ℞ *topical corticosteroidal anti-inflammatory; local anesthetic* [hydrocortisone acetate; pramoxine] 1%•1%

Epifrin eye drops ℞ *topical antiglaucoma agent* [epinephrine HCl] 0.5%, 1%, 2% ⑨ epinephrine; EpiPen

Epiject (CAN) IV infusion ℞ *anticonvulsant* [valproate sodium] 100 mg/mL

EpiLeukin ℞ *investigational (Phase III) treatment for malignant melanoma*

epilin [see: dietifen]

E-Pilo-1; E-Pilo-2; E-Pilo-4; E-Pilo-6 eye drops ℞ *topical antiglaucoma agent* [pilocarpine HCl; epinephrine bitartrate] 1%•1%; 2%•1%; 4%•1%; 6%•1%

Epilyt lotion concentrate OTC *moisturizer; emollient*

epimestrol USAN, INN, BAN *anterior pituitary activator*

Epinal eye drops ℞ *topical antiglaucoma agent* [epinephryl borate] 0.5%, 1% ⑨ Epitol

epinastine INN

epinephran [see: epinephrine]

epinephrine USP, INN *vasoconstrictor; sympathomimetic bronchodilator; topical antiglaucoma agent; vasopressor for shock* [also: adrenaline] 1:1000, 1:10 000 (1, 0.1 mg/mL) injection ⑨ Epifrin

epinephrine bitartrate USP *sympathomimetic bronchodilator; ophthalmic adrenergic; topical antiglaucoma agent*

epinephrine borate *topical antiglaucoma agent*

epinephrine & cisplatin *investigational (Phase II) injectable gel for inoperable primary liver cancer*

epinephrine HCl *sympathomimetic bronchodilator; nasal decongestant; topical antiglaucoma agent; vasopressor for shock* 0.1% eye drops; 1:1000, 1:2000, 1:10 000 (1, 0.5, 0.1 mg/mL) injection

Epinephrine Pediatric subcu injection (discontinued 2000) ℞ *bronchodilator for bronchial asthma or bronchospasm; vasopressor for shock* [epinephrine HCl] 1:100 000 (0.01 mg/mL)

epinephryl borate USAN, USP *adrenergic; topical antiglaucoma agent*

epioestriol BAN [also: epiestriol]

EpiPen; EpiPen Jr. auto-injector (automatic IM injection device) ℞ *emergency treatment of anaphylaxis; vasopressor for shock* [epinephrine] 1:1000 (1 mg/mL); 1:2000 (0.5 mg/mL) ⑨ Epifrin

epipropidine USAN, INN *antineoplastic*

epirizole USAN, INN *analgesic; anti-inflammatory*

epiroprim INN

epirubicin INN, BAN *anthracycline antibiotic antineoplastic* [also: epirubicin HCl]

epirubicin HCl USAN, JAN *anthracycline antibiotic antineoplastic for breast cancer* [also: epirubicin]

epitetracycline HCl USP *antibacterial*

epithiazide USAN, BAN *antihypertensive; diuretic* [also: epitizide]

epithioandrostanol [see: epitiostanol]

epitiostanol INN

epitizide INN *antihypertensive; diuretic* [also: epithiazide]

Epitol tablets ℞ *anticonvulsant; analgesic for trigeminal neuralgia; antipsychotic* [carbamazepine] 200 mg ⑨ Epinal

Epival (CAN) enteric-coated tablets ℞ *anticonvulsant* [divalproex sodium] 125, 250, 500 mg

Epival ER (CAN) extended-release tablets ℞ *anticonvulsant* [divalproex sodium] 500 mg

Epivir film-coated tablets, oral solution ℞ *nucleoside reverse transcriptase inhibitor (NRTI) antiviral for HIV* [lamivudine] 150 mg; 10 mg/mL

Epivir-HBV film-coated tablets, oral solution ℞ *nucleoside reverse transcriptase inhibitor (NRTI) antiviral for hepatitis B virus (HBV) infection* [lamivudine] 100 mg; 5 mg/mL

eplerenone USAN *aldosterone receptor antagonist for congestive heart failure,* *hypertension, and cirrhosis; investigational (Phase III) to improve survival after cardiovascular event*

EPO (epoetin alfa) [q.v.]

EPO (evening primrose oil) [see: evening primrose]

EPOCH (etoposide, prednisone, Oncovin, cyclophosphamide, Halotestin) *chemotherapy protocol*

epoetin alfa (EPO) USAN, INN, BAN, JAN *hematinic for anemia of chronic renal failure, HIV, and chemotherapy (orphan); to reduce blood transfusions in surgery*

epoetin beta USAN, INN, BAN, JAN *antianemic; hematinic; investigational (orphan) for anemia of end-stage renal disease*

Epogen IV or subcu injection ℞ *stimulates RBC production; for anemia of chronic renal failure, HIV, or chemotherapy (orphan)* [epoetin alfa] 2000, 3000, 4000, 10 000, 20 000 U/mL ⊠ "amp and gent" (ampicillin & gentamicin)

epoprostenol USAN, INN *platelet aggregation inhibitor and vasodilator for primary pulmonary hypertension (orphan)*

epoprostenol sodium USAN, BAN *platelet aggregation inhibitor and vasodilator for hypertension*

epostane USAN, INN, BAN *interceptive*

epoxytropine tropate methylbromide [see: methscopolamine bromide]

eprazinone INN

Eprex (name changed to Procrit in 1997)

eprinomectin USAN *veterinary antiparasitic*

epristeride USAN, INN, BAN *alpha reductase inhibitor for benign prostatic hypertrophy*

eprosartan USAN *antihypertensive; angiotensin II receptor antagonist*

eprosartan mesylate USAN *antihypertensive; angiotensin II receptor antagonist*

eprovafen INN

eproxindine INN

eprozinol INN

epsikapron [see: aminocaproic acid]

epsilon-aminocaproic acid (EACA) [see: aminocaproic acid]

epsiprantel INN, BAN

Epsom salt granules OTC *saline laxative* [magnesium sulfate]

Epsom salt [see: magnesium sulfate]

e.p.t. Quick Stick test stick for home use *in vitro diagnostic aid; urine pregnancy test*

eptacog alfa (activated) *activated recombinant human blood coagulation factor VII (rFVIIa) for hemophilia A and B*

eptaloprost INN

eptamestrol [see: etamestrol]

eptaprost [see: eptaloprost]

eptastatin sodium [see: pravastatin sodium]

eptastigmine INN *investigational treatment for Alzheimer disease*

eptazocine INN

eptifibatide *glycoprotein (GP) IIb/IIIa receptor antagonist; platelet aggregation inhibitor for acute coronary syndrome, unstable angina, myocardial infarction, and cardiac surgery*

Epulor liquid OTC *enteral nutritional therapy* [milk-based formula]

Equagesic tablets ℞ *analgesic; antipyretic; anti-inflammatory; anxiolytic; sedative* [aspirin; meprobamate] 325•200 mg

Equalactin chewable tablets OTC *bulk laxative; antidiarrheal* [calcium polycarbophil] 625 mg

Equanil tablets ℞ *anxiolytic* [meprobamate] 200, 400 mg ⊠ Aldoril; Elavil; Eldepryl; Enovil; Mellaril

Equilet chewable tablets OTC *antacid* [calcium carbonate] 500 mg

equilin USP *estrogen*

Equipoise *brand name for boldenone undecylenate, a veterinary anabolic steroid abused as a street drug*

Equisetum arvens *medicinal herb* [see: horsetail]

Eramycin film-coated tablets (discontinued 1998) ℞ *macrolide antibiotic* [erythromycin stearate] 250 mg

erbium *element (Er)*

erbulozole USAN, INN *antineoplastic adjunct*

erbumine USAN, INN, BAN *combining name for radicals or groups*

Ercaf tablets ℞ *migraine-specific vasoconstrictor* [ergotamine tartrate; caffeine] 1•100 mg

erdosteine INN

Erechtites hieracfolia *medicinal herb* [see: pilewort]

Ergamisol tablets ℞ *biological response modifier; antineoplastic adjunct for colon cancer* [levamisole HCl] 50 mg

ergocalciferol (vitamin D_2) USP, INN, BAN, JAN *fat-soluble vitamin for refractory rickets, familial hypophosphatemia, and hypoparathyroidism*

ergoloid mesylates USAN, USP *cognition adjuvant for age-related mental capacity decline* [also: co-dergocrine mesylate] 0.5, 1 mg oral

Ergomar sublingual tablets ℞ *migraine treatment; vasoconstrictor* [ergotamine tartrate] 2 mg

ergometrine INN, BAN *oxytocic for induction of labor* [also: ergonovine maleate]

ergonovine maleate USP *oxytocic for induction of labor* [also: ergometrine]

Ergoset once-daily tablets ℞ *investigational (NDA filed) dopamine agonist for hypoglycemic control in type 2 diabetes; investigational (Phase II/III) treatment for clinical obesity* [bromocriptine mesylate]

ergosterol, activated [see: ergocalciferol]

ergot (*Claviceps purpurea*) dried sclerotia *medicinal herb used as an abortifacient, emmenagogue, hemostatic, oxytocic, and vasoconstrictor; source of ergotamine and LSD*

ergot alkaloids [see: ergoloid mesylates]

ergotamine INN, BAN *migraine-specific analgesic* [also: ergotamine tartrate]

ergotamine tartrate USP *migraine-specific analgesic* [also: ergotamine]

Ergotrate Maleate IM or IV injection ℞ *oxytocic for the induction of labor and prevention of postpartum and postabortal hemorrhage* [ergonovine maleate] 0.2 mg/mL

ericolol INN

Erigeron canadensis *medicinal herb* [see: fleabane; horseweed]

eriodictyon NF

Eriodictyon californicum *medicinal herb* [see: yerba santa]

eritrityl tetranitrate INN *coronary vasodilator* [also: erythrityl tetranitrate]

erizepine INN

erlizumab USAN *monoclonal antibody to treat reperfusion injury following acute myocardial infarction*

E-R-O Ear Drops OTC *agent to emulsify and disperse ear wax* [carbamide peroxide] 6.5%

erocainide INN

errhines *a class of agents that promote nasal discharge or secretion*

ersofermin USAN, INN *wound healing agent; transglutaminase inhibitor for the treatment of scar tissue*

ertapenem sodium USAN *antibiotic*

Erwinase ℞ *investigational (orphan) antineoplastic for acute lymphocytic leukemia* [erwinia L-asparaginase]

erwinia L-asparaginase *investigational (orphan) antineoplastic for acute lymphocytic leukemia*

ERYC delayed-release capsules containing enteric-coated pellets ℞ *macrolide antibiotic* [erythromycin] 250 mg ⓢ ara-C

Erycette topical solution ℞ *topical antibiotic for acne* [erythromycin] 2% ⓢ Aricept

EryDerm 2% topical solution ℞ *topical antibiotic for acne* [erythromycin] 2%

Erygel gel ℞ *topical antibiotic for acne* [erythromycin; alcohol 92%] 2%

Erymax topical solution ℞ *topical antibiotic for acne* [erythromycin] 2%

Eryngium aquaticum *medicinal herb* [see: water eryngo]

EryPed chewable tablets, drops ℞ *macrolide antibiotic* [erythromycin ethylsuccinate] 200 mg; 100 mg/2.5 mL

EryPed granules for oral suspension (discontinued 1998) ℞ *macrolide*

antibiotic [erythromycin ethylsuccinate] 400 mg/5 mL

EryPed 200; EryPed 400 oral suspension ℞ *macrolide antibiotic* [erythromycin ethylsuccinate] 200 mg/5 mL; 400 mg/5 mL

Ery-Tab delayed-release enteric-coated tablets ℞ *macrolide antibiotic* [erythromycin] 250, 333, 500 mg

erythorbic acid

Erythra-Derm topical solution ℞ *topical antibiotic for acne* [erythromycin] 2%

Erythraea centaurium *medicinal herb* [see: centaury]

erythrityl tetranitrate USAN, USP *coronary vasodilator; antianginal* [also: eritrityl tetranitrate]

Erythrocin powder for IV injection ℞ *macrolide antibiotic* [erythromycin lactobionate] 500, 1000 mg/vial

Erythrocin Stearate Filmtabs (film-coated tablets) ℞ *macrolide antibiotic* [erythromycin stearate] 250, 500 mg

erythrol tetranitrate [now: erythrityl tetranitrate]

erythromycin USP, INN, BAN *macrolide antibiotic* 250, 500 mg oral; 0.5%, 2% topical ⓢ clarithromycin; dirithromycin

erythromycin 2′-acetate octadecanoate [see: erythromycin acistrate]

erythromycin 2′-acetate stearate [see: erythromycin acistrate]

erythromycin acistrate USAN, INN *macrolide antibiotic*

erythromycin B [see: berythromycin]

erythromycin estolate USAN, USP, BAN *macrolide antibiotic* 250 mg oral; 125, 250 mg/5 mL oral

erythromycin ethyl succinate BAN *macrolide antibiotic* [also: erythromycin ethylsuccinate]

erythromycin ethylcarbonate USP *macrolide antibiotic*

erythromycin ethylsuccinate (EES) USP *macrolide antibiotic* [also: erythromycin ethyl succinate] 400 mg oral; 200, 400 mg/5 mL oral;

erythromycin gluceptate USP *macrolide antibiotic*

erythromycin glucoheptonate [see: erythromycin gluceptate]

erythromycin lactobionate USP *macrolide antibiotic* 500, 1000 mg/vial injection

erythromycin lauryl sulfate, propionyl [now: erythromycin estolate]

erythromycin monoglucoheptonate [see: erythromycin gluceptate]

erythromycin octadecanoate [see: erythromycin stearate]

erythromycin 2′-propanoate [see: erythromycin propionate]

erythromycin propionate USAN *macrolide antibiotic*

erythromycin 2′-propionate dodecyl sulfate [see: erythromycin estolate]

erythromycin propionate lauryl sulfate [now: erythromycin estolate]

erythromycin salnacedin USAN *macrolide antibiotic for acne vulgaris*

erythromycin stearate USP, BAN *macrolide antibiotic* 250, 500 mg oral

erythromycin stinoprate INN *macrolide antibiotic*

Erythronium americanum *medicinal herb* [see: adder's tongue]

erythropoietin, gene-activated (GA-EPO) *investigational (NDA filed) gene therapy for anemia of renal failure*

erythropoietin, recombinant human (rEPO) [see: epoetin alfa; epoetin beta]

erythrosine sodium USP *dental disclosing agent*

Eryzole granules for oral suspension ℞ *antibiotic* [erythromycin ethylsuccinate; sulfisoxazole acetyl] 200•600 mg/5 mL

esafloxacin INN

esaprazole INN

escitalopram oxalate USAN *antidepressant; selective serotonin reuptake inhibitor (SSRI); isomer of citalopram*

Esclim transdermal patch ℞ *estrogen replacement therapy for postmenopausal symptoms* [estradiol] 25, 37.5, 50, 75, 100 µg/day

esculamine INN

eseridine INN

eserine [see: physostigmine]

Eserine Sulfate ophthalmic ointment (discontinued 1999) ℞ *topical antiglaucoma agent; reversible cholinesterase inhibitor miotic* [physostigmine sulfate] 0.25%

esflurbiprofen INN, BAN

Esgic caplets, capsules ℞ *analgesic; barbiturate sedative* [acetaminophen; caffeine; butalbital] 325•40•50 mg

Esgic-Plus caplets, capsules ℞ *analgesic; barbiturate sedative* [acetaminophen; caffeine; butalbital] 500•40•50 mg

ESHAP (etoposide, Solu-Medrol, high-dose ara-C, Platinol) *chemotherapy protocol for non-Hodgkin lymphoma*

ESHAP-MINE (alternating cycles of ESHAP and MINE) *chemotherapy protocol*

Esidrix tablets ℞ *antihypertensive; diuretic* [hydrochlorothiazide] 25, 50, 100 mg ⊡ Lasix

esilate INN *combining name for radicals or groups* [also: esylate]

Esimil tablets ℞ *antihypertensive; diuretic* [hydrochlorothiazide; guanethidine monosulfate] 25•10 mg ⊡ Estinyl; Isomil

Eskalith capsules, tablets ℞ *antipsychotic for manic episodes of a bipolar disorder* [lithium carbonate] 300 mg

Eskalith CR controlled-release tablets ℞ *antipsychotic for manic episodes of a bipolar disorder* [lithium carbonate] 450 mg

esmolol INN, BAN *antiadrenergic (β-blocker); antiarrhythmic* [also: esmolol HCl]

esmolol HCl USAN *antiadrenergic (β-blocker); antiarrhythmic for supraventricular tachycardia* [also: esmolol]

E-Solve OTC *lotion base*

esomeprazole magnesium USAN *proton pump inhibitor for gastric and duodenal ulcers, erosive esophagitis, GERD, and other gastroesophageal disorders; isomer of omeprazole*

esopiclone *investigational (NDA filed) non-benzodiazepine sedative and hypnotic*

esorubicin INN *antineoplastic* [also: esorubicin HCl]

esorubicin HCl USAN *antineoplastic* [also: esorubicin]

Esotérica Dry Skin Treatment lotion OTC *moisturizer; emollient*

Esotérica Facial; Esotérica Fortified; Esotérica Sunscreen cream OTC *hyperpigmentation bleaching agent; sunscreen* [hydroquinone; padimate O; oxybenzone] 2%•3.3%•2.5%

Esotérica Regular; Esotérica Sensitive Skin Formula cream OTC *hyperpigmentation bleaching agent* [hydroquinone] 2%; 1.5%

Esotérica Soap OTC *bath emollient*

Espotabs tablets (discontinued 1998) OTC *stimulant laxative* [yellow phenolphthalein] 97.2 mg

esprolol *investigational (Phase II) beta-adrenoreceptor antagonist for angina pectoris*

esproquin HCl USAN *adrenergic* [also: esproquine]

esproquine INN *adrenergic* [also: esproquin HCl]

Essential ProPlus powder OTC *oral protein supplement with vitamins and minerals* [soy protein; multiple vitamins and minerals]

Essential Protein powder OTC *oral protein supplement* [soy protein]

Estalis 140/50; Estalis 250/50 (CAN) transdermal patch ℞ *hormone replacement therapy for postmenopausal symptoms* [norethindrone acetate; estradiol-17β] 140•50 µg/day; 250•50 µg/day

Estar gel OTC *topical antipsoriatic; antiseborrheic* [coal tar] 5%

estazolam USAN, INN *hypnotic* 1, 2 mg oral

Ester-C Plus, Extra Potency tablets (name changed to Ester-C Plus Vitamin C in 1999)

Ester-C Plus Multi-Mineral capsules OTC *vitamin C/mineral supplement with multiple bioflavonoids* [vitamin C; acerola; rose hips; multiple minerals; citrus bioflavonoids; rutin] 425•12.5•12.5•±•50•5 mg

Ester-C Plus Vitamin C capsules OTC *vitamin C/calcium supplement with multiple bioflavonoids* [vitamin C; acerola; rose hips; calcium; citrus bioflavonoids; rutin] 500•10•10•62•25•5 mg; 1000•25•25•125•200•25 mg

esterified estrogens [see: estrogens, esterified]

esterifilcon A USAN *hydrophilic contact lens material*

Esterom solution ℞ *investigational (Phase III) topical treatment for acute impaired shoulder function*

estilben [see: diethylstilbestrol dipropionate]

Estinyl tablets ℞ *estrogen replacement therapy for postmenopausal symptoms; palliative therapy for inoperable prostate and breast cancers* [ethinyl estradiol] 0.02, 0.05, 0.5 mg [2] Esimil

estolate INN *combining name for radicals or groups*

estomycin sulfate [see: paromomycin sulfate]

Estorra ℞ *investigational (NDA filed) non-benzodiazepine sedative and hypnotic* [esopiclone]

Estrace tablets ℞ *estrogen replacement therapy for postmenopausal symptoms; palliative therapy for prostate and metastatic breast cancers* [estradiol] 0.5, 1, 2 mg

Estrace vaginal cream ℞ *estrogen replacement for postmenopausal atrophic vaginitis* [estradiol] 0.1 mg/g

Estraderm transdermal patch ℞ *estrogen replacement therapy for postmenopausal symptoms* [estradiol] 50, 100 µg/day [2] Estradurin

estradiol USP, INN *estrogen replacement therapy for postmenopausal disorders; palliative therapy for prostate and metastatic breast cancers* [also: oestradiol] 0.5, 1, 2 mg oral

estradiol-17β *estrogen replacement therapy for postmenopausal disorders*

estradiol benzoate USP, INN, JAN [also: oestradiol benzoate]

estradiol 17-cyclopentanepropionate [see: estradiol cypionate]

estradiol cypionate (E_2C) USP *estrogen replacement therapy for postmenopausal disorders* 5 mg/mL injection (in oil)

estradiol dipropionate NF, JAN

estradiol enanthate USAN *estrogen*

estradiol hemihydrate *topical estrogen therapy for atrophic vaginitis*

estradiol 17-heptanoate [see: estradiol enanthate]

estradiol monobenzoate [see: estradiol benzoate]

estradiol 17-nicotinate 3-propionate [see: estrapronicate]

estradiol phosphate polymer [see: polyestradiol phosphate]

Estradiol Transdermal System patch ℞ *estrogen replacement therapy for postmenopausal symptoms* [estradiol] 0.05, 0.1 mg/day

estradiol 17-undecanoate [see: estradiol undecylate]

estradiol undecylate USAN, INN *estrogen*

estradiol valerate USP, INN, JAN *estrogen replacement; hormonal antineoplastic for prostatic carcinoma* [also: oestradiol valerate] 20, 40 mg/mL IM injection

Estra-L 20 IM injection (discontinued 1998) ℞ *estrogen replacement therapy for postmenopausal symptoms; palliative therapy for inoperable prostate cancer* [estradiol valerate in oil] 20 mg/mL

Estra-L 40 IM injection ℞ *estrogen replacement therapy for postmenopausal symptoms; antineoplastic for prostatic cancer* [estradiol valerate in oil] 40 mg/mL

estramustine USAN, INN, BAN *nitrogen mustard-type alkylating antineoplastic*

estramustine phosphate sodium USAN, BAN, JAN *nitrogen mustard-type alkylating antineoplastic for palliative treatment of progressive or metastatic prostate cancer*

estramustine & vinblastine sulfate *chemotherapy protocol for prostate cancer*

estrapronicate INN

Estrasorb cream, transdermal patch ℞ *investigational (Phase II) estrogen replacement therapy for postmenopausal symptoms* [estradiol-17β]

Estratab tablets ℞ *estrogen replacement therapy for postmenopausal symptoms; palliative therapy for inoperable prostate and breast cancers* [esterified estrogens] 0.3, 0.625, 2.5 mg ⓢ Ethatab

Estratest; Estratest H.S. sugar-coated tablets ℞ *hormone replacement therapy for postmenopausal symptoms* [esterified estrogens; methyltestosterone] 1.25•2.5 mg; 0.625•1.25 mg

estrazinol INN *estrogen* [also: estrazinol hydrobromide]

estrazinol hydrobromide USAN *estrogen* [also: estrazinol]

Estrinex (name changed to Fareston upon release in 1998)

Estring vaginal ring ℞ *three-month estrogen replacement for postmenopausal atrophic vaginitis* [estradiol] 2 mg (7.5 μg/day)

estriol USP *estrogen* [also: estriol succinate; oestriol succinate]

estriol succinate INN *estrogen* [also: estriol; oestriol succinate]

estrobene [see: diethylstilbestrol]

estrobene DP [see: diethylstilbestrol dipropionate]

Estro-Cyp IM injection (discontinued 1998) ℞ *estrogen replacement therapy for postmenopausal symptoms* [estradiol cypionate in oil] 5 mg/mL

estrofurate USAN, INN *estrogen*

Estrogel ⓒⓐⓝ transdermal gel ℞ *estrogen replacement therapy for postmenopausal symptoms* [estrogen-17β] 0.06% (1.25 g/metered actuation)

Estrogenic Substance Aqueous IM injection (discontinued 1998) ℞ *estrogen replacement therapy for postmenopausal symptoms; palliative therapy for prostate and breast cancers* [estrone and other estrogens] 2 mg/mL

estrogenic substances, conjugated [see: estrogens, conjugated]

estrogenine [see: diethylstilbestrol]

estrogens *a class of female sex hormones that includes estradiol, estrone, and estriol, also used as an antineoplastic*

estrogens, conjugated USP, JAN *estrogen replacement therapy for postmenopausal disorders; palliative therapy for prostate and metastatic breast cancers*

estrogens, esterified USP *estrogen replacement therapy for postmenopausal disorders; palliative therapy for inoperable prostate and breast cancers*

estromenin [see: diethylstilbestrol]

estrone USP, INN *estrogen replacement therapy for postmenopausal disorders; palliative therapy for prostate and breast cancers* [also: oestrone]

Estrone 5 IM injection (discontinued 1998) ℞ *estrogen replacement therapy for postmenopausal symptoms; palliative therapy for prostate and breast cancers* [estrone] 5 mg/mL

Estrone Aqueous IM injection ℞ *estrogen replacement therapy for postmenopausal symptoms; palliative therapy for prostate and breast cancers* [estrone] 5 mg/mL

estrone hydrogen sulfate [see: estrone sodium sulfate]

estrone sodium sulfate

Estrophasic (trademarked/patented dosing regimen) *gradual estrogen intake with steady progestin intake*

estropipate USP *estrogen replacement therapy for postmenopausal disorders* 0.75, 1.5, 3, 6 mg oral

Estrostep 21 tablets (in packs of 21) ℞ *triphasic oral contraceptive; treatment for acne vulgaris in females* [norethindrone acetate; ethinyl estradiol] Phase 1 (5 days): 1 mg•20 μg; Phase 2 (7 days): 1 mg•30 μg; Phase 3 (9 days): 1 mg•35 μg

Estrostep Fe tablets (in packs of 28) ℞ *triphasic oral contraceptive with iron* [norethindrone acetate; ethinyl estradiol; ferrous fumarate] Phase 1: 1 mg•20 μg•75 mg;

Phase 2: 1 mg•30 µg•75 mg;
Phase 3: 1 mg•35 µg•75 mg;
Counters: 0•0•75 mg (iron only)

esuprone INN
esylate USAN, BAN *combining name for radicals or groups* [also: esilate]
etabenzarone INN
etabonate USAN, INN *combining name for radicals or groups*
etacepride INN
etacrynic acid INN, JAN *antihypertensive; loop diuretic* [also: ethacrynic acid]
etafedrine INN, BAN *adrenergic* [also: etafedrine HCl]
etafedrine HCl USAN *adrenergic* [also: etafedrine]
etafenone INN
etafilcon A USAN *hydrophilic contact lens material*
etamestrol INN
etaminile INN
etamiphyllin INN [also: etamiphylline]
etamiphyllin methesculetol [see: metescufylline]
etamiphylline BAN [also: etamiphyllin]
etamivan INN *central and respiratory stimulant* [also: ethamivan]
etamocycline INN
etamsylate INN *hemostatic* [also: ethamsylate]
etanercept USAN *soluble tumor necrosis factor receptor (sTNFR) inhibitor for rheumatoid arthritis (RA) and juvenile rheumatoid arthritis (JRA); investigational (NDA filed) for congestive heart failure*
etanidazole USAN, INN *antineoplastic; hypoxic cell radiosensitizer*
etanterol INN
etaperazine [see: perphenazine]
etaqualone INN
etarotene USAN, INN *keratolytic*
etasuline INN
etazepine INN
etazolate INN *antipsychotic* [also: etazolate HCl]
etazolate HCl USAN *antipsychotic* [also: etazolate]
etebenecid INN [also: ethebenecid]
etenzamide BAN [also: ethenzamide]
eterobarb USAN, INN, BAN *anticonvulsant*
etersalate INN
ethacridine INN [also: ethacridine lactate; acrinol] ⑨ ethacrynic
ethacridine lactate [also: ethacridine; acrinol]
ethacrynate sodium USAN, USP *antihypertensive; loop diuretic*
ethacrynic acid USAN, USP, BAN *antihypertensive; loop diuretic* [also: etacrynic acid] ⑨ ethacridine
ethambutol INN, BAN *bacteriostatic; primary tuberculostatic* [also: ethambutol HCl]
ethambutol HCl USAN, USP *bacteriostatic; primary tuberculostatic* [also: ethambutol]
ethamivan USAN, USP, BAN *central and respiratory stimulant* [also: etamivan]
Ethamolin IV injection ℞ *sclerosing agent for bleeding esophageal varices (orphan)* [ethanolamine oleate] 5%
ethamsylate USAN, BAN *hemostatic* [also: etamsylate]
ethanol JAN *topical anti-infective/antiseptic; astringent; solvent; a widely abused "legal street drug" used to produce euphoria* [also: alcohol]
ethanol, dehydrated JAN *antidote* [also: alcohol, dehydrated]
ethanolamine oleate USAN *sclerosing agent for bleeding esophageal varices (orphan)* [also: monoethanolamine oleate]
ethanolamines *a class of antihistamines that includes diphenhydramine HCl and clemastine fumarate*
ethaverine INN *peripheral vasodilator*
ethaverine HCl *peripheral vasodilator* [see: ethaverine]
ethchlorvynol USP, INN, BAN *sedative; hypnotic*
ethebenecid BAN [also: etebenecid]
ethenzamide INN, JAN [also: etenzamide]
ether USP *inhalation anesthetic*
ethiazide INN, BAN
ethidium bromide [see: homidium bromide]

ethinamate USP, INN, BAN *sedative; hypnotic* ☒ ethionamide

ethinyl estradiol USP *estrogen replacement therapy for postmenopausal disorders; palliative therapy for inoperable prostate and breast cancers; investigational (orphan) for Turner syndrome* [also: ethinylestradiol; ethinyloestradiol]

ethinylestradiol INN *estrogen replacement therapy for postmenopausal disorders; palliative therapy for inoperable prostate and breast cancers* [also: ethinyl estradiol; ethinyloestradiol]

ethinyloestradiol BAN *estrogen replacement therapy for postmenopausal disorders; palliative therapy for inoperable prostate and breast cancers* [also: ethinyl estradiol; ethinylestradiol]

ethiodized oil USP *parenteral radiopaque contrast medium (37% iodine)*

ethiodized oil (^{131}I) INN *antineoplastic; radioactive agent* [also: ethiodized oil I 131]

ethiodized oil I 131 USAN *antineoplastic; radioactive agent* [also: ethiodized oil (^{131}I)]

Ethiodol intracavitary instillation ℞ *radiopaque contrast medium for lymphography and gynecological imaging* [ethiodized oil (37% iodine)] 1284 mg/mL (475 mg/mL) ☒ ethynodiol

ethiofos [now: amifostine]

ethionamide USAN, USP, INN, BAN *bacteriostatic; tuberculosis retreatment* ☒ ethinamate

ethisterone NF, INN, BAN

Ethmozine film-coated tablets ℞ *antiarrhythmic* [moricizine HCl] 200, 250, 300 mg

ethodryl [see: diethylcarbamazine citrate]

ethoglucid BAN [also: etoglucid]

ethoheptazine BAN [also: ethoheptazine citrate]

ethoheptazine citrate NF, INN [also: ethoheptazine]

ethohexadiol USP

ethomoxane INN, BAN

ethomoxane HCl [see: ethomoxane]

ethonam nitrate USAN *antifungal* [also: etonam]

ethopabate BAN

ethopropazine BAN *anticholinergic; antiparkinsonian* [also: ethopropazine HCl; profenamine]

ethopropazine HCl USP *anticholinergic; antiparkinsonian* [also: profenamine; ethopropazine]

ethosalamide BAN [also: etosalamide]

ethosuximide USAN, USP, INN, BAN *anticonvulsant* 250 mg/5 mL oral

ethotoin USP, INN, BAN *hydantoin anticonvulsant*

ethoxarutine [see: ethoxazorutoside]

ethoxazene HCl USAN *analgesic* [also: etoxazene]

ethoxazorutoside INN

ethoxyacetanilide *(withdrawn from market)* [see: phenacetin]

***o*-ethoxybenzamide** [see: ethenzamide; etenzamide]

ethoxzolamide USP

Ethrane liquid for vaporization ℞ *inhalation general anesthetic* [enflurane]

ethybenztropine USAN, BAN *anticholinergic* [also: etybenzatropine]

ethyl acetate NF *solvent*

ethyl alcohol (EtOH; ETOH) [now: alcohol; ethanol]

ethyl aminobenzoate (ethyl *p*-aminobenzoate) JAN *topical anesthetic; nonprescription diet aid* [also: benzocaine]

ethyl 2-benzimidazolecarbamate [see: lobendazole]

ethyl N-benzylcyclopropanecarbamate [see: encyprate]

ethyl biscoumacetate NF, INN, BAN

ethyl biscumacetate [see: ethyl biscoumacetate]

ethyl carbamate [now: urethane]

ethyl carfluzepate INN

ethyl cartrizoate INN

ethyl chloride USP *topical local anesthetic; topical vapo-coolant*

ethyl dibunate USAN, INN, BAN *antitussive*

ethyl dirazepate INN

ethyl ether [see: ether]

ethyl *p*-fluorophenyl sulfone [see: fluoresone]
ethyl *p*-hydroxybenzoate [see: ethylparaben]
ethyl loflazepate INN
ethyl nitrite NF
ethyl oleate NF *vehicle*
ethyl oxide [see: ether]
ethyl vanillin NF *flavoring agent*
ethylcellulose NF *tablet binder*
ethylchlordiphene [see: etofamide]
ethyldicoumarol [see: ethyl biscoumacetate]
ethylene NF *inhalation general anesthesia*
ethylene distearate [see: glycol distearate]
ethylenediamine USP, JAN
ethylenediaminetetraacetate [see: edetate disodium]
ethylenediaminetetraacetic acid (EDTA) [see: edetate disodium]
N,N-ethylenediarsanilic acid [see: difetarsone]
ethylenedinitrilotetraacetate disodium [see: edetate disodium]
ethylestrenol USAN, INN *anabolic steroid; also abused as a street drug* [also: ethyloestrenol; ethylnandrol]
ethylhexanediol [see: ethohexadiol]
2-ethylhexyl diphenyl phosphate [see: octicizer]
2-ethylhexyl *p*-methoxycinnamate [see: octinoxate]
2-ethylhexyl salicylate [see: octisalate]
ethylhydrocupreine HCl NF
ethylmethylthiambutene INN, BAN
ethylmorphine BAN [also: ethylmorphine HCl]
ethylmorphine HCl NF [also: ethylmorphine]
ethylnandrol JAN *anabolic steroid; also abused as a street drug* [also: ethylestrenol; ethyloestrenol]
ethylnorepinephrine HCl USP *sympathomimetic bronchodilator*
ethyloestradiol BAN *estrogen* [also: ethinyl estradiol]
ethyloestrenol BAN *anabolic steroid; also abused as a street drug* [also: ethylestrenol; ethylnandrol]
ethylpapaverine HCl [see: ethaverine HCl]
ethylparaben NF *antifungal agent*
ethylphenacemide [see: pheneturide]
ethylstibamine [see: stibosamine]
2-ethylthioisonicotinamide [see: ethionamide]
ethynerone USAN, INN *progestin*
ethynodiol BAN *progestin* [also: ethynodiol diacetate; etynodiol] ⑨ Ethiodol
ethynodiol diacetate USAN, USP *progestin* [also: etynodiol; ethynodiol]
5-ethynyluracil [see: eniluracil]
Ethyol powder for IV infusion ℞ *chemoprotective agent for cisplatin and paclitaxel chemotherapy (orphan); radioprotective agent; treatment for radiation-induced xerostomia; investigational (orphan) for cyclophosphamide rescue* [amifostine] 500 mg/vial
ethypicone INN
ethypropymal sodium [see: probarbital sodium]
etibendazole USAN, INN *anthelmintic*
eticlopride INN
eticyclidine INN
etidocaine USAN, INN, BAN *injectable local anesthetic*
etidocaine HCl *injectable local anesthetic*
etidronate disodium USAN, USP *bisphosphonate bone resorption inhibitor for Paget disease, heterotopic ossification, and hypercalcemia of malignancy (orphan)*
etidronate monosodium
etidronate sodium *(this term is used only when the form of sodium cannot be more accurately identified)*
etidronate tetrasodium
etidronate trisodium
etidronic acid USAN, INN, BAN *calcium regulator*
etifelmine INN
etifenin USAN, INN, BAN *diagnostic aid*
etifoxin BAN [also: etifoxine]
etifoxine INN [also: etifoxin]
etilamfetamine INN
etilefrine INN
etilefrine pivalate INN

etintidine INN *antagonist to histamine H_2 receptors* [also: etintidine HCl]
etintidine HCl USAN *antagonist to histamine H_2 receptors* [also: etintidine]
etiocholanedione *investigational (orphan) for aplastic anemia and Prader-Willi syndrome*
etipirium iodide INN
etiproston INN
etiracetam INN
etiroxate INN
etisazole INN, BAN
etisomicin INN, BAN
etisulergine INN
etizolam INN
etobedolum [see: etonitazene]
etocarlide INN
etocrilene INN *ultraviolet screen* [also: etocrylene]
etocrylene USAN *ultraviolet screen* [also: etocrilene]
etodolac USAN, INN, BAN *analgesic; antiarthritic; nonsteroidal anti-inflammatory drug (NSAID)* [also: etodolic acid] 200, 300, 400, 500, 600 mg oral
etodolic acid INN *analgesic; antiarthritic; nonsteroidal anti-inflammatory drug (NSAID)* [also: etodolac]
etodroxizine INN
etofamide INN
etofenamate USAN, INN, BAN *analgesic; anti-inflammatory*
etofenprox INN
etofibrate INN
etoformin INN *antidiabetic* [also: etoformin HCl]
etoformin HCl USAN *antidiabetic* [also: etoformin]
etofuradine INN
etofylline INN
etofylline clofibrate INN *antihyperlipoproteinemic* [also: theofibrate]
etoglucid INN [also: ethoglucid]
EtOH; ETOH (ethyl alcohol) [now: alcohol]
etolorex INN
etolotifen INN
etoloxamine INN
etomidate USAN, INN, BAN *rapid-acting nonbarbiturate general anesthetic; hypnotic*
etomidoline INN
etomoxir INN
etonam INN *antifungal* [also: ethonam nitrate]
etonam nitrate [see: ethonam nitrate]
etonitazene INN, BAN
etonogestrel USAN, INN *progestin*
etoperidone INN *antidepressant* [also: etoperidone HCl]
etoperidone HCl USAN *antidepressant* [also: etoperidone]
etophylate [see: acepifylline]
Etopophos powder for IV injection ℞ *antineoplastic for testicular and small cell lung cancers* [etoposide phosphate diethanolate] 119.3 mg/vial
etoposide USAN, INN, BAN *antineoplastic* 20, 30 mg/mL injection
etoposide & paclitaxel & carboplatin *chemotherapy protocol for primary adenocarcinoma and small cell lung cancer*
etoposide phosphate USAN *antineoplastic*
etoprindole INN
etoprine USAN *antineoplastic*
etoricoxib USAN *antiarthritic; antipyretic; COX-2 inhibitor; nonsteroidal anti-inflammatory drug (NSAID)*
etorphine INN, BAN
etosalamide INN [also: ethosalamide]
etoxadrol INN *anesthetic* [also: etoxadrol HCl]
etoxadrol HCl USAN *anesthetic* [also: etoxadrol]
etoxazene INN *analgesic* [also: ethoxazene HCl]
etoxazene HCl [see: ethoxazene HCl]
etoxeridine INN, BAN
etozolin USAN, INN *diuretic*
etrabamine INN
Etrafon; Etrafon 2-10; Etrafon-A; Etrafon-Forte tablets ℞ *conventional (typical) antipsychotic; antidepressant* [perphenazine; amitriptyline HCl] 2•25 mg; 2•10 mg; 4•10 mg; 4•25 mg

etretin [see: acitretin]

etretinate USAN, INN, BAN, JAN *systemic antipsoriatic; retinoic acid analogue*

etryptamine INN, BAN *CNS stimulant* [also: etryptamine acetate]

etryptamine acetate USAN *CNS stimulant* [also: etryptamine]

etybenzatropine INN *anticholinergic* [also: ethybenztropine]

etymemazine INN

etymemazine HCl [see: etymemazine]

etynodiol INN *progestin* [also: ethynodiol diacetate; ethynodiol]

etyprenaline [see: isoetharine]

eucaine HCl NF

Eucalyptamint ointment, gel OTC *topical analgesic; counterirritant; antiseptic* [menthol; eucalyptus oil] 16%•?; 8%•?

eucalyptol USAN *topical bacteriostatic antiseptic/germicidal*

eucalyptus *(Eucalyptus globulus)* oil *medicinal herb for bronchitis, lung disorders, neuralgia, and skin sores; source of bioflavonoids*

eucalyptus oil NF *topical antiseptic*

eucatropine INN, BAN *ophthalmic anticholinergic* [also: eucatropine HCl]

eucatropine HCl USP *ophthalmic anticholinergic* [also: eucatropine]

Eucerin cream, lotion OTC *moisturizer; emollient*

Eucerin OTC *cream base*

Eucerin Plus lotion OTC *moisturizer; emollient* [sodium lactate; urea] 5%•5%

eucodal [see: oxycodone]

Eudal-SR sustained-release tablets ℞ *decongestant; expectorant* [pseudoephedrine HCl; guaifenesin] 120•400 mg

euflavine [see: acriflavine]

Euflex (CAN) tablets ℞ *antiandrogen antineoplastic adjunct to metastatic prostate cancer* [flutamide] 250 mg

Eugenia caryophyllata *medicinal herb* [see: cloves]

Eugenia pimenta *medicinal herb* [see: allspice]

eugenol USP *dental analgesic*

Euglucon (CAN) tablets ℞ *sulfonylurea antidiabetic* [glyburide] 2.5, 5 mg

eukadol [see: oxycodone]

Eulexin capsules ℞ *antiandrogen antineoplastic for metastatic prostate cancer* [flutamide] 125 mg

Euonymus atropurpureus *medicinal herb* [see: wahoo]

Eupatorium cannabinum *medicinal herb* [see: hemp agrimony]

Eupatorium perfoliatum *medicinal herb* [see: boneset]

Eupatorium purpureum *medicinal herb* [see: queen of the meadow]

Euphorbia poinsettia; E. pulcherrima *medicinal herb* [see: poinsettia]

euphoretics; euphoriants; euphoragens *a class of agents that produce euphoria*

Euphrasia officinalis; E. rostkoviana; E. strica *medicinal herb* [see: eyebright]

euprocin INN *topical anesthetic* [also: euprocin HCl]

euprocin HCl USAN *topical anesthetic* [also: euprocin]

euquinine [see: quinine ethylcarbonate]

Eurax cream, lotion ℞ *scabicide; antipruritic* [crotamiton] 10% ⊡ Serax; Urex

European alder; European black alder; European buckthorn *medicinal herb* [see: buckthorn]

European aspen *medicinal herb* [see: black poplar]

europium *element (Eu)*

EVA (etoposide, vinblastine, Adriamycin) *chemotherapy protocol for Hodgkin lymphoma*

Evacet ℞ *investigational (NDA filed) antibiotic antineoplastic for metastatic breast cancer* [doxorubicin, liposomal]

Evac-Q-Kit oral solution + 2 tablets + 2 suppositories (discontinued 1999) OTC *pre-procedure bowel evacuant* [Evac-Q-Mag (q.v.); Evac-Q-Tabs (q.v.); Evac-Q-Sert (q.v.)] ⊡ Evac-Q-Kwik

Evac-Q-Kwik suppositories OTC *stimulant laxative* [bisacodyl] 10 mg ⊡ Evac-Q-Kit

Evac-Q-Kwik Kit oral solution + 2 tablets + 1 suppository OTC *pre-pro-*

cedure bowel evacuant [Evac-Q-Mag (q.v.); Evac-Q-Tabs (q.v.); Evac-Q-Kwik suppository (q.v.)]

Evac-Q-Mag carbonated oral solution OTC *saline laxative* [magnesium citrate; citric acid; potassium citrate]

Evac-Q-Tabs tablets OTC *stimulant laxative* [bisacodyl] 5 mg

Evac-Q-Tabs tablets (discontinued 1998) OTC *stimulant laxative* [phenolphthalein] 130 mg

Evac-U-Gen chewable tablets (discontinued 1998) OTC *stimulant laxative* [yellow phenolphthalein] 97.2 mg

Evac-U-Lax chewable wafers (discontinued 1998) OTC *stimulant laxative* [phenolphthalein] 80 mg

Evalose syrup (discontinued 1999) ℞ *hyperosmotic laxative* [lactulose] 10 g/15 mL

evandamine INN

Evans blue USP *diagnostic aid for blood volume* [also: azovan blue] 5 mL injection

evening primrose *(Oenothera biennis)* bark, leaves, oil *medicinal herb for cardiovascular health, hypertension, mastalgia, multiple sclerosis, nerves, obesity, premenstrual syndrome, prostate disorders, rheumatoid arthritis, and skin disorders*

everlasting *(Anaphalis margaritacea; Gnaphalium polycephalum; G. uliginosum)* plant *medicinal herb used as an astringent, diaphoretic, febrifuge, pectoral, vermifuge, and vulnerary*

evernimicin USAN *investigational antibiotic*

everolimus *investigational agent for transplant rejection*

Everone 200 IM injection (discontinued 2001) ℞ *androgen replacement for delayed puberty or breast cancer* [testosterone enanthate] 200 mg/mL

Evista film-coated tablets ℞ *selective estrogen receptor modulator (SERM) for the prevention and treatment of postmenopausal osteoporosis* [raloxifene HCl] 60 mg ⊡ Avita

E-Vista IM injection (discontinued 1997) ℞ *anxiolytic; minor tranquilizer* [hydroxyzine HCl] 50 mg/mL

E-Vitamin ointment OTC *emollient* [vitamin E] 30 mg/g

E-Vitamin Succinate capsules (discontinued 1999) OTC *vitamin supplement* [vitamin E (as *d*-alpha tocopheryl acid succinate)] 165, 330 mg

E-VMAC (escalated methotrexate, vinblastine, Adriamycin, cisplatin) *chemotherapy protocol*

E-VMAC (escalated methotrexate, vinblastine, Adriamycin, cyclophosphamide) *chemotherapy protocol*

Evoxac capsules ℞ *cholinergic and muscarinic receptor agonist for treatment of dry mouth due to Sjögren syndrome* [cevimeline HCl] 30 mg

Evra [see: Ortho Evra]

Exact liquid OTC *topical keratolytic cleanser for acne* [salicylic acid] 2%

Exact vanishing cream OTC *topical keratolytic for acne* [benzoyl peroxide] 5%

exalamide INN

exametazime USAN, INN, BAN *regional cerebral perfusion imaging aid*

exaprolol INN *antiadrenergic (β-receptor)* [also: exaprolol HCl]

exaprolol HCl USAN *antiadrenergic (β-receptor)* [also: exaprolol]

exatecan mesylate USAN *antineoplastic*

Excedrin Aspirin Free caplets, geltabs OTC *analgesic; antipyretic; anti-inflammatory* [acetaminophen; caffeine] 500•65 mg

Excedrin Dual, Aspirin Free film-coated caplets (discontinued 2000) OTC *analgesic; antipyretic; antacid* [acetaminophen; calcium carbonate; magnesium carbonate; magnesium oxide] 500•111•64•30 mg

Excedrin Extra Strength caplets, tablets, geltabs OTC *analgesic; antipyretic; anti-inflammatory* [acetaminophen; aspirin; caffeine] 250•250•65 mg

Excedrin Migraine tablets OTC *analgesic for relief of migraine headache syndrome, including prodrome, pain, and*

associated symptoms [acetaminophen; aspirin; caffeine] 250•250•65 mg

Excedrin P.M. liquid, liquigels OTC *antihistaminic sleep aid; analgesic* [diphenhydramine HCl; acetaminophen] 50•1000 mg/30 mL; 25•500 mg

Excedrin P.M. tablets, caplets, geltabs OTC *antihistaminic sleep aid; analgesic* [diphenhydramine citrate; acetaminophen] 38•500 mg

Excedrin Sinus tablets, caplets OTC *decongestant; analgesic; antipyretic* [pseudoephedrine HCl; acetaminophen] 30•500 mg

Excita Extra premedicated condom OTC *spermicidal/barrier contraceptive* [nonoxynol 9] 8%

Exelderm solution ℞ *topical antifungal* [sulconazole nitrate] 1%

Exelon capsules, oral solution ℞ *acetylcholinesterase inhibitor to increase cognition in Alzheimer disease* [rivastigmine tartrate] 1.5, 3, 4.5, 6 mg; 2 mg/mL

exemestane INN *aromatase inhibitor; antihormonal antineoplastic for advanced breast cancer in postmenopausal women (orphan)*

exepanol INN

Exgest LA long-acting tablets ℞ *decongestant; expectorant* [phenylpropanolamine HCl; guaifenesin] 75•400 mg

Ex-Histine syrup ℞ *decongestant; antihistamine; anticholinergic* [phenylephrine HCl; chlorpheniramine maleate; methscopolamine bromide] 10•2•1.25 mg

Exidine Skin Cleanser; Exidine-2 Scrub; Exidine-4 Scrub liquid OTC *broad-spectrum antimicrobial; germicidal* [chlorhexidine gluconate; alcohol 4%] 4%; 2%; 4%

exifone INN

exiproben INN

exisulind *investigational (Phase III, orphan) for familial adenomatous polyposis (FAP; also known as adenomatous polyposis coli, or APC); investigational (Phase II/III) for prostate cancer*

Ex-Lax tablets, chocolated chewable tablets OTC *stimulant laxative* [sennosides] 15 mg

Ex-Lax Extra Gentle Pills tablets (discontinued 1997) OTC *stimulant laxative; stool softener* [phenolphthalein; docusate sodium] 65•75 mg

Ex-Lax Gentle Nature tablets (discontinued 1997) OTC *stimulant laxative* [sennosides] 20 mg

Ex-Lax Gentle Strength caplets OTC *stimulant laxative; stool softener* [sennosides; docusate sodium] 10•65 mg

Ex-Lax Maximum Relief tablets OTC *stimulant laxative* [sennosides] 25 mg

Ex-Lax Maximum Relief; Ex-Lax Unflavored tablets (discontinued 1997) OTC *stimulant laxative* [yellow phenolphthalein] 135 mg; 90 mg

Ex-Lax Stool Softener caplets OTC *laxative; stool softener* [docusate sodium] 100 mg

Exna tablets ℞ *diuretic; antihypertensive* [benzthiazide] 50 mg

Exocaine Medicated Rub; Exocaine Plus Rub OTC *counterirritant* [methyl salicylate] 25%; 30%

Exosurf ℞ *investigational (orphan) for adult respiratory distress syndrome (ARDS)* [colfosceril palmitate]

Exosurf Neonatal powder for injection, intratracheal suspension ℞ *pulmonary surfactant for hyaline membrane disease and respiratory distress syndrome (orphan)* [colfosceril palmitate] 108 mg

expectorants *a class of drugs that promote the ejection of mucus from the respiratory tract*

Expidet (trademarked dosage form) *fast-dissolving dose*

Exsel lotion/shampoo ℞ *antiseborrheic; antifungal* [selenium sulfide] 2.5%

exsiccated sodium arsenate [see: sodium arsenate, exsiccated]

Extencap (trademarked dosage form) *extended-release capsule*

extended insulin zinc [see: insulin zinc, extended]

Extendryl chewable tablets, syrup ℞ *decongestant; antihistamine; anticholinergic* [phenylephrine HCl; chlorpheniramine maleate; methscopolamine nitrate] 10•2•1.25 mg; 10•2•1.25 mg/5 mL

Extendryl JR sustained-release capsules ℞ *pediatric decongestant, antihistamine, and anticholinergic* [phenylephrine HCl; chlorpheniramine maleate; methscopolamine nitrate] 10•4•1.25 mg

Extendryl SR sustained-release capsules ℞ *decongestant; antihistamine; anticholinergic* [phenylephrine HCl; chlorpheniramine maleate; methscopolamine nitrate] 20•8•2.5 mg

Extentab (trademarked dosage form) *extended-release tablet*

Extra Action Cough syrup OTC *antitussive; expectorant* [dextromethorphan hydrobromide; guaifenesin; alcohol 1.4%] 10•100 mg/5 mL

"Extra Strength" products [see under product name]

Extraneal Peritoneal Dialysis Solution ℞ *investigational (orphan) for end-stage renal disease* [icodextrin] 7.5%

eye balm; eye root *medicinal herb* [see: goldenseal]

Eye Drops OTC *topical ophthalmic decongestant and vasoconstrictor* [tetrahydrozoline HCl] 0.05%

Eye Irrigating Solution OTC *extraocular irrigating solution* [sterile isotonic solution]

Eye Irrigating Wash OTC *extraocular irrigating solution* [sterile isotonic solution]

Eye Stream ophthalmic solution OTC *extraocular irrigating solution* [sterile isotonic solution]

Eye Wash ophthalmic solution OTC *extraocular irrigating solution* [sterile isotonic solution]

eyebright *(Euphrasia officinalis; E. rostkoviana; E. strica)* plant *medicinal herb for blood cleansing, cataracts, colds, conjunctivitis, eye disorders and infections, and stimulating liver function; not generally regarded as safe and effective for topical ophthalmic use*

Eye-Lube-A eye drops OTC *ophthalmic moisturizer/lubricant* [glycerin] 0.25%

Eye-Scrub premoistened pads OTC *eyelid cleanser for blepharitis or contact lenses*

Eye-Sed eye drops OTC *ophthalmic astringent* [zinc sulfate] 0.25%

Eyesine eye drops OTC *topical ophthalmic decongestant and vasoconstrictor* [tetrahydrozoline HCl] 0.05%

EZ Detect test kit for home use *in vitro diagnostic aid for fecal occult blood*

ezetimibe USAN *investigational (Phase III) antihyperlipidemic; intestinal cholesterol absorption inhibitor*

Ezide tablets ℞ *antihypertensive; diuretic* [hydrochlorothiazide] 50 mg

ezlopitant USAN *substance P receptor antagonist for emesis, pain, and inflammation*

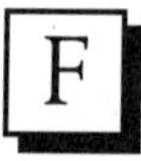

1+1-F Creme ℞ *topical corticosteroidal anti-inflammatory; antifungal; antibacterial; local anesthetic* [hydrocortisone; clioquinol; pramoxine] 1%•3%•1%

^{18}F [see: fludeoxyglucose F 18]

^{18}F [see: sodium fluoride F 18]

FABRase ℞ *investigational (orphan) enzyme replacement therapy for Fabry disease* [alpha-galactosidase A]

Fabrazyme injection ℞ *investigational (NDA filed) enzyme replacement therapy for Fabry disease* [agalsidase beta]

FAC (fluorouracil, Adriamycin, cyclophosphamide) *chemotherapy protocol for breast cancer*

FAC-LEV (fluorouracil, Adriamycin, Cytoxin, levamisole) *chemotherapy protocol*

FAC-M (fluorouracil, Adriamycin, cyclophosphamide, methotrexate) *chemotherapy protocol*

Fact Plus test kit for home use *in vitro diagnostic aid; urine pregnancy test*

Factive ℞ *investigational (NDA filed) antibiotic for respiratory tract infections* [gemifloxacin mesylate]

factor II (prothrombin)

factor III [see: thromboplastin]

factor VIIa, recombinant *coagulant for hemophilia A and B (orphan); investigational (orphan) for von Willebrand disease*

factor VIII [see: antihemophilic factor]

factor VIII (rDNA) BAN *blood coagulating factor*

factor VIII fraction BAN *blood coagulating factor*

factor VIII SQ, recombinant *investigational (orphan) for long-term hemophilia A treatment or for surgical procedures*

factor IX complex USP *systemic hemostatic; antihemophilic for hemophilia B (orphan)* [also: factor IX fraction]

factor IX fraction BAN *systemic hemostatic; antihemophilic* [also: factor IX complex]

factor XIII, plasma-derived *investigational (orphan) for congenital factor XIII deficiency*

Factrel powder for subcu or IV injection ℞ *gonad-stimulating principle; in vivo diagnostic aid for anterior pituitary function* [gonadorelin HCl] 100, 500 µg

fadrozole INN *antineoplastic; aromatase inhibitor* [also: fadrozole HCl]

fadrozole HCl USAN *antineoplastic; aromatase inhibitor* [also: fadrozole]

falintolol INN

falipamil INN

false foxglove *medicinal herb* [see: feverweed]

false unicorn ***(Chamaelirium luteum)*** *root medicinal herb used for amenorrhea, morning sickness, and preventing miscarriages; also used for colic, cough, and digestive, kidney, and prostate problems; emetic in high doses*

false valerian *medicinal herb* [see: life root]

false vervain *medicinal herb* [see: blue vervain]

FAM (fluorouracil, Adriamycin, mitomycin) *chemotherapy protocol for adenocarcinoma and gastric cancer*

FAM-CF (fluorouracil, Adriamycin, mitomycin, citrovorum factor) *chemotherapy protocol*

famciclovir USAN, INN, BAN *antiviral for herpes simplex and zoster*

FAME; FAMe (fluorouracil, Adriamycin, MeCCNU) *chemotherapy protocol*

famiraprinium chloride INN

FAMMe (fluorouracil, Adriamycin, mitomycin, MeCCNU) *chemotherapy protocol*

famotidine USAN, USP, INN, BAN *histamine H_2 antagonist for gastric ulcers* 10, 20, 40 mg oral

famotine INN *antiviral* [also: famotine HCl]

famotine HCl USAN *antiviral* [also: famotine]

fampridine USAN, INN *investigational (orphan) for multiple sclerosis and spinal cord injury*

famprofazone INN, BAN

FAM-S (fluorouracil, Adriamycin, mitomycin, streptozocin) *chemotherapy protocol*

FAMTX (fluorouracil, Adriamycin, methotrexate [with leucovorin rescue]) *chemotherapy protocol for gastric cancer*

Famvir film-coated tablets ℞ *antiviral for acute herpes zoster and genital herpes infections and suppression of recurrent episodes* [famciclovir] 125, 250, 500 mg

fananserin USAN *antipsychotic; antischizophrenic; dopamine D_2 and serotonin 5-HT_2 receptor antagonist*

fanetizole INN, BAN *immunoregulator* [also: fanetizole mesylate]

fanetizole mesylate USAN *immunoregulator* [also: fanetizole]

Fansidar tablets ℞ *antimalarial* [sulfadoxine; pyrimethamine] 500•25 mg

fanthridone BAN *antidepressant* [also: fantridone HCl; fantridone]

fantridone INN *antidepressant* [also: fantridone HCl; fanthridone]

fantridone HCl USAN *antidepressant* [also: fantridone; fanthridone]

FAP (fluorouracil, Adriamycin, Platinol) *chemotherapy protocol for gastric cancer*

Farbee with Vitamin C caplets OTC *vitamin supplement* [multiple B vitamins; vitamin C] ≛•300 mg

Fareston tablets ℞ *antiestrogen antineoplastic for estrogen-receptive metastatic breast cancer in postmenopausal women (orphan); investigational (orphan) for desmoid tumors* [toremifene citrate] 60 mg

farglitazar USAN *thiazolidinedione antidiabetic; increases cellular response to insulin without increasing insulin secretion*

farnesil INN *combining name for radicals or groups*

fasiplon INN

Faslodex ℞ *investigational antiestrogen antineoplastic for breast cancer* [fluvestrant]

Faspak (trademarked form) *flexible plastic bag*

Fastic (Japanese name for U.S. product Starlix)

Fastin capsules ℞ *anorexiant; CNS stimulant* [phentermine HCl] 30 mg

Fastlene capsules OTC *CNS stimulant; analeptic* [caffeine] 200 mg

Fast-Trak (trademarked delivery system) *quick-loading syringe*

fat, hard NF *suppository base*

fat emulsion, intravenous *parenteral essential fatty acid replacement*

Father John's Medicine Plus liquid OTC *antitussive; decongestant; antihistamine; expectorant* [dextromethorphan hydrobromide; phenylephrine HCl; chlorpheniramine maleate; guaifenesin; ammonium chloride] 7.5•2.5•1•30•83.3 mg/5 mL

Fatsia horrida *medicinal herb* [see: devil's club]

fazadinium bromide INN, BAN

fazarabine USAN, INN *antineoplastic*

5-FC (5-fluorocytosine) [see: flucytosine]

FCAP (fluorouracil, cyclophosphamide, Adriamycin, Platinol) *chemotherapy protocol*

FCE (fluorouracil, cisplatin, etoposide) *chemotherapy protocol*

F-CL (fluorouracil, leucovorin calcium [rescue]) *chemotherapy protocol for colorectal cancer* [also: FU/LV]

FCP (fluorouracil, cyclophosphamide, prednisone) *chemotherapy protocol*

FD&C Red No. 2 (Food, Drug & Cosmetic Act) [see: amaranth]

FD&C Red No. 3 (Food, Drug & Cosmetic Act) [see: erythrosine sodium]

F-ddA (fluorodideoxyadenosine) [see: lodenosine]

^{18}FDG (fludeoxyglucose) [see: fludeoxyglucose F 18]

FDh (2(3H) furanone di-hydro) *a precursor to gamma hydroxybutyrate (GHB); a formerly legal alternative to GHB, now also illegal (Schedule I); also known as gamma butyrolactone (GBL)* [see: gamma hydroxybutyrate (GHB)]

FDP (fructose-1,6-diphosphate) [q.v.]

Fe^{50} (or Fe50) extended-release caplets OTC *hematinic* [ferrous sulfate, dried (source of iron)] 160 mg (50 mg)

^{59}Fe [see: ferric chloride Fe 59]

^{59}Fe [see: ferric citrate (^{59}Fe)]

^{59}Fe [see: ferrous citrate Fe 59]

^{59}Fe [see: ferrous sulfate Fe 59]

febantel USAN, INN, BAN *veterinary anthelmintic*

febarbamate INN

febricides *a class of agents that relieve or reduce fever* [also called: antifebriles; antipyretics; antithermics; febrifuges]

febrifuges *a class of agents that relieve or reduce fever* [also called: antifebriles; antipyretics; antithermics; febricides]

febuprol INN

febuverine INN

FEC (fluorouracil, epirubicin, cyclophosphamide) *chemotherapy protocol for breast cancer*

feclemine INN

feclobuzone INN

FED (fluorouracil, etoposide, DDP) *chemotherapy protocol for non–small cell lung cancer (NSCLC)*

Fedahist tablets OTC *decongestant; antihistamine* [pseudoephedrine HCl; chlorpheniramine maleate] 60•4 mg

Fedahist Timecaps (timed-release capsules), Gyrocaps (extended-release capsules) ℞ *decongestant; antihistamine* [pseudoephedrine HCl; chlorpheniramine maleate] 120•8 mg; 65•10 mg

Fedahist Expectorant syrup (discontinued 1998) OTC *decongestant; expectorant* [pseudoephedrine HCl; guaifenesin] 20•200 mg/5 mL

fedotozine INN *investigational kappa selective opioid agonist for irritable bowel syndrome*

fedrilate INN

Feen-A-Mint chewable tablets, gum (discontinued 1997) OTC *stimulant laxative* [yellow phenolphthalein] 97.2 mg

Feen-A-Mint chocolated chewable tablets (discontinued 1997) OTC *stimulant laxative* [yellow phenolphthalein] 65 mg

Feen-A-Mint enteric-coated tablets OTC *stimulant laxative* [bisacodyl] 5 mg

Feen-A-Mint Pills tablets (discontinued 1998) OTC *stimulant laxative; stool softener* [phenolphthalein; docusate sodium] 65•100 mg

Feiba VH Immuno IV injection or drip ℞ *antihemophilic to correct factor VIII deficiency and coagulation deficiency* [anti-inhibitor coagulant complex, vapor heated and freeze-dried] (each bottle is labeled with dosage)

felbamate USAN, INN *anticonvulsant; adjunctive therapy for Lennox-Gastaut syndrome (orphan)*

Felbatol tablets, oral suspension (the FDA and the manufacturer strongly caution against its use due to adverse side effects) ℞ *anticonvulsant; adjunctive therapy for Lennox-Gastaut syndrome (orphan)* [felbamate] 400, 600 mg; 600 mg/5 mL

felbinac USAN, INN, BAN *anti-inflammatory*

Feldene capsules ℞ *antiarthritic; nonsteroidal anti-inflammatory drug (NSAID)* [piroxicam] 10, 20 mg

felipyrine INN

felodipine USAN, INN, BAN *vasodilator; antihypertensive; calcium channel blocker*

felonwood; felonwort *medicinal herb* [see: bittersweet nightshade]

felvizumab USAN *monoclonal antibody for prophylaxis and treatment of respiratory syncytial virus (RSV)*

felypressin USAN, INN, BAN *vasoconstrictor*

Fem-1 tablets OTC *analgesic; anti-inflammatory; diuretic* [acetaminophen; pamabrom] 500•25 mg

female fern *(Polypodium vulgare)* root *medicinal herb used as an anthelmintic, cholagogue, demulcent, and purgative*

female regulator *medicinal herb* [see: life root]

Femara film-coated tablets ℞ *aromatase inhibitor; hormonal antineoplastic for advanced breast cancer in postmenopausal women* [letrozole] 2.5 mg

FemBack caplets OTC *analgesic; antihistaminic sleep aid* [acetaminophen; salicylamide; phenyltoloxamine citrate] 150•150•44 mg

FemCal tablets OTC *calcium supplement* [calcium carbonate; vitamin D; multiple minerals] 250 mg•100 IU•≛

Femcet capsules (discontinued 2000) ℞ *analgesic; barbiturate sedative* [acetaminophen; caffeine; butalbital] 325•40•50 mg

Fem-Etts tablets (discontinued 1997) OTC *analgesic; anti-inflammatory; diuretic* [acetaminophen; pamabrom] 325•25 mg

femhrt 1/5 (rendered as FemHRT in Canada) tablets (in packs of 28) ℞ *hormone replacement therapy for postmenopausal symptoms* [norethindrone acetate; ethinyl estradiol] 1 mg•5 μg

Femicine vaginal suppositories (discontinued 1998) OTC *for vaginal irritations, itching, and burning* [pulsatilla 28x]

Femilax tablets (discontinued 1998) OTC *stimulant laxative; stool softener* [phenolphthalein; docusate sodium] 65•100 mg

Feminique Disposable Douche solution OTC *antiseptic; antifungal; vaginal cleanser and deodorizer; acidity modifier* [sodium benzoate; sorbic acid; lactic acid]

Feminique Disposable Douche solution OTC *vaginal cleanser and deodorizer; acidity modifier* [vinegar (acetic acid)]

Femiron tablets OTC *hematinic* [ferrous fumarate (source of iron)] 63 mg (20 mg) ⑨ Remeron

Femiron Multi-Vitamins and Iron tablets OTC *vitamin/iron supplement* [multiple vitamins; ferrous fumarate; folic acid] ≛•20•0.4 mg

Femizol-M vaginal cream OTC *antifungal* [miconazole nitrate] 2%

femoxetine INN

FemPatch transdermal patch ℞ *estrogen replacement therapy for postmenopausal symptoms* [estradiol] 25 μg/day

FemSoft urethral insert *treatment for stress urinary incontinence* [silicone plug]

Femstat 3 vaginal cream in prefilled applicator OTC *antifungal* [butoconazole nitrate] 2%

FemStat One vaginal cream (discontinued 2001) OTC *antifungal* [butoconazole nitrate] 2%

fenabutene INN

fenacetinol INN

fenaclon INN

fenadiazole INN

fenaftic acid INN

fenalamide USAN, INN *smooth muscle relaxant*

fenalcomine INN

fenamifuril INN

fenamisal INN *antibacterial; tuberculostatic* [also: phenyl aminosalicylate]

fenamole USAN, INN *anti-inflammatory*

fenaperone INN

fenarsone [see: carbarsone]

fenasprate [see: benorilate]

fenbendazole USAN, INN, BAN *anthelmintic*

fenbenicillin INN [also: phenbenicillin]

fenbufen USAN, INN, BAN *anti-inflammatory*

fenbutrazate INN [also: phenbutrazate]

fencamfamin INN, BAN

fencamfamin HCl [see: fencamfamin]

fencarbamide INN *anticholinergic* [also: phencarbamide]

fenchlorphos BAN *systemic insecticide* [also: ronnel; fenclofos]

fencilbutirol USAN, INN *choleretic*

fenclexonium metilsulfate INN

fenclofenac USAN, INN, BAN *anti-inflammatory*

fenclofos INN *systemic insecticide* [also: ronnel; fenchlorphos]

fenclonine USAN, INN *serotonin inhibitor*

fenclorac USAN, INN *anti-inflammatory*

fenclozic acid INN, BAN

fendiline INN

fendizoate INN *combining name for radicals or groups*

fendosal USAN, INN, BAN *anti-inflammatory*

feneritrol INN

Fenesin sustained-release tablets ℞ *expectorant* [guaifenesin] 600 mg

Fenesin DM tablets ℞ *antitussive; expectorant* [dextromethorphan hydrobromide; guaifenesin] 30•600 mg

fenestrel USAN, INN *estrogen*

fenethazine INN

fenethylline BAN *CNS stimulant* [also: fenethylline HCl; fenetylline]

fenethylline HCl USAN *CNS stimulant* [also: fenetylline; fenethylline]

fenetradil INN

fenetylline INN *CNS stimulant* [also: fenethylline HCl; fenethylline]

fenflumizole INN

fenfluramine INN, BAN *anorexiant; CNS depressant* [also: fenfluramine HCl]

fenfluramine HCl USAN *anorexiant; CNS depressant* [also: fenfluramine]

fenfluthrin INN, BAN

fengabine USAN, INN, BAN *mood regulator*

fenharmane INN

fenimide USAN, INN, BAN *antipsychotic*

feniodium chloride INN

fenipentol INN

fenirofibrate INN

fenisorex USAN, INN, BAN *anorectic*

fenleuton USAN *5-lipoxygenase inhibitor*

fenmetozole INN *antidepressant; narcotic antagonist* [also: fenmetozole HCl]

fenmetozole HCl USAN *antidepressant; narcotic antagonist* [also: fenmetozole]

fenmetramide USAN, INN, BAN *antidepressant*

fennel *(Anethum foeniculum; Foeniculum officinale; F. vulgare)* seeds *medicinal herb for colic, gas, intestinal problems, promoting expectoration, stimulating lactation and menses, and sedation in children*

fennel oil NF

fenobam USAN, INN *sedative*

fenocinol INN

fenoctimine INN *gastric antisecretory* [also: fenoctimine sulfate]

fenoctimine sulfate USAN *gastric antisecretory* [also: fenoctimine]

fenofibrate INN, BAN *antihyperlipidemic for primary hypercholesterolemia (types IIa and IIb hyperlipidemia), hypertriglyceridemia (types IV and V hyperlipidemia), and mixed dyslipidemia*

fenoldopam INN, BAN *vasodilator for hypertensive emergencies; dopamine agonist* [also: fenoldopam mesylate]

fenoldopam mesylate USAN *vasodilator for hypertensive emergencies; dopamine agonist* [also: fenoldopam]

fenoprofen USAN, INN, BAN *analgesic; antiarthritic; nonsteroidal anti-inflammatory drug (NSAID)*

fenoprofen calcium USAN, USP, BAN *analgesic; antiarthritic; nonsteroidal anti-inflammatory drug (NSAID)* 200, 300, 600 mg oral

fenoterol USAN, INN, BAN *bronchodilator* [also: fenoterol hydrobromide]

fenoterol hydrobromide JAN *bronchodilator* [also: fenoterol]

fenoverine INN

fenoxazol [see: pemoline]

fenoxazoline INN

fenoxazoline HCl [see: fenoxazoline]

fenoxedil INN

fenoxypropazine INN [also: phenoxypropazine]

fenozolone INN

fenpentadiol INN

fenperate INN

fenpipalone USAN, INN *anti-inflammatory*

fenpipramide INN, BAN

fenpiprane INN, BAN

fenpiprane HCl [see: fenpiprane]

fenpiverinium bromide INN

fenprinast INN *bronchodilator; antiallergic* [also: fenprinast HCl]

fenprinast HCl USAN *bronchodilator; antiallergic* [also: fenprinast]

fenproporex INN

fenprostalene USAN, INN, BAN *luteolysin*

fenquizone USAN, INN *diuretic*

fenretinide USAN, INN *investigational (Phase III) retinoid cancer chemopreventative*

fenspiride INN *bronchodilator; antiadrenergic (α-receptor)* [also: fenspiride HCl]

fenspiride HCl USAN *bronchodilator; antiadrenergic (α-receptor)* [also: fenspiride]

fentanyl INN, BAN *narcotic analgesic; also abused as a street drug* [also: fentanyl citrate] ⊠ Sentinel

fentanyl citrate USAN, USP, JAN *narcotic analgesic; also abused as a street drug* [also: fentanyl] 0.05 mg/mL injection

Fentanyl Oralet lozenges ℞ *oral transmucosal narcotic analgesic for anesthesia premedication* [fentanyl citrate] 100, 200, 300, 400 μg

fenthion BAN

fentiazac USAN, INN, BAN *anti-inflammatory*

fenticlor USAN, INN, BAN *topical anti-infective*

fenticonazole INN, BAN *antifungal* [also: fenticonazole nitrate]

fenticonazole nitrate USAN *antifungal* [also: fenticonazole]

fentonium bromide INN

fenugreek *(Trigonella foenum-graecum)* seeds *medicinal herb for boils, bronchial secretions, cellulitis, diabetes, hypercholesterolemia, kidney stones, lung infections, promoting expectoration, stomach irritation, and tuberculosis*

fenyramidol INN *analgesic; skeletal muscle relaxant* [also: phenyramidol HCl]

fenyripol INN *skeletal muscle relaxant* [also: fenyripol HCl]

fenyripol HCl USAN *skeletal muscle relaxant* [also: fenyripol]

Feocyte prolonged-action tablets ℞ *hematinic* [ferrous fumarate; ferrous gluconate; ferrous sulfate; liver, desiccated; vitamins B_6, B_{12}, and C; folic acid] 110 mg (total iron)•15 mg•2 mg•50 μg•100 mg•0.8 mg

Fe-O.D. timed-release tablets (discontinued 1998) OTC *hematinic* [ferrous fumarate; ascorbic acid] 100•500 mg

Feosol caplets OTC *hematinic; iron supplement* [carbonyl iron] 50 mg

Feosol elixir OTC *hematinic* [ferrous sulfate (source of iron)] 220 mg/5 mL (44 mg/5 mL) ⊠ Feostat; Fer-In-Sol; Festal

Feosol tablets OTC *hematinic* [ferrous sulfate, dried (source of iron)] 200 mg (65 mg)

Feosol timed-release capsules (discontinued 1998) OTC *hematinic* [ferrous sulfate, dried (source of iron)] 159 mg (50 mg)

Feostat chewable tablets, suspension, drops OTC *hematinic* [ferrous fumarate (source of iron)] 100 mg (33 mg); 100 mg/5 mL (33 mg/5 mL); 45 mg/0.6 mL (15 mg/0.6 mL) ⊠ Feosol

fepentolic acid INN

fepitrizol INN

fepradinol INN

feprazone INN, BAN

fepromide INN

feprosidnine INN

Ferancee chewable tablets (discontinued 1998) OTC *hematinic* [ferrous fumarate; ascorbic acid] 67•150 mg

Ferancee-HP film-coated tablets (discontinued 1998) OTC *hematinic* [ferrous fumarate; ascorbic acid] 110•600 mg

Feratab tablets OTC *hematinic* [ferrous sulfate, dried (source of iron)] 187 mg (60 mg)

Fer-gen-sol drops OTC *hematinic* [ferrous sulfate (source of iron)] 75 mg/0.6 mL (15 mg/0.6 mL)

Fergon elixir (discontinued 1998) OTC *hematinic* [ferrous gluconate (source of iron)] 300 mg/5 mL (34 mg/5 mL)

Fergon tablets OTC *hematinic* [ferrous gluconate (source of iron)] 240 mg (27 mg)

Feridex IV injection ℞ *contrast agent for MRI of the liver* [ferumoxides] (11.2 mg iron)

Fer-In-Sol capsules (discontinued 1997) OTC *hematinic* [ferrous sulfate, dried (source of iron)] 190 mg (60 mg) ⊠ Feosol

Fer-In-Sol drops, syrup OTC *hematinic* [ferrous sulfate (source of iron)] 75 mg/0.6 mL (15 mg/0.6 mL); 90 mg/5 mL (18 mg/5 mL)

Fer-Iron drops OTC *hematinic* [ferrous sulfate (source of iron)] 75 mg/0.6 mL (15 mg/0.6 mL)

fermium *element (Fm)*

fern; fern brake *medicinal herb* [see: buckhorn brake; female fern]

fern, flowering; king's fern; water fern *medicinal herb* [see: buckhorn brake]

fern-leaved foxglove *medicinal herb* [see: feverweed]

Ferocyl sustained-release tablets (discontinued 1998) OTC *hematinic* [ferrous fumarate; docusate sodium] 150•100 mg

Fero-Folic-500 controlled-release Filmtabs (film-coated tablets) ℞ *hematinic* [ferrous sulfate; ascorbic acid; folic acid] 105•500•0.8 mg

Fero-Grad-500 timed-release tablets OTC *hematinic; iron/vitamin C supplement* [iron (from ferrous sulfate); sodium ascorbate] 105•500 mg

Fero-Gradumet timed-release Filmtabs (film-coated tablets) (discontinued 1998) OTC *hematinic* [ferrous sulfate (source of iron)] 525 mg (105 mg)

Ferospace capsules (discontinued 1998) OTC *hematinic* [ferrous sulfate (source of iron)] 250 mg (50 mg)

Ferotrinsic capsules ℞ *hematinic* [ferrous fumarate; cyanocobalamin; ascorbic acid; intrinsic factor concentrate; folic acid] 110 mg•15 μg•75 mg•240 mg•0.5 mg

Ferralet tablets (discontinued 1998) OTC *hematinic* [ferrous gluconate (source of iron)] 320 mg (37 mg)

Ferralet Plus tablets OTC *hematinic* [ferrous gluconate; cyanocobalamin; ascorbic acid; folic acid] 46 mg•25 μg•400 mg•0.8 mg

Ferralet S.R. sustained-release tablets (discontinued 1998) OTC *hematinic* [ferrous gluconate (source of iron)] 320 mg (37 mg)

Ferralyn Lanacaps (timed-release capsules) (discontinued 1998) OTC *hematinic* [ferrous sulfate, dried (source of iron)] 250 mg (50 mg)

Ferra-TD timed-release capsules (discontinued 1998) OTC *hematinic* [ferrous sulfate, dried (source of iron)] 250 mg (50 mg)

Ferretts tablets (discontinued 1997) OTC *hematinic* [ferrous fumarate] 325 mg

Ferrex 150 capsules OTC *hematinic; iron supplement* [polysaccharide iron complex] 150 mg iron

Ferrex 150 Forte capsules ℞ *antianemic* [polysaccharide iron complex; vitamin B_{12}; folic acid] 150 mg iron•25 μg•1 mg

Ferrex PC; Ferrex PC Forte film-coated tablets ℞ *vitamin/mineral/iron supplement for pregnancy and lactation* [multiple vitamins & minerals; polysaccharide iron complex; folic acid] ≛•60 mg iron•1 mg

ferric ammonium citrate NF

ferric ammonium sulfate

ferric cacodylate NF

ferric chloride

ferric chloride Fe 59 USAN *radioactive agent*

ferric citrate (^{59}Fe) INN

ferric citrochloride NF

ferric fructose USAN, INN *hematinic*

ferric glycerophosphate NF

ferric hydroxide sucrose complex [see: iron sucrose; saccharated ferric oxide]

ferric hypophosphite NF

ferric oxide NF *coloring agent*

ferric oxide, red NF

ferric oxide, yellow NF

ferric pyrophosphate, soluble NF

ferric subsulfate NF

ferricholinate [see: ferrocholinate]

ferriclate calcium sodium USAN *hematinic* [also: calcium sodium ferriclate]

ferristene USAN *paramagnetic imaging agent for MRI*

Ferrlecit IV infusion ℞ *hematinic for iron deficiency of chronic hemodialysis with erythropoietin therapy* [sodium ferric gluconate] 62.5 mg/5 mL

Ferro Dok TR timed-release capsules (discontinued 1998) OTC *hematinic*

[ferrous fumarate; docusate sodium] 150•100 mg

ferrocholate [see: ferrocholinate]

ferrocholinate INN

Ferro-Docusate T.R. timed-release capsules (discontinued 1998) OTC *hematinic* [ferrous fumarate; docusate sodium] 150•100 mg

Ferro-DSS S.R. timed-release capsules (discontinued 1998) OTC *hematinic* [ferrous fumarate; docusate sodium] 150•100 mg

Ferromar sustained-release caplets OTC *hematinic* [ferrous fumarate; vitamin C] 201.5•200 mg

ferropolimaler INN

Ferro-Sequels timed-release tablets OTC *hematinic; iron supplement* [ferrous fumarate; docusate sodium] 50•≟ mg

ferrotrenine INN

ferrous citrate Fe 59 USAN, USP *radioactive agent*

ferrous fumarate USP *hematinic (33% elemental iron)* 200, 325 mg oral

ferrous gluconate USP *hematinic (11.6% elemental iron)* 325 mg oral

ferrous lactate NF

ferrous orotate JAN

ferrous sulfate USP, JAN *hematinic (20% elemental iron)* 250, 325 mg oral; 220 mg/5 mL oral; 75 mg/0.6 mL oral

ferrous sulfate, dried USP *hematinic (30% elemental iron)*

ferrous sulfate, exsiccated [see: ferrous sulfate, dried]

ferrous sulfate Fe 59 USAN *radioactive agent*

Fertinex subcu injection ℞ *follicle-stimulating hormone (FSH); ovulation stimulant for polycystic ovary disease (orphan) and assisted reproductive technologies (ART); investigational (orphan) for spermatogenesis in hormone-deficient males* [urofollitropin] 75, 150 IU

fertirelin INN, BAN *veterinary gonadotropin-releasing hormone* [also: fertirelin acetate]

fertirelin acetate USAN *veterinary gonadotropin-releasing hormone* [also: fertirelin]

ferucarbotran USAN *superparamagnetic diagnostic aid*

Ferula assafoetida; F. foetida; F. rubricaulis *medicinal herb* [see: asafetida; asafoetida]

ferumoxides USAN *diagnostic aid for magnetic resonance imaging of the liver*

ferumoxsil USAN *oral MRI contrast medium for upper GI tract imaging*

ferumoxtran-10 USAN *superparamagnetic diagnostic aid*

Fetal Fibronectin Test kit for professional use *in vitro diagnostic aid for fetal fibronectin in vaginal secretions at 24–34 weeks, a predictor of preterm delivery*

fetal neural cells [see: neural cells, porcine fetal]

fetid hellebore *(Helleborus foetidus)* [see: hellebore]

fetid hellebore *(Helleborus foetidus)* [see: hellebore]

Fe-Tinic 150 capsules OTC *antianemic* [polysaccharide iron complex] 150 mg iron

Fe-Tinic 150 Forte capsules ℞ *antianemic* [polysaccharide iron complex; vitamin B_{12}; folic acid] 150 mg iron•25 µg•1 mg

fetoxilate INN *smooth muscle relaxant* [also: fetoxylate HCl; fetoxylate]

fetoxylate BAN *smooth muscle relaxant* [also: fetoxylate HCl; fetoxilate]

fetoxylate HCl USAN *smooth muscle relaxant* [also: fetoxilate; fetoxylate]

fever root *medicinal herb* [see: coral root]

fever twig *medicinal herb* [see: bittersweet nightshade]

Feverall, Children's; Infant's Feverall; Junior Feverall suppositories OTC *analgesic; antipyretic* [acetaminophen] 120 mg; 80 mg; 325 mg

Feverall, Children's; Junior Feverall Sprinkle Caps (powder) OTC *analgesic; antipyretic* [acetaminophen] 80 mg; 160 mg ⑨ Fiberall

feverbush *medicinal herb* [see: winterberry]

feverfew (*Chrysanthemum parthenium; Leucanthemum parthenium; Pyrethrum parthenium; Tanacetum parthenium*) leaves and flowers *medicinal herb used as an aspirin substitute for chills, colds, fever, inflammation, and migraine and sinus headache* 125, 400 mg oral (CAN)

feverweed (*Gerardia pedicularia*) plant *medicinal herb used as an antiseptic, diaphoretic, febrifuge, and sedative*

fexicaine INN, DCF

Fexicam (CAN) suppositories ℞ *nonsteroidal anti-inflammatory drug (NSAID) for rheumatoid arthritis, osteoarthritis, ankylosing spondylitis, and primary dysmenorrhea* [piroxicam] 20 mg

fexinidazole INN

fexofenadine HCl USAN *second-generation piperidine antihistamine for allergic rhinitis and chronic idiopathic urticaria*

fezatione INN

fezolamine INN *antidepressant* [also: fezolamine fumarate]

fezolamine fumarate USAN *antidepressant* [also: fezolamine]

FGN-1 *investigational (Phase III, orphan) for familial adenomatous polyposis (FAP; also known as adenomatous polyposis coli, or APC)* [now: exisulind]

fiacitabine (FIAC) USAN, INN *antiviral; investigational (Phase I/II) for HIV and AIDS*

fialuridine (FIAU) USAN, INN *antiviral; investigational (Phase II) for HIV; investigational (orphan) for chronic active hepatitis B*

Fiberall chewable tablets (discontinued 1999) OTC *bulk laxative; antidiarrheal* [calcium polycarbophil] 1250 mg ⑨ Feverall

Fiberall powder OTC *bulk laxative* [psyllium hydrophilic mucilloid] 3.5 g/tsp.

Fiberall wafers (discontinued 1999) OTC *bulk laxative* [psyllium hydrophilic mucilloid] 3.4 g

FiberCon tablets OTC *bulk laxative; antidiarrheal* [calcium polycarbophil] 500 mg

Fiberlan liquid OTC *enteral nutritional therapy* [lactose-free formula]

Fiber-Lax tablets OTC *bulk laxative; antidiarrheal* [calcium polycarbophil] 625 mg

FiberNorm tablets OTC *bulk laxative; antidiarrheal* [calcium polycarbophil] 625 mg

Fiblast ℞ *investigational (Phase II/III) basic fibroblast growth factor (bFGF) for stroke and coronary artery disease* [trafermin]

fibracillin INN

Fibrad powder (discontinued 1997) OTC *oral dietary fiber supplement* [pea, oat and sugar beet fiber] 7 g total fiber per serving

Fibrillex ℞ *investigational (orphan) agent for the treatment of secondary amyloidosis*

Fibrimage ℞ *investigational (Phase III) imaging agent for deep vein thrombosis* [technetium Tc 99m]

fibrin INN

fibrinase [see: factor XIII]

fibrinogen (^{125}I) INN [also: fibrinogen I 125]

fibrinogen, human USP *investigational (orphan) to control bleeding in fibrinogen-deficient patients*

fibrinogen I 125 USAN *vascular patency test; radioactive agent* [also: fibrinogen (^{125}I)]

fibrinoligase [see: factor XIII]

fibrinolysin, human INN [also: plasmin]

fibrinolysin & desoxyribonuclease *topical enzymes for necrotic tissue debridement*

fibrin-stabilizing factor (FSF) [see: factor XIII]

fibroblast growth factor, basic (bFGF) [see: ersofermin]

fibroblast interferon [now: interferon beta]

Fibrogammin P ℞ *investigational (orphan) for congenital factor XIII deficiency* [factor XIII, plasma-derived]

fibronectin *investigational (orphan) for nonhealing corneal ulcers or epithelial defects*

Ficus carica *medicinal herb* [see: fig]

fiduxosin HCl USAN α_{1a}*-adrenoceptor antagonist for benign prostatic hyperplasia (BPH)*

50% Dextrose with Electrolyte Pattern A (or N) IV infusion ℞ *intravenous nutritional/electrolyte therapy* [combined electrolyte solution; dextrose]

fig *(Ficus carica)* fruit *medicinal herb used as a demulcent, emollient, and laxative*

figwort *(Scrophularia nodosa)* leaves, stems, and roots *medicinal herb for abrasions, athlete's foot, cradle cap, fever, impetigo, restlessness, skin diseases, and skin tumors*

filaminast USAN *selective phosphodiesterase IV inhibitor for asthma*

filenadol INN

filgrastim USAN, INN, BAN *hematopoietic stimulant for severe chronic neutropenia (orphan); investigational (Phase III, orphan) cytokine for AIDS-related cytomegalovirus retinitis*

filgrastim & methionyl stem cell factor, recombinant human *investigational adjunct to myelosuppressive or myeloablative therapy; orphan status withdrawn 1998*

Filipendula ulmaria *medicinal herb* [see: meadowsweet]

filipin USAN, INN *antifungal*

Filmix ℞ *investigational (orphan) neurosonographic contrast medium for intracranial tumors* [microbubble contrast agent]

Filmlok (trademarked dosage form) *film-coated tablet*

Filmseal (trademarked dosage form) *film-coated tablet*

Filmtabs (trademarked dosage form) *film-coated tablets*

FIME (fluorouracil, ICRF-159, MeCCNU) *chemotherapy protocol*

Finac lotion OTC *topical acne treatment* [salicylic acid; isopropyl alcohol] 2%•22.5%

Finajet; Finaplix *brand names for trenbolone acetate, a European veterinary anabolic steroid abused as a street drug*

finasteride USAN, INN, BAN *α-reductase inhibitor; androgen hormone inhibitor for benign prostatic hypertension and androgenic alopecia in men*

Finevin cream ℞ *antimicrobial and keratolytic for inflammatory acne vulgaris* [azelaic acid] 20%

finger leaf *medicinal herb* [see: cinquefoil]

Fiorgen PF tablets (discontinued 1998) ℞ *analgesic; sedative* [aspirin; caffeine; butalbital] 325•40•50 mg

Fioricet tablets ℞ *analgesic; barbiturate sedative* [acetaminophen; caffeine; butalbital] 325•40•50 mg ⊡ Lorcet

Fioricet with Codeine capsules ℞ *narcotic analgesic; barbiturate sedative* [codeine phosphate; acetaminophen; caffeine; butalbital] 30•325•40•50 mg

Fiorinal capsules ℞ *analgesic; barbiturate sedative* [aspirin; caffeine; butalbital] 325•40•50 mg ⊡ Florinef

Fiorinal tablets (discontinued 2000) ℞ *analgesic; barbiturate sedative* [aspirin; caffeine; butalbital] 325•40•50 mg ⊡ Florinef

Fiorinal with Codeine capsules ℞ *narcotic analgesic; barbiturate sedative* [codeine phosphate; aspirin; caffeine; butalbital] 30•325•40•50 mg

Fiorinal-C ¼; Fiorinal-C ½ (CAN) capsules ℞ *narcotic analgesic; barbiturate sedative* [codeine phosphate; aspirin; caffeine; butalbital] 15•330•40•50 mg; 30•330•40•50 mg

Fiorpap tablets (discontinued 2000) ℞ *analgesic; barbiturate sedative* [acetaminophen; caffeine; butalbital] 325•40•50 mg

Fiortal capsules ℞ *analgesic; barbiturate sedative* [aspirin; caffeine; butalbital] 325•40•50 mg

fipexide INN

fire ant venom allergenic extract *investigational (orphan) skin test and immunotherapy for fire ant reactions*

fireweed *medicinal herb* [see: pilewort]

First Choice reagent strips for home use *in vitro diagnostic aid for blood glucose*

First Response; First Response Early Result test stick for home use *in vitro diagnostic aid; urine pregnancy test*

First Response Ovulation Predictor test kit for home use *in vitro diagnostic aid to predict ovulation time*

fisalamine [see: mesalamine]

fit root (*Monotropa uniflora*) *medicinal herb used as an antispasmodic, febrifuge, nervine, and sedative*

FIV-ASA suppositories ℞ *anti-inflammatory for distal ulcerative colitis (DUC) and ulcerative proctitis* [mesalamine (5-aminosalicylic acid)] 500 mg

5 + 2 protocol (cytarabine, daunorubicin) *chemotherapy protocol for acute myelocytic leukemia (AML)*

5 + 2 protocol (cytarabine, mitoxantrone) *chemotherapy protocol for acute myelocytic leukemia (AML)*

5-ALA HCl; ALA [see: aminolevulinic acid HCl]

5% Alcohol and 5% Dextrose in Water; 10% Alcohol and 5% Dextrose in Water IV infusion ℞ *for caloric replacement and rehydration* [dextrose; alcohol] 5%•5%; 10%•5%

5 Benzagel; 10 Benzagel gel ℞ *topical keratolytic for acne* [benzoyl peroxide] 5%; 10%

5% Travert and Electrolyte No. 2; 10% Travert and Electrolyte No. 2 IV infusion ℞ *intravenous nutritional/electrolyte therapy* [combined electrolyte solution; invert sugar (50% dextrose + 50% fructose)]

520C9x22 [see: bispecific antibody 520C9x22]

5-FC (5-fluorocytosine) [see: flucytosine]

five-finger grass; five fingers *medicinal herb* [see: cinquefoil]

five-fingers root *medicinal herb* [see: ginseng]

5-HT (5-hydroxytryptamine) [see: serotonin]

5-HT$_3$ (hydroxytryptamine) receptor antagonists *a class of antiemetic and antinauseant agents used primarily after emetogenic cancer chemotherapy* [also called: selective serotonin 5-HT$_3$ blockers]

5-HTP (5-hydroxytryptophan) [see: L-5 hydroxytryptophan]

FK-565 *investigational (Phase I) immunomodulator for cancer and HIV*

FL (flutamide, leuprolide acetate) *chemotherapy protocol for prostate cancer*

FLAC (fluorouracil, leucovorin [rescue], Adriamycin, cyclophosphamide) *chemotherapy protocol*

flag, sweet; myrtle flag *medicinal herb* [see: calamus]

flag lily; poison flag; water flag *medicinal herb* [see: blue flag]

Flagyl film-coated tablets, capsules ℞ *antibiotic; antiprotozoal; amebicide* [metronidazole] 250, 500 mg; 375 mg

Flagyl ER film-coated extended-release tablets ℞ *once-daily antibiotic for bacterial vaginosis* [metronidazole] 750 mg

Flagyl IV powder for injection ℞ *antibiotic; antiprotozoal; amebicide* [metronidazole HCl] 500 mg

Flagyl IV RTU (ready-to-use) injection ℞ *antibiotic; antiprotozoal; amebicide* [metronidazole] 500 mg/100 mL

flamenol INN

Flanders Buttocks ointment OTC *topical diaper rash treatment* [zinc oxide; peruvian balsam]

flannel flower *medicinal herb* [see: mullein]

FLAP (fluorouracil, leucovorin [rescue], Adriamycin, Platinol) *chemotherapy protocol*

Flarex Drop-Tainers (eye drop suspension) ℞ *topical ophthalmic corticosteroidal anti-inflammatory* [fluorometholone acetate] 0.1%

Flatulex drops OTC *antiflatulent* [simethicone] 40 mg/0.6 mL

Flatulex tablets OTC *adsorbent; detoxicant; antiflatulent* [activated charcoal; simethicone] 250•80 mg

flavamine INN

flavine [see: acriflavine HCl]

flavivirus vaccine, chimeric *investigational vaccine*

flavodic acid INN

flavodilol INN *antihypertensive* [also: flavodilol maleate]

flavodilol maleate USAN *antihypertensive* [also: flavodilol]

flavonoid [see: troxerutin]

Flavons tablets OTC *dietary supplement* [mixed bioflavonoids] 500 mg

Flavons-500 tablets OTC *dietary supplement* [citrus bioflavonoids] 500 mg

Flavorcee chewable tablets (discontinued 1999) OTC *vitamin C supplement* [ascorbic acid] 100, 250, 500 mg

flavoxate INN, BAN *smooth muscle relaxant; urinary antispasmodic* [also: flavoxate HCl]

flavoxate HCl USAN *smooth muscle relaxant; urinary antispasmodic* [also: flavoxate]

flaxseed *(Linum usitatissimum)* *medicinal herb for arthritis, autoimmune diseases, colds, constipation, cough, heart disease, lowering cholesterol levels, skin disorders, and urinary tract infections*

flazalone USAN, INN, BAN *anti-inflammatory*

FLe (fluorouracil, levamisole) *chemotherapy protocol for colorectal cancer*

flea seed; fleawort *medicinal herb* [see: plantain]

fleabane; horseweed *(Erigeron canadensis)* plant *medicinal herb used as an astringent, diuretic, and hemostatic*

fleawort; flea seed *medicinal herb* [see: plantain]

flecainide INN, BAN *antiarrhythmic* [also: flecainide acetate]

flecainide acetate USAN *antiarrhythmic* [also: flecainide] 50, 100, 150 mg

Fleet disposable enema OTC *saline laxative* [sodium phosphate, monobasic; sodium phosphate, dibasic] 7•19 g/118 mL dose

Fleet Babylax rectal liquid OTC *hyperosmolar laxative* [glycerin] 4 mL/dose

Fleet Bisacodyl disposable enema OTC *stimulant laxative* [bisacodyl] 10 mg/30 mL dose

Fleet Bisacodyl Prep enema (discontinued 1999) OTC *stimulant laxative* [bisacodyl] 10 mg/packet

Fleet Flavored Castor Oil oral emulsion (discontinued 1999) OTC *stimulant laxative* [castor oil] 67%

Fleet Laxative enteric-coated tablets, suppositories OTC *stimulant laxative* [bisacodyl] 5 mg; 10 mg

Fleet Medicated Wipes cleansing pads OTC *moisturizer and cleanser for external rectal/vaginal areas; astringent; antiseptic; antifungal* [hamamelis water; glycerin; alcohol] 50%•10%•7%

Fleet Mineral Oil disposable enema OTC *emollient laxative* [mineral oil] 118 mL dose

Fleet Pain Relief anorectal wipes OTC *topical local anesthetic* [pramoxine HCl; glycerin] 1%•12%

Fleet Phospho-Soda oral solution OTC *saline laxative* [sodium phosphate, monobasic; sodium phosphate, dibasic] 2.4•0.9 g/5 mL

Fleet Prep Kits No. 1 to No. 3 OTC *pre-procedure bowel evacuant* [other Fleet products in combination kits]

Fleet Prep Kits No. 4 to No. 6 (discontinued 1999) OTC *pre-procedure bowel evacuant* [other Fleet products in combination kits]

FLEP (fluorouracil, leucovorin, etoposide, Platinol) *chemotherapy protocol*

flerobuterol INN

fleroxacin USAN, INN *antibacterial*

flesinoxan INN *investigational (Phase III) antidepressant and anxiolytic*

flestolol INN *antiadrenergic (β-receptor)* [also: flestolol sulfate]

flestolol sulfate USAN *antiadrenergic (β-receptor)* [also: flestolol]

fletazepam USAN, INN, BAN *skeletal muscle relaxant*

Fletcher's Castoria oral liquid OTC *stimulant laxative* [senna concentrate] 33.3 mg/mL

fleur-de-lis *medicinal herb* [see: blue flag]

Flex-all 454 gel OTC *topical analgesic; antipruritic; counterirritant; topical local anesthetic* [menthol; methyl salicylate] 16%•?

Flexaphen capsules ℞ *skeletal muscle relaxant; analgesic* [chlorzoxazone; acetaminophen] 250•300 mg

Flex-Care Especially for Sensitive Eyes solution OTC *chemical disinfecting solution for soft contact lenses* [note: soft contact indication different from RGP contact indication for same product]

Flex-Care Especially for Sensitive Eyes solution OTC *disinfecting/wetting/soaking solution for rigid gas permeable contact lenses* [note: RGP contact indication different from soft contact indication for same product]

Flexderm sheets *absorbent wound dressing* [hydrogel polymer]

Flexeril film-coated tablets ℞ *skeletal muscle relaxant* [cyclobenzaprine HCl] 10 mg ⊠ Flaxedil

Flexoject IV or IM injection ℞ *skeletal muscle relaxant* [orphenadrine citrate] 30 mg/mL

Flexon IV or IM injection ℞ *skeletal muscle relaxant* [orphenadrine citrate] 30 mg/mL

FlexPack HP test for professional use *diagnostic aid for serum IgG antibodies to H. pylori (for peptic ulcers)*

Flextra-DS tablets ℞ *analgesic; antipyretic; antihistaminic sleep aid* [acetaminophen; phenyltoloxamine citrate] 500•50 mg

Flexzan; Flexzan Extra adhesive sheets *absorbent, semi-occlusive wound dressing* [polyurethane foam]

flibanserin USAN *antidepressant*

Flintstones Children's; Flintstones Plus Calcium; Flintstones Plus Extra C Children's chewable tablets OTC *vitamin supplement* [multiple vitamins; folic acid] *•0.3 mg

Flintstones Complete chewable tablets OTC *vitamin/mineral/iron supplement* [multiple vitamins & minerals; iron; folic acid; biotin] *•18 mg•0.4 mg•40 μg

Flintstones Plus Iron chewable tablets OTC *vitamin/iron supplement* [multiple vitamins; iron; folic acid] *•15•0.3 mg

Flo-Coat oral/rectal suspension ℞ *radiopaque contrast medium for gastrointestinal imaging* [barium sulfate] 100%

Flocor ℞ *investigational (Phase III, orphan) coagulation inhibitor for treatment of sickle cell vaso-occlusive crisis; investigational (orphan) for severe burns and for vasospasm following cerebral aneurysm repair* [poloxamer 188]

floctafenine USAN, INN, BAN *analgesic*

Flolan IV infusion ℞ *platelet aggregation inhibitor and vasodilator for primary pulmonary hypertension (orphan)* [epoprostenol] 0.5, 1.5 mg

Flomax capsules ℞ *α_1 antagonist for benign prostatic hypertrophy (BPH)* [tamsulosin HCl] 0.4 mg ⊠ Slow-Mag; Zomig

flomoxef INN

Flonase nasal spray ℞ *corticosteroidal anti-inflammatory for seasonal or perennial rhinitis* [fluticasone propionate] 50 μg/dose

Flo-Pack (trademarked packaging form) *vial for IV drip*

flopropione INN

florantyrone INN, BAN

flordipine USAN, INN *antihypertensive*

floredil INN

Florentine iris *medicinal herb* [see: orris root]

floretione [see: fluoresone]

florfenicol USAN, INN, BAN *veterinary antibacterial*

Florical capsules, tablets OTC *calcium/fluoride supplement* [calcium carbonate; sodium fluoride] 364•8.3 mg

Florida Sunburn Relief lotion OTC *topical analgesic; antipruritic; counterirritant* [phenol; camphor; menthol; benzyl alcohol] 0.4%•0.2%•0.15%•3%

florifenine INN

Florinef Acetate tablets ℞ *adrenocortical insufficiency in Addison disease* [fludrocortisone acetate] 0.1 mg ⓢ Fiorinal

Florone cream, ointment ℞ *topical corticosteroidal anti-inflammatory* [diflorasone diacetate] 0.05%

Florone E cream ℞ *topical corticosteroidal anti-inflammatory; emollient* [diflorasone diacetate] 0.05%

floropipamide [now: pipamperone]

floropipeton [see: propyperone]

Florvite drops ℞ *pediatric vitamin supplement and dental caries preventative* [multiple vitamins; sodium fluoride] ≛•0.25, ≛•0.5 mg/mL

Florvite; Florvite Half Strength chewable tablets ℞ *pediatric vitamin supplement and dental caries preventative* [multiple vitamins; sodium fluoride; folic acid] ≛•1•0.3 mg; ≛•0.5•0.3 mg

Florvite + Iron drops ℞ *pediatric vitamin/iron supplement and dental caries preventative* [multiple vitamins & minerals; sodium fluoride; ferrous sulfate] ≛•0.25•10, ≛•0.5•10 mg/mL

Florvite + Iron; Half Strength Florvite + Iron chewable tablets ℞ *pediatric vitamin/iron supplement and dental caries preventative* [multiple vitamins & minerals; sodium fluoride; ferrous sulfate; folic acid] ≛•1•12•0.3 mg; ≛•0.5•12•0.3 mg

flosequinan USAN, INN, BAN *antihypertensive; vasodilator*

flotrenizine INN

Flovent metered dose inhaler, Rotadisk (inhalation powder), Diskus (powder inhalation device) ℞ *corticosteroidal antiasthmatic* [fluticasone propionate] 44, 110, 220 µg/dose; 50, 100, 250 µg/dose; 50, 100, 250 µg/dose

floverine INN

flower velure *medicinal herb* [see: coltsfoot]

flower-de-luce *medicinal herb* [see: blue flag]

floxacillin USAN *antibacterial* [also: flucloxacillin]

floxacrine INN

Floxin film-coated tablets, UroPak (3-day supply), IV injection ℞ *broad-spectrum fluoroquinolone antibiotic* [ofloxacin] 200, 300, 400 mg; 6 tablets×200 mg; 200, 400 mg/vial

Floxin Otic ear drops ℞ *broad-spectrum fluoroquinolone antibiotic* [ofloxacin] 0.3%

floxuridine USAN, USP, INN *antimetabolic antineoplastic for GI adenocarcinoma metastatic to the liver* 500 mg injection

FLT (fluorothymidine) [q.v.]

Flu, Cold & Cough Medicine powder for oral solution OTC *antitussive; decongestant; antihistamine; analgesic* [dextromethorphan hydrobromide; pseudoephedrine HCl; chlorpheniramine maleate; acetaminophen] 20•60•4•500 mg/packet

Flu OIA (Optical ImmunoAssay) test for professional use *rapid (less than 20 minutes) diagnostic aid for influenza A and B in sputum, nasal aspirate, or nasopharyngeal swab*

fluacizine INN

flualamide INN

fluanisone INN, BAN

fluazacort USAN, INN *anti-inflammatory*

flubanilate INN *CNS stimulant* [also: flubanilate HCl]

flubanilate HCl USAN *CNS stimulant* [also: flubanilate]

flubendazole USAN, INN, BAN *antiprotozoal*

flubenisolone [see: betamethasone]

flubepride INN

flubuperone [see: melperone]

flucarbril INN

flucetorex INN

flucindole USAN, INN *antipsychotic*

fluciprazine INN

fluclorolone acetonide INN, BAN *corticosteroid; anti-inflammatory* [also: flucloronide]
flucloronide USAN *corticosteroid; anti-inflammatory* [also: fluclorolone acetonide]
flucloxacillin INN, BAN *antibacterial* [also: floxacillin]
fluconazole USAN, INN, BAN *systemic triazole antifungal*
flucrilate INN *tissue adhesive* [also: flucrylate]
flucrylate USAN *tissue adhesive* [also: flucrilate]
flucytosine USAN, USP, INN, BAN *systemic antifungal*
fludalanine USAN, INN *antibacterial*
Fludara powder for IV injection ℞ *antineoplastic for chronic lymphocytic leukemia and non-Hodgkin lymphoma (orphan)* [fludarabine phosphate] 50 mg
fludarabine INN *antimetabolite antineoplastic* [also: fludarabine phosphate]
fludarabine phosphate USAN *antimetabolite antineoplastic for chronic lymphocytic leukemia and non-Hodgkin lymphoma (orphan)* [also: fludarabine]
fludazonium chloride USAN, INN *topical anti-infective*
fludeoxyglucose (^{18}F) INN *diagnostic aid; radioactive agent* [also: fludeoxyglucose F 18]
fludeoxyglucose F 18 USAN, USP *diagnostic aid; radioactive agent* [also: fludeoxyglucose (^{18}F)]
fludiazepam INN
fludorex USAN, INN *anorectic; antiemetic*
fludoxopone INN
fludrocortisone INN, BAN *salt-regulating adrenocortical steroid; mineralocorticoid* [also: fludrocortisone acetate]
fludrocortisone acetate USP *salt-regulating adrenocortical steroid; mineralocorticoid* [also: fludrocortisone]
fludroxicortide [see: flurandrenolide]
fludroxycortide INN *topical corticosteroid* [also: flurandrenolide; flurandrenolone]
flufenamic acid USAN, INN, BAN *anti-inflammatory*
flufenisal USAN, INN *analgesic*
flufosal INN
flufylline INN
flugestone INN, BAN *progestin* [also: flurogestone acetate]
flugestone acetate [see: flurogestone acetate]
Fluimucil ℞ *investigational (Phase I) immunomodulator for HIV and AIDS* [acetylcysteine]
fluindarol INN
fluindione INN
Flumadine film-coated tablets, syrup ℞ *antiviral for prophylaxis and treatment of influenza A infections* [rimantadine HCl] 100 mg; 50 mg/5 mL
flumazenil USAN, INN, BAN *benzodiazepine antagonist/antidote*
flumazepil [see: flumazenil]
flumecinol INN *investigational (orphan) for neonatal hyperbilirubinemia*
flumedroxone INN, BAN
flumequine USAN, INN, BAN *antibacterial*
flumeridone USAN, INN, BAN *antiemetic*
flumetasone INN *corticosteroid; anti-inflammatory* [also: flumethasone]
flumethasone USAN, BAN *topical corticosteroidal anti-inflammatory* [also: flumetasone]
flumethasone pivalate USAN, USP, BAN *topical corticosteroidal anti-inflammatory*
flumethiazide INN, BAN
flumethrin BAN
flumetramide USAN, INN *skeletal muscle relaxant*
flumexadol INN
flumezapine USAN, INN, BAN *antipsychotic; neuroleptic*
fluminorex USAN, INN *anorectic*
FluMist ℞ *investigational (NDA filed) intranasal influenza virus vaccine*
flumizole USAN, INN *anti-inflammatory*
flumoxonide USAN, INN *adrenocortical steroid*
flunamine INN
flunarizine INN, BAN *vasodilator; investigational (orphan) for alternating hemiplegia* [also: flunarizine HCl]

flunarizine HCl USAN *vasodilator* [also: flunarizine]

flunidazole USAN, INN *antiprotozoal*

flunisolide USAN, USP, INN, BAN *corticosteroidal anti-inflammatory for chronic asthma and rhinitis*

flunisolide acetate USAN *anti-inflammatory*

flunitrazepam USAN, INN, BAN, JAN *benzodiazepine sedative and hypnotic; also abused as a "date rape" street drug*

flunixin USAN, INN, BAN *anti-inflammatory; analgesic*

flunixin meglumine USAN *anti-inflammatory; analgesic*

flunoprost INN

flunoxaprofen INN

fluocinolide [now: fluocinonide]

fluocinolone BAN *topical corticosteroidal anti-inflammatory* [also: fluocinolone acetonide]

fluocinolone acetonide USAN, USP, INN *topical corticosteroidal anti-inflammatory* [also: fluocinolone] 0.01%, 0.025% topical

fluocinonide USAN, USP, INN, BAN *topical corticosteroidal anti-inflammatory* 0.05% topical

fluocortin INN *anti-inflammatory* [also: fluocortin butyl]

fluocortin butyl USAN, BAN *anti-inflammatory* [also: fluocortin]

fluocortolone USAN, INN, BAN *corticosteroid; anti-inflammatory*

fluocortolone caproate USAN *corticosteroid; anti-inflammatory*

Fluogen IM injection in vials and disposable syringes ℞ *flu vaccine* [influenza split-virus vaccine] 0.5 mL/dose

Fluonex cream ℞ *topical corticosteroidal anti-inflammatory* [fluocinonide] 0.05%

Fluonid topical solution ℞ *topical corticosteroidal anti-inflammatory* [fluocinolone acetonide] 0.01%

fluopromazine BAN *antipsychotic* [also: triflupromazine]

Fluoracaine eye drops ℞ *topical ophthalmic anesthetic; corneal disclosing agent* [proparacaine HCl; fluorescein sodium] 0.5%•0.25%

fluoracizine [see: fluacizine]

fluorescein USP, BAN, JAN *ophthalmic diagnostic aid*

fluorescein, soluble [now: fluorescein sodium]

fluorescein sodium USP, BAN, JAN *ophthalmic diagnostic aid* 2% eye drops

fluorescein sodium & proparacaine HCl *corneal disclosing agent; topical ophthalmic anesthetic* 0.25%•0.5%

Fluorescite antecubital venous injection ℞ *ophthalmic diagnostic agent* [fluorescein sodium] 10%, 25%

Fluoresoft eye drops ℞ *diagnostic aid in fitting contact lenses* [fluorexon] 0.35%

fluoresone INN

Fluorets ophthalmic strips OTC *corneal disclosing agent* [fluorescein sodium] 1 mg

fluorexon *diagnosis and fitting aid for contact lenses*

fluorhydrocortisone acetate [see: fludrocortisone acetate]

Fluoride tablets OTC *dental caries preventative* [sodium fluoride] 2.21 mg

Fluoride Loz lozenges ℞ *topical dental caries preventative* [sodium fluoride] 2.21 mg

Fluorigard oral rinse OTC *topical dental caries preventative* [sodium fluoride; alcohol 6%] 0.05%

Fluori-Methane spray ℞ *topical vapocoolant anesthetic* [trichloromonofluoromethane; dichlorodifluoromethane] 85%•15%

fluorine *element (F)*

fluorine F 18 fluorodeoxyglucose [see: fludeoxyglucose F 18]

Fluorinse oral rinse ℞ *topical dental caries preventative* [sodium fluoride] 0.2%

Fluor-I-Strip; Fluor-I-Strip A.T. ophthalmic strips ℞ *corneal disclosing agent* [fluorescein sodium] 9 mg; 1 mg

Fluoritab chewable tablets, drops ℞ *dental caries preventative* [sodium fluoride] 1.1, 2.2 mg; 0.55 mg/drop

fluormethylprednisolone [see: dexamethasone]

5-fluorocytosine (5-FC) [see: flucytosine]

fluorodeoxyglucose F 18 [see: fludeoxyglucose F 18]

fluorodideoxyadenosine (F-ddA) [see: lodenosine]

fluorometholone USP, INN, BAN *topical ophthalmic corticosteroidal anti-inflammatory* 0.1% eye drops

fluorometholone acetate USAN *topical ophthalmic corticosteroidal anti-inflammatory*

fluoromethylene deoxycytidine (FMdC) [now: tezacitabine]

Fluor-Op eye drop suspension ℞ *topical ophthalmic corticosteroidal anti-inflammatory* [fluorometholone] 0.1%

Fluoroperm 32 ℞ *hydrophobic contact lens material* [paflufocon C]

Fluoroperm 62 ℞ *hydrophobic contact lens material* [paflufocon B]

Fluoroperm 92 ℞ *hydrophobic contact lens material* [paflufocon A]

Fluoroperm 151 ℞ *hydrophobic contact lens material* [paflufocon D]

Fluoroplex cream, topical solution ℞ *antimetabolite antineoplastic for actinic keratoses and basal cell carcinomas* [fluorouracil] 1%

fluoroquinolones *a class of synthetic, broad-spectrum, antimicrobial, bactericidal antibiotics*

fluorosalan USAN *disinfectant* [also: flusalan]

fluorothymidine (FLT) *investigational (Phase II) antiviral for HIV and AIDS*

fluorouracil (5-FU) USAN, USP, INN, BAN *antimetabolite antineoplastic for colorectal, breast, stomach, and pancreatic cancers; investigational (NDA filed) microsponge delivery system for actinic keratosis* 50 mg/mL injection

fluorouracil & interferon alfa-2a *investigational (orphan) for esophageal and advanced colorectal carcinoma*

fluorouracil & leucovorin *antineoplastic for metastatic colorectal cancer (orphan)*

fluoruridine deoxyribose [see: floxuridine]

fluostigmine [see: isoflurophate]

Fluothane liquid for vaporization ℞ *inhalation general anesthetic* [halothane]

fluotracen INN *antipsychotic; antidepressant* [also: fluotracen HCl]

fluotracen HCl USAN *antipsychotic; antidepressant* [also: fluotracen]

fluoxetine USAN, INN, BAN *selective serotonin reuptake inhibitor (SSRI) for depression, obsessive-compulsive disorder, bulimia nervosa, and premenstrual dysphoric disorder*

fluoxetine HCl USAN *selective serotonin reuptake inhibitor (SSRI) for depression, obsessive-compulsive disorder, bulimia nervosa, and premenstrual dysphoric disorder* 10, 20, 40 mg oral; 20 mg/5 mL oral

fluoximesterone [see: fluoxymesterone]

Flu-Oxinate eye drops ℞ *topical ophthalmic anesthetic; corneal disclosing agent* [benoxinate HCl; fluorescein sodium] 0.4%•0.25%

fluoxiprednisolone [see: triamcinolone]

fluoxymesterone USP, INN, BAN *oral androgen replacement for hypogonadism or testosterone deficiency in men, delayed puberty in boys, and metastatic breast cancer in women* 10 mg oral

fluparoxan INN, BAN *antidepressant* [also: fluparoxan HCl]

fluparoxan HCl USAN *antidepressant* [also: fluparoxan]

flupenthixol BAN *thioxanthene antipsychotic* [also: flupentixol]

flupentixol INN *thioxanthene antipsychotic* [also: flupenthixol]

fluperamide USAN, INN *antiperistaltic*

fluperlapine INN

fluperolone INN, BAN *corticosteroid; anti-inflammatory* [also: fluperolone acetate]

fluperolone acetate USAN *corticosteroid; anti-inflammatory* [also: fluperolone]

fluphenazine INN, BAN *phenothiazine antipsychotic* [also: fluphenazine enanthate]

fluphenazine decanoate *phenothiazine antipsychotic; prolonged parenteral neuroleptic therapy* 25 mg/mL injection

fluphenazine enanthate USP *phenothiazine antipsychotic; prolonged parenteral neuroleptic therapy* [also: fluphenazine]
fluphenazine HCl USP, BAN *phenothiazine antipsychotic* 1, 2.5, 5, 10 mg oral; 5 mg/mL oral; 2.5 mg/mL injection
flupimazine INN
flupirtine INN, BAN *analgesic* [also: flupirtine maleate]
flupirtine maleate USAN *analgesic* [also: flupirtine]
flupranone INN
fluprazine INN
fluprednidene INN, BAN
fluprednisolone USAN, NF, INN, BAN *corticosteroid; anti-inflammatory*
fluprednisolone valerate USAN *corticosteroid; anti-inflammatory*
fluprofen INN, BAN
fluprofylline INN
fluproquazone USAN, INN, BAN *analgesic*
fluprostenol INN, BAN *prostaglandin* [also: fluprostenol sodium]
fluprostenol sodium USAN *prostaglandin* [also: fluprostenol]
fluquazone USAN, INN *anti-inflammatory*
Flura tablets ℞ *dental caries preventative* [sodium fluoride] 2.2 mg
fluracil [see: fluorouracil]
fluradoline INN *analgesic* [also: fluradoline HCl]
fluradoline HCl USAN *analgesic* [also: fluradoline]
Flura-Drops ℞ *dental caries preventative* [sodium fluoride] 0.55 mg/drop
Flura-Loz lozenges ℞ *topical dental caries preventative* [sodium fluoride] 2.2 mg
flurandrenolide USAN, USP *topical corticosteroid* [also: fludroxycortide; flurandrenolone] 0.05% topical
flurandrenolone BAN *topical corticosteroid* [also: flurandrenolide; fludroxycortide]
flurantel INN
Flurate eye drops ℞ *topical ophthalmic anesthetic; corneal disclosing agent* [benoxinate HCl; fluorescein sodium] 0.4%•0.25%
flurazepam INN, BAN *anticonvulsant; hypnotic; muscle relaxant; sedative; also abused as a street drug* [also: flurazepam HCl]
flurazepam HCl USAN, USP *anticonvulsant; hypnotic; muscle relaxant; sedative; also abused as a street drug* [also: flurazepam] 15, 30 mg oral
flurbiprofen USAN, USP, INN, BAN *antiarthritic; nonsteroidal anti-inflammatory drug (NSAID)* 50, 100 mg oral
flurbiprofen sodium USP *prostaglandin synthesis inhibitor; antimiotic; ophthalmic nonsteroidal anti-inflammatory drug (NSAID)* 0.03% eye drops
Fluress eye drops ℞ *topical ophthalmic anesthetic; corneal disclosing agent* [benoxinate HCl; fluorescein sodium] 0.4%•0.25%
fluretofen USAN, INN *anti-inflammatory; antithrombotic*
flurfamide [now: flurofamide]
flurithromycin INN
flurocitabine USAN, INN *antineoplastic*
Fluro-Ethyl aerosol spray ℞ *topical refrigerant anesthetic* [ethyl chloride; dichlorotetrafluoroethane] 25%•75%
flurofamide USAN, INN *urease enzyme inhibitor*
flurogestone acetate USAN *progestin* [also: flugestone]
Flurosyn ointment, cream ℞ *topical corticosteroidal anti-inflammatory* [fluocinolone acetonide] 0.025%; 0.01, 0.025%
flurothyl USAN, USP, BAN *CNS stimulant* [also: flurotyl]
flurotyl INN *CNS stimulant* [also: flurothyl]
fluroxene USAN, NF, INN *inhalation anesthetic*
fluroxyspiramine [see: spiramide]
flusalan INN *disinfectant* [also: fluorosalan]
FluShield IM injection in vials and Tubex (cartridge-needle unit) ℞ *flu vaccine* [influenza purified split-virus vaccine] 0.5 mL/dose
flusoxolol INN, BAN
fluspiperone USAN, INN *antipsychotic*

fluspirilene USAN, INN, BAN *diphenylbutylpiperidine antipsychotic*
flutamide USAN, INN, BAN *antiandrogen antineoplastic for metastatic prostate cancer* 125 mg oral
flutazolam INN
flutemazepam INN
Flutex ointment, cream ℞ *topical corticosteroidal anti-inflammatory* [triamcinolone acetonide] 0.025%, 0.1%, 0.5%
flutiazin USAN, INN *veterinary anti-inflammatory*
fluticasone INN, BAN *corticosteroidal anti-inflammatory for chronic asthma or rhinitis* [also: fluticasone propionate]
fluticasone propionate USAN *corticosteroidal anti-inflammatory for chronic asthma or rhinitis* [also: fluticasone]
flutizenol INN
flutomidate INN
flutonidine INN
flutoprazepam INN
flutrimazole INN
flutroline USAN, INN *antipsychotic*
flutropium bromide INN
fluvastatin INN, BAN *HMG-CoA reductase inhibitor for hypercholesterolemia and atherosclerosis* [also: fluvastatin sodium]
fluvastatin sodium USAN *HMG-CoA reductase inhibitor for hypercholesterolemia, hypertriglyceridemia, and atherosclerosis* [also: fluvastatin]
fluvestrant USAN *investigational antiestrogen antineoplastic for breast cancer*
Fluvirin IM injection in vials and prefilled syringes ℞ *flu vaccine* [influenza purified surface antigen] 0.5 mL/dose
fluvoxamine INN, BAN *selective serotonin reuptake inhibitor (SSRI) for obsessive-compulsive disorder* [also: fluvoxamine maleate]
fluvoxamine maleate USAN *selective serotonin reuptake inhibitor (SSRI) for obsessive-compulsive disorder; investigational (Phase III) for depression and panic disorder* [also: fluvoxamine] 25, 50, 100 mg oral
flux root *medicinal herb* [see: pleurisy root]
fluzinamide USAN, INN *anticonvulsant*
Fluzone IM injection in vials and prefilled syringes ℞ *flu vaccine* [influenza split-virus or whole-virus vaccine] 0.5 mL/dose
fluzoperine INN
flytrap *medicinal herb* [see: dogbane]
FMdC (fluoromethylene deoxycytidine) [now: tezacitabine]
FML; FML Forte eye drop suspension ℞ *topical ophthalmic corticosteroidal anti-inflammatory* [fluorometholone] 0.1%; 0.25%
FML S.O.P. ophthalmic ointment ℞ *topical ophthalmic corticosteroidal anti-inflammatory* [fluorometholone] 0.1%
FML-S eye drop suspension ℞ *topical ophthalmic corticosteroidal anti-inflammatory; antibiotic* [fluorometholone; sulfacetamide sodium] 0.1%•10%
FMS (fluorouracil, mitomycin, streptozocin) *chemotherapy protocol*
FMV (fluorouracil, MeCCNU, vincristine) *chemotherapy protocol*
FNC (fluorouracil, Novantrone, cyclophosphamide) *chemotherapy protocol for breast cancer* [also: CFN; CNF]
FNM (fluorouracil, Novantrone, methotrexate) *chemotherapy protocol*
foal's foot *medicinal herb* [see: coltsfoot]
FOAM (fluorouracil, Oncovin, Adriamycin, mitomycin) *chemotherapy protocol*
Foamicon chewable tablets OTC *antacid* [aluminum hydroxide; magnesium trisilicate] 80•20 mg
focofilcon A USAN *hydrophilic contact lens material*
fodipir USAN *excipient*
Foeniculum officinale; F. vulgare *medicinal herb* [see: fennel]
fohy030 gene *investigational gene that encodes the protein melastatin, a metastasis suppressor in malignant melanoma*
Foille spray OTC *topical local anesthetic; antiseptic* [benzocaine; chloroxylenol] 5%•0.63%

Foille Medicated First Aid ointment, aerosol spray OTC *topical local anesthetic; antiseptic* [benzocaine; chloroxylenol] 5%•0.1%; 5%•0.6%

Foille Plus aerosol spray OTC *topical local anesthetic; antiseptic* [benzocaine; chloroxylenol; alcohol 57.33%] 5%•0.6%

folacin [see: folic acid] ⊡ Fulvicin

folate [see: folic acid]

folate sodium USP

Folergot-DF tablets ℞ *GI anticholinergic; sedative; analgesic* [belladonna alkaloids; phenobarbital; ergotamine tartrate] 0.2•40•0.6 mg

folescutol INN

Folex PFS powder for IV or IM injection (discontinued 1999) ℞ *antimetabolite antineoplastic for leukemia; systemic antipsoriatic; antirheumatic* [methotrexate sodium] 25 mg/mL

Folgard tablets OTC *vitamin B supplement* [vitamins B_6 and B_{12}; folic acid] 10 mg•115 µg•800 µg

folic acid USP, INN, BAN *vitamin B_c; vitamin M; hematopoietic* 0.4, 0.8, 1 mg oral; 5 mg/mL injection

folinate-SF calcium [see: leucovorin calcium]

folinic acid [see: leucovorin calcium]

follicle-stimulating hormone (FSH) BAN [also: menotropins]

follidrin [see: estradiol benzoate]

Follistim subcu or IM injection ℞ *recombinant follicle-stimulating hormone (FSH) for the induction of ovulation* [follitropin beta] 75 IU

follitropin alfa INN *recombinant follicle-stimulating hormone (FSH) for the induction of ovulation or spermatogenesis*

follitropin beta INN *recombinant follicle-stimulating hormone (FSH) for the induction of ovulation*

follotropin [see: menotropins]

Follow-Up [see: Carnation Follow-Up]

Foloxatine ℞ *investigational (orphan) alkylating antineoplastic for ovarian and colorectal cancers* [oxaliplatin]

Foltrin capsules ℞ *hematinic* [ferrous fumarate; cyanocobalamin; ascorbic acid; intrinsic factor concentrate; folic acid] 110 mg•15 µg•75 mg•240 mg•0.5 mg

Foltx tablets ℞ *vitamin B therapy for arteriosclerosis, cardiovascular and peripheral vascular disease, and neurological disorders* [vitamins B_6 and B_{12}; folic acid] 25•1•2.5 mg

Folvite IM injection ℞ *antianemic* [folic acid] 5 mg/mL

fomepizole USAN, INN *antidote; alcohol dehydrogenase inhibitor for methanol or ethylene glycol poisoning (orphan)*

FOMI; FOMi (fluorouracil, Oncovin, mitomycin) *chemotherapy protocol*

fomidacillin INN, BAN

fominoben INN [also: fominoben HCl]

fominoben HCl JAN [also: fominoben]

fomivirsen sodium *antisense drug for AIDS-related CMV retinitis*

fomocaine INN, BAN

fonatol [see: diethylstilbestrol]

fonazine mesylate USAN *serotonin inhibitor* [also: dimetotiazine; dimethothiazine]

fondaparinux sodium *investigational (NDA filed) selective factor Xa inhibitor for prevention of deep vein thrombosis (DVT) following orthopedic surgery*

fontarsol [see: dichlorophenarsine HCl]

fopirtoline INN

Foradil encapsulated powder for inhalation (used with an Aerolizer device) ℞ *β_2 agonist; twice-daily bronchodilator for asthma, COPD, and emphysema* [formoterol fumarate] 12 µg/dose

Forane liquid for vaporization ℞ *inhalation general anesthetic* [isoflurane]

forasartan USAN *antihypertensive; CHF treatment; angiotensin II receptor antagonist*

Forcaltonin nasal spray ℞ *investigational (Phase III) agent for osteoporosis*

foreign colombo *medicinal herb* [see: colombo]

forfenimex INN

formaldehyde solution USP *disinfectant; anhidrotic*

Formalyde-10 spray ℞ *drying agent for hyperhidrosis and bromhidrosis* [formaldehyde] 10%

formebolone INN, BAN

formetamide [see: formetorex]

formetorex INN

formidacillin [see: fomidacillin]

forminitrazole INN, BAN

formocortal USAN, INN, BAN *corticosteroid; anti-inflammatory*

formoterol INN *bronchodilator for asthma, COPD, and emphysema* [also: eformoterol; formoterol fumarate]

formoterol fumarate USAN, JAN *bronchodilator for asthma, COPD, and emphysema* [also: formoterol; eformoterol fumarate]

Formula 44 Cough Control Disks; Formula 44 Cough Silencers lozenges OTC *antitussive; topical oral anesthetic* [dextromethorphan hydrobromide; benzocaine] 5•1.25 mg; 2.5•1 mg

Formula 405 cleansing bar OTC *therapeutic skin cleanser*

Formula B tablets ℞ *vitamin supplement* [multiple B vitamins; vitamin C; folic acid] ≛•500•0.5 mg

Formula B Plus tablets ℞ *vitamin/mineral/iron supplement* [multiple vitamins & minerals; ferrous fumarate; folic acid; biotin] ≛•27•0.8•0.15 mg

Formula VM-2000 tablets OTC *dietary supplement* [multiple vitamins & minerals; multiple amino acids; iron; folic acid; biotin] ≛•5 mg•0.2 mg•50 µg

4'-formylacetanilide thiosemicarbazone [see: thioacetazone; thiacetazone]

foropafant INN

forskolin [see: colforsin]

Forta Drink powder OTC *enteral nutritional therapy* [lactose-free formula]

Forta Shake powder OTC *enteral nutritional therapy* [milk-based formula]

Fortaz powder or frozen premix for IV or IM injection ℞ *cephalosporin antibiotic* [ceftazidime] 0.5, 1, 2, 6 g

Fortel Midstream test stick for professional use *in vitro diagnostic aid; urine pregnancy test*

Fortel Plus test kit for home use *in vitro diagnostic aid; urine pregnancy test*

Fortéo ℞ *investigational (Phase III) agent for osteoporosis* [parathyroid hormone]

Fortical injection ℞ *investigational (Phase III) calcium regulator for hypercalcemia, Paget disease, and postmenopausal osteoporosis* [calcitonin (salmon), recombinant]

fortimicin A [now: astromicin sulfate]

Fortovase soft gelatin capsules ℞ *antiretroviral protease inhibitor for HIV infection* [saquinavir] 200 mg

40 winks capsules OTC *antihistaminic sleep aid* [diphenhydramine HCl] 50 mg

.44 Magnum capsules OTC *CNS stimulant; analeptic* [caffeine] 200 mg

Forvade gel ℞ *investigational (Phase I/II) nucleoside antiviral for AIDS-related genital herpes* [cidofovir]

Fosamax tablets ℞ *bisphosphonate bone resorption inhibitor for Paget disease and corticosteroid-induced or age-related osteoporosis in men and women* [alendronate sodium] 5, 10, 35, 40, 70 mg

fosamprenavir calcium USAN *antiviral; HIV protease inhibitor*

fosamprenavir sodium USAN *antiviral; HIV protease inhibitor*

fosarilate USAN, INN *antiviral*

fosazepam USAN, INN, BAN *hypnotic*

Foscan ℞ *investigational (NDA filed) photodynamic therapy for head and neck cancer* [temoporfin]

foscarnet sodium USAN, INN, BAN *antiviral for cytomegalovirus (CMV) and various herpes viruses (HSV-1, HSV-2)*

Foscavir IV injection ℞ *antiviral for cytomegalovirus (CMV) retinitis and herpes simplex virus (HSV) infections in immunocompromised patients* [foscarnet sodium] 24 mg/mL

foscolic acid INN

fosenazide INN

fosenopril sodium [see: fosinopril sodium]

fosfestrol INN, BAN *antineoplastic; estrogen* [also: diethylstilbestrol diphosphate]

fosfocreatinine INN

fosfomycin USAN, INN, BAN *antibacterial* [also: fosfomycin calcium; fosfomycin sodium]

fosfomycin calcium JAN *antibacterial* [also: fosfomycin; fosfomycin sodium]

fosfomycin sodium JAN *antibacterial* [also: fosfomycin; fosfomycin calcium]

fosfomycin tromethamine USAN *broad-spectrum bactericidal antibiotic for urinary tract infections*

fosfonet sodium USAN, INN *antiviral*

fosfosal INN

Fosfree tablets OTC *vitamin/iron supplement* [multiple vitamins; iron] ≛ • 29 mg

fosinopril INN, BAN *antihypertensive; angiotensin-converting enzyme (ACE) inhibitor* [also: fosinopril sodium]

fosinopril sodium USAN *antihypertensive; angiotensin-converting enzyme (ACE) inhibitor* [also: fosinopril]

fosinoprilat USAN, INN *antihypertensive*

fosmenic acid INN

fosmidomycin INN

fosphenytoin INN *hydantoin anticonvulsant* [also: fosphenytoin sodium]

fosphenytoin sodium USAN *hydantoin anticonvulsant for grand mal status epilepticus (orphan)* [also: fosphenytoin]

fospirate USAN, INN *veterinary anthelmintic*

fosquidone USAN, INN, BAN *antineoplastic*

fostedil USAN, INN *vasodilator; calcium channel blocker*

Fostex cleansing bar OTC *topical keratolytic for acne* [benzoyl peroxide] 10% ⊡ pHisoHex

Fostex 10% BPO gel OTC *topical keratolytic for acne* [benzoyl peroxide] 10%

Fostex 10% Wash liquid OTC *topical keratolytic for acne* [benzoyl peroxide] 10%

Fostex Acne Cleansing cream OTC *topical keratolytic for acne* [salicylic acid] 2%

Fostex Acne Medication Cleansing bar OTC *medicated cleanser for acne* [salicylic acid] 2%

Fostex Medicated Cleansing Shampoo OTC *antiseborrheic; keratolytic* [sulfur; salicylic acid] 2% • 2%

fostriecin INN *antineoplastic* [also: fostriecin sodium]

fostriecin sodium USAN *antineoplastic* [also: fostriecin]

Fostril lotion OTC *topical acne treatment* [sulfur; zinc oxide]

fosveset USAN *ligant excipient*

fotemustine INN, BAN

fo-ti; ho-shou-wu ***(Polygonum multiflorum)*** root *medicinal herb for atherosclerosis, blood cleansing, constipation, improving liver and kidney function, insomnia, malaria, muscle aches, TB, and weak bones; also used to increase fertility, prevent aging, and promote longevity*

Fototar cream OTC *topical antipsoriatic; antiseborrheic* [coal tar] 2%

fotretamine INN

Fouchet reagent (solution)

4 Hair softgel capsules OTC *vitamin/mineral/iron supplement* [multiple vitamins & minerals; iron; folic acid; biotin] ≛ • 2.5 • 33.3 • 0.25 mg

4 Nails softgel capsules OTC *vitamin/mineral/calcium/iron supplement* [multiple vitamins & minerals; calcium; iron; folic acid; biotin] ≛ • 167 • 3 • 0.333 • 0.0083 mg

4-Way Fast Acting nasal spray OTC *nasal decongestant; antihistamine* [phenylephrine HCl; naphazoline HCl; pyrilamine maleate] 0.5% • 0.05% • 0.2%

4-Way Long Lasting nasal spray OTC *nasal decongestant* [oxymetazoline HCl] 0.05%

4B5 antibody *investigational (Phase I) fully human monoclonal antibody for immunotherapy in melanoma patients*

Fourneau 309 (available only from the Centers for Disease Control) ℞ *antiparasitic for African trypanosomiasis and onchocerciasis* [suramin sodium]

foxglove *(Digitalis ambigua; D. ferriginea; D. grandiflora; D. lanata; D. lutea; D. purpurea)* leaves *medicinal herb for asthma, burns, congestive heart failure, edema, promoting wound healing, and sedation; not generally regarded as safe for children as ingestion can be fatal*

foxglove, American; false foxglove; fern-leaved foxglove *medicinal herb* [see: feverweed]

foxtail *medicinal herb* [see: club moss]

frabuprofen INN

Fractar (trademarked ingredient) OTC *antipsoriatic; antiseborrheic* [crude coal tar]

Fragaria vesca *medicinal herb* [see: strawberry]

Fragmin deep subcu injection, prefilled syringes ℞ *anticoagulant/antithrombotic for prevention of deep vein thrombosis (DVT) after abdominal or hip replacement surgery, unstable angina, and myocardial infarction* [dalteparin sodium] 2500, 5000, 10 000 IU/0.2 mL (16, 32, 64 mg/0.2 mL)

framycetin INN, BAN *anti-infective wound dressing*

francium *element (Fr)*

Frangula purshiana *medicinal herb* [see: cascara sagrada]

frankincense *(Boswellia serrata)* leaves and bark *medicinal herb for anaphylaxis, arthritis, asthma, blood cleansing, bronchial disorders, dysentery, rheumatism, skin ailments, ulcers, and wound healing*

fraxinella *(Dictamnus albus)* root, plant, and seed *medicinal herb used as an anthelmintic, diuretic, emmenagogue, expectorant, and febrifuge*

Fraxiparine (CAN) subcu injection, prefilled syringes ℞ *anticoagulant/antithrombotic for prevention of deep vein thrombosis (DVT) after surgery and clotting during hemodialysis; treatment for unstable angina and myocardial infarction* [nadroparin calcium] 9500 IU/mL; 0.2, 0.3, 0.4, 0.6, 0.8, 1 mL

Fraxiparine Forte (CAN) subcu injection, prefilled syringes ℞ *anticoagulant/antithrombotic for prevention of deep vein thrombosis (DVT) after surgery, clotting during hemodialysis, unstable angina, and myocardial infarction* [nadroparin calcium] 19 000 IU/mL; 0.6, 0.8, 1 mL

FreAmine III 3% (8.5%) with Electrolytes IV infusion ℞ *total parenteral nutrition (8.5% only); peripheral parenteral nutrition (both)* [multiple essential and nonessential amino acids; electrolytes]

FreAmine III 8.5%; FreAmine III 10% IV infusion ℞ *total parenteral nutrition; peripheral parenteral nutrition* [multiple essential and nonessential amino acids]

FreAmine HBC 6.9% IV infusion ℞ *nutritional therapy for high metabolic stress* [multiple branched-chain essential and nonessential amino acids; electrolytes]

Free & Clear shampoo OTC *soap-free therapeutic cleanser*

Freedavite tablets OTC *vitamin/mineral/iron supplement* [multiple vitamins & minerals; ferrous fumarate6400.2] ≛ •10 mg

Freedox solution ℞ *investigational (Phase III) lazaroid for subarachnoid hemorrhage, ischemic stroke, spinal cord and head injury* [tirilazad mesylate]

Freezone liquid OTC *topical keratolytic* [salicylic acid in a collodion-like vehicle] 13.6%

frentizole USAN, INN, BAN *immunoregulator*

fringe tree *(Chionanthus virginica)* bark *medicinal herb used as an aperient, diuretic, febrifuge, and tonic*

Frisium ℞ *investigational benzodiazepine tranquilizer; anxiolytic* [clobazam]

fronepidil INN

frost plant; frost weed; frostwort *medicinal herb* [see: rock rose]

frovatriptan succinate USAN *investigational (NDA filed) serotonin 5-HT$_{1B/1D}$ agonist for acute treatment of migraine*

froxiprost INN

β-fructofuranosidase [see: sacrosidase]

fructose (D-fructose) USP *nutrient; caloric replacement* [also: levulose]

fructose-1,6-diphosphate (FDP) *investigational (Phase III) adjunct to coronary artery bypass graft (CABG) surgery; investigational (Phase III, orphan) cytoprotective agent for vaso-occlusive episodes of sickle cell disease; investigational asthma treatment*

Fruit C 100; Fruit C 200; Fruit C 500 chewable tablets OTC *vitamin C supplement* [ascorbic acid and calcium ascorbate] 100 mg; 200 mg; 500 mg

Fruity Chews chewable tablets OTC *vitamin supplement* [multiple vitamins; folic acid] ≛•0.3 mg

Fruity Chews with Iron chewable tablets OTC *vitamin/iron supplement* [multiple vitamins; iron; folic acid] ≛•12•0.3 mg

frusemide BAN *antihypertensive; loop diuretic* [also: furosemide]

FS Shampoo (name changed to Capex in 2001)

FSF (fibrin-stabilizing factor) [see: factor XIII]

FSH (follicle-stimulating hormone) [see: menotropins]

ftalofyne INN *veterinary anthelmintic* [also: phthalofyne]

ftaxilide INN

FTC [see: emtricitabine]

ftivazide INN

ftormetazine INN

ftorpropazine INN

FTY-720 *investigational (Phase II) immunosuppressant for transplant rejection and autoimmune disease*

5-FU (5-fluorouracil) [see: fluorouracil]

fubrogonium iodide INN

fuchsin, basic USP *topical antibacterial/antifungal*

Fucidin (CAN) cream, ointment ℞ *topical antibiotic* [fusidic acid] 2%

Fucidin H (CAN) cream OTC *topical antibiotic and corticosteroidal anti-inflammatory* [fusidic acid; hydrocortisone] 2•1 mg/g

Fucus versiculosus *medicinal herb* [see: kelp]

FUDR powder for intra-arterial infusion ℞ *antimetabolic antineoplastic for GI adenocarcinoma metastatic to the liver* [floxuridine] 500 mg

FUDR; FUdR (5-fluorouracil deoxyribonucleoside) [see: floxuridine]

fuge, devil's *medicinal herb* [see: mistletoe]

Ful-Glo ophthalmic strips ℞ *corneal disclosing agent* [fluorescein sodium] 0.6 mg

fulmicoton [see: pyroxylin]

FU/LV (fluorouracil, leucovorin calcium [rescue]) *chemotherapy protocol for colorectal cancer* [also: F-CL]

Fulvicin P/G tablets ℞ *systemic antifungal* [griseofulvin (ultramicrosize)] 125, 165, 250, 330 mg ⑨ folacin; Furacin

Fulvicin U/F tablets ℞ *systemic antifungal* [griseofulvin (microsize)] 250, 500 mg

FUM (fluorouracil, methotrexate) *chemotherapy protocol*

fumagillin INN, BAN

Fumaria officinalis *medicinal herb* [see: fumitory]

fumaric acid NF *acidifier*

Fumasorb tablets (discontinued 1998) OTC *hematinic* [ferrous fumarate (source of iron)] 200 mg (66 mg)

Fumatinic sustained-release capsules ℞ *hematinic* [ferrous fumarate; cyanocobalamin; ascorbic acid] 200 mg•5 µg•60 mg

Fumerin sugar-coated tablets (discontinued 1998) OTC *hematinic* [ferrous fumarate (source of iron)] 195 mg (64 mg)

fumitory (*Fumaria officinalis*) plant *medicinal herb for cardiovascular disorders, constipation, eczema, edema, and hepatobiliary disorders*

fumoxicillin USAN, INN *antibacterial*

Funduscein-10; Funduscein-25 antecubital venous injection ℞ *ophthalmic diagnostic agent* [fluorescein sodium] 10%; 25%
fungicidin [see: nystatin]
fungimycin USAN *antifungal*
Fungi-Nail liquid OTC *topical antifungal; keratolytic; anesthetic* [resorcinol; salicylic acid; chloroxylenol; benzocaine; alcohol 50%] 1%•2%•2%•0.5%
Fungizone cream, lotion, ointment ℞ *topical antifungal* [amphotericin B] 3%
Fungizone oral suspension ℞ *systemic antifungal; "swish and swallow" treatment for oral candidiasis* [amphotericin B] 100 mg/mL
Fungizone powder for IV infusion ℞ *systemic polyene antifungal* [amphotericin B deoxycholate] 50 mg/vial
Fung-O liquid OTC *topical keratolytic* [salicylic acid] 17%
Fungoid cream (discontinued 2000) ℞ *topical antifungal* [clotrimazole] 1%
Fungoid solution (became OTC and name changed to Fungoid AF in 1997) ℞ *topical antifungal* [undecylenic acid] 25%
Fungoid solution (discontinued 2000) ℞ *topical antifungal* [clotrimazole] 1%
Fungoid tincture OTC *topical antifungal* [miconazole nitrate] 2%
Fungoid AF solution (discontinued 2000) OTC *topical antifungal* [undecylenic acid] 25%
Fungoid-HC cream ℞ *topical corticosteroidal anti-inflammatory; antipruritic; antifungal; antibacterial* [miconazole nitrate; hydrocortisone] 2%•1%
fuprazole INN
furacilin [see: nitrofurazone]
Furacin topical solution, cream ℞ *broad-spectrum antibacterial; adjunct to burn therapy and skin grafting* [nitrofurazone] 0.2% ⑨ Fulvicin
Furacin Soluble Dressing ointment ℞ *broad-spectrum antibacterial; adjunct to burn therapy and skin grafting* [nitrofurazone] 0.2%
furacrinic acid INN, BAN
Furadantin oral suspension ℞ *urinary antibiotic* [nitrofurantoin] 25 mg/5 mL
furafylline INN
Furalan tablets ℞ *urinary antibiotic* [nitrofurantoin] 50, 100 mg
furalazine INN
furaltadone INN, BAN
Furamide (available only from the Centers for Disease Control) ℞ *investigational anti-infective for amebiasis* [diloxanide furoate]
2(3H) furanone di-hydro (FDh) *a precursor to gamma hydroxybutyrate (GHB); a formerly legal alternative to GHB, now also illegal (Schedule I); also known as gamma butyrolactone (GBL)* [see: gamma hydroxybutyrate (GHB)]
furaprofen USAN, INN *anti-inflammatory*
furazabol INN
furazolidone USP, INN, BAN *bactericidal; antiprotozoal (Trichomonas); antidiarrheal*
furazolium chloride USAN, INN *antibacterial*
furazolium tartrate USAN *antibacterial*
furbucillin INN
furcloprofen INN
furegrelate INN *thromboxane synthetase inhibitor* [also: furegrelate sodium]
furegrelate sodium USAN *thromboxane synthetase inhibitor* [also: furegrelate]
furethidine INN, BAN
furfenorex INN
furfuryltrimethylammonium iodide [see: furtrethonium iodide]
furidarone INN
furmethoxadone INN
furobufen USAN, INN *anti-inflammatory*
furodazole USAN, INN *anthelmintic*
furofenac INN
furomazine INN
furosemide USAN, USP, INN, JAN *antihypertensive; loop diuretic* [also: frusemide] 20, 40, 80 mg oral; 10 mg/mL oral; 40 mg/5 mL oral; 10 mg/mL injection
furostilbestrol INN
furoxicillin [see: fumoxicillin]
Furoxone tablets, liquid ℞ *antibacterial* [furazolidone] 100 mg; 50 mg/15 mL

fursalan USAN, INN *disinfectant*
fursultiamine INN
furterene INN
furtrethonium iodide INN
furtrimethonium iodide [see: furtrethonium iodide]
fusafungine INN, BAN
fusidate sodium USAN *antibacterial*
fusidic acid USAN, INN, BAN *topical antibacterial*
fusidic acid, sodium salt [see: fusidate sodium]
FUVAC (5-FU, vinblastine, Adriamycin, cyclophosphamide) *chemotherapy protocol*
fuzlocillin INN, BAN
fytic acid INN
FZ (flutamide, Zoladex) *chemotherapy protocol for prostate cancer*

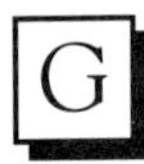

G-3139 *investigational (Phase III) adjunct used with docetaxel for malignant melanoma, breast cancer, and other malignancies; investigational (Phase I/II) for AIDS-related non-Hodgkin lymphoma*
^{67}Ga [see: gallium citrate Ga 67]
GABA (gamma-aminobutyric acid) [see: γ-aminobutyric acid]
gabapentin USAN, INN *anticonvulsant; investigational (orphan) for amyotrophic lateral sclerosis*
Gabbromicina ℞ *investigational (orphan) for tuberculosis,* Mycobacterium avium *complex, and visceral leishmaniasis* [aminosidine]
gabexate INN
Gabitril Filmtabs (film-coated tablets) ℞ *anticonvulsant adjunct for partial seizures* [tiagabine HCl] 2, 4, 12, 16, 20 mg ⓢ Carbatrol
gaboxadol INN
gadobenate dimeglumine USAN *MRI diagnostic aid* [also: gadobenic acid]
gadobenic acid INN *MRI diagnostic aid* [also: gadobenate dimeglumine]
gadobutrol INN *investigational aid for MRI*
gadodiamide USAN, INN, BAN *parenteral MRI contrast medium*
gadofosveset trisodium USAN *parenteral MRI contrast medium*
gadolinium *element (Gd)*
gadolinium texaphyrin (Gd-Tex) [now: motexafin gadolinium]
Gadolite oral suspension ℞ *investigational diagnostic aid*
gadopenamide INN
gadopentetate dimeglumine USAN *parenteral MRI contrast medium* [also: gadopentetic acid]
gadopentetic acid INN, BAN *parenteral MRI contrast medium* [also: gadopentetate dimeglumine]
gadoteric acid INN
gadoteridol USAN, INN, BAN *MRI contrast medium*
gadoversetamide USAN, INN *MRI contrast medium for imaging of the brain, head, and spine and liver structure and vascularity*
gadoxanum USAN *gadolinium-xanthan gum complex; diagnostic aid*
gadozelite USAN *gadolinium zeolite complex; diagnostic aid*
GA-EPO (gene-activated erythropoietin) [see: erythropoietin, gene-activated]
gaiactamine [see: guaiactamine]
gaietamine [see: guaiactamine]
galactagogues *a class of agents that promote or increase the flow of breast milk* [also called: lactagogues]
galactochitosan *investigational immune system stimulant and anticancer therapy*
α-D-galactopyranose [see: galactose]

galactose USAN *ultrasound contrast medium for echocardiography*
α-galactosidase [see: agalsidase alfa]
galamustine INN
galangal (*Alpinia galanga; A. officinarum*) rhizomes *medicinal herb for diuresis, fungal infections, gas, hypertension, tumors, ulcers, and worms; also used as an antiplatelet agent*
galantamine USAN, INN *acetylcholinesterase inhibitor to increase cognition in Alzheimer disease*
galantamine hydrobromide USAN *acetylcholinesterase inhibitor to increase cognition in Alzheimer disease*
galanthamine [see: galantamine]
Galardin ℞ *investigational (orphan) matrix metalloproteinase (MMP) inhibitor for corneal ulcers* [ilomastat]
galdansetron INN, BAN *antiemetic* [also: galdansetron HCl]
galdansetron HCl USAN *antiemetic* [also: galdansetron]
Galeopsis tetrahit *medicinal herb* [see: hemp nettle]
Galium aparine; G. verum *medicinal herb* [see: bedstraw]
Galium odoratum *medicinal herb* [see: sweet woodruff]
gallamine BAN *neuromuscular blocker* [also: gallamine triethiodide]
gallamine triethiodide USP, INN *neuromuscular blocker; muscle relaxant* [also: gallamine]
gallamone triethiodide [see: gallamine triethiodide]
gallic acid NF
gallic acid, bismuth basic salt [see: bismuth subgallate]
gallium *element (Ga)*
gallium (^{67}Ga) citrate INN *radiopaque contrast medium; radioactive agent* [also: gallium citrate Ga 67]
gallium citrate Ga 67 USAN, USP *radiopaque contrast medium; radioactive agent* [also: gallium (^{67}Ga) citrate]
gallium nitrate USAN *bone resorption inhibitor for hypercalcemia of malignancy (orphan); investigational (Phase II) agent for AIDS-related non-Hodgkin lymphoma*
gallium nitrate nonahydrate [see: gallium nitrate]
gallopamil INN, BAN
gallotannic acid [see: tannic acid]
gallstone solubilizing agents *a class of drugs that dissolve gallstones*
galosemide INN
galtifenin INN
Galzin capsules ℞ *copper blocking/complexing agent for Wilson disease (orphan)* [zinc acetate] 25, 50 mg
gamfexine USAN, INN *antidepressant*
Gamimune N IV infusion ℞ *passive immunizing agent for HIV, ITP, and BMT; infection prophylaxis in pediatric HIV (orphan); investigational (orphan) for myocarditis and juvenile rheumatoid arthritis* [immune globulin, solvent/detergent treated] 5%, 10%
gamma benzene hexachloride [now: lindane]
gamma butyraldehyde (GHB-aldehyde) *a precursor to gamma hydroxybutyrate (GHB)* [see: gamma hydroxybutyrate (GHB)]
gamma butyrolactone (GBL) *a precursor to gamma hydroxybutyrate (GHB); a formerly legal alternative to GHB, now also illegal (Schedule I); also known as 2(3H) furanone dihydro (FDh)* [see: gamma hydroxybutyrate (GHB)]
gamma globulin [see: globulin, immune]
gamma hydroxybutyrate (GHB) *a CNS depressant used as an anesthetic in some countries, produced and abused as a "date rape" street drug in the U.S.; illegal in the U.S. (Schedule I); investigational (orphan) for narcolepsy, cataplexy, sleep paralysis, and hypnagogic hallucinations* [the sodium salt is medically known as sodium oxybate]
gamma oryzanol; gamma-oz *medicinal herb* [see: rice bran oil]
gamma-aminobutyric acid (GABA) [see: γ-aminobutyric acid]

Gammagard S/D freeze-dried powder for IV infusion ℞ *passive immunizing agent for HIV, idiopathic thrombocytopenic purpura (ITP), B-cell chronic lymphocytic leukemia, and Kawasaki syndrome* [immune globulin, solvent/detergent treated] 50 mg/mL

gamma-hydroxybutyrate sodium [see: sodium oxybate]

gamma-linolenic acid (GLA) *investigational (orphan) for juvenile rheumatoid arthritis*

Gamma-OH (commercially available in Europe) ℞ *sedative; hypnotic; antidepressant* [gamma hydroxybutyrate (GHB)] 2.5 g

gammaphos [now: ethiofos]

Gammar-P I.V. (pasteurized) powder for IV infusion ℞ *passive immunizing agent and immunomodulator for HIV; pediatric treatment of primary immune deficiency (PID)* [immune globulin, heat treated] 5%

gamma-vinyl GABA (gamma-aminobutyric acid) [see: vigabatrin]

gamolenic acid INN, BAN

Gamulin Rh IM injection (discontinued 2001) ℞ *obstetric Rh factor immunity suppressant* [Rh_0(D) immune globulin] 300 µg

ganaxolone USAN *neuroactive steroid for migraine and adult epilepsy; investigational (orphan) for infantile spasms*

ganciclovir USAN, INN, BAN *antiviral; ocular implant for cytomegalovirus retinitis (orphan); investigational (Phase I/II) for HIV prophylaxis* [also: ganciclovir sodium]

ganciclovir sodium USAN *antiviral* [also: ganciclovir]

ganciclovir sodium & cytomegalovirus immune globulin intravenous (CMV-IGIV) *investigational (orphan) for cytomegalovirus pneumonia in bone marrow transplant patients*

ganglefene INN

ganirelix INN *gonadotropin-releasing hormone (Gn-RH) antagonist for infertility* [also: ganirelix acetate]

ganirelix acetate USAN *gonadotropin-releasing hormone (Gn-RH) antagonist for infertility* [also: ganirelix]

Ganite IV infusion ℞ *bone resorption inhibitor for hypercalcemia of malignancy (orphan)* [gallium nitrate] 25 mg/mL

Gantanol tablets (discontinued 2001) ℞ *broad-spectrum sulfonamide bacteriostatic* [sulfamethoxazole] 500 mg

Gantrisin pediatric suspension ℞ *broad-spectrum sulfonamide antibiotic* [sulfisoxazole acetyl; alcohol 0.3%] 500 mg/5 mL

gapicomine INN

gapromidine INN

Garamicina (Mexican name for U.S. product Garamycin)

Garamycin cream, ointment ℞ *topical antibiotic* [gentamicin sulfate] 0.1% ⑨ Gamastan; kanamycin; Terramycin; Theramycin

Garamycin eye drops, ophthalmic ointment ℞ *topical ophthalmic antibiotic* [gentamicin sulfate] 3 mg/mL; 3 mg/g

Garamycin intrathecal injection (discontinued 1998) ℞ *aminoglycoside antibiotic* [gentamicin sulfate] 2 mg/mL

Garamycin IV or IM injection ℞ *aminoglycoside antibiotic* [gentamicin sulfate] 40 mg/mL

Garamycin Pediatric IV or IM injection (discontinued 1998) ℞ *aminoglycoside antibiotic* [gentamicin sulfate] 10 mg/mL

garcinia (*Garcinia cambogia*) fruit *medicinal herb for appetite suppressant, thermogenesis, and weight control*

garden nightshade *medicinal herb* [see: bittersweet nightshade]

garden patience *medicinal herb* [see: yellow dock]

Gardrin ℞ *investigational treatment for acute peptic ulcers* [enprostil]

Garfield; Garfield Plus Extra C chewable tablets OTC *vitamin supplement* [multiple vitamins; folic acid] ≛•0.3 mg

Garfield Complete with Minerals chewable tablets OTC *vitamin/mineral/iron supplement* [multiple vitamins & minerals; iron; folic acid; biotin] ≛ •18•0.4•0.04 mg

Garfield Plus Iron chewable tablets OTC *vitamin/iron supplement* [multiple vitamins; iron; folic acid] ≛ •15•0.3 mg

garget *medicinal herb* [see: pokeweed]

garlic (*Allium sativum*) bulb *medicinal herb for asthma, cancer immunity, diabetes, digestive disorders, ear infections, flatulence, hypercholesterolemia, hypertension, and infectious diseases*

GAS (group A streptococcal) vaccine *investigational vaccine*

gas gangrene antitoxin, pentavalent

gas gangrene antitoxin, polyvalent [see: gas gangrene antitoxin, pentavalent]

Gas Permeable Daily Cleaner solution OTC *cleaning solution for rigid gas permeable contact lenses*

Gas Relief chewable tablets, drops OTC *antiflatulent* [simethicone] 80, 125 mg; 40 mg/0.6 mL

Gas-Ban tablets OTC *antacid; antiflatulent* [calcium carbonate; simethicone] 300•40 mg

Gas-Ban DS liquid OTC *antacid; antiflatulent* [aluminum hydroxide; magnesium hydroxide; simethicone] 400•400•40 mg/5 mL

gastric acid inhibitors [see: proton pump inhibitors]

gastric mucin BAN

Gastrimmune ℞ *investigational (Phase III) synthetic peptide vaccine for gastrointestinal cancers*

Gastroccult slide test for professional use *in vitro diagnostic aid for gastric occult blood*

Gastrocrom capsules (discontinued 1999) ℞ *mastocytosis treatment (orphan)* [cromolyn sodium] 100 mg

Gastrocrom oral solution ℞ *mastocytosis treatment (orphan); investigational prophylactic treatment for food allergies* [cromolyn sodium] 100 mg/5 mL

Gastrografin oral solution ℞ *radiopaque contrast medium for gastrointestinal imaging* [diatrizoate meglumine; diatrizoate sodium (48.29% total iodine)] 660•100 mg/mL (367 mg/mL)

GastroMARK oral suspension ℞ *MRI contrast medium for upper GI tract imaging* [ferumoxsil] 175 µg iron/mL

Gastrosed drops, tablets ℞ *GI/GU antispasmodic; antiparkinsonian; anticholinergic "drying agent" for allergic rhinitis and hyperhidrosis* [hyoscyamine sulfate] 0.125 mg/mL; 0.125 mg

Gastro-Test string capsules for professional use *in vitro diagnostic aid for GI disorders*

Gastrozepine ℞ *investigational (NDA filed) treatment for peptic ulcers* [pirenzepine HCl]

Gas-X chewable tablets, softgels OTC *antiflatulent* [simethicone] 80, 125 mg; 125 mg

gatifloxacin USAN *broad-spectrum fluoroquinolone antibiotic*

gaultheria oil [see: methyl salicylate]

Gaultheria procumbens *medicinal herb* [see: wintergreen]

gauze, absorbent USP *surgical aid*

gauze, petrolatum USP *surgical aid*

gauze bandage [see: bandage, gauze]

gavestinel USAN *N-methyl-D-aspartate (NMDA) receptor antagonist for stroke*

Gaviscon liquid OTC *antacid* [aluminum hydroxide; magnesium carbonate] 31.7•119.3 mg/5 mL

Gaviscon; Gaviscon-2 chewable tablets OTC *antacid* [aluminum hydroxide; magnesium trisilicate] 80•20 mg; 160•40 mg

Gaviscon Relief Formula chewable tablets, liquid OTC *antacid* [aluminum hydroxide; magnesium carbonate] 160•105 mg; 254•237.5 mg/5 mL

GBC-590 *investigational (Phase I/II) antineoplastic*

GBH *a mistaken acronym for gamma hydroxybutyrate (GHB)* [see: gamma hydroxybutyrate (GHB)]

GBL (gamma butyrolactone) *a precursor to gamma hydroxybutyrate (GHB); a formerly legal alternative to GHB, now also illegal (Schedule I); also known as 2(3H) furanone di-*

hydro (FDh) [see: gamma hydroxybutyrate (GHB)]

G-CSF (granulocyte colony-stimulating factor) [see: filgrastim]

Gd texaphyrin [see: motexafin gadolinum]

Gd-Tex ℞ *investigational (Phase III) radiosensitizer for brain metastasis* [motexafin gadolinium]

gedocarnil INN *investigational treatment of central nervous system disorders*

Gee-Gee tablets OTC *expectorant* [guaifenesin] 200 mg

gefarnate INN, BAN

gelatin NF *encapsulating, suspending, binding and coating agent*

gelatin film, absorbable USP *topical local hemostat for surgery*

gelatin powder, absorbable *topical local hemostat for surgery*

gelatin solution, special intravenous [see: polygeline]

gelatin sponge, absorbable USP *topical local hemostat for surgery*

gelcaps (dosage form) *soft gelatin capsules*

Gelfilm; Gelfilm Ophthalmic ℞ *topical local hemostat for surgery* [absorbable gelatin film]

Gelfoam powder ℞ *topical local hemostat for surgery* [absorbable gelatin powder] ㉿ Ger-O-Foam

Gelfoam sponge, packs, dental packs, prostatectomy cones ℞ *topical local hemostat for surgery* [absorbable gelatin sponge] ㉿ Ger-O-Foam

Gelhist pediatric oral suspension ℞ *decongestant; antihistamine* [phenylephrine tannate; chlorpheniramine tannate; pyrilamine tannate] 5•2•12.5 mg/5 mL

Gel-Kam gel ℞ *topical dental caries preventative* [stannous fluoride] 0.4%

Gelpirin tablets (discontinued 2000) OTC *analgesic; antipyretic; anti-inflammatory* [acetaminophen; aspirin, buffered; caffeine] 125•240•32 mg

Gelpirin-CCF tablets OTC *decongestant; antihistamine; analgesic; expectorant* [phenylpropanolamine HCl; chlorpheniramine maleate; acetaminophen; guaifenesin] 12.5•1•325•25 mg

Gelseal (trademarked dosage form) *soft gelatin capsule*

gelsemium *(Bignonia sempervirens; Gelsemium nitidum; G. sempervirens)* plant *medicinal herb for asthma, neuralgia, and respiratory disorders; not generally regarded as safe, as it is highly toxic*

gelsolin, recombinant human *investigational (orphan) for respiratory symptoms of cystic fibrosis and bronchiectasis*

Gel-Tin gel OTC *topical dental caries preventative* [stannous fluoride] 0.4%

Gelusil chewable tablets OTC *antacid; antiflatulent* [aluminum hydroxide; magnesium hydroxide; simethicone] 200•200•25 mg

GEM 123 *investigational (Phase II) antisense oligonucleotide for AIDS-related cytomegalovirus retinitis*

GEM 231 *investigational (Phase I) anticancer agent for treatment of solid tumors*

GEM-92 tablets ℞ *investigational mixed backbone antisense compound for AIDS and HIV infection*

gemazocine INN

gemcadiol USAN, INN *antihyperlipoproteinemic*

gemcitabine USAN, INN,BAN *antimetabolite antineoplastic*

gemcitabine HCl USAN *antineoplastic for advanced or metastatic pancreatic and non–small cell lung cancers (NSCLC)*

gemcitabine-cis (gemcitabine, cisplatin) *chemotherapy protocol for non–small cell lung cancer (NSCLC)*

Gemcor film-coated tablets ℞ *antihyperlipidemic for hypercholesterolemia* [gemfibrozil] 600 mg

gemeprost USAN, INN, BAN *prostaglandin*

gemfibrozil USAN, USP, INN, BAN *triglyceride-lowering antihyperlipidemic for hypertriglyceridemia (types IV and V hyperlipidemia) and coronary heart disease* 600 mg oral

gemifloxacin mesylate USAN *investigational (NDA filed) antibiotic for respiratory tract infections*

gemopatrilat USAN *vasopeptidase inhibitor (VPI); angiotensin-converting enzyme (ACE) inhibitor for hypertension and congestive heart failure*

gemtuzumab ozogamicin *antibody-targeted chemotherapy agent for acute myeloid leukemia (AML)*

Gemzar powder for IV infusion ℞ *antineoplastic for advanced or metastatic pancreatic and non–small cell lung cancers (NSCLC)* [gemcitabine HCl] 20 mg/mL

Genabid timed-release capsules (discontinued 1997) ℞ *peripheral vasodilator; smooth muscle relaxant for cerebral, myocardial, and peripheral ischemias* [papaverine HCl] 150 mg

Genac tablets OTC *decongestant; antihistamine* [pseudoephedrine HCl; triprolidine HCl] 60•2.5 mg

Gen-Acebutolol (CAN) film-coated tablets ℞ *antihypertensive; antianginal* [acebutolol HCl] 100, 200, 400 mg

Genacol tablets OTC *antitussive; decongestant; antihistamine; analgesic* [dextromethorphan hydrobromide; phenylpropanolamine HCl; chlorpheniramine maleate; acetaminophen] 10•30•2•325 mg

Genahist capsules, tablets (discontinued 1997) ℞ *antihistamine* [diphenhydramine HCl] 25 mg; 25 mg

Genahist liquid OTC *antihistamine* [diphenhydramine HCl] 12.5 mg/5 mL

Gen-Allerate tablets OTC *antihistamine* [chlorpheniramine maleate] 4 mg

Genamin Cold syrup OTC *decongestant; antihistamine* [phenylpropanolamine HCl; chlorpheniramine maleate] 6.25•1 mg/5 mL

Gen-Amiodarone (CAN) tablets ℞ *antiarrhythmic* [amiodarone HCl] 200 mg

Gen-Amoxicillin (CAN) capsules ℞ *antibiotic* [amoxicillin trihydrate] 250, 500 mg

Genapap tablets, caplets OTC *analgesic; antipyretic* [acetaminophen] 325, 500 mg; 500 mg

Genapap, Children's chewable tablets, elixir OTC *analgesic; antipyretic* [acetaminophen] 80 mg; 160 mg/5 mL

Genapap, Infants' drops OTC *analgesic; antipyretic* [acetaminophen] 100 mg/mL

Genaphed tablets OTC *nasal decongestant* [pseudoephedrine HCl] 30 mg

Genasal nasal spray OTC *nasal decongestant* [oxymetazoline HCl] 0.05%

Genasense ℞ *investigational (orphan) antineoplastic*

Genasoft softgels OTC *laxative; stool softener* [docusate sodium] 100 mg

Genasoft Plus softgels OTC *stimulant laxative; stool softener* [casanthranol; docusate sodium] 30•100 mg

Genaspor cream OTC *topical antifungal* [tolnaftate] 1%

Genatap elixir OTC *decongestant; antihistamine* [phenylpropanolamine HCl; brompheniramine maleate] 12.5•2 mg/5 mL ⓢ Genapap

Genaton chewable tablets OTC *antacid* [aluminum hydroxide; magnesium trisilicate] 80•20 mg

Genaton liquid OTC *antacid* [aluminum hydroxide; magnesium carbonate] 31.7•137.3 mg/5 mL

Genaton, Extra Strength chewable tablets OTC *antacid* [aluminum hydroxide; magnesium carbonate] 160•105 mg

Genatuss syrup OTC *expectorant* [guaifenesin; alcohol 3.5%] 100 mg/5 mL

Genatuss DM syrup OTC *antitussive; expectorant* [dextromethorphan hydrobromide; guaifenesin] 10•100 mg/5 mL

Gen-bee with C caplets OTC *vitamin supplement* [multiple B vitamins; vitamin C] ≛•300 mg

Gencalc 600 film-coated tablets OTC *calcium supplement* [calcium carbonate] 1.5 g

Gen-Carbamazepine CR (CAN) film-coated tablets ℞ *anticonvulsant;*

analgesic for trigeminal neuralgia; antimanic [carbamazepine] 200, 400 mg

Gencold sustained-release capsules OTC *decongestant; antihistamine* [phenylpropanolamine HCl; chlorpheniramine maleate] 75•8 mg

Gen-Cyproterone (CAN) tablets ℞ *antiandrogen* [cyproterone acetate] 50 mg

Gendecon tablets OTC *decongestant; antihistamine; analgesic* [phenylephrine HCl; chlorpheniramine maleate; acetaminophen] 5•2•325 mg

Gendex 75 IV infusion ℞ *plasma volume expander for shock due to hemorrhage, burns, or surgery* [dextran 75] 6%

Gen-Doxazosin (CAN) tablets ℞ *antihypertensive (α-blocker); treatment for benign prostatic hyperplasia* [doxazosin mesylate] 1, 2, 4, 8 mg

Genebs tablets, caplets OTC *analgesic; antipyretic* [acetaminophen] 325, 500 mg; 500 mg

Generet-500 timed-release tablets OTC *hematinic* [ferrous sulfate; multiple B vitamins; sodium ascorbate] 105•≛•500 mg ⓢ Gentap

Generix-T tablets OTC *vitamin/mineral/iron supplement* [multiple vitamins & minerals; iron] ≛•15 mg

GenESA computer-controlled IV infusion device ("GenESA System") ℞ *cardiac stressor for diagnosis of coronary artery disease* [arbutamine HCl] 0.05 mg/mL

Gen-Etodolac (CAN) capsules ℞ *analgesic; antiarthritic; nonsteroidal anti-inflammatory drug (NSAID)* [etodolac] 200, 300 mg

Genevax-HIV ℞ *investigational (Phase I/II) vaccine for HIV*

Geneye eye drops OTC *topical ophthalmic decongestant and vasoconstrictor* [tetrahydrozoline HCl] 0.05%

Geneye AC Allergy Formula eye drops (discontinued 1997) OTC *topical ophthalmic decongestant and astringent* [tetrahydrozoline HCl; zinc sulfate] 0.05%•0.25%

Geneye Extra eye drops OTC *topical ophthalmic decongestant, vasoconstrictor, and lubricant* [tetrahydrozoline HCl; polytheylene glycol 400] 0.05%•1%

Gen-Fenofibrate Micro (CAN) capsules ℞ *antihyperlipidemic* [fenofibrate, micronized] 200 mg

Genfiber powder OTC *bulk laxative* [psyllium hydrophilic mucilloid] 3.4 g/tsp.

Gen-Fluoxetine (CAN) capsules ℞ *selective serotonin reuptake inhibitor (SSRI) for depression and obsessive-compulsive disorder (OCD)* [fluoxetine HCl] 10, 20 mg

Gen-Fluvoxamine (CAN) film-coated tablets ℞ *selective serotonin reuptake inhibitor (SSRI) for depression and obsessive-compulsive disorder (OCD)* [fluvoxamine maleate] 50, 100 mg

Gen-Gliclazide (CAN) tablets ℞ *antidiabetic* [gliclazide] 80 mg

Gen-Glybe (CAN) tablets ℞ *sulfonylurea antidiabetic* [glyburide] 2.5, 5 mg

Gengraf capsules ℞ *immunosuppressant for allogenic kidney, liver, and heart transplants, rheumatoid arthritis, and psoriasis* [cyclosporine; alcohol 12.8%] 25, 100 mg

Gen-Ipratropium (CAN) inhalation solution ℞ *bronchodilator for asthma* [ipratropium bromide] 0.025%

Genista tinctoria *medicinal herb* [see: dyer's broom]

genistein *investigational antineoplastic for breast cancer; investigational for amyotrophic lateral sclerosis and stroke*

Genite liquid OTC *antitussive; decongestant; antihistamine; analgesic* [dextromethorphan hydrobromide; pseudoephedrine HCl; doxylamine succinate; acetaminophen; alcohol 25%] 5•10•1.25•167 mg/5 mL

Gen-K powder ℞ *potassium supplement* [potassium chloride] 20 mEq/packet

Gen-Metformin (CAN) film-coated tablets ℞ *biguanide antidiabetic* [metformin HCl] 500, 850 mg

Gen-Metoprolol (CAN) film-coated tablets ℞ *antihypertensive; antianginal* [metoprolol tartrate] 50, 100 mg

Gen-Naproxen EC (CAN) enteric-coated tablets ℞ *antiarthritic; nonsteroidal anti-inflammatory drug (NSAID)* [naproxen] 500 mg

genophyllin [see: aminophylline]

Genoptic eye drops ℞ *topical ophthalmic antibiotic* [gentamicin sulfate] 3 mg/mL

Genoptic S.O.P. ophthalmic ointment ℞ *topical ophthalmic antibiotic* [gentamicin sulfate] 3 mg/g

Genora 0.5/35; Genora 1/35 tablets (discontinued 1999) ℞ *monophasic oral contraceptive* [norethindrone; ethinyl estradiol] 0.5 mg•35 µg; 1 mg•35 µg

Genora 1/50 tablets (discontinued 1999) ℞ *monophasic oral contraceptive* [norethindrone; mestranol] 1 mg•50 µg

Genotropin powder for subcu injection ℞ *growth hormone for adults or children with congenital or endogenous growth hormone deficiency, children with Turner syndrome or renal-induced growth failure* [somatropin] 1.5, 5.8, 13.3 mg (4.5, 17.4, 41.4 IU) per cartridge

Genotropin MiniQuick subcu injection (prefilled syringe in packs of 7) ℞ *growth hormone for children or adults with congenital or endogenous growth hormone deficiency, children with Turner syndrome or renal-induced growth failure, or AIDS-wasting syndrome (orphan)* [somatropin] 0.2, 0.4, 0.6, 0.8, 1, 1.2, 1.4, 1.6, 1.8, 2 mg/syringe

Genpril film-coated tablets OTC *analgesic; antiarthritic; antipyretic; nonsteroidal anti-inflammatory drug (NSAID)* [ibuprofen] 200 mg

Genprin tablets OTC *analgesic; antipyretic; anti-inflammatory; antirheumatic* [aspirin] 325 mg

Gen-Ranitidine (CAN) film-coated tablets ℞ *histamine H_2 antagonist for gastric and duodenal ulcers* [ranitidine HCl] 150, 300 mg

Gensan tablets (discontinued 2000) OTC *analgesic; antipyretic; anti-inflammatory* [aspirin; caffeine] 400•32 mg

Gentacidin eye drops ℞ *topical ophthalmic antibiotic* [gentamicin sulfate] 0.3%

Gentacidin ophthalmic ointment (discontinued 2001) ℞ *topical ophthalmic antibiotic* [gentamicin sulfate] 3 mg/g

Gentak eye drops, ophthalmic ointment ℞ *topical ophthalmic antibiotic* [gentamicin sulfate] 3 mg/mL; 3 mg/g

gentamicin BAN *aminoglycoside antibiotic* [also: gentamicin sulfate] ▯ Jenamicin; kanamycin

gentamicin sulfate USAN, USP *aminoglycoside antibiotic* [also: gentamicin] 3 mg/mL eye drops; 3 mg/g topical; 0.1% topical; 10, 40 mg/mL injection

gentamicin sulfate, liposomal *investigational (orphan) for disseminated Mycobacterium avium-intracellulare infection*

gentamicin-impregnated polymethyl methacrylate (PMMA) beads *investigational (orphan) for chronic osteomyelitis*

GenTeal; GenTeal Mild eye drops OTC *ophthalmic moisturizer/lubricant* [hydroxypropyl methylcellulose]

GenTeal gel OTC *ophthalmic moisturizer/lubricant* [hydroxypropyl methylcellulose; carbopol 980]

gentian *(Gentiana lutea)* root *medicinal herb for aiding digestion, appetite stimulation, arthritis, hysteria, jaundice, liver disorders, and sore throat*

gentian violet USP *topical anti-infective/antifungal* [also: methylrosanilinium chloride] 1%, 2%

Gen-Ticlodipine (CAN) tablets ℞ *platelet aggregation inhibitor* [ticlodipine HCl] 250 mg

gentisic acid ethanolamide NF *complexing agent*

Gentlax granules (discontinued 1999) OTC *stimulant laxative* [senna concentrate] 326 mg/tsp.

Gentlax S tablets (discontinued 1999) OTC *stimulant laxative; stool softener* [sennosides; docusate sodium] 8.6•50 mg

Gentran 40 IV injection ℞ *plasma volume expander for shock due to hemorrhage, burns, or surgery* [dextran 40] 10%

Gentran 70 IV infusion ℞ *plasma volume expander for shock due to hemorrhage, burns, or surgery* [dextran 70] 6%

Gen-Verapamil (CAN) film-coated tablets ℞ *antianginal; antiarrhythmic; antihypertensive* [verapamil HCl] 80, 120 mg

Genvir ℞ *investigational (Phase III) controlled-release form for acute genital herpes* [acyclovir]

Gen-Xene tablets ℞ *anxiolytic; minor tranquilizer; anticonvulsant adjunct; alcohol withdrawal aid* [chlorazepate dipotassium] 3.75, 7.5, 15 mg

Gen-Zopiclone (CAN) tablets ℞ *sedative; hypnotic* [zopiclone] 7.5 mg

Geocillin film-coated tablets ℞ *extended-spectrum penicillin antibiotic* [carbenicillin indanyl sodium] 382 mg

Geodon capsules ℞ *serotonin and dopamine antagonist; atypical antipsychotic for schizophrenia* [ziprasidone HCl] 20, 40, 60, 80 mg

Geodon IM injection ℞ *serotonin and dopamine antagonist; atypical antipsychotic for schizophrenia* [ziprasidone mesylate]

gepefrine INN

gepirone INN *tranquilizer; anxiolytic; antidepressant* [also: gepirone HCl]

gepirone HCl USAN *tranquilizer; anxiolytic; antidepressant* [also: gepirone]

Geranium maculatum *medicinal herb* [see: alum root]

2-geranylhydroquinone [see: geroquinol]

Gerardia pedicularia *medicinal herb* [see: feverweed]

Geravim elixir OTC *vitamin/mineral supplement* [multiple B vitamins & minerals] ≛

Geravite elixir OTC *geriatric vitamin supplement* [multiple B vitamins] ≛

Gerber Baby Formula with Iron liquid, powder (discontinued 1997) OTC *total or supplementary infant feeding*

Gerber Baby Low Iron Formula liquid, powder OTC *total or supplementary infant feeding*

Gerber Soy Formula liquid (discontinued 1997) OTC *hypoallergenic infant formula* [soy protein formula]

Gerber Soy Formula powder OTC *hypoallergenic infant formula* [soy protein formula]

Geref powder for IV injection ℞ *diagnostic aid for pituitary function; treatment for growth hormone deficiency (orphan), anovulation, and AIDS-related weight loss* [sermorelin acetate] 50 µg

Geridium tablets (discontinued 1997) ℞ *urinary analgesic* [phenazopyridine HCl] 100, 200 mg

Gerimal sublingual tablets, tablets ℞ *cognition adjuvant for age-related mental capacity decline* [ergoloid mesylates] 0.5, 1 mg; 1 mg

Gerimed film-coated tablets OTC *geriatric vitamin/mineral supplement* [multiple vitamins & minerals] ≛

Geriot film-coated tablets OTC *hematinic; vitamin/mineral supplement* [carbonyl iron; multiple vitamins & minerals; folic acid; biotin] 50 mg•≛•0.4 mg•45 µg

Geritol Complete tablets OTC *vitamin/mineral/iron supplement* [multiple vitamins & minerals; ferrous fumarate; folic acid; biotin] ≛•18 mg•0.4 mg•45 µg

Geritol Extend caplets OTC *vitamin/mineral/iron supplement* [multiple vitamins & minerals; ferrous fumarate; folic acid] ≛•10•0.2 mg

Geritol Tonic liquid OTC *hematinic* [ferric pyrophosphate; multiple B vitamins; alcohol 12%] 18•≛ mg/15 mL

Geritonic liquid OTC *hematinic* [ferric ammonium citrate; liver fraction 1; multiple B vitamins & minerals; alcohol 20%] 105•375•≛ mg/15 mL

Gerivite liquid OTC *geriatric vitamin/mineral supplement* [multiple B vitamins & minerals; alcohol 18%] ≛

Gerivites tablets OTC *hematinic; vitamin/mineral supplement* [ferrous sulfate; multiple vitamins & minerals; folic acid] 50•≛•0.4 mg

German valerian *medicinal herb* [see: valerian]

Germanin (available only from the Centers for Disease Control) ℞ *antiparasitic for African trypanosomiasis and onchocerciasis* [suramin sodium]

germanium *element (Ge)*

germicides *a class of agents that destroy micro-organisms* [see also: antiseptics; disinfectants]

geroquinol INN

Geroton Forte liquid OTC *geriatric vitamin/mineral supplement* [multiple B vitamins & minerals; alcohol 13.5%] ≛

gesarol [see: chlorophenothane]

gestaclone USAN, INN *progestin*

gestadienol INN

gestanin [see: allyloestrenol]

gestodene USAN, INN, BAN *progestin*

gestonorone caproate USAN, INN *progestin* [also: gestronol]

gestrinone USAN, INN *progestin*

gestronol BAN *progestin* [also: gestonorone caproate]

Get Better Bear Sore Throat Pops OTC *throat emollient and protectant* [pectin] 19 mg

Gets-It liquid OTC *topical keratolytic* [salicylic acid; zinc chloride; alcohol 28%]

gevotroline INN *antipsychotic* [also: gevotroline HCl]

gevotroline HCl USAN *antipsychotic* [also: gevotroline]

Gevrabon liquid OTC *vitamin/mineral supplement* [multiple B vitamins & minerals; alcohol 18%] ≛

Gevral tablets OTC *vitamin/mineral/iron supplement* [multiple vitamins & minerals; ferrous fumarate; folic acid] ≛•18 mg•0.4 mg

Gevral Protein powder OTC *oral protein supplement* [calcium caseinate; sucrose]

G-F 20 [see: hylan G-F 20]

GFN (guaifenesin) [q.v.]

GFN/PSE tablets ℞ *expectorant; decongestant* [guaifenesin; pseudoephedrine HCl] 1200•120 mg

GG-Cen capsules (discontinued 2000) OTC *expectorant* [guaifenesin] 200 mg

GHB (gamma hydroxybutyrate) *a CNS depressant used as an anesthetic in some countries, produced and abused as a "date rape" street drug in the U.S.; illegal in the U.S. (Schedule I)* [the sodium salt is medically known as sodium oxybate]

GHB-aldehyde (gamma butyraldehyde) *a precursor to gamma hydroxybutyrate (GHB)* [see: gamma hydroxybutyrate (GHB)]

GH-RF; GHRF (growth hormone-releasing factor) [q.v.]

Gilead, balm of *medicinal herb* [see: balm of Gilead]

ginger (*Zingiber officinale*) root *medicinal herb for childhood diseases, colds, colic, dizziness, fever, flu, gas pains, headache, indigestion, morning sickness, nausea, poor circulation, toothache, and vestibular disorders*

ginger, wild *medicinal herb* [see: wild ginger]

ginkgo (*Ginkgo biloba*) leaves *medicinal herb for Alzheimer disease, antioxidant, anxiety, asthma, attention-deficit disorder, chilblains, cerebral insufficiency, dementia, dizziness, memory loss, poor circulation, Raynaud disease, stroke, and tinnitus*

ginseng (*Panax* spp.) root *medicinal herb for age spots, blood diseases, depression, hemorrhage, increasing endurance and longevity, and stress; also used as an aphrodisiac* [also see: Siberian ginseng]

ginseng, blue; yellow ginseng *medicinal herb* [see: blue cohosh]

giparmen INN

giractide INN

girisopam INN
gitalin NF [also: gitalin amorphous]
gitalin amorphous INN [also: gitalin]
gitaloxin INN
gitoformate INN
gitoxin 16-formate [see: gitaloxin]
gitoxin pentaacetate [see: pengitoxin]
GLA (gamma-linolenic acid)
glacial acetic acid [see: acetic acid, glacial]
glafenine INN, DCF, JAN
Glandosane oral spray (discontinued 2000) OTC *saliva substitute*
glaphenine [see: glafenine]
glatiramer acetate USAN *immunomodulator for relapsing-remitting multiple sclerosis (orphan)* [formerly known as copolymer 1]
Glauber salt [see: sodium sulfate]
glaucarubin
Glaucon Drop-Tainers (eye drops) ℞ *topical antiglaucoma agent* [epinephrine HCl] 1%, 2%
GlaucTabs tablets ℞ *carbonic anhydrase inhibitor for glaucoma* [methazolamide] 25, 50 mg
glaze, pharmaceutical NF *tablet-coating agent*
glaziovine INN
Gleevec capsules ℞ *antineoplastic for chronic myeloid leukemia (CML) (orphan); investigational for gastrointestinal stromal tumors (GIST)* [imatinib mesylate] 100 mg
glemanserin USAN, INN *anxiolytic*
gleptoferron USAN, INN, BAN *veterinary hematinic*
Gliadel wafers ℞ *nitrosourea-type alkylating antineoplastic cerebral implants for excised brain tumors (orphan)* [carmustine in a polifeprosan 20 carrier] 7.7 mg
gliamilide USAN, INN *antidiabetic*
glibenclamide INN, BAN *sulfonylurea antidiabetic* [also: glyburide]
glibornuride USAN, INN, BAN *antidiabetic*
glibutimine INN
glicaramide INN
glicetanile INN *antidiabetic* [also: glicetanile sodium]
glicetanile sodium USAN *antidiabetic* [also: glicetanile]
gliclazide INN, BAN *sulfonylurea antidiabetic*
glicondamide INN
glidazamide INN
gliflumide USAN, INN *antidiabetic*
glimepiride USAN, INN, BAN *sulfonylurea antidiabetic*
glipentide [see: glisentide]
glipizide USAN, INN, BAN *sulfonylurea antidiabetic* 5, 10 mg oral
gliquidone INN, BAN
glisamuride INN
glisentide INN
glisindamide INN
glisolamide INN
glisoxepide INN, BAN
Glivec (foreign name for U.S. product Gleevec)
globin zinc insulin INN [also: insulin, globin zinc]
globulin, immune USP *passive immunizing agent for HIV, ITP, B-cell CLL, and BMT; infection prophylaxis in pediatric HIV (orphan); investigational (orphan) for myocarditis and juvenile rheumatoid arthritis*
globulin, immune human serum [now: globulin, immune]
Glossets (trademarked form) *sublingual or rectal administration*
gloxazone USAN, INN, BAN *veterinary anaplasmodastat*
gloximonam USAN, INN *antibacterial*
GlucaGen Diagnostic Kit IV injection ℞ *agent to inhibit movement of the gastrointestinal tract during radiographic procedures* [glucagon, recombinant] 1 mg
GlucaGen Emergency Kit subcu, IV, or IM injection ℞ *emergency treatment of hypoglycemic crisis* [glucagon, recombinant] 1 mg
glucagon USP, INN, BAN *antidiabetic; glucose elevating agent; diagnostic aid for GI imaging*
Glucagon Diagnostic Kit IM or IV injection ℞ *to inhibit GI tract move-*

ment during radiographic procedures [glucagon, recombinant] 1 mg (1 U)

Glucagon Emergency Kit subcu, IM, or IV injection ℞ *emergency treatment for hypoglycemic crisis* [glucagon, recombinant] 1 mg (1 U)

glucalox INN [also: glycalox]

glucametacin INN

glucan synthesis inhibitors *a class of antifungals* [also: echinocandins]

D-glucaric acid, calcium salt tetrahydrate [see: calcium saccharate]

gluceptate USAN, USP, INN, BAN *combining name for radicals or groups*

gluceptate sodium USAN *pharmaceutic aid*

Glucerna ready-to-use liquid OTC *enteral nutritional therapy for abnormal glucose tolerance*

D-glucitol [see: sorbitol]

D-glucitol hexanicotinate [see: sorbinicate]

β-glucocerebrosidase, macrophage-targeted [see: alglucerase]

glucocerebrosidase, recombinant retroviral vector *investigational (orphan) enzyme replacement for types I, II, or III Gaucher disease*

glucocerebrosidase-β-glucosidase [see: alglucerase]

glucocorticoids *a class of adrenal cortical steroids that modify the body's immune response*

Glucofilm reagent strips for home use *in vitro diagnostic aid for blood glucose*

glucoheptonic acid, calcium salt [see: calcium gluceptate]

glucomannan ***(Amorphophallus konjac)*** root *medicinal herb for constipation, diverticular disease, hemorrhoids, hypercholesterolemia, and obesity; not generally regarded as safe for diabetics, as it may result in altered insulin requirements or hypoglycemia*

Glucometer Encore; Glucometer Elite reagent strips for home use *in vitro diagnostic aid for blood glucose*

D-gluconic acid, calcium salt [see: calcium gluconate]

D-gluconic acid, magnesium salt [see: magnesium gluconate]

D-gluconic acid, monopotassium salt [see: potassium gluconate]

D-gluconic acid, monosodium salt [see: sodium gluconate]

GlucoNorm (CAN) tablets ℞ *oral antidiabetic agent that stimulates release of insulin from the pancreas for type 2 diabetes* [repaglinide] 0.5, 1, 2 mg

Glucophage film-coated tablets ℞ *biguanide antidiabetic* [metformin HCl] 500, 850, 1000 mg

Glucophage XR extended-release tablets ℞ *once-daily biguanide antidiabetic* [metformin HCl] 500 mg

β-D-glucopyranuronamide [see: glucuronamide]

glucosamine USAN, INN *pharmaceutic aid*

glucosamine sulfate *natural remedy for osteoarthritis*

***d*-glucose** [see: dextrose]

glucose, liquid NF *tablet binder and coating agent; antihypoglycemic; diagnostic aid for diabetes* ⑨ Glutose

***d*-glucose monohydrate** [see: dextrose]

glucose oxidase

glucose polymers *caloric replacement*

Glucose-40 ophthalmic ointment (discontinued 1999) ℞ *corneal edema-reducing agent* [glucose] 40%

Glucostix reagent strips for home use *in vitro diagnostic aid for blood glucose*

glucosulfamide INN

glucosulfone INN

glucosylceramidase [see: alglucerase]

Glucotrol tablets ℞ *sulfonylurea antidiabetic* [glipizide] 5, 10 mg

Glucotrol XL extended-release tablets ℞ *sulfonylurea antidiabetic* [glipizide] 2.5, 5, 10 mg

Glucovance film-coated tablets ℞ *antidiabetic combination for type 2 diabetes* [glyburide; metformin HCl] 1.25•250, 2.5•500, 5•500 mg

glucurolactone INN

glucuronamide INN, BAN

glunicate INN

gluside [see: saccharin]

gluside, soluble [see: saccharin sodium]

glusoferron INN
Glustat ℞ *investigational α-glucosidase inhibitor for diabetes* [voglibose]
glutamic acid (L-glutamic acid) USAN, INN *nonessential amino acid; symbols:* Glu, E 340, 500 mg oral
glutamic acid HCl *gastric acidifier*
glutamine (L-glutamine) *nonessential amino acid; symbols:* Gln, Q [see: levoglutamide]
glutamine & somatropin *investigational (orphan) for GI malabsorption due to short bowel syndrome*
glutaral USAN, USP, INN *disinfectant*
glutaraldehyde [see: glutaral]
Glutarex-1 powder OTC *formula for infants with glutaric aciduria type I*
Glutarex-2 powder OTC *enteral nutritional therapy for glutaric aciduria type I*
glutasin [see: glutamic acid HCl]
glutathione *endogenous antioxidant produced in the liver; unstable as a supplement, so levels are increased by supplementing its precursors,* MSM *and* NAC *(q.v.)*
L-glutathione, reduced *investigational (orphan) for AIDS-related cachexia*
glutaurine INN
glutethimide USP, INN, BAN *sedative; sometimes abused as a street drug* 250, 500 mg oral
Glutofac tablets OTC *vitamin/mineral supplement* [multiple vitamins & minerals]
Glutose gel OTC *glucose elevating agent* [glucose] 40% ⊠ glucose
Glyate syrup OTC *expectorant* [guaifenesin; alcohol 3.5%] 100 mg/5 mL
glyburide USAN *sulfonylurea antidiabetic* [also: glibenclamide] 1.25, 1.5, 2.5, 3, 4.5, 5, 6 mg oral
glybutamide [see: carbutamide]
glybuthiazol INN
glybuthizol [see: glybuthiazol]
glybuzole INN
glycalox BAN [also: glucalox]
glycerides oleiques polyoxyethylenes [see: peglicol 5 oleate]
glycerin USP *humectant; solvent; osmotic diuretic; hyperosmotic laxative; emollient/protectant; ophthalmic moisturizer* [also: glycerol]
glycerol INN *humectant; solvent; osmotic diuretic; hyperosmotic laxative; emollient/protectant; monoctanoin component D* [also: glycerin]
glycerol, iodinated USAN, BAN *(disapproved for use as an expectorant in 1991)*
glycerol 1-decanoate *monoctanoin component B* [see: monoctanoin]
glycerol 1,2-dioctanoate *monoctanoin component C* [see: monoctanoin]
glycerol 1-octanoate *monoctanoin component A* [see: monoctanoin]
glycerol phosphate, manganese salt [see: manganese glycerophosphate]
glyceryl behenate NF *tablet and capsule lubricant*
glyceryl borate [see: boroglycerin]
glyceryl guaiacolate [now: guaifenesin]
glyceryl monostearate NF *emulsifying agent*
glyceryl triacetate [now: triacetin]
glyceryl trierucate *investigational (orphan) for adrenoleukodystrophy* [also: glyceryl trioleate]
glyceryl trinitrate BAN *coronary vasodilator* [also: nitroglycerin]
glyceryl trioleate *investigational (orphan) for adrenoleukodystrophy* [also: glyceryl trierucate]
glycerylaminophenaquine [see: glafenine]
Glyceryl-T capsules, liquid ℞ *antiasthmatic; bronchodilator; expectorant* [theophylline; guaifenesin] 150•90 mg; 150•90 mg/15 mL
glycinato dihydroxyaluminum hydrate [see: dihydroxyaluminum aminoacetate]
glycine USP, INN *nonessential amino acid; urologic irrigant; symbols:* Gly, G [also: aminoacetic acid] 1.5%
glycine aluminum-zirconium complex [see: aluminum zirconium tetrachlorohydrex gly; aluminum zirconium trichlorohydrex gly]
Glycine max *medicinal herb* [see: soy]
glyclopyramide INN

glycobiarsol USP, INN [also: bismuth glycollylarsanilate]
glycocholate sodium [see: sodium glycocholate]
glycocoll [see: glycine]
Glycofed tablets OTC *decongestant; expectorant* [pseudoephedrine HCl; guaifenesin] 30•100 mg
glycol distearate USAN *thickening agent*
glycolic acid *mild exfoliant and keratolytic*
***p*-glycolophenetidide** [see: fenacetinol]
glycopeptides *a class of antibiotic antineoplastics*
glycophenylate [see: mepenzolate bromide]
glycoprotein (GP) IIb/IIIa receptor antagonists *a class of platelet aggregation inhibitors for acute coronary syndrome, unstable angina, myocardial infarction, and cardiac surgery*
glycopyrrolate USAN, USP *GI antispasmodic; antisecretory; peptic ulcer adjunct* [also: glycopyrronium bromide] 0.2 mg/mL injection
glycopyrrone bromide [see: glycopyrrolate]
glycopyrronium bromide INN, BAN *GI antispasmodic; antisecretory; peptic ulcer adjunct* [also: glycopyrrolate]
glycosaminoglycans *a class of anticoagulants used for the prophylaxis of postoperative deep vein thrombosis (DVT)*
glycosides, cardiac *a class of cardiovascular drugs that increase the force of cardiac contractions* [also called: digitalis glycosides]
Glycotuss tablets OTC *expectorant* [guaifenesin] 100 mg ⑨ Glytuss
Glycotuss-dM tablets OTC *antitussive; expectorant* [dextromethorphan hydrobromide; guaifenesin] 10•100 mg
glycyclamide INN, BAN
glycyrrhetinic acid [see: enoxolone]
glycyrrhiza NF
Glycyrrhiza glabra; G. palidiflora; G. uralensis *medicinal herb* [see: licorice]
glydanile sodium [now: glicetanile sodium]
glyhexamide USAN, INN *antidiabetic*
glyhexylamide [see: metahexamide]
Glylorin ℞ *investigational (Phase III, orphan) for non-bullous congenital ichthyosiform erythroderma* [monolaurin]
glymidine BAN *antidiabetic* [also: glymidine sodium]
glymidine sodium USAN, INN *antidiabetic* [also: glymidine]
glymol [see: mineral oil]
Glynase PresTabs (micronized tablets) ℞ *sulfonylurea antidiabetic* [glyburide] 1.5, 3, 6 mg
glyoctamide USAN, INN *antidiabetic*
Gly-Oxide oral solution OTC *oral anti-inflammatory and anti-infective* [carbamide peroxide] 10%
glyparamide USAN *antidiabetic*
glyphylline [see: dyphylline]
glypinamide INN
Glypressin ℞ *investigational (orphan) for bleeding esophageal ulcers* [terlipressin]
glyprothiazol INN
glyprothizol [see: glyprothiazol]
Glyquin cream ℞ *hyperpigmentation bleaching agent* [hydroquinone (in a base containing glycolic acid and vitamins C and E)] 4%
Glyset tablets ℞ *antidiabetic agent for type 2 diabetes; α-glucosidase inhibitor that delays the digestion of dietary carbohydrates* [miglitol] 25, 50, 100 mg
glysobuzole INN [also: isobuzole]
Glytuss film-coated tablets OTC *expectorant* [guaifenesin] 200 mg ⑨ Glycotuss
GM-CSF (granulocyte-macrophage colony-stimulating factor) [see: regramostim; sargramostim; molgramostim]
GMK *investigational (Phase III) GM2 ganglioside protein vaccine for malignant melanoma*
G-myticin cream, ointment ℞ *topical antibiotic* [gentamicin sulfate] 1 mg
Gnaphalium polycephalum; G. uliginosum *medicinal herb* [see: everlasting]
Gn-RH (gonadotropin-releasing hormone) *an endogenous hormone, produced in the hypothalamus, which stimulates the release of luteinizing hormone (LH) and follicle-stimulating*

hormone (FSH) from the pituitary [also known as: luteinizing hormone–releasing hormone (LH-RH)]

goatweed *medicinal herb* [see: St. John wort]

Go-Evac powder for oral solution (discontinued 1999) ℞ *pre-procedure bowel evacuant* [polyethylene glycol–electrolyte solution; electrolytes] 59 g/L

gold *element (Au)*

gold Au 198 USAN, USP *antineoplastic; liver imaging aid; radioactive agent*

gold sodium thiomalate USP *antirheumatic (50% gold)* [also: sodium aurothiomalate] 50 mg/mL injection

gold sodium thiosulfate NF [also: sodium aurotiosulfate]

gold thioglucose [see: aurothioglucose]

gold thread *(Coptis trifolia)* root *medicinal herb used as an antiphlogistic, bitter tonic, and sedative*

golden senecio *medicinal herb* [see: life root]

goldenrod *(Solidago nemoralis; S. odora; S. virgaurea)* leaves and flowering tops *medicinal herb used as an astringent, carminative, diaphoretic, diuretic, and stimulant*

goldenseal *(Hydrastis canadensis)* rhizome and root *medicinal herb used as an antibiotic and antiseptic and for internal bleeding, colon inflammation, eye infections, liver disorders, menorrhagia, mouth sores, muscular pain, sciatic pain, and vaginitis*

GoLYTELY powder for oral solution ℞ *pre-procedure bowel evacuant* [polyethylene glycol–electrolyte solution (PEG 3350)] 60 g/L

gonacrine [see: acriflavine]

Gonadimmune *investigational anti-gonadotropin-releasing hormone for prostate, breast, and endometrial cancer and endometriosis*

gonadorelin INN, BAN *gonad-stimulating principle* [also: gonadorelin acetate]

gonadorelin acetate USAN *gonad-stimulating principle for hypothalamic amenorrhea (orphan); diagnostic aid for fertility* [also: gonadorelin]

gonadorelin HCl USAN *gonad-stimulating principle; synthetic luteinizing hormone–releasing hormone (LH-RH); in vivo diagnostic aid for anterior pituitary function*

gonadotrophin, chorionic INN, BAN *gonad-stimulating principle* [also: gonadotropin, chorionic]

gonadotrophin, serum INN

gonadotropin, chorionic USP *gonad-stimulating principle* [also: gonadotrophin, chorionic] 500, 1000, 2000 U/mL injection

gonadotropin, serum [see: gonadotrophin, serum]

gonadotropin-releasing hormone (Gn-RH) *an endogenous hormone, produced in the hypothalamus, which stimulates the release of luteinizing hormone (LH) and follicle-stimulating hormone (FSH) from the pituitary* [also known as: luteinizing hormone–releasing hormone (LH-RH)]

gonadotropin-releasing hormone analogs *a class of hormonal antineoplastics*

gonadotropins *a class of hormones that stimulate the ovaries, including follicle-stimulating hormone (FSH) and luteinizing hormone (LH)*

Gonak ophthalmic solution OTC *gonioscopic examination aid* [hydroxypropyl methylcellulose] 2.5% ⑨ Gonic

Gonal-F subcu injection ℞ *recombinant follicle-stimulating hormone (FSH) for induction of ovulation or spermatogenesis* [follitropin alfa] 37.5, 75, 150 IU

Gonic powder for IM injection ℞ *hormone for prepubertal cryptorchidism and hypogonadism; ovulation stimulant* [chorionic gonadotropin] 1000 U/mL ⑨ Gonak

***Goniopora* spp.** *natural material* [see: coral]

Gonioscopic Prism Solution Drop-Tainers (eye drops) OTC *agent for*

bonding gonioscopic prisms to eye [hydroxyethyl cellulose]

Goniosol ophthalmic solution OTC *gonioscopic examination aid* [hydroxypropyl methylcellulose] 2.5%

Gonozyme Diagnostic reagent kit for professional use *in vitro diagnostic aid for Neisseria gonorrhoeae*

GoodStart [see: Carnation Good Start]

Goody's Body Pain powder OTC *analgesic; antipyretic; anti-inflammatory* [acetaminophen; aspirin] 325•500 mg/dose

Goody's Extra Strength Headache powder OTC *analgesic; antipyretic; anti-inflammatory* [acetaminophen; aspirin; caffeine] 250•520•32.5 mg/dose

goose grass *medicinal herb* [see: bedstraw; cinquefoil]

goose hair; gosling weed *medicinal herb* [see: bedstraw]

Gordobalm OTC *topical analgesic; counterirritant; antiseptic* [methyl salicylate; menthol; camphor; alcohol 16%]

Gordochom solution OTC *topical antifungal; antiseptic* [undecylenic acid; chloroxylenol] 25%•3%

Gordofilm liquid ℞ *topical keratolytic* [salicylic acid in flexible collodion] 16.7%

Gordogesic Creme OTC *counterirritant* [methyl salicylate] 10%

Gordon's Urea 40% cream ℞ *for removal of dystrophic nails* [urea] 40%

Gormel Creme OTC *moisturizer; emollient; keratolytic* [urea] 20%

goserelin USAN, INN, BAN *hormonal antineoplastic for prostate and breast cancer; luteinizing hormone–releasing hormone (LH-RH) agonist* [also: goserelin acetate]

goserelin acetate JAN *hormonal antineoplastic for prostatic carcinoma and breast cancer; luteinizing hormone–releasing hormone (LH-RH) agonist for endometriosis and endometrial thinning* [also: goserelin]

gosling weed; goose grass; goose hair *medicinal herb* [see: bedstraw]

gossypol (*Gossypium* spp.) seed oil *medicinal herb for male and female contraception; not generally regarded as safe, as male sterility may be irreversible; investigational for metastatic endometrial carcinoma; investigational antiviral/interferon inducer for AIDS; investigational (orphan) for adrenal cortex cancer*

gotu kola (*Centella asiatica; Hydrocotyle asiatica*) entire plant *medicinal herb for abscesses, hypertension, contraception, leprosy, nervous breakdown, physical and mental fatigue, promoting wound healing, and rheumatism*

goutberry *medicinal herb* [see: blackberry]

govafilcon A USAN *hydrophilic contact lens material*

GP IIb/IIIa inhibitors [see: glycoprotein (GP) IIb/IIIa receptor antagonists]

gp100 adenoviral gene therapy *investigational (orphan) for metastatic melanoma*

gp120 (glycoprotein 120) antigens *investigational (Phase III) vaccine for HIV* [also: AIDS vaccine]

gp160 (glycoprotein 160) antigens *investigational (orphan) antiviral (therapeutic, Phase II) and vaccine (preventative, Phase I) for HIV and AIDS*

GP-500 tablets ℞ *decongestant; expectorant* [pseudoephedrine HCl; guaifenesin] 120•500 mg

GPI-1046 *investigational neurotrophic agent for treatment of Parkinson disease*

GPI-5000 *investigational for stroke*

grace, herb of *medicinal herb* [see: rue]

Gradumet (trademarked dosage form) *controlled-release tablet*

graftskin *a living, bilayered skin construct for diabetic foot ulcers and pressure sores (the epidermal layer is living human keratinocytes; the dermal layer is living human fibroblasts)*

gramicidin USP, INN *antibacterial antibiotic*

gramicidin & neomycin sulfate & polymyxin B sulfate *topical antibi-*

otic 0.025 mg•1.75 mg•10 000 U per mL eye drops

gramicidin S INN

Graminis rhizoma *medicinal herb* [see: couch grass]

granisetron USAN, INN, BAN *serotonin 5-HT$_3$ receptor antagonist; antiemetic for nausea following chemotherapy, radiation, or surgery*

granisetron HCl USAN *serotonin 5-HT$_3$ receptor antagonist; antiemetic for nausea following chemotherapy, radiation, or surgery*

Granulderm aerosol spray ℞ *topical enzyme for wound debridement; capillary bed stimulant* [trypsin; peruvian balsam; castor oil] 0.1•72.5•650 mg/0.82 mL

Granulex aerosol ℞ *topical enzyme for wound debridement; capillary bed stimulant* [trypsin; peruvian balsam; castor oil] 0.12•87•788 mg/g

granulocyte colony-stimulating factor (G-CSF), recombinant [see: filgrastim]

granulocyte-macrophage colony-stimulating factor (GM-CSF) [see: regramostim; sargramostim; molgramostim]

GranuMed aerosol spray ℞ *topical enzyme for wound debridement* [trypsin; peruvian balsam] 0.1•72.5 mg/0.82 mL

grape, bear's *medicinal herb* [see: uva ursi]

grape, Rocky Mountain; wild Oregon grape *medicinal herb* [see: Oregon grape]

grape seed *(Vitis coigetiae; V. vinifera)* oil *medicinal herb for dental caries; also used as a dietary source of essential fatty acids and tocopherols*

grape seed extract *natural free radical scavenger for inflammatory collagen disease and peripheral vascular disease; contains 92%–95% procyanidolic oligomers (PCOs)*

grapefruit *(Citrus paradisi)* *medicinal herb for potassium replacement; the pectin is used to help reduce cholesterol and promote regression of atherosclerosis*

grass burdock *medicinal herb* [see: burdock]

grass myrtle *medicinal herb* [see: calamus]

Gratiola officinalis *medicinal herb* [see: hedge hyssop]

gravelroot *medicinal herb* [see: queen of the meadow]

graybeard tree *medicinal herb* [see: fringe tree]

great wild valerian *medicinal herb* [see: valerian]

greater celandine *medicinal herb* [see: celandine]

green broom; greenweed *medicinal herb* [see: dyer's broom]

green hellebore *(Veratrum viride)* *medicinal herb* [see: hellebore]

green soap [see: soap, green]

green tea *(Camellia sinensis)* leaves *medicinal herb used as an antihyperlipidemic, antimicrobial, antineoplastic, and antioxidant; also used to promote longevity by attenuating severe fatal diseases*

greenweed; green broom *medicinal herb* [see: dyer's broom]

grepafloxacin INN *broad-spectrum fluoroquinolone antibiotic*

grepafloxacin HCl USAN *broad-spectrum fluoroquinolone antibiotic*

GRF1-44 *investigational (Phase III) human growth hormone releasing factor in slow-release implant form for growth disorders*

Grifola frondosa *medicinal herb* [see: maitake mushrooms]

Grifulvin V tablets, oral suspension ℞ *systemic antifungal* [griseofulvin (microsize)] 250, 500 mg; 125 mg/5 mL

Grindelia squarrosia *medicinal herb* [see: gum weed]

Grisactin 250 capsules ℞ *systemic antifungal* [griseofulvin (microsize)] 250 mg

Grisactin 500 tablets ℞ *systemic antifungal* [griseofulvin (microsize)] 500 mg

Grisactin Ultra tablets ℞ *systemic antifungal* [griseofulvin (ultramicrosize)] 250 mg

griseofulvin USP, INN, BAN *systemic antifungal* 125, 165, 250, 330 mg oral

Gris-PEG film-coated tablets ℞ *systemic antifungal* [griseofulvin (ultramicrosize)] 125, 250 mg

ground apple *medicinal herb* [see: chamomile]

ground berry *medicinal herb* [see: wintergreen]

ground holly *medicinal herb* [see: pipsissewa]

ground lemon *medicinal herb* [see: mandrake]

ground lily *medicinal herb* [see: birthroot]

ground raspberry *medicinal herb* [see: goldenseal]

ground squirrel pea *medicinal herb* [see: twin leaf]

ground thistle *medicinal herb* [see: carline thistle]

group A streptococcal (GAS) vaccine *investigational vaccine*

group C meningococcal conjugate vaccine *investigational vaccine*

growth hormone, human (hGH) [see: somatropin]

growth hormone-releasing factor (GHRF; GH-RF) *investigational (orphan) for inadequate endogenous growth hormone in children*

GS 393 *investigational (Phase I/II) antiviral for HIV* [also: PMEA]

G-strophanthin [see: ouabain]

guabenxan INN

guacetisal INN

guafecainol INN

guaiac

guaiacol NF

***p*-guaiacol** [see: mequinol]

guaiacol carbonate NF

guaiacol glyceryl ether [see: guaifenesin]

guaiactamine INN

guaiapate USAN, INN *antitussive*

guaiazulene soluble [see: sodium gualenate]

guaietolin INN

Guaifed syrup OTC *decongestant; expectorant* [pseudoephedrine HCl; guaifenesin] 30•200 mg

Guaifed timed-release capsules ℞ *decongestant; expectorant* [pseudoephedrine HCl; guaifenesin] 120•250 mg

Guaifed-PD timed-release capsules ℞ *pediatric decongestant and expectorant* [pseudoephedrine HCl; guaifenesin] 60•300 mg

guaifenesin USAN, USP, INN *expectorant* [also: guaiphenesin] 100 mg/5 mL oral ⑨ guanfacine

guaifenesin & codeine phosphate *expectorant; antitussive; narcotic analgesic* 300•10 mg oral; 100•10 mg/5 mL oral

Guaifenesin DAC liquid OTC *narcotic antitussive; decongestant; expectorant* [codeine phosphate; pseudoephedrine HCl; guaifenesin; alcohol 1.9%] 10•30•100 mg

guaifenesin & dyphylline *expectorant; bronchodilator* 200•200 mg

guaifenesin & hydrocodone bitartrate *expectorant; antitussive* 100•5 mg/5 mL oral

guaifenesin & phenylephrine HCl & phenylpropanolamine HCl *expectorant; nasal decongestant* 200•5•45 mg oral

Guaifenex liquid ℞ *decongestant; expectorant* [phenylpropanolamine HCl; phenylephrine HCl; guaifenesin] 20•5•100 mg/5 mL

Guaifenex DM extended-release tablets ℞ *antitussive; expectorant* [dextromethorphan hydrobromide; guaifenesin] 30•600 mg

Guaifenex LA extended-release tablets ℞ *expectorant* [guaifenesin] 600 mg

Guaifenex PPA 75 extended-release tablets ℞ *decongestant; expectorant* [phenylpropanolamine HCl; guaifenesin] 75•600 mg

Guaifenex PSE 60; Guaifenex PSE 120; Guaifenex Rx DM extended-release tablets ℞ *decongestant; expectorant* [pseudoephedrine HCl; guaifenesin] 60•600 mg; 120•600 mg; 60•600 mg

Guaifenex Rx extended-release tablets (AM and PM) ℞ *decongestant; expectorant* [pseudoephedrine HCl + guaifenesin (AM); guaifenesin (PM)] 60•600 mg; 600 mg

guaifylline INN *bronchodilator; expectorant* [also: guaithylline]

GuaiMAX-D extended-release tablets ℞ *decongestant; expectorant* [pseudoephedrine HCl; guaifenesin] 120•600 mg

guaimesal INN

Guaipax sustained-release tablets ℞ *decongestant; expectorant* [phenylpropanolamine HCl; guaifenesin] 75•400 mg

guaiphenesin BAN *expectorant* [also: guaifenesin]

guaisteine INN

Guaitab tablets OTC *decongestant; expectorant* [pseudoephedrine HCl; guaifenesin] 60•400 mg

Guaitex capsules, liquid ℞ *decongestant; expectorant* [phenylephrine HCl; phenylpropanolamine HCl; guaifenesin] 5•45•200 mg; 5•20•100 mg/5 mL

Guaitex LA sustained-release tablets ℞ *decongestant; expectorant* [phenylpropanolamine HCl; guaifenesin] 75•400 mg

Guaitex PSE tablets ℞ *decongestant; expectorant* [pseudoephedrine HCl; guaifenesin] 120•500 mg

guaithylline USAN *bronchodilator; expectorant* [also: guaifylline]

Guaivent capsules ℞ *decongestant; expectorant* [pseudoephedrine HCl; guaifenesin] 120•250 mg

Guaivent PD capsules ℞ *pediatric decongestant and expectorant* [pseudoephedrine HCl; guaifenesin] 60•300 mg

Guai-Vent/PSE sustained-release tablets ℞ *decongestant; expectorant* [pseudoephedrine HCl; guaifenesin] 120•600 mg

guamecycline INN, BAN

guanabenz USAN, INN *centrally acting antiadrenergic antihypertensive*

guanabenz acetate USAN, USP, JAN *centrally acting antiadrenergic antihypertensive* 4, 8 mg oral

guanacline INN, BAN *antihypertensive* [also: guanacline sulfate]

guanacline sulfate USAN *antihypertensive* [also: guanacline]

guanadrel INN *antihypertensive* [also: guanadrel sulfate]

guanadrel sulfate USAN, USP *antihypertensive* [also: guanadrel]

guanatol HCl [see: chloroguanide HCl]

guanazodine INN

guancidine INN *antihypertensive* [also: guancydine]

guancydine USAN *antihypertensive* [also: guancidine]

guanethidine INN, BAN *antihypertensive* [also: guanethidine monosulfate] ⑨ guanidine

guanethidine monosulfate USAN, USP *antihypertensive; investigational (orphan) for reflex sympathetic dystrophy and causalgia* [also: guanethidine]

guanethidine sulfate USAN, USP, JAN *antihypertensive*

guanfacine INN, BAN *antihypertensive; antiadrenergic* [also: guanfacine HCl] ⑨ guaifenesin

guanfacine HCl USAN *antihypertensive; antiadrenergic* [also: guanfacine] 1, 2 mg oral

guanidine HCl *cholinergic muscle stimulant* 125 mg oral ⑨ guanethidine

guanisoquin sulfate USAN *antihypertensive* [also: guanisoquine]

guanisoquine INN *antihypertensive* [also: guanisoquin sulfate]

guanoclor INN, BAN *antihypertensive* [also: guanoclor sulfate]

guanoclor sulfate USAN *antihypertensive* [also: guanoclor]

guanoctine INN *antihypertensive* [also: guanoctine HCl]

guanoctine HCl USAN *antihypertensive* [also: guanoctine]

guanoxabenz USAN, INN *antihypertensive*

guanoxan INN, BAN *antihypertensive* [also: guanoxan sulfate]
guanoxan sulfate USAN *antihypertensive* [also: guanoxan]
guanoxyfen INN *antihypertensive; antidepressant* [also: guanoxyfen sulfate]
guanoxyfen sulfate USAN *antihypertensive; antidepressant* [also: guanoxyfen]
guar gum NF *tablet binder and disintegrant*
guarana *(Paullinia cupana; P. sorbilis)* seed paste *medicinal herb for dysentery, malaria, and weight reduction*
guaranine [see: caffeine]
guggul *(Commiphora mukul)* plant *medicinal herb for hypercholesterolemia and for arthritis and weight reduction in Ayurvedic medicine*
GuiaCough CF liquid (discontinued 2000) OTC *antitussive; decongestant; expectorant* [dextromethorphan hydrobromide; phenylpropanolamine HCl; guaifenesin; alcohol 4.75%] 10•12.5•100 mg/5 mL
GuiaCough PE syrup (discontinued 2000) OTC *decongestant; expectorant* [pseudoephedrine HCl; guaifenesin; alcohol 1.4%] 30•100 mg/5 mL
Guiatex LA tablets ℞ *decongestant; expectorant* [phenylpropanolamine HCl; guaifenesin] 75•400 mg
Guiatex PSE tablets ℞ *decongestant; expectorant* [pseudoephedrine HCl; guaifenesin] 120•500 mg
Guiatuss syrup OTC *expectorant* [guaifenesin] 100 mg/5 mL ⊠ Guiatussin
Guiatuss AC syrup ℞ *narcotic antitussive; expectorant* [codeine phosphate; guaifenesin; alcohol] 10•100 mg/5 mL
Guiatuss CF liquid OTC *antitussive; decongestant; expectorant* [dextromethorphan hydrobromide; phenylpropanolamine HCl; guaifenesin; alcohol 4.75%] 10•12.5•100 mg/5 mL
Guiatuss DAC liquid ℞ *narcotic antitussive; decongestant; expectorant* [codeine phosphate; pseudoephedrine HCl; guaifenesin; alcohol] 10•30•100 mg/5 mL
Guiatuss DM liquid OTC *antitussive; expectorant* [dextromethorphan hydrobromide; guaifenesin] 10•100 mg/5 mL
Guiatuss PE liquid OTC *decongestant; expectorant* [pseudoephedrine HCl; guaifenesin; alcohol 1.4%] 30•100 mg/5 mL
Guiatussin DAC syrup ℞ *narcotic antitussive; decongestant; expectorant* [codeine phosphate; pseudoephedrine HCl; guaifenesin; alcohol 1.6%] 10•30•100 mg/5 mL ⊠ Guiatuss
Guiatussin with Codeine Expectorant liquid ℞ *narcotic antitussive; expectorant* [codeine phosphate; guaifenesin; alcohol 3.5%] 10•100 mg/5 mL
Guiatussin with Dextromethorphan liquid OTC *antitussive; expectorant* [dextromethorphan hydrobromide; guaifenesin; alcohol 1.4%] 15•100 mg/5 mL
gum Arabic *medicinal herb* [see: acacia]
gum arabic [see: acacia]
gum ivy *medicinal herb* [see: English ivy]
gum myrrh tree *medicinal herb* [see: myrrh]
gum plant *medicinal herb* [see: comfrey; yerba santa]
gum senegal [see: acacia]
gum tree, hemlock *medicinal herb* [see: hemlock]
gum weed *(Grindelia squarrosia)* flowering top and leaves *medicinal herb for asthma, bronchitis, bladder infection, poison ivy and oak, and psoriasis and other skin disorders*
guncotton, soluble [see: pyroxylin]
gusperimus INN *immunosuppressant; investigational (orphan) for acute renal graft rejection* [also: gusperimus trihydrochloride; gusperimus HCl]
gusperimus HCl JAN *immunosuppressant* [also: gusperimus trihydrochloride; gusperimus]
gusperimus trihydrochloride USAN *immunosuppressant* [also: gusperimus; gusperimus HCl]

Gustase tablets OTC *digestive enzymes* [amylase; protease; cellulase] 30•6•2 mg

Gustase Plus tablet ℞ *digestive enzymes; sedative* [amylase; protease; cellulase; homatropine methylbromide; phenobarbital] 30•6•2•2.5•8 mg

gutta percha USP *dental restoration agent*

GVAX ℞ *investigational (Phase I/II) theraccine for prostate cancer; investigational (Phase I) for pancreatic cancer*

GW-2570 *investigational (Phase III) antidiabetic*

GW275175 *investigational (Phase I) DNA maturation inhibitor for AIDS-related cytomegalovirus retinitis*

G-Well lotion, shampoo ℞ *pediculicide for lice; scabicide* [lindane] 1%

gymnema (*Gymnema melicida; G. sylvestre*) leaves and roots *medicinal herb for diabetes, hyperactivity, and hypoglycemia*

Gynazole-1 vaginal cream in prefilled applicator ℞ *antifungal* [butoconazole nitrate] 2%

Gynecort 5 cream (discontinued 1997) OTC *topical corticosteroidal anti-inflammatory* [hydrocortisone acetate] 0.5%

Gynecort 10 (name changed to Gynecort Female Creme in 1997)

Gynecort Female Creme cream OTC *topical corticosteroidal anti-inflammatory* [hydrocortisone acetate] 1%

Gyne-Lotrimin combination pack (name changed to Gyne-Lotrimin 7 in 1999 [with 100 mg inserts], then to Gyne-Lotrimin 3 in 2000 [with 200 mg inserts])

Gyne-Lotrimin vaginal inserts, vaginal cream (name changed to Gyne-Lotrimin 3 in 1999)

Gyne-Lotrimin 3 vaginal inserts, vaginal cream, combination pack (inserts + cream) OTC *antifungal* [clotrimazole] 200 mg; 2%; 200 mg + 1%

Gyne-Lotrimin 3 vaginal inserts, combination pack (discontinued 2000 [replaced by 200 mg inserts]) OTC *antifungal* [clotrimazole] 100 mg; 100 mg + 1%

Gyne-Lotrimin 7 combination pack (name changed to Gyne-Lotrimin 3 in 2000 [with 200 mg inserts]) OTC *antifungal* [clotrimazole] 100 mg + 1%

Gyne-Lotrimin 7 vaginal cream OTC *antifungal* [clotrimazole] 1%

Gyne-Moistrin vaginal gel (discontinued 1998) OTC *lubricant* [propylene glycol]

gynergon [see: estradiol]

Gyne-Sulf vaginal cream (discontinued 2001) ℞ *broad-spectrum bacteriostatic* [sulfathiazole; sulfacetamide; sulfabenzamide] 3.42%•2.86%•3.7%

Gynodiol tablets ℞ *estrogen replacement therapy for postmenopausal symptoms* [estradiol, micronized] 0.5, 1, 1.5, 2 mg

gynoestryl [see: estradiol]

Gynogen L.A. 20 IM injection ℞ *estrogen replacement therapy for postmenopausal symptoms; antineoplastic for prostatic cancer* [estradiol valerate in oil] 20 mg/mL

Gynol II Contraceptive vaginal gel, vaginal jelly OTC *spermicidal contraceptive (for use with a diaphragm)* [nonoxynol 9] 2%; 3%

Gynostemma pentaphyllum *medicinal herb* [see: jiaogulan]

Gynovite Plus tablets OTC *vitamin/mineral/calcium/iron supplement* [multiple vitamins & minerals; calcium; iron; folic acid; biotin] ≛•83•3•0.067•≟ mg

Gy-Pak (trademarked packaging form) *unit-of-issue package*

gypsy weed *medicinal herb* [see: speedwell]

Gyrocap (trademarked dosage form) *timed-release capsule*

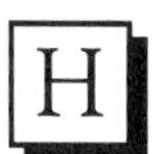

H_1 blockers *a class of antihistamines* [also called: histamine H_1 antagonists]

H_2 blockers *a class of gastrointestinal antisecretory agents* [also called: histamine H_2 antagonists]

^2H (deuterium) [see: deuterium oxide]

$H_2{}^{15}O$ [see: water O 15]

^3H (tritium) [see: tritiated water]

HAART (highly active antiretroviral therapy) *multi-drug therapy given to HIV-positive patients to prevent progression to AIDS; a generic term applied to several different anti-HIV protocols*

Habitrol transdermal patch ℞ *smoking deterrent; nicotine withdrawal aid* [nicotine] 7, 14, 21 mg/day

hachimycin INN, BAN

HAD (hexamethylmelamine, Adriamycin, DDP) *chemotherapy protocol*

hafnium *element (Hf)*

Hair Booster Vitamin tablets OTC *vitamin/mineral/iron supplement* [multiple B vitamins & minerals; iron; folic acid] ≛ •18•0.4 mg

halarsol [see: dichlorophenarsine HCl]

halazepam USAN, USP, INN, BAN *anxiolytic; sedative*

halazone USP, INN *disinfectant; water purifier*

halcinonide USAN, USP, INN, BAN *topical corticosteroidal anti-inflammatory*

Halcion tablets ℞ *benzodiazepine sedative; hypnotic* [triazolam] 0.125, 0.25 mg

Haldol oral concentrate, IM injection ℞ *conventional (typical) antipsychotic; antidyskinetic for Tourette syndrome* [haloperidol lactate] 2 mg/mL; 5 mg/mL ⑨ Halenol; Halog

Haldol tablets ℞ *conventional (typical) antipsychotic; antidyskinetic for Tourette syndrome* [haloperidol] 0.5, 1, 2, 5, 10, 20 mg

Haldol Decanoate 50; Haldol Decanoate 100 long-acting IM injection ℞ *conventional (typical) antipsychotic* [haloperidol decanoate] 50 mg/mL; 100 mg/mL

Halenol, Children's liquid OTC *analgesic; antipyretic* [acetaminophen] 160 mg/5 mL

haletazole INN [also: halethazole]

halethazole BAN [also: haletazole]

Haley's M-O oral liquid OTC *saline/emollient laxative* [magnesium hydroxide; mineral oil] 900 mg•3.75 mL per 15 mL

Halfan tablets ℞ *antimalarial (orphan)* [halofantrine HCl] 250 mg

Halfprin; Halfprin 81 enteric-coated tablets OTC *analgesic; antipyretic; anti-inflammatory; antirheumatic* [aspirin] 165 mg; 81 mg

Hall's Plus lozenges OTC *topical oral analgesic; counterirritant; mild local anesthetic; antiseptic* [menthol] 10 mg

Hall's Sugar Free Mentho-Lyptus lozenges OTC *topical oral analgesic; counterirritant; mild local anesthetic; antiseptic* [menthol; eucalyptus oil] 5•2.8, 6•2.8 mg

Halls Zinc Defense lozenges OTC *topical anti-infective to relieve sore throat* [zinc acetate] 5 mg

hallucinogens *a class of agents that induce hallucinations*

halobetasol propionate USAN *topical corticosteroidal anti-inflammatory* [also: ulobetasol]

halocarban INN *disinfectant* [also: cloflucarban]

halocortolone INN

halocrinic acid [see: brocrinat]

halofantrine INN, BAN *antimalarial* [also: halofantrine HCl]

halofantrine HCl USAN *antimalarial (orphan)* [also: halofantrine]

Halofed tablets OTC *nasal decongestant* [pseudoephedrine HCl] 30, 60 mg

halofenate USAN, INN, BAN *antihyperlipoproteinemic; uricosuric*

halofuginone INN, BAN *antiprotozoal* [also: halofuginone hydrobromide]

halofuginone hydrobromide USAN *antiprotozoal; investigational (orphan) for scleroderma* [also: halofuginone]

Halog ointment, cream, solution ℞ *topical corticosteroidal anti-inflammatory* [halcinonide] 0.1%; 0.025%, 0.1%; 0.1% ⊠ Haldol

Halog-E cream ℞ *topical corticosteroidal anti-inflammatory; emollient* [halcinonide] 0.1%

halometasone INN

halonamine INN

halopemide USAN, INN *antipsychotic*

halopenium chloride INN, BAN

haloperidol USAN, USP, INN, BAN *butyrophenone antipsychotic; antidyskinetic for Tourette syndrome* 0.5, 1, 2, 5, 10, 20 mg oral

haloperidol decanoate USAN, BAN *butyrophenone antipsychotic* 5, 50, 100 mg/mL injection

Haloperidol LA (CAN) long-acting IM injection ℞ *conventional (typical) antipsychotic* [haloperidol decanoate] 50, 100 mg/mL

haloperidol lactate *butyrophenone antipsychotic; antidyskinetic for Tourette syndrome* 2 mg/mL oral; 5 mg/mL injection

halopone chloride [see: halopenium chloride]

halopredone INN *topical anti-inflammatory* [also: halopredone acetate]

halopredone acetate USAN *topical anti-inflammatory* [also: halopredone]

haloprogesterone USAN, INN *progestin*

haloprogin USAN, USP, INN, JAN *antibacterial; antifungal*

halopyramine BAN [also: chloropyramine]

Halotestin tablets ℞ *androgen for hypogonadism or testosterone deficiency in men, delayed puberty in boys, and metastatic breast cancer in women* [fluoxymesterone] 2, 5, 10 mg ⊠ Halotex; Halotussin

Halotex cream, solution ℞ *topical antifungal* [haloprogin] 1% ⊠ Halotestin

halothane USP, INN, BAN *inhalation general anesthetic*

Halotussin syrup OTC *expectorant* [guaifenesin; alcohol 3.5%] 100 mg/5 mL ⊠ Halotestin

Halotussin-DM liquid, sugar-free liquid OTC *antitussive; expectorant* [dextromethorphan hydrobromide; guaifenesin] 10•100 mg/5 mL

haloxazolam INN

haloxon INN, BAN

halquinol BAN *topical anti-infective* [also: halquinols]

halquinols USAN *topical anti-infective* [also: halquinol]

Haltran tablets OTC *analgesic; antiarthritic; antipyretic; nonsteroidal anti-inflammatory drug (NSAID)* [ibuprofen] 200 mg

HAM (hexamethylmelamine, Adriamycin, melphalan) *chemotherapy protocol*

HAM (hexamethylmelamine, Adriamycin, methotrexate) *chemotherapy protocol*

Hamamelis virginiana *medicinal herb* [see: witch hazel]

hamamelis water *medicinal herb* [see: witch hazel]

hamycin USAN, INN *antifungal*

hard fat [see: fat, hard]

hardock *medicinal herb* [see: burdock]

hareburr *medicinal herb* [see: burdock]

Harpagophytum procumbens *medicinal herb* [see: devil's claw]

hashish *(Cannabis sativa)* *euphoric/hallucinogenic street drug made from the resin of the flowering tops of the cannabis plant*

Havrix IM injection, prefilled syringe ℞ *immunization against hepatitis A virus (HAV)* [hepatitis A vaccine, inactivated] 720 EL.U./0.5 mL (pediatric), 1440 EL.U./mL (adult)

haw *medicinal herb* [see: hawthorn]

Hawaiian Tropic Cool Aloe with I.C.E. gel OTC *topical local anesthetic; analgesic; counterirritant* [lidocaine; menthol] ?•?

hawthorn *(Crataegus laevigata; C. monogyna; C. oxyacantha)* flowers, leaves, and berries *medicinal herb for angina pectoris, arrhythmias, arteriosclerosis, enlarged heart, high or low blood pressure, hypoglycemia, palpita-*

tions, and tachycardia; also used as an antiseptic

Hayfebrol liquid OTC *decongestant; antihistamine* [pseudoephedrine HCl; chlorpheniramine maleate] 30•2 mg/5 mL

hazel, snapping; hazelnut *medicinal herb* [see: witch hazel]

H-BIG IM injection (discontinued 2000) ℞ *hepatitis B immunizing agent* [hepatitis B immune globulin] 4, 5 mL

H-BIG IV injection *investigational (orphan) prophylaxis against hepatitis B reinfection in liver transplant patients* [hepatitis B immune globulin]

HBIG (hepatitis B immune globulin) [q.v.]

hBNP (human B-type natriuretic peptide) [see: nesiritide; nesiritide citrate]

HBY097 *investigational (Phase II) nonnucleoside reverse transcriptase inhibitor (NNRTI) for HIV infection*

1% HC ointment ℞ *topical corticosteroidal anti-inflammatory* [hydrocortisone] 1%

HC (hydrocortisone) [q.v.]

4-HC (4-hydroperoxycyclophosphamide) [q.v.]

HC Derma-Pax liquid OTC *topical corticosteroidal anti-inflammatory; antihistamine; antiseptic* [hydrocortisone; pyrilamine maleate; chlorpheniramine maleate; chlorobutanol] 0.5%•0.44%•0.06%•25%

HCA (hydrocortisone acetate) [q.v.]

H-CAP (hexamethylmelamine, cyclophosphamide, Adriamycin, Platinol) *chemotherapy protocol*

hCG (human chorionic gonadotropin) [see: gonadotropin, chorionic]

HCT (hydrochlorothiazide) [q.v.]

HCTZ (hydrochlorothiazide) [q.v.]

HD 85 oral/rectal suspension ℞ *radiopaque contrast medium for gastrointestinal imaging* [barium sulfate] 85%

HD 200 Plus powder for oral suspension ℞ *radiopaque contrast medium for gastrointestinal imaging* [barium sulfate] 98%

HDCV (human diploid cell vaccine) [see: rabies vaccine]

HDMTX (high-dose methotrexate [with leucovorin rescue]) *chemotherapy protocol for bone sarcoma*

HDMTX-CF (high-dose methotrexate, citrovorum factor) *chemotherapy protocol*

HDMTX/LV (high-dose methotrexate, leucovorin [rescue]) *chemotherapy protocol*

HDPEB (high-dose PEB protocol) *chemotherapy protocol* [see: PEB]

HD-VAC (high-dose [methotrexate], vinblastine, Adriamycin, cisplatin) *chemotherapy protocol*

HE-200 *investigational (Phase I/II) cellular energy regulator for HIV and AIDS*

Head & Shoulders cream shampoo, lotion shampoo OTC *antiseborrheic; antibacterial; antifungal* [pyrithione zinc] 1%

Head & Shoulders Dry Scalp shampoo OTC *antiseborrheic; antibacterial; antifungal* [pyrithione zinc] 1%

Head & Shoulders Intensive Treatment Dandruff Shampoo OTC *antiseborrheic* [selenium sulfide] 1%

heal-all *medicinal herb* [see: figwort; stone root; woundwort]

healing herb *medicinal herb* [see: comfrey]

Healon; Healon GV intraocular injection ℞ *viscoelastic agent for ophthalmic surgery* [hyaluronate sodium] 10 mg/mL; 14 mg/mL

Healon Yellow intraocular injection ℞ *viscoelastic agent for ophthalmic surgery; diagnostic agent* [hyaluronate sodium; fluorescein sodium] 10•0.005 mg/mL

Healon5 (CAN) intraocular injection in preloaded syringes ℞ *viscoelastic agent for ophthalmic surgery* [hyaluronate sodium 5000] 23 mg/0.6 mL

heart, mother's; shepherd's heart *medicinal herb* [see: shepherd's purse]

Heartline enteric-coated tablets OTC *analgesic; antipyretic; anti-inflammatory; antirheumatic* [aspirin] 81 mg

heather *(Calluna vulgaris)* flowering shoots *medicinal herb used as an antiseptic, cholagogue, diaphoretic, diuretic, expectorant, and vasoconstrictor*

heavy liquid petrolatum [see: mineral oil]

heavy water (D_2O) [see: deuterium oxide]

Heb Cream Base (discontinued 1998) OTC *cream base*

Hectorol softgels ℞ *synthetic vitamin D analogue; calcium regulator for hyperparathyroidism secondary to chronic renal dialysis* [doxercalciferol] 2.5 µg

hedaquinium chloride INN, BAN

Hedeoma pulegeoides *medicinal herb* [see: pennyroyal]

Hedera helix *medicinal herb* [see: English ivy]

hedge bindweed *(Convolvulus sepium)* flowering plant and roots *medicinal herb used as a cholagogue, febrifuge, and purgative*

hedge garlic *(Sisymbrium alliaria)* *medicinal herb* [see: garlic]

hedge hyssop *(Gratiola officinalis)* plant *medicinal herb used as a cardiac, diuretic, purgative, and vermifuge*

hedge-burs *medicinal herb* [see: bedstraw]

"hedgehog" proteins *a class of novel human proteins that induce the formation of regenerative tissue*

Heet Liniment OTC *counterirritant; topical antiseptic* [methyl salicylate; camphor; capsaicin; alcohol 70%] 15%•3.6%•0.025%

hefilcon A USAN *hydrophilic contact lens material*

hefilcon B USAN *hydrophilic contact lens material*

hefilcon C USAN *hydrophilic contact lens material*

helenien [see: xantofyl palmitate]

Helianthemum canadense *medicinal herb* [see: rock rose]

Helicide ℞ *investigational (Phase III) combination therapy for H. pylori infection*

helicon [see: aspirin]

Helicosol powder for oral solution ℞ *diagnostic aid for detection of H. pylori in the stomach* [carbon C 13 urea]

Helidac 14-day dose-pack ℞ *combination treatment for active duodenal ulcer with H. pylori infection* [bismuth subsalicylate (chewable tablets); metronidazole (tablets); tetracycline HCl (capsules)] 262.4 mg; 250 mg; 500 mg

heliomycin INN

heliox *helium-oxygen mixture used for respiratory distress* (usually an 80%•20% mix)

Helistat sponge ℞ *topical local hemostat for surgery* [absorbable collagen sponge]

helium USP *diluent for gases; element (He)*

Helivax ℞ *investigational (Phase II) H. pylori vaccine*

Helixate powder for IV injection ℞ *antihemophilic to correct coagulation deficiency* [antihemophilic factor VIII, recombinant] 250, 500, 1000 IU

hellebore (*Helleborus* spp.; *Veratrum* spp.) rhizome *medicinal herb used as an antihypertensive; not generally regarded as safe for internal consumption due to toxicity*

***Helleborus* species** *medicinal herb* [see: hellebore]

helmet flower *medicinal herb* [see: aconite; sandalwood; skullcap]

helmet pod *medicinal herb* [see: twin leaf]

HEMA (2-hydroxyethyl methacrylate) *contact lens material* [see: ocufilcon A–F]

Hemabate IM injection ℞ *prostaglandin-type abortifacient; oxytocic for postpartum uterine bleeding* [carboprost tromethamine] 250 µg/mL

Hema-Check slide tests for home use *in vitro diagnostic aid for fecal occult blood*

Hema-Combistix reagent strips *in vitro diagnostic aid for multiple urine products*

Hemaseel HMN ℞ *investigational (Phase III) fibrin sealant for surgery*

Hemaspan timed-release tablets OTC *hematinic; iron/vitamin C supplement* [iron (from ferrous fumarate); ascorbic acid; docusate sodium] 110•200•20 mg

HemAssist *investigational (Phase III) blood substitute for perfusion deficit disorders and blood loss from severe trauma* [hemoglobin crosfumaril]

Hemastix reagent strips for professional use *in vitro diagnostic aid for urine occult blood*

Hematest reagent tablets for professional use *in vitro diagnostic aid for fecal occult blood*

hematinics *a class of iron-containing agents for the prevention and treatment of iron-deficiency anemia*

hematopoietics *a class of antianemic agents that promote the formation of red blood cells*

heme arginate *investigational (orphan) for acute symptomatic porphyria and myelodysplastic syndrome*

HemeSelect Collection kit for home use *in vitro diagnostic aid for fecal occult blood* [for use with HemeSelect Reagent kit]

HemeSelect Reagent kit for professional use *in vitro diagnostic aid for fecal occult blood* [for use with HemeSelect Collection kit]

Hemex ℞ *investigational (orphan) for acute porphyric syndromes* [hemin; zinc mesoporphyrin]

hemiacidrin [see: citric acid, glucono-delta-lactone & magnesium carbonate]

hemin *enzyme inhibitor for acute intermittent porphyria (AIP), porphyria variegata, and hereditary coproporphyria (orphan)*

hemin & zinc mesoporphyrin *investigational (orphan) for acute porphyric syndromes*

hemlock *(Tsuga canadensis)* bark *medicinal herb used as an astringent, diaphoretic, and diuretic*

Hemoccult slide tests for professional use, test tape for professional use *in vitro diagnostic aid for fecal occult blood*

Hemoccult II slide tests for professional use *in vitro diagnostic aid for fecal occult blood*

Hemoccult II Dispenserpak; Hemoccult II Dispenserpak Plus slide tests for home use *in vitro diagnostic aid for fecal occult blood*

Hemoccult SENSA; Hemoccult II SENSA slide tests for professional use *in vitro diagnostic aid for fecal occult blood*

Hemocitrate *investigational (orphan) adjunct to leukapheresis procedures* [sodium citrate]

Hemocyte tablets OTC *hematinic* [ferrous fumarate (source of iron)] 324 mg (106 mg)

Hemocyte Plus elixir ℞ *hematinic* [polysaccharide-iron complex; multiple B vitamins & minerals; folic acid] 12•≛•0.33 mg

Hemocyte Plus tablets ℞ *hematinic* [ferrous fumarate; multiple B vitamins & minerals; sodium ascorbate; folic acid] 106•≛•200•1 mg

Hemocyte-F tablets ℞ *hematinic* [ferrous fumarate; folic acid] 106•1 mg

Hemofil M IV injection ℞ *antihemophilic to correct coagulation deficiency* [antihemophilic factor VIII] 10, 20, 30 mL

hemoglobin, recombinant human (rHb1.1) *investigational agent for chronic anemia*

hemoglobin crosfumaril USAN, INN *investigational (Phase III) blood substitute for perfusion deficit disorders and blood loss due to severe trauma*

Hemokine *investigational progenitor cell stimulator for neutropenia and thrombocytopenia* [muplestim]

Hemolink ℞ *investigational (Phase III) human blood substitute for surgery and chronic anemia associated with kidney failure*

Hemonyne IV infusion ℞ *antihemophilic to correct factor IX deficiency*

(Christmas disease) [coagulation factors II, VII, IX, and X, heat treated] 20, 40 mL

Hemopad fiber ℞ *topical hemostatic aid in surgery* [microfibrillar collagen hemostat]

Hemophilus b conjugate vaccine *active bacterin for Haemophilus influenzae type b*

Hemopure ℞ *investigational (Phase III) oxygen-carrier blood substitute* [hemoglobin glutamer 250 bovine]

Hemorid for Women cream OTC *topical local anesthetic and vasoconstrictor for hemorrhoids* [pramoxine HCl; phenylephrine HCl] 1%•0.25%

Hemorid for Women lotion OTC *topical emollient and protectant for hemorrhoids* [mineral oil; petrolatum; glycerin]

Hemorid for Women rectal suppositories OTC *vasoconstrictor and astringent for hemorrhoids* [zinc oxide; phenylephrine HCl] 11%•0.25%

Hemorrhoidal HC rectal suppositories ℞ *corticosteroidal anti-inflammatory for hemorrhoids* [hydrocortisone acetate] 25 mg

hemostatics *a class of therapeutic blood modifiers that arrest the flow of blood* [see also: astringents; styptics]

Hemotene fiber ℞ *topical hemostatic aid in surgery* [microfibrillar collagen hemostat] 1 g

hemp *medicinal herb* [see: marijuana]

hemp agrimony *(Eupatorium cannabinum)* plant *medicinal herb used as a cholagogue, diaphoretic, diuretic, emetic, expectorant, and purgative*

hemp nettle *(Galeopsis tetrahit)* plant *medicinal herb used as an astringent, diuretic, and expectorant*

Hem-Prep anorectal ointment, rectal suppositories OTC *temporary relief of hemorrhoidal symptoms; topical vasoconstrictor; astringent* [phenylephrine HCl; zinc oxide] 0.025%•11%; 0.25%•11%

Hemril Uniserts (rectal suppositories) OTC *temporary relief of hemorrhoidal symptoms* [bismuth subgallate; bismuth resorcin compound; benzyl benzoate; peruvian balsam; zinc oxide] 2.25%•1.75%•1.2%•1.8%•11%

Hemril-HC Uniserts (suppositories) ℞ *corticosteroidal anti-inflammatory for hemorrhoids* [hydrocortisone acetate] 25 mg

henbane *(Hyoscyamus niger)* plant *medicinal herb used as an anodyne, antispasmodic, calmative, and narcotic; primarily used externally because of its high toxicity*

heneicosafluorotripropylamine [see: perfluamine]

henna *(Alkanna tinctoria)* root *medicinal herb used as an astringent, antibiotic, and cosmetic dye; not generally regarded as safe and effective*

henna *(Lawsonia inermis)* leaves *medicinal herb used as an astringent*

HEOD (hexachloro-epoxy-octahydro-dimethanonaphthalene) [see: dieldrin]

Hepagene ℞ *investigational (NDA filed) hepatitis B vaccine and treatment for chronic carriers*

Hepandrin ℞ *anabolic steroid for weight gain; investigational (orphan) for muscular dystrophy, AIDS-wasting syndrome, and alcoholic hepatitis; also abused as a street drug* [oxandrolone]

heparin BAN *anticoagulant; antithrombotic* [also: heparin calcium]

heparin, 2-0-desulfated *investigational (orphan) for cystic fibrosis*

heparin calcium USP *anticoagulant; antithrombotic* [also: heparin]

Heparin Lock Flush solution ℞ *IV flush for catheter patency (not therapeutic)* [heparin sodium] 10, 100 U/mL

heparin sodium USP, INN, BAN *anticoagulant; antithrombotic* 1000, 2000, 2500, 5000, 7500, 10 000, 20 000, 40 000 U/mL injection

heparin sodium & sodium chloride 0.45% *anticoagulant; antithrombotic* 12 500 U•250 mL, 25 000 U•250 mL, 25 000 U•500 mL

heparin sodium & sodium chloride 0.9% *anticoagulant; antithrombotic* 1000 U•500 mL, 2000 U•1000 mL

heparin sulfate [see: danaparoid sodium]

heparin whole blood [see: blood, whole]

heparinase 1 *investigational (Phase III) agent for the reversal of heparin-induced anticoagulation*

heparinase III *investigational cardioprotective agent*

HepatAmine IV infusion ℞ *nutritional therapy for hepatic failure and hepatic encephalopathy* [multiple branched-chain essential and nonessential amino acids; electrolytes]

hepatica *(Hepatica acutiloba; H. triloba)* leaves and flowers *medicinal herb used as a diuretic and pectoral*

Hepatic-Aid II Instant Drink powder OTC *enteral nutritional treatment for chronic liver disease* [multiple branched chain amino acids]

hepatics *a class of agents that affect the liver (a term used in folk medicine)*

hepatitis A vaccine, inactivated *active immunizing agent for the hepatitis A virus (HAV)*

hepatitis B immune globulin (HBIG) USP *passive immunizing agent; investigational (orphan) prophylaxis against hepatitis B reinfection in liver transplant patients*

hepatitis B surface antigen [see: hepatitis B virus vaccine, inactivated]

hepatitis B virus vaccine, inactivated USP *active immunizing agent for hepatitis B and D*

hepatitis C vaccine *investigational (Phase I) immunizing agent for hepatitis C*

Hepflush-10 solution ℞ *IV flush for catheter patency (not therapeutic)* [heparin sodium] 10 U/mL

Hep-Forte capsules OTC *geriatric dietary supplement* [multiple vitamins & food products; folic acid; biotin] ≛•60•≟ μg

Hep-Lock; Hep-Lock U/P solution ℞ *IV flush for catheter patency (not therapeutic)* [heparin sodium] 10, 100 U/mL

HEPP (H-chain ε [IgE] pentapeptide) [see: pentigetide]

hepronicate INN

heptabarb INN [also: heptabarbitone]

heptabarbital [see: heptabarb; heptabarbitone]

heptabarbitone BAN [also: heptabarb]

Heptalac syrup (discontinued 1999) ℞ *hyperosmotic laxative* [lactulose] 10 g/15 mL

heptaminol INN, BAN

heptaminol HCl [see: heptaminol]

2-heptanamine [see: tuaminoheptane]

2-heptanamine sulfate [see: tuaminoheptane sulfate]

heptaverine INN

heptolamide INN

Heptovir (CAN) tablets, oral solution ℞ *antiviral nucleoside reverse transcriptase inhibitor for hepatitis B virus (HBV)* [lamivudine] 100 mg; 5 mg/mL

hepzidine INN

HER2 (human epidermal growth factor receptor 2) MAb [see: trastuzumab]

Heracleum lanatum *medicinal herb* [see: masterwort]

herb of grace *medicinal herb* [see: rue]

Herbal Laxative tablets (discontinued 1999) OTC *stimulant laxative* [senna leaves; cascara sagrada bark] 125•20 mg

HercepTest test kit *diagnostic aid for the HER2 protein, used to screen patients who may benefit from treatment with Herceptin*

Herceptin powder for IV infusion ℞ *anti-HER2 monoclonal antibody for metastatic breast cancer; investigational (NDA filed) for ovarian and female genital tract cancers* [trastuzumab] 440 mg

Hercules woundwort *medicinal herb* [see: woundwort]

heroin *potent narcotic analgesic street drug which is highly addictive; banned in the U.S.* [medically known as diacetylmorphine HCl and diamorphine]

heroin HCl *(banned in the U.S.)* [see: diacetylmorphine HCl]

Herpecin-L lip balm OTC *vulnerary; sunblock* [allantoin; padimate O]

herpes simplex virus gene *investigational (orphan) for primary and metastatic brain tumors*

Herpetrol tablets OTC *dietary supplement; claimed to prevent and treat herpes simplex infections* [L-lysine; multiple vitamins; zinc]

Herplex eye drops (discontinued 1997) ℞ *ophthalmic antiviral* [idoxuridine] 0.1%

Herrick Lacrimal Plug ℞ *blocks the puncta and canaliculus to eliminate tear loss in keratitis sicca* [silicone plug]

HES (hydroxyethyl starch) [see: hetastarch]

Hespan IV infusion ℞ *plasma volume expander for shock due to hemorrhage, burns, surgery* [hetastarch] 6 g/100 mL ⊠ Histatan

hesperidin *a bioflavonoid (q.v.)*

hesperidin methyl chalcone [see: bioflavonoids]

hetacillin USAN, USP, INN, BAN *antibacterial*

hetacillin potassium USAN, USP *antibacterial*

hetaflur USAN, INN, BAN *dental caries prophylactic*

hetastarch USAN, BAN *plasma volume extender* [also: hydroxyethylstarch] 6% in normal saline

heteronium bromide USAN, INN, BAN *anticholinergic*

Hetrazan tablets (available for compassionate use only) ℞ *anthelmintic for Bancroft filariasis, onchocerciasis, tropical eosinophilia, and loiasis* [diethylcarbamazine citrate] 50 mg

hexaammonium molybdate tetrahydrate [see: ammonium molybdate]

Hexabrix injection ℞ *radiopaque contrast medium* [ioxaglate meglumine; ioxaglate sodium (54.3% total iodine)] 393•196 mg/mL (320 mg/mL)

HexaCAF; Hexa-CAF (hexamethylmelamine, cyclophosphamide, amethopterin, fluorouracil) *chemotherapy protocol for ovarian cancer*

hexacarbacholine bromide INN [also: carbolonium bromide]

hexachlorane [see: lindane]

hexachlorocyclohexane [see: lindane]

hexachlorophane BAN *topical anti-infective; detergent* [also: hexachlorophene]

hexachlorophene USP, INN *topical anti-infective; detergent* [also: hexachlorophane]

hexacyclonate sodium INN

hexacyprone INN

hexadecanoic acid, methylethyl ester [see: isopropyl palmitate]

hexadecanol [see: cetyl alcohol]

hexadecylamine hydrofluoride [see: hetaflur]

hexadecylpyridinium chloride [see: cetylpyridinium chloride]

hexadecyltrimethylammonium bromide [see: cetrimonium bromide]

hexadecyltrimethylammonium chloride [see: cetrimonium chloride]

2,4-hexadienoic acid, potassium salt [see: potassium sorbate]

hexadiline INN

hexadimethrine bromide INN, BAN

hexadiphane [see: prozapine]

Hexadrol tablets, elixir ℞ *corticosteroid; anti-inflammatory* [dexamethasone] 1.5, 4 mg; 0.5 mg/5 mL ⊠ Hexalol

Hexadrol Phosphate intra-articular, intralesional, soft tissue, or IM injection ℞ *corticosteroid; anti-inflammatory* [dexamethasone sodium phosphate] 4, 10, 20 mg/mL

hexadylamine [see: hexadiline]

hexafluorenium bromide USAN, USP *skeletal muscle relaxant; succinylcholine synergist* [also: hexafluronium bromide]

hexafluorodiethyl ether [see: flurothyl]

hexaflurone bromide [see: hexafluorenium bromide]

hexafluronium bromide INN *skeletal muscle relaxant; succinylcholine synergist* [also: hexafluorenium bromide]

Hexalen capsules ℞ *antineoplastic for advanced ovarian adenocarcinoma (orphan)* [altretamine] 50 mg ⓓ Hexalol
hexamarium bromide [see: distigmine bromide]
hexametazime BAN
hexamethone bromide [see: hexamethonium bromide]
hexamethonium bromide INN, BAN
hexamethylenamine [now: methenamine]
hexamethylenamine mandelate [see: methenamine mandelate]
hexamethylenetetramine [see: methenamine]
hexamethylmelamine (HMM; HXM) [see: altretamine]
hexamidine INN
hexamine hippurate BAN *urinary antibacterial* [also: methenamine hippurate]
hexamine mandelate [see: methenamine mandelate]
hexapradol INN
hexaprofen INN, BAN
hexapropymate INN, BAN
hexasonium iodide INN
hexavitamin USP
Hexavitamin tablets OTC *vitamin supplement* [multiple vitamins] ≛
hexcarbacholine bromide INN [also: carbolonium bromide]
hexedine USAN, INN *antibacterial*
hexemal [see: cyclobarbital]
hexestrol NF, INN
hexetidine BAN
hexicide [see: lindane]
hexinol [see: cyclomenol]
hexobarbital USP, INN
hexobarbital sodium NF
hexobendine USAN, INN, BAN *vasodilator*
hexocyclium methylsulfate *peptic ulcer adjunct* [also: hexocyclium metilsulfate; hexocyclium methylsulphate]
hexocyclium methylsulphate BAN [also: hexocyclium methylsulfate; hexocyclium metilsulfate]
hexocyclium metilsulfate INN [also: hexocyclium methylsulfate; hexocyclium methylsulphate]
hexoprenaline INN, BAN *tocolytic; bronchodilator* [also: hexoprenaline sulfate]
hexoprenaline sulfate USAN, JAN *tocolytic; bronchodilator* [also: hexoprenaline]
hexopyrimidine [see: hexetidine]
hexopyrrolate [see: hexopyrronium bromide]
hexopyrronium bromide INN
Hextend ℞ *investigational (NDA filed) blood plasma volume expander for surgical blood loss*
hexydaline [see: methenamine mandelate]
hexylcaine INN *local anesthetic* [also: hexylcaine HCl]
hexylcaine HCl USP *local anesthetic* [also: hexylcaine]
hexylene glycol NF *humectant; solvent*
hexylresorcinol USP *anthelmintic; topical antiseptic*
1-hexyltheobromine [see: pentifylline]
H-F Gel ℞ *investigational (orphan) emergency treatment for hydrofluoric acid burns* [calcium gluconate]
HFA-134a (hydrofluoroalkane) *propellant used in CFC-free aerosol delivery systems*
hFSH (human follicle-stimulating hormone) [now: menotropins]
HFZ (homofenazine) [q.v.]
^{197}Hg [see: chlormerodrin Hg 197]
^{197}Hg [see: merisoprol acetate Hg 197]
^{197}Hg [see: merisoprol Hg 197]
^{203}Hg [see: chlormerodrin Hg 203]
^{203}Hg [see: merisoprol acetate Hg 203]
hGH (human growth hormone) [see: somatropin]
HGP-30W *investigational (Phase II) vaccine for HIV*
HGP-30W & sargramostim *investigational (Phase I) combination for HIV infection*
HI-236 *investigational for multidrug-resistant HIV infection*

hibenzate INN *combining name for radicals or groups* [also: hybenzate]

Hibiclens sponge/brush OTC *broad-spectrum antimicrobial; germicidal* [chlorhexidine gluconate; alcohol 4%] 4%

Hibiclens Antiseptic/AntiMicrobial Skin Cleanser liquid OTC *broad-spectrum antimicrobial; germicidal* [chlorhexidine gluconate; alcohol 4%] 4%

hibiscus (*Hibiscus sabdariffa* and other species) flowers and leaves *medicinal herb for cancer, edema, heart problems and nervous disorders; also used topically as an emollient; not generally regarded as safe and effective*

Hibistat Germicidal Hand Rinse liquid OTC *broad-spectrum antimicrobial; germicidal* [chlorhexidine gluconate; alcohol 70%] 0.5%

Hibistat Towelette OTC *broad-spectrum antimicrobial; germicidal* [chlorhexidine gluconate; alcohol 70%] 0.5%

HibTITER IM injection ℞ *pediatric (2–71 months) vaccine for Haemophilus influenzae type b (HIB)* [Hemophilus b conjugate vaccine (with a diphtheria CRM_{197} carrier)] 10•(25) µg/0.5 mL

Hi-Cal VM nutrition bar OTC *enteral nutritional therapy for HIV and AIDS*

Hi-Cor 1.0; Hi-Cor 2.5 cream ℞ *topical corticosteroidal anti-inflammatory* [hydrocortisone] 1%; 2.5%

HIDA (hepatoiminodiacetic acid) [see: lidofenin]

HiDAC (high-dose ara-C) *chemotherapy protocol*

Hieracium pilosella *medicinal herb* [see: mouse ear]

high angelica *medicinal herb* [see: angelica]

high molecular weight dextran [see: dextran 70]

high osmolar contrast media (HOCM) *a class of older radiopaque agents that have a high osmolar concentration of iodine (the contrast agent), which corresponds to a higher incidence of adverse reactions* [also called: ionic contrast media]

High Potency N-Vites tablets OTC *vitamin supplement* [multiple B vitamins; vitamin C] ≛•500 mg

High Potency Tar gel shampoo OTC *antiseborrheic; antipsoriatic; antipruritic; antibacterial* [coal tar] 25%

hilafilcon A USAN *hydrophilic contact lens material*

hilafilcon B USAN *hydrophilic contact lens material*

hillberry *medicinal herb* [see: wintergreen]

Himalayan ginseng (*Panax pseudoginseng*) *medicinal herb* [see: ginseng]

hindheel *medicinal herb* [see: tansy]

hini *medicinal herb* [see: Culver root]

hioxifilcon A USAN *hydrophilic contact lens material*

Hipotest tablets OTC *dietary supplement* [multiple vitamins & minerals; multiple food products; calcium; iron; biotin] ≛•53.5•50•0.001 mg

Hi-Po-Vites tablets OTC *dietary supplement* [multiple vitamins & minerals; multiple food products; iron; folic acid; biotin] ≛•6•0.4•1 mg

Hiprex tablets ℞ *urinary antibiotic* [methenamine hippurate] 1 g

Hirudo medicinalis *natural treatment* [see: leeches]

Hirulog ℞ *investigational (NDA filed) antithrombotic for DVT and unstable angina, and to prevent reocclusion in MI and angioplasty* [bivalirudin]

Hismanal tablets (discontinued 1999) ℞ *nonsedating antihistamine for allergic rhinitis and chronic idiopathic urticaria* [astemizole] 10 mg

Histade extended-release capsules ℞ *decongestant; antihistamine* [phenylpropanolamine HCl; chlorpheniramine maleate] 75•12 mg

Histagesic Modified tablets OTC *decongestant; antihistamine; analgesic* [phenylephrine HCl; chlorpheniramine maleate; acetaminophen] 10•4•324 mg

Histalet syrup ℞ *decongestant; antihistamine* [pseudoephedrine HCl; chlorpheniramine maleate] 45•3 mg/5 mL

Histalet Forte tablets ℞ *decongestant; antihistamine* [phenylpropanolamine HCl; phenylephrine HCl; chlorpheniramine maleate; pyrilamine maleate] 50•10•4•25 mg

Histalet X tablets, syrup ℞ *decongestant; expectorant* [pseudoephedrine HCl; guaifenesin] 120•400 mg; 45•200 mg/5 mL

histamine dihydrochloride USAN

histamine H_1 antagonists *a class of antihistamines* [also called: H_1 blockers]

histamine H_2 antagonists *a class of antihistamines* [also called: H_2 blockers]

histamine phosphate USP *gastric secretory stimulant; diagnostic aid for pheochromocytoma*

histantin [see: chlorcyclizine HCl]

histapyrrodine INN

Histatab Plus tablets OTC *decongestant; antihistamine* [phenylephrine HCl; chlorpheniramine maleate] 5•2 mg

Hista-Vadrin tablets ℞ *decongestant; antihistamine* [phenylpropanolamine HCl; phenylephrine HCl; chlorpheniramine maleate] 40•5•6 mg

Histerone 100 IM injection (discontinued 2001) ℞ *androgen replacement for delayed puberty or breast cancer* [testosterone] 100 mg/mL

Histex HC syrup ℞ *narcotic antitussive; decongestant; antihistamine* [hydrocodone bitartrate; pseudoephedrine maleate; carbinoxamine maleate] 2.5•30•2 mg/5 mL

Histex PD oral liquid ℞ *antihistamine for allergic rhinitis* [carbinoxamine maleate] 2 mg/5 mL

Histex SR film-coated, sustained-release tablets ℞ *decongestant; antihistamine; analgesic* [phenylephrine HCl; chlorpheniramine maleate; acetaminophen] 40•8•500 mg

histidine (L-histidine) USAN, USP, INN *amino acid (essential in infants and in renal failure, nonessential otherwise); symbols: His, H*

histidine monohydrochloride NF

495-L-histidineglucosylceramidase [see: imiglucerase]

Histine DM; Histinex DM syrup ℞ *antitussive; decongestant; antihistamine* [dextromethorphan hydrobromide; phenylpropanolamine HCl; brompheniramine maleate] 10•12.5•2 mg/5 mL

Histinex HC syrup ℞ *narcotic antitussive; decongestant; antihistamine* [hydrocodone bitartrate; phenylephrine HCl; chlorpheniramine maleate] 2.5•5•2 mg/5 mL

Histinex PV syrup ℞ *narcotic antitussive; decongestant; antihistamine* [hydrocodone bitartrate; pseudoephedrine HCl; chlorpheniramine maleate] 2.5•30•2 mg/5 mL

Histolyn-CYL intradermal injection ℞ *diagnostic aid for histoplasmosis* [histoplasmin (mycelial derivative)] 1:100

histoplasmin USP *dermal histoplasmosis test; Histoplasma capsulatum cultures in mycelial or yeast lysate form* 1:100 injection (yeast lysate form)

Histor-D syrup ℞ *decongestant; antihistamine* [phenylephrine HCl; chlorpheniramine maleate; alcohol 2%] 5•2 mg/5 mL

Histosal tablets OTC *decongestant; antihistamine; analgesic* [phenylpropanolamine HCl; pyrilamine maleate; acetaminophen; caffeine] 20•12.5•324•30 mg

histrelin USAN, INN *LH-RH agonist; investigational (orphan) for acute intermittent porphyria, hereditary coproporphyria, and variegate porphyria*

histrelin acetate *LH-RH agonist; central precocious puberty treatment (orphan)*

Histussin D oral liquid ℞ *narcotic antitussive; decongestant* [hydrocodone bitartrate; pseudoephedrine HCl] 5•60 mg/5 mL

Histussin HC syrup ℞ *narcotic antitussive; decongestant; antihistamine* [hydrocodone bitartrate; phenylephrine HCl; chlorpheniramine maleate] 2.5•5•2 mg/5 mL

HIV immune globulin (HIVIG) *investigational (Phase III, orphan)*

immunomodulator for AIDS and maternal/fetal HIV transfer

HIV immunotherapeutic (HIV-IT); HIV therapeutic *investigational (Phase II) gene therapy for HIV; investigational (Phase I–III) antiviral for symptomatic HIV*

HIV protease inhibitors *a class of antivirals that block HIV replication*

HIV vaccine [see: AIDS vaccine]

HIV-1 LA test [see: Recombigen HIV-1 LA]

HIV-1 peptide vaccine *investigational (Phase I) vaccine for HIV*

HIVAB HIV-1 EIA; HIVAB HIV-1/HIV-2 EIA; HIVAB HIV-2 EIA reagent kit for professional use *in vitro diagnostic aid for HIV antibodies* [enzyme immunoassay (EIA)]

HIVAG-1 reagent kit for professional use *in vitro diagnostic aid for HIV antibodies* [enzyme immunoassay (EIA)]

hive vine *medicinal herb* [see: squaw vine]

Hi-Vegi-Lip tablets OTC *digestive enzymes* [pancreatin; lipase; protease; amylase] 2400 mg•4800 U•60 000 U•60 000 U

Hivid film-coated tablets ℞ *nucleoside reverse transcriptase inhibitor (NRTI) antiviral for HIV infection (orphan)* [zalcitabine] 0.375, 0.75 mg

HIV-IG ℞ *investigational (Phase III, orphan) immunomodulator for AIDS and maternal/fetal HIV transfer* [HIV immune globulin]

HIV-neutralizing antibodies *orphan status withdrawn 1997*

HK-Cardiosol *investigational heart preservation solution*

HMB (homatropine methylbromide) [q.v.]

HMDP (hydroxymethylene diphosphonate) [see: oxidronic acid]

hMG (human menopausal gonadotropin) [see: menotropins]

HMG-CoA (3-hydroxy-3-methylglutaryl-coenzyme A) reductase inhibitors *a class of antihyperlipidemics that reduce serum LDL, VLDL, and triglycerides, but increase HDL* [also called: "statins"]

HMM (hexamethylmelamine) [see: altretamine]

HMR 3480 *investigational anti-inflammatory agent*

HMR 4004 *investigational (Phase II) gene-modified T-lymphocytes for HIV and AIDS*

HMR-3647 *investigational (Phase III) ketolide antibiotic for community-acquired pneumonia (CAP)*

HMS eye drop suspension ℞ *corticosteroidal anti-inflammatory* [medrysone] 1%

HN_2 (nitrogen mustard) [see: mechlorethamine HCl]

HNK-20 *investigational (Phase III) monoclonal IgA antibody for respiratory syncytial virus (RSV) infections in infants; investigational (Phase III) nose drops for prevention of viral pneumonia in infants*

HOAP-BLEO (hydroxydaunomycin, Oncovin, ara-C, prednisone, bleomycin) *chemotherapy protocol*

hoarhound *medicinal herb* [see: horehound]

hock heal *medicinal herb* [see: woundwort]

hog apple *medicinal herb* [see: mandrake; noni]

hogweed *medicinal herb* [see: broom; masterwort]

Hold DM; Children's Hold lozenges OTC *antitussive* [dextromethorphan hydrobromide] 5 mg

holly *(Ilex aquifolium; I. opaca; I. vomitoria)* leaves and berries *medicinal herb used as a CNS stimulant and emetic; not generally regarded as safe and effective*

holly, ground *medicinal herb* [see: pipsissewa]

holly bay *medicinal herb* [see: magnolia]

holly-leaved barberry; holly mahonia *medicinal herb* [see: Oregon grape]

holmium *element (Ho)*

holmium-166 DOTMP *investigational (Phase III) skeletal targeted radiotherapy agent for treatment of multiple myeloma*

holy thistle; blessed cardus *medicinal herb* [see: blessed thistle]

homarylamine INN

homatropine BAN *ophthalmic anticholinergic* [also: homatropine hydrobromide]

homatropine hydrobromide USP *ophthalmic anticholinergic; cycloplegic; mydriatic* [also: homatropine] 5% eye drops

homatropine methylbromide USP, INN, BAN *anticholinergic*

Home Access; Home Access Express test kit for home use *in vitro diagnostic aid for HIV in the blood*

Home Access Hepatitis C Check test kit for home use *in vitro diagnostic aid for hepatitis C in the blood*

homidium bromide INN, BAN

Hominex-1 powder OTC *formula for infants with homocystinuria or hypermethioninemia*

Hominex-2 powder OTC *enteral nutritional therapy for homocystinuria or hypermethioninemia*

homochlorcyclizine INN, BAN

homofenazine (HFZ) INN

homomenthyl salicylate [see: homosalate]

homopipramol INN

homosalate USAN, INN *ultraviolet sunscreen*

4-homosulfanilamide [see: mafenide]

homprenorphine INN, BAN

honey *natural remedy used as an antibacterial and wound healing agent and as a gargle to promote expectoration; not generally regarded as safe for infants because of possible Clostridium botulinum contamination*

honeybee venom *natural remedy* [see: bee venom]

honeybloom *medicinal herb* [see: dogbane]

hoodwart *medicinal herb* [see: skullcap]

HOP (hydroxydaunomycin, Oncovin, prednisone) *chemotherapy protocol*

hopantenic acid INN

hops *(Humulus lupulus)* flower *medicinal herb for aiding digestion, appetite stimulation, bronchitis, cystitis, delirium, edema, headache, hyperactivity, insomnia, intestinal cramps, menstrual disorders, nervousness, pain, excessive sexual desire, and TB*

hoquizil INN *bronchodilator* [also: hoquizil HCl]

hoquizil HCl USAN *bronchodilator* [also: hoquizil]

Hordeum vulgare *medicinal herb* [see: barley]

horehound *(Marrubium vulgare)* plant *medicinal herb for asthma, colds and cough, croup, inducing diaphoresis and diuresis, intestinal parasites, lung disorders, promoting expectoration, and respiratory disorders*

horse chestnut *(Aesculus californica; A. glabra; A. hippocastanum)* leaves and nuts *medicinal herb for arthritis, colds and congestion, hemorrhoids, rheumatism, and varicose veins; not generally regarded as safe for internal use, as it is highly toxic*

horse-elder; horseheal *medicinal herb* [see: elecampane]

horsefoot; horsehoof *medicinal herb* [see: coltsfoot]

horsemint *(Monarda punctata)* leaves and flowering tops *medicinal herb used as a cardiac, carminative, diaphoretic, diuretic, emmenagogue, stimulant, and sudorific*

horseradish *(Armoracia lapathiofolia; A. rusticana)* root *medicinal herb for appetite stimulation, colic, cough, edema, expelling afterbirth, hay fever, poor circulation, sciatic pain, sinus disorders, and skin and internal tumors; also used as a vermifuge*

horsetail *(Equisetum arvens)* plant *medicinal herb for bladder disorders, brittle nails, glandular disorders, inter-*

nal bleeding, nosebleeds, poor circulation, tuberculosis, and urinary disorders

horseweed; fleabane *(Erigeron canadensis)* plant *medicinal herb used as an astringent, diuretic, and hemostatic*

ho-shou-wu; fo-ti *(Polygonum multiflorum)* root *medicinal herb for atherosclerosis, blood cleansing, constipation, improving liver and kidney function, insomnia, malaria, muscle aches, TB, and weak bones; also used to increase fertility, prevent aging, and promote longevity*

H.P. Acthar Gel IM or subcu injectable gel ℞ *corticosteroid; anti-inflammatory* [corticotropin repository] 40, 80 U/mL

HP-3 *investigational (Phase II) treatment for cystic fibrosis and chronic obstructive pulmonary disease*

HP-4 *investigational (Phase II) treatment for benign prostatic hyperplasia*

HPMCP (hydroxypropyl methylcellulose phthalate) [q.v.]

HPMPC (3-hydroxy-2-phosphonomethoxypropyl cytosine [dihydrate]) [see: cidofovir]

Hp-PAC (CAN) blister packs for daily administration ℞ *multiple products for the eradication of H. pylori* [lansoprazole (delayed-release capsules); clarithromycin (tablets); amoxicillin trihydrate (capsules)] 30•500•500 mg

H-R Lubricating vaginal jelly OTC *lubricant* [hydroxypropyl methylcellulose]

HspE7 *investigational (Phase III, orphan) agent for human papilloma virus–related diseases, including anal dysplasia and recurrent respiratory papillomatosis*

5-HT (5-hydroxytryptamine) [see: serotonin]

HT (human thrombin) [see: thrombin]

HT; 3-HT (3-hydroxytyramine) [see: dopamine]

5-HTP (5-hydroxytryptophan) [see: L-5 hydroxytryptophan]

H-Tuss-D liquid ℞ *narcotic antitussive; decongestant* [hydrocodone bitartrate; pseudoephedrine HCl; alcohol 5%] 5•60 mg/5 mL

HU-1124 *investigational (Phase III) monoclonal antibody for the treatment for psoriasis; investigational (Phase I/II) for transplant rejection*

Hu23F2G *investigational (Phase II) cell adhesion inhibitor for ischemic stroke, acute myocardial infarction, and trauma-induced hemorrhagic shock* [now: rovelizumab]

huckleberry *medicinal herb* [see: bilberry]

HuM291 (human-mouse monoclonal antibody) [now: visilizumab]

Humalog subcu injection, prefilled syringe cartridges, disposable pen injectors ℞ *insulin analogue for diabetes* [insulin lispro, human (rDNA)] 100 U/mL; 150 U/1.5 mL; 300 U/3 mL

Humalog Mix 50/50 subcu injection, prefilled syringe cartridges, disposable pen injectors ℞ *insulin analogue for diabetes* [insulin lispro protamine; insulin lispro, human (rDNA)] 50%•50% (100 U/mL total)

Humalog Mix 75/25 vials, disposable pen injectors ℞ *insulin analogue for diabetes* [insulin lispro protamine; insulin lispro, human (rDNA)] 75%•25% (100 U/mL total)

Humalog Mix25 (CAN) prefilled syringe cartridges, disposable pen injectors ℞ *insulin analogue for diabetes* [insulin lispro protamine; insulin lispro, human (rDNA)] 75%•25% (100 U/mL total)

human acid alpha-glucosidase *investigational (orphan) for glycogen storage disease type II*

human albumin [see: albumin, human]

human amniotic fluid-derived surfactant [see: surfactant, human amniotic-fluid derived]

human antihemophilic factor [see: antihemophilic factor]

human B-type natriuretic peptide (hBNP) [see: nesiritide; nesiritide citrate]

human chorionic gonadotropin (hCG) [see: gonadotropin, chorionic]

human complement receptor [see: complement receptor type I, soluble recombinant human]

human cytomegalovirus immune globulin [see: cytomegalovirus immune globulin, human]

human diploid cell vaccine (HDCV) [see: rabies vaccine]

human epidermal growth factor [see: epidermal growth factor, human]

human fibrinogen [see: fibrinogen, human]

human fibrinolysin [see: fibrinolysin, human]

human follicle-stimulating hormone (hFSH) [now: menotropins]

human growth hormone (hGH) JAN *growth hormone* [also: somatropin]

human growth hormone, recombinant (rhGH) [see: somatropin]

human growth hormone releasing factor (hGH-RF) [see: growth hormone-releasing factor (GH-RF)]

human immunodeficiency virus (HIV-1) immune globulin (HIVIG) [see: HIV immune globulin]

human insulin [see: insulin, human]

human luteinizing hormone, recombinant & menotropins *investigational for chronic anovulation due to hypogonadotropic hypogonadism; orphan status withdrawn 1998*

human menopausal gonadotropin (hMG) [see: menotropins]

human respiratory syncytial virus immune globulin [see: respiratory syncytial virus immune globulin, human]

human serum albumin diethylenetriaminepentaacetic acid (DTPA) technetium (^{99m}Tc) JAN *radioactive agent* [also: technetium Tc 99m pentetate]

human superoxide dismutase (SOD) [see: superoxide dismutase, human]

human T-cell inhibitor [see: muromonab-CD3]

human T-cell lymphotrophic virus type III (HTLV-III) [now: human immunodeficiency virus (HIV)]

Human T-Lymphotropic Virus Type I EIA reagent kit for professional use *in vitro diagnostic aid for HTLV I antibody in serum or plasma* [enzyme immunoassay (EIA)]

Humate-P IV injection ℞ *antihemophilic for von Willebrand disease (orphan)* [antihemophilic factor VIII]

Humatin capsules ℞ *aminoglycoside antibiotic; amebicide* [paromomycin sulfate] 250 mg

Humatrope powder for subcu or IM injection; prefilled cartridges for HumatroPen (self-injection device) ℞ *growth hormone for adults or children with congenital or endogenous growth hormone deficiency, children with Turner syndrome or renal-induced growth failure* [somatropin] 5 mg (15 IU) per vial; 6, 12, 24 mg (18, 36, 72 IU) per cartridge

HumatroPen (trademarked device) *subcu self-injector for Humatrope*

Humegon powder for IM injection ℞ *ovulation stimulant for women; spermatogenesis stimulant for men* [menotropins] 75, 150 IU

Humibid DM sustained-release tablets ℞ *antitussive; expectorant* [dextromethorphan hydrobromide; guaifenesin] 30•600 mg

Humibid DM Sprinkle sustained-release capsules ℞ *antitussive; expectorant* [dextromethorphan hydrobromide; guaifenesin] 15•300 mg

Humibid L.A. sustained-release tablets ℞ *expectorant* [guaifenesin] 600 mg

Humibid Sprinkle sustained-release capsules ℞ *expectorant* [guaifenesin] 300 mg

HuMist nasal mist OTC *nasal moisturizer* [sodium chloride (saline solution)] 0.65%

Humorsol Ocumeter (eye drops) ℞ *antiglaucoma agent; reversible cholinesterase inhibitor miotic* [demecarium bromide] 0.125%, 0.25%

Humulin 30/70 (CAN) subcu injection, prefilled syringe cartridges OTC *antidiabetic* [insulin; isophane insulin] 100 U/mL; 1.5, 3 mL

Humulin 50/50 subcu injection (prefilled cartridges available in Canada) OTC *antidiabetic* [isophane human insulin (rDNA); human insulin (rDNA)] 100 U/mL; (1.5, 3 mL)

Humulin 70/30 subcu injection, prefilled syringe cartridges, disposable pen injectors OTC *antidiabetic* [isophane human insulin (rDNA); human insulin (rDNA)] 100 U/mL; 150 U/1.5 mL; 300 U/3 mL

Humulin L subcu injection OTC *antidiabetic* [human insulin zinc (rDNA)] 100 U/mL

Humulin N subcu injection, prefilled syringe cartridges, disposable pen injectors OTC *antidiabetic* [isophane human insulin (rDNA)] 100 U/mL; 100 U/1.5 mL; 300 U/3 mL

Humulin R subcu injection OTC *antidiabetic* [human insulin (rDNA)] 100 U/mL; 1.5 mL

Humulin R Regular U-500 (concentrated) subcu injection ℞ *antidiabetic* [human insulin (rDNA)] 500 U/mL

Humulin U Ultralente subcu injection OTC *antidiabetic* [extended human insulin zinc (rDNA)] 100 U/mL

Humulin-U (CAN) subcu injection OTC *antidiabetic* [extended insulin zinc (ultralente)] 100 U/mL

Humulus lupulus *medicinal herb* [see: hops]

hurr-burr *medicinal herb* [see: burdock]

Hurricaine spray, liquid, gel OTC *mucous membrane anesthetic* [benzocaine] 20%

HXM (hexamethylmelamine) [see: altretamine]

Hyacne ℞ *investigational (Phase III) acne treatment*

Hyalgan intra-articular injection ℞ *viscoelastic lubricant and "shock absorber" for osteoarthritis and temporomandibular joint syndrome* [hyaluronate sodium] 20 mg/2 mL

hyalosidase INN, BAN

hyaluronate sodium USAN, JAN *ophthalmic surgical aid; treatment for osteoarthritis and TMJ syndrome; veterinary synovitis agent* [also: hyaluronic acid]

hyaluronate sodium & diclofenac potassium *investigational (Phase III) topical treatment for actinic keratosis; clinical trials as a topical analgesic discontinued 1996*

hyaluronic acid BAN *ophthalmic surgical aid; treatment for osteoarthritis and TMJ syndrome; veterinary synovitis agent* [also: hyaluronate sodium]

hyaluronidase USP, INN, BAN *dispersion aid; absorption facilitator*

hyaluronoglucosaminidase [see: hyalosidase]

hyamate [see: buramate]

hybenzate USAN *combining name for radicals or groups* [also: hibenzate]

Hybolin Decanoate-50; Hybolin Decanoate-100 IM injection (discontinued 2000) ℞ *anabolic steroid for anemia of renal insufficiency* [nandrolone decanoate (in oil)] 50 mg/mL; 100 mg/mL

Hybolin Improved IM injection (discontinued 2000) ℞ *anabolic steroid for metastatic breast cancer in women* [nandrolone phenpropionate (in oil)] 50 mg/mL

Hybri-CEAker *orphan status withdrawn 1997* [indium In 111 altumomab pentetate]

Hybrid Capture II Chlamydia Test reagent kit for professional use *in vitro diagnostic aid for Chlamydia trachomatis*

Hycamtin powder for IV injection ℞ *topoisomerase I inhibitor; antineoplastic for ovarian and small cell lung cancers* [topotecan HCl] 4 mg/vial

hycanthone USAN, INN *antischistosomal*

hycanthone mesylate *antischistosomal*

hyclate INN *combining name for radicals or groups*

HyClinda ℞ *investigational (Phase III) antibiotic delivery system* [clindamycin]

HycoClear Tuss syrup ℞ *narcotic antitussive; expectorant* [hydrocodone bitartrate; guaifenesin] 5•100 mg/5 mL

Hycodan tablets, syrup ℞ *narcotic antitussive; anticholinergic* [hydrocodone bitartrate; homatropine methylbromide] 5•1.5 mg; 5•1.5 mg/5 mL ⊠ Hycomine; Vicodin

Hycomine syrup, pediatric syrup ℞ *narcotic antitussive; decongestant* [hydrocodone bitartrate; phenylpropanolamine HCl] 5•25 mg/5 mL; 2.5•12.5 mg/5 mL ⊠ Byclomine; Hycodan; Vicodin

Hycomine Compound tablets ℞ *narcotic antitussive; decongestant; antihistamine; analgesic* [hydrocodone bitartrate; phenylephrine HCl; chlorpheniramine maleate; acetaminophen; caffeine] 5•10•2•250•30 mg

Hycort cream, ointment ℞ *topical corticosteroidal anti-inflammatory* [hydrocortisone] 1%

Hycotuss Expectorant syrup ℞ *narcotic antitussive; expectorant* [hydrocodone bitartrate; guaifenesin; alcohol 10%] 5•100 mg/5 mL

hydantoins *a class of anticonvulsants*

Hydeltrasol IV, IM injection ℞ *corticosteroid; anti-inflammatory* [prednisolone sodium phosphate] 20 mg/mL

Hydeltra-T.B.A. intra-articular, intralesional, or soft tissue injection (discontinued 1997) ℞ *corticosteroid; anti-inflammatory* [prednisolone tebutate] 20 mg/mL

Hydergine sublingual tablets, tablets, liquid ℞ *cognition adjuvant for age-related mental capacity decline* [ergoloid mesylates] 0.5, 1 mg; 1 mg; 1 mg/mL ⊠ Hydramine

Hydergine LC liquid capsules ℞ *cognition adjuvant for age-related mental capacity decline* [ergoloid mesylates] 1 mg

hydracarbazine INN

hydragogues *a class of purgatives that produce abundant watery discharge from the bowels*

hydralazine INN, BAN *antihypertensive; peripheral vasodilator* [also: hydralazine HCl]

hydralazine HCl USP, JAN *antihypertensive; peripheral vasodilator* [also: hydralazine] 10, 25, 50, 100 mg oral; 20 mg/mL injection

hydralazine polistirex USAN *antihypertensive*

Hydramyn syrup (discontinued 1997) ℞ *antihistamine; antitussive* [diphenhydramine HCl; alcohol 5%] 12.5 mg/5 mL ⊠ Hydramine; Hytramyn

hydrangea ***(Hydrangea arborescens)*** leaves and root *medicinal herb for arthritis, bladder infections, gallstones, gonorrhea, gout, kidney stones, rheumatism, and urinary disorders*

Hydrap-ES tablets ℞ *antihypertensive; vasodilator; diuretic* [hydrochlorothiazide; reserpine; hydralazine HCl] 15•0.1•25 mg

hydrargaphen INN, BAN

hydrastine USP

hydrastine HCl USP

hydrastinine HCl NF

Hydrastis canadensis *medicinal herb* [see: goldenseal]

Hydrate IV or IM injection ℞ *antinauseant; antiemetic; antivertigo; motion sickness preventative* [dimenhydrinate] 50 mg/mL

hydrazinecarboximidamide monohydrochloride [see: pimagedine HCl]

hydrazinoxane [see: domoxin]

Hydrea capsules ℞ *antineoplastic for melanoma, ovarian carcinoma, myelocytic leukemia, and squamous cell carcinoma; sickle cell anemia treatment (orphan)* [hydroxyurea] 500 mg

Hydrisea lotion OTC *moisturizer; emollient* [Dead Sea salts]

Hydrisinol cream, lotion OTC *moisturizer; emollient*

Hydro Cobex IM injection ℞ *antianemic; vitamin B_{12} supplement* [hydroxocobalamin] 1000 µg/mL

hydrobentizide INN

hydrobutamine [see: butidrine]

Hydrocare Cleaning and Disinfecting solution OTC *chemical disinfecting solution for soft contact lenses*

Hydrocare Preserved Saline solution OTC *rinsing/storage solution for soft contact lenses* [sodium chloride (preserved saline solution)]

Hydrocet capsules ℞ *narcotic analgesic* [hydrocodone bitartrate; acetaminophen] 5•500 mg

hydrochloric acid NF *acidifying agent*

hydrochloric acid, diluted NF *acidifying agent*

hydrochlorothiazide (HCT; HCTZ) USP, INN, BAN *antihypertensive; diuretic* 12.5, 25, 50, 100 mg oral; 50 mg/5 mL oral; 100 mg/mL oral

hydrochlorothiazide & bisoprolol fumarate *antihypertensive; diuretic; β-blocker* 6.5•2.5, 6.5•5, 6.5•10 mg oral

hydrochlorothiazide & captopril *antihypertensive; diuretic; angiotensin-converting enzyme (ACE) inhibitor* 15•25, 25•25, 15•50, 25•50 mg oral

hydrochlorothiazide & enalapril maleate *antihypertensive; diuretic; angiotensin-converting enzyme (ACE) inhibitor* 12.5•5, 25•10 mg oral

hydrochlorothiazide & triamterene *antihypertensive; potassium-sparing diuretic* 25•37.5 mg oral

hydrocholeretics *a class of gastrointestinal drugs that exert laxative effects and increase volume and water content of bile actions*

Hydrocil Instant powder OTC *bulk laxative* [psyllium hydrophilic mucilloid] 3.5 g/scoop

hydrocodone INN, BAN *antitussive* [also: hydrocodone bitartrate]

hydrocodone bitartrate USAN, USP *antitussive* [also: hydrocodone]

hydrocodone bitartrate & acetaminophen *antitussive; analgesic* 7.5•650, 10•325, 10•500, 10•650, 10•660 mg oral; 2.5•167 mg/5 mL oral

hydrocodone bitartrate & guaifenesin *antitussive; expectorant* 5•100 mg/5 mL oral

Hydrocodone Compound syrup ℞ *narcotic antitussive; anticholinergic* [hydrocodone bitartrate; homatropine hydrobromide] 5•1.5 mg/5 mL

Hydrocodone CP; Hydrocodone HD oral liquid ℞ *narcotic antitussive; decongestant; antihistamine* [hydrocodone bitartrate; phenylephrine HCl; chlorpheniramine maleate] 2.5•5•2 mg/5 mL; 1.67•5•2 mg/5 mL

Hydrocodone GF syrup ℞ *narcotic antitussive; expectorant* [hydrocodone bitartrate; guaifenesin] 5•100 mg/5 mL

Hydrocodone PA syrup, pediatric syrup ℞ *narcotic antitussive; decongestant* [hydrocodone bitartrate; phenylpropanolamine HCl] 5•25 mg/5 mL; 2.5•12.5 mg/5 mL

hydrocodone polistirex USAN *antitussive*

Hydrocol adhesive dressings *occlusive wound dressing* [hydrocolloid gel]

hydrocolloid gel *dressings for wet wounds*

Hydrocort cream ℞ *topical corticosteroidal anti-inflammatory* [hydrocortisone] 2.5%

hydrocortamate INN

hydrocortamate HCl [see: hydrocortamate]

hydrocortisone (HC) USP, INN, BAN *corticosteroid; anti-inflammatory* 5, 10, 20 mg oral; 0.5%, 1%, 2.5% topical

hydrocortisone aceponate INN *corticosteroid; anti-inflammatory*

hydrocortisone acetate (HCA) USP, BAN *corticosteroid; anti-inflammatory* 25, 50 mg/mL injection; 1% topical

hydrocortisone buteprate USAN *topical corticosteroidal anti-inflammatory*

hydrocortisone butyrate BAN *topical corticosteroidal anti-inflammatory* [also: hydrocortisone probutate]

hydrocortisone cyclopentylpropionate *corticosteroid; anti-inflammatory* [see: hydrocortisone cypionate]

hydrocortisone cypionate USP *corticosteroid; anti-inflammatory*

hydrocortisone hemisuccinate USP *corticosteroid; anti-inflammatory*

Hydrocortisone Iodoquinol 1% cream ℞ *corticosteroidal anti-inflammatory; amebicide; antimicrobial* [hydrocortisone; iodoquinol] 1%•1%

hydrocortisone probutate USAN, USP *topical corticosteroidal anti-inflammatory* [also: hydrocortisone buteprate]

hydrocortisone sodium phosphate USP, BAN *corticosteroid; anti-inflammatory*

hydrocortisone sodium succinate USP, BAN *corticosteroid; anti-inflammatory*

hydrocortisone valerate USAN, USP *topical corticosteroidal anti-inflammatory* 0.2% topical

Hydrocortone tablets ℞ *corticosteroid; anti-inflammatory* [hydrocortisone] 10, 20 mg

Hydrocortone Acetate intralesional, intra-articular, or soft tissue injection ℞ *corticosteroid; anti-inflammatory* [hydrocortisone acetate] 25, 50 mg/mL

Hydrocortone Phosphate IV, subcu, or IM injection ℞ *corticosteroid; anti-inflammatory* [hydrocortisone sodium phosphate] 50 mg/mL

Hydrocotyle asiatica *medicinal herb* [see: gotu kola]

Hydrocream Base OTC *cream base*

Hydro-Crysti 12 IM injection ℞ *antianemic; vitamin B_{12} supplement* [hydroxocobalamin] 1000 µg/mL

HydroDIURIL tablets ℞ *antihypertensive; diuretic* [hydrochlorothiazide] 25, 50, 100 mg

hydrofilcon A USAN *hydrophilic contact lens material*

hydroflumethiazide USP, INN, BAN *antihypertensive; diuretic* 50 mg oral

hydrofluoric acid *dental caries prophylactic*

hydrofluoroalkane (HFA) *propellant used in CFC-free aerosol delivery systems* [usually HFA-134a]

hydrogen *element (H)*

hydrogen peroxide USP *topical anti-infective*

hydrogen tetrabromoaurate [see: bromauric acid]

hydrogenated ergot alkaloids [now: ergoloid mesylates]

hydrogenated vegetable oil [see: vegetable oil, hydrogenated]

Hydrogesic capsules ℞ *narcotic analgesic* [hydrocodone bitartrate; acetaminophen] 5•500 mg

hydromadinone INN

Hydromet syrup ℞ *narcotic antitussive; anticholinergic* [hydrocodone bitartrate; homatropine methylbromide] 5•1.5 mg/5 mL

hydromorphinol INN, BAN

hydromorphone INN, BAN *narcotic analgesic; widely abused as a street drug* [also: hydromorphone HCl]

hydromorphone HCl USP *narcotic analgesic; widely abused as a street drug* [also: hydromorphone] 2, 4, 8 mg oral; 5 mg/5 mL oral; 3 mg rectal; 1, 2, 4, 10 mg/mL injection

hydromorphone sulfate

Hydromox tablets ℞ *diuretic; antihypertensive* [quinethazone] 50 mg

Hydro-Par tablets ℞ *antihypertensive; diuretic* [hydrochlorothiazide] 25, 50 mg

Hydro-PC oral liquid ℞ *narcotic antitussive; decongestant; antihistamine* [hydrocodone bitartrate; phenylephrine HCl; chlorpheniramine maleate] 2•5•2 mg/5 mL

Hydropel ointment OTC *skin protectant* [silicone; hydrophobic starch derivative] 30%•10%

Hydrophed tablets ℞ *antiasthmatic; bronchodilator; decongestant; antihistamine* [theophylline; ephedrine sulfate; hydroxyzine HCl] 130•25•10 mg

Hydrophilic OTC *ointment base*

hydrophilic ointment [see: ointment, hydrophilic]

hydrophilic petrolatum [see: petrolatum, hydrophilic]

Hydropres-50 tablets ℞ *antihypertensive; diuretic* [hydrochlorothiazide; reserpine] 50•0.125 mg

hydroquinone USP *hyperpigmentation bleaching agent* 3%, 4% topical

hydroquinone methyl ether [see: mequinol]

Hydro-Serp tablets ℞ *antihypertensive; diuretic* [hydrochlorothiazide; reserpine] 50•0.125 mg

Hydroserpine #1; Hydroserpine #2 tablets ℞ *antihypertensive; diuretic* [hydrochlorothiazide; reserpine] 25•0.125 mg; 50•0.125 mg

HydroSkin cream, ointment, lotion OTC *topical corticosteroidal anti-inflammatory* [hydrocortisone acetate] 1%

HydroStat IR tablets (discontinued 1999) ℞ *narcotic analgesic* [hydromorphone HCl] 1, 2, 3, 4 mg

hydrotalcite INN, BAN

HydroTex cream ℞ *topical corticosteroidal anti-inflammatory* [hydrocortisone] 0.5%

hydroxamethocaine BAN [also: hydroxytetracaine]

hydroxidione sodium succinate [see: hydroxydione sodium succinate]

hydroxindasate INN

hydroxindasol INN

hydroxizine chloride [see: hydroxyzine HCl]

hydroxocobalamin USAN, USP, INN, BAN, JAN *vitamin B_{12}; hematopoietic* [also: hydroxocobalamin acetate] 1 mg/mL injection

hydroxocobalamin acetate JAN *vitamin B_{12}; hematopoietic* [also: hydroxocobalamin]

hydroxocobalamin & sodium thiosulfate *investigational (orphan) for severe acute cyanide poisoning*

hydroxocobemine [see: hydroxocobalamin]

3-hydroxy-2-phosphonomethoxypropyl cytosine (HPMPC) dihydrate [see: cidofovir]

N-hydroxyacetamide [see: acetohydroxamic acid]

4′-hydroxyacetanilide [see: acetaminophen]

4′-hydroxyacetanilide salicylate [see: acetaminosalol]

hydroxyamfetamine INN *ophthalmic adrenergic; mydriatic* [also: hydroxyamphetamine hydrobromide; hydroxyamphetamine]

hydroxyamphetamine BAN *ophthalmic adrenergic; mydriatic* [also: hydroxyamphetamine hydrobromide; hydroxyamfetamine]

hydroxyamphetamine hydrobromide USP *ophthalmic adrenergic/vasoconstrictor; mydriatic* [also: hydroxyamfetamine; hydroxyamphetamine]

4-hydroxyanisole (4HA); *p*-hydroxyanisole [see: mequinol]

hydroxyapatite BAN *prosthetic aid* [also: durapatite; calcium phosphate, tribasic]

2-hydroxybenzamide [see: salicylamide]

2-hydroxybenzoic acid [see: salicylic acid]

***o*-hydroxybenzyl alcohol** [see: salicyl alcohol]

hydroxybutanedioic acid [see: malic acid]

4-hydroxybutanoic acid [see: gamma hydroxybutyrate (GHB)]

4-hydroxybutanoic acid, sodium salt [see: sodium oxybate]

hydroxybutyrate sodium, gamma [see: sodium oxybate]

hydroxycarbamide INN *antineoplastic* [also: hydroxyurea]

hydroxychloroquine INN, BAN *antimalarial; lupus erythematosus suppressant* [also: hydroxychloroquine sulfate]

hydroxychloroquine sulfate USP *antimalarial; antirheumatic; lupus erythematosus suppressant* [also: hydroxychloroquine] 200 mg oral

25-hydroxycholecalciferol [see: calcifediol]

hydroxycincophene [see: oxycinchophen]

hydroxydaunomycin [see: doxorubicin]

14-hydroxydihydromorphine [see: hydromorphinol]

hydroxydione sodium succinate INN, BAN

1α-hydroxyergocalciferol [see: doxercalciferol]

hydroxyethyl cellulose NF *suspending and viscosity-increasing agent; ophthalmic aid*

2-hydroxyethyl methacrylate (HEMA) *contact lens material* [see: ocufilcon A–F]

hydroxyethyl starch (HES) [see: hetastarch]

hydroxyethylstarch JAN *plasma volume extender* [also: hetastarch]

hydroxyhexamide

hydroxylapatite [see: durapatite; calcium phosphate, tribasic]

hydroxymagnesium aluminate [see: magaldrate]

hydroxymesterone [see: medrysone]

hydroxymethylene diphosphonate (HMDP) [see: oxidronic acid]

hydroxymethylgramicidin [see: methocidin]

N-hydroxynaphthalimide diethyl phosphate [see: naftalofos]

hydroxypethidine INN, BAN

hydroxyphenamate USAN *minor tranquilizer* [also: oxyfenamate]

N-4-hydroxyphenylretinamide [see: fenretinide]

hydroxyprocaine INN, BAN

hydroxyprogesterone INN, BAN *progestin for amenorrhea, metrorrhagia, and dysfunctional uterine bleeding* [also: hydroxyprogesterone caproate]

hydroxyprogesterone caproate USP, INN, JAN *progestin for amenorrhea, metrorrhagia, and dysfunctional uterine bleeding* [also: hydroxyprogesterone] 125, 250 mg/mL IM injection (in oil)

2-hydroxypropanoic acid, calcium salt, hydrate [see: calcium lactate]

hydroxypropyl cellulose NF *topical protectant; emulsifying and coating agent* [also: hydroxypropylcellulose]

hydroxypropyl methylcellulose USP *suspending and viscosity-increasing agent; ophthalmic moisturizer and surgical aid* [also: hypromellose; hydroxypropylmethylcellulose]

hydroxypropyl methylcellulose 1828 USP

hydroxypropyl methylcellulose phthalate (HPMCP) NF *tablet-coating agent* [also: hydroxypropylmethylcellulose phthalate]

hydroxypropyl methylcellulose phthalate 200731 NF *tablet-coating agent*

hydroxypropyl methylcellulose phthalate 220824 NF *tablet-coating agent*

hydroxypropylcellulose JAN *topical protectant; emulsifying and coating agent* [also: hydroxypropyl cellulose]

hydroxypropylmethylcellulose JAN *suspending and viscosity-increasing agent; ophthalmic surgical aid* [also: hydroxypropyl methylcellulose; hypromellose]

hydroxypropylmethylcellulose phthalate JAN *tablet-coating agent* [also: hydroxypropyl methylcellulose phthalate]

hydroxypyridine tartrate INN

hydroxyquinoline *topical antiseptic*

4′-hydroxysalicylanilide [see: osalmid]

hydroxystearin sulfate NF

hydroxystenozole INN

hydroxystilbamidine INN, BAN *antileishmanial* [also: hydroxystilbamidine isethionate]

hydroxystilbamidine isethionate USP *antileishmanial* [also: hydroxystilbamidine]

hydroxysuccinic acid [see: malic acid]

hydroxytetracaine INN [also: hydroxamethocaine]

hydroxytoluic acid INN, BAN

5-hydroxytryptamine$_1$ (5-HT$_1$) [see: serotonin]

5-hydroxytryptamine$_3$ (5-HT$_3$) receptor antagonists *a class of antinauseant and antiemetic agents used primarily after emetogenic cancer chemotherapy*

5-hydroxytryptophan (5-HTP) [see: L-5 hydroxytryptophan]

3-hydroxytyramine (HT; 3-HT) [see: dopamine]

hydroxyurea USAN, USP, BAN *antimetabolite antineoplastic; sickle cell anemia treatment (orphan); investigational adjunctive therapy for HIV* [also: hydroxycarbamide] 250, 500 mg oral

1α-hydroxyvitamin D_2 [see: doxercalciferol]

hydroxyzine INN, BAN *anxiolytic; minor tranquilizer; antiemetic; piperazine antihistamine; antipruritic* [also: hydroxyzine HCl]

hydroxyzine HCl USP *anxiolytic; minor tranquilizer; antiemetic; piperazine antihistamine; antipruritic* [also: hydroxyzine] 10, 25, 50 mg oral; 10 mg/5 mL oral; 25, 50 mg/mL injection

hydroxyzine pamoate USP *anxiolytic; minor tranquilizer; antiemetic; piperazine antihistamine; antipruritic* 25, 50, 100 mg oral

Hygenic Cleansing anorectal pads OTC *moisturizer and cleanser for external rectal/vaginal areas; astringent* [witch hazel] 50%

Hygroton tablets ℞ *antihypertensive; diuretic* [chlorthalidone] 25, 50, 100 mg ⊠ Regroton

Hylagel Uro ℞ *investigational (Phase I) hylan B gel tissue augmentation agent for the treatment of urge urinary incontinence*

hylan G-F 20 *hylan gel-fluid polymer mixture for osteoarthritis and TMJ syndrome*

Hylorel tablets ℞ *antihypertensive* [guanadrel sulfate] 10, 25 mg

Hylutin IM injection ℞ *progestin for amenorrhea, metrorrhagia, and dysfunctional uterine bleeding* [hydroxyprogesterone caproate in oil] 125, 250 mg/mL

hymecromone USAN, INN *choleretic*

hyoscine hydrobromide BAN *GI antispasmodic; prevent motion sickness; cycloplegic; mydriatic* [also: scopolamine hydrobromide]

hyoscine methobromide BAN *anticholinergic* [also: methscopolamine bromide]

hyoscyamine (L-hyoscyamine) USP, BAN *anticholinergic; urinary antispasmodic*

hyoscyamine hydrobromide USP *GI antispasmodic; anticholinergic*

hyoscyamine sulfate USP *GI/GU antispasmodic; antiparkinsonian; anticholinergic "drying agent" for allergic rhinitis and hyperhidrosis* [also: hyoscyamine sulphate] 0.375 mg oral; 0.125 mg/mL oral

hyoscyamine sulphate BAN *GI/GU antispasmodic; antiparkinsonian; anticholinergic "drying agent" for allergic rhinitis and hyperhidrosis* [also: hyoscyamine sulfate]

Hyoscyamus niger *medicinal herb* [see: henbane]

Hyosophen tablets, elixir ℞ *GI antispasmodic; anticholinergic; sedative* [atropine sulfate; scopolamine hydrobromide; hyoscyamine hydrobromide; phenobarbital] 0.0194•0.0065•0.1037•16.2 mg; 0.0194•0.0065•0.1037•16.2 mg/5 mL

Hypaque Meglumine 30%; Hypaque Meglumine 60% injection ℞ *radiopaque contrast medium* [diatrizoate meglumine (46.67% iodine)] 300 mg/mL (141 mg/mL); 600 mg/mL (282 mg/mL)

Hypaque Sodium oral/rectal solution, powder for oral/rectal solution ℞ *radiopaque contrast medium for gastrointestinal imaging* [diatrizoate sodium (59.87% iodine)] 416.7 mg (249 mg); 1002 mg (600 mg)

Hypaque Sodium 20% intracavitary instillation ℞ *radiopaque contrast medium for urological imaging* [diatrizoate sodium (59.87% iodine)] 200 mg/mL (120 mg/mL)

Hypaque Sodium 25%; Hypaque Sodium 50% injection ℞ *radiopaque contrast medium* [diatrizoate sodium (46.67% iodine)] 250 mg/mL (150 mg/mL); 500 mg/mL (300 mg/mL)

Hypaque-76 injection ℞ *radiopaque contrast medium* [diatrizoate meglumine; diatrizoate sodium (48.7% total iodine)] 660•100 mg/mL (370 mg/mL)

Hypaque-Cysto intracavitary instillation ℞ *radiopaque contrast medium for urological imaging* [diatrizoate meglumine (46.67% iodine)] 300 mg/mL (141 mg/mL)

Hypaque-M 75; Hypaque-M 90 injection (discontinued 1999) ℞ *radiopaque contrast medium* [diatrizoate meglumine; diatrizoate sodium (51.1% total iodine)] 50%•25% (38.3%); 60%•30% (46%)

HyperHep IM injection (name changed to BayHep B in 2000) ⊠ Hyper-Tet; Hyperstat

hypericin *investigational (Phase I) antiviral for HIV and AIDS*

Hypericum perforatum *medicinal herb* [see: St. John's wort]

Hyperlyte; Hyperlyte CR; Hyperlyte R IV admixture ℞ *intravenous electrolyte therapy* [combined electrolyte solution]

Hypermune RSV ℞ *preventative for respiratory syncytial virus (RSV) infections in high-risk infants (orphan); investigational (orphan) treatment for RSV* [respiratory syncytial virus immune globulin (RSV-IG)]

hyperosmotic laxatives *a subclass of laxatives that use the osmotic effect to retain water in the intestines, lowering colonic pH and increasing peristalsis* [see also: laxatives]

HyperRab IM injection (name changed to BayRab in 2000)

Hyperstat IV injection ℞ *vasodilator for hypertensive emergency* [diazoxide] 15 mg/mL ⊠ Hyper-Tet; HyperHep; Nitrostat

Hyper-Tet IM injection (name changed to BayTet in 2000) ⊠ HyperHep; Hyperstat

Hyphed syrup ℞ *narcotic antitussive; decongestant; antihistamine* [hydrocodone bitartrate; pseudoephedrine HCl; chlorpheniramine maleate; alcohol ≟%] 2.5•30•2 mg/5 mL

Hy-Phen tablets ℞ *narcotic analgesic* [hydrocodone bitartrate; acetaminophen] 5•500 mg

hyphylline [see: dyphylline]

hypnogene [see: barbital]

hypnotics *a class of agents that induce sleep*

hypochlorous acid, sodium salt [see: sodium hypochlorite]

β-hypophamine [see: vasopressin]

α-hypophamine [see: oxytocin]

hypophosphorous acid NF *antioxidant*

Hyporet (trademarked delivery system) *prefilled disposable syringe*

HypoTears ophthalmic ointment OTC *ocular moisturizer/lubricant* [white petrolatum; mineral oil]

HypoTears; HypoTears PF eye drops OTC *ophthalmic moisturizer/lubricant* [polyvinyl alcohol] 1%

HypRho-D; HypRho-D Mini-Dose IM injection (name changed to BayRho-D Full Dose/BayRho-D Mini-Dose in 2000)

Hyprogest 250 IM injection (discontinued 1997) ℞ *progestin for amenorrhea, metrorrhagia, and dysfunctional uterine bleeding* [hydroxyprogesterone caproate in oil] 250 mg/mL

hyprolose [see: hydroxypropyl cellulose]

hypromellose INN, BAN *suspending and viscosity-increasing agent* [also: hydroxypropyl methylcellulose; hydroxypropylmethylcellulose]

Hyrexin-50 injection ℞ *antihistamine; motion sickness preventative; sleep aid; antiparkinsonian* [diphenhydramine HCl] 50 mg/mL

Hyskon uterine infusion ℞ *hysteroscopy aid* [dextran 70; dextrose] 32%•10%

Hysone cream OTC *topical corticosteroidal anti-inflammatory; antifungal; antibacterial* [hydrocortisone; clioquinol] 10•30 mg/g

hyssop *(Hyssopus officinalis)* leaves *medicinal herb for chronic hay fever, congestion, cough, lung ailments, promoting expectoration, and sore throat*

hyssop, hedge *medicinal herb* [see: hedge hyssop]

hyssop, Indian; wild hyssop *medicinal herb* [see: blue vervain]

hyssop, prairie *medicinal herb* [see: wild hyssop]

Hytakerol capsules ℞ *vitamin D therapy for tetany and hypoparathyroidism* [dihydrotachysterol] 0.125 mg

Hytinic capsules, elixir OTC *hematinic; iron supplement* [polysaccharide-iron complex] 150 mg; 100 mg/5 mL

Hytinic IM injection ℞ *hematinic* [ferrous gluconate; multiple B vitamins; procaine HCl] 3 mg/mL•≛•2%

Hytone cream, lotion, ointment ℞ *topical corticosteroidal anti-inflammatory* [hydrocortisone] 1%, 2.5%; 1%, 2.5%; 2.5% ⊡ Vytone

Hytone 1% ointment, spray ℞ *topical corticosteroidal anti-inflammatory* [hydrocortisone] 1%

Hytrin soft capsules ℞ *antihypertensive (α-blocker); treatment for benign prostatic hyperplasia (BPH)* [terazosin HCl] 1, 2, 5, 10 mg

Hytrin (CAN) tablets, starter pack ℞ *antihypertensive (α-blocker); treatment for benign prostatic hyperplasia (BPH)* [terazosin HCl] 1, 2, 5, 10 mg; 1 mg ×7 + 2 mg×7 + 5 mg×14

Hytuss tablets OTC *expectorant* [guaifenesin] 100 mg

Hytuss 2X capsules OTC *expectorant* [guaifenesin] 200 mg

Hyzaar film-coated tablets ℞ *antihypertensive; angiotensin II receptor antagonist; diuretic* [losartan potassium; hydrochlorothiazide] 50•12.5, 100•25 mg

Hyzine-50 IM injection (discontinued 1998) ℞ *anxiolytic; antiemetic* [hydroxyzine HCl] 50 mg/mL

I

^{123}I [see: iodohippurate sodium I 123]

^{123}I [see: sodium iodide I 123]

^{125}I [see: albumin, iodinated I 125 serum]

^{125}I [see: diatrizoate sodium I 125]

^{125}I [see: diohippuric acid I 125]

^{125}I [see: diotyrosine I 125]

^{125}I [see: fibrinogen I 125]

^{125}I [see: insulin I 125]

^{125}I [see: iodohippurate sodium I 125]

^{125}I [see: iodopyracet I 125]

^{125}I [see: iomethin I 125]

^{125}I [see: iothalamate sodium I 125]

^{125}I [see: liothyronine I 125]

^{125}I [see: oleic acid I 125]

^{125}I [see: povidone I 125]

^{125}I [see: rose bengal sodium I 125]

^{125}I [see: sodium iodide I 125]

^{125}I [see: thyroxine I 125]

^{125}I [see: triolein I 125]

^{131}I [see: albumin, aggregated iodinated I 131 serum]

^{131}I [see: albumin, iodinated I 131 serum]

^{131}I [see: diatrizoate sodium I 131]

^{131}I [see: diohippuric acid I 131]

^{131}I [see: diotyrosine I 131]

^{131}I [see: ethiodized oil I 131]

^{131}I [see: insulin I 131]

^{131}I [see: iodipamide sodium I 131]

^{131}I [see: iodoantipyrine I 131]

^{131}I [see: iodocholesterol I 131]

^{131}I [see: iodohippurate sodium I 131]

^{131}I [see: iodopyracet I 131]

^{131}I [see: iomethin I 131]

^{131}I [see: iothalamate sodium I 131]

^{131}I [see: iotyrosine I 131]

^{131}I [see: liothyronine I 131]

^{131}I [see: macrosalb (^{131}I)]

^{131}I [see: oleic acid I 131]

^{131}I [see: povidone I 131]

^{131}I [see: rose bengal sodium I 131]

^{131}I [see: sodium iodide I 131]

^{131}I [see: thyroxine I 131]

^{131}I [see: tolpovidone I 131]

^{131}I [see: triolein I 131]

Iamin ℞ *investigational (Phase II) immunostimulating gel for peptic ulcers, surgical wound repair, venous leg ulcers, and bone healing* [prezatide copper acetate]

IB-367 *investigational (Phase III) antimicrobial rinse for oral mucositis*

ibacitabine INN

ibafloxacin USAN, INN, BAN *antibacterial*

ibandronate sodium USAN *bone resorption inhibitor for postmenopausal osteoporosis, metastatic bone disease, hypercalcemia of malignancy, and Paget disease*

ibazocine INN

IBC (isobutyl cyanoacrylate) [see: bucrylate]

Iberet; Iberet-500 controlled-release Filmtabs (film-coated tablets) OTC *hematinic* [ferrous sulfate; multiple B vitamins; sodium ascorbate] 105•≛•150 mg; 105•≛•500 mg

Iberet; Iberet-500 liquid OTC *hematinic* [ferrous sulfate; multiple B vitamins] 78.75•≛ mg/15 mL

Iberet-Folic-500 controlled-release Filmtabs (film-coated tablets) ℞ *hematinic* [ferrous sulfate; multiple B vitamins; sodium ascorbate; folic acid] 105•≛•500•0.8 mg

iboga *(Tabernanthe iboga)* *euphoric/hallucinogenic street drug, the root of which is chewed or chopped into a fine powder and mixed with other drugs; doses high enough to induce hallucinations are also likely to cause death*

ibopamine USAN, INN, BAN *peripheral dopaminergic agent; vasodilator*

ibritumomab tiuxetan USAN *investigational radioimmunotherapy for non-Hodgkin B-cell lymphoma*

ibrotal [see: ibrotamide]

ibrotamide INN

Ibu film-coated tablets (discontinued 2000) ℞ *analgesic; antiarthritic; antipyretic; nonsteroidal anti-inflammatory drug (NSAID)* [ibuprofen] 400, 600, 800 mg

ibudilast INN

ibufenac USAN, INN, BAN *analgesic; anti-inflammatory*

Ibuprin tablets (discontinued 2000) OTC *analgesic; antiarthritic; antipyretic; nonsteroidal anti-inflammatory drug (NSAID)* [ibuprofen] 200 mg

ibuprofen USAN, USP, INN, BAN *analgesic; antiarthritic; antipyretic; nonsteroidal anti-inflammatory drug (NSAID); investigational (orphan) IV treatment for patent ductus arteriosus* 200, 400, 600, 800 mg oral; 100 mg/5 mL oral; 40 mg/mL oral

ibuprofen aluminum USAN *anti-inflammatory*

ibuprofen piconol USAN *topical anti-inflammatory*

Ibuprohm caplets, tablets (discontinued 2000) OTC *analgesic; antiarthritic; antipyretic; nonsteroidal anti-inflammatory drug (NSAID)* [ibuprofen] 200 mg

Ibuprohm tablets ℞ *nonsteroidal anti-inflammatory drug (NSAID); antiarthritic; analgesic* [ibuprofen] 400 mg

ibuproxam INN

ibutamoren mesylate USAN *growth hormone for congenital growth hormone deficiency, musculoskeletal impairment, and hip fractures*

ibuterol INN

ibutilide INN *antiarrhythmic* [also: ibutilide fumarate]

ibutilide fumarate USAN *antiarrhythmic for atrial fibrillation/flutter* [also: ibutilide]

ibuverine INN

ibylcaine chloride [see: butethamine HCl]

ICAPS timed-release tablets OTC *vitamin/mineral supplement* [multiple vitamins & minerals] ≛

ICAPS Plus tablets OTC *vitamin/mineral supplement* [multiple vitamins & minerals] ≛

Icar pediatric suspension OTC *hematinic; iron supplement* [carbonyl iron] 15 mg/1.25 mL

icatibant acetate USAN *antiasthmatic*

ICE (ifosfamide [with mesna rescue], carboplatin, etoposide) *chemother-*

apy protocol for sarcoma, osteosarcoma, and lung cancer [also: MICE]

Iceland moss *(Cetraria islandica)* plant *medicinal herb for anemia, bronchitis, hay fever, congestion, cough, digestive disorders, and lung disorders*

ICE-T (ifosfamide [with mesna rescue], carboplatin, etoposide, Taxol) *chemotherapy protocol for sarcoma, breast cancer, and non–small cell lung cancer (NSCLC)*

ichthammol USP, BAN *topical anti-infective* 10%, 20%

iclazepam INN

icodextrin INN, BAN *investigational (orphan) peritoneal dialysis agent for end-stage renal disease*

icopezil maleate USAN *acetylcholinesterase inhibitor; cognition adjuvant for Alzheimer disease*

icosapent INN *omega-3 marine triglyceride* [also: eicosapentaenoic acid (EPA)]

icospiramide INN

icotidine USAN *antagonist to histamine* H_1 *and* H_2 *receptors*

ictasol USAN *disinfectant*

Ictotest reagent tablets for professional use *in vitro diagnostic aid for bilirubin in the urine*

Icy Hot balm, cream, stick OTC *topical analgesic; counterirritant* [methyl salicylate; menthol] 29%•7.6%; 30%•10%; 30%•10%

Idamycin powder for IV injection ℞ *anthracycline antibiotic antineoplastic for acute myeloid and other leukemias (orphan); investigational (orphan) for pediatric use* [idarubicin HCl] 5, 10, 20 mg

Idamycin PFS powder for IV injection ℞ *anthracycline antibiotic antineoplastic for acute myeloid and other leukemias (orphan); investigational (orphan) for pediatric use* [idarubicin HCl] 1 mg/mL

idarubicin INN, BAN *anthracycline antibiotic antineoplastic* [also: idarubicin HCl]

idarubicin HCl USAN, INN *anthracycline antibiotic antineoplastic for acute myeloid and other leukemias (orphan); investigational (orphan) for pediatric use* [also: idarubicin]

idaverine INN

idazoxan INN, BAN

idebenone INN, JAN *investigational treatment for Alzheimer disease*

IDEC-CE9.1 *investigational (Phase III) anti-CD4 antibody for rheumatoid arthritis* [also: SB-210396]

idenast INN

Identi-Dose (trademarked dosage form) *unit dose package*

idoxifene USAN *antihormone antineoplastic; osteoporosis treatment; estrogen receptor antagonist for hormone replacement therapy*

idoxuridine (IDU) USAN, USP, INN, BAN, JAN *ophthalmic antiviral; investigational (orphan) for nonparenchymatous sarcomas*

idralfidine INN

idrobutamine [see: butidrine]

idrocilamide INN

idropranolol INN

IDU (idoxuridine) [q.v.]

iduronidase, recombinant [now: laronidase]

IE (ifosfamide [with mesna rescue], etoposide) *chemotherapy protocol for soft tissue sarcoma*

ifenprodil INN

ifetroban USAN *antithrombotic; anti-ischemic; antivasospastic*

ifetroban sodium USAN *antithrombotic; anti-ischemic; antivasospastic*

Ifex powder for IV injection ℞ *nitrogen mustard-type alkylating antineoplastic for testicular cancer (orphan); investigational (orphan) for bone and soft tissue sarcomas* [ifosfamide] 1, 3 g

IFN (interferon) [q.v.]

IFN-alpha 2 (interferon alfa-2) [see: interferon alfa-2b, recombinant]

ifosfamide USAN, USP, INN, BAN *nitrogen mustard-type alkylating antineoplastic for testicular cancer (orphan); investigational (orphan) for bone and soft tissue sarcomas*

IfoVP (ifosfamide [with mesna rescue], VePesid) *chemotherapy protocol for sarcoma and osteosarcoma*

ifoxetine INN

IG (immune globulin) [see: globulin, immune]

IgE pentapeptide [see: pentigetide]

Igel 56 *hydrophilic contact lens material* [hefilcon C]

IGF-1 (insulin-like growth factor-1) [now: mecasermin]

IGF-1/BP3 complex *investigational (Phase II) treatment for muscle degradation following severe burns and hip fracture surgery; investigational (Phase II) for type 1 diabetes*

IgG 1 [see: immunoglobulin G 1]

IGIM (immune globulin intramuscular) [see: globulin, immune]

IGIV (immune globulin intravenous) [see: globulin, immune]

igmesine HCl USAN *sigma receptor ligand antidepressant*

IL-1, IL-2, etc. [see: interleukin-1, interleukin-2, etc.]

IL-2 (interleukin-2) [see: aldesleukin; teceleukin; celmoleukin]

IL-4R (interleukin-4 receptor) [q.v.]

IL-13-PE38QQR protein *investigational novel chimeric human protein for kidney cancer therapy*

ilepcimide USAN, INN *anticonvulsant; investigational (orphan) for drug-resistant generalized tonic-clonic epilepsy*

Iletin (U.S. products) [see under: Regular, NPH, and Lente]

Iletin (CAN) subcu injection (discontinued 2001) OTC *antidiabetic* [insulin (beef-pork)] 100 U/mL

Iletin (CAN) subcu injection (discontinued 2001) OTC *antidiabetic* [insulin zinc (beef-pork)] 100 U/mL

Iletin NPH (CAN) subcu injection (discontinued 2001) OTC *antidiabetic* [insulin (beef-pork)] 100 U/mL

Iletin II Pork Lente (CAN) subcu injection OTC *antidiabetic* [insulin zinc (pork)] 100 U/mL

Iletin II Pork NPH (CAN) subcu injection OTC *antidiabetic* [insulin (pork)] 100 U/mL

Iletin II Pork Regular (CAN) subcu injection OTC *antidiabetic* [insulin (pork)] 100 U/mL

Ilex aquifolium; I. opaca; I. vomitoria *medicinal herb* [see: holly]

Ilex paraguariensis *medicinal herb* [see: yerba maté]

Ilex verticillata *medicinal herb* [see: winterberry]

Illicium anisatum; I. verum *medicinal herb* [see: star anise]

ilmofosine USAN, INN *antineoplastic*

ilomastat USAN *matrix metalloproteinase (MMP) inhibitor for corneal ulcers, inflammation, and cancers*

ilonidap USAN, INN *anti-inflammatory*

Ilopan IM injection, IV infusion ℞ *postoperative ileus prophylactic* [dexpanthenol] 250 mg/mL

Ilopan-Choline tablets ℞ *antiflatulent for splenic flexure syndrome* [dexpanthenol; choline bitartrate] 50•25 mg

iloperidone USAN, INN *investigational (Phase III) novel antipsychotic for schizophrenia*

iloprost INN, BAN *prostacyclin analogue for cardiovascular disorders; orphan status withdrawn 1996*

Ilosone tablets, Pulvules (capsules), oral suspension ℞ *macrolide antibiotic* [erythromycin estolate] 500 mg; 250 mg; 125, 250 mg/5 mL ⑨ inosine

Ilotycin ophthalmic ointment ℞ *topical ophthalmic antibiotic* [erythromycin] 0.5%

Ilotycin Gluceptate IV injection ℞ *macrolide antibiotic* [erythromycin gluceptate] 1 g/vial

Ilozyme tablets ℞ *digestive enzymes* [lipase; protease; amylase] 11 000•30 000•30 000 U

I-L-X elixir OTC *hematinic* [ferrous gluconate; liver concentrate 1:20; multiple B vitamins] 70•98•≛ mg/15 mL

I-L-X B_{12} caplets OTC *hematinic* [carbonyl iron; liver, desiccated; multiple B vitamins; ascorbic acid] 37.5•130•≟•120 mg

I-L-X B_{12} elixir OTC *hematinic* [ferric ammonium citrate; liver fraction 1; multiple B vitamins] 102•98•≟ mg/15 mL

IM-862 *investigational (Phase III) antineoplastic for Kaposi sarcoma*

imafen INN *antidepressant* [also: imafen HCl]

imafen HCl USAN *antidepressant* [also: imafen]

Imagent BP ℞ *investigational imaging agent for CT and ultrasound scans of the liver and spleen*

Imagent US ℞ *investigational (NDA filed) ultrasound contrast medium for cardiac imaging* [perflexane]

Imager ac rectal suspension ℞ *radiopaque contrast medium for gastrointestinal imaging* [barium sulfate] 100%

imanixil INN

imatinib mesylate *antineoplastic for chronic myeloid leukemia (CML) (orphan)*

imazodan INN *cardiotonic* [also: imazodan HCl]

imazodan HCl USAN *cardiotonic* [also: imazodan]

imcarbofos USAN, INN *veterinary anthelmintic*

imciromab INN *antimyosin monoclonal antibody* [also: imciromab pentetate]

imciromab pentetate USAN, BAN *antimyosin monoclonal antibody; investigational (orphan) diagnostic aid for myocarditis and cardiac transplant rejection* [also: imciromab]

Imdur extended-release tablets ℞ *antianginal; vasodilator* [isosorbide mononitrate] 30, 60, 120 mg

imexon INN *investigational (orphan) for multiple myeloma*

IMF (ifosfamide [with mesna rescue], methotrexate, fluorouracil) *chemotherapy protocol*

imiclopazine INN

imidapril INN, BAN

imidazole carboxamide [see: dacarbazine]

imidazole salicylate INN

imidecyl iodine USAN *topical anti-infective*

imidocarb INN, BAN *antiprotozoal (Babesia)* [also: imidocarb HCl]

imidocarb HCl USAN *antiprotozoal (Babesia)* [also: imidocarb]

imidoline INN *antipsychotic* [also: imidoline HCl]

imidoline HCl USAN *antipsychotic* [also: imidoline]

imidurea NF *antimicrobial*

imiglucerase USAN, INN *glucocerebrosidase enzyme replacement for types I, II, and III Gaucher disease (orphan)*

Imigran (foreign name for U.S. product Imitrex)

imiloxan INN *antidepressant* [also: imiloxan HCl]

imiloxan HCl USAN *antidepressant* [also: imiloxan]

iminophenimide INN

iminostilbene [see: carbamazepine]

imipemide [now: imipenem]

imipenem USAN, USP, INN, BAN, JAN *carbapenem antibiotic*

imipramine INN, BAN *tricyclic antidepressant* [also: imipramine HCl] ⊡ Imferon; Norpramin; trimipramine

imipramine HCl USP *tricyclic antidepressant; treatment for childhood enuresis* [also: imipramine] 10, 25, 50 mg oral ⊡ Imferon; Norpramin; trimipramine

imipramine pamoate *tricyclic antidepressant* ⊡ Imferon; Norpramin; trimipramine

imipraminoxide INN

imiquimod USAN, INN *topical immunomodulator for external genital and perianal warts*

imirestat INN

Imitrex film-coated tablets, nasal spray ℞ *vascular serotonin 5-HT_1 receptor agonist for migraine headache* [sumatriptan succinate] 25, 50, 100 mg; 5, 20 mg/100 µL dose

Imitrex subcu injection in vials, prefilled syringes, or STATdose kits (two prefilled syringes) ℞ *vascular*

serotonin 5-HT$_1$ receptor agonist for migraine and cluster headaches [sumatriptan succinate] 12 mg/mL

ImmStat ℞ *investigational gene therapy for HIV infection*

ImmTher ℞ *investigational (orphan) immunostimulant for pulmonary and hepatic metastases of colorectal adenocarcinoma and osteosarcoma; investigational (Phase II, orphan) for Ewing sarcoma* [disaccharide tripeptide glycerol dipalmitoyl]

ImmuCyst (CAN) powder for intravesical instillation ℞ *antineoplastic for urinary bladder cancer* [BCG vaccine, live] 81 mg/vial

ImmuDyn *investigational (orphan) agent to increase platelet count in immune thrombocytopenic purpura* [*Pseudomonas aeruginosa* purified extract]

Immun-Aid powder OTC *enteral nutritional therapy for immunocompromised patients*

immune globulin (IG) [see: globulin, immune]

immune globulin intramuscular [see: globulin, immune]

immune globulin intravenous (IGIV) [see: globulin, immune]

immune globulin intravenous pentetate USAN *radiodiagnostic imaging agent for inflammation and infection* [also: indium In 111 IGIV pentetate]

immune serum globulin (ISG) [see: globulin, immune]

Immunex CRP test kit for professional use *in vitro diagnostic aid for C-reactive protein (CRP) in blood to diagnose inflammatory conditions* [latex agglutination test]

Immuno-C ℞ *investigational (Phase II, orphan) treatment of cryptosporidiosis in immunocompromised patients* [*Cryptosporidium parvum* bovine colostrum IgG concentrate]

Immunocal powder OTC *enteral nutritional therapy* [milk-based formula] 10 g packet

ImmunoCAP Specific IgE blood test kit for professional use *in vitro diagnostic aid for IgE detection* [tests 316 different allergens]

immunoglobulin G1 (mouse monoclonal 7E11-C5.3 antihuman prostatic carcinoma cell) disulfide [see: capromab pendetide]

immunoglobulin G1 (mouse monoclonal ZCE025 antihuman antigen CEA) disulfide [see: indium In 111 altumomab pentetate; altumomab]

immunoglobulin G2 (human-mouse monoclonal HuM291 anti-CD3 antigen) disulfide [now: visilizumab]

immunosuppressants *a class of drugs used to suppress the immune response, used primarily after organ transplantation surgery*

Immupath *orphan status withdrawn 1997* [HIV-neutralizing antibodies]

ImmuRAID-AFP ℞ *investigational (orphan) for diagnostic aid for AFP-producing tumors, hepatoblastoma, and hepatocellular carcinoma* [technetium Tc 99m murine MAb to human alpha-fetoprotein (AFP)]

ImmuRAID-hCG ℞ *investigational (orphan) for diagnostic aid for hCG-producing tumors* [technetium Tc 99m murine MAb to human chorionic gonadotropin (hCG)]

ImmuRAIT-LL2 ℞ *investigational (orphan) treatment for B-cell leukemia and lymphoma* [iodine I 131 murine MAb IgG$_2$a to B cell]

Imodium capsules ℞ *antidiarrheal* [loperamide HCl] 2 mg

Imodium (CAN) quick-dissolving lingual tablets OTC *antidiarrheal* [loperamide HCl] 2 mg

Imodium A-D caplets, liquid OTC *antidiarrheal* [loperamide HCl] 1 mg; 1 mg/5 mL

Imodium Advanced (CAN) chewable tablets OTC *antidiarrheal; antiflatulent* [loperamide HCl; simethicone] 2 • 125 mg

Imogam IM injection (discontinued 2001; replaced by Imogam Rabies-HT) ℞ *passive immunizing agent for rabies prophylaxis and treatment* [rabies immune globulin] 150 IU/mL

Imogam Rabies-HT IM injection ℞ *passive immunizing agent for rabies prophylaxis and treatment* [rabies immune globulin, heat treated] 150 IU/mL

imolamine INN, BAN

Imovane (CAN) tablets ℞ *sedative; hypnotic* [zopiclone] 7.5 mg

Imovax intradermal (ID) injection, IM injection ℞ *rabies prophylaxis* [rabies vaccine (HDCV)] 0.25 IU/0.1 mL; 2.5 IU/mL

imoxiterol INN

impacarzine INN

Impact ready-to-use liquid OTC *enteral nutritional therapy* [lactose-free formula]

Impact Rubella slide test for professional use *in vitro diagnostic aid for detection of rubella virus antibodies in serum* [latex agglutination test]

Impatiens balsamina; I. biflora; I. capensis *medicinal herb* [see: jewelweed]

IMPE [see: etipirium iodide]

impromidine INN, BAN *gastric secretion indicator* [also: impromidine HCl]

impromidine HCl USAN *gastric secretion indicator* [also: impromidine]

improsulfan INN

Improved Analgesic ointment OTC *topical analgesic; counterirritant* [methyl salicylate; menthol] 18.3%•16%

Improved Congestant tablets OTC *antihistamine; analgesic* [chlorpheniramine maleate; acetaminophen] 2•325 mg

Imreg-1 ℞ *investigational (Phase III) immunomodulator for HIV*

imuracetam INN

Imuran IV injection ℞ *immunosuppressant for organ transplantation and rheumatoid arthritis* [azathioprine sodium] 100 mg ⊡ Enduron; Imferon

Imuran tablets ℞ *immunosuppressant for organ transplantation and rheumatoid arthritis* [azathioprine] 50 mg

Imuthiol ℞ *investigational (Phase II/III, orphan) immunomodulator for HIV and AIDS* [diethyldithiocarbamate]

Imuvert ℞ *investigational (orphan) for primary brain malignancies* [*Serratia marcescens* extract (polyribosomes)]

^{111}**In** [see: indium In 111 altumomab pentetate]

^{111}**In** [see: indium In 111 imciromab pentetate]

^{111}**In** [see: indium In 111 murine anti-CEA monoclonal antibody]

^{111}**In** [see: indium In 111 murine monoclonal antibody]

^{111}**In** [see: indium In 111 oxyquinoline]

^{111}**In** [see: indium In 111 pentetate]

^{111}**In** [see: indium In 111 pentetreotide]

^{111}**In** [see: indium In 111 satumomab pendetide]

^{111}**In** [see: pentetate indium disodium In 111]

^{113m}**In** [see: indium chlorides In 113m]

inactivated mumps vaccine [see: mumps virus vaccine, inactivated]

inactivated poliomyelitis vaccine (IPV) [see: poliovirus vaccine, inactivated]

inactivated poliovirus vaccine (IPV) [see: poliovirus vaccine, inactivated]

Inactivin ℞ *investigational (Phase I/II) cellular energy regulator for HIV and AIDS* [HE-200 (code name—generic name not yet assigned)]

inamrinone USAN *cardiotonic* [also: amrinone]

inamrinone lactate *vasodilator for congestive heart failure* [previously known as amrinone lactate; name changed 2000] 5 mg/mL injection

inaperisone INN

Inapsine IV or IM injection ℞ *general anesthetic; antiemetic* [droperidol] 2.5 mg/mL

Incel ℞ *investigational (Phase II) multi–drug-resistance inhibitor for prostate and ovarian cancers* [biricodar dicitrate] ⊡ Enbrel

indacrinic acid [see: indacrinone]

indacrinone USAN, INN *antihypertensive; diuretic*

indalpine INN, BAN

indanazoline INN

indanediones *a class of anticoagulants that interfere with vitamin K–dependent clotting factors*

indanidine INN

indanorex INN

indapamide USAN, INN, BAN *antihypertensive; diuretic* 1.25, 2.5 mg oral

indatraline INN

indecainide INN *antiarrhythmic* [also: indecainide HCl]

indecainide HCl USAN *antiarrhythmic* [also: indecainide]

indeloxazine INN *antidepressant* [also: indeloxazine HCl]

indeloxazine HCl USAN *antidepressant* [also: indeloxazine]

indenolol INN, BAN

Inderal tablets, IV injection ℞ *antiarrhythmic; antihypertensive; antianginal; antiadrenergic (β-blocker); migraine prophylaxis* [propranolol HCl] 10, 20, 40, 60, 80 mg; 1 mg/mL ⧉ Enduron; Enduronyl; Inderide

Inderal LA long-acting capsules ℞ *antiarrhythmic; antihypertensive; antianginal; antiadrenergic (β-blocker); migraine prophylaxis* [propranolol HCl] 60, 80, 120, 160 mg

Inderide 40/25; Inderide 80/25 tablets ℞ *antihypertensive; β-blocker; diuretic* [propranolol HCl; hydrochlorothiazide] 40•25 mg; 80•25 mg ⧉ Inderal

Inderide LA 80/50; Inderide LA 120/50; Inderide LA 160/50 long-acting capsules ℞ *antihypertensive; β-blocker; diuretic* [propranolol HCl; hydrochlorothiazide] 80•50 mg; 120•50 mg; 160•50 mg

Indian apple *medicinal herb* [see: mandrake]

Indian arrow; Indian arrow wood *medicinal herb* [see: wahoo]

Indian bark *medicinal herb* [see: magnolia]

Indian bay *medicinal herb* [see: laurel]

Indian corn *(Zea mays)* styles (silk) *medicinal herb used as an analgesic, diuretic, demulcent, and litholytic*

Indian cress *(Tropaeolum majus)* flowers, leaves, and seeds *medicinal herb used as an antiseptic and expectorant*

Indian elm *medicinal herb* [see: slippery elm]

Indian frankincense *medicinal herb* [see: frankincense]

Indian hemp *medicinal herb* [see: marijuana]

Indian hyssop *medicinal herb* [see: blue vervain]

Indian paint, red *medicinal herb* [see: bloodroot]

Indian paint, yellow *medicinal herb* [see: goldenseal]

Indian pipe *medicinal herb* [see: fit root]

Indian plant *medicinal herb* [see: bloodroot; goldenseal]

Indian poke *(Veratrum viride)* *medicinal herb* [see: hellebore]

Indian root *medicinal herb* [see: spikenard; wahoo]

Indian shamrock *medicinal herb* [see: birthroot]

Indian tobacco *medicinal herb* [see: lobelia]

Indiana protocol *chemotherapy protocol for ovarian cancer* [see: PAC-I]

indigo (*Indigofera* spp.) plant *medicinal herb for fever, hemorrhoids, inducing emesis, inflammation, liver cleansing, ovarian and stomach cancer, pain, scorpion bites, and worms; not generally regarded as safe and effective*

indigo, wild *medicinal herb* [see: wild indigo]

indigo carmine BAN *cystoscopy aid* [also: indigotindisulfonate sodium]

indigotindisulfonate sodium USP *cystoscopy aid* [also: indigo carmine]

indinavir USAN *antiviral; HIV-1 protease inhibitor*

indinavir sulfate USAN *antiviral; HIV-1 protease inhibitor*

indinavir sulfate & amprenavir *investigational (Phase II) protease inhibitor combination for AIDS*

indium *element (In)*
indium (^{111}In) diethylenetriamine pentaacetate JAN *radionuclide cisternography aid; radioactive agent* [also: indium In 111 pentetate]
indium chlorides In 113m USAN, USP *radioactive agent*
indium In 111 altumomab pentetate USAN *radiodiagnostic monoclonal antibody for colorectal carcinoma; anticarcinoembryonic antigen; orphan status withdrawn 1997* [also: altumomab]
indium In 111 antimelanoma antibody XMMME-0001-DTPA [see: antimelanoma antibody]
indium In 111 CYT-103 [now: indium In 111 satumomab pendetide]
indium In 111 IGIV pentetate *radiodiagnostic imaging agent for inflammation and infection* [also: immune globulin intravenous pentetate]
indium In 111 imciromab pentetate *radioactive diagnostic aid for cardiac imaging*
indium In 111 murine anti-CEA MAb type ZCE 025 *orphan status withdrawn 1997*
indium In 111 murine MAb (2B8-MXDTPA) & yttrium Y 90 murine MAb (2B8-MXDTPA) *investigational (orphan) for non-Hodgkin B-cell lymphoma*
indium In 111 murine MAb Fab to myosin [now: imciromab pentetate]
indium In 111 oxyquinoline USAN, USP *radioactive agent; diagnostic aid*
indium In 111 pentetate USP *radionuclide cisternography aid; radioactive agent* [also: indium (^{111}In) diethylenetriamine pentaacetate]
indium In 111 pentetreotide USAN *radioactive imaging agent for SPECT scans of neuroendocrine tumors*
indium In 111 satumomab pendetide USAN *radiodiagnostic imaging aid for ovarian (orphan) and colorectal carcinoma* [also: satumomab]
indobufen INN
indocate INN
Indochron E-R extended-release tablets (discontinued 2000) ℞ *antiarthritic; nonsteroidal anti-inflammatory drug (NSAID) for ankylosing spondylitis and acute bursitis/tendinitis* [indomethacin] 75 mg
Indocin capsules, oral suspension, suppositories ℞ *antiarthritic; nonsteroidal anti-inflammatory drug (NSAID) for ankylosing spondylitis and acute bursitis/tendinitis* [indomethacin] 25, 50 mg; 25 mg/5 mL; 50 mg ⊡ Lincocin; Minocin
Indocin I.V. powder for IV injection ℞ *prostaglandin synthesis inhibitor for neonatal closure of patent ductus arteriosus* [indomethacin sodium trihydrate] 1 mg
Indocin SR sustained-release capsules ℞ *antiarthritic; nonsteroidal anti-inflammatory drug (NSAID) for ankylosing spondylitis and acute bursitis/tendinitis* [indomethacin] 75 mg
indocyanine green USP, JAN *cardiac output test; hepatic function test; ophthalmic angiography*
indolapril INN *antihypertensive* [also: indolapril HCl]
indolapril HCl USAN *antihypertensive* [also: indolapril]
indolidan USAN, INN, BAN *cardiotonic*
indolones *a class of dopamine receptor antagonists with conventional (typical) antipsychotic activity* [also called: dihydroindolones]
indometacin INN, JAN *antiarthritic; nonsteroidal anti-inflammatory drug (NSAID)* [also: indomethacin]
indometacin farnecil JAN *antiarthritic; nonsteroidal anti-inflammatory drug (NSAID)* [also: indomethacin]
indomethacin USAN, USP, BAN *antiarthritic; nonsteroidal anti-inflammatory drug (NSAID) for ankylosing spondylitis and acute bursitis/tendinitis* [also: indometacin; indometacin farnecil] 25, 50, 75 mg oral
indomethacin sodium USAN *anti-inflammatory*
indomethacin sodium trihydrate *neonatal closure of patent ductus arteriosus*

indopanolol INN

indopine INN

indoprofen USAN, INN, BAN *analgesic; anti-inflammatory*

indoramin USAN, INN, BAN *antihypertensive*

indoramin HCl USAN, BAN *antihypertensive*

indorenate INN *antihypertensive* [also: indorenate HCl]

indorenate HCl USAN *antihypertensive* [also: indorenate]

indoxole USAN, INN *antipyretic; anti-inflammatory*

indriline INN *CNS stimulant* [also: indriline HCl]

indriline HCl USAN *CNS stimulant* [also: indriline]

inductin [see: diphoxazide]

Infalyte oral solution OTC *electrolyte replacement* [sodium, potassium, and chloride electrolytes]

Infanrix IM injection ℞ *active immunizing agent for diphtheria, tetanus, and pertussis* [diphtheria & tetanus toxoids & acellular pertussis (DTaP) vaccine, adsorbed] 25 LfU•10 LfU•25 μg per 0.5 mL

Infasurf intratracheal suspension ℞ *agent for prophylaxis and treatment of respiratory distress syndrome (RDS) in premature infants* [calfactant] 6 mL

Infatab (trademarked dosage form) *pediatric chewable tablet*

InFeD IV or IM injection ℞ *hematinic* [iron dextran] 50 mg/mL ⓢ NSAID

Infergen subcu injection, SingleJect (prefilled syringe) ℞ *consensus interferon for the treatment of chronic hepatitis* C [interferon alfacon-1] 9, 15 μg

Inflamase Mild; Inflamase Forte eye drops ℞ *topical ophthalmic corticosteroidal anti-inflammatory* [prednisolone sodium phosphate] 0.125%; 1%

infliximab *anti-inflammatory; anti-TNFα (tumor necrosis factor alpha) monoclonal antibody for Crohn disease (orphan) and rheumatoid arthritis*

influenza purified surface antigen [see: influenza split-virus vaccine]

influenza split-virus vaccine *subcategory of influenza virus vaccine*

influenza subvirion vaccine [see: influenza split-virus vaccine]

influenza vaccine, intranasal *investigational (Phase III) delivery form for the vaccine*

influenza virus vaccine USP *active immunizing agent for influenza* [see web update for specific strains given in the 2001/2002 season]

influenza whole-virus vaccine *subcategory of influenza virus vaccine*

infraRUB cream OTC *topical analgesic; counterirritant* [methyl salicylate; menthol] 35%•10%

Infumorph concentrate for continuous microinfusion ℞ *narcotic analgesic; intraspinal microinfusion for intractable chronic pain (orphan)* [morphine sulfate] 10, 25 mg/mL

Infurfer (CAN) IV or IM injection ℞ *hematinic; iron supplement* [iron dextran] 50 mg/mL

infusible platelet membranes *investigational platelet alternative*

Infuvite Pediatric IV infusion ℞ *multivitamin adjunct for infants and children receiving parenteral nutrition* [multiple vitamins]

INGN-201 *investigational (Phase I/II) adenoviral-p53 gene therapy for various cancers; investigational (Phase III) for head and neck cancers* [also: adenoviral p53 gene; p53 adenoviral gene]

INH (isonicotinic acid hydrazide) [see: isoniazid]

Inhal-Aid (trademarked form) *portable inhalation device*

inhalants *a class of street drugs that include nitrous oxide, volatile nitrites, and petroleum distillates* [see: nitrous oxide; volatile nitrites; petroleum distillate inhalants]

inicarone INN

Inject-all (trademarked delivery system) *prefilled disposable syringe*

Inlay-Tabs (trademarked dosage form) *tablets with contrasting inlay*

InnoGel Plus gel packs + comb OTC *pediculicide for lice* [pyrethrins; piperonyl butoxide technical] 0.3%•3%

Innohep deep subcu injection ℞ *anticoagulant/antithrombotic for prevention of deep vein thrombosis (DVT)* [tinzaparin sodium] 20 000 IU anti–factor Xa/mL

Innovar injection (discontinued 2001) ℞ *narcotic analgesic; major tranquilizer* [fentanyl citrate; droperidol] 0.05•2.5 mg/mL

Inocor IV injection (discontinued 2000) ℞ *vasodilator for congestive heart failure* [inamrinone lactate] 5 mg/mL

inocoterone INN *anti-acne* [also: inocoterone acetate]

inocoterone acetate USAN *anti-acne* [also: inocoterone]

INOmax inhalation gas ℞ *vasodilator for neonatal hypoxic respiratory failure due to persistent pulmonary hypertension (orphan); investigational (orphan) for acute adult respiratory distress syndrome (ARDS)* [nitric oxide] 100, 800 ppm

inosine INN, JAN ⑨ Ilosone

inosine pranobex BAN, JAN *investigational antiviral/immunomodulator for AIDS; investigational (orphan) for subacute sclerosing panencephalitis*

inosiplex [now: inosine pranobex]

inositol NF *dietary lipotropic supplement* 250, 500, 650 mg oral

inositol niacinate USAN *peripheral vasodilator* [also: inositol nicotinate]

inositol nicotinate INN, BAN *peripheral vasodilator* [also: inositol niacinate]

inotropes *a class of drugs that affect the force or energy of muscle contractions*

inprochone [see: inproquone]

inproquone INN, BAN

INS-1 *investigational (Phase II) treatment for type 2 diabetes*

INSH (isonicotinoyl-salicylidene-hydrazine) [see: salinazid]

InspirEase (trademarked form) *portable inhalation device*

Insta-Glucose gel OTC *glucose elevating agent* [glucose] 40%

insulin USP, JAN *antidiabetic* ⑨ inulin

insulin, biphasic INN, BAN *antidiabetic*

insulin, biphasic isophane BAN *antidiabetic*

insulin, dalanated USAN, INN *antidiabetic*

insulin, globin zinc USP [also: globin zinc insulin]

insulin, isophane USP, BAN, INN, JAN *antidiabetic*

insulin, neutral USAN, JAN *antidiabetic* [also: neutral insulin]

insulin, NPH (neutral protamine Hagedorn) [see: insulin, isophane]

insulin, protamine zinc (PZI) USP *antidiabetic* [also: insulin zinc protamine; protamine zinc insulin]

insulin argine INN *antidiabetic*

insulin aspart USAN, INN *antidiabetic; rapid-acting insulin analogue*

insulin defalan INN *antidiabetic*

insulin detemir USAN *antidiabetic*

insulin glargine INN *antidiabetic; long-acting, once-daily basal insulin analogue*

insulin human USAN, USP, INN, BAN, JAN *antidiabetic*

insulin human, isophane USP *antidiabetic*

insulin human zinc USP *antidiabetic*

insulin human zinc, extended USP *antidiabetic*

insulin I 125 USAN *radioactive agent*

insulin I 131 USAN *radioactive agent*

insulin lispro USAN, INN, BAN *antidiabetic*

insulin lispro protamine *antidiabetic*

Insulin Reaction gel OTC *glucose elevating agent* [glucose] 40%

insulin zinc USP, INN, BAN, JAN *antidiabetic*

insulin zinc, extended USP *antidiabetic* [also: insulin zinc suspension (crystalline)]

insulin zinc, prompt USP *antidiabetic* [also: insulin zinc suspension (amorphous)]

insulin zinc protamine JAN *antidiabetic* [also: insulin, protamine zinc; protamine zinc insulin]

insulin zinc suspension (amorphous) INN, BAN, JAN *antidiabetic* [also: insulin zinc, prompt]

insulin zinc suspension (crystalline) INN, BAN, JAN *antidiabetic* [also: insulin zinc, extended]

insulin-like growth factor-1, recombinant human (rhIGF-1) [now: mecasermin]

Intal solution for nebulization, aerosol spray ℞ *anti-inflammatory; mast cell stabilizer for prophylactic treatment of allergy, asthma, and bronchospasm* [cromolyn sodium] 20 mg/ampule; 800 μg/dose ⊡ Endal

Integra (commercially available in 21 countries) *investigational artificial skin*

Integrilin IV injection ℞ *GP IIb/IIIa platelet aggregation inhibitor for acute coronary syndrome, unstable angina, myocardial infarction, and cardiac surgery* [eptifibatide] 0.75, 2 mg/mL

Intensol (trademarked form) *concentrated oral solution*

α-2-interferon [see: interferon alfa-2b, recombinant]

interferon, fibroblast [now: interferon beta]

interferon, leukocyte [now: interferon alfa-n3]

interferon α2b [see: interferon alfa-2b]

interferon αA [see: interferon alfa-2a]

interferon alfa JAN *investigational (Phase III) oral treatment for Sjögren syndrome; investigational (Phase II) for AIDS-related xerostomia; investigational (Phase I) cytokine for AIDS and hepatitis*

interferon alfa (BALL-1) JAN

interferon alfa-2a (IFN-αA; rIFN-A) USAN, INN, BAN, JAN *antineoplastic/antiviral for hairy cell leukemia, Kaposi sarcoma (orphan), and chronic myelogenous leukemia (orphan); investigational (orphan) for renal cell carcinoma*

interferon alfa-2a & fluorouracil *investigational (orphan) for esophageal carcinoma and advanced colorectal cancer*

interferon alfa-2a & teceleukin *investigational (orphan) for metastatic renal cell carcinoma and metastatic malignant melanoma*

interferon alfa-2b (IFN-α2) USAN, INN, BAN *antineoplastic for hairy-cell leukemia, malignant melanoma, AIDS-related Kaposi sarcoma (orphan), and various other cancers; antiviral for condylomata acuminata and chronic hepatitis B and C; investigational (Phase I/II) cytokine for AIDS*

interferon alfacon-1 USAN *bioengineered consensus interferon for the treatment of chronic hepatitis C*

interferon alfa-n1 USAN, INN, BAN *antineoplastic; biological response modifier for chronic hepatitis C (orphan); investigational (Phase III) cytokine for HIV; investigational (orphan) for human papillomavirus in severe respiratory papillomatosis*

interferon alfa-n3 USAN *immunomodulator and antiviral for condylomata acuminata; investigational (Phase III) cytokine for HIV, AIDS, ARC, and hepatitis C*

interferon & alitretinoin *investigational (Phase I/II) combination treatment for AIDS-related Kaposi sarcoma*

interferon beta (IFN-B) BAN, JAN *antineoplastic; antiviral; immunomodulator*

interferon beta-1a USAN *immunomodulator for relapsing multiple sclerosis (orphan); investigational (orphan) for non-A, non-B hepatitis, Kaposi sarcoma, brain tumors, and various other cancers*

interferon beta-1b USAN *immunomodulator for relapsing-remitting multiple sclerosis (orphan); investigational (Phase II/III) cytokine for AIDS; investigational (Phase III) for atopic dermatitis*

interferon gamma-1a JAN

interferon gamma-1b USAN, INN, BAN *antineoplastic; antiviral; immunoregulator for chronic granulomatous disease (orphan) and severe congenital osteopetrosis (orphan); investigational (orphan) for renal cell carcinoma*

interferon gamma-2a [see: interferon gamma-1b]

α-interferons [see: interferon alfa-n1 and -n3]

interleukin-1 beta *investigational antineoplastic for melanoma; investigational liposome-encapsulated formulation for influenza A*

interleukin-1 receptor, soluble *investigational (Phase I) antiviral for HIV*

interleukin-1 receptor antagonist, recombinant human [now: anakinra]

interleukin-2, liposome-encapsulated recombinant *investigational (orphan) for brain, central nervous system, kidney, and pelvic cancers*

interleukin-2, recombinant (IL-2) [see: aldesleukin; teceleukin; celmoleukin]

interleukin-2 PEG [see: PEG-interleukin-2]

interleukin-2 receptor (IL-2R) fusion protein *investigational (NDA filed) for cutaneous T-cell lymphoma (CTCL); investigational (Phase II) for other lymphomas and leukemias; investigational (Phase II) for squamous cell carcinoma of the head and neck*

interleukin-3, recombinant human *investigational (Phase I) cytokine for HIV with cytopenia; investigational adjunct to bone marrow transplants; orphan status withdrawn 1996*

interleukin-4 (IL-4) Pseudomonas toxin fusion protein *investigational (orphan) antineoplastic for astrocytic glioma* [also: NBI-3001]

interleukin-4 receptor (IL-4R) *investigational (Phase II) treatment for allergy, asthma, transplant rejection, and infectious diseases*

interleukin-6, recombinant human (rhIL-6) *investigational (Phase III) bone marrow/platelet stimulant adjunct for chemotherapy*

interleukin-10 (IL-10) *investigational (Phase I) immunomodulator for HIV infection*

interleukin-11, recombinant human (rhIL-11) *platelet growth factor for thrombocytopenia of chemotherapy or radiation (orphan)* [also: oprelvekin]

interleukin-12 (IL-12) [see: edodekin alfa]

intermedine INN

intoplicine INN *investigational (Phase I) antineoplastic and topoisomerase I and II inhibitor*

Intrachol ℞ *investigational (orphan) for choline deficiency of long-term parenteral nutrition* [choline chloride]

IntraDose injectable gel ℞ *investigational (NDA filed, orphan) alkylating antineoplastic for squamous cell carcinoma of the head and neck* [cisplatin; epinephrine]

Intralipid 10%; Intralipid 20% IV infusion ℞ *nutritional therapy* [fat emulsion]

IntraSite gel OTC *wound dressing* [graft T starch copolymer] 2%

intravascular perfluorochemical emulsion *synthetic blood oxygen carrier for PTCA*

intravenous fat emulsion [see: fat emulsion, intravenous]

intravenous immunoglobulin (IVIG) *investigational IV solution of concentrated antibodies for AIDS*

intrazole USAN, INN *anti-inflammatory*

intrifiban [now: eptifibatide]

intrinsic factor concentrate *antianemic to enhance the body's utilization of vitamin B_{12}*

intriptyline INN *antidepressant* [also: intriptyline HCl]

intriptyline HCl USAN *antidepressant* [also: intriptyline]

Introlan Half-Strength liquid OTC *enteral nutritional therapy* [lactose-free formula]

Introlite liquid OTC *enteral nutritional therapy* [lactose-free formula]

Intron A subcu or IM injection ℞ *antineoplastic for hairy cell leukemia, malignant melanoma, Kaposi sarcoma (orphan), and various other cancers; antiviral for condylomata acuminata and chronic hepatitis B and C; investigational (Phase I/II) cytokine for AIDS* [interferon alfa-2b] 3, 5, 10, 18, 25, 50 million IU/vial

Intropaste oral paste ℞ *radiopaque contrast medium for esophageal imaging* [barium sulfate] 70%

Intropin IV injection ℞ *vasopressor for cardiac, pulmonary, traumatic, septic, or renal shock* [dopamine HCl] 40, 80, 160 mg/mL ⊠ Ditropan; Isoptin

Inula helenium *medicinal herb* [see: elecampane]

inulin USP *diagnostic aid for renal function* 100 mg/mL injection ⊠ insulin

invenol [see: carbutamide]

Inversine tablets ℞ *nicotinic receptor antagonist for hypertension* [mecamylamine HCl] 2.5 mg

invert sugar [see: sugar, invert]

Invicorp intracavernosal injection ℞ *investigational (NDA filed) treatment for organic-based erectile dysfunction* [vasoactive intestinal polypeptide; phentolamine mesylate]

Invirase capsules (this product is being replaced by Fortovase) ℞ *antiretroviral protease inhibitor for HIV infection* [saquinavir mesylate] 200 mg

iobenguane (^{131}I) INN *radioactive agent* [also: iobenguane I 131]

iobenguane I 123 USP *radioactive agent*

iobenguane I 131 USAN *radioactive agent* [also: iobenguane (^{131}I)]

iobenguane sulfate I 123 USAN *radiopharmaceutical diagnostic aid for adrenomedullary disorders and neuroendocrine tumors*

iobenguane sulfate I 131 USAN *diagnostic aid for pheochromocytoma (orphan)*

iobenzamic acid USAN, INN, BAN *radiopaque contrast medium for cholecystography*

Iobid DM sustained-release tablets ℞ *antitussive; expectorant* [dextromethorphan hydrobromide; guaifenesin] 30•600 mg

iobutoic acid INN

iocanlidic acid I 123 USAN *cardiac diagnostic aid*

Iocare Balanced Salt ophthalmic solution OTC *intraocular irrigating solution* [sodium chloride (balanced saline solution)]

iocarmate meglumine USAN *radiopaque contrast medium* [also: meglumine iocarmate]

iocarmic acid USAN, INN, BAN *radiopaque contrast medium*

iocetamic acid USAN, USP, INN, BAN *oral radiopaque contrast medium for cholecystography (62% iodine)*

Iocon shampoo OTC *antiseborrheic; antipsoriatic; antipruritic; antibacterial* [coal tar; alcohol]

Iodal HD liquid ℞ *narcotic antitussive; decongestant; antihistamine* [hydrocodone bitartrate; phenylephrine HCl; chlorpheniramine maleate] 1.67•5•2 mg/5 mL

iodamide USAN, INN, BAN *radiopaque contrast medium*

iodamide meglumine USAN *radiopaque contrast medium*

iodecimol INN

iodecol [see: iodecimol]

iodetryl INN

Iodex; Iodex-P ointment OTC *broad-spectrum antimicrobial* [povidone-iodine] 4.7%; 10%

Iodex with Methyl Salicylate salve OTC *counterirritant; topical anti-infective* [methyl salicylate; iodine; oil of wintergreen] ≟•4.7%•4.8%

iodinated (^{125}I) human serum albumin INN *radioactive agent; blood volume test* [also: albumin, iodinated I 125 serum]

iodinated (^{131}I) human serum albumin INN, JAN *radioactive agent; intrathecal imaging agent; blood volume test* [also: albumin, iodinated I 131 serum]

iodinated glycerol [see: glycerol, iodinated]

iodinated I 125 albumin [see: albumin, iodinated I 125]

iodinated I 131 aggregated albumin [see: albumin, iodinated I 131 aggregated]

iodinated I 131 albumin [see: albumin, iodinated I 131]

iodine USP *broad-spectrum topical anti-infective; element (I)* 2% topical

iodine I 123 murine MAb to alpha-fetoprotein (AFP) *investigational (orphan) diagnostic aid for AFP-producing tumors, hepatocellular carcinoma, and hepatoblastoma*

iodine I 123 murine MAb to human chorionic gonadotropin (hCG) *investigational (orphan) diagnostic aid for hCG-producing tumors*

iodine I 131 6B-iodomethyl-19-norcholesterol *investigational (orphan) for adrenal cortical imaging*

iodine I 131 Lym-1 MAb *investigational (Phase III, orphan) treatment for non-Hodgkin B-cell lymphoma*

iodine I 131 metaiodobenzylguanidine sulfate [now: iobenguane sulfate I 131]

iodine I 131 murine MAb IgG_2a to B cell *investigational (orphan) for B-cell leukemia and lymphoma*

iodine I 131 murine MAb to alpha-fetoprotein (AFP) *investigational (orphan) treatment for AFP-producing tumors, hepatocellular carcinoma, and hepatoblastoma*

iodine I 131 murine MAb to human chorionic gonadotropin (hCG) *investigational (orphan) treatment for hCG-producing tumors*

iodine I 131 radiolabeled B1 MAb *investigational (orphan) for non-Hodgkin B-cell lymphoma*

iodine I 131 tositumomab *investigational (NDA filed) treatment for low-grade non-Hodgkin lymphoma*

iodipamide USP, BAN *parenteral radiopaque contrast medium* [also: adipiodone]

iodipamide meglumine USP, BAN *parenteral radiopaque contrast medium (49.42% iodine)* [also: adipiodone meglumine]

iodipamide methylglucamine [see: iodipamide meglumine]

iodipamide sodium USP *parenteral radiopaque contrast medium*

iodipamide sodium I 131 USAN *radioactive agent*

iodisan [see: prolonium iodide]

iodixanol USAN, INN, BAN *parenteral radiopaque contrast medium (49.1% iodine)*

iodized oil NF

iodoalphionic acid NF [also: pheniodol sodium]

iodoantipyrine I 131 USAN *radioactive agent*

iodobehenate calcium NF

***m*-iodobenzylguanidine sulfate I 123** [see: iobenguane sulfate I 123]

iodocetylic acid (^{123}I) INN *diagnostic aid* [also: iodocetylic acid I 123]

iodocetylic acid I 123 USAN *diagnostic aid* [also: iodocetylic acid (^{123}I)]

iodochlorhydroxyquin [now: clioquinol]

iodocholesterol (^{131}I) INN *radioactive agent* [also: iodocholesterol I 131]

iodocholesterol I 131 USAN *radioactive agent* [also: iodocholesterol (^{131}I)]

iodoform NF

iodohippurate sodium I 123 USAN, USP *renal function test; radioactive agent*

iodohippurate sodium I 125 USAN *radioactive agent*

iodohippurate sodium I 131 USAN, USP *renal function test; radioactive agent* [also: sodium iodohippurate (^{131}I)]

iodohydroxyquin [see: clioquinol]

iodol USP

iodomethamate sodium NF

iodopanoic acid [see: iopanoic acid]

Iodopen IV injection ℞ *intravenous nutritional therapy* [sodium iodide] 118 μg/mL

iodophthalein, soluble [now: iodophthalein sodium]

iodophthalein sodium NF, INN

iodopyracet NF [also: diodone]

iodopyracet I 125 USAN *radioactive agent*

iodopyracet I 131 USAN *radioactive agent*

iodoquinol USAN, USP *amebicide; antimicrobial* [also: diiodohydroxyquinoline]

Iodosorb (CAN) paste, ointment OTC *antibacterial; antiulcerative wound dressing* [cadexomer iodine] 0.9%
iodothiouracil INN, BAN
iodothymol [see: thymol iodide]
Iodotope capsules, oral solution ℞ *radioactive agent for hyperthyroidism and thyroid carcinoma* [sodium iodide I 131] 1–50 mCi; 7.05 mCi/mL
iodoxamate meglumine USAN, BAN *radiopaque contrast medium*
iodoxamic acid USAN, INN, BAN *radiopaque contrast medium*
iodoxyl [see: iodomethamate sodium]
Iofed extended-release capsules ℞ *decongestant; antihistamine* [pseudoephedrine HCl; brompheniramine maleate] 120•12 mg
Iofed PD extended-release capsules ℞ *pediatric decongestant and antihistamine* [pseudoephedrine HCl; brompheniramine maleate] 60•6 mg
iofendylate INN *radiopaque contrast medium* [also: iophendylate]
iofetamine (^{123}I) INN *diagnostic aid; radioactive agent* [also: iofetamine HCl I 123]
iofetamine HCl I 123 USAN *diagnostic aid; radioactive agent* [also: iofetamine (^{123}I)]
Iofoam (trademarked form) *foaming skin cleanser*
IoGen ℞ *investigational (Phase II) oral treatment for fibrocystic breast disease*
ioglicic acid USAN, INN, BAN *radiopaque contrast medium*
ioglucol USAN, INN *radiopaque contrast medium*
ioglucomide USAN, INN *radiopaque contrast medium*
ioglunide INN
ioglycamic acid USAN, INN, BAN *radiopaque contrast medium for cholecystography*
iogulamide USAN *radiopaque contrast medium*
iohexol USAN, INN, BAN *parenteral radiopaque contrast medium (46.36% iodine)*
Iohist D elixir ℞ *decongestant; antihistamine* [phenylpropanolamine HCl; phenyltoloxamine citrate; pyrilamine maleate; pheniramine maleate] 25•4•4•4 mg/5 mL
Iohist DM syrup ℞ *antitussive; decongestant; antihistamine* [dextromethorphan hydrobromide; phenylpropanolamine HCl; brompheniramine maleate] 10•12.5•2 mg/5 mL
iolidonic acid INN
iolixanic acid INN
iomeglamic acid INN
iomeprol USAN, INN, BAN *radiopaque contrast medium*
iomethin I 125 USAN *neoplasm test; radioactive agent* [also: iometin (^{125}I)]
iomethin I 131 USAN *neoplasm test; radioactive agent* [also: iometin (^{131}I)]
iometin (^{125}I) INN *neoplasm test; radioactive agent* [also: iomethin I 125]
iometin (^{131}I) INN *neoplasm test; radioactive agent* [also: iomethin I 131]
iometopane I 123 USAN *diagnostic imaging aid for dopamine and serotonin transporter sites*
iomorinic acid INN
Ionamin capsules ℞ *anorexiant; CNS stimulant* [phentermine HCl resin complex] 15, 30 mg
Ionax foam OTC *medicated cleanser for acne* [benzalkonium chloride]
Ionax Astringent Skin Cleanser liquid OTC *topical keratolytic cleanser for acne* [salicylic acid; isopropyl alcohol]
Ionax Scrub OTC *abrasive medicated cleanser for acne* [benzalkonium chloride]
ionic contrast media *a class of older radiopaque agents that, in general, have a high osmolar concentration of iodine (the contrast agent), which corresponds to a higher incidence of adverse reactions* [also called: high osmolar contrast media (HOCM)]
Ionil shampoo OTC *antiseborrheic; keratolytic; antiseptic* [salicylic acid; benzalkonium chloride]
Ionil Plus shampoo OTC *antiseborrheic; keratolytic* [salicylic acid] 2%

Ionil T shampoo OTC *antiseborrheic; antipsoriatic; keratolytic; antiseptic* [coal tar; salicylic acid; benzalkonium chloride]

Ionil-T Plus shampoo OTC *antiseborrheic; antipsoriatic; antipruritic; antibacterial* [coal tar] 2%

ionphylline [see: aminophylline]

iopamidol USAN, USP, INN, BAN *parenteral radiopaque contrast medium (49% iodine)*

iopanoic acid USP, INN, BAN *oral radiopaque contrast medium for cholecystography (66.68% iodine)*

iopentol USAN, INN, BAN *radiopaque contrast medium*

Iophen tablets, elixir, drops ℞ *expectorant* [iodinated glycerol] 30 mg; 60 mg/5 mL; 50 mg/mL

Iophen-C liquid ℞ *narcotic antitussive; expectorant* [codeine phosphate; iodinated glycerol] 10•30 mg/5 mL

Iophen-DM liquid ℞ *antitussive; expectorant* [dextromethorphan hydrobromide; iodinated glycerol] 10•30 mg/5 mL

iophendylate USP, BAN *radiopaque contrast medium* [also: iofendylate]

iophenoic acid INN [also: iophenoxic acid]

iophenoxic acid USP [also: iophenoic acid]

Iophylline elixir ℞ *antiasthmatic; bronchodilator; expectorant* [theophylline; iodinated glycerol] 120•30 mg/15 mL

Iopidine Drop-Tainer (eye drops) ℞ *topical sympathomimetic antiglaucoma agent* [apraclonidine HCl] 0.5%, 1%

ioprocemic acid USAN, INN *radiopaque contrast medium*

iopromide USAN, INN, BAN *parenteral radiopaque contrast medium (39% iodine)*

iopronic acid USAN, INN, BAN *radiopaque contrast medium for cholecystography*

iopydol USAN, INN, BAN *radiopaque contrast medium for bronchography*

iopydone USAN, INN, BAN *radiopaque contrast medium for bronchography*

Iosal II extended-release tablets ℞ *decongestant; expectorant* [pseudoephedrine HCl; guaifenesin] 60•600 mg

iosarcol INN

iosefamic acid USAN, INN *radiopaque contrast medium*

ioseric acid USAN, INN *radiopaque contrast medium*

iosimide INN

iosulamide INN *radiopaque contrast medium* [also: iosulamide meglumine]

iosulamide meglumine USAN *radiopaque contrast medium* [also: iosulamide]

iosulfan blue *parenteral radiopaque contrast medium for lymphography*

iosumetic acid USAN, INN *radiopaque contrast medium*

iotalamic acid INN *radiopaque contrast medium* [also: iothalamic acid]

iotasul USAN, INN *radiopaque contrast medium*

iotetric acid USAN, INN *radiopaque contrast medium*

iothalamate meglumine USP *parenteral radiopaque contrast medium (47% iodine)* [also: meglumine iothalamate]

iothalamate sodium USP *parenteral radiopaque contrast medium (59.9% iodine)* [also: sodium iothalamate]

iothalamate sodium I 125 USAN *radioactive agent* [also: sodium iotalamate (^{125}I)]

iothalamate sodium I 131 USAN *radioactive agent* [also: sodium iotalamate (^{131}I)]

iothalamic acid USP, BAN *radiopaque contrast medium* [also: iotalamic acid]

iothiouracil sodium

iotranic acid INN

iotriside INN

iotrizoic acid INN

iotrol [now: iotrolan]

iotrolan USAN, INN, BAN *parenteral radiopaque contrast medium*

iotroxic acid USAN, INN, BAN *radiopaque contrast medium*
Iotussin HC syrup ℞ *narcotic antitussive; decongestant; antihistamine* [hydrocodone bitartrate; phenylephrine HCl; chlorpheniramine maleate] 2.5•5•2 mg/5 mL
iotyrosine I 131 USAN *radioactive agent*
ioversol USAN, INN, BAN *parenteral radiopaque contrast medium (47.3% iodine)*
ioxabrolic acid INN
ioxaglate meglumine USAN *radiopaque contrast medium* [also: meglumine ioxaglate]
ioxaglate sodium USAN *radiopaque contrast medium* [also: sodium ioxaglate]
ioxaglic acid USAN, INN, BAN *radiopaque contrast medium*
ioxilan USAN, INN *diagnostic aid*
ioxitalamic acid INN
ioxotrizoic acid USAN, INN *radiopaque contrast medium*
iozomic acid INN
IPA (ifosfamide, Platinol, Adriamycin) *chemotherapy protocol for pediatric hepatoblastoma*
ipazilide fumarate USAN *antiarrhythmic*
ipecac USP *emetic*
ipecac, milk *medicinal herb* [see: birthroot; dogbane]
ipecac, powdered USP
ipexidine INN *dental caries prophylactic* [also: ipexidine mesylate]
ipexidine mesylate USAN, INN *dental caries prophylactic* [also: ipexidine]
IPL-423 *investigational agent for rheumatoid arthritis*
IPL-576 *investigational phospholipase A2 inhibitor*
ipodate calcium USP *oral radiopaque contrast medium for cholecystography (61.7% iodine)*
ipodate sodium USAN, USP *oral radiopaque contrast medium for cholecystography (61.4% iodine)* [also: sodium ipodate; sodium iopodate]
IPOL subcu injection ℞ *poliomyelitis vaccine* [poliovirus vaccine, inactivated] 0.5 mL
Ipomoea pandurata *medicinal herb* [see: wild jalap]
***Ipomoea violacea* (morning glory)** seeds *contain lysergic acid amide, chemically similar to LSD, which produces hallucinations when ingested as a street drug* [see also: LSD]
ipragratine INN
ipramidil INN
ipratropium bromide USAN, INN, BAN *anticholinergic bronchodilator for bronchospasm; antisecretory for rhinorrhea* 0.02% inhalation
Ipravent [see: Apo-Ipravent]
iprazochrome INN
iprazone [see: isoprazone]
ipriflavone INN
iprindole USAN, INN, BAN *antidepressant*
iprocinodine HCl USAN, BAN *veterinary antibacterial*
iproclozide INN, BAN
iprocrolol INN
iprofenin USAN *hepatic function test*
iproheptine INN
iproniazid INN, BAN
ipronidazole USAN, INN, BAN *antiprotozoal (Histomonas)*
ipropethidine [see: properidine]
iproplatin USAN, INN, BAN *antineoplastic*
iprotiazem INN
iproxamine INN *vasodilator* [also: iproxamine HCl]
iproxamine HCl USAN *vasodilator* [also: iproxamine]
iprozilamine INN
ipsalazide INN, BAN
ipsapirone INN, BAN *anxiolytic* [also: ipsapirone HCl]
ipsapirone HCl USAN *anxiolytic* [also: ipsapirone]
Ipsatol Cough Formula for Children; Ipsatol Cough Formula for Adults liquid OTC *antitussive; decongestant; expectorant* [dextromethorphan hydrobromide; phenylpropanolamine HCl; guaifenesin] 10•9•100 mg/5 mL
IPTD (isopropyl-thiadiazol) [see: glyprothiazol]

IPV (inactivated poliomyelitis vaccine) [see: poliovirus vaccine, inactivated]
IPV (inactivated poliovaccine) [see: poliovirus vaccine, inactivated]
iquindamine INN
^{192}Ir [see: iridium Ir 192]
IR-501 *investigational (Phase II) rheumatoid arthritis vaccine*
IR-502 *investigational (Phase II) T-cell receptor peptide vaccine for psoriasis*
irbesartan USAN *antihypertensive; angiotensin II receptor antagonist*
Ircon tablets OTC *hematinic* [ferrous fumarate (source of iron)] 200 mg (66 mg)
Ircon-FA tablets OTC *hematinic* [ferrous fumarate; folic acid] 82•0.8 mg
irgasan [see: triclosan]
iridium *element (Ir)*
iridium Ir 192 USAN *radioactive agent*
irindalone INN
irinotecan INN *topoisomerase I inhibitor; antineoplastic for metastatic colon and rectal cancers* [also: irinotecan HCl]
irinotecan HCl USAN, JAN *topoisomerase I inhibitor; antineoplastic for metastatic colon and rectal cancers* [also: irinotecan]
Iris florentina *medicinal herb* [see: orris root]
Iris versicolor *medicinal herb* [see: blue flag]
Irish broom *medicinal herb* [see: broom]
Irish moss *(Chondrus crispus)* plant *medicinal herb used as a demulcent*
irloxacin INN
irolapride INN
Iromin-G tablets OTC *vitamin/iron supplement* [multiple vitamins; ferrous gluconate; folic acid] ≛•30•0.8 mg
iron *element (Fe)*
iron carbohydrate complex [see: polyferose]
iron dextran USP *hematinic*
iron heptonate [see: gleptoferron]
iron hydroxide sucrose complex [see: iron sucrose; saccharated ferric oxide]
iron oxide, saccharated [see: iron sucrose; saccharated ferric oxide]
iron perchloride [see: ferric chloride]
iron polymalether [see: ferropolimaler]
iron saccharate [see: iron sucrose; saccharated ferric oxide]
iron sorbitex USAN, USP *hematinic*
iron sucrose USAN *hematinic for iron deficiency anemia in patients undergoing chronic dialysis* [also: saccharated ferric oxide]
iron sugar [see: iron sucrose; saccharated ferric oxide]
Iron-Folic 500 timed-release tablets OTC *hematinic* [ferrous sulfate; multiple B vitamins; sodium ascorbate; folic acid] 105•≛•500•0.8 mg
Irospan timed-release tablets, timed-release capsules (name changed to Vitelle Irospan in 2000)
Irrigate eye wash OTC *extraocular irrigating solution* [sterile isotonic solution]
irritant laxatives *a subclass of laxatives that work by direct action on the intestinal mucosa and nerve plexus to increase peristaltic action* [more commonly called stimulant laxatives]
irsogladine INN
irtemazole USAN, INN, BAN *uricosuric*
IS 5-MN (isosorbide 5-mononitrate) [see: isorbide mononitrate]
isaglidole INN
isamfazone INN
isamoltan INN
isamoxole USAN, INN, BAN *antiasthmatic*
isaxonine INN
isbogrel INN
iscador *investigational (Phase I) antiviral for HIV and AIDS*
isepamicin USAN, INN, BAN *aminoglycoside antibiotic*
isethionate USAN, BAN *combining name for radicals or groups* [also: isetionate]
isetionate INN *combining name for radicals or groups* [also: isethionate]
ISG (immune serum globulin) [see: globulin, immune]
ISIS 2302 *investigational (Phase II) antisense inhibitor for Crohn disease*
ISIS 2503 *investigational (Phase II) Ha-ras selective antisense inhibitor for*

colon, breast, pancreatic, and non–small cell lung cancers (NSCLC)

ISIS 3521 *investigational (Phase I) antisense anticancer compound*

ISIS 5132 *investigational (Phase II) anticancer agent for solid tumors*

ISIS 13312 *investigational (Phase I/II) second-generation antisense agent for cytomegalovirus retinitis*

ISIS-3521 *investigational (Phase III) antineoplastic*

ISIS-5132 *investigational (Phase III) antineoplastic*

Ismelin tablets ℞ *antihypertensive; investigational (orphan) for reflex sympathetic dystrophy and causalgia* [guanethidine monosulfate] 25 mg 🔊 Ritalin

Ismo film-coated tablets ℞ *antianginal; vasodilator* [isosorbide mononitrate] 20 mg

Ismotic solution ℞ *osmotic diuretic* [isosorbide] 45%

iso-alcoholic elixir NF

isoaminile INN, BAN

isoamyl *p*-methoxycinnamate [see: amiloxate]

isoamyl nitrate [see: amyl nitrite]

Iso-B capsules OTC *vitamin supplement* [multiple B vitamins; folic acid; biotin] ≛ • 200 • 100 μg

isobromindione INN

isobucaine HCl USP

isobutamben USAN, INN *topical anesthetic*

isobutane NF *aerosol propellant*

isobutyl *p*-aminobenzoate [see: isobutamben]

isobutyl α-phenylcyclohexaneglycolate [see: ibuverine]

isobutyl 2-cyanoacrylate (IBC) [see: bucrylate]

isobutyl nitrite; butyl nitrite *amyl nitrite substitutes, sold as euphoric street drugs, which produce a quick but short-lived "rush"* [see also: amyl nitrite; volatile nitrites]

***p*-isobutylhydratropohydroxamic acid** [see: ibuproxam]

isobutylhydrochlorothiazide [see: buthiazide]

isobutyramide *investigational (orphan) for sickle cell disease, beta-thalassemia syndrome, and beta-hemoglobinopathies*

isobuzole BAN [also: glysobuzole]

Isocaine HCl injection ℞ *injectable local anesthetic* [mepivacaine HCl] 3%

Isocaine HCl injection ℞ *injectable local anesthetic* [mepivacaine HCl; levonordefrin] 2% • 1:20 000

Isocal liquid OTC *enteral nutritional therapy* [lactose-free formula]

Isocal HCN ready-to-use liquid OTC *enteral nutritional therapy* [lactose-free formula]

Isocal HN liquid OTC *enteral nutritional therapy* [lactose-free formula]

isocarboxazid USP, INN, BAN *antidepressant; MAO inhibitor*

Isocet tablets (discontinued 2000) ℞ *analgesic; barbiturate sedative* [acetaminophen; caffeine; butalbital] 325 • 40 • 50 mg

Isoclor Expectorant liquid ℞ *narcotic antitussive; decongestant; expectorant* [codeine phosphate; pseudoephedrine HCl; guaifenesin; alcohol 5%] 10 • 30 • 100 mg/5 mL

Isocom capsules ℞ *vasoconstrictor; sedative; analgesic (for migraine)* [isometheptene mucate; dichloralphenazone; acetaminophen] 65 • 100 • 325 mg

isoconazole USAN, INN, BAN *antibacterial; antifungal*

isocromil INN

Isocult for Bacteriuria culture paddles for professional use *in vitro diagnostic aid for nitrate, uropathogens, or bacteria in the urine*

Isocult for Candida culture paddles for professional use *in vitro diagnostic aid for Candida albicans in the vagina*

Isocult for N gonorrhoeae and Candida culture test for professional use *in vitro diagnostic aid for gonorrhea and Candida in various specimens*

Isocult for Neisseria gonorrhoeae culture paddles for professional use *in vitro diagnostic aid for Neisseria gonorrhoeae*

Isocult for Staphylococcus aureus culture paddles for professional use *in vitro diagnostic aid for Staphylococcus aureus in exudate*

Isocult for Streptococcal pharyngitis culture paddles for professional use *in vitro diagnostic test for streptococcal pharyngitis in throat swabs*

Isocult for T vaginalis and Candida culture test for professional use *in vitro diagnostic aid for Trichomonas and Candida in vaginal or urethral cultures*

isodapamide [see: zidapamide]

***d*-isoephedrine HCl** [see: pseudoephedrine HCl]

isoetarine INN *sympathomimetic bronchodilator* [also: isoetharine]

isoethadione [see: paramethadione]

isoetharine USAN, BAN *sympathomimetic bronchodilator* [also: isoetarine]

isoetharine HCl USP, BAN *sympathomimetic bronchodilator* 1% inhalation

isoetharine mesylate USP, BAN *sympathomimetic bronchodilator*

isofezolac INN

isoflupredone INN, BAN *anti-inflammatory* [also: isoflupredone acetate]

isoflupredone acetate USAN *anti-inflammatory* [also: isoflupredone]

isoflurane USAN, USP, INN, BAN *inhalation general anesthetic*

isoflurophate USP *antiglaucoma agent; irreversible cholinesterase inhibitor miotic* [also: dyflos]

Isoject (trademarked delivery system) *prefilled disposable syringe*

Isolan liquid OTC *enteral nutritional therapy* [lactose-free formula]

isoleucine (L-isoleucine) USAN, USP, INN, JAN *essential amino acid; symbols: Ile, I*

isoleucine & leucine & valine *investigational (orphan) for hyperphenylalaninemia*

Isollyl Improved tablets, capsules (discontinued 1998) ℞ *analgesic; sedative* [aspirin; caffeine; butalbital] 325•40•50 mg

Isolyte E (G; H; M; P; R; S) with 5% Dextrose IV infusion ℞ *intravenous nutritional/electrolyte therapy* [combined electrolyte solution; dextrose]

Isolyte E; Isolyte S; Isolyte S pH 7.4 IV infusion ℞ *intravenous electrolyte therapy* [combined electrolyte solution]

Isolyte S pH 7.4 IV infusion ℞ *intravenous electrolyte therapy* [combined electrolyte solution]

isomazole INN *cardiotonic* [also: isomazole HCl]

isomazole HCl USAN *cardiotonic* [also: isomazole]

isomeprobamate [see: carisoprodol]

isomerol USAN *antiseptic*

isometamidium BAN [also: isometamidium chloride]

isometamidium chloride INN [also: isometamidium]

isomethadone INN, BAN

isomethepdrine chloride [see: isometheptene]

isometheptene INN, BAN

isometheptene HCl [see: isometheptene]

isometheptene mucate USP *cerebral vasoconstrictor; "possibly effective" for migraine headaches*

Isomil liquid, powder OTC *hypoallergenic infant food* [soy protein formula] ⑨ Esimil

Isomil DF ready-to-use liquid OTC *hypoallergenic infant food for management of diarrhea* [soy protein formula]

Isomil SF liquid OTC *hypoallergenic infant food* [soy protein formula, sucrose free]

isomylamine HCl USAN *smooth muscle relaxant*

isoniazid USP, INN, BAN *bactericidal; primary tuberculostatic* 100, 300 mg oral; 50 mg/5 mL oral

isonicophen [see: aconiazide]

isonicotinic acid hydrazide (INH) [see: isoniazid]

isonicotinic acid vanillylidenehydrazide [see: ftivazide]

1-isonicotinoyl-2-salicylidenehydrazine (INSH) [see: salinazid]

isonicotinylhydrazine [see: isoniazid]

isonixin INN
isooctadecanol [see: isostearyl alcohol]
isooctadecyl alcohol [see: isostearyl alcohol]
Isopan liquid OTC *antacid* [magaldrate] 540 mg/5 mL
Isopan Plus liquid OTC *antacid; antiflatulent* [magaldrate; simethicone] 540•40 mg/5 mL
Isopap capsules ℞ *vasoconstrictor; sedative; analgesic (for migraine)* [isometheptene mucate; dichloralphenazone; acetaminophen] 65•100•325 mg
isopentyl *p*-methoxycinnamate [see: amiloxate]
isopentyl nitrite [see: amyl nitrite]
isophenethanol [see: nifenalol]
isoprazone INN, BAN
isoprednidene INN, BAN
isopregnenone [see: dydrogesterone]
isoprenaline INN, BAN *sympathomimetic bronchodilator; vasopressor for shock* [also: isoproterenol HCl]
L-isoprenaline [see: levisoprenaline]
isoprenaline HCl [see: isoproterenol HCl]
Isoprinosine ℞ *investigational (NDA filed) antiviral/immunomodulator for AIDS; investigational (orphan) for subacute sclerosing panencephalitis* [inosine pranobex]
isoprofen INN
isopropamide iodide USP, INN, BAN *peptic ulcer adjunct*
isopropanol [see: isopropyl alcohol]
isopropicillin INN
isoproponum iodide [see: isopropamide iodide]
7-isopropoxyisoflavone [see: ipriflavone]
isopropyl alcohol USP *topical anti-infective/antiseptic; solvent*
isopropyl alcohol, rubbing USP *rubefacient*
N-isopropyl meprobamate [see: carisoprodol]
isopropyl myristate NF *emollient*
isopropyl palmitate NF *oleaginous vehicle*
isopropyl sebacate
isopropyl unoprostone [see: unoprostone isopropyl]
isopropylantipyrine [see: propyphenazone]
isopropylarterenol HCl [see: isoproterenol HCl]
isopropylarterenol sulfate [see: isoproterenol sulfate]
isoproterenol HCl USP *sympathomimetic bronchodilator; vasopressor for shock* [also: isoprenaline] 1:5000, 1:50 000 (0.2, 0.02 mg/mL) injection
isoproterenol sulfate USP *sympathomimetic bronchodilator*
Isoptin film-coated tablets (discontinued 2001) ℞ *antianginal; antiarrhythmic; antihypertensive; calcium channel blocker* [verapamil HCl] 40, 80, 120 mg ⊠ Intropin
Isoptin IV injection ℞ *antitachyarrhythmic; calcium channel blocker* [verapamil HCl] 5 mg/2 mL
Isoptin SR film-coated sustained-release tablets ℞ *antihypertensive; antianginal; antiarrhythmic; calcium channel blocker* [verapamil HCl] 120, 180, 240 mg
Isopto Atropine Drop-Tainers (eye drops) ℞ *cycloplegic; mydriatic* [atropine sulfate] 0.5%, 1%
Isopto Carbachol Drop-Tainers (eye drops) ℞ *topical antiglaucoma agent; direct-acting miotic* [carbachol] 0.75%, 1.5%, 2.25%, 3%
Isopto Carpine Drop-Tainers (eye drops) ℞ *topical antiglaucoma agent; direct-acting miotic* [pilocarpine HCl] 0.25%, 0.5%, 1%, 2%, 3%, 4%, 5%, 6%, 8%, 10% ⊠ Isopto Eserine
Isopto Cetamide Drop-Tainers (eye drops) ℞ *topical ophthalmic antibiotic* [sulfacetamide sodium] 15%
Isopto Cetapred eye drop suspension ℞ *topical ophthalmic corticosteroidal anti-inflammatory; antibiotic* [prednisolone acetate; sulfacetamide sodium] 0.25%•10%
Isopto Homatropine Drop-Tainers (eye drops) ℞ *cycloplegic; mydriatic* [homatropine hydrobromide] 2%, 5%

Isopto Hyoscine Drop-Tainers (eye drops) ℞ *cycloplegic; mydriatic* [scopolamine hydrobromide] 0.25%

Isopto Plain; Isopto Tears Drop-Tainers (eye drops) OTC *ophthalmic moisturizer/lubricant* [hydroxypropyl methylcellulose] 0.5%

Isordil Titradose (tablets), Tembid (sustained-release capsules and tablets), sublingual ℞ *antianginal; vasodilator* [isosorbide dinitrate] 5, 10, 20, 30, 40 mg; 40 mg; 2.5, 5, 10 mg ⓢ Isuprel

isosorbide USAN, USP, INN, BAN *osmotic diuretic*

isosorbide dinitrate USAN, USP, INN, BAN *coronary vasodilator; antianginal* 2.5, 5, 10, 20, 30, 40 mg oral

isosorbide mononitrate USAN, INN, BAN *coronary vasodilator; antianginal* 20, 30, 60, 120 mg oral

Isosource; Isosource HN liquid OTC *enteral nutritional therapy* [lactose-free formula]

isospaglumic acid INN

isospirilene [see: spirilene]

isostearyl alcohol USAN *emollient; solvent*

isosulfamerazine [see: sulfaperin]

isosulfan blue USAN *lymphangiography aid* [also: sulphan blue]

isosulpride INN

Isotein HN powder OTC *enteral nutritional therapy* [lactose-free formula]

3-isothiocyanato-1-propene [see: allyl isothiocyanate]

isothiocyanic acid, allyl ester [see: allyl isothiocyanate]

isothipendyl INN, BAN

isothipendyl HCl [see: isothipendyl]

isotiquimide USAN, INN, BAN *antiulcerative*

Isotrate ER extended-release tablets ℞ *antianginal; vasodilator* [isosorbide dinitrate] 60 mg

isotretinoin USAN, USP, INN, BAN *keratolytic for severe recalcitrant nodular acne*

isotretinoin anisatil USAN *keratolytic for acne vulgaris*

Isovorin ℞ *chemotherapy "rescue" agent (orphan)* [L-leucovorin]

Isovue-128; Isovue-200; Isovue-250; Isovue-300; Isovue-370 injection ℞ *radiopaque contrast medium* [iopamidol (49% iodine)] 261 mg/mL (128 mg/mL); 408 mg/mL (200 mg/mL); 510 mg/mL (250 mg/mL); 612 mg/mL (300 mg/mL); 755 mg/mL (370 mg/mL)

Isovue-M 200; Isovue-M 300 intrathecal injection ℞ *radiopaque contrast medium for myelography* [iopamidol (49% iodine)] 408 mg/mL (200 mg/mL); 612 mg/mL (300 mg/mL)

isoxaprolol INN

isoxepac USAN, INN, BAN *anti-inflammatory*

isoxicam USAN, INN, BAN *nonsteroidal anti-inflammatory drug (NSAID); antiarthritic; analgesic; antipyretic*

isoxsuprine INN, BAN *peripheral vasodilator* [also: isoxsuprine HCl]

isoxsuprine HCl USP, JAN *peripheral vasodilator* [also: isoxsuprine] 10, 20 mg oral

I-Soyalac liquid OTC *hypoallergenic infant food* [soybean protein formula]

isradipine USAN, INN, BAN *antihypertensive; dihydropyridine calcium channel blocker*

isrodipine [see: isradipine]

Istin (European name for U.S. product Norvasc)

Isuprel intracardiac, IV, IM, or subcu injection ℞ *vasopressor for cardiac, hypovolemic, or septic shock; sympathomimetic bronchodilator* [isoproterenol HCl] 1:5000, 1:50 000 (0.2, 0.02 mg/mL) ⓢ Isordil

Isuprel Mistometer (metered-dose inhalation aerosol), solution for inhalation ℞ *sympathomimetic bronchodilator* [isoproterenol HCl] 103 µg/dose; 0.5% (1:200), 1% (1:100)

ISV-205 *investigational (Phase II) cyclooxygenase inhibitor for glaucoma*

ISV-208 *investigational (Phase I) ophthalmic beta blocker for elevated intraocular pressure*

itanoxone INN

itasetron USAN *anxiolytic; antidepressant; antiemetic; serotonin 5-HT_3 receptor antagonist*

itazigrel USAN, INN *platelet antiaggregatory agent*

itazogrel [see: itazigrel]

itchweed *(Veratrum viride)* *medicinal herb* [see: hellebore]

Itch-X spray, gel OTC *topical local anesthetic* [pramoxine HCl] 1%

itobarbital [see: butalbital]

itraconazole USAN, INN, BAN *systemic triazole antifungal*

itramin tosilate INN [also: itramin tosylate]

itramin tosylate BAN [also: itramin tosilate]

itrocainide INN

iturelix USAN *gonadotropin releasing hormone antagonist; ovarian and testicular steroid suppressant*

I-Valex-1 powder OTC *formula for infants with leucine catabolism disorder*

I-Valex-2 powder OTC *enteral nutritional therapy for leucine catabolism disorder*

Ivanaz injection ℞ *investigational (NDA filed) broad-spectrum carbapenem antibiotic* [MK-826 (code name—generic name not yet assigned)]

Ivarest cream OTC *topical poison ivy treatment* [calamine; diphenhydramine HCl] 14%•2%

Ivarest cream, lotion (discontinued 2001) OTC *topical poison ivy treatment* [calamine; benzocaine] 14%•5%

ivarimod INN

Iveegam freeze-dried powder for IV infusion ℞ *passive immunizing agent for HIV and Kawasaki syndrome; investigational (orphan) for acute myocarditis and juvenile rheumatoid arthritis* [immune globulin; glucose] 50•50 mg/mL

ivermectin USAN, INN, BAN *antiparasitic; anthelmintic for strongyloidiasis and onchocerciasis*

ivermectin component B_{1a}

ivermectin component B_{1b}

IVIG (intravenous immunoglobulin) [q.v.]

Ivomec-SR (name changed to Stromectol upon marketing release in 1997)

ivoqualine INN

ivy *medicinal herb* [see: American ivy; English ivy; poison ivy]

Ivy Shield cream OTC *skin protectant*

IvyBlock OTC *topical treatment for poison ivy, poison oak, and poison sumac* [bentoquatam] 5%

Ivy-Chex spray OTC *topical poison ivy treatment* [polyvinylpyrrolidone-vinylacetate copolymers; methyl salicylate; benzalkonium chloride]

Ivy-Dry lotion OTC *topical poison ivy treatment* [zinc acetate; isopropanol] 2%•12.5%

Ivy-Rid spray OTC *topical poison ivy treatment* [polyvinylpyrrolidone-vinylacetate copolymers; benzalkonium chloride]

izonsteride USAN *antineoplastic 5α-reductase inhibitor for prostate cancer*

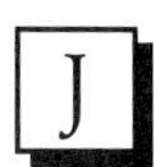

jalap *(Ipomoea jalapa)* *medicinal herb* [see: wild jalap]

Jamaica mignonette *medicinal herb* [see: henna *(Lawsonia)*]

Jamaica pepper *medicinal herb* [see: allspice]

Jamaica sarsaparilla *medicinal herb* [see: sarsaparilla]

Jamaica sorrel *medicinal herb* [see: hibiscus]

Japanese encephalitis (JE) virus vaccine *active immunization vaccine*

jasmine *(Jasminum officinale)* flowers *medicinal herb used as a calmative*

jaundice berry *medicinal herb* [see: barberry]

jaundice root *medicinal herb* [see: goldenseal]

java pepper *medicinal herb* [see: cubeb]

Jeffersonia diphylla *medicinal herb* [see: twin leaf]

Jenamicin IV or IM injection (discontinued 1998) ℞ *aminoglycoside antibiotic* [gentamicin sulfate] 40 mg/mL

Jenest-28 tablets (in packs of 28) ℞ *biphasic oral contraceptive* [norethindrone; ethinyl estradiol]
Phase 1 (7 days): 0.5 mg•35 µg;
Phase 2 (14 days): 1 mg•35 µg

Jersey tea *medicinal herb* [see: New Jersey tea]

Jerusalem cowslip; Jerusalem sage *medicinal herb* [see: lungwort]

jessamine, yellow *medicinal herb* [see: gelsemium]

Jesuit's bark *medicinal herb* [see: quinine]

Jets chewable tablets OTC *dietary supplement* [lysine; multiple vitamins] 300•≛ mg

JE-VAX powder for subcu injection ℞ *active immunizing agent* [Japanese encephalitis virus vaccine] 0.5 mL

Jevity liquid OTC *enteral nutritional therapy* [lactose-free formula]

Jevity Plus (CAN) liquid OTC *enteral nutritional therapy* [lactose-free formula] 235 mL

jewelweed *(Impatiens balsamina; I. biflora; I. capensis)* juice *medicinal herb for prophylaxis and treatment of poison ivy rash*

Jew's harp plant *medicinal herb* [see: birthroot]

jiaogulan *(Gynostemma pentaphyllum)* leaves *medicinal herb used to regulate blood pressure and strengthen the immune system, and for its adaptogenic, antihyperlipidemic, antineoplastic, antioxidant, and cardio- and cerebrovascular protective effects*

jimsonweed *(Datura stramonium)* leaves and flowering tops *medicinal herb used as an analgesic, antiasthmatic, antispasmodic, hypnotic, and narcotic; also abused as a street drug*

jodphthalein sodium [see: iodophthalein sodium]

joe-pye weed *medicinal herb* [see: queen of the meadow]

jofendylate [see: iophendylate]

Johnswort *medicinal herb* [see: St. John wort]

jopanoic acid [see: iopanoic acid]

josamycin USAN, INN *antibacterial*

jotrizoic acid [see: iotrizoic acid]

JTT-501 *investigational (Phase II) insulin sensitizer for type 2 diabetes*

Juglans cinerea *medicinal herb* [see: butternut]

Juglans nigra *medicinal herb* [see: black walnut]

Juglans regia *medicinal herb* [see: English walnut]

"Junior Strength" products [see under product name]

juniper *(Juniperus communis)* berries *medicinal herb for arthritis, bleeding, bronchitis, colds, edema, infections, kidney infections, pancreatic disorders, uric acid build-up, urinary disorders, and water retention*

juniper, prickly *(Juniperus oxycedrus)* *medicinal herb* [see: juniper]

juniper tar USP *antieczematic*

Just Tears eye drops OTC *ophthalmic moisturizer/lubricant* [polyvinyl alcohol] 1.4%

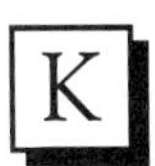

K+ 8; K+ 10 film-coated extended-release tablets ℞ *potassium supplement* [potassium chloride] 8 mEq (600 mg); 10 mEq (750 mg)

K+ Care powder ℞ *potassium supplement* [potassium chloride] 15, 20, 25 mEq/packet

K+ Care ET effervescent tablets ℞ *potassium supplement* [potassium bicarbonate] 20, 25 mEq

^{42}K [see: potassium chloride K 42]

k82 ImmunoCap test kit for professional use *in vitro diagnostic aid for specific latex allergies*

Kabikinase powder for IV or intracoronary infusion (discontinued 2000) ℞ *thrombolytic enzyme for lysis of thrombi and catheter clearance* [streptokinase] 250 000, 600 000, 750 000, 1 500 000 IU

Kadian polymer-coated sustained-release pellets in capsules ℞ *narcotic analgesic* [morphine sulfate] 20, 50, 100 mg

kainic acid INN

Kala tablets OTC *dietary supplement; fever blister treatment; not generally regarded as safe and effective as an antidiarrheal* [Lactobacillus acidophilus (soy-based)] 200 million U

kalafungin USAN, INN *antifungal*

Kaletra soft capsules, oral solution ℞ *antiviral protease inhibitor for HIV infection* [lopinavir; ritonavir] 133.3•33.3 mg; 80•20 mg/mL

kallidinogenase INN, BAN

Kalmia latifolia *medicinal herb* [see: mountain laurel]

kalmopyrin [see: calcium acetylsalicylate]

kalsetal [see: calcium acetylsalicylate]

Kaltostat; Kaltostat Fortex pads OTC *wound dressing* [calcium alginate fiber]

kalumb *medicinal herb* [see: colombo]

kanamycin INN, BAN *aminoglycoside antibiotic; tuberculosis retreatment* [also: kanamycin sulfate] ⊡ Garamycin; gentamicin

kanamycin B [see: bekanamycin]

kanamycin sulfate USP *aminoglycoside antibiotic; tuberculosis retreatment* [also: kanamycin] 75, 500, 1000 mg/vial injection

Kank-a liquid/film OTC *topical oral anesthetic* [benzocaine] 20%

Kantrex capsules, IV or IM injection, pediatric injection ℞ *aminoglycoside antibiotic* [kanamycin sulfate] 500 mg; 500, 1000 mg; 75 mg

Kao Lectrolyte powder for oral solution OTC *pediatric electrolyte replenisher*

Kaochlor 10%; Kaochlor S-F liquid ℞ *potassium supplement* [potassium chloride; alcohol 5%] 20 mEq/15 mL ⊡ K-Lor

Kaodene Non-Narcotic liquid OTC *antidiarrheal; GI adsorbent; antacid* [kaolin; pectin; bismuth subsalicylate] 3.9 g•194.4 mg•≟ per 30 mL ⊡ codeine

Kaodene Non-Narcotic oral liquid OTC *antidiarrheal; GI adsorbent; antacid* [kaolin; pectin; bismuth subsalicylate] 130•6.48•≟ mg/mL

kaolin USP clay *natural material used topically as an emollient and drying agent and ingested for binding gastrointestinal toxins and controlling diarrhea* ⊡ Calan; Kaon

Kaon elixir ℞ *potassium supplement* [potassium gluconate] 20 mEq/15 mL ⊡ Calan; kaolin

Kaon-Cl; Kaon-Cl 10 extended-release tablets ℞ *potassium supplement* [potassium chloride] 500 mg (6.7 mEq); 750 mg (10 mEq) ⊡ Calan; kaolin

Kaon-Cl 20% liquid ℞ *potassium supplement* [potassium chloride; alcohol 5%] 40 mEq/15 mL ⊡ Calan; kaolin

Kaopectate, Children's liquid OTC *antidiarrheal; GI adsorbent* [attapulgite] 600 mg/15 mL ⊡ Kapectalin

Kaopectate II caplets OTC *antidiarrheal* [loperamide HCl] 2 mg

Kaopectate Advanced Formula oral liquid OTC *antidiarrheal; GI adsorbent* [attapulgite] 750 mg/15 mL

Kaopectate Maximum Strength caplets OTC *antidiarrheal; GI adsorbent* [attapulgite] 750 mg

Kao-Spen oral suspension OTC *GI adsorbent; antidiarrheal* [kaolin; pectin] 5.2 g•260 mg per 30 mL

Kapectolin liquid OTC *GI adsorbent; antidiarrheal* [kaolin; pectin] 90•2 g/30 mL ⓢ Kaopectate

Kapseal (trademarked dosage form) *capsules sealed with a band*

karaya gum *(Sterculia tragacantha; S. urens; S. villosa)* *medicinal herb used as a topical astringent and bulk laxative*

Karidium tablets, chewable tablets, drops ℞ *dental caries preventative* [sodium fluoride] 2.2 mg; 2.2 mg; 0.275 mg/drop

Karigel; Karigel-N gel ℞ *topical dental caries preventative* [sodium fluoride] 1.1%

karyocyte growth factor [see: pegylated megakaryocyte growth and development factor, recombinant human]

kasal USAN *food additive*

Kasof capsules (discontinued 1999) OTC *laxative; stool softener* [docusate potassium] 240 mg

kava kava *(Piper methysticum)* root *medicinal herb for insomnia and nervousness*

Kay Ciel liquid, powder ℞ *potassium supplement* [potassium chloride] 20 mEq/15 mL; 20 mEq/packet ⓢ KCl

Kayexalate powder ℞ *potassium-removing agent for hyperkalemia* [sodium polystyrene sulfonate]

Kaylixir liquid ℞ *potassium supplement* [potassium gluconate; alcohol 5%] 20 mEq/15 mL

K-C oral suspension OTC *antidiarrheal; GI adsorbent; antacid* [kaolin; pectin; bismuth subcarbonate] 5 g•260 mg•260 mg per 30 mL

KCl (potassium chloride) [q.v.] ⓢ Kay Ciel

K-Dur 10; K-Dur 20 controlled-release tablets ℞ *potassium supplement* [potassium chloride] 750 mg (10 mEq); 1500 mg (20 mEq)

kebuzone INN

Keep Alert caplets OTC *CNS stimulant; analeptic* [caffeine] 200 mg

Keep Going caplets OTC *CNS stimulant; analeptic* [caffeine] 200 mg

Keflex Pulvules (capsules), oral suspension ℞ *cephalosporin antibiotic* [cephalexin] 250, 500 mg; 125, 250 mg/5 mL ⓢ Keflet; Keflin

Keftab tablets ℞ *cephalosporin antibiotic* [cephalexin HCl] 500 mg

Kefurox powder for IV or IM injection ℞ *cephalosporin antibiotic* [cefuroxime sodium] 0.75, 1.5, 7.5 g

Kefzol powder or frozen premix for IV or IM injection ℞ *cephalosporin antibiotic* [cefazolin sodium] 0.5, 1, 10, 20 g ⓢ Cefzil

kellofylline [see: visnafylline]

kelp *(Fucus versiculosus)* plant *medicinal herb for brittle fingernails, cleaning arteries, colitis, eczema, goiter, obesity, and toning adrenal, pituitary, and thyroid glands*

kelp *(Laminaria digitata; L. japonica)* plant *medicinal herb for cervical dilation and cervical ripening*

Kemadrin tablets ℞ *anticholinergic; antiparkinsonian* [procyclidine HCl] 5 mg ⓢ Coumadin

Kemsol (CAN) topical solution ℞ *anti-inflammatory for scleroderma* [dimethyl sulfoxide (DMSO)] 70%

Kenacort tablets, syrup (discontinued 2000) ℞ *corticosteroid; anti-inflammatory* [triamcinolone] 4, 8 mg; 4 mg/5 mL

Kenaject-40 IM, intra-articular, intrabursal, intradermal injection ℞ *corticosteroid; anti-inflammatory* [triamcinolone acetonide] 40 mg/mL

Kenalog ointment, cream, lotion, aerosol spray ℞ *topical corticosteroidal anti-inflammatory* [triamcinolone acetonide] 0.025%, 0.1%, 0.5%;

0.025%, 0.1%, 0.5%; 0.025%, 0.1%; ⩟ ⊡ Ketalar

Kenalog in Orabase oral paste ℞ *topical corticosteroidal anti-inflammatory* [triamcinolone acetonide] 0.1%

Kenalog-10; Kenalog-40 IM, intra-articular, intrabursal, intradermal injection ℞ *corticosteroid; anti-inflammatory* [triamcinolone acetonide] 10 mg/mL; 40 mg/mL

Kenalog-H cream ℞ *topical corticosteroidal anti-inflammatory* [triamcinolone acetonide] 0.1%

Kendall compound A [see: dehydrocorticosterone]

Kendall compound B [see: corticosterone]

Kendall compound E [see: cortisone acetate]

Kendall compound F [see: hydrocortisone]

Kendall desoxy compound B [see: desoxycorticosterone acetate]

Kenonel cream ℞ *topical corticosteroidal anti-inflammatory* [triamcinolone acetonide] 1%

Kenral-MPA (CAN) [see: Alti-MPA]

Kenwood Therapeutic liquid OTC *vitamin/mineral supplement* [multiple vitamins & minerals] ≛

keoxifene HCl [now: raloxifene HCl]

Keppra film-coated tablets ℞ *anticonvulsant for partial-onset seizures* [levetiracetam] 250, 500, 750 mg

keracyanin INN

keratinocyte growth factor-2 (KGF-2) *investigational (Phase I) vulnerary*

keratolytics *a class of agents that cause sloughing of the horny layer of the epidermis and softening of the skin*

Keri; Keri Light lotion OTC *moisturizer; emollient*

Keri Creme OTC *moisturizer; emollient*

KeriCort-10 cream OTC *topical corticosteroidal anti-inflammatory* [hydrocortisone] 1%

Kerlone film-coated tablets ℞ *antihypertensive; antiadrenergic (β-blocker)* [betaxolol HCl] 10, 20 mg

kernelwort *medicinal herb* [see: figwort]

Kerodex #51 cream OTC *skin protectant for dry or oily work*

Kerodex #71 cream OTC *water repellant skin protectant for wet work*

Kestrone 5 IM injection ℞ *estrogen replacement therapy for postmenopausal symptoms; palliative therapy for inoperable prostatic and breast cancer* [estrone] 5 mg/mL

Ketalar IV or IM injection ℞ *rapid-acting general anesthetic; sometimes abused as a street drug due to its "dissociative state" effects* [ketamine HCl] 10, 50, 100 mg/mL ⊡ Kenalog

ketamine INN, BAN *a rapid-acting general anesthetic; sometimes abused as a street drug due to its "dissociative state" effects* [also: ketamine HCl]

ketamine HCl USAN, USP, JAN *a rapid-acting general anesthetic; sometimes abused as a street drug due to its "dissociative state" effects* [also: ketamine]

ketanserin USAN, INN, BAN *serotonin antagonist*

ketazocine USAN, INN *analgesic*

ketazolam USAN, INN, BAN *minor tranquilizer*

Ketek oral solution ℞ *investigational (NDA filed) broad-spectrum ketolide antibiotic*

kethoxal USAN *antiviral* [also: ketoxal]

ketimipramine INN *antidepressant* [also: ketipramine fumarate]

ketimipramine fumarate [see: ketipramine fumarate]

ketipramine fumarate USAN *antidepressant* [also: ketimipramine]

7-KETO DHEA *investigational dehydroepiandrosterone (DHEA) derivative for Alzheimer disease*

ketobemidone INN, BAN

ketocaine INN

ketocainol INN

ketocholanic acid [see: dehydrocholic acid]

ketoconazole USAN, USP, INN, BAN *broad-spectrum imidazole antifungal* 200 mg oral; 2% topical

ketoconazole & cyclosporine *orphan status withdrawn 1996*

Keto-Diastix reagent strips *in vitro diagnostic aid for multiple urine products*

ketohexazine [see: cetohexazine]

ketolides *a class of investigational (NDA filed) antibiotics*

Ketonex-1 powder OTC *formula for infants with maple syrup urine disease*

Ketonex-2 powder OTC *enteral nutritional therapy for maple syrup urine disease (MSUD)*

ketoprofen USAN, INN, BAN, JAN *analgesic; antiarthritic; antipyretic; nonsteroidal anti-inflammatory drug (NSAID)* 50, 75, 100, 150, 200 mg oral

ketorfanol USAN, INN *analgesic*

ketorolac INN, BAN *analgesic; nonsteroidal anti-inflammatory drug (NSAID)* [also: ketorolac tromethamine]

ketorolac tromethamine USAN *analgesic; nonsteroidal anti-inflammatory drug (NSAID)* [also: ketorolac] 10 mg oral; 15, 30 mg/mL injection

Ketostix reagent strips for home use *in vitro diagnostic aid for acetone (ketones) in the urine*

ketotifen INN, BAN *antihistamine; mast cell stabilizer* [also: ketotifen fumarate]

ketotifen fumarate USAN, JAN *antihistamine; mast cell stabilizer* [also: ketotifen]

ketotrexate INN

ketoxal INN *antiviral* [also: kethoxal]

Key-Plex injection ℞ *parenteral vitamin therapy* [multiple B vitamins; vitamin C] ≛•50 mg/mL

Key-Pred 25; Key-Pred 50 IM injection ℞ *corticosteroid; anti-inflammatory* [prednisolone acetate] 25 mg/mL; 50 mg/mL

Key-Pred-SP IV or IM injection ℞ *corticosteroid; anti-inflammatory* [prednisolone sodium phosphate] 20 mg/mL

K-G Elixir ℞ *potassium supplement* [potassium gluconate] 20 mEq/15 mL

KGF-2 (keratinocyte growth factor-2) [q.v.]

KGHB (potassium gamma hydroxybutyrate) [see: gamma hydroxybutyrate (GHB)]

khellin INN

khelloside INN

Kid Kare Children's Cough/Cold oral liquid OTC *antitussive; decongestant; antihistamine* [dextromethorphan hydrobromide; pseudoephedrine HCl; chlorpheniramine maleate] 5•15•1 mg/5 mL

Kid Kare Nasal Decongestant oral drops OTC *nasal decongestant* [pseudoephedrine HCl] 7.5 mg/0.8 mL

kidney root *medicinal herb* [see: queen of the meadow]

KIE syrup ℞ *decongestant; expectorant* [ephedrine HCl; potassium iodide] 8•150 mg/5 mL

Kindercal liquid OTC *enteral nutritional therapy* [lactose-free formula]

Kinerase cream, lotion OTC *moisturizer; emollient* [N^6-furfuryladenine] 0.1%

Kineret ℞ *investigational (NDA filed) nonsteroidal anti-inflammatory drug (NSAID) for rheumatoid arthritis (RA)* [anakinra]

Kinevac powder for IV injection ℞ *diagnostic aid for gallbladder function* [sincalide] 1 µg/mL

king's clover *medicinal herb* [see: melilot]

king's cure *medicinal herb* [see: pipsissewa]

king's fern *medicinal herb* [see: buckhorn brake]

kininase II inhibitors [see: angiotensin-converting enzyme inhibitors]

kinnikinnik *medicinal herb* [see: uva ursi]

kitasamycin USAN, INN, BAN, JAN *antibacterial* [also: acetylkitasamycin; kitasamycin tartrate]

kitasamycin tartrate JAN *antibacterial* [also: kitasamycin; acetylkitasamycin]

KL4 surfactant *investigational (Phase II/III, orphan) for respiratory distress syndrome in adults and premature infants and meconium aspiration in newborn infants* [also: lucinactant]

Klamath weed *medicinal herb* [see: St. John wort]

Klaron lotion ℞ *topical antibiotic for acne* [sulfacetamide sodium] 10%

KLB6; Ultra KLB6 softgels OTC *dietary supplement* [vitamin B_6; multiple food supplements] 3.5•≛ mg; 16.7•≛ mg

K-Lease extended-release capsules ℞ *potassium supplement* [potassium chloride] 750 mg (10 mEq)

Kleen-Handz solution OTC *topical antiseptic* [ethyl alcohol] 62%

Klerist-D tablets, sustained-release capsules ℞ *decongestant; antihistamine* [pseudoephedrine HCl; chlorpheniramine maleate] 60•4 mg; 120•8 mg

Klonopin tablets, Rx Pak (prescription package), Tel-E-Dose (unit dose package) ℞ *anticonvulsant; investigational (orphan) for hyperexplexia (startle disease)* [clonazepam] 0.5, 1, 2 mg ⊡ clonidine

K-Lor powder ℞ *potassium supplement* [potassium chloride] 15, 20 mEq/packet ⊡ Kaochlor

Klor-Con; Klor-Con/25 powder ℞ *potassium supplement* [potassium chloride] 20 mEq/packet; 25 mEq/packet

Klor-Con 8; Klor-Con 10; Klor-Con M10; Klor-Con M20 film-coated extended-release tablets ℞ *potassium supplement* [potassium chloride] 600 mg (8 mEq); 750 mg (10 mEq); 750 mg (10 mEq); 1500 mg (20 mEq)

Klor-Con/EF effervescent tablets ℞ *potassium supplement* [potassium bicarbonate; potassium citrate] 25 mEq (K)

Klorvess liquid, effervescent granules, effervescent tablets ℞ *potassium supplement* [potassium chloride] 20 mEq/15 mL; 20 mEq/packet; 20 mEq

Klotrix film-coated controlled-release tablets ℞ *potassium supplement* [potassium chloride] 750 mg (10 mEq) ⊡ Liotrix

Klout liquid OTC *pesticide-free lice removal agent* [acetic acid; isopropanol; sodium laureth sulfate]

K-Lyte (CAN) effervescent tablets ℞ *urinary alkalizer for hypocitruria* [potassium citrate] 2.5 g (25 mEq K)

K-Lyte; K-Lyte DS effervescent tablets ℞ *potassium supplement* [potassium bicarbonate; potassium citrate] 25 mEq; 50 mEq (K)

K-Lyte/Cl powder ℞ *potassium supplement* [potassium chloride] 1.86 g (25 mEq K) per dose

K-Lyte/Cl; K-Lyte/Cl 50 effervescent tablets ℞ *potassium supplement* [potassium chloride] 25 mEq; 50 mEq

knitback; knitbone *medicinal herb* [see: comfrey]

knob grass; knob root *medicinal herb* [see: stone root]

K-Norm controlled-release capsules ℞ *potassium supplement* [potassium chloride] 750 mg (10 mEq)

knotted marjoram *medicinal herb* [see: marjoram]

knotweed *(Polygonum aviculare; P. hydropiper; P. persicaria; P. punctatum)* plant *medicinal herb used as an antiseptic, astringent, diaphoretic, diuretic, emmenagogue, rubefacient, and stimulant*

Koāte-DVI (double viral inactivation) powder for IV injection ℞ *antihemophilic to correct coagulation deficiency* [antihemophilic factor VIII, solvent/detergent and dry heat treated] 250, 500, 1000 IU/dose

Koāte-HP powder for IV injection (discontinued 2001) ℞ *antihemophilic to correct coagulation deficiency* [antihemophilic factor VIII] 250, 500, 1000, 1500 IU

Kof-Eze lozenges OTC *topical analgesic; counterirritant; mild local anesthetic* [menthol] 6 mg

Kogenate powder for IV injection (discontinued 2001) ℞ *antihemophilic for treatment of hemophilia A and presurgical prophylaxis of hemophiliacs (orphan)* [antihemophilic factor VIII, recombinant]

Kogenate FS powder for IV injection ℞ *antihemophilic for treatment of hemophilia A* [antihemophilic factor VIII; sucrose] 500 IU•28 mg

KOH (potassium hydroxide) [q.v.]

kola nut *(Cola acuminata)* seed *medicinal herb used as a stimulant; natural source of caffeine*

Kolephrin caplets OTC *decongestant; antihistamine; analgesic* [pseudoephedrine HCl; chlorpheniramine maleate; acetaminophen] 30•2•325 mg

Kolephrin GG/DM liquid OTC *antitussive; expectorant* [dextromethorphan hydrobromide; guaifenesin] 10•150 mg/5 mL

Kolephrin/DM caplets OTC *antitussive; decongestant; antihistamine; analgesic* [dextromethorphan hydrobromide; pseudoephedrine HCl; chlorpheniramine maleate; acetaminophen] 10•30•2•325 mg

kolfocon A USAN *hydrophobic contact lens material*

kolfocon B USAN *hydrophobic contact lens material*

kolfocon C USAN *hydrophobic contact lens material*

kolfocon D USAN *hydrophobic contact lens material*

Kolyum liquid ℞ *potassium supplement* [potassium gluconate; potassium chloride] 20 mEq/15 mL (K)

kombucha (yeast/bacteria/fungus symbiont) fermented tea *natural treatment for aging, cancer, intestinal disorders, and rheumatism*

Konakion IM injection (discontinued 1997) ℞ *coagulant; correct anticoagulant-induced prothrombin deficiency; vitamin K supplement* [phytonadione] 2 mg/mL

Kondon's Nasal jelly OTC *nasal decongestant* [ephedrine] 1%

Kondremul Plain emulsion OTC *emollient laxative* [mineral oil]

Kondremul with Phenolphthalein emulsion (discontinued 1998) OTC *stimulant/emollient laxative* [mineral oil; phenolphthalein] 55%•150 mg/15 mL

Konsyl powder OTC *bulk laxative* [psyllium] 6 g/tsp. or packet

Konsyl Easy Mix Formula powder OTC *bulk laxative with electrolytes* [psyllium; electrolytes] 6•≛ g/tsp. or packet

Konsyl Fiber tablets OTC *bulk laxative; antidiarrheal* [calcium polycarbophil] 625 mg

Konsyl Orange powder OTC *bulk laxative* [psyllium] 3.4 g/tbsp. or packet

Konsyl-D powder OTC *bulk laxative* [psyllium] 3.4 g/tsp.

Konyne 80 IV infusion ℞ *antihemophilic to correct factor VIII (hemophilia A) and factor IX (hemophilia B; Christmas disease) deficiencies* [coagulation factors II, VII, IX, and X, heat treated] 20, 40 mL

Kophane Cough & Cold Formula liquid OTC *antitussive; decongestant; antihistamine* [dextromethorphan hydrobromide; phenylpropanolamine HCl; chlorpheniramine maleate] 10•12.5•2 mg/5 mL

Korean ginseng *(Panax ginseng; P. shin-seng)* *medicinal herb* [see: ginseng]

Koromex vaginal cream OTC *spermicidal contraceptive (for use with a diaphragm)* [octoxynol 9] 3%

Koromex vaginal foam, vaginal jelly OTC *spermicidal contraceptive* [nonoxynol 9] 12.5%; 3% ⊡ Komex

Koromex Crystal Clear vaginal gel OTC *spermicidal contraceptive (for use with a diaphragm)* [nonoxynol 9] 2%

Kovitonic liquid OTC *hematinic* [ferric pyrophosphate; multiple B vitamins; lysine; folic acid] 42•≛•10•0.1 mg/15 mL

K-Pek oral suspension OTC *antidiarrheal; GI adsorbent* [attapulgite] 600 mg/15 mL

K-Phen-50 injection (discontinued 1997) ℞ *antihistamine; sedative; antiemetic; motion sickness relief* [promethazine HCl] 50 mg/mL

K-Phos M.F. tablets ℞ *urinary acidifier* [potassium acid phosphate; sodium acid phosphate] 155•350 mg (1.1 mEq potassium, 2.9 mEq sodium)

K-Phos Neutral film-coated tablets ℞ *urinary acidifier; phosphorus supplement* [sodium phosphate, dibasic;

potassium phosphate, monobasic; sodium phosphate, monobasic] 852•155•130 mg (1.1 mEq potassium, 13.0 mEq sodium)

K-Phos No. 2 tablets ℞ *urinary acidifier* [potassium acid phosphate; sodium acid phosphate] 305•700 mg (2.3 mEq potassium, 5.8 mEq sodium)

K-Phos Original tablets ℞ *urinary acidifier* [potassium acid phosphate] 500 mg (3.7 mEq potassium)

K.P.N. tablets OTC *vitamin/mineral/calcium/iron supplement* [multiple vitamins & minerals; calcium; iron; folic acid] ≛•333•11•0.27 mg

^{81m}Kr [see: krypton Kr 81m]

^{85}Kr [see: krypton clathrate Kr 85]

Kredex (European name for U.S. product Coreg)

Kristalose crystals for oral solution ℞ *hyperosmotic laxative* [lactulose] 10, 20 g/packet

Kronocap (trademarked dosage form) *sustained-release capsule*

Kronofed-A sustained-release capsules ℞ *decongestant; antihistamine* [pseudoephedrine HCl; chlorpheniramine maleate] 120•8 mg

Kronofed-A Jr. Kronocaps (sustained-release capsules) ℞ *pediatric decongestant and antihistamine* [pseudoephedrine HCl; chlorpheniramine maleate] 60•4 mg

krypton *element (Kr)*

krypton clathrate Kr 85 USAN *radioactive agent*

krypton Kr 81m USAN, USP *radioactive agent*

K-Tab film-coated extended-release tablets ℞ *potassium supplement* [potassium chloride] 750 mg (10 mEq)

Kudrox oral suspension OTC *antacid* [aluminum hydroxide; magnesium hydroxide; simethicone] 500•450•40 mg/5 mL

kudzu ***(Pueraria lobata; P. thunbergiana)*** root *medicinal herb for the management of alcoholism*

Kutapressin subcu or IM injection ℞ *claimed to be an anti-inflammatory for multiple dermatoses* [liver derivative complex] 25.5 mg/mL

Kutrase capsules ℞ *digestive enzymes; GI antispasmodic; sedative* [amylase; protease; lipase] 30 000•30 000•2400 USP units

Ku-Zyme capsules ℞ *digestive enzymes* [amylase; protease; lipase] 15 000•15 000•1200 USP units

Ku-Zyme HP capsules ℞ *digestive enzymes* [lipase; protease; amylase] 8000•30 000•30 000 U

K-vescent effervescent powder ℞ *potassium supplement* [potassium chloride] 20 mEq/packet

Kwelcof liquid ℞ *narcotic antitussive; expectorant* [hydrocodone bitartrate; guaifenesin] 5•100 mg/5 mL

Kwellada-P (CAN) creme rinse OTC *pediculicide for lice; scabicide* [permethrin] 1%

Kwellada-P (CAN) lotion OTC *pediculicide for lice; scabicide* [permethrin] 5%

K-Y vaginal jelly OTC *lubricant* [glycerin; hydroxyethyl cellulose]

K-Y Plus vaginal gel OTC *spermicidal contraceptive (for use with a diaphragm)* [nonoxynol 9] 2.2%

kyamepromazin [see: cyamemazine]

Kybernin IV ℞ *for thrombosis and pulmonary emboli of congenital AT-III deficiency (orphan)* [antithrombin III]

Kytril film-coated tablets, IV infusion, oral solution ℞ *serotonin 5-HT_3 receptor antagonist; antiemetic for nausea following chemotherapy, radiation, or surgery* [granisetron HCl] 1 mg; 1 mg/mL;

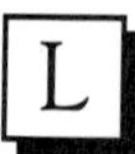

L-5 hydroxytryptophan (L-5HTP) *natural precursor to serotonin; investigational (orphan) for postanoxic intention myoclonus*

LA-12 IM injection ℞ *antianemic; vitamin B_{12} supplement* [hydroxocobalamin] 1000 μg/mL

LAAM (*l*-acetyl-α-methadol [or] *l*-alpha-acetyl-methadol) [see: levomethadyl acetate]

labetalol INN, BAN *antihypertensive; antiadrenergic (α- and β-receptor)* [also: labetalol HCl]

labetalol HCl USAN, USP *antihypertensive; antiadrenergic (α- and β-receptor)* [also: labetalol] 100, 200, 300 mg oral; 5 mg/mL injection

Labrador tea *(Ledum groenlandicum; L. latifolium; L. palustre)* leaves *medicinal herb for bronchial infections, cough, diarrhea, headache, kidney disorders, lung infections, malignancies, rheumatism, and sore throat*

Labstix reagent strips *in vitro diagnostic aid for multiple urine products*

Lac-Hydrin cream, lotion ℞ *moisturizer; emollient* [ammonium lactate] 12%

Lac-Hydrin Five lotion OTC *moisturizer; emollient* [lactic acid]

LACI (lipoprotein-associated coagulation inhibitor) [see: tifacogin]

lacidipine USAN, INN, BAN *antihypertensive; calcium channel blocker*

Lacipil (commercially available in Europe) ℞ *investigational antihypertensive; calcium channel blocker* [lacidipine]

Lacril eye drops OTC *ophthalmic moisturizer/lubricant* [hydroxypropyl methylcellulose] 0.5%

Lacri-Lube NP; Lacri-Lube S.O.P. ophthalmic ointment OTC *ocular moisturizer/lubricant* [white petrolatum; mineral oil; lanolin]

Lacrisert ophthalmic insert OTC *ophthalmic moisturizer/lubricant* [hydroxypropyl cellulose] 5 mg

lactagogues *a class of agents that promote or increase the flow of breast milk* [also called: galactagogues]

LactAid liquid, tablets OTC *digestive aid for lactose intolerance* [lactase enzyme] 250 U/drop; 3000 U

lactalfate INN

lactase enzyme *digestive enzyme for lactose intolerance*

lactated potassic saline [see: potassic saline, lactated]

lactated Ringer (LR) injection [see: Ringer injection, lactated]

lactated Ringer (LR) solution [see: Ringer injection, lactated]

lactic acid USP *pH adjusting agent*

LactiCare lotion OTC *emollient; moisturizer* [lactic acid]

LactiCare-HC lotion ℞ *topical corticosteroidal anti-inflammatory* [hydrocortisone] 1%, 2.5%

Lactinex granules, chewable tablets OTC *dietary supplement; fever blister treatment; not generally regarded as safe and effective as an antidiarrheal* [*Lactobacillus acidophilus; Lactobacillus bulgaricus*]

Lactinol lotion ℞ *emollient; moisturizer* [lactic acid] 10%

Lactinol-E cream ℞ *emollient; moisturizer* [lactic acid; vitamin E] 10%•116.67 IU/g

lactitol INN, BAN

Lactobacillus acidophilus *natural bacteria* [see: acidophilus]

Lactobacillus bulgaricus *dietary supplement; not generally regarded as safe and effective as an antidiarrheal*

lactobin *investigational (orphan) for AIDS-related diarrhea*

lactobionic acid, calcium salt, dihydrate [see: calcium lactobionate]

Lactocal-F film-coated tablets ℞ *vitamin/mineral/calcium/iron supplement* [multiple vitamins & minerals; calcium; iron; folic acid] ≛•200•65•1 mg

lactoflavin [see: riboflavin]

Lactofree liquid, powder OTC *hypoallergenic infant formula* [milk-based formula, lactose free]

β-lactone [see: propiolactone]

γ-lactone D-glucofuranuronic acid [see: glucurolactone]

lactose NF *tablet and capsule diluent; dietary supplement*

Lactrase capsules OTC *digestive aid for lactose intolerance* [lactase enzyme] 250 mg

Lactuca sativa *medicinal herb* [see: lettuce]

Lactuca virosa *medicinal herb* [see: wild lettuce]

lactulose USAN, USP, INN, BAN *hyperosmotic laxative; synthetic disaccharide used to prevent and treat portal-systemic encephalopathy* 10 g/15 mL oral or rectal

ladakamycin [now: azacitidine]

Lady Esther cream OTC *moisturizer; emollient* [mineral oil]

lady's mantle *(Alchemilla xanthochlora; A. vulgaris)* plant *medicinal herb for diarrhea and other digestive disorders; also used as an astringent, anti-inflammatory agent, menstrual cycle regulator, and muscle relaxant*

lady's slipper *(Cypripedium pubescens)* root *medicinal herb for chorea, hysteria, insomnia, nervousness, and restlessness*

laidlomycin INN *veterinary growth stimulant* [also: laidlomycin propionate potassium]

laidlomycin propionate potassium USAN *veterinary growth stimulant* [also: laidlomycin]

Laki-Lorand factor [see: factor XIII]

lamb mint *medicinal herb* [see: peppermint; spearmint]

Lambda ℞ *investigational (Phase III) treatment for hyperphosphatemia in chronic renal failure* [lanthanum carbonate]

lamb's quarter *medicinal herb* [see: birthroot]

Lamictal tablets, chewable/dispersible tablets ℞ *phenyltriazine anticonvulsant; adjunctive treatment for Lennox-Gastaut syndrome (orphan)* [lamotrigine] 25, 100, 150, 200 mg; 2, 5, 25 mg

lamifiban USAN, INN *glycoprotein (GP) IIb/IIIa receptor inhibitor; antiplatelet/antithrombotic agent for unstable angina*

lamifiban HCl USAN *glycoprotein (GP) IIb/IIIa receptor inhibitor; antiplatelet/antithrombotic agent for unstable angina*

Laminaria digitata; L. japonica *medicinal herb* [see: kelp]

Lamisil cream (became OTC and name changed to Lamisil AT in 1999)

Lamisil spray (became OTC and name changed to Lamisil AT in 2000)

Lamisil tablets ℞ *systemic allylamine antifungal for onychomycosis* [terbinafine HCl] 250 mg

Lamisil AT cream, spray, drops OTC *topical allylamine antifungal* [terbinafine HCl] 1%

Lamisil DermGel gel ℞ *topical allylamine antifungal* [terbinafine HCl] 1%

Lamium album *medicinal herb* [see: blind nettle]

lamivudine USAN, INN, BAN *nucleoside reverse transcriptase inhibitor (NRTI) antiviral for HIV and chronic hepatitis B*

lamivudine & saquinavir mesylate & ritonavir *investigational (Phase II) reverse transcriptase inhibitor and protease inhibitor combination for HIV infection*

lamivudine & zidovudine & amprenavir *investigational (Phase III) second-generation protease inhibitor combination for AIDS*

lamivudine & zidovudine & efavirenz *investigational (Phase III) antiviral combination for HIV and AIDS*

lamotrigine USAN, INN, BAN *phenyltriazine anticonvulsant; adjunctive treatment for Lennox-Gastaut syndrome (orphan)*

Lampit (available only from the Centers for Disease Control) ℞ *investigational anti-infective for Chagas disease* [nifurtimox]

Lamprene capsules ℞ *bactericidal; tuberculostatic; leprostatic (orphan)* [clofazimine] 50 mg

lamtidine INN, BAN

Lanabiotic ointment OTC *topical antibiotic; anesthetic* [polymyxin B sulfate; neomycin sulfate; bacitracin; lidocaine] 10 000 U•3.5 mg•500 U•40 mg per g

Lanacane spray, cream OTC *topical local anesthetic; antiseptic* [benzocaine; benzethonium chloride] 20%•0.1%; 6%•0.1%

Lanacaps (dosage form) *timed-release capsules*

Lanacort 5 cream, ointment OTC *topical corticosteroidal anti-inflammatory* [hydrocortisone acetate] 0.5%

Lanacort 10 cream OTC *topical corticosteroidal anti-inflammatory* [hydrocortisone acetate] 1%

Lanacort 10 ointment (discontinued 1997) OTC *topical corticosteroidal anti-inflammatory* [hydrocortisone acetate] 1%

Lanaphilic cream OTC *moisturizer; emollient; keratolytic* [urea] 20%

Lanaphilic OTC *ointment base*

Lanaphilic with Urea OTC *ointment base* [urea] 10%

Lanatabs (dosage form) *sustained-release tablets*

lanatoside NF, INN, BAN

Laniazid syrup (discontinued 1998) ℞ *tuberculostatic* [isoniazid] 50 mg/5 mL

Laniazid tablets ℞ *tuberculostatic* [isoniazid] 50 mg

Laniazid C.T. tablets ℞ *tuberculostatic* [isoniazid] 300 mg

lanolin USP *ointment base; water-in-oil emulsion; emollient/protectant* 🗩 Lanoline

lanolin, anhydrous USP *absorbent ointment base*

lanolin alcohols *ointment base ingredient*

Lanolor cream OTC *moisturizer; emollient*

Lanophyllin elixir ℞ *antiasthmatic; bronchodilator* [theophylline] 80 mg/15 mL

Lanorinal tablets, capsules (discontinued 2000) ℞ *analgesic; barbiturate sedative* [aspirin; caffeine; butalbital] 325•40•50 mg

lanoteplase USAN *investigational (Phase III) thrombolytic and tissue plasminogen activator (tPA)*

Lanoxicaps capsules ℞ *cardiac glycoside to increase cardiac output; antiarrhythmic* [digoxin] 0.05, 0.1, 0.2 mg

Lanoxin tablets, pediatric elixir, IV or IM injection ℞ *cardiac glycoside to increase cardiac output; antiarrhythmic* [digoxin] 0.125, 0.25 mg; 0.05 mg/mL; 0.1, 0.25 mg/mL

lanreotide acetate USAN *antineoplastic*

lansoprazole USAN, INN, BAN *proton pump inhibitor for gastric and duodenal ulcers, erosive esophagitis, GERD, and other gastroesophageal disorders*

lanthanum *element (La)*

lanthanum carbonate *investigational (Phase III) treatment for hyperphosphatemia in chronic renal failure*

Lantus subcu injection, prefilled cartridges for OptiPen One device ℞ *human insulin analogue; long-acting, once-daily antidiabetic* [insulin glargine (rDNA)] 100 IU/mL; 300 IU/3 mL

Lapacho colorado; L. morado *medicinal herb* [see: pau d'arco]

lapirium chloride INN *surfactant* [also: lapyrium chloride]

LAPOCA (L-asparaginase, Oncovin, cytarabine, Adriamycin) *chemotherapy protocol*

laprafylline INN

lapyrium chloride USAN *surfactant* [also: lapirium chloride]

laramycin [see: zorbamycin]

larch *(Larix americana; L. europaea)* bark, resin, young shoots, and needles *medicinal herb used as an anthelmintic, diuretic, laxative, and vulnerary*

Largon IV or IM injection ℞ *sedative; analgesic adjunct* [propiomazine HCl] 20 mg/mL

Lariam tablets ℞ *antimalarial for acute chloroquine-resistant malaria (orphan)* [mefloquine HCl] 250 mg

Larix americana; L. europaea *medicinal herb* [see: larch]
Larodopa capsules ℞ *dopamine precursor; antiparkinsonian* [levodopa] 100, 250, 500 mg
Larodopa tablets ℞ *dopamine precursor; antiparkinsonian* [levodopa] 100, 250, 500 mg
laronidase USAN *investigational (Phase III, orphan) enzyme replacement therapy for mucopolysaccharidosis-1 (MPS-1)*
Larrea divaricata; L. glutinosa; L. tridentata *medicinal herb* [see: chaparral]
lasalocid USAN, INN, BAN *coccidiostat for poultry*
Lasan cream, ointment ℞ *topical antipsoriatic* [anthralin] 0.1%, 0.2%, 0.4%; 0.4%
Lasan HP-1 cream ℞ *topical antipsoriatic* [anthralin] 1%
Lasix tablets, oral solution, IM or IV injection ℞ *antihypertensive; loop diuretic* [furosemide] 20, 40, 80 mg; 10 mg/mL; 10 mg/mL ⑨ Esidrix; Lidex
lasofoxifene tartrate USAN *tissue-selective estrogen agonist/antagonist for osteoporosis and breast cancer and for reduction of cardiovascular risk*
Lassar paste [betanaphthol (q.v.) + zinc oxide (q.v.)]
latamoxef INN, BAN *anti-infective* [also: moxalactam disodium]
latamoxef disodium [see: moxalactam disodium]
latanoprost USAN, INN *prostaglandin agonist for glaucoma and ocular hypertension*
latex agglutination test *in vitro diagnostic aid*
laudexium methylsulfate [see: laudexium metilsulfate; laudexium methylsulphate]
laudexium methylsulphate BAN [also: laudexium metilsulfate]
laudexium metilsulfate INN [also: laudexium methylsulphate]
lauralkonium chloride INN
laurel *(Laurus nobilis)* leaves and fruit *medicinal herb used as an aromatic, astringent, carminative, and stomachic*
laurel, mountain; rose laurel; sheep laurel *medicinal herb* [see: mountain laurel]
laurel, red; swamp laurel *medicinal herb* [see: magnolia]
laurel, spurge; spurge olive *medicinal herb* [see: mezereon]
laureth 4 USAN *surfactant*
laureth 9 USAN *spermaticide; surfactant*
laureth 10S USAN *spermaticide*
lauril INN *combining name for radicals or groups*
laurilsulfate INN *combining name for radicals or groups* [also: sodium lauryl sulfate]
laurixamine INN
laurocapram USAN, INN *excipient*
laurocapram & methotrexate *investigational (orphan) for topical treatment of Mycosis fungoides*
lauroguadine INN
laurolinium acetate INN, BAN
lauromacrogol 400 INN
Laurus nobilis *medicinal herb* [see: laurel]
Laurus persea *medicinal herb* [see: avocado]
lauryl isoquinolinium bromide USAN *anti-infective*
lavender (*Lavandula* spp.) flowers, leaves, and oil *medicinal herb for acne, bile flow stimulation, diabetes, edema, flatulence, hyperactivity, insomnia, intestinal spasms, migraine headache, and stimulating menstrual flow*
lavender oil NF
lavoltidine INN *antiulcerative; histamine H_2-receptor blocker* [also: lavoltidine succinate; loxtidine]
lavoltidine succinate USAN *antiulcerative; histamine H_2-receptor blocker* [also: lavoltidine; loxtidine]
lawrencium *element (Lr)*
Lawsonia inermis *medicinal herb* [see: henna]
Lax Pills tablets (discontinued 1998) OTC *stimulant laxative* [yellow phenolphthalein] 90 mg
Laxative Pills tablets (discontinued 1998) OTC *stimulant laxative* [yellow phenolphthalein] 90 mg

Laxative & Stool Softener softgels OTC *stimulant laxative; stool softener* [casanthranol; docusate sodium] 30•100 mg

laxatives *a class of agents that promote evacuation of the bowels or have a mild purgative effect; subclasses: saline, stimulant, bulk-producing, emollient, stool-softening, and hyperosmotic* [see also: cathartics; purgatives; various subclasses]

lazabemide USAN, INN *antiparkinsonian*

lazabemide HCl USAN *investigational treatment for Alzheimer disease*

lazaroids *a class of potent antioxidants that can protect against oxygen radical–mediated lipid peroxidation and progressive neuronal degeneration following brain or spinal trauma, subarachnoid hemorrhage, or stroke* [also called: 21-aminosteroids]

Lazer Creme OTC *moisturizer; emollient* [vitamins A and E] 3333.3•116.67 U/g

Lazer Formalyde solution ℞ *drying agent for hyperhidrosis and bromhidrosis* [formaldehyde] 10%

LazerSporin-C ear drops ℞ *topical corticosteroidal anti-inflammatory; antibiotic* [hydrocortisone; neomycin sulfate; polymyxin B sulfate] 1%•5 mg•10 000 U per mL

LC-65 solution OTC *cleaning solution for hard, soft, or rigid gas permeable contact lenses*

LCD (liquor carbonis detergens) [see: coal tar]

LCR (leurocristine) [see: vincristine]

LCx *Neisseria gonorrhoeae* Assay reagent kit for professional use *in vitro diagnostic aid for Neisseria gonorrhoeae*

LDI-200 *investigational (Phase III) apoptosis inducer for myelodysplastic syndrome*

LDP-02 *investigational (Phase II) agent for inflammatory bowel disease*

lead *element (Pb)*

lecimibide USAN *hypocholesterolemic; antihyperlipidemic*

lecithin NF *emulsifier; surfactant; natural phospholipid mixture of various phosphatidylcholines used as an antihypercholesterolemic and cognition enhancer for Alzheimer and other dementias* 420, 1200 mg oral

lecithol *natural remedy* [see: lecithin]

LED (liposome-encapsulated doxorubicin) [see: doxorubicin HCl, liposome-encapsulated]

Ledercillin VK tablets, powder for oral solution (discontinued 1997) ℞ *natural penicillin antibiotic* [penicillin V potassium] 250, 500 mg; 250 mg/5 mL

Lederject (trademarked delivery system) *prefilled disposable syringe*

ledoxantrone trihydrochloride USAN *antineoplastic; topoisomerase II inhibitor* [previously: sedoxantrone trihydrochloride]

Ledum groenlandicum; L. latifolium; L. palustre *medicinal herb* [see: Labrador tea]

leeches *(Hirudo medicinalis)* *natural adjunct to postsurgical wound management*

leek *(Allium porrum)* bulb, lower stem, and leaves *medicinal herb used as an appetite stimulant, decongestant, and diuretic*

lefetamine INN

leflunomide USAN, INN *anti-inflammatory for rheumatoid arthritis; investigational (orphan) for malignant glioma, ovarian cancer, and prevention of rejection of organ transplants; investigational (Phase II) for prostate and non–small cell lung cancers; investigational (Phase III) for first relapse glioblastoma multiforme*

Legalon *orphan status withdrawn 1997* [disodium silibinin dihemisuccinate]

Legatrin PM caplets OTC *prevention and treatment of nocturnal leg cramps* [diphenhydramine HCl; acetaminophen] 50•500 mg

legs, red *medicinal herb* [see: bistort]

leiopyrrole INN

lemidosul INN

lemon *(Citrus limon)* fruit and peel *medicinal herb used as an astringent, refrigerant, and source of vitamin C*

lemon, ground; wild lemon *medicinal herb* [see: mandrake]
lemon balm *(Melissa officinalis)* plant *medicinal herb used as an antispasmodic and sedative; also used for Graves disease and cold sores*
lemon oil NF
lemon verbena (*Aloysiatriphylla* spp.) leaves and flowers *medicinal herb for fever, flatulence, gastrointestinal spasms and other disorders, and sedation*
lemon walnut *medicinal herb* [see: butternut]
lemongrass *(Andropogon citratus; Cymbopogon citratus)* leaves *medicinal herb for colds, cough, fever, gastrointestinal spasm and other disorders, nervousness, pain, and rheumatism; also used as an antiemetic*
lenampicillin INN
lenercept USAN *tumor necrosis factor (TNF) receptor antagonist for septic shock, multiple sclerosis, inflammatory bowel disease, and rheumatoid arthritis*
leniquinsin USAN, INN *antihypertensive*
lenitzol [see: amitriptyline]
lenograstim USAN, INN, BAN *immunomodulator; antineutropenic; hematopoietic stimulant*
lenperone USAN, INN *antipsychotic*
Lens Drops solution OTC *rewetting solution for hard or soft contact lenses*
Lens Lubricant solution OTC *rewetting solution for hard or soft contact lenses*
Lens Plus Daily Cleaner solution OTC *surfactant cleaning solution for soft contact lenses*
Lens Plus Oxysept products [see: Oxysept]
Lens Plus Rewetting Drops OTC *rewetting solution for soft contact lenses*
Lens Plus Sterile Saline aerosol solution OTC *rinsing/storage solution for soft contact lenses* [sodium chloride (saline solution)]
Lente Iletin I subcu injection (discontinued 1999) OTC *antidiabetic* [insulin zinc (beef-pork)] 100 U/mL
Lente Iletin II subcu injection OTC *antidiabetic* [insulin zinc (pork)] 100 U/mL
Lente Insulin subcu injection (discontinued 1997) OTC *antidiabetic* [insulin zinc (beef)] 100 U/mL
Lente L subcu injection (discontinued 2000) OTC *antidiabetic* [insulin zinc (pork)] 100 U/mL
lentin [see: carbachol]
lentinan JAN *investigational (Phase II/III) immunomodulator for HIV and AIDS*
Lentinula edodes *medicinal herb* [see: shiitake mushrooms]
Leontodon taraxacum *medicinal herb* [see: dandelion]
Leonurus cardiaca *medicinal herb* [see: motherwort]
leopard's bane *medicinal herb* [see: arnica]
Lepidium meyenii *medicinal herb* [see: maca]
lepirudin *anticoagulant for heparin-induced thrombocytopenia (orphan)*
leprostatics *a class of drugs effective against leprosy*
leptacline INN
leptandra; purple leptandra *medicinal herb* [see: Culver root]
lercanidipine *investigational calcium channel blocker*
lergotrile USAN, INN *prolactin enzyme inhibitor*
lergotrile mesylate USAN *prolactin enzyme inhibitor*
leridistim USAN *interleukin-3 and granulocyte colony-stimulating factor (G-CSF) receptor agonist for chemotherapy-induced neutropenia and thrombocytopenia*
Lescol capsules ℞ *HMG-CoA reductase inhibitor for hypercholesterolemia, hypertriglyceridemia, and atherosclerosis* [fluvastatin sodium] 20, 40 mg
Lescol XL film-coated extended-release tablets ℞ *HMG-CoA reductase inhibitor for hypercholesterolemia, hypertriglyceridemia, and atherosclerosis* [fluvastatin sodium] 80 mg
lesopitron INN *investigational anxiolytic*

lesser centaury *medicinal herb* [see: centaury]

leteprinim potassium USAN *investigational (Phase II) nerve growth factor for Alzheimer disease, spinal cord injury, and stroke*

letimide INN *analgesic* [also: letimide HCl]

letimide HCl USAN *analgesic* [also: letimide]

letosteine INN

letrazuril INN *investigational (Phase II) treatment for AIDS-related cryptosporidial diarrhea*

letrozole USAN, INN *aromatase inhibitor; hormone antagonist antineoplastic for advanced breast cancer in postmenopausal women*

lettuce *(Lactuca sativa)* juice and leaves *medicinal herb used as an anodyne, antispasmodic, expectorant, and sedative (for herbal medical use, common garden lettuce is harvested after it has gone to seed, and a milky juice is extracted)*

Leucanthemum parthenium *medicinal herb* [see: feverfew]

leucarsone [see: carbarsone]

leucine (L-leucine) USAN, USP, INN, JAN *essential amino acid; symbols: Leu, L*

leucine & isoleucine & valine *investigational (orphan) for hyperphenylalaninemia*

leucinocaine INN

leucocianidol INN

Leucomax (commercially available in 36 foreign countries) ℞ *antineutropenic; hematopoietic stimulant; investigational (Phase II/III) cytokine for AIDS* [molgramostim]

leucomycin [see: kitasamycin; spiramycin]

Leucotropin ℞ *investigational (Phase III) granulocyte-macrophage colony-stimulating factor (GM-CSF) for white cell rescue following chemotherapy (trial discontinued 2000)* [regramostim]

L-leucovorin *chemotherapy "rescue" agent (orphan)*

leucovorin calcium USP *antianemic; folate replenisher; antidote to folic acid antagonist; chemotherapy "rescue" agent (orphan)* [also: calcium folinate] 5, 15, 25 mg oral; 3, 10 mg injection; 50, 100, 350 mg/vial injection

leucovorin & fluorouracil *antineoplastic for metastatic colorectal cancer (orphan)*

leucovorin & methotrexate *antineoplastic for osteosarcoma (orphan)*

LeukArrest ℞ *immunomodulator; investigational (Phase III) cell adhesion inhibitor for acute ischemic stroke (trial discontinued 2000)* [rovelizumab]

Leukeran tablets ℞ *nitrogen mustard-type alkylating antineoplastic for multiple leukemias, lymphomas, and neoplasms* [chlorambucil] 2 mg

Leukine IV infusion ℞ *myeloid reconstitution after autologous bone marrow transplant (orphan); investigational (Phase III) for malignant melanoma; investigational (Phase III) cytokine for HIV infection* [sargramostim] 250, 500 µg

leukocyte interferon [now: interferon alfa-n3]

leukocyte protease inhibitor [see: secretory leukocyte protease inhibitor]

leukocyte typing serum USP *in vitro blood test*

leukopoietin [see: sargramostim]

LeukoScan *investigational (Phase III) diagnostic aid for osteomyelitis; investigational (NDA filed) diagnostic aid for infectious lesions* [technetium Tc 99m sulesomab]

leukotriene receptor antagonists (LTRAs); leukotriene receptor inhibitors *a class of antiasthmatics that inhibit bronchoconstriction when used prophylactically (will not reverse bronchospasm)*

LeukoVAX ℞ *investigational (Phase I/II) white blood cell formulation for treatment of rheumatoid arthritis*

leupeptin *investigational (orphan) aid to microsurgical peripheral nerve repair*

Leuprogel sustained-release subcu injection ℞ *investigational (Phase III) antihormonal antineoplastic for advanced prostate cancer* [leuprolide acetate]

leuprolide acetate USAN *testosterone suppressant; antihormonal antineoplastic for various cancers; LH-RH agonist for endometriosis and central precocious puberty (CPP) (orphan)* [also: leuprorelin] 5 mg/mL injection

leuprorelin INN, BAN *testosterone suppressant; antihormonal antineoplastic for various cancers* [also: leuprolide acetate]

leurocristine (LCR) [see: vincristine]

leurocristine sulfate [see: vincristine sulfate]

Leustatin IV infusion ℞ *antineoplastic for hairy-cell leukemia (orphan); investigational (orphan) for chronic lymphocytic leukemia, multiple sclerosis, and non-Hodgkin lymphoma* [cladribine] 1 mg/mL

LeuTech *investigational (NDA filed) radiolabeled infection imaging agent for equivocal appendicitis*

leutetium texaphyrin *investigational light-activated agent for dissolving arterial plaque*

Leuvectin ℞ *investigational (Phase I/II) gene-based therapy for advanced metastatic renal cell carcinoma; investigational (Phase I/II) for prostate cancer*

levacetylmethadol INN *narcotic analgesic* [also: levomethadyl acetate]

levalbuterol *sympathomimetic bronchodilator; single-isomer albuterol*

levalbuterol HCl USAN *sympathomimetic bronchodilator; single-isomer albuterol*

levalbuterol sulfate USAN *sympathomimetic bronchodilator; single-isomer albuterol*

Levall 5.0 syrup ℞ *narcotic antitussive; decongestant; expectorant* [hydrocodone bitartrate; phenylephrine HCl; guaifenesin] 5•15•100 mg/5 mL

levallorphan INN, BAN [also: levallorphan tartrate] ⑨ levorphanol

levallorphan tartrate USP [also: levallorphan]

levamfetamine INN *anorectic* [also: levamfetamine succinate; levamphetamine]

levamfetamine succinate USAN *anorectic* [also: levamfetamine; levamphetamine]

levamisole INN, BAN *biological response modifier; antineoplastic; veterinary anthelmintic* [also: levamisole HCl]

levamisole HCl USAN, USP *biological response modifier; antineoplastic; veterinary anthelmintic* [also: levamisole]

levamphetamine BAN *anorectic* [also: levamfetamine succinate; levamfetamine]

levant berry *(Anamirta cocculus; A. paniculata)* leaves and berries *medicinal herb for epilepsy, lice, malaria, morphine poisoning, and worms; not generally regarded as safe for ingestion or topical application on abraded skin*

Levaquin film-coated tablets, IV infusion ℞ *broad-spectrum fluoroquinolone antibiotic* [levofloxacin] 250, 500, 750 mg; 250, 500, 750 mg/vial

levarterenol [see: norepinephrine bitartrate]

levarterenol bitartrate [now: norepinephrine bitartrate]

Levatol caplets ℞ *antihypertensive; antiadrenergic (β-blocker)* [penbutolol sulfate] 20 mg

Levbid extended-release tablets ℞ *GI/GU antispasmodic; antiparkinsonian; anticholinergic "drying agent" for allergic rhinitis or hyperhidrosis* [hyoscyamine sulfate] 0.375 mg

levcromakalim USAN, INN, BAN *antiasthmatic; antihypertensive*

levcycloserine USAN, INN *enzyme inhibitor*

levdobutamine INN *cardiotonic* [also: levdobutamine lactobionate]

levdobutamine lactobionate USAN *cardiotonic* [also: levdobutamine]

levdropropizine INN

levemopamil INN *investigational treatment for stroke*

levetiracetam INN *anticonvulsant for partial-onset seizures*

levisoprenaline INN

Levisticum officinale *medicinal herb* [see: lovage]

Levlen tablets (in Slidecases of 21 or 28) ℞ *monophasic oral contraceptive; emergency postcoital contraceptive* [levonorgestrel; ethinyl estradiol] 0.15 mg•30 µg

Levlite tablets (in Slidecases of 21 or 28) ℞ *monophasic oral contraceptive; emergency postcoital contraceptive* [levonorgestrel; ethinyl estradiol] 0.1 mg•20 µg

levlofexidine INN

levobetaxolol INN *topical antiglaucoma agent (β-blocker)* [also: levobetaxolol HCl]

levobetaxolol HCl USAN *topical antiglaucoma agent (β-blocker)* [also: levobetaxolol]

levobunolol INN, BAN *topical antiglaucoma agent (β-blocker)* [also: levobunolol HCl]

levobunolol HCl USAN, USP *topical antiglaucoma agent (β-blocker)* [also: levobunolol] 0.25%, 0.5% eye drops

levobupivacaine HCl USAN *long-acting local anesthetic*

levocabastine INN, BAN *antihistamine* [also: levocabastine HCl]

levocabastine HCl USAN *antihistamine* [also: levocabastine]

levocarbinoxamine tartrate [see: rotoxamine tartrate]

levocarnitine USAN, USP, INN *dietary amino acid for primary and secondary genetic carnitine deficiency (orphan) and end-stage renal disease (orphan); investigational (orphan) for pediatric cardiomyopathy* 250 mg oral

levodopa USAN, USP, INN, BAN, JAN *antiparkinsonian; dopamine precursor* ⑨ methyldopa

levodopa & carbidopa *antiparkinsonian* 100•10, 100•25, 200•50, 250•25 mg oral

Levo-Dromoran tablets, subcu or IV injection ℞ *narcotic analgesic* [levorphanol tartrate] 2 mg; 2 mg/mL

levofacetoperane INN

levofenfluramine INN

levofloxacin USAN, INN, JAN *broad-spectrum fluoroquinolone antibiotic*

levofuraltadone USAN, INN *antibacterial; antiprotozoal*

levoglutamide INN *nonessential amino acid*

levoleucovorin calcium USAN *antidote to folic acid antagonists*

levomenol INN

levomepate [see: atromepine]

levomepromazine INN *analgesic* [also: methotrimeprazine]

levomethadone INN

levomethadyl acetate USAN *narcotic analgesic* [also: levacetylmethadol]

levomethadyl acetate HCl USAN *narcotic analgesic for management of opiate addiction (orphan)*

levomethorphan INN, BAN

levometiomeprazine INN

levomoprolol INN

levomoramide INN, BAN

levonantradol INN, BAN *analgesic* [also: levonantradol HCl]

levonantradol HCl USAN *analgesic* [also: levonantradol]

levonordefrin USP *adrenergic; vasoconstrictor* [also: corbadrine]

levonorgestrel USAN, USP, INN, BAN *progestin; intrauterine contraceptive (IUD); emergency postcoital oral contraceptive*

Levophed IV infusion ℞ *vasopressor for acute hypotensive shock* [norepinephrine bitartrate] 1 mg/mL

levophenacylmorphan INN, BAN

Levoprome IM injection ℞ *central analgesic; CNS depressant* [methotrimeprazine HCl] 20 mg/mL

levopropicillin INN *antibacterial* [also: levopropylcillin potassium]

levopropicillin potassium [see: levopropylcillin potassium]

levopropoxyphene INN, BAN *antitussive* [also: levopropoxyphene napsylate]

levopropoxyphene napsylate USAN *antitussive* [also: levopropoxyphene]

levopropylcillin potassium USAN *antibacterial* [also: levopropicillin]

levopropylhexedrine INN

levoprotiline INN

Levora 0.15/30 tablets (in packs of 21 or 28) ℞ *monophasic oral contraceptive; emergency postcoital contraceptive* [levonorgestrel; ethinyl estradiol] 0.15 mg•30 μg

levorin INN

levormeloxifene *investigational (Phase III) partial estrogen receptor agonist for osteoporosis (clinical trials discontinued 1998)*

levorphanol INN, BAN *narcotic analgesic* [also: levorphanol tartrate] ⊠ levallorphan

levorphanol tartrate USP *narcotic analgesic* [also: levorphanol] 2 mg oral

levosimendan USAN *investigational cardiotonic and vasodilator for congestive heart failure*

Levo-T tablets ℞ *synthetic thyroid* T_4 *hormone* [levothyroxine sodium] 25, 50, 75, 100, 125, 150, 200, 300 μg

Levothroid (CAN) tablets ℞ *synthetic thyroid* T_4 *hormone* [levothyroxine sodium] 25, 50, 75, 100, 112, 125, 150, 175, 200, 300 μg

Levothroid tablets, powder for injection ℞ *synthetic thyroid* T_4 *hormone* [levothyroxine sodium] 25, 50, 75, 88, 100, 112, 125, 137, 150, 175, 200, 300 μg; 200, 500 μg

levothyroxine sodium (T_4) USP, INN *synthetic thyroid hormone* [also: thyroxine] 0.1, 0.15, 0.2, 0.3 mg oral; 200, 500 μg/vial injection ⊠ liothyronine

levothyroxine sodium & tiratricol *investigational (orphan) to suppress thyroid-stimulating hormone (TSH) in thyroid cancer*

Levovist (CAN) powder for IV injection ℞ *ultrasound contrast medium for echocardiography* [galactose; palmitic acid]

levoxadrol INN *local anesthetic; smooth muscle relaxant* [also: levoxadrol HCl]

levoxadrol HCl USAN *local anesthetic; smooth muscle relaxant* [also: levoxadrol]

Levoxyl tablets ℞ *synthetic thyroid* T_4 *hormone* [levothyroxine sodium] 25, 50, 75, 88, 100, 112, 125, 137, 150, 175, 200, 300 μg

Levsin IV, IM, or subcu injection ℞ *GI/GU antispasmodic to reduce motility during radiologic imaging; preoperative antimuscarinic to reduce salivary and gastric secretions* [hyoscyamine sulfate] 0.5 mg/mL

Levsin tablets, drops, elixir ℞ *GI/GU antispasmodic; antiparkinsonian; anticholinergic "drying agent" for allergic rhinitis and hyperhidrosis* [hyoscyamine sulfate] 0.125 mg; 0.125 mg/mL; 0.125 mg/5 mL

Levsin PB drops ℞ *GI/GU antispasmodic; anticholinergic; sedative* [hyoscyamine sulfate; phenobarbital; alcohol 5%] 0.125•15 mg/mL

Levsin with Phenobarbital tablets ℞ *GI/GU antispasmodic; anticholinergic; sedative* [hyoscyamine sulfate; phenobarbital] 0.125•15 mg

Levsinex Timecaps (timed-release capsules) ℞ *GI/GU antispasmodic; antiparkinsonian; anticholinergic "drying agent" for allergic rhinitis or hyperhidrosis* [hyoscyamine sulfate] 0.375 mg

Levsin/SL sublingual tablets (also may be chewed or swallowed) ℞ *GI/GU antispasmodic; anticholinergic* [hyoscyamine sulfate] 0.125 mg

Levulan Kerastick topical solution ℞ *photosensitizer for photodynamic therapy of precancerous actinic keratoses of the face and scalp (for use with the BLU-U Blue Light Photodynamic Therapy Illuminator)* [aminolevulinic acid HCl] 20%

levulose BAN *nutrient; caloric replacement* [also: fructose]

LEX-032 *investigational (Phase II) serine protease inhibitor for treatment of reperfusion injury*

lexipafant USAN *platelet activating factor (PAF) antagonist; investigational (Phase III) treatment for acute pancreatitis*

lexithromycin USAN, INN *antibacterial*

lexofenac INN

Lexxel film-coated combination-release tablets ℞ *antihypertensive; angiotensin-converting enzyme (ACE) inhibitor; calcium channel blocker* [enalapril maleate (immediate release); felodipine (extended release)] 5•5, 5•2.5 mg

LH-RF (luteinizing hormone-releasing factor) acetate hydrate [see: gonadorelin acetate]

LH-RF diacetate tetrahydrate [now: gonadorelin acetate]

LH-RF dihydrochloride [now: gonadorelin HCl]

LH-RF HCl [see: gonadorelin HCl]

LH-RH (luteinizing hormone–releasing hormone) *an endogenous hormone, produced in the hypothalamus, which stimulates the release of luteinizing hormone (LH) and follicle-stimulating hormone (FSH) from the pituitary* [also known as: gonadotropin-releasing hormone (Gn-RH)]

liarozole INN, BAN *antipsoriatic; aromatase inhibitor* [also: liarozole fumarate]

liarozole fumarate USAN *antipsoriatic; aromatase inhibitor* [also: liarozole]

liarozole HCl USAN *antineoplastic for prostate cancer; aromatase inhibitor*

liatermin USAN *dopaminergic neuronal growth stimulator for Parkinson disease*

Liatris scariosa; L. spicata; L. squarrosa *medicinal herb* [see: blazing star]

libecillide INN

libenzapril USAN, INN *angiotensin-converting enzyme (ACE) inhibitor*

Librax capsules ℞ *GI anticholinergic; anxiolytic* [clidinium bromide; chlordiazepoxide HCl] 2.5•5 mg

Libritabs film-coated tablets ℞ *benzodiazepine anxiolytic* [chlordiazepoxide] 10, 25 mg

Librium capsules, powder for injection ℞ *benzodiazepine anxiolytic; sometimes abused as a street drug* [chlordiazepoxide HCl] 5, 10, 25 mg; 100 mg

Lice-Enz foam shampoo OTC *pediculicide for lice* [pyrethrins; piperonyl butoxide] 0.3%•3%

licorice (*Glycyrrhiza glabra; G. pallidiflora; G. uralensis*) root *medicinal herb for Addison disease, blood cleansing, colds, cough, drug withdrawal, female disorders, hoarseness, hypoglycemia, lung disorders, sore throat, and stomach ulcers; also used as an expectorant and to increase energy*

licostinel USAN *investigational (Phase I) NMDA receptor antagonist for stroke*

licryfilcon A USAN *hydrophilic contact lens material*

licryfilcon B USAN *hydrophilic contact lens material*

Lid Wipes-SPF solution, pads OTC *eyelid cleansing wipes for blepharitis or contact lenses*

Lidakol cream ℞ *investigational (Phase II) antiviral lipase inhibitor for HIV infection and AIDS-related Kaposi sarcoma* [docosanol] 10%

Lida-Mantle-HC cream ℞ *local anesthetic; topical corticosteroidal anti-inflammatory* [lidocaine; hydrocortisone acetate] 3%•0.5%

lidamidine INN *antiperistaltic* [also: lidamidine HCl]

lidamidine HCl USAN *antiperistaltic* [also: lidamidine]

Lidex cream, ointment, topical solution ℞ *topical corticosteroidal anti-inflammatory* [fluocinonide] 0.05% ⑨ Lasix; Lidox; Wydase

Lidex gel (discontinued 2000) ℞ *topical corticosteroidal anti-inflammatory* [fluocinonide] 0.05% ⑨ Lasix; Lidox; Wydase

Lidex-E cream ℞ *topical corticosteroidal anti-inflammatory; emollient* [fluocinonide] 0.05%

lidimycin INN *antifungal* [also: lydimycin]

lidocaine USP, INN *topical local anesthetic; investigational (orphan) trans-*

dermal delivery for post-herpetic neuralgia [also: lignocaine]

lidocaine benzyl benzoate [see: denatonium benzoate]

lidocaine HCl USP *local anesthetic; antiarrhythmic* [also: lignocaine HCl] 2%, 4%, 5% topical; 1%, 1.5%, 2% injection; 4%, 10%, 20% IV admixture

Lidoderm transdermal patch ℞ *topical anesthetic for post-herpetic neuralgia (orphan)* [lidocaine] 5%

lidofenin USAN, INN *hepatic function test*

lidofilcon A USAN *hydrophilic contact lens material*

lidofilcon B USAN *hydrophilic contact lens material*

lidoflazine USAN, INN, BAN *coronary vasodilator*

Lidoject-1; Lidoject-2 injection ℞ *injectable local anesthetic* [lidocaine HCl] 1%; 2%

LidoPen auto-injector (automatic IM injection device) ℞ *emergency injection for cardiac arrhythmias* [lidocaine HCl] 10%

LID-Pack (CAN) ophthalmic ointment + towelettes OTC *antibiotic* [polymyxin B sulfate; bacitracin zinc] 10 000•500 U/g

lifarizine USAN, INN, BAN *platelet aggregation inhibitor*

life everlasting *medicinal herb* [see: everlasting]

life root (*Senecio aureus; S. jacoboea; S. vulgaris*) *medicinal herb for childbirth pain, diaphoresis, edema, fever, and stimulation of labor and menses; not generally regarded as safe for ingestion because of hepatotoxicity*

life-of-man *medicinal herb* [see: spikenard]

lifibrate USAN, INN *antihyperlipoproteinemic*

lifibrol USAN, INN *antihyperlipidemic*

LIG (lymphocyte immune globulin) [q.v.]

light mineral oil [see: mineral oil, light]

lignocaine BAN *topical local anesthetic* [also: lidocaine]

lignocaine HCl BAN *local anesthetic; antiarrhythmic* [also: lidocaine HCl]

lignosulfonic acid, sodium salt [see: polignate sodium]

lilopristone INN

lily, conval; May lily *medicinal herb* [see: lily of the valley]

lily, ground *medicinal herb* [see: birthroot]

lily, white pond; sweet water lily; sweet-scented pond lily; sweet-scented water lily; white water lily; toad lily *medicinal herb* [see: white pond lily]

lily of the valley (*Convallaria majalis*) flower, leaves, and rhizome *medicinal herb for arrhythmias, edema, epilepsy, and heart disorders*

limaprost INN

limarsol [see: acetarsone]

Limbitrol DS 10-25 tablets ℞ *antidepressant; anxiolytic* [chlordiazepoxide; amitriptyline HCl] 10•25 mg

lime USP *pharmaceutic necessity*

lime, sulfurated (calcium polysulfide, calcium thiosulfate) USP *wet dressing/soak for cystic acne and seborrhea*

lime tree *medicinal herb* [see: linden tree]

Lin-Amox (CAN) capsules, oral suspension ℞ *antibiotic* [amoxicillin trihydrate] 250, 500 mg; 125, 250 mg/5 mL

linarotene USAN, INN *antikeratinizing agent*

Lin-Buspirone (CAN) tablets ℞ *azaspirone anxiolytic* [buspirone HCl] 10 mg

Lincocin capsules, IV or IM injection ℞ *lincosamide antibiotic* [lincomycin HCl] 500 mg; 300 mg/mL ⊡ Cleocin; Indocin

Lincocin pediatric capsules (discontinued 1998) ℞ *lincosamide antibiotic* [lincomycin HCl] 250 mg ⊡ Cleocin; Indocin

lincomycin USAN, INN, BAN *lincosamide antibiotic*

lincomycin HCl USP *lincosamide antibiotic* 300 mg/mL injection

Lincorex IV or IM injection ℞ *lincosamide antibiotic* [lincomycin HCl] 300 mg/mL

lincosamides *a class of antimicrobial antibiotics with potentially serious side effects, to which bacterial resistance has been shown*

lindane USAN, USP, INN, BAN *pediculicide for lice; scabicide* 1% topical

linden tree *(Tilia americana; T. cordata; T. europaea; T. platyphyllos)* flowers *medicinal herb for diaphoresis, diarrhea, headache, hypertension, indigestion, nasal congestion, nervousness, skin moisturizer, stomach disorders, and throat irritation*

linezolid USAN *oxazolidinone antibiotic for gram-positive bacterial infections*

Linguets (trademarked form) *buccal tablets*

Linker protocol (daunorubicin, vincristine, prednisone, asparaginase, teniposide, cytarabine, methotrexate [with leucovorin rescue]) *chemotherapy protocol for acute lymphocytic leukemia (ALL)*

Lin-Megestrol (CAN) tablets ℞ *progestin; hormonal antineoplastic for advanced carcinoma of the breast or endometrium* [megestrol acetate] 40, 160 mg

linogliride USAN, INN *antidiabetic*

linogliride fumarate USAN *antidiabetic*

linolexamide [see: clinolamide]

Linomide ℞ *investigational (Phase II) immunomodulator for HIV; investigational for bone marrow transplant for leukemia; clinical trials for MS discontinued 1997; orphan status withdrawn 1998* [roquinimex]

linopiridine USAN, INN *cognition enhancer for Alzheimer disease*

Lin-Pravastatin (CAN) tablets ℞ *HMG-CoA reductase inhibitor for hyperlipidemia and hypertriglyceridemia* [pravastatin sodium] 10, 20, 40 mg

linseed *medicinal herb* [see: flaxseed]

linsidomine INN

lint bells *medicinal herb* [see: flaxseed]

lintopride INN

Linum usitatissimum *medicinal herb* [see: flaxseed]

lion's ear; lion's tail *medicinal herb* [see: motherwort]

lion's tooth *medicinal herb* [see: dandelion]

Lioresal intrathecal injection ℞ *skeletal muscle relaxant for intractable spasticity due to spinal cord injury or disease (orphan); investigational (orphan) for trigeminal neuralgia* [baclofen] 10 mg/20 mL (500 µg/mL), 10 mg/5 mL (2000 µg/mL)

Lioresal tablets ℞ *skeletal muscle relaxant* [baclofen] 10, 20 mg

liothyronine INN, BAN *radioactive agent* [also: liothyronine I 125] ⓢ levothyroxine

liothyronine I 125 USAN *radioactive agent* [also: liothyronine]

liothyronine I 131 USAN *radioactive agent*

liothyronine sodium (T_3) USP, BAN *synthetic thyroid hormone; treatment of myxedema coma or precoma (orphan)* 25 µg oral

liotrix USAN, USP *synthetic thyroid hormone (T_4 and T_3 in a 4:1 ratio)* ⓢ Klotrix

Lip Medex ointment OTC *topical antipruritic/counterirritant; mild local anesthetic* [camphor; phenol] 1%•0.54%

lipancreatin [see: pancrelipase]

lipase *digestive enzyme* [24 IU/mg in pancrelipase; 2 IU/mg in pancreatin]

lipase of pancreas [see: pancrelipase]

lipase triacylglycerol [see: pancrelipase]

Lipidil Supra (CAN) film-coated tablets ℞ *antihyperlipidemic for hypercholesterolemia and hypertriglyceridemia* [fenofibrate] 100, 160 mg

Lipisorb powder OTC *enteral nutritional therapy* [lactose-free formula]

Lipitor film-coated tablets ℞ *HMG-CoA reductase inhibitor for hypercholesterolemia, dysbetalipoproteinemia, and hypertriglyceridemia* [atorvastatin calcium] 10, 20, 40, 80 mg

Lipoflavonoid capsules OTC *dietary lipotropic with vitamin supplementation*

[choline; inositol; multiple B vitamins; vitamin C; lemon bioflavonoids] 111.3•111.3•≛•100•100 mg

Lipogen capsules, caplets OTC *dietary lipotropic with vitamin supplementation* [choline; inositol; multiple vitamins] 111•111•≛ mg

α-lipoic acid; lipoicin *natural antioxidant* [see: alpha lipoic acid]

Lipomul liquid OTC *dietary fat supplement* [corn oil] 10 g/15 mL

Liponol capsules OTC *dietary lipotropic with vitamin supplementation* [choline; inositol; methionine; multiple B vitamins] 115•83•110•≛ mg

lipoprotein OspA, recombinant *active immunizing agent against Lyme disease*

lipoprotein-associated coagulation inhibitor (LACI) [see: tifacogin]

liposomal gentamicin [see: gentamicin liposome]

liposome-encapsulated doxorubicin HCl (LED) [see: doxorubicin HCl, liposome-encapsulated]

liposome-encapsulated recombinant interleukin-2 [see: interleukin-2, liposome-encapsulated recombinant]

liposome-encapsulated T4 endonuclease V [see: T4 endonuclease V, liposome encapsulated]

Liposyn II 20%; Liposyn III 20% IV infusion ℞ *nutritional therapy* [fat emulsion]

Lipotriad caplets OTC *dietary lipotropic with vitamin supplementation* [choline; inositol; multiple vitamins] 111•≟•≛ mg

lipotropics *a class of oral nutritional supplements*

Lipram-CR20 capsules ℞ *digestive enzymes* [lipase; amylase; protease] 20 000•66 400•75 000 U

Lipram-PN10 capsules ℞ *digestive enzymes* [lipase; amylase; protease] 10 000•30 000•30 000 U

Lipram-PN16 capsules ℞ *digestive enzymes* [lipase; amylase; protease] 16 000•48 000•48 000 U

Lipram-UL12 capsules ℞ *digestive enzymes* [lipase; amylase; protease] 12 000•39 000•39 000 U

Lipram-UL18 capsules ℞ *digestive enzymes* [lipase; amylase; protease] 18 000•58 500•58 500 U

Lipram-UL20 capsules ℞ *digestive enzymes* [lipase; amylase; protease] 20 000•65 000•65 000 U

Liquaemin Sodium IV or deep subcu injection (discontinued 1997) ℞ *anticoagulant* [heparin sodium] 1000, 5000, 10 000, 20 000, 40 000 U/mL

liquefied phenol [see: phenol, liquefied]

Liquibid; Liquibid-1200 sustained-release tablet ℞ *expectorant* [guaifenesin] 600 mg; 1200 mg

Liquibid-D sustained-release tablets ℞ *decongestant; expectorant* [phenylephrine HCl; guaifenesin] 40•600 mg

Liqui-Char oral liquid OTC *adsorbent antidote for poisoning* [activated charcoal] 12.5 g/60 mL, 15 g/75 mL, 25 g/120 mL, 30 g/120 mL, 50 g/240 mL

Liqui-Coat HD concentrated oral suspension ℞ *radiopaque contrast medium for gastrointestinal imaging* [barium sulfate] 210%

Liquid Caps (dosage form) *soft liquid-filled capsules*

liquid glucose [see: glucose, liquid]

liquid petrolatum [see: mineral oil]

Liquid Pred syrup ℞ *corticosteroid; anti-inflammatory* [prednisone; alcohol 5%] 5 mg/5 mL

Liquid Tabs (dosage form) *liquid-filled tablets*

Liquidambar orientalis; L. styraciflua *medicinal herb* [see: storax]

Liqui-Doss emulsion OTC *emollient laxative* [mineral oil]

Liquifilm Tears; Liquifilm Forte eye drops OTC *ophthalmic moisturizer/lubricant* [polyvinyl alcohol] 1.4%; 3%

Liquifilm Wetting solution OTC *wetting solution for hard contact lenses*

Liqui-Gels (trademarked dosage form) *soft liquid-filled gelatin capsules*

Liqui-Histine DM syrup ℞ *antitussive; decongestant; antihistamine* [dextromethorphan hydrobromide; phenylpropanolamine HCl; brompheniramine maleate] 10•12.5•2 mg/5 mL

Liqui-Histine-D elixir ℞ *decongestant; antihistamine* [phenylpropanolamine HCl; phenyltoloxamine citrate; pyrilamine maleate; pheniramine maleate] 12.5•4•4•4 mg/5 mL

Liquimat lotion OTC *antibacterial and exfoliant for acne* [sulfur] 4%

Liquipake oral/rectal suspension (discontinued 1999) ℞ *radiopaque contrast medium for gastrointestinal imaging* [barium sulfate] 100%

Liquiprin elixir (discontinued 1997) OTC *analgesic; antipyretic* [acetaminophen] 160 mg/5 mL

Liquiprin Drops for Children OTC *analgesic; antipyretic* [acetaminophen] 80 mg/1.66 mL

Liquitab (trademarked dosage form) *chewable tablet*

LiquiVent ℞ *investigational (Phase III) blood substitute; investigational (Phase III) treatment for pediatric acute respiratory distress syndrome (ARDS); investigational (Phase II/III) agent for adults with acute lung injury or ARDS* [perflubron]

liquor carbonis detergens (LCD) [see: coal tar]

liroldine INN

lisadimate USAN, INN *sunscreen*

lisinopril USAN, INN, BAN *antihypertensive; angiotensin-converting enzyme (ACE) inhibitor*

lisofylline (LSF) USAN *acetyltransferase inhibitor; investigational (Phase III) immunomodulator and cytokine inhibitor for acute myeloid leukemia and bone marrow transplants; investigational agent for prevention of GI tract damage during chemotherapy; investigational (Phase II/III) for ARDS and acute lung injury*

Listerine; Cool-Mint Listerine; FreshBurst Listerine mouthwash/gargle OTC *topical oral antiseptic; analgesic* [thymol; eucalyptol; methyl salicylate; menthol; alcohol 22%–26%] 0.06%•0.09%•0.06%•0.04%

Listermint Arctic Mint mouthwash/gargle OTC

lisuride INN [also: lysuride]

Lithane (CAN) capsules ℞ *antipsychotic for manic episodes of a bipolar disorder* [lithium carbonate] 150, 300 mg

lithium *element (Li)*

lithium benzoate NF

lithium carbonate USAN, USP *antimanic; immunity booster in chemotherapy and AIDS* 150, 300, 600 mg oral

lithium citrate USP *antimanic; immunity booster in chemotherapy and AIDS* 300 mg/5 mL oral

lithium hydroxide USP *antimanic*

lithium hydroxide monohydrate [see: lithium hydroxide]

lithium salicylate NF

Lithobid slow-release tablets ℞ *antipsychotic for manic episodes of a bipolar disorder* [lithium carbonate] 300 mg

litholytics *a class of agents that dissolve stones or calculi* [see also: antilithics]

Lithonate capsules ℞ *antipsychotic for manic episodes of a bipolar disorder* [lithium carbonate] 300 mg

Lithostat tablets ℞ *adjunctive therapy in chronic urea-splitting urinary tract infections* [acetohydroxamic acid] 250 mg

Lithotabs film-coated tablets ℞ *antipsychotic for manic episodes of a bipolar disorder* [lithium carbonate] 300 mg

litracen INN

liver, desiccated; liver extracts *source of vitamin B_{12}*

Liver Combo No. 5 IM injection ℞ *antianemic; vitamin supplement* [liver extracts; vitamin B_{12}; folic acid] 10 µg•100 µg•0.4 mg per mL

liver derivative complex *claimed to be an anti-inflammatory for various dermatological conditions*

liver lily *medicinal herb* [see: blue flag]

liverleaf; liverwort *medicinal herb* [see: hepatica]

Livial (commercially available in Europe, Asia, and South America) ℞ *investigational (NDA filed) syn-*

thetic steroid for osteoporosis and other postmenopausal symptoms [tibolone]

lividomycin INN

Livitrinsic-f capsules ℞ *hematinic* [ferrous fumarate; cyanocobalamin; ascorbic acid; intrinsic factor concentrate; folic acid] 110 mg•15 µg•75 mg•240 mg•0.5 mg

Livostin eye drop suspension ℞ *topical antihistamine for allergic conjunctivitis* [levocabastine HCl] 0.05%

Livostin (CAN) nasal spray ℞ *antihistamine for seasonal allergic rhinitis* [levocabastine HCl] 0.05%

lixazinone sulfate USAN *cardiotonic; phosphodiesterase inhibitor*

LKV Infant Drops powder + liquid OTC *vitamin supplement* [multiple vitamins; biotin] ≛•75 µg/0.6 mL

LLD factor [see: cyanocobalamin]

10% LMD IV injection ℞ *plasma volume expander for shock due to hemorrhage, burns, or surgery* [dextran 40] 10%

LMD (low molecular weight dextran) [see: dextran 40]

LMF (Leukeran, methotrexate, fluorouracil) *chemotherapy protocol*

LMWD (low molecular weight dextran) [see: dextran 40]

Lobac capsules ℞ *skeletal muscle relaxant; analgesic* [salicylamide; phenyltoloxamine; acetaminophen] 200•20•300 mg

Lobana Body lotion OTC *moisturizer; emollient*

Lobana Body Shampoo; Lobana Liquid Lather liquid OTC *soap-free therapeutic skin cleanser* [chloroxylenol]

Lobana Derm-Ade cream OTC *moisturizer; emollient* [vitamins A, D, and E]

Lobana Peri-Garde ointment OTC *moisturizer; emollient; antiseptic* [vitamins A, D, and E; chloroxylenol]

lobelia *(Lobelia inflata)* plant (tincture) *medicinal herb for arthritis, asthma, bronchitis, hay fever, colds, cough, ear infections, epilepsy, fever, food poisoning, lockjaw, nervousness, pain, pneumonia, preventing miscarriage, whooping cough, and worms*

lobeline INN *nicotine withdrawal aid* [also: lobeline HCl]

lobeline HCl JAN *nicotine withdrawal aid* [also: lobeline]

lobeline sulfate *investigational (Phase III) nicotine withdrawal aid; clinical trials discontinued 1997*

lobendazole USAN, INN *veterinary anthelmintic*

lobenzarit INN *antirheumatic* [also: lobenzarit sodium]

lobenzarit sodium USAN *antirheumatic* [also: lobenzarit]

lobradimil USAN *receptor-mediated permeabilizer; investigational (Phase II) blood-brain barrier permeability-enhancing agent for carrying carboplatin to brain tumors*

lobucavir USAN, INN *antiviral; investigational (Phase III) for AIDS-related asymptomatic cytomegalovirus (clinical trials discontinued 1999)*

lobuprofen INN

LoCholest; LoCholest Light powder for oral suspension ℞ *cholesterol-lowering antihyperlipidemic; also used for biliary obstruction* [cholestyramine resin] 4 g/dose

locicortolone dicibate INN

locicortone [see: locicortolone dicibate]

Locilex ℞ *investigational (NDA filed) broad-spectrum antibiotic for impetigo and diabetic foot ulcers* [pexiganan acetate]

Locoid cream, ointment, solution ℞ *topical corticosteroidal anti-inflammatory* [hydrocortisone butyrate] 0.1%

locust plant *medicinal herb* [see: senna]

lodaxaprine INN

lodazecar INN

lodelaben USAN, INN *antiarthritic; emphysema therapy adjunct*

lodenosine USAN *investigational (Phase II) reverse transcriptase antiviral for HIV infection*

Lodine film-coated tablets, capsules ℞ *analgesic; antiarthritic; nonsteroidal* *anti-inflammatory drug (NSAID)* [etodolac] 400, 500 mg; 200, 300 mg

Lodine XL film-coated extended-release tablets ℞ *once-daily analgesic and antiarthritic; nonsteroidal anti-inflammatory drug (NSAID)* [etodolac] 400, 500, 600 mg

lodinixil INN

lodiperone INN

Lodosyn tablets ℞ *decarboxylase inhibitor; antiparkinsonian adjunct (used with levodopa; no effect when given alone)* [carbidopa] 25 mg

lodoxamide INN, BAN *antiallergic; antiasthmatic* [also: lodoxamide ethyl]

lodoxamide ethyl USAN *antiallergic; antiasthmatic* [also: lodoxamide]

lodoxamide trometamol BAN *antiallergic; antiasthmatic* [also: lodoxamide tromethamine]

lodoxamide tromethamine USAN *antiasthmatic; antiallergic for vernal keratoconjunctivitis (orphan)* [also: lodoxamide trometamol]

Lodrane LD sustained-release capsules ℞ *decongestant; antihistamine* [pseudoephedrine HCl; brompheniramine maleate] 60•6 mg

Loestrin 21 1/20; Loestrin 21 1.5/30 tablets (in packs of 21) ℞ *monophasic oral contraceptive* [norethindrone acetate; ethinyl estradiol] 1 mg•20 µg; 1.5 mg•30 µg

Loestrin Fe 1/20; Loestrin Fe 1.5/30 tablets (in packs of 28) ℞ *monophasic oral contraceptive; iron supplement* [norethindrone acetate; ethinyl estradiol; ferrous fumarate] 1 mg•20 µg•75 mg; 1.5 mg•30 µg•75 mg

lofemizole INN *anti-inflammatory; analgesic; antipyretic* [also: lofemizole HCl]

lofemizole HCl USAN *anti-inflammatory; analgesic; antipyretic* [also: lofemizole]

Lofenalac powder OTC *special diet for infants with phenylketonuria*

lofendazam INN, BAN

lofentanil INN, BAN *narcotic analgesic* [also: lofentanil oxalate]

lofentanil oxalate USAN *narcotic analgesic* [also: lofentanil]

lofepramine INN, BAN *antidepressant* [also: lofepramine HCl]

lofepramine HCl USAN *antidepressant* [also: lofepramine]

lofexidine INN, BAN *centrally acting antiadrenergic antihypertensive* [also: lofexidine HCl]

lofexidine HCl USAN *centrally acting antiadrenergic antihypertensive; investigational (Phase III) treatment for opiate withdrawal syndrome* [also: lofexidine]

loflucarban INN

Logen tablets ℞ *antidiarrheal* [diphenoxylate HCl; atropine sulfate] 2.5•0.025 mg

LOMAC (leucovorin, Oncovin, methotrexate, Adriamycin, cyclophosphamide) *chemotherapy protocol*

Lomanate liquid ℞ *antidiarrheal* [diphenoxylate HCl; atropine sulfate] 2.5•0.025 mg/5 mL

lombazole INN, BAN

lomefloxacin USAN, INN, BAN *broad-spectrum fluoroquinolone antibiotic*

lomefloxacin HCl USAN *broad-spectrum fluoroquinolone antibiotic*

lomefloxacin mesylate USAN *antibacterial*

lometraline INN *antipsychotic; antiparkinsonian* [also: lometraline HCl]

lometraline HCl USAN *antipsychotic; antiparkinsonian* [also: lometraline]

lometrexol INN *antineoplastic* [also: lometrexol sodium]

lometrexol sodium USAN *antineoplastic* [also: lometrexol]

lomevactone INN

lomifylline INN

lomofungin USAN *antifungal*

Lomotil tablets, liquid ℞ *antidiarrheal* [diphenoxylate HCl; atropine sulfate] 2.5•0.025 mg; 2.5•0.025 mg/5 mL

lomustine USAN, INN, BAN *nitrosourea-type alkylating antineoplastic for brain tumors and Hodgkin disease*

Lonalac powder OTC *enteral nutritional therapy* [milk-based formula]

lonapalene USAN *antipsoriatic*

lonaprofen INN

lonazolac INN

lonidamine INN

Loniten tablets ℞ *antihypertensive; vasodilator* [minoxidil] 2.5, 10 mg ⊡ clonidine

Lonox tablets ℞ *antidiarrheal* [diphenoxylate HCl; atropine sulfate] 2.5•0.025 mg ⊡ Lovenox

loop diuretics *a class of diuretic agents that inhibit the reabsorption of sodium and chloride*

Lo/Ovral tablets (in Pilpaks of 21) ℞ *monophasic oral contraceptive; emergency postcoital contraceptive* [norgestrel; ethinyl estradiol] 0.3 mg•30 μg

loperamide INN, BAN *antiperistaltic; antidiarrheal* [also: loperamide HCl]

loperamide HCl USAN, USP, JAN *antiperistaltic; antidiarrheal* [also: loperamide] 2 mg oral; 1 mg/5 mL oral

loperamide oxide INN, BAN *antiperistaltic; antidiarrheal*

Lophophora williamsii *a flowering Mexican cactus whose heads (mescal buttons) are used to produce mescaline, a hallucinogenic street drug*

Lopid film-coated tablets ℞ *triglyceride-lowering antihyperlipidemic for hypertriglyceridemia (types IV and V hyperlipidemia) and coronary heart disease* [gemfibrozil] 600 mg (300 mg capsules available in Canada)

lopinavir USAN *antiviral protease inhibitor for HIV infection*

lopirazepam INN

loprazolam INN, BAN

lopremone [now: protirelin]

Lopressor caplets, IV injection ℞ *antihypertensive; antianginal; antiadrenergic (β-blocker)* [metoprolol tartrate] 50, 100 mg; 1 mg/mL

Lopressor HCT 50/25; Lopressor HCT 100/25; Lopressor HCT 100/50 tablets ℞ *antihypertensive; β-blocker; diuretic* [metoprolol tartrate; hydrochlorothiazide] 50•25 mg; 100•25 mg; 100•50 mg

loprodiol INN

Loprox cream, lotion, gel ℞ *topical antifungal* [ciclopirox olamine] 1%

Lorabid Pulvules (capsules), powder for oral suspension ℞ *carbacephem antibiotic* [loracarbef] 200, 400 mg; 100, 200 mg/5 mL

loracarbef USAN, INN *carbacephem antibiotic*

lorajmine INN *antiarrhythmic* [also: lorajmine HCl]

lorajmine HCl USAN *antiarrhythmic* [also: lorajmine]

lorapride INN

loratadine USAN, INN, BAN *second-generation piperidine antihistamine for allergic rhinitis and chronic idiopathic urticaria*

lorazepam USAN, USP, INN, BAN *benzodiazepine anxiolytic; minor tranquilizer* 0.5, 1, 2 mg oral; 2 mg/mL oral; 2, 4 mg/mL injection

lorbamate USAN, INN *muscle relaxant*

lorcainide INN, BAN *antiarrhythmic* [also: lorcainide HCl]

lorcainide HCl USAN *antiarrhythmic* [also: lorcainide]

Lorcet tablets (discontinued 1997) ℞ *narcotic analgesic* [hydrocodone bitartrate; acetaminophen] 5•500 mg

Lorcet Plus; Lorcet 10/650 tablets ℞ *narcotic analgesic* [hydrocodone bitartrate; acetaminophen] 7.5•650 mg; 10•650 mg

Lorcet-HD capsules ℞ *narcotic analgesic* [hydrocodone bitartrate; acetaminophen] 5•500 mg ⊡ Fioricet

lorcinadol USAN, INN, BAN *analgesic*

loreclezole USAN, INN, BAN *antiepileptic*

Lorenzo oil (erucic acid and oleic acid) *natural treatment for childhood adrenoleukodystrophy and adrenomyeloneuropathy in adults*

lorglumide INN

lormetazepam USAN, INN, BAN *sedative; hypnotic*

lornoxicam USAN, INN, BAN *analgesic; anti-inflammatory*

Lorothidol (available only from the Centers for Disease Control) ℞

investigational anti-infective for paragonimiasis and fascioliasis [bithionol]

Loroxide lotion OTC *topical keratolytic for acne* [benzoyl peroxide] 5.5%

lorpiprazole INN

Lortab elixir ℞ *narcotic analgesic* [hydrocodone bitartrate; acetaminophen] 2.5•167 mg/5 mL

Lortab 2.5/500; Lortab 5/500; Lortab 7.5/500; Lortab 10/500 tablets ℞ *narcotic analgesic* [hydrocodone bitartrate; acetaminophen] 2.5•500 mg; 5•500 mg; 7.5•500 mg; 10•500 mg

Lortab ASA tablets ℞ *narcotic analgesic* [hydrocodone bitartrate; aspirin] 5•500 mg

lortalamine USAN, INN *antidepressant*

lorzafone USAN, INN *minor tranquilizer*

losartan INN *antihypertensive; angiotensin II receptor antagonist* [also: losartan potassium]

losartan potassium USAN *antihypertensive; angiotensin II receptor antagonist* [also: losartan]

Losec (CAN) delayed-release tablets ℞ *proton pump inhibitor for gastric and duodenal ulcers and other gastroesophageal disorders* [omeprazole magnesium] 10, 20 mg

Losec 1-2-3 A (CAN) ℞ *7-day regimen for eradication of H. pylori–associated peptic ulcer disease* [Losec, 20 mg b.i.d; amoxicillin, 1000 mg b.i.d; clarithromycin, 500 mg b.i.d.]

Losec 1-2-3 M (CAN) ℞ *7-day regimen for eradication of H. pylori–associated peptic ulcer disease* [Losec, 20 mg b.i.d; metronidazole, 500 mg b.i.d; clarithromycin, 250 mg b.i.d.]

losigamone INN

losindole INN

losmiprofen INN

losoxantrone INN *antineoplastic* [also: losoxantrone HCl]

losoxantrone HCl USAN *antineoplastic* [also: losoxantrone]

losulazine INN *antihypertensive* [also: losulazine HCl]

losulazine HCl USAN *antihypertensive* [also: losulazine]

Lotemax eye drop suspension ℞ *corticosteroidal anti-inflammatory* [loteprednol etabonate] 0.5%

Lotensin tablets ℞ *antihypertensive; angiotensin-converting enzyme (ACE) inhibitor* [benazepril HCl] 5, 10, 20, 40 mg

Lotensin HCT 5/6.25; Lotensin HCT 10/12.5; Lotensin HCT 20/12.5; Lotensin HCT 20/25 tablets ℞ *antihypertensive; angiotensin-converting enzyme (ACE) inhibitor; diuretic* [benazepril HCl; hydrochlorothiazide] 5•6.25 mg; 10•12.5 mg; 20•12.5 mg; 20•25 mg

loteprednol INN *corticosteroidal anti-inflammatory* [also: loteprednol etabonate]

loteprednol etabonate USAN *ophthalmic corticosteroidal anti-inflammatory* [also: loteprednol]

lotifazole INN

lotrafiban HCl USAN *platelet aggregation inhibitor; GP IIb/IIIa receptor antagonist*

Lotrel capsules ℞ *antihypertensive; angiotensin-converting enzyme (ACE) inhibitor; calcium channel blocker* [amlodipine besylate; benazepril HCl] 2.5•10, 5•10, 5•20 mg

lotrifen INN

Lotrimin cream, solution, lotion ℞ *topical antifungal* [clotrimazole] 1% ⑨ Otrivin

Lotrimin AF cream, solution, lotion OTC *topical antifungal* [clotrimazole] 1%

Lotrimin AF powder, spray powder, spray liquid OTC *topical antifungal* [miconazole nitrate] 2%

Lotrisone cream, lotion ℞ *topical corticosteroidal anti-inflammatory; antifungal* [betamethasone dipropionate; clotrimazole] 0.05%•1%

Lotronex film-coated tablets (discontinued 2000) ℞ *serotonin 5-HT_3 receptor antagonist for irritable bowel syndrome* [alosetron HCl] 1 mg

lotucaine INN

lousewort *medicinal herb* [see: betony; feverweed]

lovage (*Angelica levisticum; Levisticum officinale*) leaves and roots *medicinal herb for bad breath, boils, edema, flatulence, and sore throat; also used topically as a skin emollient*

lovastatin USAN, INN, BAN *HMG-CoA reductase inhibitor for hypercholesterolemia and coronary heart disease* 10, 20, 40 mg oral

Lovenox deep subcu injection in prefilled syringes ℞ *anticoagulant/antithrombotic for prevention of deep vein thrombosis (DVT) following knee, hip, or abdominal surgery, unstable angina, and myocardial infarction* [enoxaparin sodium] 30 mg/0.3 mL, 40 mg/0.4 mL, 60, 90 mg/0.6 mL, 80, 120 mg/0.8 mL, 100, 150 mg/mL ⊡ Lonox

loviride USAN, INN *investigational nonnucleoside reverse transcriptase inhibitor (NNRTI) antiviral for HIV*

low molecular weight dextran (LMD; LMWD) [see: dextran 40]

low molecular weight heparins *a class of anticoagulants used for the prophylaxis or treatment of thromboembolic complications of surgery and ischemic complications of unstable angina or myocardial infarction*

low osmolar contrast media (LOCM) *a class of newer radiopaque agents that have a low osmolar concentration of iodine (the contrast agent), which corresponds to a lower incidence of adverse reactions* [also called: nonionic contrast media]

Lowila Cake bar OTC *soap-free therapeutic skin cleanser*

Low-Ogestrel tablets (in packs of 21 or 28) ℞ *monophasic oral contraceptive; emergency postcoital contraceptive* [norgestrel; ethinyl estradiol] 0.3 mg•30 µg

Lowsium Plus oral suspension OTC *antacid; antiflatulent* [magaldrate; simethicone] 540•40 mg/5 mL

loxanast INN

Loxapac (CAN) oral concentrate, IM injection (discontinued 2001) ℞ *conventional (typical) antipsychotic* [loxapine HCl] 25 mg/mL; 50 mg/mL

Loxapac (CAN) tablets (discontinued 2001) ℞ *conventional (typical) antipsychotic* [loxapine] 5, 10, 25, 50 mg

loxapine USAN, INN, BAN *minor tranquilizer; dibenzoxazepine antipsychotic*

loxapine HCl *minor tranquilizer; dibenzoxazepine antipsychotic*

loxapine succinate USAN *minor tranquilizer; dibenzoxazepine antipsychotic* 5, 10, 25, 50 mg oral

loxiglumide INN

Loxitane capsules ℞ *conventional (typical) antipsychotic* [loxapine succinate] 5, 10, 25, 50 mg ⊡ doxepin

Loxitane C oral concentrate ℞ *conventional (typical) antipsychotic* [loxapine HCl] 25 mg/mL

Loxitane IM injection ℞ *conventional (typical) antipsychotic* [loxapine HCl] 50 mg/mL

loxoprofen INN

loxoribine USAN, INN *immunostimulant; vaccine adjuvant; orphan status withdrawn 1996*

loxotidine [now: lavoltidine succinate]

loxtidine BAN *antiulcerative; histamine H_2-receptor blocker* [also: lavoltidine succinate; lavoltidine]

lozilurea INN

Lozi-Tabs (trademarked form) *lozenges*

Lozol film-coated tablets ℞ *antihypertensive; diuretic* [indapamide] 1.25, 2.5 mg

LP-2307 *investigational (Phase I/II) melanoma vaccine*

L-PAM (L-phenylalanine mustard) [see: melphalan]

LR (lactated Ringer) solution [see: Ringer injection, lactated]

LSD (lysergic acid diethylamide) *hallucinogenic street drug associated with disorders of sensory and temporal perception, depersonalization, and ataxia* [medically known as lysergide]

LSF (lisofylline) [q.v.]

LTRAs (leukotriene receptor antagonists) *a class of antiasthmatics*

Lu texaphyrin [see: motexafin lutetium]
lubeluzole USAN, INN *investigational neural protective for ischemic stroke*
LubraSol Bath Oil OTC *bath emollient*
Lubricating Gel (name changed to WHF Lubricating Gel in 1998)
Lubricating Jelly OTC *vaginal lubricant* [glycerin; propylene glycol]
Lubriderm cream, lotion OTC *moisturizer; emollient*
Lubriderm Bath Oil OTC *bath emollient*
Lubrin vaginal inserts OTC *lubricant for sexual intercourse* [glycerin; caprylic triglyceride]
LubriTears eye drops OTC *ophthalmic moisturizer/lubricant* [hydroxypropyl methylcellulose] 0.3%
LubriTears ophthalmic ointment OTC *ocular moisturizer/lubricant* [white petrolatum; mineral oil; lanolin]
lucanthone INN, BAN *antischistosomal* [also: lucanthone HCl]
lucanthone HCl USAN, USP *antischistosomal* [also: lucanthone]
lucartamide INN
lucensomycin [see: lucimycin]
Lucilia caesar *natural treatment* [see: maggots]
lucimycin INN
lucinactant *investigational (Phase II/III, orphan) for respiratory distress syndrome in adults and premature infants and meconium aspiration in newborn infants* [also: KL4 surfactant]
Ludiomil coated tablets (discontinued 2001) ℞ *tetracyclic antidepressant* [maprotiline HCl] 25, 50, 75 mg
lufironil USAN, INN *collagen inhibitor*
lufuradom INN
Lufyllin tablets, elixir, IM injection ℞ *antiasthmatic; bronchodilator* [dyphylline] 200 mg; 100 mg/15 mL; 250 mg/mL
Lufyllin 400 tablets ℞ *antiasthmatic; bronchodilator* [dyphylline] 400 mg
Lufyllin-EPG tablets, elixir ℞ *antiasthmatic; bronchodilator; decongestant; expectorant; sedative* [dyphylline; ephedrine HCl; guaifenesin; phenobarbital] 100•16•200•16 mg; 150•24•300•24 mg/15 mL
Lufyllin-GG tablets, elixir ℞ *antiasthmatic; bronchodilator; expectorant* [dyphylline; guaifenesin] 200•200 mg; 100•100 mg/15 mL
Lugol solution ℞ *thyroid-blocking therapy; topical antimicrobial* [iodine; potassium iodide] 5%•10%
Lumigan eye drops ℞ *synthetic prostamide analogue for glaucoma and ocular hypertension* [bimatoprost] 0.03%
Luminal Sodium IV or IM injection ℞ *long-acting barbiturate sedative, hypnotic, and anticonvulsant; also abused as a street drug* [phenobarbital sodium] 130 mg/mL ⑨ Tuinal
Lunelle IM injection ℞ *once-monthly injectable contraceptive* [estradiol cypionate; medroxyprogesterone acetate] 5•25 mg/0.5 mL
lung surfactant, synthetic [see: colfosceril palmitate]
lungwort *(Pulmonaria officinalis)* flowering plant *medicinal herb used as an astringent, demulcent, emollient, expectorant, and pectoral*
2,6-lupetidine [see: nanofin]
lupitidine INN *veterinary antagonist to histamine H_2 receptors* [also: lupitidine HCl]
lupitidine HCl USAN *veterinary antagonist to histamine H_2 receptors* [also: lupitidine]
Lupron; Lupron Pediatric subcu injection (daily) ℞ *hormonal antineoplastic for prostatic cancer; LH-RH agonist for central precocious puberty (CPP) (orphan)* [leuprolide acetate] 5 mg/mL ⑨ Mepron; Napron
Lupron Depot microspheres for IM injection (monthly) ℞ *hormonal antineoplastic for prostatic cancer, endometriosis, and uterine fibroids* [leuprolide acetate] 3.75, 7.5 mg ⑨ Mepron; Napron
Lupron Depot–3 month; Lupron Depot–4 month microspheres for IM injection ℞ *hormonal antineoplastic for prostatic cancer, endometriosis,*

and uterine fibroids [leuprolide acetate] 11.5, 22.5 mg; 30 mg ⑨ Mepron; Napron

Lupron Depot-Ped microspheres for IM injection (monthly) ℞ *hormonal antineoplastic for central precocious puberty (CPP) (orphan)* [leuprolide acetate] 7.5, 11.25, 15 mg ⑨ Mepron; Napron

luprostiol INN, BAN

Luride Lozi-Tabs (chewable tablets), drops, gel ℞ *dental caries preventative* [sodium fluoride] 0.25, 1.1, 2.2 mg; 1.1 mg/mL; 1.2%

Luride SF Lozi-Tabs (lozenges) ℞ *topical dental caries preventative* [sodium fluoride] 2.2 mg

Lurline PMS tablets (name changed to Vitelle Lurline PMS in 2000)

lurosetron mesylate USAN *antiemetic*

lurtotecan dihydrochloride USAN *antineoplastic; topoisomerase I inhibitor*

Lustra; Lustra-AF cream ℞ *hyperpigmentation bleaching agent* [hydroquinone (in a base containing glycolic acid and vitamins C and E); (AF also contains sunscreens)] 4% ⑨ Alustra

lutein *natural carotenoid used to prevent and treat age-related macular degeneration (AMD), retinitis pigmentosa (RP), and other retinal dysfunction*

luteinizing hormone-releasing factor acetate hydrate [see: gonadorelin acetate]

luteinizing hormone-releasing factor diacetate tetrahydrate [now: gonadorelin acetate]

luteinizing hormone-releasing factor dihydrochloride [now: gonadorelin HCl]

luteinizing hormone-releasing factor HCl [see: gonadorelin HCl]

luteinizing hormone–releasing hormone (LH-RH) *an endogenous hormone, produced in the hypothalamus, which stimulates the release of luteinizing hormone (LH) and follicle-stimulating hormone (FSH) from the pituitary* [also known as: gonadotropin-releasing hormone (Gn-RH)]

lutetium *element (Lu)*

lutetium texaphyrin [now: motexafin lutetium]

Lu-Tex ℞ *investigational for the photodynamic treatment of cancer; investigational (Phase I/II) photosensitizer for ophthalmologic indications including age-related macular degeneration* [motexafin lutetium]

lutrelin INN *luteinizing hormone–releasing hormone (LH-RH) agonist* [also: lutrelin acetate]

lutrelin acetate USAN *luteinizing hormone–releasing hormone (LH-RH) agonist* [also: lutrelin]

Lutrepulse powder for continuous ambulatory infusion ℞ *gonadotropin-releasing hormone for hypothalamic amenorrhea (orphan)* [gonadorelin acetate] 0.8, 3.2 mg

Lutrin ℞ *investigational photodynamic therapy for recurrent breast cancer* [motexafin lutetium]

Luvox film-coated tablets ℞ *selective serotonin reuptake inhibitor (SSRI) for obsessive-compulsive disorder (OCD); investigational (Phase III) for depression and panic disorder* [fluvoxamine maleate] 25, 50, 100 mg

luxabendazole INN, BAN

Luxiq foam ℞ *topical corticosteroidal anti-inflammatory for scalp dermatoses* [betamethasone valerate] 0.12%

L-VAM (leuprolide acetate, vinblastine, Adriamycin, mitomycin) *chemotherapy protocol*

LY-315535 *investigational (Phase I) for functional bowel disorders*

lyapolate sodium USAN *anticoagulant* [also: sodium apolate]

lycetamine USAN *topical antimicrobial*

lycine HCl [see: betaine HCl]

lycopene *natural substance found in high concentration in ripe tomatoes; a member of the carotene family; used as an antineoplastic and antioxidant*

Lycopodium clavatum *medicinal herb* [see: club moss]

Lycopus virginicus *medicinal herb* [see: bugleweed]

Lyderm (CAN) cream, ointment, gel ℞ *topical corticosteroidal anti-inflammatory* [fluocinonide] 0.05%

lydimycin USAN *antifungal* [also: lidimycin]

Lyme borreliosis vaccine [see: lipoprotein OspA, recombinant]

lymecycline INN, BAN

LYMErix IM injection ℞ *active immunizing agent against Lyme disease* [lipoprotein OspA, recombinant] 30 µg/0.5 mL

Lymphazurin 1% subcu injection ℞ *radiopaque contrast medium for lymphography* [isosulfan blue] 10 mg/mL (1%)

LymphoCide ℞ *investigational (Phase I/II, orphan) for AIDS-related non-Hodgkin lymphoma* [monoclonal antibody CD22 antigen on B-cells, radiolabeled]

lymphocyte immune globulin (LIG) *passive immunizing agent to prevent allograft rejection of renal transplants; treatment for aplastic anemia; investigational (orphan) for organ and bone marrow transplants* [also: antithymocyte globulin (ATG)]

lymphogranuloma venereum antigen USP

lymphoma antibody, humanized *investigational*

LymphoScan ℞ *investigational (Phase III, orphan) for diagnostic aid for non-Hodgkin B-cell lymphoma, AIDS-related lymphomas, and other acute and chronic B-cell leukemias* [technetium Tc 99m bectumomab]

lynestrenol USAN, INN *progestin* [also: lynoestrenol]

lynoestrenol BAN *progestin* [also: lynestrenol]

Lyo-Ject (trademarked delivery system) *prefilled dual-chambered syringe with lyophilized powder and diluent*

Lyphocin powder for IV or IM injection (discontinued 1998) ℞ *tricyclic glycopeptide antibiotic* [vancomycin HCl] 0.5, 1, 5 g

Lypholized Vitamin B Complex & Vitamin C with B_{12} injection ℞ *parenteral vitamin therapy* [multiple B vitamins; vitamin C] ≛•50 mg/mL

Lypholyte; Lypholyte II IV admixture ℞ *intravenous electrolyte therapy* [combined electrolyte solution]

lypressin USAN, USP, INN, BAN *posterior pituitary hormone; antidiuretic; vasoconstrictor*

lysergic acid diethylamide (LSD) *street drug* [see: LSD; lysergide]

lysergide INN, BAN, DCF

lysine (L-lysine) USAN, INN *essential amino acid; symbols: Lys, K; natural remedy for the prophylaxis and treatment of recurrent oral and genital herpes simplex outbreaks; inhibits HSV replication* 312, 500, 1000 mg oral

lysine acetate USP *amino acid*

DL-lysine acetylsalicylate [see: aspirin DL-lysine]

lysine HCl USAN, USP *amino acid*

L-lysine monoacetate [see: lysine acetate]

L-lysine monohydrochloride [see: lysine HCl]

8-L-lysine vasopressin [see: lypressin]

Lysodase ℞ *investigational (orphan) chronic enzyme replacement therapy for Gaucher disease* [PEG-glucocerebrosidase]

Lysodren tablets ℞ *antibiotic antineoplastic for inoperable adrenal cortical carcinoma* [mitotane] 500 mg

lysostaphin USAN *antibacterial enzyme; investigational agent for methicillin-resistant Staphylococcus aureus (MRSA) endocarditis*

lysuride BAN [also: lisuride]

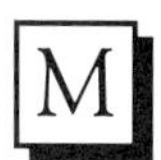

M-CSF (macrophage colony-stimulating factor) [now: cilmostim]

M-2 protocol (vincristine, carmustine, cyclophosphamide, prednisone, melphalan) *chemotherapy protocol for multiple myeloma*

MAA (macroaggregated albumin) [see: albumin, aggregated]

Maalox chewable tablets (discontinued 2001) OTC *antacid* [aluminum hydroxide; magnesium hydroxide] 200•200, 350•350 mg ⑨ Marax

Maalox oral suspension OTC *antacid* [aluminum hydroxide; magnesium hydroxide] 225•200 mg/5 mL ⑨ Marax

Maalox, Extra Strength oral suspension (name changed to Maalox Anti-Gas Extra Strength in 2001)

Maalox Antacid caplets (discontinued 2001) OTC *antacid* [calcium carbonate] 1 g

Maalox Antacid/Calcium Supplement chewable tablets OTC *antacid; calcium supplement* [calcium carbonate] 600 mg

Maalox Anti-Diarrheal caplets (discontinued 2001) OTC *antidiarrheal* [loperamide HCl] 2 mg

Maalox Anti-Gas chewable tablets OTC *antiflatulent* [simethicone] 80, 150 mg

Maalox Anti-Gas Extra Strength oral suspension OTC *antacid; antiflatulent* [aluminum hydroxide; magnesium hydroxide; simethicone] 500•450•40 mg/5 mL

Maalox Daily Fiber Therapy powder (discontinued 1999) OTC *bulk laxative* [psyllium hydrophilic mucilloid] 3.4 g/dose

Maalox H2 Acid Controller (CAN) film-coated tablets OTC *histamine H_2 antagonist for heartburn and acid indigestion* [famotidine] 10 mg

Maalox HRF (Heartburn Relief Formula) liquid (discontinued 2001) OTC *antacid* [aluminum hydroxide; magnesium carbonate] 140•175 mg/5 mL

Maalox Plus chewable tablets, oral suspension (discontinued 2001) OTC *antacid; antiflatulent* [aluminum hydroxide; magnesium hydroxide; simethicone] 200•200•25 mg; 500•450•40 mg/5 mL

Maalox Quick Dissolve chewable tablets OTC *antacid* [calcium carbonate] 600, 1000 mg

Maalox TC oral suspension OTC *antacid* [aluminum hydroxide; magnesium hydroxide] 600•300 mg/5 mL

Maalox Therapeutic Concentrate oral suspension (name changed to Maalox TC in 2001)

MAb; MAB (monoclonal antibody)

MABOP (Mustargen, Adriamycin, bleomycin, Oncovin, prednisone) *chemotherapy protocol*

MabThera (European name for U.S. product Rituxan)

mabuterol INN

MAC (methotrexate, actinomycin D, chlorambucil) *chemotherapy protocol*

MAC; MAC III (methotrexate, actinomycin D, cyclophosphamide) *chemotherapy protocol for gestational trophoblastic neoplasm*

MAC (mitomycin, Adriamycin, cyclophosphamide) *chemotherapy protocol*

maca *(Lepidium meyenii)* root *medicinal herb used as an adaptogen, aphrodisiac in males, fertility aid in females, and to relieve stress*

MACC (methotrexate, Adriamycin, cyclophosphamide, CCNU) *chemotherapy protocol for non–small cell lung cancer (NSCLC)*

mace *(Myristica fragrans)* dried nutmeg aril (the fleshy network surrounding the seed) *medicinal herb* [see: nutmeg]

MACHO (methotrexate, asparaginase, cyclophosphamide, hydroxydaunomycin, Oncovin) *chemotherapy protocol*

MACOP-B (methotrexate, Adriamycin, cyclophosphamide, Oncovin, prednisone, bleomycin) *chemotherapy protocol for non-Hodgkin lymphoma*

Macritonin injection, intranasal ℞ *investigational (Phase III) oral treatment for osteoporosis* [calcitonin (salmon)]

macroaggregated albumin (MAA) [see: albumin, aggregated]

macroaggregated iodinated (^{131}I) human albumin [see: macrosalb (^{131}I)]

Macrobid capsules ℞ *urinary antibiotic* [nitrofurantoin (macrocrystals); nitrofurantoin monohydrate] 25•75 mg

Macrodantin capsules ℞ *urinary antibiotic* [nitrofurantoin (macrocrystals)] 25, 50, 100 mg

Macrodex IV infusion ℞ *plasma volume expander for shock due to hemorrhage, burns, or surgery* [dextran 70] 6%

macrogol 4000 INN, BAN [also: polyethylene glycol 4000]

macrogol ester 2000 INN *surfactant* [also: polyoxyl 40 stearate]

macrogol ester 400 INN *surfactant* [also: polyoxyl 8 stearate]

macrolides *a class of antibiotics that are bacteriostatic or bactericidal, depending on drug concentration*

macrophage colony-stimulating factor (M-CSF) [now: cilmostim]

macrophage-targeted β-glucocerebrosidase [now: alglucerase]

macrosalb (^{131}I) INN, BAN

macrosalb (^{99m}Tc) INN, BAN [also: technetium (^{99m}Tc) labeled macroaggregated human ...]

Macroscint ℞ *investigational inflammation and infection imaging aid* [indium In 111 IGIV pentetate]

Macrotys actaeoides *medicinal herb* [see: black cohosh]

Macrulin *investigational (Phase I) oral agent for type 2 diabetes* [insulin]

Macstim ℞ *hematopoietic; macrophage colony-stimulating factor; investigational antineoplastic for various cancers; investigational antihyperlipidemic* [cilmostim]

MAD (MeCCNU, Adriamycin) *chemotherapy protocol*

mad-dog weed; mad weed *medicinal herb* [see: skullcap]

MADDOC (mechlorethamine, Adriamycin, dacarbazine, DDP, Oncovin, cyclophosphamide) *chemotherapy protocol*

madnep; madness *medicinal herb* [see: masterwort]

maduramicin USAN, INN *anticoccidal*

mafenide USAN, INN, BAN *bacteriostatic; adjunct to burn therapy*

mafenide acetate USP *broad-spectrum bacteriostatic to prevent meshed autograft loss on second- and third-degree burns (orphan)*

mafenide HCl

mafilcon A USAN *hydrophilic contact lens material*

mafoprazine INN

mafosfamide INN

Mag-200 tablets OTC *magnesium supplement* [magnesium oxide] 400 mg

magaldrate USAN, USP, INN *antacid* 540 mg/5 mL oral

Magaldrate Plus oral suspension OTC *antacid; antiflatulent* [magaldrate; simethicone] 540•40 mg/5 mL

Magalox Plus chewable tablets OTC *antacid; antiflatulent* [aluminum hydroxide; magnesium hydroxide; simethicone] 200•200•25 mg

Magan tablets ℞ *analgesic; antirheumatic* [magnesium salicylate] 545 mg

Mag-Cal tablets OTC *dietary supplement* [calcium carbonate; vitamin D; multiple minerals] 416.7 mg•66.7 IU•≛

Mag-Cal Mega tablets OTC *mineral supplement* [magnesium; calcium] 800•400 mg

Mag-G tablets OTC *magnesium supplement* [magnesium gluconate] 500 mg

maggots *(Lucilia caesar; Phaenicia sericata; Pharmia regina)* *natural treatment for debriding necrotic tissue in abscesses, burns, cellulitis, gangrene, osteomyelitis, and ulcers*

Magnacal ready-to-use liquid OTC *enteral nutritional therapy* [lactose-free formula]

Magnalox liquid (discontinued 2000) OTC *antacid* [aluminum hydroxide; magnesium hydroxide] 225•220 mg/5 mL

Magnaprin; Magnaprin Arthritis Strength Captabs film-coated tablets OTC *analgesic; antipyretic; anti-inflammatory; antirheumatic* [aspirin (buffered with aluminum hydroxide, magnesium hydroxide, and calcium carbonate)] 325 mg

MagneBind 200; MagneBind 300 tablets OTC *calcium/magnesium supplement that binds dietary phosphate* [magnesium carbonate; calcium carbonate] 200•400 mg; 300•250 mg

MagneBind 400 Rx tablets ℞ *calcium/magnesium supplement that binds dietary phosphate* [magnesium carbonate; calcium carbonate; folic acid] 400•200•1 mg

magnesia, milk of USP *antacid; saline laxative* [also: magnesium hydroxide] 400 mg/5 mL oral

magnesia magma [now: magnesia, milk of]

magnesium *element (Mg)* 27 mg oral

magnesium aluminosilicate hydrate [see: almasilate]

magnesium aluminum silicate NF *suspending agent*

magnesium amino acid chelate *dietary magnesium supplement*

magnesium aspartate [see: potassium aspartate & magnesium aspartate]

magnesium carbonate USP *antacid; dietary magnesium supplement*

magnesium carbonate hydrate [see: magnesium carbonate]

magnesium chloride USP *electrolyte replenisher* 1.97 mEq/mL (20%) injection

magnesium chloride hexahydrate [see: magnesium chloride]

magnesium citrate USP *saline laxative* 1.75 g/30 mL oral

magnesium clofibrate INN

magnesium D-gluconate dihydrate [see: magnesium gluconate]

magnesium D-gluconate hydrate [see: magnesium gluconate]

magnesium gluconate USP *magnesium replenisher*

magnesium glycinate USAN

magnesium hydroxide USP *antacid; saline laxative* [also: magnesia, milk of]

magnesium hydroxycarbonate *antiurolithic*

magnesium oxide USP *antacid; sorbent* 400, 500 mg oral

magnesium phosphate USP *antacid*

magnesium phosphate pentahydrate [see: magnesium phosphate]

magnesium salicylate USP *analgesic; antipyretic; anti-inflammatory; antirheumatic*

magnesium salicylate tetrahydrate [see: magnesium salicylate]

magnesium silicate NF *tablet excipient*

magnesium silicate hydrate [see: magnesium trisilicate]

magnesium stearate NF *tablet and capsule lubricant*

magnesium sulfate USP, JAN *anticonvulsant; saline laxative; electrolyte replenisher* 0.8, 1, 4 mEq/mL (10%, 12.5%, 50%) injection

magnesium sulfate heptahydrate [see: magnesium sulfate]

magnesium trisilicate USP *antacid*

Magnevist IV injection, prefilled syringes ℞ *MRI contrast medium* [gadopentetate dimeglumine] 469 mg/mL

magnolia *(Magnolia glauca)* bark *medicinal herb used as an antiperiodic, aromatic, astringent, diaphoretic, febrifuge, stimulant, and tonic*

Magnox oral suspension OTC *antacid* [aluminum hydroxide; magnesium hydroxide] 225•200 mg/5 mL

Magonate tablets, liquid OTC *magnesium supplement* [magnesium gluconate] 500 mg; 1000 mg/5 mL

Mag-Ox 400 tablets OTC *antacid; magnesium supplement* [magnesium oxide] 400 mg

Magsal tablets ℞ *analgesic; antipyretic; anti-inflammatory; antihistaminic sleep aid* [magnesium salicylate; phenyltoloxamine citrate] 600•25 mg

Mag-Tab SR sustained-release caplets OTC *magnesium supplement* [magnesium lactate] 7 mEq (84 mg)

Magtrate tablets OTC *magnesium supplement* [magnesium gluconate] 500 mg

mahogany birch; mountain mahogany *medicinal herb* [see: birch]

Mahonia aquifolium *medicinal herb* [see: Oregon grape]

ma-huang *medicinal herb* [see: ephedra]

MAID (mesna [rescue], Adriamycin, ifosfamide, dacarbazine) *chemotherapy protocol for soft tissue and bone sarcomas*

maitake mushrooms *(Grifola frondosa)* cap and stem *medicinal herb for cancer, diabetes, hypercholesterolemia, hypertension, obesity, and stimulation of the immune system*

maitansine INN *antineoplastic* [also: maytansine]

Maitec injection ℞ *investigational (orphan) for disseminated* Mycobacterium avium-intracellulare *infection* [gentamicin sulfate, liposomal]

Majorana hortensis *medicinal herb* [see: marjoram]

Major-Con chewable tablets OTC *antiflatulent* [simethicone] 80 mg

Major-gesic tablets OTC *antihistamine; analgesic* [phenyltoloxamine citrate; acetaminophen] 30•325 mg

MAK 195 F *investigational therapy for graft vs. host disease* [monoclonal antibodies]

malaleuca *medicinal herb* [see: tea tree oil]

Malarone; Malarone Pediatric film-coated tablets ℞ *malaria prophylaxis and treatment* [atovaquone; proguanil HCl (chloroguanide HCl)] 250•100 mg; 62.5•25 mg

Malatal tablets (discontinued 1997) ℞ *GI antispasmodic; anticholinergic; sedative* [atropine sulfate; scopolamine hydrobromide; hyoscyamine hydrobromide; phenobarbital] 0.0194•0.0065•0.1037•16.2 mg

malathion USP, BAN *pediculicide*

maletamer INN *antiperistaltic* [also: malethamer]

malethamer USAN *antiperistaltic* [also: maletamer]

maleylsulfathiazole INN

malic acid NF *acidifying agent*

malidone [see: aloxidone]

Mallamint chewable tablets OTC *antacid* [calcium carbonate] 420 mg

Mallazine eye drops OTC *topical ophthalmic decongestant and vasoconstrictor* [tetrahydrozoline HCl] 0.05%

Mallisol ointment (discontinued 1999) OTC *broad-spectrum antimicrobial* [povidone-iodine]

mallow *(Malva rotundifolia; M. sylvestris)* plant *medicinal herb used as an astringent, demulcent, emollient, and expectorant*

mallow, marsh *(Althaea officinalis)* *medicinal herb* [see: marsh mallow]

malonal [see: barbital]

malotilate USAN, INN *liver disorder treatment*

Malpighia glabra; M. punicifolia *medicinal herb* [see: acerola]

Maltsupex coated tablets, powder, liquid OTC *bulk laxative* [barley malt soup extract] 750 mg; 8 g/scoop; 16 g/tbsp.

Malva rotundifolia; M. sylvestris *medicinal herb* [see: mallow]

Mammol ointment OTC *emollient for nipples of nursing mothers* [bismuth subnitrate] 40%

***m*-AMSA (acridinylamine methanesulphon anisidide)** [see: amsacrine]

Mandameth enteric-coated tablets ℞ *urinary antibiotic* [methenamine mandelate] 0.5, 1 g

Mandelamine film-coated tablets ℞ *urinary antibiotic* [methenamine mandelate] 0.5, 1 g

mandelic acid NF

Mandol powder for IV or IM injection ℞ *cephalosporin antibiotic* [cefamandole nafate] 1 g ⑨ nadolol

mandrake (*Mandragora officinarium; Podophyllum peltatum*) root and resin *medicinal herb for cancer, condylomata, constipation, fever, indigestion, liver disorders, lower bowel disorders, warts, and worms; not generally regarded as safe for children or pregnant women*

Manerix (CAN) film-coated tablets ℞ *antidepressant; MAO inhibitor* [moclobemide] 150, 300 mg

mangafodipir trisodium USAN *paramagnetic contrast agent for MRI of the liver*

manganese *element (Mn)*

manganese chloride USP *dietary manganese supplement* 0.1 mg/mL injection

manganese chloride tetrahydrate [see: manganese chloride]

manganese gluconate (manganese D-gluconate) USP *dietary manganese supplement*

manganese glycerophosphate NF

manganese hypophosphite NF

manganese phosphinate [see: manganese hypophosphite]

manganese sulfate USP *dietary manganese supplement* 0.1 mg/mL injection

manganese sulfate monohydrate [see: manganese sulfate]

mangofodipir trisodium *MRI contrast medium for liver imaging*

manidipine 6300 INN

manna sugar [see: mannitol]

mannite [see: mannitol]

mannitol (D-mannitol) USP *renal function test aid; antihypertensive; osmotic diuretic; urologic irrigant* 10%, 15%, 20%, 25% injection

mannitol hexanitrate INN

mannityl nitrate [see: mannitol hexanitrate]

mannomustine INN, BAN

mannosulfan INN

manozodil INN

Mantadil cream (discontinued 1997) ℞ *topical corticosteroidal anti-inflammatory; antihistamine* [hydrocortisone acetate; chlorcyclizine HCl] 0.5%•2%

Mantoux test [see: tuberculin]

MAO inhibitors (monoamine oxidase inhibitors) [q.v.]

Maolate tablets ℞ *skeletal muscle relaxant* [chlorphenesin carbamate] 400 mg

Maox 420 tablets OTC *antacid* [magnesium oxide] 420 mg

MAP (mitomycin, Adriamycin, Platinol) *chemotherapy protocol*

Mapap tablets OTC *analgesic; antipyretic* [acetaminophen] 325, 500 mg

Mapap, Children's liquid OTC *analgesic; antipyretic* [acetaminophen] 160 mg/5 mL

Mapap Cold Formula tablets OTC *antitussive; decongestant; antihistamine; analgesic* [dextromethorphan hydrobromide; pseudoephedrine HCl; chlorpheniramine maleate; acetaminophen] 15•30•2•325 mg

Mapap Infant Drops OTC *analgesic; antipyretic* [acetaminophen] 100 mg/mL

maple lungwort *medicinal herb* [see: lungwort]

maprotiline USAN, INN *tetracyclic antidepressant*

maprotiline HCl USP *tetracyclic antidepressant* 25, 50, 75 mg oral

Maranox tablets OTC *analgesic; antipyretic* [acetaminophen] 325 mg

Marax tablets ℞ *antiasthmatic; bronchodilator; decongestant* [theophylline; ephedrine sulfate] 130•25 mg ⓢ Atarax; Maalox

Marax-DF pediatric syrup ℞ *antiasthmatic; bronchodilator; decongestant; antihistamine* [theophylline; ephedrine sulfate; hydroxyzine HCl] 97.5•18.75•7.5 mg/15 mL

Marblen tablets, liquid OTC *antacid* [calcium carbonate; magnesium carbonate] 520•400 mg; 540•400 mg/5 mL

Marcaine HCl injection ℞ *injectable local anesthetic* [bupivacaine HCl] 0.25%, 0.5%, 0.75%

Marcaine HCl injection ℞ *injectable local anesthetic* [bupivacaine HCl; epinephrine bitartrate] 0.25%•1:200 000, 0.5%•1:200 000, 0.75%•1:200 000 ⓢ Narcan

Marcaine Spinal injection ℞ *injectable local anesthetic* [bupivacaine HCl] 0.75%

Marcillin capsules ℞ *aminopenicillin antibiotic* [ampicillin] 500 mg

Marcillin powder for oral suspension (discontinued 1998) ℞ *aminopenicillin antibiotic* [ampicillin] 250 mg/100 mL

Marcof Expectorant syrup ℞ *narcotic antitussive; expectorant* [hydrocodone bitartrate; potassium guaiacolsulfonate] 5•300 mg/5 mL

mare's tail *medicinal herb* [see: fleabane; horseweed]

Marezine tablets OTC *antiemetic; anticholinergic; antihistamine; motion sickness preventative* [cyclizine HCl] 50 mg

Margesic capsules ℞ *analgesic; barbiturate sedative* [acetaminophen; caffeine; butalbital] 325•40•50 mg

Margesic H capsules ℞ *narcotic analgesic* [hydrocodone bitartrate; acetaminophen] 5•500 mg

maribavir USAN *antiviral for cytomegalovirus infections*

maridomycin INN

marigold ***(Calendula officinalis)*** florets *medicinal herb for bruises, cuts, dysmenorrhea, eye infections, fever, and skin diseases; not generally regarded as safe and effective*

marijuana; marihuana ***(Cannabis sativa)*** *euphoric/hallucinogenic street drug made from the dried leaves and flowering tops of the cannabis plant; medicinal herb for asthma, analgesia, leprosy, and loss of appetite*

marijuana (CAN) *approved for compassionate use in terminally ill patients*

marimastat USAN *investigational (Phase III) antineoplastic; matrix metalloproteinase (MMP) inhibitor*

Marine Lipid Concentrate softgels OTC *dietary supplement* [omega-3 fatty acids] 1200 mg

Marinol soft gelatin capsules ℞ *antiemetic for nausea following chemotherapy; appetite stimulant for AIDS patients (orphan)* [dronabinol] 2.5, 5, 10 mg

mariptiline INN

marjoram ***(Majorana hortensis; Origanum vulgare)*** plant *medicinal herb for abdominal cramps, colic, headache, indigestion, respiratory problems, and violent cough*

Marlin Salt System tablets OTC *rinsing/storage solution for soft contact lenses* [sodium chloride (normal saline solution)] 250 mg

Marlin Salt System II tablets OTC *rinsing/storage solution for soft contact lenses* [sodium chloride (normal saline solution)] 250 mg

Marmine IV or IM injection ℞ *antinauseant; antiemetic; antivertigo; motion sickness preventative* [dimenhydrinate] 50 mg/mL

Marmine tablets OTC *antinauseant; antiemetic; antivertigo; motion sickness preventative* [dimenhydrinate] 50 mg

Marnal tablets, capsules (discontinued 1998) ℞ *analgesic; sedative* [aspirin; caffeine; butalbital] 325•40•50 mg

Marnatal-F film-coated tablets ℞ *vitamin/mineral/calcium/iron supplement* [multiple vitamins & minerals; calcium; iron; folic acid] ≛•250•60•1 mg

Marogen ℞ *investigational substitute for blood transfusion; investigational (orphan) for anemia of end-stage renal disease* [epoetin beta]

maroxepin INN

Marplan tablets ℞ *antidepressant; monoamine oxidase (MAO) inhibitor* [isocarboxazid] 10 mg

Marpres tablets ℞ *antihypertensive; vasodilator; diuretic* [hydrochlorothiazide; reserpine; hydralazine HCl] 15•0.1•25 mg

Marrubium vulgare *medicinal herb* [see: horehound]

marsh clover; marsh trefoil *medicinal herb* [see: buckbean]

marsh mallow ***(Althaea officinalis)*** root *medicinal herb for asthma, boils, bronchial infections, cough, emphysema, infected wounds, kidney disorders, lung congestion, sore throat, and urinary bleeding*

MART-1 adenoviral gene therapy *investigational (orphan) for metastatic malignant melanoma*

Marten-Tab caplets ℞ *analgesic; barbiturate sedative* [acetaminophen; butalbital] 325•50 mg

Marthritic tablets ℞ *analgesic; antipyretic; anti-inflammatory; antirheumatic* [salsalate] 750 mg

Marvelon (CAN) tablets (in packs of 21 or 28) ℞ *monophasic oral contraceptive* [desogestrel; ethinyl estradiol] 0.15 mg•30 μg

masoprocol USAN, INN *antineoplastic for actinic keratoses (AK)*

Massé Breast cream OTC *moisturizer and emollient for nipples of nursing women*

Massengill Baking Soda Freshness solution OTC *vaginal cleanser and deodorizer; acidity modifier* [sodium bicarbonate]

Massengill Disposable Douche solution OTC *antiseptic/germicidal; vaginal cleanser and deodorizer; acidity modifier* [cetylpyridinium chloride; lactic acid; sodium lactate]

Massengill Disposable Douche; Massengill Vinegar & Water Extra Mild solution OTC *vaginal cleanser and deodorizer; acidity modifier* [vinegar (acetic acid)]

Massengill Douche powder OTC *astringent; analgesic; counterirritant; vaginal cleanser and deodorizer* [ammonium alum; phenol; methyl salicylate; menthol; thymol]

Massengill Douche solution concentrate OTC *vaginal cleanser and deodorizer; acidity modifier* [lactic acid; sodium lactate; sodium bicarbonate]

Massengill Feminine Cleansing Wash liquid OTC *for external perivaginal cleansing*

Massengill Medicated towelettes OTC *topical corticosteroidal anti-inflammatory* [hydrocortisone] 0.5%

Massengill Medicated Douche with Cepticin; Massengill Medicated Disposable Douche with Cepticin solution OTC *antiseptic/germicidal; vaginal cleanser and deodorizer* [povidone-iodine] 12%; 10%

Massengill Vinegar & Water Extra Cleansing with Puraclean solution OTC *antiseptic/germicidal; vaginal cleanser and deodorizer; acidity modifier* [cetylpyridinium chloride; vinegar (acetic acid)]

mast cell stabilizers *a class of topical agents that inhibit the antigen-induced release of inflammatory mediators (e.g., various histamines and leukotrienes) from human mast cells; used on nasal, ophthalmological, and gastrointestinal mucosa* [also known as: mediator release inhibitors]

masterwort ***(Heracleum lanatum)*** root and seed *medicinal herb used as an antispasmodic, carminative, and stimulant*

maté *medicinal herb* [see: yerba maté]

Materna tablets (discontinued 1997) ℞ *vitamin/mineral/calcium/iron supplement* [multiple vitamins & minerals; calcium; iron; folic acid; biotin] ≛•250•60•1•0.03 mg

Matricaria chamomilla *medicinal herb* [see: chamomile]

matrix metalloproteinase (MMP) inhibitors *a class of investigational (Phase III) antineoplastics and investigational (orphan) agents to treat corneal ulcers*

Matulane capsules ℞ *antineoplastic for Hodgkin disease; investigational for lymphoma, brain and lung cancer* [procarbazine HCl] 50 mg

Mavik (CAN) capsules ℞ *antihypertensive; angiotensin-converting enzyme (ACE) inhibitor* [trandolapril] 0.5, 1, 2 mg

Mavik tablets ℞ *antihypertensive; angiotensin-converting enzyme (ACE) inhibitor* [trandolapril] 1, 2, 4 mg

maxacalcitol USAN *investigational vitamin D_3 analogue for the topical treatment of psoriasis*

Maxair Autohaler (breath-activated metered-dose inhaler) ℞ *sympathomimetic bronchodilator* [pirbuterol acetate] 0.2 mg/dose

Maxalt caplets ℞ *vascular serotonin 5-HT$_1$ receptor agonist for migraine headache* [rizatriptan benzoate] 5, 10 mg

Maxalt-MLT orally disintegrating tablets ℞ *vascular serotonin 5-HT$_1$ receptor agonist for migraine headache* [rizatriptan benzoate] 5, 10 mg

Maxalt-RPD (CAN) orally disintegrating tablets ℞ *vascular serotonin 5-HT$_1$ receptor agonist for migraine headache* [rizatriptan benzoate] 5, 10 mg

Maxamine ℞ *investigational (NDA filed, orphan) adjuvant to interleukin-2 for stage IV malignant melanoma and acute myelogenous leukemia; investigational (Phase II) adjunct to interferon alfa-2b for chronic hepatitis* C [aldesleukin]

Maxaquin film-coated tablets ℞ *broad-spectrum fluoroquinolone antibiotic* [lomefloxacin HCl] 400 mg

MaxEPA soft capsules OTC *dietary supplement* [omega-3 fatty acids; multiple vitamins & minerals] 1000•≛ mg

Maxibolin *an anabolic steroid abused as a street drug* [see: ethylestrenol]

Maxicam ℞ *investigational (NDA filed) nonsteroidal anti-inflammatory drug (NSAID); antiarthritic; analgesic; antipyretic* [isoxicam]

Maxidex Drop-Tainers (eye drop suspension) ℞ *topical ophthalmic corticosteroidal anti-inflammatory* [dexamethasone] 0.1%

Maxidex ophthalmic ointment (discontinued 1998) ℞ *topical ophthalmic corticosteroidal anti-inflammatory* [dexamethasone] 0.05%

Maxidone caplets ℞ *narcotic analgesic* [hydrocodone bitartrate; acetaminophen] 10•750 mg

Maxifed; Maxifed-G tablets OTC *decongestant; expectorant* [pseudoephedrine HCl; guaifenesin] 80•700 mg; 60•550 mg

Maxifed DM sustained-release caplets OTC *antitussive; decongestant; expectorant* [dextromethorphan hydrobromide; phenylpropanolamine HCl; guaifenesin] 30•60•550 mg

Maxiflor cream, ointment ℞ *topical corticosteroidal anti-inflammatory* [diflorasone diacetate] 0.05%

Maxilube jelly OTC *vaginal lubricant*

Maximum Blue Label; Maximum Green Label tablets OTC *vitamin/mineral supplement* [multiple vitamins & minerals; folic acid; biotin] ≛•130•50 μg

Maximum Red Label tablets OTC *vitamin/mineral/iron supplement* [multiple vitamins & minerals; iron; folic acid; biotin] ≛•3.3 mg•0.13 mg•50 μg

"Maximum Strength" products [see under product name]

Maxipime powder for IV or IM injection ℞ *cephalosporin antibiotic* [cefepime HCl] 0.5, 1, 2 g

Maxitrol eye drop suspension, ophthalmic ointment ℞ *topical ophthalmic corticosteroidal anti-inflammatory; antibiotic* [dexamethasone; neomycin sulfate; polymyxin B sulfate] 0.1%•0.35%•10 000 U/mL; 0.1%•0.35%•10 000 U/g

Maxivate ointment, cream, lotion ℞ *topical corticosteroidal anti-inflammatory* [betamethasone dipropionate] 0.05%

Maxi-Vite tablets OTC *vitamin/mineral/calcium/iron supplement* [multiple vitamins & minerals; calcium; iron; folic acid; biotin] ≛•53.5•1.5•0.4•0.001 mg

Maxolon tablets ℞ *antidopaminergic; antiemetic for chemotherapy; peristaltic* [metoclopramide HCl] 10 mg

Maxovite sustained-release tablets OTC *vitamin/mineral supplement* [multiple vitamins & minerals; folic acid; biotin] ≛•330•11.7 μg

Maxzide tablets ℞ *antihypertensive; diuretic* [triamterene; hydrochlorothiazide] 37.5•25, 75•50 mg ⓢ Microzide

May apple *medicinal herb* [see: mandrake]

May bells; May lily *medicinal herb* [see: lily of the valley]

May bush; May tree *medicinal herb* [see: hawthorn]

May lily *medicinal herb* [see: lily of the valley]

maytansine USAN *antineoplastic* [also: maitansine]

May-Vita elixir ℞ *vitamin supplement* [multiple B vitamins; folic acid] ≛•0.1 mg

Mazanor tablets ℞ *anorexiant; CNS stimulant* [mazindol] 1 mg

mazapertine succinate USAN *antipsychotic; dopamine receptor antagonist*

mazaticol INN

MAZE (*m*-AMSA, azacitidine, etoposide) *chemotherapy protocol*

mazindol USAN, USP, INN, BAN *anorexiant; CNS stimulant; investigational (orphan) treatment for Duchenne muscular dystrophy* ⑨ mebendazole

mazipredone INN

MB (methylene blue) [q.v.]

m-BACOD; M-BACOD (methotrexate, bleomycin, Adriamycin, cyclophosphamide, Oncovin, dexamethasone) *chemotherapy protocol for non-Hodgkin lymphoma* ("m" is 200 mg/m^2; "M" is 3 g/m^2)

M-BACOS (methotrexate, bleomycin, Adriamycin, cyclophosphamide, Oncovin, Solu-Medrol) *chemotherapy protocol*

MBC (methotrexate, bleomycin, cisplatin) *chemotherapy protocol for head and neck cancer*

MBD (methotrexate, bleomycin, DDP) *chemotherapy protocol*

MBR (methylene blue, reduced) [see: methylene blue]

MC (mitoxantrone, cytarabine) *chemotherapy protocol for acute myelocytic leukemia (AML)*

M-Caps capsules ℞ *urinary acidifier to control ammonia production* [racemethionine] 200 mg

MCBP (melphalan, cyclophosphamide, BCNU, prednisone) *chemotherapy protocol*

MCH (microfibrillar collagen hemostat) [q.v.]

MCP (melphalan, cyclophosphamide, prednisone) *chemotherapy protocol*

M-CSF (macrophage colony-stimulating factor) [now: cilmostim]

MCT oil OTC *dietary fat supplement* [medium chain triglycerides from coconut oil]

MCT (medium chain triglycerides) [q.v.]

MCV (methotrexate, cisplatin, vinblastine) *chemotherapy protocol*

MD-60; MD-76 injection (discontinued 1999) ℞ *radiopaque contrast medium* [diatrizoate meglumine; diatrizoate sodium (48.7% total iodine)] 52%•8% (29.3%); 66%•10% (37%)

MD-76 R injection ℞ *radiopaque contrast medium* [diatrizoate meglumine; diatrizoate sodium (48.7% total iodine)] 660•100 mg/mL (370 mg/mL)

MDA (methylenedioxyamphetamine) [see: MDMA, MDEA]

mda-7 *investigational tumor suppressor gene for cancer therapy*

MDEA (3,4-methylenedioxyethamphetamine) *a hallucinogenic amphetamine derivative closely related to MDMA, abused as a street drug, which causes dependence* [also see: amphetamines; MDMA]

MD-Gastroview oral solution ℞ *radiopaque contrast medium for gastrointestinal imaging* [diatrizoate meglumine; diatrizoate sodium (48.29% total iodine)] 660•100 mg/mL (367 mg/mL)

MDI (dosage form) *metered-dose inhaler*

MDMA (3,4-methylenedioxymethamphetamine) *widely abused hallucinogenic street drug that is chemically related to amphetamines and mescaline and causes dependence* [see also: amphetamines; mescaline; MDEA]

MDP (methylene diphosphonate) [now: medronate disodium]

MDX-210 *investigational (Phase II) HER-2 receptor antibody for prostate cancer*

MDX-240 *investigational (Phase II) virus-specific antibody for AIDS*
MDX-447 *investigational (Phase I/II) anticancer antibody*
MDX-RA *investigational (Phase III) immunotoxin for the prevention of secondary cataracts (clinical trials discontinued 1998)*
MEA (mercaptoethylamine) [see: mercaptamine]
meadow cabbage *medicinal herb* [see: skunk cabbage]
meadow sorrel *medicinal herb* [see: sorrel]
meadowsweet *(Filipendula ulmaria)* plant *medicinal herb used for ulcers and upper respiratory problems; also used as an astringent, diaphoretic, and diuretic*
mealberry *medicinal herb* [see: uva ursi]
mealy starwort *medicinal herb* [see: star grass]
measles, mumps & rubella virus vaccine, live USP *active immunizing agent for measles (rubeola), mumps and rubella*
measles immune globulin USP
measles & rubella virus vaccine, live USP *active immunizing agent for measles (rubeola) and rubella*
measles virus vaccine, live USP *active immunizing agent for measles (rubeola)*
Mebadin (available only from the Centers for Disease Control) ℞ *investigational anti-infective for amebiasis and amebic dysentery* [dehydroemetine]
meballymal [see: secobarbital]
mebamoxine [see: benmoxin]
mebanazine INN, BAN
Mebaral tablets ℞ *long-acting barbiturate sedative, hypnotic, and anticonvulsant* [mephobarbital] 32, 50, 100 mg 🔊 Medrol
mebendazole USAN, USP, INN *anthelmintic for trichuriasis, enterobiasis, ascariasis, and uncinariasis* 100 mg oral 🔊 mazindol
mebenoside INN
mebeverine INN *smooth muscle relaxant* [also: mebeverine HCl]
mebeverine HCl USAN *smooth muscle relaxant* [also: mebeverine]
mebezonium iodide INN, BAN
mebhydrolin INN, BAN
mebiquine INN
mebolazine INN
mebrofenin USAN, INN *hepatobiliary function test*
mebrophenhydramine HCl [see: embramine HCl]
mebubarbital [see: pentobarbital]
mebumal [see: pentobarbital]
mebutamate USAN, INN *antihypertensive*
mebutizide INN
mecamylamine INN *nicotinic receptor antagonist for hypertension* [also: mecamylamine HCl]
mecamylamine HCl USP *nicotinic receptor antagonist for hypertension* [also: mecamylamine]
mecamylamine HCl & nicotine *investigational (Phase III) transdermal patch for smoking cessation*
mecarbinate INN
mecarbine [see: mecarbinate]
mecasermin USAN, INN, BAN *investigational (NDA filed, orphan) for amyotrophic lateral sclerosis, type 1 and type 2 diabetes, growth hormone insufficiency, and post-poliomyelitis syndrome* [previously known as insulin-like growth factor 1 (IGF-1)]
MeCCNU (methyl chloroethylcyclohexyl-nitrosourea) [see: semustine]
mecetronium ethylsulfate USAN *antiseptic* [also: mecetronium etilsulfate]
mecetronium etilsulfate INN *antiseptic* [also: mecetronium ethylsulfate]
mechlorethamine HCl USP *nitrogen mustard-type alkylating antineoplastic* [also: chlormethine; mustine; nitrogen mustard *N*-oxide HCl]
meciadanol INN
mecillinam INN, BAN *antibacterial* [also: amdinocillin]
mecinarone INN

Meclan cream ℞ *topical antibiotic for acne* [meclocycline sulfosalicylate] 1% ⊡ Meclomen; Mezlin

meclizine HCl USP *antiemetic; antihistamine; anticholinergic; motion sickness relief* [also: meclozine] 12.5, 25, 50 mg oral ⊡ mescaline

meclocycline USAN, INN, BAN *topical antibiotic*

meclocycline sulfosalicylate USAN, USP *topical antibiotic*

meclofenamate sodium USAN, USP *analgesic; antiarthritic; nonsteroidal anti-inflammatory drug (NSAID)* 50, 100 mg oral

meclofenamic acid USAN, INN *nonsteroidal anti-inflammatory drug (NSAID)*

meclofenoxate INN, BAN

meclonazepam INN

mecloqualone USAN, INN *sedative; hypnotic*

mecloralurea INN

meclorisone INN, BAN *topical anti-inflammatory* [also: meclorisone dibutyrate]

meclorisone dibutyrate USAN *topical anti-inflammatory* [also: meclorisone]

mecloxamine INN

meclozine INN, BAN *antiemetic; antihistamine; anticholinergic; motion sickness relief* [also: meclizine HCl] ⊡ mescaline

mecobalamin USAN, INN *vitamin; hematopoietic*

mecrilate INN *tissue adhesive* [also: mecrylate]

mecrylate USAN *tissue adhesive* [also: mecrilate]

MECY (methotrexate, cyclophosphamide) *chemotherapy protocol*

mecysteine INN

Med Timolol (CAN) eye drops (discontinued 1998) ℞ *topical antiglaucoma agent (β-blocker)* [timolol maleate] 0.25%, 0.5%

Meda Cap capsules OTC *analgesic; antipyretic* [acetaminophen] 500 mg

Meda Tab tablets OTC *analgesic; antipyretic* [acetaminophen] 325 mg

Medacote lotion OTC *topical antihistamine; astringent; antipruritic* [pyrilamine maleate; zinc oxide] 1%•?

Medalone 40; Medalone 80 [see: depMedalone 40; depMedalone 80]

medazepam INN *minor tranquilizer* [also: medazepam HCl]

medazepam HCl USAN *minor tranquilizer* [also: medazepam]

medazomide INN

medazonamide [see: medazomide]

Medebar Plus rectal suspension ℞ *radiopaque contrast medium for gastrointestinal imaging* [barium sulfate] 100%

Mederma gel OTC *moisturizer and emollient for scars* [PEG-4; onion extract; xanthan gum; allantoin]

Medescan oral suspension ℞ *radiopaque contrast medium for gastrointestinal imaging* [barium sulfate] 2.3%

medetomidine INN, BAN *veterinary analgesic; veterinary sedative* [also: medetomidine HCl]

medetomidine HCl USAN *veterinary analgesic; veterinary sedative* [also: medetomidine]

mediator release inhibitors *a class of topical agents that inhibit the antigen-induced release of inflammatory mediators (e.g., various histamines and leukotrienes) from human mast cells; used on nasal, ophthalmological, and gastrointestinal mucosa* [also known as: mast cell stabilizers]

medibazine INN

Medicago sativa *medicinal herb* [see: alfalfa]

medical air [see: air, medical]

Medicated Acne Cleanser OTC *topical acne treatment* [colloidal sulfur; resorcinol] 4%•2%

medicinal zinc peroxide [see: zinc peroxide, medicinal]

Medicone anorectal ointment OTC *topical local anesthetic* [benzocaine] 20%

Medicone rectal suppositories OTC *topical vasoconstrictor for hemorrhoids* [phenylephrine HCl] 0.25%

medifoxamine INN

Medigesic capsules ℞ *analgesic; barbiturate sedative* [acetaminophen; caffeine; butalbital] 325•40•50 mg

Medihaler-Iso inhalation aerosol ℞ *sympathomimetic bronchodilator* [isoproterenol sulfate] 80 µg/dose

Medilax chewable tablets (discontinued 1998) OTC *stimulant laxative* [phenolphthalein] 120 mg

medinal [see: barbital sodium]

Medipain 5 capsules (discontinued 1997) ℞ *narcotic analgesic* [hydrocodone bitartrate; acetaminophen] 5•500 mg

Mediplast plaster OTC *topical keratolytic* [salicylic acid] 40%

Mediplex Tabules (tablets) OTC *vitamin/mineral supplement* [multiple vitamins & minerals] ≛

Medi-Quik ointment OTC *topical antibiotic* [polymyxin B sulfate; neomycin; bacitracin] 5000 U•3.5 mg•400 U per g

Medi-Quik spray OTC *topical local anesthetic; antiseptic* [lidocaine; benzalkonium chloride] 2%•0.13%

medium chain triglycerides (MCT) *dietary lipid supplement*

medorinone USAN, INN *cardiotonic*

medorubicin INN

Medotar ointment OTC *topical antipsoriatic; antiseborrheic; astringent; antiseptic* [coal tar; zinc oxide] 1%•?

Medralone 40; Medralone 80 intralesional, soft tissue, and IM injection ℞ *corticosteroid; anti-inflammatory; immunosuppressant* [methylprednisolone acetate] 40 mg/mL; 80 mg/mL

medrogestone USAN, INN, BAN *progestin*

Medrol tablets, Dosepak (unit of use package) ℞ *corticosteroid; anti-inflammatory; immunosuppressant* [methylprednisolone] 2, 4, 8, 16, 24, 32 mg ⊡ Mebaral

medronate disodium USAN *pharmaceutic aid*

medronic acid USAN, INN, BAN *pharmaceutic aid*

medroxalol USAN, INN, BAN *antihypertensive*

medroxalol HCl USAN *antihypertensive*

medroxiprogesterone acetate [see: medroxyprogesterone acetate]

medroxyprogesterone INN, BAN *progestin for secondary amenorrhea, abnormal uterine bleeding, and endometrial hyperplasia; hormonal antineoplastic* [also: medroxyprogesterone acetate]

medroxyprogesterone acetate (MPA) USP *progestin for secondary amenorrhea, abnormal uterine bleeding, and endometrial hyperplasia; hormonal antineoplastic for endometrial or renal carcinoma* [also: medroxyprogesterone] 2.5, 5, 10 mg oral

MED-Rx controlled-release tablets (14-day, 56-tablet regimen) ℞ *decongestant; expectorant* [pseudoephedrine HCl + guaifenesin (blue tablets); guaifenesin (white tablets)] 60•600 mg; 600 mg

MED-Rx DM controlled-release tablets (14-day, 56-tablet regimen) ℞ *decongestant; expectorant; antitussive* [pseudoephedrine HCl + guaifenesin (blue tablets); dextromethorphan hydrobromide + guaifenesin (green tablets)] 60•600 mg; 30•600 mg

medrylamine INN

medrysone USAN, USP, INN *ophthalmic corticosteroidal anti-inflammatory*

mefeclorazine INN

mefenamic acid USAN, USP, INN, BAN *analgesic; nonsteroidal anti-inflammatory drug (NSAID)*

mefenidil USAN, INN *cerebral vasodilator*

mefenidil fumarate USAN *cerebral vasodilator*

mefenidramium metilsulfate INN

mefenorex INN *anorectic* [also: mefenorex HCl]

mefenorex HCl USAN *anorectic* [also: mefenorex]

mefeserpine INN

mefexamide USAN, INN *CNS stimulant*

mefloquine USAN, INN, BAN *antimalarial*

mefloquine HCl USAN *antimalarial for acute chloroquine-resistant malaria (orphan)*

Mefoxin powder or frozen premix for IV or IM injection ℞ *cephamycin antibiotic* [cefoxitin sodium] 1, 2, 10 g

mefruside USAN, INN *diuretic*

Mega AO (CAN) tablets OTC *antioxidant/vitamin supplement* [multiple vitamins; coenzyme Q_{10}; folic acid; biotin] ≛ •4•0.333•0.167 mg

Mega VM-80 tablets OTC *geriatric vitamin/mineral supplement* [multiple vitamins & minerals; folic acid; biotin] ≛ •400•80 µg

Mega-B tablets OTC *vitamin supplement* [multiple B vitamins; folic acid; biotin] ≛ •100•100 µg

Megace oral suspension ℞ *progestin; hormonal antineoplastic for AIDS-related anorexia and cachexia (orphan)* [megestrol acetate] 40 mg/mL

Megace tablets ℞ *progestin; hormonal antineoplastic for advanced carcinoma of the breast or endometrium* [megestrol acetate] 20, 40 mg

Megagen ℞ *investigational (orphan) adjunct to hematopoietic stem cell transplantation* [megakaryocyte growth and development factor, pegylated, recombinant human]

megakaryocyte growth and development factor, pegylated, recombinant human *investigational (orphan) adjunct to hematopoietic stem cell transplantation*

megallate INN *combining name for radicals or groups*

megalomicin INN *antibacterial* [also: megalomicin potassium phosphate]

megalomicin potassium phosphate USAN *antibacterial* [also: megalomicin]

Megaton elixir ℞ *vitamin/mineral supplement* [multiple B vitamins & minerals; folic acid] ≛ •0.1 mg

megestrol INN, BAN *progestin; hormonal antineoplastic for breast or endometrial cancer* [also: megestrol acetate]

megestrol acetate USAN, USP *progestin; hormonal antineoplastic for breast or endometrial cancer; therapy for AIDS-related anorexia and cachexia (orphan)* [also: megestrol] 20, 40 mg oral

meglitinide INN

meglucycline INN

meglumine USP, INN *radiopaque contrast medium*

meglumine diatrizoate BAN *oral/parenteral radiopaque contrast medium (46.67% iodine)* [also: diatrizoate meglumine]

meglumine iocarmate BAN *radiopaque contrast medium* [also: iocarmate meglumine]

meglumine iothalamate BAN *parenteral radiopaque contrast medium (47% iodine)* [also: iothalamate meglumine]

meglumine ioxaglate BAN *radiopaque contrast medium* [also: ioxaglate meglumine]

meglutol USAN, INN *antihyperlipoproteinemic*

mel B [see: melarsoprol]

mel W [see: melarsonyl potassium]

Melacine ℞ *investigational (NDA filed, orphan) theraccine for invasive stage III–IV melanoma; investigational (Phase III) for early-stage melanoma* [melanoma vaccine]

meladrazine INN, BAN

melafocon A USAN *hydrophobic contact lens material*

Melaleuca alternifolia *medicinal herb* [see: tea tree oil]

Melanex solution ℞ *hyperpigmentation bleaching agent* [hydroquinone] 3%

melanoma vaccine *investigational (NDA filed, orphan) therapeutic vaccine for invasive stage III–IV melanoma; investigational (Phase III) for early-stage melanoma*

melarsonyl potassium INN, BAN

melarsoprol INN, BAN, DCF *investigational anti-infective for trypanosomiasis*

melatonin *natural sleep aid; investigational (orphan) for circadian rhythm sleep disorders in blind people with no light perception*

melengestrol INN *antineoplastic; progestin* [also: melengestrol acetate]

melengestrol acetate USAN *antineoplastic; progestin* [also: melengestrol]

meletimide INN

melfalan [see: melphalan]

Melfiat-105 Unicelles (sustained-release capsules) ℞ *anorexiant; CNS stimulant* [phendimetrazine tartrate] 105 mg

Melia azedarach *medicinal herb* [see: pride of China]

melilot *(Melilotus alba; M. officinalis)* flowering plant *medicinal herb used as an antispasmodic, diuretic, emollient, expectorant, and vulnerary*

Melimmune *investigational (orphan) for non-Hodgkin B-cell lymphoma* [indium In 111 murine MAb (2B8-MXDTPA); yttrium Y 90 murine MAB (2B8-MXDTPA)]

melinamide INN

Melissa officinalis *medicinal herb* [see: lemon balm]

melitracen INN *antidepressant* [also: melitracen HCl]

melitracen HCl USAN *antidepressant* [also: melitracen]

melizame USAN, INN *sweetener*

Mellaril tablets, oral concentrate ℞ *conventional (typical) antipsychotic* [thioridazine HCl] 10, 15, 25, 50, 100, 150, 200 mg; 30, 100 mg/mL ⊠ Aldoril; Elavil; Eldepryl; Enovil; Equanil; Moderil

Mellaril-S oral suspension ℞ *conventional (typical) antipsychotic* [thioridazine HCl] 25, 100 mg/5 mL (10 mg/5 mL available in Canada)

meloxicam USAN, INN, BAN *analgesic; antiarthritic; antipyretic; COX-2 inhibitor; nonsteroidal anti-inflammatory drug (NSAID)*

Melpaque HP cream ℞ *hyperpigmentation bleaching agent; sunscreen* [hydroquinone in a sunblock base] 4%

melperone INN, BAN

melphalan (MPL) USAN, USP, INN, BAN, JAN *nitrogen mustard-type alkylating antineoplastic for multiple myeloma (orphan) and ovarian cancer; investigational (orphan) for metastatic melanoma*

Melquin HP cream ℞ *hyperpigmentation bleaching agent* [hydroquinone] 4%

memantine INN *NMDA antagonist; neuroprotective agent; investigational (Phase II/III) for chronic pain of peripheral diabetic neuropathy; investigational (Phase III) cognition adjuvant for for vascular dementia and Alzheimer disease; investigational (Phase II) for AIDS dementia*

Memorette (trademarked packaging form) *patient compliance package*

memotine INN *antiviral* [also: memotine HCl]

memotine HCl USAN *antiviral* [also: memotine]

menabitan INN *analgesic* [also: menabitan HCl]

menabitan HCl USAN *analgesic* [also: menabitan]

menadiol BAN *vitamin K_4; prothrombogenic* [also: menadiol sodium diphosphate]

menadiol sodium diphosphate USP *vitamin K_4; prothrombogenic* [also: menadiol]

menadiol sodium sulfate INN

menadione USP *vitamin K_3; prothrombogenic*

menadione sodium bisulfite USP, INN

Menadol captabs OTC *analgesic; antiarthritic; antipyretic; nonsteroidal anti-inflammatory drug (NSAID)* [ibuprofen] 200 mg

menaphthene [see: menadione]

menaphthone [see: menadione]

menaphthone sodium bisulfite [see: menadione sodium bisulfite]

menaquinone *vitamin K_2; prothrombogenic*

menatetrenone INN

menbutone INN, BAN

mendelevium *element (Md)*

Menest film-coated tablets ℞ *estrogen replacement therapy for postmenopausal symptoms; palliative therapy for inoperable prostatic and breast cancer* [esterified estrogens] 0.3, 0.625, 1.25, 2.5 mg

menfegol INN

menglytate INN

menichlopholan [see: niclofolan]

Meni-D capsules ℞ *anticholinergic; antivertigo agent; motion sickness preventative* [meclizine HCl] 25 mg

meningococcal polysaccharide vaccine, group A USP *active bacterin for meningitis (Neisseria meningitidis)*

meningococcal polysaccharide vaccine, group C USP *active bacterin for meningitis (Neisseria meningitidis)*

meningococcal polysaccharide vaccine, group W-135 *active bacterin for meningitis (Neisseria meningitidis)*

meningococcal polysaccharide vaccine, group Y *active bacterin for meningitis (Neisseria meningitidis)*

Menispermum cocculus; M. lacunosum *medicinal herb* [see: levant berry]

menitrazepam INN

menoctone USAN, INN *antimalarial*

menogaril USAN, INN *antibiotic antineoplastic*

Menogen; Menogen H.S. tablets (discontinued 1999) ℞ *hormone replacement therapy for postmenopausal symptoms* [esterified estrogens; methyltestosterone] 1.25•2.5 mg; 0.625•1.25 mg

Menomune-A/C/Y/W-135 powder for subcu injection ℞ *meningitis vaccine* [meningococcal polysaccharide vaccine, groups A, C, Y, and W-135] 50 µg of each group per 0.5 mL dose

Menoplex tablets (discontinued 2000) OTC *analgesic; antipyretic; antihistaminic sleep aid* [acetaminophen; phenyltoloxamine citrate] 325•30 mg

Menorest transdermal patch ℞ *investigational estrogen replacement therapy for postmenopausal symptoms* [estradiol]

menotropins USAN, USP *gonadotropin; gonad-stimulating principle for the induction of ovulation in women and the stimulation of spermatogenesis in men*

menotropins & human luteinizing hormone (hLH), recombinant *investigational for chronic anovulation due to hypogonadotropic hypogonadism; orphan status withdrawn 1998*

Menrium 5-2; Menrium 5-4; Menrium 10-4 tablets (discontinued 1997) ℞ *estrogen replacement therapy for postmenopausal symptoms; anxiolytic* [chlordiazepoxide; esterified estrogens] 5•0.2 mg; 5•0.4 mg; 10•0.4 mg

Mentax cream ℞ *topical benzylamine antifungal* [butenafine HCl] 1%

Mentha piperita *medicinal herb* [see: peppermint]

Mentha pulegium *medicinal herb* [see: pennyroyal]

Mentha spicata *medicinal herb* [see: spearmint]

menthol USP *topical analgesic and antipruritic; counterirritant; mild local anesthetic*

MenthoRub vaporizing ointment (discontinued 2000) OTC *topical analgesic; counterirritant* [menthol; camphor; eucalyptus oil; oil of turpentine] 2.6%•4.73%•?•?

menthyl anthranilate [see: meradimate]

Menyanthes trifoliata *medicinal herb* [see: buckbean]

meobentine INN *antiarrhythmic* [also: meobentine sulfate]

meobentine sulfate USAN *antiarrhythmic* [also: meobentine]

mepacrine INN *anthelmintic; antimalarial* [also: quinacrine HCl]

mepacrine HCl [see: quinacrine HCl]

meparfynol [see: methylpentynol]

mepartricin USAN, INN *antifungal; antiprotozoal*

mepazine acetate [see: pecazine]

mepenzolate bromide USP, INN *peptic ulcer adjunct*

mepenzolate methylbromide [see: mepenzolate bromide]

mepenzolone bromide [see: mepenzolate bromide]

Mepergan injection ℞ *narcotic analgesic; sedative* [meperidine HCl; promethazine HCl] 25•25 mg/mL

Mepergan Fortis capsules ℞ *narcotic analgesic; sedative* [meperidine HCl; promethazine HCl] 50•25 mg

meperidine HCl USP *narcotic analgesic; also abused as a street drug* [also: pethidine] 50, 100 mg oral; 50 mg/5 mL oral; 10, 25, 50, 75, 100 mg/mL injection ⑨ meprobamate

Mephaquin ℞ *antimalarial for acute chloroquine-resistant malaria (orphan)* [mefloquine HCl]
mephenesin NF, INN
mephenhydramine [see: moxastine]
mephenoxalone INN
mephentermine INN *adrenergic; vasoconstrictor; vasopressor for hypotensive shock* [also: mephentermine sulfate]
mephentermine sulfate USP *adrenergic; vasoconstrictor; vasopressor for hypotensive shock* [also: mephentermine]
mephenytoin USAN, USP, INN *hydantoin anticonvulsant* [also: methoin] ⓢ Mephyton; Mesantoin (D/C 2000)
mephobarbital USP, JAN *anticonvulsant; sedative* [also: methylphenobarbital; methylphenobarbitone]
Mephyton tablets ℞ *coagulant to correct anticoagulant-induced prothrombin deficiency; vitamin K supplement* [phytonadione] 5 mg ⓢ mephenytoin; methadone
mepicycline [see: pipacycline]
MEPIG (mucoid exopolysaccharide *Pseudomonas* [hyper]-immune globulin) [q.v.]
mepindolol INN, BAN
mepiperphenidol bromide
mepiprazole INN, BAN
mepirizole [see: epirizole]
mepiroxol INN
mepitiostane INN
mepivacaine INN *local anesthetic* [also: mepivacaine HCl]
mepivacaine HCl USP *local anesthetic* [also: mepivacaine] 1%, 2% injection
mepixanox INN
mepramidil INN
meprednisone USAN, USP, INN
meprobamate USP, INN, BAN, JAN *anxiolytic; sedative; hypnotic; minor tranquilizer; also abused as a street drug* 200, 400 mg oral ⓢ meperidine
Mepron oral suspension ℞ *antiprotozoal for Pneumocystis carinii pneumonia (orphan); investigational (orphan) for Toxoplasma gondii encephalitis* [atovaquone] 750 mg/5 mL ⓢ Lupron; Napron
meproscillarin INN, BAN
Meprospan sustained-release capsules (discontinued 1997) ℞ *anxiolytic* [meprobamate] 200, 400 mg ⓢ Naprosyn
meprothixol BAN [also: meprotixol]
meprotixol INN [also: meprothixol]
meprylcaine INN *local anesthetic* [also: meprylcaine HCl]
meprylcaine HCl USP *local anesthetic* [also: meprylcaine]
meptazinol INN, BAN *analgesic* [also: meptazinol HCl]
meptazinol HCl USAN *analgesic* [also: meptazinol]
mepyramine INN, BAN *antihistamine* [also: pyrilamine maleate]
mepyramine maleate [see: pyrilamine maleate]
mepyrium [see: amprolium]
mepyrrotazine [see: dimelazine]
mequidox USAN, INN *antibacterial*
mequinol USAN, INN *hyperpigmentation bleaching agent*
mequitamium iodide INN
mequitazine INN, BAN
mequitazium iodide [see: mequitamium iodide]
meradimate USAN *ultraviolet A sunscreen*
meragidone sodium
meralein sodium USAN, INN *topical anti-infective*
meralluride NF, INN
merbaphen USP
merbromin NF, INN *general antiseptic*
mercaptamine INN *antiurolithic* [also: cysteamine]
mercaptoarsenical [see: arsthinol]
mercaptoarsenol [see: arsthinol]
mercaptoethylamine (MEA) [see: mercaptamine]
mercaptomerin (MT6) INN [also: mercaptomerin sodium]
mercaptomerin sodium USP [also: mercaptomerin]
mercaptopurine (6-MP) USP, INN *antimetabolite antineoplastic*
mercuderamide INN

mercufenol chloride USAN *topical anti-infective*
mercumatilin sodium INN
mercuric oxide, yellow NF *ophthalmic antiseptic (FDA ruled it "not safe and effective" in 1992)*
mercuric salicylate NF
mercuric succinimide NF
mercurobutol INN
Mercurochrome solution (discontinued 2000) OTC *antiseptic* [merbromin] 2%
mercurophylline NF, INN
mercurous chloride [see: calomel]
mercury *element (Hg)*
mercury, ammoniated USP *topical anti-infective; antipsoriatic*
mercury amide chloride [see: mercury, ammoniated]
mercury oleate NF
merethoxylline procaine
mergocriptine INN
Meridia capsules ℞ *anorexiant for the treatment of obesity* [sibutramine HCl] 5, 10, 15 mg
merisoprol acetate Hg 197 USAN *radioactive agent*
merisoprol acetate Hg 203 USAN *radioactive agent*
merisoprol Hg 197 USAN *renal function test; radioactive agent*
Meritene powder OTC *enteral nutritional therapy* [milk-based formula]
meropenem USAN, INN, BAN *broad-spectrum carbapenem antibiotic for intra-abdominal infections and bacterial meningitis*
Merrem powder for IV infusion ℞ *broad-spectrum carbapenem antibiotic for intra-abdominal infections and bacterial meningitis* [meropenem] 500, 1000 mg
mersalyl INN
mersalyl sodium [see: mersalyl]
Mersol solution, tincture OTC *antiseptic; antibacterial; antifungal* [thimerosal] 1:1000
mertiatide INN
Meruvax II powder for subcu injection ℞ *rubella vaccine* [rubella virus vaccine, live] 0.5 mL
mesabolone INN
mesalamine USAN *anti-inflammatory; treatment of ulcerative colitis and proctitis* [also: mesalazine]
mesalazine INN, BAN *anti-inflammatory; treatment of ulcerative colitis and proctitis* [also: mesalamine]
Mesantoin tablets (discontinued 2000) ℞ *hydantoin anticonvulsant* [mephenytoin] 100 mg ⑨ mephenytoin; Mestinon; Metatensin
mescaline *hallucinogenic street drug derived from the flowering heads (mescal buttons) of a Mexican cactus* ⑨ meclizine
Mescolor sustained-release film-coated tablets ℞ *decongestant; antihistamine; anticholinergic* [pseudoephedrine HCl; chlorpheniramine maleate; methscopolamine nitrate] 120•8•2.5 mg
meseclazone USAN, INN *anti-inflammatory*
mesifilcon A USAN *hydrophilic contact lens material*
mesilate INN *combining name for radicals or groups* [also: mesylate]
M-Eslon (CAN) capsules ℞ *narcotic analgesic* [morphine sulfate] 10, 15, 30, 60, 100, 200 mg
mesna USAN, INN, BAN *prophylaxis for ifosfamide-induced hemorrhagic cystitis (orphan); investigational (orphan) for cyclophosphamide-induced hemorrhagic cystitis*
Mesnex IV injection ℞ *prophylaxis for ifosfamide-induced hemorrhagic cystitis (orphan); investigational (orphan) for cyclophosphamide-induced hemorrhagic cystitis* [mesna] 100 mg/mL
mesocarb INN
meso-inositol [see: inositol]
meso-NDGA (nordihydroguaiaretic acid) [see: masoprocol]
meso-nordihydroguaiaretic acid (NDGA) [see: masoprocol]
mesoridazine USAN, INN *phenothiazine antipsychotic*
mesoridazine besylate USP *phenothiazine antipsychotic*

mespiperone C 11 USAN *radiopharmaceutical imaging aid for PET scans of the brain (produced at bedside for immediate administration)*
mespirenone INN
mestanolone INN, BAN
mestenediol [see: methandriol]
mesterolone USAN, INN, BAN *androgen; also abused as a street drug*
Mestinon tablets, Timespan (sustained-release tablets), syrup, IM or IV injection ℞ *cholinergic/anticholinesterase muscle stimulant; muscle relaxant reversal; treatment for myasthenia gravis* [pyridostigmine bromide] 60 mg; 180 mg; 60 mg/5 mL; 5 mg/mL ⓢ Mesantoin; Metatensin
mestranol USAN, USP, INN *estrogen*
mesudipine INN
mesulergine INN
mesulfamide INN
mesulfen INN [also: mesulphen]
mesulphen BAN [also: mesulfen]
mesuprine INN *vasodilator; smooth muscle relaxant* [also: mesuprine HCl]
mesuprine HCl USAN *vasodilator; smooth muscle relaxant* [also: mesuprine]
mesuximide INN *anticonvulsant* [also: methsuximide]
mesylate USAN, USP, BAN *combining name for radicals or groups* [also: mesilate]
metabromsalan USAN, INN *disinfectant*
metabutethamine HCl NF
metabutoxycaine HCl NF
metacetamol INN, BAN
metaclazepam INN
metacycline INN *antibacterial* [also: methacycline]
Metadate CD extended-release capsules ℞ *CNS stimulant; once-daily treatment for attention-deficit hyperactivity disorder (ADHD)* [methylphenidate HCl] 20 mg
Metadate ER extended-release tablets ℞ *CNS stimulant for attention-deficit hyperactivity disorder (ADHD)* [methylphenidate HCl] 10, 20 mg
Metadol (CAN) oral liquid ℞ *narcotic analgesic; treatment for opioid dependence* [methadone HCl] 10 mg/mL
metaglycodol INN
metahexamide INN
metahexanamide [see: metahexamide]
Metahydrin tablets ℞ *diuretic; antihypertensive* [trichlormethiazide] 4 mg ⓢ Metandren
metalkonium chloride INN
metallibure INN *anterior pituitary activator for swine* [also: methallibure]
metalol HCl USAN *antiadrenergic (β-receptor)*
metamelfalan INN
metamfazone INN [also: methamphazone]
metamfepramone INN [also: dimepropion]
metamfetamine INN *CNS stimulant; widely abused as a street drug* [also: methamphetamine HCl]
metamizole sodium INN *analgesic; antipyretic* [also: dipyrone]
metampicillin INN
Metamucil effervescent powder OTC *bulk laxative; antacid* [psyllium hydrophilic mucilloid; sodium bicarbonate; potassium bicarbonate] 3.4•?•? g/packet
Metamucil wafers OTC *bulk laxative* [psyllium husk] 3.4 g
Metamucil Original Texture; Metamucil Smooth Texture powder OTC *bulk laxative* [psyllium husk] 3.4 g/dose
metandienone INN [also: methandrostenolone; methandienone]
metanixin INN
metaoxedrine chloride [see: phenylephrine HCl]
metaphosphoric acid, potassium salt [see: potassium metaphosphate]
metaphosphoric acid, trisodium salt [see: sodium trimetaphosphate]
metaphyllin [see: aminophylline]
metapramine INN
Metaprel syrup (discontinued 1999) ℞ *sympathomimetic bronchodilator* [metaproterenol sulfate] 10 mg/5 mL

metaproterenol polistirex USAN *sympathomimetic bronchodilator* [also: orciprenaline] ⊡ metoprolol

metaproterenol sulfate USAN, USP *sympathomimetic bronchodilator* 10, 20 mg oral; 10 mg/5 mL oral; 0.4%, 0.6%, 5% inhalation

metaradrine bitartrate [see: metaraminol bitartrate]

metaraminol INN *adrenergic; vasopressor for acute hypotensive shock, anaphylaxis, or traumatic shock* [also: metaraminol bitartrate]

metaraminol bitartrate USP *adrenergic; vasopressor for acute hypotensive shock, anaphylaxis, or traumatic shock* [also: metaraminol]

Metaret injection ℞ *investigational (NDA filed, orphan) growth factor antagonist for prostate cancer* [suramin hexasodium] 600 mg

Metastat (name changed to Metadol upon marketing approval in 2001)

Metastron IV injection ℞ *analgesic for metastatic bone pain* [strontium chloride Sr 89] 10.9–22.6 mg/mL (4 mCi)

Metatensin #2; Metatensin #4 tablets ℞ *antihypertensive* [trichlormethiazide; reserpine] 2•0.1 mg; 4•0.1 mg ⊡ Mesantoin; Mestinon

metaterol INN

metaxalone USAN, INN, BAN *skeletal muscle relaxant* ⊡ metolazone

metazamide INN

metazepium iodide [see: buzepide metiodide]

metazide INN

metazocine INN, BAN

metbufen INN

metcaraphen HCl

metembonate INN *combining name for radicals or groups*

meteneprost USAN, INN *oxytocic; prostaglandin*

metenolone INN *anabolic steroid; also abused as a street drug* [also: methenolone acetate; methenolone; metenolone acetate]

metenolone acetate JAN *anabolic steroid; also abused as a street drug* [also: methenolone acetate; metenolone; methenolone]

metenolone enanthate JAN *anabolic steroid; also abused as a street drug* [also: methenolone enanthate]

Metered Solution Inhaler (MSI) *investigational (Phase I/II) pulmonary delivery device for asthma*

metergoline INN, BAN

metergotamine INN

metescufylline INN

metesculetol INN

metesind glucuronate USAN *specific thymidylate synthase (TS) inhibitor antineoplastic* ⊡ medicine

metethoheptazine INN

metetoin INN *anticonvulsant* [also: methetoin]

metformin USAN, INN, BAN *biguanide antidiabetic* [also: metformin HCl]

metformin HCl USAN, JAN *biguanide antidiabetic* [also: metformin]

Metformin XT ℞ *investigational (Phase III) once-daily treatment for diabetes* [metformin HCl]

methacholine bromide NF

methacholine chloride USP, INN *cholinergic; bronchoconstrictor for pulmonary challenge tests*

methacrylic acid copolymer NF *tablet-coating agent*

methacycline USAN *antibacterial* [also: metacycline]

methacycline HCl USP *gram-negative and gram-positive bacteriostatic; antirickettsial*

methadol [see: dimepheptanol]

methadone INN *narcotic analgesic; treatment for opioid dependence; often abused as a street drug* [also: methadone HCl] ⊡ Mephyton

methadone HCl USP *narcotic analgesic; treatment for opioid dependence; often abused as a street drug* [also: methadone] 5, 10, 40 mg oral; 5, 10 mg/5 mL oral; 10 mg/mL oral

methadonium chloride [see: methadone HCl]

Methadose tablets, oral concentrate, powder ℞ *narcotic analgesic; treat-*

ment for opioid dependence; often abused as a street drug [methadone HCl] 5, 10, 40 mg; 10 mg/mL; 50, 100, 500, 1000 g

methadyl acetate USAN *narcotic analgesic* [also: acetylmethadol]

methafilcon B USAN *hydrophilic contact lens material*

Methagual OTC *counterirritant* [methyl salicylate; guaiacol] 8%•2%

Methalgen cream OTC *topical analgesic; counterirritant* [methyl salicylate; menthol; camphor; mustard oil]

methallenestril INN

methallenestrol [see: methallenestril]

methallibure USAN *anterior pituitary activator for swine* [also: metallibure]

methalthiazide USAN *diuretic; antihypertensive*

methamoctol

methamphazone BAN [also: metamfazone]

methamphetamine HCl USP *CNS stimulant; widely abused as a street drug* [also: metamfetamine]

methampyrone [now: dipyrone]

methanabol [see: methandriol]

methandienone BAN [also: methandrostenolone; metandienone]

methandriol

methandrostenolone USP *steroid; discontinued for human use, but the veterinary product is still available and sometimes abused as a street drug* [also: metandienone; methandienone]

methaniazide INN

methanol [see: methyl alcohol]

methantheline bromide USP *peptic ulcer adjunct* [also: methanthelinium bromide]

methanthelinium bromide INN, BAN *anticholinergic* [also: methantheline bromide]

methaphenilene INN, BAN [also: methaphenilene HCl]

methaphenilene HCl NF [also: methaphenilene]

methapyrilene INN [also: methapyrilene fumarate]

methapyrilene fumarate USP [also: methapyrilene]

methapyrilene HCl USP

methaqualone USAN, USP, INN, BAN *hypnotic; sedative; widely abused as a street drug, which leads to dependence*

methaqualone HCl USP

metharbital USP, INN, JAN *anticonvulsant* [also: metharbitone]

metharbitone BAN *anticonvulsant* [also: metharbital]

methastyridone INN

Methatropic capsules OTC *dietary lipotropic with vitamin supplementation* [choline; inositol; methionine; multiple B vitamins] 115•83•110•≛ mg

methazolamide USP, INN *carbonic anhydrase inhibitor for glaucoma* 25, 50 mg oral

Methblue 65 tablets ℞ *urinary anti-infective and antiseptic; antidote to cyanide poisoning* [methylene blue] 65 mg

methcathinone *a highly addictive manufactured street drug similar to cathinone, with amphetamine-like effects* [see also: cathinone; *Catha edulis*]

methdilazine USP, INN *phenothiazine antihistamine; antipruritic*

methdilazine HCl USP *phenothiazine antihistamine; antipruritic*

methenamine USP, INN *urinary antibiotic* ⑨ methionine

methenamine hippurate USAN, USP *urinary antibiotic* [also: hexamine hippurate]

methenamine mandelate USP *urinary antibiotic* 0.5, 1 g oral; 0.5 g/5 mL oral

methenamine sulfosalicylate *topical antipsoriatic*

methenolone BAN *anabolic steroid; also abused as a street drug* [also: methenolone acetate; metenolone; metenolone acetate]

methenolone acetate USAN *anabolic steroid; also abused as a street drug* [also: metenolone; methenolone; metenolone acetate]

methenolone enanthate USAN *anabolic steroid; also abused as a street drug* [also: metenolone enanthate]

metheptazine INN
Methergine coated tablets, IV or IM injection ℞ *oxytocic for induction of labor, control of postpartum uterine atony, and postpartum hemorrhage* [methylergonovine maleate] 0.2 mg; 0.2 mg/mL
methestrol INN
methetharimide [see: bemegride]
methetoin USAN *anticonvulsant* [also: metetoin]
methicillin sodium USAN, USP *penicillinase-resistant penicillin antibiotic* [also: meticillin]
methimazole USP *thyroid inhibitor* [also: thiamazole] 5, 10 mg oral
methindizate BAN [also: metindizate]
methiodal sodium USP, INN
methiomeprazine INN
methiomeprazine HCl [see: methiomeprazine]
methionine (DL-methionine) NF, JAN *urinary acidifier* [also: racemethionine] 500 mg oral
methionine (L-methionine) USAN, USP, INN, JAN *essential amino acid; symbols: Met, M; investigational (orphan) for AIDS myelopathy* ⓢ methenamine
methionyl neurotropic factor, brain-derived, recombinant *investigational (orphan) for amyotrophic lateral sclerosis*
methionyl stem cell factor, recombinant human *investigational (orphan) for progressive bone marrow failure*
methionyl stem cell factor, recombinant human & filgrastim *investigational adjunct to myelosuppressive or myeloablative therapy; orphan status withdrawn 1998*
N-methionylleptin (human) [see: metreleptin]
methiothepin [see: metitepine]
methisazone USAN *antiviral* [also: metisazone]
methisoprinol [now: inosine pranobex]
Methitest tablets ℞ *androgen replacement for hypogonadism or testosterone deficiency in men, delayed puberty in boys, and metastatic breast cancer in women; also abused as a street drug* [methyltestosterone] 10 mg; 25 mg
methitural INN
methixene HCl USAN *smooth muscle relaxant* [also: metixene] ⓢ methoxsalen
methocamphone methylsulfate [see: trimethidinium methosulfate]
methocarbamol USP, INN, BAN, JAN *skeletal muscle relaxant* 500, 750 mg oral; 100 mg/mL injection
methocidin INN
methohexital USP, INN *barbiturate general anesthetic* [also: methohexitone]
methohexital sodium USP *barbiturate general anesthetic*
methohexitone BAN *barbiturate general anesthetic* [also: methohexital]
methoin BAN *anticonvulsant* [also: mephenytoin]
methonaphthone [see: menbutone]
methophedrine [see: methoxyphedrine]
methophenazine [see: metofenazate]
methopholine USAN *analgesic* [also: metofoline]
methoprene INN
methopromazine INN
methopromazine maleate [see: methopromazine]
methopyrimazole [see: epirizole]
***d*-methorphan** [see: dextromethorphan]
***d*-methorphan hydrobromide** [see: dextromethorphan hydrobromide]
methoserpidine INN, BAN
methotrexate (MTX) USAN, USP, INN, BAN, JAN *antimetabolite antineoplastic; antirheumatic; systemic antipsoriatic; investigational (orphan) for juvenile rheumatoid arthritis* 2.5 mg oral; 1 g injection
methotrexate & laurocapram *investigational (orphan) for topical treatment of Mycosis fungoides*
methotrexate & leucovorin *antineoplastic for osteosarcoma (orphan)*
methotrexate sodium USP *antirheumatic; systemic antipsoriatic; antimetabolite antineoplastic for osteogenic sarcoma (orphan)* 2.5 mg oral; 20,

1000 mg/vial injection; 2.5, 25 mg/mL injection

methotrimeprazine USAN, USP *central analgesic; CNS depressant* [also: levomepromazine]

methotrimeprazine maleate *CNS depressant; neuroleptic*

methoxamine INN *adrenergic; vasoconstrictor; vasopressor for hypotensive shock during surgery* [also: methoxamine HCl]

methoxamine HCl USP *adrenergic; vasoconstrictor; vasopressor for hypotensive shock during surgery* [also: methoxamine]

methoxiflurane [see: methoxyflurane]

methoxsalen (8-methoxsalen) USP *repigmentation agent for vitiligo; antipsoriatic; palliative treatment for cutaneous T-cell lymphoma (CTCL); investigational (orphan) for diffuse systemic sclerosis and cardiac allografts* ⑨ methixene

methoxy polyethylene glycol [see: polyethylene glycol monomethyl ether]

8-methoxycarbonyloctyl oligosaccharides *investigational (Phase III) E. coli neutralizer for traveler's diarrhea and hemolytic uremic syndrome (HUS)*

methoxyfenoserpin [see: mefeserpine]

methoxyflurane USAN, USP, INN, BAN *inhalation general anesthetic*

methoxyphedrine INN

***p*-methoxyphenacyl** [see: anisatil]

methoxyphenamine INN [also: methoxyphenamine HCl]

methoxyphenamine HCl USP [also: methoxyphenamine]

4-methoxyphenol [see: mequinol]

***o*-methoxyphenyl salicylate acetate** [see: guacetisal]

methoxypromazine maleate [see: methopromazine]

8-methoxypsoralen (8-MOP) [see: methoxsalen]

5-methoxyresorcinol [see: flamenol]

methphenoxydiol [see: guaifenesin]

methscopolamine bromide USP *GI antispasmodic; peptic ulcer adjunct* [also: hyoscine methobromide]

methscopolamine nitrate *anticholinergic*

methsuximide USP, BAN *succinimide anticonvulsant* [also: mesuximide]

methyclothiazide USAN, USP, INN *diuretic; antihypertensive* 2.5, 5 mg oral

methydromorphine [see: methyldihydromorphine]

methyl alcohol NF *solvent*

methyl benzoquate BAN *coccidiostat for poultry* [also: nequinate]

methyl cresol [see: cresol]

methyl cysteine [see: mecysteine]

methyl *p*-hydroxybenzoate [see: methylparaben]

methyl isobutyl ketone NF *alcohol denaturant*

methyl nicotinate USAN

methyl palmoxirate USAN *antidiabetic*

methyl phthalate [see: dimethyl phthalate]

methyl salicylate NF *flavoring agent; counterirritant; topical anesthetic*

methyl sulfoxide [see: dimethyl sulfoxide]

methyl violet [see: gentian violet]

***l*-methylaminoethanolcatechol** [see: epinephrine]

methylaminopterin [see: methotrexate]

methylandrostenediol [see: methandriol]

methylatropine nitrate USAN *anticholinergic* [also: atropine methonitrate]

methylbenactyzium bromide INN

methylbenzethonium chloride USP, INN *topical anti-infective/antiseptic*

α-methylbenzylhydrazine [see: mebanazine]

methylcarbamate of salicylanilide [see: anilamate]

methyl-CCNU (chloroethyl-cyclohexyl-nitrosourea) [see: semustine]

methylcellulose USP, INN *ophthalmic moisturizer; suspending and viscosity-increasing agent; bulk laxative*

methylcellulose, propylene glycol ether of [see: hydroxypropyl methylcellulose]
methylchromone INN, BAN
methyldesorphine INN, BAN
methyldigoxin [see: metildigoxin]
methyldihydromorphine INN
methyldihydromorphinone HCl [see: metopon]
methyldinitrobenzamide [see: dinitolmide]
methyldioxatrine [see: meletimide]
N-methyldiphenethylamine [see: demelverine]
α-methyl-DL-thyroxine ethyl ester [see: etiroxate]
methyldopa USAN, USP, INN, BAN, JAN *centrally acting antiadrenergic antihypertensive* 125, 250, 500 mg oral ⓢ levodopa
α-methyldopa [now: methyldopa]
methyldopate BAN *centrally acting antiadrenergic antihypertensive* [also: methyldopate HCl]
methyldopate HCl USAN, USP *centrally acting antiadrenergic antihypertensive* [also: methyldopate] 50 mg/mL injection
methylene blue (MB) USP *antimethemoglobinemic; GU antiseptic; antidote to cyanide poisoning; diagnostic aid for gastric secretions* [also: methylthioninium chloride] 65 mg oral; 10 mg/mL injection
methylene chloride NF *solvent*
methylene diphosphonate (MDP) [now: medronate disodium]
methylenedioxyamphetamine (MDA) [see: MDMA, MDEA]
3,4-methylenedioxyethamphetamine (MDEA) [q.v.]
3,4-methylenedioxymethamphetamine (MDMA) [q.v.]
6-methyleneoxytetracycline (MOTC) [see: methacycline]
methylenprednisolone [see: prednylidene]
methylergometrine INN *oxytocic* [also: methylergonovine maleate]
methylergometrine maleate [see: methylergonovine maleate]
methylergonovine maleate USP *oxytocic for induction of labor* [also: methylergometrine]
methylergonovinium bimaleate [see: methylergonovine maleate]
methylergotamine [see: metergotamine]
methylestrenolone [see: normethandrone]
methyl-GAG (methylglyoxal-*bis*-guanylhydrazone) [see: mitoguazone]
methylglyoxal-*bis*-guanylhydrazone (methyl-GAG; MGBG) [see: mitoguazone]
1-methylhexylamine [see: tuaminoheptane]
1-methylhexylamine sulfate [see: tuaminoheptane sulfate]
N-methylhydrazine [see: procarbazine]
Methylin tablets ℞ *CNS stimulant for attention-deficit hyperactivity disorder (ADHD); also abused as a street drug* [methylphenidate HCl] 5, 10, 20 mg
Methylin ER extended-release tablets ℞ *CNS stimulant for attention-deficit hyperactivity disorder (ADHD)* [methylphenidate HCl] 10, 20 mg
methylmorphine [see: codeine]
methylnaltrexone *investigational treatment for chronic opioid-induced constipation; orphan status withdrawn 1998*
methyl-nitro-imidazole [see: carnidazole]
methylnortestosterone [see: normethandrone]
methylparaben USAN, NF *antifungal agent; preservative*
methylparaben sodium USAN, NF *antimicrobial preservative*
methylparafynol [see: meparfynol]
methylpentynol INN, BAN
methylperidol [see: moperone]
(+)-methylphenethylamine [see: dextroamphetamine]
(–)-methylphenethylamine [see: levamphetamine]

methylphenethylamine HCl [see: amphetamine HCl]

methylphenethylamine phosphate [see: amphetamine phosphate]

(–)-methylphenethylamine succinate [see: levamfetamine succinate]

methylphenethylamine sulfate [see: amphetamine sulfate]

(+)-methylphenethylamine sulfate [see: dextroamphetamine sulfate]

methylphenidate INN, BAN *CNS stimulant for attention-deficit hyperactivity disorder (ADHD) and narcolepsy; also abused as a street drug* [also: methylphenidate HCl]

d-methylphenidate HCl (d-MPH) *investigational (Phase III) stimulant for attention-deficit hyperactivity disorder (ADHD)*

methylphenidate HCl (MPH) USP, JAN *CNS stimulant for attention-deficit hyperactivity disorder (ADHD) and narcolepsy; also abused as a street drug* [also: methylphenidate] 5, 10, 20 mg oral

methylphenobarbital INN *anticonvulsant; sedative* [also: mephobarbital; methylphenobarbitone]

methylphenobarbitone BAN *anticonvulsant; sedative* [also: mephobarbital; methylphenobarbital]

***d*-methylphenylamine sulfate** [see: dextroamphetamine sulfate]

methylphytyl napthoquinone [see: phytonadione]

methylprednisolone USP, INN, BAN, JAN *corticosteroid; anti-inflammatory; immunosuppressant* 4, 16 mg oral

methylprednisolone aceponate INN

methylprednisolone acetate USP, JAN *corticosteroid; anti-inflammatory; immunosuppressant* 20, 40, 80 mg/mL injection

methylprednisolone hemisuccinate USP *corticosteroid; anti-inflammatory*

methylprednisolone sodium phosphate USAN *corticosteroid; anti-inflammatory* 40, 125, 500, 1000 mg/vial injection

methylprednisolone sodium succinate USP, JAN *corticosteroid; anti-inflammatory; immunosuppressant*

methylprednisolone suleptanate USAN, INN *corticosteroid; anti-inflammatory*

methylpromazine

4-methylpyrazole (4-MP) [see: fomepizole]

methylrosaniline chloride [now: gentian violet]

methylrosanilinium chloride INN *topical anti-infective* [also: gentian violet]

methylscopolamine bromide [see: methscopolamine bromide]

methylsulfate USP *combining name for radicals or groups* [also: metilsulfate]

methylsulfonylmethane (MSM) *natural source of sulfur; promotes an increase in collagen and the endogenous antioxidant glutathione*

methyltestosterone USP, INN, BAN *androgen replacement for hypogonadism or testosterone deficiency in men, delayed puberty in boys, and metastatic breast cancer in women; also abused as a street drug* 10, 25 mg oral

methyltheobromine [see: caffeine]

methylthionine chloride [see: methylene blue]

methylthionine HCl [see: methylene blue]

methylthioninium chloride INN *antimethemoglobinemic; antidote to cyanide poisoning* [also: methylene blue]

methylthiouracil USP, INN

methyltrienolone [see: metribolone]

methynodiol diacetate USAN *progestin* [also: metynodiol]

methyprylon USP, INN *sedative; hypnotic* [also: methprylone]

methyprylone BAN *sedative* [also: methyprylon]

methyridene BAN [also: metyridine]

methysergide USAN, INN, BAN *migraine-specific vasoconstrictor and peripheral serotonin antagonist for the prophylaxis of vascular headaches*

methysergide maleate USP *migraine-specific vasoconstrictor and peripheral* *serotonin antagonist for the prophylaxis of vascular headaches*

metiamide USAN, INN *antagonist to histamine H_2 receptors*

metiapine USAN, INN *antipsychotic*

metiazinic acid INN

metibride INN

meticillin INN *penicillinase-resistant penicillin antibiotic* [also: methicillin sodium]

meticillin sodium *penicillinase-resistant penicillin antibiotic* [see: methicillin sodium]

Meticorten tablets ℞ *corticosteroid; anti-inflammatory; immunosuppressant* [prednisone] 1 mg

meticrane INN

metildigoxin INN

metilsulfate INN *combining name for radicals or groups* [also: methylsulfate]

Metimyd eye drop suspension, ophthalmic ointment ℞ *topical ophthalmic corticosteroidal anti-inflammatory; antibiotic* [prednisolone acetate; sulfacetamide sodium] 0.5%•10%

metindizate INN [also: methindizate]

metioprim USAN, INN, BAN *antibacterial*

metioxate INN

metipirox INN

metipranolol USAN, INN, BAN *topical antiglaucoma agent (β-blocker)*

metipranolol HCl *topical antiglaucoma agent (β-blocker)*

metiprenaline INN

metirosine INN *antihypertensive* [also: metyrosine]

metisazone INN *antiviral* [also: methisazone]

metitepine INN

metixene INN *smooth muscle relaxant* [also: methixene HCl]

metixene HCl [see: methixene HCl]

metizoline INN *adrenergic; vasoconstrictor* [also: metizoline HCl]

metizoline HCl USAN *adrenergic; vasoconstrictor* [also: metizoline]

metkefamide INN *analgesic* [also: metkephamid acetate]

metkefamide acetate [see: metkephamid acetate]

metkephamid acetate USAN *analgesic* [also: metkefamide]

metochalcone INN

metocinium iodide INN

metoclopramide INN, BAN, JAN *antiemetic for chemotherapy; GI stimulant; antidopaminergic; radiosensitizer* [also: metoclopramide HCl]

metoclopramide HCl USAN, USP, JAN *antiemetic for chemotherapy; GI stimulant; antidopaminergic; radiosensitizer* [also: metoclopramide] 5, 10 mg oral; 5, 10 mg/5 mL oral; 10 mg/mL oral; 5 mg/mL injection

metoclopramide monohydrochloride monohydrate [see: metoclopramide HCl]

metocurine iodide USAN, USP *neuromuscular blocker; muscle relaxant* 2 mg/mL injection

metofenazate INN

metofoline INN *analgesic* [also: methopholine]

metogest USAN, INN *hormone*

metolazone USAN, INN *antihypertensive; diuretic* ⑨ metaxalone

metomidate INN, BAN

metopimazine USAN, INN *antiemetic*

Metopirone softgels ℞ *diagnostic aid for pituitary function* [metyrapone] 250 mg ⑨ metyrapone

metopon INN

metopon HCl [see: metopon]

metoprine USAN *antineoplastic*

metoprolol USAN, INN, BAN *antihypertensive; antianginal; antiadrenergic (β-blocker)* ⑨ metaproterenol

metoprolol fumarate USAN *antihypertensive; antianginal; antiadrenergic (β-blocker)*

metoprolol succinate USAN *antihypertensive; antianginal; antiadrenergic (β-blocker)*

metoprolol tartrate USAN, USP *antihypertensive; antianginal; antiadrenergic (β-blocker)* 1 mg/mL injection

metoquizine USAN, INN *anticholinergic*

metoserpate INN *veterinary sedative* [also: metoserpate HCl]

metoserpate HCl USAN *veterinary sedative* [also: metoserpate]
metostilenol INN
metoxepin INN
metoxiestrol [see: moxestrol]
metrafazoline INN
metralindole INN
metrazifone INN
metreleptin USAN *metabolic regulator for obesity*
metrenperone USAN, INN, BAN *veterinary myopathic*
metribolone INN
metrifonate INN *veterinary anthelmintic; investigational (NDA filed) acetylcholinesterase inhibitor for Alzheimer dementia* [also: trichlorfon; metriphonate]
metrifudil INN
metriphonate BAN *veterinary anthelmintic* [also: trichlorfon; metrifonate]
metrizamide USAN, INN *parenteral radiopaque contrast medium (48.25% iodine)*
metrizoate sodium USAN *radiopaque contrast medium* [also: sodium metrizoate]
Metro I.V. ready-to-use injection ℞ *antibiotic; antiprotozoal; amebicide* [metronidazole] 500 mg/100 mL
MetroCream ℞ *topical antibiotic for rosacea* [metronidazole] 0.75%
Metrodin powder for IM injection (discontinued 1997) ℞ *ovulation stimulant in polycystic ovary disease (orphan)* [urofollitropin] 0.83, 1.66 mg/ampule
MetroGel; MetroLotion ℞ *antibacterial for rosacea (orphan); investigational (orphan) for decubitus ulcers and perioral dermatitis* [metronidazole] 0.75%
MetroGel Vaginal gel ℞ *antibacterial for bacterial vaginosis* [metronidazole] 0.75%
metronidazole USAN, USP, INN, BAN *antibiotic; antiprotozoal/amebicide; acne rosacea treatment (orphan); investigational (orphan) for decubitus ulcers and perioral dermatitis* 250, 500 mg oral; 500 mg/100 mL injection
metronidazole benzoate *antiprotozoal (Trichomonas)*
metronidazole HCl USAN *antibiotic; antiprotozoal; amebicide*
metronidazole phosphate USAN *antibacterial; antiprotozoal*
MET-Rx food bar, powder for drink OTC *enteral nutritional therapy* 100 g; 72 g
Metubine Iodide IV injection ℞ *neuromuscular blocker; anesthesia adjunct* [metocurine iodide] 2 mg/mL
metuclazepam [see: metaclazepam]
meturedepa USAN, INN *antineoplastic*
metynodiol INN *progestin* [also: methynodiol diacetate]
metynodiol diacetate [see: methynodiol diacetate]
metyrapone USAN, USP, INN *diagnostic aid for pituitary function* ⊡ Metopirone; metyrosine
metyrapone tartrate USAN *pituitary function test*
metyridine INN [also: methyridene]
metyrosine USAN, USP *antihypertensive; pheochromocytomic agent* ⊡ metyrapone
Mevacor tablets ℞ *HMG-CoA reductase inhibitor for hypercholesterolemia and coronary heart disease* [lovastatin] 10, 20, 40 mg
mevastatin INN
mevinolin [now: lovastatin]
mexafylline INN
mexazolam INN
mexenone INN, BAN
mexiletine INN, BAN *antiarrhythmic* [also: mexiletine HCl]
mexiletine HCl USAN, USP *antiarrhythmic* [also: mexiletine] 150, 200, 250 mg oral
mexiprostil INN
Mexitil capsules ℞ *antiarrhythmic* [mexiletine HCl] 150, 200, 250 mg
mexoprofen INN
Mexoryl SX *investigational UVA sunscreen* [ecamsule]
mexrenoate potassium USAN, INN *aldosterone antagonist*
Mexsana Medicated powder OTC *topical diaper rash treatment* [kaolin; zinc

oxide; eucalyptus oil; camphor; corn starch]

mezacopride INN

mezepine INN

mezereon *(Daphne mezereum)* bark *medicinal herb used as a cathartic, diuretic, emetic, and rubefacient; eating the berries can be fatal, and people have been poisoned by eating birds that ate the berries*

mezilamine INN

Mezlin powder for IV or IM injection ℞ *extended-spectrum penicillin antibiotic* [mezlocillin sodium] 1, 2, 3, 4, 20 g/vial Meclan

mezlocillin USAN, INN *extended-spectrum penicillin antibiotic*

mezlocillin sodium USP *extended-spectrum penicillin antibiotic*

MF (methotrexate [with leucovorin rescue], fluorouracil) *chemotherapy protocol for breast cancer*

MF (mitomycin, fluorouracil) *chemotherapy protocol*

MFP (melphalan, fluorouracil, medroxyprogesterone acetate) *chemotherapy protocol*

MG Cold Sore Formula solution OTC *topical oral anesthetic; antipruritic/counterirritant* [lidocaine; menthol] ?•1%

MG217 Dual Treatment lotion (name changed to MG217 Medicated Tar in 2000)

MG217 Medicated conditioner OTC *topical antipsoriatic; antiseborrheic* [coal tar solution] 2%

MG217 Medicated ointment OTC *topical antipsoriatic; antiseborrheic; antifungal; keratolytic* [coal tar solution; colloidal sulfur; salicylic acid] 2%•1.1%•1.5%

MG217 Medicated shampoo OTC *topical antipsoriatic; antiseborrheic; antifungal; keratolytic* [coal tar solution; salicylic acid] 5%•2%

MG217 Medicated Tar lotion, ointment, shampoo OTC *topical antipsoriatic; antiseborrheic* [coal tar solution] 5%; 10%; 15%

MG217 Medicated Tar-Free shampoo OTC *antiseborrheic; keratolytic* [sulfur; salicylic acid] 5%•3%

MG217 Sal-Acid ointment OTC *antipsoriatic; keratolytic* [salicylic acid] 3%

MG400 shampoo OTC *antiseborrheic; keratolytic* [salicylic acid; sulfur] 3%•5%

MGA (melengestrol acetate) [q.v.]

MGBG (methylglyoxal-*bis*-guanylhydrazone) [see: mitoguazone]

MGI-114 *investigational (Phase II) antineoplastic for hormone-refractory prostate and ovarian cancers*

MGW (magnesium sulfate + glycerin + water) enema [q.v.]

Miacalcin nasal spray ℞ *calcium regulator for postmenopausal osteoporosis (only)* [calcitonin (salmon)] 200 IU/0.09 mL dose

Miacalcin subcu or IM injection ℞ *calcium regulator for hypercalcemia, Paget disease, and postmenopausal osteoporosis* [calcitonin (salmon)] 200 IU/mL

Mi-Acid gelcaps OTC *antacid* [calcium carbonate; magnesium carbonate] 311•232 mg

Mi-Acid; Mi-Acid II liquid OTC *antacid; antiflatulent* [aluminum hydroxide; magnesium hydroxide; simethicone] 200•200•20 mg/5 mL; 400•400•40 mg/5 mL

mianserin INN, BAN *serotonin inhibitor; antihistamine* [also: mianserin HCl]

mianserin HCl USAN, JAN *serotonin inhibitor; antihistamine* [also: mianserin]

mibefradil INN *vasodilator and calcium channel blocker for hypertension and chronic stable angina* [also: mibefradil dihydrochloride]

mibefradil dihydrochloride USAN *vasodilator and calcium channel blocker for hypertension and chronic stable angina* [also: mibefradil]

M^{131}IBG [now: iobenguane sulfate I 131]

MIBG-I-123 [see: iobenguane sulfate I 123]

mibolerone USAN, INN *anabolic; androgen*

micafungin *investigational (Phase III) echinocandin antifungal agent*

Micanol (CAN) cream OTC *topical antipsoriatic* [anthralin] 1%, 3%

Micardis tablets ℞ *long-acting antihypertensive; angiotensin II receptor antagonist* [telmisartan] 40, 80 mg

Micardis HCT tablets ℞ *long-acting antihypertensive; angiotensin II receptor antagonist; diuretic* [telmisartan; hydrochlorothiazide] 40•12.5, 80•12.5 mg

Micardis Plus (CAN) tablets ℞ *long-acting antihypertensive; angiotensin II receptor antagonist; diuretic* [telmisartan; hydrochlorothiazide] 80•12.5 mg

Micatin cream, powder, aerosol powder, liquid spray OTC *topical antifungal* [miconazole nitrate] 2%

MICE (mesna [rescue], ifosfamide, carboplatin, etoposide) *chemotherapy protocol for sarcoma, osteosarcoma, and lung cancer* [also: ICE]

micinicate INN

Miconal cream ℞ *topical antipsoriatic* [anthralin] 1%

miconazole USP, INN, BAN, JAN *fungicidal*

Miconazole 7 vaginal inserts OTC *antifungal* [miconazole nitrate] 100 mg

miconazole nitrate USAN, USP, JAN *antifungal* 2% topical/vaginal

Micrainin tablets ℞ *analgesic; antipyretic; anti-inflammatory; anxiolytic; sedative* [aspirin; meprobamate] 325•200 mg

MICRhoGAM IM injection ℞ *obstetric Rh factor immunity suppressant* [Rh_0(D) immune globulin] 50 µg ⑨ microgram

microbubble contrast agent *investigational (orphan) neurosonographic diagnostic aid for intracranial tumors*

Microcaps (trademarked dosage form) *fast-melting tablets*

microcrystalline cellulose [see: cellulose, microcrystalline]

microcrystalline wax [see: wax, microcrystalline]

microfibrillar collagen hemostat (MCH) *topical local hemostatic*

Microgestin Fe 1/20; Microgestin Fe 1.5/30 tablets (in packs of 28) ℞ *monophasic oral contraceptive; iron supplement* [norethindrone acetate; ethinyl estradiol; ferrous fumarate] 1 mg•20 µg•75 mg; 1.5 mg•30 µg•75 mg

Micro-K; Micro-K 10 Extencaps (controlled-release capsules) ℞ *potassium supplement* [potassium chloride] 600 mg (8 mEq); 750 mg (10 mEq)

Micro-K LS extended-release powder ℞ *potassium supplement* [potassium chloride] 20 mEq/packet

Microlipid emulsion OTC *dietary fat supplement* [safflower oil] 50%

Micronase tablets ℞ *sulfonylurea antidiabetic* [glyburide] 1.25, 2.5, 5 mg

microNefrin solution for inhalation OTC *sympathomimetic bronchodilator for bronchial asthma and COPD* [racepinephrine HCl] 2.25%

micronized aluminum *astringent*

Micronized Glyburide tablets ℞ *sulfonylurea antidiabetic* [glyburide] 1.5, 3 mg

micronomicin INN

Micronor tablets (in Dialpaks of 28) ℞ *oral contraceptive (progestin only)* [norethindrone] 0.35 mg

Microstix-3 reagent strips for professional use *in vitro diagnostic aid for nitrate, uropathogens, or bacteria in the urine*

MicroTrak Chlamydia trachomatis slide test for professional use *in vitro diagnostic aid for Chlamydia trachomatis*

MicroTrak HSV 1/HSV 2 Culture Identification/Typing Test culture test for professional use *in vitro diagnostic aid for herpes simplex virus in tissue cultures*

MicroTrak HSV 1/HSV 2 Direct Specimen Identification/Typing Test slide test for professional use *in vitro diagnostic aid for herpes simplex virus in external lesions*

MicroTrak Neisseria gonorrhoeae Culture Confirmation Test reagent kit for professional use *in vitro diagnostic aid for Neisseria gonorrhoeae*

Microzide capsules ℞ *once-daily antihypertensive; thiazide diuretic* [hydrochlorothiazide] 12.5 mg ⑨ Maxzide

mictine [see: aminometradine]

midaflur USAN, INN *sedative*

midaglizole INN

midalcipran [see: milnacipran]

midamaline INN

Midamor tablets ℞ *antihypertensive; potassium-sparing diuretic* [amiloride HCl] 5 mg

midazogrel INN

midazolam INN, BAN, JAN *short-acting benzodiazepine general anesthetic* [also: midazolam HCl]

midazolam HCl USAN *short-acting benzodiazepine general anesthetic* [also: midazolam] 1, 5 mg/mL injection

midazolam maleate USAN *intravenous anesthetic*

Midchlor capsules (discontinued 2000) ℞ *vasoconstrictor; sedative; analgesic (for migraine)* [isometheptene mucate; dichloralphenazone; acetaminophen] 65•100•325 mg

midecamycin INN

midodrine INN, BAN *antihypotensive; vasoconstrictor; vasopressor for orthostatic hypotension (OH)* [also: midodrine HCl]

midodrine HCl USAN, JAN *antihypotensive; vasoconstrictor; vasopressor for orthostatic hypotension (orphan)* [also: midodrine]

Midol, Maximum Strength Cramp Formula tablets OTC *analgesic; antiarthritic; antipyretic; nonsteroidal anti-inflammatory drug (NSAID)* [ibuprofen] 200 mg

Midol IB tablets (name changed to Maximum Strength Midol in 1999)

Midol Maximum Strength Menstrual caplets, gelcaps OTC *analgesic; anti-inflammatory; antihistaminic sleep aid* [acetaminophen; caffeine; pyrilamine maleate] 500•60•15 mg

Midol Multi-Symptom Formula caplets (discontinued 2000) OTC *analgesic; anti-inflammatory; antihistaminic sleep aid* [acetaminophen; pyrilamine maleate] 325•12.5 mg

Midol Multi-Symptom Menstrual caplets (name changed to Midol Maximum Strength Menstrual in 2000)

Midol PM caplets OTC *analgesic; antipyretic; antihistaminic sleep aid* [acetaminophen; diphenhydramine] 500•25 mg

Midol PMS caplets, gelcaps OTC *analgesic; anti-inflammatory; diuretic; antihistaminic sleep aid* [acetaminophen; pamabrom; pyrilamine maleate] 500•25•15 mg

Midol Teen caplets OTC *analgesic; anti-inflammatory; diuretic* [acetaminophen; pamabrom] 500•25 mg

Midrin capsules ℞ *vasoconstrictor; sedative; analgesic (for migraine)* [isometheptene mucate; dichloralphenazone; acetaminophen] 65•100•325 mg ⑨ Mydfrin

Midstream Pregnancy Test kit for home use *in vitro diagnostic aid; urine pregnancy test*

MIFA (mitomycin, fluorouracil, Adriamycin) *chemotherapy protocol*

mifarmonab [see: imciromab pentetate]

Mifegyne (European name for U.S. product Mifeprex)

mifentidine INN

Mifeprex tablets ℞ *abortifacient; emergency postcoital contraceptive; progesterone antagonist investigational for meningioma, endometriosis, and Cushing syndrome* [mifepristone] 200 mg (note: not available to pharmacies; must be obtained from a physician in an office, clinic, or hospital setting)

mifepristone USAN, INN, BAN *abortifacient; emergency postcoital oral contraceptive; progesterone antagonist investigational for meningioma, endometriosis, and Cushing syndrome*

mifobate USAN, INN *antiatherosclerotic*

miglitol USAN, INN, BAN *antidiabetic agent for type 2 diabetes; α-glucosidase* *inhibitor that delays the digestion of dietary carbohydrates*

mignonette, Jamaica *medicinal herb* [see: henna *(Lawsonia)*]

Migranal nasal spray ℞ *rapid-acting antimigraine agent* [dihydroergotamine mesylate] 0.05 mg/spray

Migratine capsules ℞ *vasoconstrictor; sedative; analgesic (for migraine)* [isometheptene mucate; dichloralphenazone; acetaminophen] 65•100•325 mg

Miguard, Migard film-coated tablets ℞ *investigational (NDA filed) 5-HT$_{1B/1D}$ agonist for acute treatment of migraine* [frovatriptan succinate] 2.5 mg

mikamycin INN, BAN

MiKasome ℞ *investigational (Phase II) antibiotic liposomal formulation for complicated urinary tract infections and AIDS-related mycobacterial infections* [amikacin]

milacemide INN *anticonvulsant; antidepressant* [also: milacemide HCl]

milacemide HCl USAN *anticonvulsant; antidepressant* [also: milacemide]

milameline HCl USAN *partial muscarinic agonist for Alzheimer disease*

mild silver protein [see: silver protein, mild]

milenperone USAN, INN, BAN *antipsychotic*

Miles Nervine caplets OTC *antihistaminic sleep aid* [diphenhydramine HCl] 25 mg

milfoil *medicinal herb* [see: yarrow]

milipertine USAN, INN *antipsychotic*

milk ipecac *medicinal herb* [see: birthroot; dogbane]

milk of bismuth [see: bismuth, milk of]

milk of magnesia [see: magnesia, milk of]

Milk of Magnesia-Cascara, Concentrated oral suspension OTC *antacid; saline/stimulant laxative* [milk of magnesia; aromatic cascara fluidextract; alcohol 7%] 30•5 mL/15 mL

milk thistle *(Silybum marianum)* seeds *medicinal herb for Amanita mushroom poisoning, bronchitis, gallbladder disorders, hemorrhage, liver damage, peritonitis, spleen disorders, stomach disorders, and varicose veins*

Milkinol emulsion (discontinued 2000) OTC *emollient laxative* [mineral oil]

milkweed *(Asclepias syriaca)* roots *medicinal herb used as a diuretic, emetic, purgative, and tonic*

milnacipran INN *investigational antidepressant*

milodistim USAN *antineutropenic; hematopoietic stimulant; granulocyte macrophage colony-stimulating factor (GM-CSF) + interleukin 3*

Milontin Kapseals (capsules) ℞ *succinimide anticonvulsant* [phensuximide] 500 mg 🔊 Dilantin; Miltown; Mylanta

Milophene tablets ℞ *ovulation stimulant* [clomiphene citrate] 50 mg

miloxacin INN

milrinone USAN, INN, BAN *cardiotonic*

milrinone lactate *vasodilator for congestive heart failure*

miltefosine INN

Miltown tablets ℞ *anxiolytic; also abused as a street drug* [meprobamate] 200, 400 mg 🔊 Milontin

Miltown-600 tablets (discontinued 2001) ℞ *anxiolytic; also abused as a street drug* [meprobamate] 600 mg 🔊 Milontin

milverine INN

MIM D2A21 *investigational for sexually transmitted diseases*

mimbane INN *analgesic* [also: mimbane HCl]

mimbane HCl USAN *analgesic* [also: mimbane]

minalrestat USAN *aldose reductase inhibitor for diabetic neuropathy and other long-term diabetic complications*

minaprine USAN, INN, BAN *psychotropic*

minaprine HCl USAN *antidepressant*

minaxolone USAN, INN *anesthetic*

mindodilol INN

mindolic acid [see: clometacin]

mindoperone INN

MINE (mesna [rescue], ifosfamide, Novantrone, etoposide) *chemotherapy protocol for non-Hodgkin lymphoma*

MINE-ESHAP (alternating cycles of MINE and ESHAP) *chemotherapy protocol for non-Hodgkin lymphoma*

minepentate INN, BAN

Mineral Ice [see: Therapeutic Mineral Ice]

mineral oil USP *emollient/protectant; laxative; solvent*

mineral oil, light NF *tablet and capsule lubricant; vehicle*

mineralocorticoids *a class of adrenal cortical steroids that are used for partial replacement therapy in adrenocortical insufficiency*

Minesse ℞ *investigational low-dose oral contraceptive in a 24-day regimen* [ethinyl estradiol; gestodene]

Mini Thin Asthma Relief tablets (discontinued 2000) OTC *decongestant; expectorant* [ephedrine HCl; guaifenesin] 25•100, 25•200 mg

Mini Thin Pseudo tablets (discontinued 2000) OTC *nasal decongestant* [pseudoephedrine HCl] 60 mg

mini-BEAM (BCNU, etoposide, ara-C, melphalan) *chemotherapy protocol for Hodgkin lymphoma*

mini-COAP (cyclophosphamide, Oncovin, ara-C, prednisone) *chemotherapy protocol*

Minidyne solution OTC *broad-spectrum antimicrobial* [povidone-iodine] 10%

Mini-Gamulin Rh IM injection (discontinued 2000) ℞ *obstetric Rh factor immunity suppressant* [Rh_0(D) immune globulin] 50 µg

Miniguard disposable pads *adhesive foam pad to seal urethral opening for stress urinary incontinence in women*

Min-I-Mix (delivery system) *dual-chambered prefilled syringe*

Minipress capsules ℞ *antihypertensive; α-blocker* [prazosin HCl] 1, 2, 5 mg

Minitran transdermal patch ℞ *antianginal; vasodilator* [nitroglycerin] 9, 18, 36, 54 mg (0.1, 0.2, 0.4, 0.6 mg/hr.)

Minit-Rub OTC *topical analgesic; counterirritant* [methyl salicylate; menthol; camphor] 15%•3.5%•2.3%

Minizide 1; Minizide 2; Minizide 5 capsules ℞ *antihypertensive; α-blocker; diuretic* [prazosin HCl; polythiazide] 1•0.5 mg; 2•0.5 mg; 5•0.5 mg

Minocin pellet-filled capsules, oral suspension, powder for IV injection ℞ *tetracycline antibiotic* [minocycline HCl] 50, 100 mg; 50 mg/5 mL; 100 mg ⓓ Indocin; Mithracin; niacin

minocromil USAN, INN, BAN *prophylactic antiallergic*

minocycline USAN, INN, BAN *gram-negative and gram-positive bacteriostatic; antirickettsial*

minocycline HCl USP *gram-negative and gram-positive bacteriostatic; antirickettsial; adjunct to scaling and root planing for periodontitis* 50, 100 mg oral

Minox (CAN) topical solution OTC *hair growth stimulant* [minoxidil] 2%

minoxidil USAN, USP, INN, BAN *antihypertensive; peripheral vasodilator; hair growth stimulant* 2.5, 10 mg oral

Minoxidil for Men topical solution OTC *hair growth stimulant* [minoxidil; alcohol 60%] 2%

mint; lamb mint; mackerel mint; Our Lady's mint *medicinal herb* [see: spearmint]

mint, brandy; lamb mint *medicinal herb* [see: peppermint]

mint, mountain *medicinal herb* [see: marjoram; Oswego tea]

mint, squaw *medicinal herb* [see: pennyroyal]

Mintezol chewable tablets, oral suspension ℞ *anthelmintic for strongyloidiasis (threadworm), larva migrans, and trichinosis* [thiabendazole] 500 mg; 500 mg/5 mL

Mintox chewable tablets, oral suspension OTC *antacid* [aluminum hydroxide; magnesium hydroxide] 200•200 mg; 225•200 mg/5 mL

Mintox Plus liquid OTC *antacid; antiflatulent* [aluminum hydroxide; magnesium hydroxide; simethicone] 500•450•40 mg/5 mL

Minute-Gel ℞ *topical dental caries preventative* [acidulated phosphate fluoride] 1.23%

Miochol-E solution ℞ *direct-acting miotic for ophthalmic surgery* [acetylcholine chloride] 1:100

mioflazine INN, BAN *coronary vasodilator* [also: mioflazine HCl]

mioflazine HCl USAN *coronary vasodilator* [also: mioflazine]

Miostat solution ℞ *direct-acting miotic for ophthalmic surgery* [carbachol] 0.01%

miotics *a class of drugs that cause the pupil of the eye to contract*

mipafilcon A USAN *hydrophilic contact lens material*

mipimazole INN

Miradon tablets ℞ *indandione-derivative anticoagulant* [anisindione] 50 mg

MiraFlow solution OTC *cleaning solution for hard or soft contact lenses*

MiraLax powder for oral solution ℞ *hyperosmotic laxative; pre-procedure bowel evacuant* [polyethylene glycol 3350] 17 g/dose

Miraluma ℞ *investigational radioactive imaging aid for mammography* [technetium Tc 99m sestamibi]

Mirapex tablets ℞ *dopamine agonist; antiparkinsonian* [pramipexole dihydrochloride] 0.125, 0.25, 0.5, 1, 1.5 mg

MiraSept Step 2 solution OTC *rinsing/storage solution for soft contact lenses* [sodium chloride (preserved saline solution)]

MiraSept System solutions OTC *two-step chemical disinfecting system for soft contact lenses* [hydrogen peroxide based] 3%

Mircette tablets (in packs of 28) ℞ *biphasic oral contraceptive* [desogestrel; ethinyl estradiol]
Phase 1 (21 days): 0.15 mg•20 µg;
Phase 2 (5 days): 0•10 µg

Mirena intrauterine device (IUD) ℞ *long-term (5 year) contraceptive insert* [levonorgestrel] 20 µg/day

Mireze (CAN) eye drops (name changed to Alocril in 2001)

mirfentanil INN *analgesic* [also: mirfentanil HCl]

mirfentanil HCl USAN *analgesic* [also: mirfentanil]

mirincamycin INN *antibacterial; antimalarial* [also: mirincamycin HCl]

mirincamycin HCl USAN *antibacterial; antimalarial* [also: mirincamycin]

mirisetron maleate USAN *anxiolytic*

miristalkonium chloride INN

miroprofen INN

mirosamicin INN

mirostipen USAN *myeloprotectant*

mirtazapine USAN, INN *tetracyclic antidepressant; serotonin 5-HT$_{1A}$ agonist*

misonidazole USAN, INN *antiprotozoal (Trichomonas)*

misoprostol USAN, INN, BAN *prevents NSAID-induced gastric ulcers*

Mission Prenatal; Mission Prenatal F.A.; Mission Prenatal H.P. tablets OTC *vitamin/iron supplement* [multiple vitamins; ferrous gluconate; folic acid] ≛•30•0.4 mg; ≛•30•0.8 mg; ≛•30•0.8 mg

Mission Prenatal Rx tablets ℞ *vitamin/calcium/iron supplement* [multiple vitamins; calcium; iron; folic acid] ≛•175•29.5•1 mg

Mission Surgical Supplement tablets OTC *vitamin/iron supplement* [multiple vitamins; ferrous gluconate] ≛•27 mg

mistletoe *(Phoradendron flavescens; P. serotinum; P. tomentosum; Viscum album)* plant *medicinal herb for cancer, chorea, epilepsy, hypertension, internal hemorrhages, menstrual disorders, nervousness, poor circulation, and spleen disorders; not generally regarded as safe for ingestion, as it is highly toxic*

Mistometer (trademarked form) *metered-dose inhalation aerosol*

Mitchella repens *medicinal herb* [see: squaw vine]

Mithracin powder for IV infusion ℞ *antibiotic antineoplastic for testicular cancer* [plicamycin] 2.5 mg ⊠ Minocin

mithramycin [now: plicamycin] ⊠ mitomycin

mitindomide USAN, INN *antineoplastic*
mitobronitol INN, BAN
mitocarcin USAN, INN *antineoplastic*
mitoclomine INN, BAN
mitocromin USAN *antineoplastic*
mitoflaxone INN
mitogillin USAN, INN *antineoplastic*
mitoguazone INN *investigational antineoplastic for multiple myeloma and head, esophagus, and prostate cancer; investigational (orphan) for non-Hodgkin lymphoma*
mitolactol INN *investigational (orphan) antineoplastic for brain tumors and recurrent or metastatic cervical squamous cell carcinoma*
mitomalcin USAN, INN *antineoplastic*
mitomycin USAN, USP, INN, BAN *antibiotic antineoplastic; investigational (orphan) for refractory glaucoma and glaucoma surgery* ⊡ mithramycin; Mutamycin
mitomycin C (MTC) [see: mitomycin]
mitonafide INN
mitopodozide INN, BAN
mitoquidone INN, BAN
mitosper USAN, INN *antineoplastic*
mitotane USAN, USP, INN *antibiotic antineoplastic for inoperable adrenal cortical carcinoma*
mitotenamine INN, BAN
mitotic inhibitors *a class of antineoplastics that inhibit cell division (mitosis)*
mitoxantrone INN *antibiotic antineoplastic* [also: mitoxantrone HCl; mitozantrone]
mitoxantrone HCl USAN *antibiotic antineoplastic for prostate cancer and acute nonlymphocytic leukemia (ANL) (orphan); treatment for progressive and relapsing-remitting multiple sclerosis* [also: mitoxantrone; mitozantrone]
mitozantrone BAN *antineoplastic* [also: mitoxantrone HCl; mitoxantrone]
mitozolomide INN, BAN
Mitran capsules ℞ *benzodiazepine anxiolytic* [chlordiazepoxide HCl] 10 mg
Mitrolan chewable tablets OTC *bulk laxative; antidiarrheal* [calcium polycarbophil] 625 mg
mitronal [see: cinnarizine]
mitumomab USAN *antineoplastic for* G_{D3} *ganglioside–expressing tumors; investigational (Phase III) for small cell lung cancer*
MIV (mitoxantrone, ifosfamide, VePesid) *chemotherapy protocol*
Mivacron IV infusion ℞ *muscle relaxant; adjunct to anesthesia* [mivacurium chloride] 0.5, 2 mg/mL
mivacurium chloride USAN, INN, BAN *neuromuscular blocking agent*
mivobulin isethionate USAN *antineoplastic; mitotic inhibitor; tubulin binder*
Mixed E 400; Mixed E 1000 softgels OTC *vitamin supplement* [vitamin E] 400 IU; 1000 IU
mixed respiratory vaccine (MRV) *active bacterin for respiratory tract infections*
mixed tocopherols [see: vitamin E]
mixidine USAN, INN *coronary vasodilator*
Mix-O-Vial (trademarked packaging form) *two-compartment vial*
mizoribine INN
MK-663 *investigational (Phase III) agent for osteoarthritis*
MK-826 *investigational (NDA filed) broad-spectrum carbapenem antibiotic*
MK-869 *investigational (Phase III) antiemetic for chemotherapy-induced emesis*
MKC-442 *investigational (Phase III) non-nucleoside reverse transcriptase inhibitor (NNRTI) for HIV and AIDS*
ML-3000 *investigational (Phase II) anti-inflammatory and analgesic*
MM (mercaptopurine, methotrexate) *chemotherapy protocol*
MMOPP (methotrexate, mechlorethamine, Oncovin, procarbazine, prednisone) *chemotherapy protocol*
MMP (matrix metalloproteinase) inhibitors [q.v.]
MMR (measles, mumps & rubella vaccines) [q.v.]
M-M-R II powder for subcu injection ℞ *measles, mumps and rubella vaccine* [measles, mumps, and rubella virus vaccine, live] 0.5 mL

MOB (mechlorethamine, Oncovin, bleomycin) *chemotherapy protocol*

MOB-III (mitomycin, Oncovin, bleomycin, cisplatin) *chemotherapy protocol*

Moban tablets, oral concentrate ℞ *conventional (typical) antipsychotic* [molindone HCl] 5, 10, 25, 50, 100 mg; 20 mg/mL ⊡ Mobidin; Modane

mobecarb INN

mobenzoxamine INN

Mobic tablets ℞ *once-daily analgesic, antiarthritic, and antipyretic; COX-2 inhibitor; nonsteroidal anti-inflammatory drug (NSAID)* [meloxicam] 7.5, 15 mg

Mobicox (CAN) tablets ℞ *once-daily analgesic, antiarthritic, and antipyretic; COX-2 inhibitor; nonsteroidal anti-inflammatory drug (NSAID)* [meloxicam] 7.5, 15 mg

Mobidin tablets ℞ *analgesic; antipyretic; anti-inflammatory; antirheumatic* [magnesium salicylate] 600 mg ⊡ Moban

Mobigesic tablets OTC *analgesic; antipyretic; anti-inflammatory; antihistaminic sleep aid* [magnesium salicylate; phenyltoloxamine citrate] 325•30 mg

Mobist ℞ *investigational neuroprotectant*

Mobisyl Creme OTC *topical analgesic* [trolamine salicylate] 10%

MOBP (mitomycin, Oncovin, bleomycin, Platinol) *chemotherapy protocol for cervical cancer*

moccasin snake antivenin [see: antivenin (Crotalidae) polyvalent]

mocimycin INN

mociprazine INN

mock pennyroyal *medicinal herb* [see: pennyroyal]

moclobemide USAN, INN, BAN *antidepressant; MAO inhibitor*

moctamide INN

Moctanin biliary infusion ℞ *anticholelithogenic for dissolution of cholesterol gallstones (orphan)* [monoctanoin]

modafinil USAN, INN *analeptic for excessive daytime sleepiness of narcolepsy (orphan)*

modaline INN *antidepressant* [also: modaline sulfate]

modaline sulfate USAN *antidepressant* [also: modaline]

Modane enteric-coated tablets OTC *stimulant laxative* [bisacodyl] 5 mg ⊡ Moban; Mudrane

Modane tablets (discontinued 1998) OTC *stimulant laxative* [white phenolphthalein] 130 mg ⊡ Moban; Mudrane

Modane Bulk powder OTC *bulk laxative* [psyllium husk] 3.4 g/tsp.

Modane Plus tablets (discontinued 1998) OTC *stimulant laxative; stool softener* [white phenolphthalein; docusate sodium] 65•100 mg

Modane Soft capsules OTC *laxative; stool softener* [docusate sodium] 100 mg

modecainide USAN, INN *antiarrhythmic*

Modecate; Modecate Concentrate (CAN) subcu or IM injection ℞ *conventional (typical) antipsychotic* [fluphenazine decanoate] 25 mg/mL; 100 mg/mL

Modicon tablets (in Dialpaks of 21 or 28; in Veridates of 28) ℞ *monophasic oral contraceptive* [norethindrone; ethinyl estradiol] 0.5 mg•35 µg ⊡ Mylicon

modified Bagshawe protocol *chemotherapy protocol* [see: CHAMOCA]

modified bovine lung surfactant extract [see: beractant]

modified Burow solution [see: aluminum acetate solution]

modified cellulose gum [now: croscarmellose sodium]

modified Shohl solution (sodium citrate & citric acid) *urinary alkalinizer; compounding agent*

Modiodal (foreign name for U.S. product Provigil)

Moditen Enanthate (CAN) subcu or IM injection ℞ *conventional (typical) antipsychotic* [fluphenazine enanthate] 25 mg/mL

Moditen HCl (CAN) tablets ℞ *conventional (typical) antipsychotic* [fluphenazine HCl] 10 mg

Modivid ℞ *investigational cephalosporin antibiotic* [cefodizime]

Moducal powder OTC *carbohydrate caloric supplement* [glucose polymers]
Moduretic tablets ℞ *antihypertensive; diuretic* [amiloride HCl; hydrochlorothiazide] 5•50 mg
moexipril INN, BAN *antihypertensive; angiotensin-converting enzyme (ACE) inhibitor*
moexipril HCl USAN *antihypertensive; angiotensin-converting enzyme (ACE) inhibitor*
moexiprilat INN
MOF (MeCCNU, Oncovin, fluorouracil) *chemotherapy protocol*
mofebutazone INN
mofedione [see: oxazidione]
mofegiline INN *antiparkinsonian* [also: mofegiline HCl]
mofegiline HCl USAN *antiparkinsonian* [also: mofegiline]
mofetil USAN, INN *combining name for radicals or groups*
mofloverine INN
mofoxime INN
MOF-STREP; MOF-Strep (MeCCNU, Oncovin, fluorouracil, streptozocin) *chemotherapy protocol*
Mogadon ℞ *investigational benzodiazepine tranquilizer; anxiolytic; anticonvulsant; hypnotic* [nitrazepam]
moguisteine INN
Moist Again vaginal gel OTC *lubricant* [glycerin; aloe vera]
Moi-Stir oral spray, Swabsticks OTC *saliva substitute* [carboxymethylcellulose sodium] ⊡ moisture
Moisture Drops eye drops OTC *ophthalmic moisturizer/lubricant* [hydroxypropyl methylcellulose] 0.5%
Moisture Eyes eye drops OTC *ocular moisturizer/lubricant* [propylene glycol] 0.95%
Moisturel lotion (discontinued 1997) OTC *moisturizer; emollient* [dimethicone] 3%
molfarnate INN
molgramostim USAN, INN, BAN *antineutropenic; hematopoietic stimulant; investigational (Phase II/III) cytokine to AIDS*
Molie capsules OTC *CNS stimulant; analeptic* [caffeine] 200 mg
molinazone USAN, INN *analgesic*
molindone INN *dihydroindolone antipsychotic* [also: molindone HCl]
molindone HCl USAN *dihydroindolone antipsychotic* [also: molindone]
Mol-Iron tablets (discontinued 1998) OTC *hematinic* [ferrous sulfate (source of iron)] 195 mg (39 mg)
Mol-Iron with Vitamin C tablets (discontinued 1998) OTC *hematinic* [iron (from ferrous sulfate); ascorbic acid] 39•75 mg
Mollifene Ear Wax Removing Formula drops OTC *agent to emulsify and disperse ear wax* [carbamide peroxide] 6.5%
molracetam INN
molsidomine USAN, INN *antianginal; coronary vasodilator*
molybdenum *element (Mo)*
Molypen IV injection ℞ *intravenous nutritional therapy* [ammonium molybdate tetrahydrate] 25 µg/mL
Momentum caplets OTC *analgesic; antipyretic; anti-inflammatory; antihistamine* [aspirin; phenyltoloxamine citrate] 500•15 mg
Momentum Muscular Backache Formula caplets OTC *analgesic; antipyretic; anti-inflammatory* [magnesium salicylate] 580 mg
mometasone INN, BAN *topical corticosteroidal anti-inflammatory* [also: mometasone furoate]
mometasone furoate USAN *topical corticosteroidal anti-inflammatory; investigational (NDA filed) inhalation powder for asthma and seasonal allergic rhinitis* [also: mometasone]
Momordica charantia *medicinal herb* [see: bitter melon]
MOMP (mechlorethamine, Oncovin, methotrexate, prednisone) *chemotherapy protocol*
Monafed sustained-release tablets ℞ *expectorant* [guaifenesin] 600 mg

Monafed DM tablets ℞ *antitussive; expectorant* [dextromethorphan hydrobromide; guaifenesin] 30•600 mg

monalazone disodium INN

monalium hydrate [see: magaldrate]

Monarda didyma *medicinal herb* [see: Oswego tea]

Monarda fistulosa *medicinal herb* [see: wild bergamot]

Monarda punctata *medicinal herb* [see: horsemint]

monascus yeast *(Monascus purpureus)* *natural remedy for gastric disorders, indigestion, lowering cholesterol, and poor circulation*

monatepil INN *antianginal; antihypertensive* [also: monatepil maleate]

monatepil maleate USAN *antianginal; antihypertensive* [also: monatepil]

monensin USAN, INN *antiprotozoal; antibacterial; antifungal*

Monistat cream OTC *topical antifungal* [miconazole nitrate] 2%

Monistat 1 vaginal ointment in prefilled applicator OTC *antifungal* [tioconazole] 6.5%

Monistat 3 vaginal cream, combination pack (vaginal inserts + cream), cream combination pak (vaginal cream in prefilled applicators + external cream) OTC *antifungal* [miconazole nitrate] 2%; 200 mg + 2%; 4% + 2%

Monistat 3 vaginal inserts (discontinued 2001) OTC *antifungal* [miconazole nitrate] 200 mg

Monistat 7 vaginal inserts, vaginal cream, combination pack (inserts + cream) OTC *antifungal* [miconazole nitrate] 100 mg; 2%; 100 mg + 2%

Monistat Dual-Pak vaginal inserts + cream ℞ *antifungal* [miconazole nitrate] 200 mg + 2%

Monistat i.v. intrathecal or IV injection (discontinued 1999) ℞ *systemic antifungal* [miconazole] 10 mg/mL

Monistat-Derm cream ℞ *topical antifungal* [miconazole nitrate] 2%

mono- & di-acetylated monoglycerides NF *plasticizer*

mono- & di-glycerides NF *emulsifying agent*

monoamine oxidase inhibitors (MAOIs) *a class of antidepressants that increase CNS monoamine neurotransmitters (epinephrine, norepinephrine, and serotonin)*

monobactams *a class of bactericidal antibiotics effective against gram-negative aerobic pathogens*

monobasic potassium phosphate [see: potassium phosphate, monobasic]

monobasic sodium phosphate [see: sodium phosphate, monobasic]

monobenzone USP, INN *depigmenting agent for vitiligo*

monobenzyl ether of hydroquinone [see: monobenzone]

monobromated camphor [see: camphor, monobromated]

monocalcium phosphate [see: calcium phosphate, dibasic]

Monocaps tablets OTC *vitamin/mineral/iron supplement* [multiple vitamins & minerals; ferrous fumerate; folic acid; biotin] ≛•14 mg•0.1 mg•15 μg ⑨ Monoclate; Monoket

Mono-Chlor liquid ℞ *cauterant; keratolytic* [monochloroacetic acid] 80%

monochloroacetic acid *strong keratolytic/cauterant*

monochlorothymol [see: chlorothymol]

monochlorphenamide [see: clofenamide]

Monocid powder for IV or IM injection ℞ *cephalosporin antibiotic* [cefonicid sodium] 1, 10 g ⑨ Monocete

Monoclate P powder for IV injection ℞ *antihemophilic to correct coagulation deficiency* [antihemophilic factor VIII:C] ⑨ Monocaps; Monoket

monoclonal antibody 17-1A *orphan status withdrawn 1997* [now: edrecolomab]

monoclonal antibody 5A8 to CD4 *investigational (orphan) for post-exposure prophylaxis to occupational HIV exposure*

monoclonal antibody 5c8, recombinant humanized *investigational (orphan) for systemic lupus erythematosus (SLE) and immune thrombocytopenic purpura*

monoclonal antibody 5G1.1, humanized *investigational (orphan) C5 complement inhibitor for dermatomyositis*

monoclonal antibody 5G1.1-SC *investigational (Phase I/II) C5 complement inhibitor for rheumatoid arthritis; investigational (Phase II) for cardiopulmonary bypass during coronary artery bypass graft surgery*

monoclonal antibody 7E3 [see: abciximab]

monoclonal antibody anti-idiotype melanoma assorted antigen, murine *orphan status withdrawn 1997*

monoclonal antibody B43.13 *investigational (orphan) for epithelial ovarian cancer*

monoclonal antibody to CD147, murine *investigational (Phase III, orphan) monoclonal antibody for steroid-resistant graft vs. host disease that reverses unwanted immune response without general immune system suppression* [also: ABX-CBL]

monoclonal antibody to CD22 antigen on B-cells, radiolabeled *investigational (Phase I/II, orphan) for AIDS-related non-Hodgkin lymphoma* [also: monoclonal antibody LL2, humanized]

monoclonal antibody to CEA, humanized *investigational (orphan) antineoplastic for pancreatic and small cell lung cancer*

monoclonal antibody to cytomegalovirus, human *investigational (orphan) prophylaxis for CMV retinitis and CMV disease in solid organ transplants*

monoclonal antibody E5 [now: edobacomab]

monoclonal antibody to hepatitis B virus, human *investigational (orphan) hepatitis B prophylaxis for liver transplant*

monoclonal antibody LL2, humanized *investigational (Phase I/II) for AIDS-related non-Hodgkin lymphoma* [also: monoclonal antibody to CD22 antigen on B-cells, radiolabeled]

monoclonal antibody to lupus nephritis *investigational (orphan) for immunization against lupus nephritis*

monoclonal antibody PM-81 *investigational (orphan) for acute myelogenous leukemia*

monoclonal antibody PM-81 & AML-2-23 *investigational (orphan) for bone marrow transplant for acute myelogenous leukemia*

monoclonal antiendotoxin antibody XMMEN-OE5 *orphan status withdrawn 1994; clinical trials discontinued 1997* [now: edobacomab]

monoclonal factor IX [see: factor IX complex]

Monocor (CAN) film-coated tablets ℞ *antihypertensive; antiadrenergic (β-blocker)* [bisoprolol fumarate] 5, 10 mg

monoctanoin USAN, BAN *anticholelithogenic for dissolution of cholesterol gallstones (orphan)*

monoctanoin component A

monoctanoin component B

monoctanoin component C

monoctanoin component D

Mono-Diff reagent kit for professional use *in vitro diagnostic aid for mononucleosis*

Monodox capsules ℞ *antibiotic* [doxycycline] 50, 100 mg

Mono-Drop (trademarked delivery system) *prefilled eye drop dispenser*

monoethanolamine NF *surfactant*

monoethanolamine oleate INN *sclerosing agent* [also: ethanolamine oleate]

Mono-Gesic film-coated tablets ℞ *analgesic; antipyretic; anti-inflammatory; antirheumatic* [salsalate] 750 mg

Monoket tablets ℞ *antianginal; vasodilator* [isosorbide mononitrate] 10, 20 mg ⓢ Monocete

Mono-Latex reagent kit for professional use *in vitro diagnostic aid for mononucleosis*

monolaurin *investigational (Phase III, orphan) for nonbullous congenital ichthyosiform erythroderma*

monometacrine INN

Mononine powder for IV infusion ℞ *antihemophilic for factor IX deficiency (hemophilia B; Christmas disease) (orphan)* [coagulation factor IX complex] 100 IU/mL

monooctanoin [see: monoctanoin]

monophenylbutazone [see: mofebutazone]

monophosphothiamine INN

Mono-Plus reagent kit for professional use *in vitro diagnostic aid for mononucleosis*

monopotassium 4-aminosalicylate [see: aminosalicylate potassium]

monopotassium carbonate [see: potassium bicarbonate]

monopotassium D-gluconate [see: potassium gluconate]

monopotassium monosodium tartrate tetrahydrate [see: potassium sodium tartrate]

monopotassium phosphate [see: potassium phosphate, monobasic]

Monopril tablets ℞ *antihypertensive; angiotensin-converting enzyme (ACE) inhibitor* [fosinopril sodium] 10, 20, 40 mg

Monopril-HCT tablets ℞ *antihypertensive; angiotensin-converting enzyme (ACE) inhibitor; diuretic* [fosinopril sodium; hydrochlorothiazide] 10•12.5, 20•12.5 mg

monosodium *p*-aminohippurate [see: aminohippurate sodium]

monosodium 4-aminosalicylate dihydrate [see: aminosalicylate sodium]

monosodium carbonate [see: sodium bicarbonate]

monosodium D-gluconate [see: sodium gluconate]

monosodium D-thyroxine hydrate [see: dextrothyroxine sodium]

monosodium glutamate NF *flavoring agent; perfume*

monosodium L-ascorbate [see: sodium ascorbate]

monosodium L-thyroxine hydrate [see: levothyroxine sodium]

monosodium phosphate dihydrate [see: sodium phosphate, monobasic]

monosodium phosphate monohydrate [see: sodium phosphate, monobasic]

monosodium salicylate [see: sodium salicylate]

monosodium sulfite [see: sodium bisulfite]

Monospot slide test for professional use *in vitro diagnostic aid for mononucleosis*

monostearin [see: glyceryl monostearate]

Monosticon Dri-Dot slide test for professional use *in vitro diagnostic aid for mononucleosis*

monosulfiram BAN [also: sulfiram]

Mono-Sure slide test for professional use *in vitro diagnostic aid for mononucleosis*

Mono-Test slide test for professional use *in vitro diagnostic aid for mononucleosis*

monothioglycerol NF *preservative*

Monotropa uniflora *medicinal herb* [see: fit root]

Mono-Vacc Test (O.T.) single-use intradermal puncture test device *tuberculosis skin test* [old tuberculin] 5 U

monoxerutin INN

montelukast sodium USAN *antiasthmatic; leukotriene receptor inhibitor*

monteplase INN

montirelin INN

montmorillonite (redmond clay) *natural remedy for bug bites and stings and other skin problems*

Monuril (foreign name for U.S. product Monurol)

Monurol granules for oral solution ℞ *broad-spectrum bactericidal antibiotic for urinary tract infections* [fosfomycin tromethamine] 3 g per packet

moose elm *medicinal herb* [see: slippery elm]

8-MOP capsules ℞ *systemic psoralens for repigmentation of idiopathic vitiligo;*

used to increase tolerance to sunlight and enhance pigmentation [methoxsalen] 10 mg

MOP (mechlorethamine, Oncovin, prednisone) *chemotherapy protocol*

MOP (mechlorethamine, Oncovin, procarbazine) *chemotherapy protocol for pediatric brain tumors*

8-MOP (8-methoxypsoralen) [see: methoxsalen]

MOP-BAP (mechlorethamine, Oncovin, procarbazine, bleomycin, Adriamycin, prednisone) *chemotherapy protocol*

moperone INN

mopidamol INN

mopidralazine INN

MOPP (mechlorethamine, Oncovin, procarbazine, prednisone) *chemotherapy protocol for Hodgkin lymphoma*

MOPP (mustine HCl, Oncovin, procarbazine, prednisone) *chemotherapy protocol*

MOPP/ABV (mechlorethamine, Oncovin, procarbazine, prednisone, Adriamycin, bleomycin, vinblastine) *chemotherapy protocol for Hodgkin lymphoma*

MOPP/ABVD (alternating cycles of MOPP and ABVD) *chemotherapy protocol for Hodgkin lymphoma*

MOPP-BLEO; MOPP-Bleo (mechlorethamine, Oncovin, procarbazine, prednisone, bleomycin) *chemotherapy protocol*

MOPPHDB (mechlorethamine, Oncovin, procarbazine, prednisone, high-dose bleomycin) *chemotherapy protocol*

MOPPLDB (mechlorethamine, Oncovin, procarbazine, prednisone, low-dose bleomycin) *chemotherapy protocol*

MOPr (mechlorethamine, Oncovin, procarbazine) *chemotherapy protocol*

moprolol INN

moquizone INN

moracizine INN, BAN *antiarrhythmic* [also: moricizine]

morantel INN *anthelmintic* [also: morantel tartrate]

morantel tartrate USAN *anthelmintic* [also: morantel]

Moranyl (available only from the Centers for Disease Control) ℞ *antiparasitic for African trypanosomiasis and onchocerciasis* [suramin sodium]

morazone INN, BAN

morclofone INN

More-Dophilus powder OTC *dietary supplement; fever blister treatment; not generally regarded as safe and effective as an antidiarrheal* [*Lactobacillus acidophilus*] 4 billion U/g

morforex INN

moricizine USAN *antiarrhythmic* [also: moracizine]

moricizine HCl *antiarrhythmic*

morinamide INN

Morinda citrifolia *medicinal herb* [see: noni]

Mormon tea *medicinal herb* [see: ephedra]

morniflumate USAN, INN *anti-inflammatory*

morning glory (*Ipomoea violacea*) *seeds contain lysergic acid amide, chemically similar to LSD, which produce hallucinations when ingested as a street drug* [see also: LSD]

morocromen INN

moroxydine INN, BAN

morphazinamide [see: morinamide]

Morphelan extended-release capsules ℞ *investigational (NDA filed) rapid-onset narcotic analgesic for treatment of pain in oncology and HIV-infected patients* [morphine]

morpheridine INN, BAN

MorphiDex ℞ *investigational (NDA filed) opioid analgesic for the relief of moderate to severe cancer pain* [morphine sulfate; dextromethorphan]

morphine BAN *narcotic analgesic; widely abused as a street drug, which leads to dependence* [also: morphine sulfate]

morphine dinicotinate ester [see: nicomorphine]

morphine HCl USP *narcotic analgesic preferred in Germany and England; widely abused as a street drug, which leads to dependence*

morphine sulfate (MS) USP *narcotic analgesic preferred in the U.S.; intraspinal microinfusion for intractable chronic pain (orphan); widely abused as a street drug, which leads to dependence* [also: morphine] 10, 15, 30, 60 mg oral; 10, 20 mg/5 mL oral; 0.5, 1, 2, 4, 5, 10, 15, 25, 50 mg/mL injection; 5, 10, 20, 30 mg rectal

4-morpholinecarboximidoylguanidine [see: moroxydine]

2-morpholinoethylrutin [see: ethoxazorutoside]

3-morpholinosydnoneimine [see: linsidomine]

morpholinyl succinimide [see: morsuximide]

morpholinylethyl morphine [see: pholcodine]

morrhuate sodium USP *sclerosing agent* [also: sodium morrhuate] 50 mg/mL injection

morsuximide INN

morsydomine [see: molsidomine]

mortification root *medicinal herb* [see: marsh mallow]

Morton Salt Substitute; Morton Seasoned Salt Substitute OTC *salt substitute* [potassium chloride] 64 mEq/5 g; 56 mEq/5 g

Morus nigra; M. rubra *medicinal herb* [see: mulberry]

Moschus moschiferus *natural remedy* [see: deer musk]

Mosco liquid OTC *topical keratolytic* [salicylic acid in flexible collodion] 17.6%

mosquito plant *medicinal herb* [see: pennyroyal]

motapizone INN

MOTC (methyleneoxytetracycline) [see: methacycline]

motexafin gadolinium USAN *investigational (Phase III) radiosensitizer for brain metastases*

motexafin lutetium USAN *investigational photo-antineoplastic for recurrent breast cancer; investigational photoangioplastic for atherosclerosis; investigational (Phase I/II) photosensitizer for ophthalmic therapy and imaging*

mother of thyme *medicinal herb* [see: thyme]

motherwort (*Leonurus cardiaca*) flowering tops and leaves *medicinal herb used as an antispasmodic, astringent, calmative, cardiac, emmenagogue, hepatic, laxative, nervine, and stomachic*

Motilium (CAN) film-coated tablets ℞ *antiemetic for diabetic gastroparesis and chronic gastritis* [domperidone maleate] 10 mg

Motofen tablets ℞ *antidiarrheal* [difenoxin HCl; atropine sulfate] 1•0.025 mg

motrazepam INN

motretinide USAN, INN *keratolytic*

Motrin chewable tablets, oral suspension (name changed to Children's Motrin in 1999)

Motrin tablets ℞ *analgesic; antiarthritic; antipyretic; nonsteroidal anti-inflammatory drug (NSAID)* [ibuprofen] 400, 600, 800 mg

Motrin, Children's chewable tablets, oral suspension OTC *analgesic; antiarthritic; antipyretic; nonsteroidal anti-inflammatory drug (NSAID)* [ibuprofen] 50 mg; 100 mg/5 mL

Motrin, Children's drops (name changed to Infants' Motrin in 1999)

Motrin, Infants' oral drops OTC *analgesic; antipyretic; nonsteroidal anti-inflammatory drug (NSAID)* [ibuprofen] 40 mg/mL

Motrin, Junior Strength tablets, chewable tablets OTC *analgesic; antiarthritic; antipyretic; nonsteroidal anti-inflammatory drug (NSAID)* [ibuprofen] 100 mg

Motrin Cold, Children's oral suspension OTC *decongestant; analgesic; antipyretic* [pseudoephedrine HCl; ibuprofen] 15•100 mg/5 mL

Motrin IB tablets, gelcaps OTC *analgesic, antiarthritic; antipyretic; nonste-*

roidal anti-inflammatory drug (NSAID) [ibuprofen] 200 mg

Motrin IB Sinus caplets OTC *decongestant; analgesic* [pseudoephedrine HCl; ibuprofen] 30•200 mg

Motrin Migraine Pain caplets OTC *analgesic; nonsteroidal anti-inflammatory drug (NSAID)* [ibuprofen] 200 mg

mountain ash *(Sorbus americana; S. aucuparia)* fruit *medicinal herb used as an aperient, astringent, and diuretic*

mountain balm *medicinal herb* [see: yerba santa]

mountain box; mountain cranberry *medicinal herb* [see: uva ursi]

mountain laurel *(Kalmia latifolia)* leaves *medicinal herb used as an astringent and sedative*

mountain mahogany *medicinal herb* [see: birch]

mountain mint *medicinal herb* [see: marjoram; Oswego tea]

mountain snuff; mountain tobacco *medicinal herb* [see: arnica]

mountain sorrel *medicinal herb* [see: wood sorrel]

mountain strawberry *medicinal herb* [see: strawberry]

mountain sumach *medicinal herb* [see: sumach]

mountain sweet *medicinal herb* [see: New Jersey tea]

mountain tea *medicinal herb* [see: wintergreen]

mouse ear *(Hieracium pilosella)* plant *medicinal herb used as an astringent, cholagogue, and diuretic*

MouthKote oral spray OTC *saliva substitute*

MouthKote F/R oral rinse (discontinued 1997) OTC *topical dental caries preventative* [sodium fluoride] 0.04%

MouthKote O/R mouthwash OTC *anesthetic and antimicrobial throat irrigation* [benzyl alcohol; menthol]

MouthKote O/R oral solution OTC *topical antihistamine* [diphenhydramine] 1.25%

MouthKote P/R oral solution, ointment OTC *topical antihistamine* [diphenhydramine HCl] 1.25%; 25%

mouthroot *medicinal herb* [see: gold thread]

moveltipril INN

moxadolen INN

moxalactam disodium USAN, USP *bactericidal antibiotic* [also: latamoxef]

moxantrazole [now: teloxantrone HCl]

moxaprindine INN

moxastine INN

moxaverine INN, BAN

moxazocine USAN, INN *analgesic; antitussive*

moxestrol INN

moxicoumone INN

moxidectin USAN, INN *veterinary antiparasitic*

moxifloxacin HCl USAN *broad-spectrum fluoroquinolone antibiotic*

moxilubant maleate USAN *leukotriene* B_4 *receptor antagonist for rheumatoid arthritis and psoriasis*

moxipraquine INN, BAN

moxiraprine INN

moxisylyte INN [also: thymoxamine]

moxnidazole USAN, INN *antiprotozoal (Trichomonas)*

moxonidine USAN, INN *centrally acting sympatholytic for hypertension, congestive heart failure, and type 2 diabetes*

M-oxy tablets ℞ *narcotic analgesic* [oxycodone HCl] 5 mg

MP (melphalan, prednisone) *chemotherapy protocol for multiple myeloma*

MP (mitoxantrone, prednisone) *chemotherapy protocol for prostate cancer*

MP-351 *investigational 2-5A antisense drug for A and B strains of respiratory syncytial virus*

4-MP (4-methylpyrazole) [see: fomepizole]

6-MP (6-mercaptopurine) [see: mercaptopurine]

MPA (medroxyprogesterone acetate) [q.v.]

MPF [see: Mucoprotective Factor]

m-PFL (methotrexate, Platinol, fluorouracil, leucovorin [rescue]) *chemotherapy protocol*

MPH (methylphenidate HCl) [q.v.]

MPIF-1 (myeloid progenitor inhibitory factor 1) [see: mirostipen]

MPL (melphalan) [q.v.]

MPL + PRED (melphalan, prednisone) *chemotherapy protocol*

M-Prednisol-40; M-Prednisol-80 intralesional, soft tissue, and IM injection ℞ *corticosteroid; anti-inflammatory; immunosuppressant* [methylprednisolone acetate] 40 mg/mL; 80 mg/mL

MPTS (minocycline periodontal therapeutic system) ℞ *investigational (NDA filed) system used in conjunction with scaling and root planing for periodontitis* [minocycline]

MRV subcu injection (discontinued 2000) ℞ *active respiratory bacteria immunizing agent* [mixed respiratory vaccine]

MRV (mixed respiratory vaccine) [q.v.]

M-R-Vax II powder for subcu injection ℞ *measles and rubella vaccine* [measles and rubella virus vaccine, live] 0.5 mL

MS (magnesium salicylate) [q.v.]

MS (morphine sulfate) [q.v.]

MS Contin controlled-release tablets ℞ *narcotic analgesic; preoperative sedative and anxiolytic* [morphine sulfate] 15, 30, 60, 100, 200 mg

MS-325 *investigational (Phase II) injectable MRI contrast medium for multiple cardiovascular indications*

MSD Enteric-Coated ASA (CAN) tablets OTC *analgesic; antipyretic; anti-inflammatory; antirheumatic* [aspirin] 325, 650 mg

MSI (Metered Solution Inhaler) [q.v.]

MSIR tablets, capsules, oral solution, oral concentrate ℞ *narcotic analgesic; preoperative sedative and anxiolytic* [morphine sulfate] 15, 30 mg; 15, 30 mg; 10, 20 mg/5 mL; 20 mg/mL

MS/L; MS/L Concentrate oral liquid (discontinued 1999) ℞ *narcotic analgesic; preoperative sedative and anxiolytic; also abused as a street drug* [morphine sulfate] 10 mg/5 mL; 100 mg/5 mL

MSM (methylsulfonylmethane) *natural source of sulfur; promotes an increase in collagen and the endogenous antioxidant glutathione*

MS/S suppositories (discontinued 1998) ℞ *narcotic analgesic; preoperative sedative and anxiolytic* [morphine sulfate] 5, 10, 20, 30 mg

MSTA (Mumps Skin Test Antigen) intradermal injection ℞ *diagnostic aid to assess immune system competency (not effective in testing immunity to mumps virus)* [mumps skin test antigen] 0.1 mL (4 U/0.1 mL)

MT6 (mercaptomerin) [q.v.]

MTC (mitomycin C) [see: mitomycin]

MTC-DOX (trademarked delivery system) *investigational (Phase I/II) magnetic targeted carrier for the treatment of primary liver cancer* [doxorubicin]

MTC-DOX (magnetically targeted carrier with doxorubicin) *investigational (orphan) delivery method for liver cancer chemotherapy*

M.T.E.-4; M.T.E.-5; M.T.E.-6; M.T.E.-7; M.T.E.-4 Concentrated; M.T.E.-5 Concentrated; M.T.E.-6 Concentrated IV injection ℞ *intravenous nutritional therapy* [multiple trace elements (metals)]

mTHPC [see: temoporfin]

MTX (methotrexate) [q.v.]

MTX + MP + CTX (methotrexate, mercaptopurine, cyclophosphamide) *chemotherapy protocol*

MTX/6-MP (methotrexate, mercaptopurine) *chemotherapy protocol for acute lymphocytic leukemia (ALL); a daily and weekly dosing protocol* [also: 1DMTX/6-MP (a 1-day dosing protocol)]

MTX/6-MP/VP (methotrexate, mercaptopurine, vincristine, prednisone) *chemotherapy protocol for acute lymphocytic leukemia (ALL)*

MTX-CDDPAdr (methotrexate [with leucovorin rescue], CDDP, Adriamycin) *chemotherapy protocol for pediatric osteosarcoma*

MUC-1 *investigational cancer vaccine*

Muco-Fen-DM timed-release tablets ℞ *antitussive; expectorant* [dextromethorphan hydrobromide; guaifenesin] 30•600 mg

Muco-Fen-LA timed-release tablets ℞ *expectorant* [guaifenesin] 600 mg

mucoid exopolysaccharide *Pseudomonas* hyperimmune globulin (MEPIG) *investigational (orphan) for pulmonary infections of cystic fibrosis*

mucolytics *a class of respiratory inhalant drugs that destroy or inhibit mucin*

Mucomyst solution for nebulization or intratracheal instillation ℞ *mucolytic; investigational (orphan) for severe acetaminophen overdose* [acetylcysteine sodium] 10%, 20%

Mucomyst 10 IV ℞ *mucolytic; investigational (orphan) for severe acetaminophen overdose* [acetylcysteine]

Mucoprotective Factor (MPF) (trademarked ingredient) *aromatic flavored syrup* [eriodictyon]

Mucosil-10; Mucosil-20 solution for nebulization or intratracheal instillation ℞ *mucolytic* [acetylcysteine sodium] 10%; 20%

Mudrane tablets ℞ *antiasthmatic; bronchodilator; decongestant; expectorant; sedative* [aminophylline; ephedrine HCl; potassium iodide; phenobarbital] 111•16•195•8 mg ⧉ Modane

Mudrane GG tablets ℞ *antiasthmatic; decongestant; expectorant; sedative* [theophylline; ephedrine HCl; guaifenesin; phenobarbital] 111•16•100•8 mg

Mudrane GG-2 tablets ℞ *antiasthmatic; bronchodilator; expectorant* [theophylline; guaifenesin] 111•100 mg

mugwort (*Artemisia vulgaris*) root and plant *medicinal herb used as a diaphoretic, emmenagogue, and laxative*

mulberry (*Morus nigra; M. rubra*) bark *medicinal herb used as an anthelmintic and cathartic*

mullein (*Verbascum nigrum; V. phlomoides; V. thapsiforme; V. thapsus*) plant *medicinal herb for asthma, bleeding in bowel and lungs, bronchitis, bruises, cough, croup, diarrhea, earache, gout, hemorrhoids, insomnia, lymphatic system, nervousness, pain, pleurisy, sinus congestion, and tuberculosis*

MulTE-Pak-4; MulTE-Pak-5 IV injection ℞ *intravenous nutritional therapy* [multiple trace elements (metals)] ≛

Multi 75 timed-release tablets OTC *vitamin/mineral supplement* [multiple vitamins & minerals; folic acid; biotin] ≛•0.4•≟ mg

Multi Vit with Iron drops OTC *vitamin/iron supplement* [multiple vitamins; iron] ≛•10 mg/mL

Multi Vitamin Concentrate injection ℞ *parenteral vitamin supplement* [multiple vitamins] ≛

Multi-12; Multi-12 Pediatric (CAN) IV infusion ℞ *vitamin supplement* [multiple vitamins]

Multi-Day tablets OTC *vitamin supplement* [multiple vitamins; folic acid] ≛•0.4 mg

Multi-Day Plus Iron tablets OTC *vitamin/iron supplement* [multiple vitamins; iron; folic acid] ≛•18•0.4 mg

Multi-Day Plus Minerals tablets OTC *vitamin/mineral/iron supplement* [multiple vitamins & minerals; iron; folic acid; biotin] ≛•18 mg•0.4 mg•30 µg

Multi-Day with Calcium and Extra Iron tablets OTC *vitamin/calcium/iron supplement* [multiple vitamins; calcium; iron; folic acid] ≛•≟•27•0.4 mg

MultiKine injection ℞ *investigational (Phase III) antineoplastic for prostate cancer; investigational (Phase I) immunotherapeutic agent for HIV infection; investigational for cancer of the oral cavity* [multiple leukocytes and interleukins]

Multilex; Multilex-T & M tablets OTC *vitamin/mineral/iron supplement* [multiple vitamins & minerals; iron] ≛•15 mg

Multilyte-20; Multilyte-40 IV admixture ℞ *intravenous electrolyte therapy* [combined electrolyte solution]

Multi-Mineral tablets OTC *mineral supplement* [multiple minerals]

Multiple Trace Element; Multiple Trace Element Concentrated; Multiple Trace Element Neonatal; Multiple Trace Element Pediatric IV injection ℞ *intravenous nutritional therapy* [multiple trace elements (metals)]

Multiple Trace Element with Selenium; Multiple Trace Element with Selenium Concentrated IV injection ℞ *intravenous nutritional therapy* [multiple trace elements (metals)]

Multistix; Multistix 2; Multistix 7; Multistix 8 SG; Multistix 9; Multistix 9 SG; Multistix 10 SG; Multistix SG reagent strips *in vitro diagnostic aid for multiple urine products*

Multitest CMI single-use intradermal skin test device *skin test for multiple allergen sensitivity* [skin test antigens (seven different); glycerin (one for test control)]

Multitrace-5 Concentrate IV injection ℞ *intravenous nutritional therapy* [multiple trace elements (metals)] ≛

multivitamin infusion, neonatal formula *investigational (orphan) total parenteral nutrition for very low birthweight infants*

Multi-Vitamin Mineral with Beta-Carotene tablets OTC *vitamin/mineral/iron supplement* [multiple vitamins & minerals; ferrous fumarate; folic acid; biotin] ≛•27•0.4•0.45 mg

Multivitamin with Fluoride drops ℞ *pediatric vitamin supplement and dental caries preventative* [multiple vitamins; fluoride] ≛•0.25, ≛•0.5 mg/mL

Multivitamins capsules OTC *vitamin supplement* [multiple vitamins] ≛

Mulvidren-F Softabs (chewable tablets) ℞ *pediatric vitamin supplement and dental caries preventative* [multiple vitamins; fluoride] ≛•1 mg

mumps skin test antigen (MSTA) USP *diagnostic aid to assess immune system competency*

mumps vaccine [see: mumps virus vaccine, inactivated]

mumps virus vaccine, inactivated NF

mumps virus vaccine, live USP *active immunizing agent for mumps*

Mumpsvax powder for subcu injection ℞ *mumps vaccine* [mumps virus vaccine, live] 0.5 mL

mupirocin USAN, INN, BAN *topical antibacterial antibiotic*

mupirocin calcium USAN *topical antibacterial antibiotic*

muplestim USAN *progenitor cell stimulator for neutropenia and thrombocytopenia*

murabutide INN

Murine eye drops OTC *ophthalmic moisturizer/lubricant* [polyvinyl alcohol] 0.5%

Murine Ear Drops OTC *agent to emulsify and disperse ear wax* [carbamide peroxide; alcohol] 6.5%•6.3%

murine MAb [see: muromonab-CD3]

Murine Plus eye drops OTC *topical ophthalmic decongestant and vasoconstrictor* [tetrahydrozoline HCl] 0.05%

Muro 128 eye drops, ophthalmic ointment OTC *corneal edema-reducing agent* [sodium chloride (hypertonic saline solution)] 2%, 5%; 5%

murocainide INN

Murocel eye drops OTC *ophthalmic moisturizer/lubricant* [methylcellulose] 1%

Murocoll-2 eye drops ℞ *cycloplegic; mydriatic* [scopolamine hydrobromide; phenylephrine HCl] 0.3%•10%

murodermin INN

muromonab-CD3 USAN, INN *monoclonal antibody immunosuppressive for renal, hepatic, and cardiac transplants*

Muroptic-5 eye drops OTC *corneal edema-reducing agent* [sodium chloride (hypertonic saline solution)] 5%

muscarinic agonists *a class of investigational analgesics*

MuscleRub ointment (discontinued 2000) OTC *topical analgesic; counterirritant* [methyl salicylate; menthol] 15%•10%

Muse single-use intraurethral suppository ℞ *vasodilator for erectile dysfunction* [alprostadil] 125, 150, 500, 1000 µg

musk *natural remedy* [see: deer musk]

mustaral oil [see: allyl isothiocyanate]

mustard *(Brassica alba; Sinapis alba)* seeds and oil *medicinal herb for indigestion and liver and lung disorders; also used as an appetizer, diuretic, emetic, and soak for aching feet, arthritis, and rheumatism*

mustard oil [see: allyl isothiocyanate]

Mustargen powder for IV or intracavitary injection ℞ *nitrogen mustard-type alkylating antineoplastic for multiple myelomas, lymphomas and leukemias, and breast, lung, and ovarian cancers* [mechlorethamine HCl] 10 mg

Musterole Deep Strength Rub OTC *topical analgesic; counterirritant* [methyl salicylate; methyl nicotinate; menthol] 30%•0.5%•3%

Musterole Extra Strength OTC *topical analgesic; counterirritant* [camphor; menthol] 5%•3%

mustine BAN *nitrogen mustard-type alkylating antineoplastic* [also: mechlorethamine HCl; chlormethine; nitrogen mustard *N*-oxide HCl]

mustine HCl [see: mechlorethamine HCl]

Mutamycin powder for IV injection ℞ *antibiotic antineoplastic for stomach, pancreatic, breast, colon, head, neck, and lung cancers* [mitomycin] 5, 20, 40 mg ⑨ mitomycin

muzolimine USAN, INN *diuretic; antihypertensive*

MV (mitomycin, vinblastine) *chemotherapy protocol for breast cancer*

MV (mitoxantrone, VePesid) *chemotherapy protocol for acute myelocytic leukemia (ALL)*

MVAC; M-VAC (methotrexate, vinblastine, Adriamycin, cisplatin) *chemotherapy protocol for bladder cancer*

M-Vax ℞ *investigational (Phase III, orphan) theraccine for postsurgical stage III malignant melanoma*

MVF (mitoxantrone, vincristine, fluorouracil) *chemotherapy protocol*

M.V.I. Neonatal IV infusion ℞ *investigational (orphan) total parenteral nutrition for very low birthweight infants* [multiple vitamins]

M.V.I. Pediatric injection ℞ *parenteral vitamin supplement* [multiple vitamins; folic acid; biotin] ≛•140•20 µg/5 mL

M.V.I.-12 injection ℞ *parenteral vitamin supplement* [multiple vitamins; folic acid; biotin] ≛•400•60 µg/5 mL

M.V.M. capsules OTC *vitamin/mineral/iron supplement* [multiple vitamins & minerals; iron; folic acid; biotin] ≛•3.6 mg•0.08 mg•160 µg

MVP (mitomycin, vinblastine, Platinol) *chemotherapy protocol for non–small cell lung cancer (NSCLC)*

MVPP (mechlorethamine, vinblastine, procarbazine, prednisone) *chemotherapy protocol for Hodgkin lymphoma*

MVT (mitoxantrone, VePesid, thiotepa) *chemotherapy protocol*

MVVPP (mechlorethamine, vincristine, vinblastine, procarbazine, prednisone) *chemotherapy protocol*

MX-6 *investigational (Phase III) treatment for cervical intraepithelial neoplasia (CIN)*

Myadec tablets OTC *vitamin/mineral/iron supplement* [multiple vitamins & minerals; iron; folic acid; biotin] ≛•18 mg•0.4 mg•30 µg

Myambutol film-coated tablets ℞ *tuberculostatic* [ethambutol HCl] 100, 400 mg ⑨ Nembutal

Myapap drops (discontinued 1997) ℞ *analgesic; antipyretic* [acetaminophen] 100 mg/mL

Mycelex cream, solution (discontinued 2000) ℞ *topical antifungal* [clotrimazole] 1%

Mycelex troches ℞ *antifungal; oral candidiasis prophylaxis or treatment* [clotrimazole] 10 mg

Mycelex OTC cream, solution (discontinued 2000) OTC *topical antifungal* [clotrimazole] 1%

Mycelex Twin Pack vaginal inserts + cream (discontinued 2001) ℞ *antifungal* [clotrimazole] 500 mg; 1%

Mycelex-3 vaginal cream in prefilled applicator OTC *antifungal* [butoconazole nitrate] 2%

Mycelex-7 vaginal cream, combination pack (vaginal inserts + cream) OTC *antifungal* [clotrimazole] 1%; 100 mg + 1%

Mycelex-7 vaginal inserts (discontinued 2001) OTC *antifungal* [clotrimazole] 100 mg

Mycelex-G vaginal inserts (discontinued 2001) ℞ *antifungal* [clotrimazole] 500 mg

Mycifradin Sulfate oral solution ℞ *aminoglycoside antibiotic* [neomycin sulfate] 125 mg/5 mL

Myciguent ointment, cream OTC *topical antibiotic* [neomycin sulfate] 3.5 mg/g

Mycinette throat spray OTC *topical anesthetic; oral antiseptic; astringent* [phenol; alum] 1.4%•0.3%

Mycinettes lozenges OTC *topical oral anesthetic* [benzocaine] 15 mg

Myci-Spray nasal spray OTC *nasal decongestant; antihistamine* [phenylephrine HCl; pyrilamine maleate] 0.25%•0.15%

Mycitracin Plus ointment OTC *topical antibiotic; local anesthetic* [polymyxin B sulfate; neomycin sulfate; bacitracin; lidocaine] 5000 U•3.5 mg•500 U•40 mg per g

Mycitracin Triple Antibiotic ointment OTC *topical antibiotic* [polymyxin B sulfate; neomycin sulfate; bacitracin] 5000 U•3.5 mg•500 U per g

***Mycobacterium avium* sensitin RS-10** *investigational (orphan) diagnostic aid for Mycobacterium avium infection in immunocompromised patients*

Myco-Biotic II cream ℞ *topical corticosteroidal anti-inflammatory; antifungal* [triamcinolone acetonide; neomycin sulfate; nystatin] 0.1%•0.5%•100 000 U per g

Mycobutin capsules ℞ *antiviral/antibacterial for prevention of Mycobacterium avium complex (MAC) in advanced HIV patients (orphan)* [rifabutin] 150 mg

Mycocide NS solution OTC *topical antiseptic* [benzalkonium chloride]

Mycogen II cream, ointment ℞ *topical corticosteroidal anti-inflammatory; antifungal* [triamcinolone acetonide; nystatin] 0.1%•100 000 U per g

Mycolog-II cream, ointment ℞ *topical corticosteroidal anti-inflammatory; antifungal* [triamcinolone acetonide; nystatin] 0.1%•100 000 U per g

Myconel cream ℞ *topical corticosteroidal anti-inflammatory; antifungal* [triamcinolone acetonide; nystatin] 0.1%•100 000 U per g

mycophenolate mofetil USAN *immunosuppressant for allogenic heart, liver, and kidney transplants; purine biosynthesis inhibitor*

mycophenolate mofetil HCl USAN *immunosuppressant for allogenic heart, liver, and kidney transplants; purine biosynthesis inhibitor*

mycophenolic acid USAN, INN *antineoplastic*

Mycostatin cream, ointment, powder ℞ *topical antifungal* [nystatin] 100 000 U/g

Mycostatin film-coated tablets ℞ *systemic antifungal* [nystatin] 500 000 U

Mycostatin oral suspension, Pastilles (troches) ℞ *antifungal; oral candidiasis treatment* [nystatin] 100 000 U/mL; 200 000 U

Mycostatin vaginal inserts (discontinued 2001) ℞ *topical antifungal* [nystatin] 100 000 U

Myco-Triacet II cream, ointment ℞ *topical corticosteroidal anti-inflamma-*

tory; antifungal [triamcinolone acetonide; nystatin] 0.1%•100 000 U per g

mydeton [see: tolperisone]

Mydfrin 2.5% eye drops ℞ *topical ophthalmic decongestant and vasoconstrictor; mydriatic* [phenylephrine HCl] 2.5% ⑨ Midrin; Myfedrine

Mydriacyl Drop-Tainers (eye drops) ℞ *cycloplegic; mydriatic* [tropicamide] 0.5%, 1%

mydriatics *a class of drugs that cause the pupil of the eye to dilate*

myelin *investigational (orphan) for multiple sclerosis*

myeloid progenitor inhibitory factor 1 (MPIF-1) [see: mirostipen]

myelosan [see: busulfan]

myfadol INN

Mygel; Mygel II oral suspension OTC *antacid; antiflatulent* [aluminum hydroxide; magnesium hydroxide; simethicone] 200•200•20 mg/5 mL; 400•400•40 mg/5 mL

Myidyl syrup (discontinued 1997) ℞ *antihistamine* [triprolidine HCl] 1.25 mg/5 mL

Mykrox tablets ℞ *antihypertensive; diuretic* [metolazone] 0.5 mg

Mylagen gelcaps OTC *antacid* [calcium carbonate; magnesium carbonate] 311•232 mg

Mylagen; Mylagen II liquid OTC *antacid; antiflatulent* [aluminum hydroxide; magnesium hydroxide; simethicone] 200•200•20 mg/5 mL; 400•400•40 mg/5 mL

Mylanta chewable tablets, oral liquid OTC *antacid; antiflatulent* [aluminum hydroxide; magnesium hydroxide; simethicone] 200•200•20, 400•400•40 mg; 200•200•20, 400•400•40 mg/5 mL ⑨ Dilantin; Milontin

Mylanta gelcaps OTC *antacid* [calcium carbonate; magnesium carbonate] 311•232 mg

Mylanta lozenges OTC *antacid* [calcium carbonate] 600 mg

Mylanta, Children's oral liquid, chewable tablets OTC *antacid* [calcium carbonate] 400 mg/5 mL; 400 mg

Mylanta AR ("acid reducer") tablets OTC *histamine H_2 antagonist for heartburn and acid indigestion* [famotidine] 10 mg

Mylanta Gas chewable tablets OTC *antiflatulent* [simethicone] 40, 80, 125 mg

Mylanta Natural Fiber Supplement powder (discontinued 1999) OTC *bulk laxative* [psyllium hydrophilic mucilloid] 3.4 g/tsp.

Mylanta Supreme oral liquid OTC *antacid* [calcium carbonate; magnesium hydroxide] 400•135 mg/5 mL

Myleran tablets ℞ *alkylating antineoplastic for chronic myelogenous leukemia (CML)* [busulfan] 2 mg ⑨ Mylicon

Mylicon drops OTC *antiflatulent* [simethicone] 40 mg/0.6 mL ⑨ Modicon; Myleran

Mylocel film-coated tablets ℞ *antineoplastic for melanoma, ovarian carcinoma, myelocytic leukemia, and squamous cell carcinoma* [hydroxyurea] 1 g

Myloral ℞ *investigational (Phase III) oral treatment for multiple sclerosis* [bovine myelin]

Mylotarg powder for IV injection ℞ *antibody-targeted chemotherapy for acute myeloid leukemia (AML)* [gemtuzumab ozogamicin] 5 mg/vial

Myminic Expectorant liquid OTC *decongestant; expectorant* [phenylpropanolamine HCl; guaifenesin; alcohol 5%] 12.5•100 mg/5 mL

Myminicol liquid OTC *antitussive; decongestant; antihistamine* [dextromethorphan hydrobromide; phenylpropanolamine HCl; chlorpheniramine maleate] 10•12.5•2 mg/5 mL

Mynatal capsules ℞ *vitamin/mineral/calcium/iron supplement* [multiple vitamins & minerals; calcium; iron; folic acid; biotin] ≛•300•65•1•0.03 mg

Mynatal FC caplets ℞ *vitamin/mineral/calcium/iron supplement* [multiple vitamins & minerals; calcium; iron; folic acid; biotin] ≛•250•60•1•0.03 mg

Mynatal P.N. captabs ℞ *vitamin/calcium/iron supplement* [multiple vitamins; calcium; iron; folic acid] ≛•125•60•1 mg

Mynatal P.N. Forte caplets ℞ *vitamin/mineral/calcium/iron supplement* [multiple vitamins & minerals; calcium; iron; folic acid] ≛•250•60•1 mg

Mynatal Rx caplets ℞ *vitamin/mineral/calcium/iron supplement* [multiple vitamins & minerals; calcium; iron; folic acid; biotin] ≛•200•60•1•0.03 mg

Mynate 90 Plus delayed-release caplets ℞ *vitamin/calcium/iron supplement* [multiple vitamins; calcium; iron; folic acid] ≛•250•90•1 mg

Myobloc injection ℞ *neurotoxin complex for symptomatic treatment of cervical dystonia (orphan)* [botulinum toxin, type B] 5000 U/mL

Myocide NS solution OTC *topical antiseptic* [benzalkonium chloride]

Myoflex Creme OTC *topical analgesic* [trolamine salicylate] 10%

Myolin IV or IM injection ℞ *skeletal muscle relaxant* [orphenadrine citrate] 30 mg/mL

Myoscint (commercially available in Europe) *investigational (orphan) imaging agent for cardiac necrosis and myocarditis* [imciromab pentetate]

Myotonachol tablets (discontinued 2001) ℞ *cholinergic urinary stimulant for postsurgical and postpartum urinary retention* [bethanechol chloride] 10, 25 mg

Myotrophin injection ℞ *investigational (NDA filed, orphan) for amyotrophic lateral sclerosis, type 1 and type 2 diabetes, growth hormone insufficiency, and post-poliomyelitis syndrome* [mecasermin]

Myoview ℞ *cardiovascular imaging aid* [technetium Tc 99m tetrofosmin]

Myphetane DC Cough syrup ℞ *narcotic antitussive; decongestant; antihistamine* [codeine phosphate; phenylpropanolamine HCl; brompheniramine maleate; alcohol 1.2%] 10•12.5•2 mg/5 mL

Myphetane DX Cough syrup ℞ *antitussive; decongestant; antihistamine* [dextromethorphan hydrobromide; pseudoephedrine HCl; brompheniramine maleate; alcohol 1%] 10•30•2 mg/5 mL

myralact INN, BAN

Myrica cerifera *medicinal herb* [see: bayberry]

myricodine [see: myrophine]

Myristica fragrans *medicinal herb* [see: nutmeg; mace]

myristica oil [see: nutmeg oil]

myristyl alcohol NF *stiffening agent*

myristyltrimethylammonium bromide *antiseborrheic*

myrophine INN, BAN

Myroxylon balsamum; M. pereirae *medicinal herb* [see: Peruvian balsam]

myrrh *(Commiphora abssynica; C. molmol; C. myrrha)* seeds *medicinal herb for bad breath, bronchitis, cancer, constipation, hay fever, hemorrhoids, leprosy, lung diseases, mouth and skin sores, sore throat, syphilis, and stimulating menses; also used as an antiseptic and astringent*

myrtecaine INN

Myrtilli fructus *medicinal herb* [see: bilberry]

myrtle *medicinal herb* [see: periwinkle]

myrtle, bog *medicinal herb* [see: buckbean]

myrtle, wax *medicinal herb* [see: bayberry]

myrtle flag; grass myrtle; sweet myrtle *medicinal herb* [see: calamus]

Mysoline tablets, oral suspension ℞ *anticonvulsant for grand mal, psychomotor, or focal epileptic seizures* [primidone] 50, 250 mg; 250 mg/5 mL

myspamol [see: proquamezine]

Mytelase caplets ℞ *anticholinesterase muscle stimulant; myasthenia gravis treatment* [ambenonium chloride] 10 mg

Mytrex cream, ointment ℞ *topical corticosteroidal anti-inflammatory; antifungal* [triamcinolone acetonide; nystatin] 0.1%•100 000 U/g

Mytussin syrup OTC *expectorant* [guaifenesin; alcohol 3.5%] 100 mg/5 mL

Mytussin AC Cough syrup ℞ *narcotic antitussive; expectorant* [codeine phosphate; guaifenesin; alcohol 3.5%] 10•100 mg/5 mL

Mytussin DAC syrup ℞ *narcotic antitussive; decongestant; expectorant* [codeine phosphate; pseudoephedrine HCl; guaifenesin; alcohol 1.7%] 10•30•100 mg/5 mL

Mytussin DM liquid OTC *antitussive; expectorant* [dextromethorphan hydrobromide; guaifenesin; alcohol 1.6%] 10•100 mg/5 mL

myuizone [see: thioacetazone; thiacetazone]

My-Vitalife capsules OTC *vitamin/mineral/calcium/iron supplement* [multiple vitamins & minerals; calcium; iron; folic acid; biotin] ≛•130•27•0.4•0.03 mg

MZM tablets ℞ *carbonic anhydrase inhibitor for glaucoma* [methazolamide] 25, 50 mg

MZM (methazolamide) [q.v.]

M-Zole 3 Combination Pack vaginal inserts + cream OTC *antifungal* [miconazole nitrate] 200 mg + 2%

M-Zole 7 Dual Pack vaginal inserts + cream OTC *antifungal* [miconazole nitrate] 100 mg + 2%

N-0923 *investigational (Phase II) dopamine agonist in a transdermal patch for Parkinson disease*

N_2 (nitrogen) [q.v.]

N-3 polyunsaturated fatty acids [see: doconexent; icosapent; omega-3 marine triglycerides]

^{22}Na [see: sodium chloride Na 22]

nabazenil USAN, INN *anticonvulsant*

Nabi-HB IM injection ℞ *hepatitis B immunizing agent* [hepatitis B immune globulin, solvent/detergent treated] 1, 5 mL

nabilone USAN, INN, BAN *minor tranquilizer*

nabitan INN *analgesic* [also: nabitan HCl]

nabitan HCl USAN *analgesic* [also: nabitan]

naboctate INN *antiglaucoma agent; antinauseant* [also: naboctate HCl]

naboctate HCl USAN *antiglaucoma agent; antinauseant* [also: naboctate]

nabumetone USAN, INN, BAN *antiarthritic; nonsteroidal anti-inflammatory drug (NSAID)*

nabutan HCl [now: nabitan HCl]

NAC (N-acetyl cysteine) *natural source of cysteine; promotes an increase in the endogenous antioxidant glutathione*

NAC (nitrogen mustard, Adriamycin, CCNU) *chemotherapy protocol*

nacartocin INN

NaCl (sodium chloride) [q.v.]

NAD (nicotinamide-adenine dinucleotide) [see: nadide]

nadide USAN, INN *antagonist to alcohol and narcotics*

nadisan [see: carbutamide]

nadolol USAN, USP, INN, BAN *antianginal; antihypertensive; antiadrenergic (β-blocker)* 20, 40, 80, 120, 160 mg oral ⑨ Nandol

nadoxolol INN

nadroparin calcium INN, BAN *anticoagulant; low molecular weight heparin*

naepaine HCl NF

nafamostat INN *anticoagulant; antifibrinolytic* [also: nafamostat mesylate; nafamostat mesilate]

nafamostat mesilate JAN *anticoagulant; antifibrinolytic* [also: nafamostat mesylate; nafamostat]

nafamostat mesylate USAN *anticoagulant; antifibrinolytic* [also: nafamostat; nafamostat mesilate]

nafarelin INN, BAN *luteinizing hormone–releasing hormone (LH-RH) agonist* [also: nafarelin acetate]

nafarelin acetate USAN *luteinizing hormone–releasing hormone (LH-RH) agonist for central precocious puberty (orphan) and endometriosis* [also: nafarelin]

Nafazair eye drops ℞ *topical ophthalmic decongestant and vasoconstrictor* [naphazoline HCl] 0.1%

nafazatrom INN, BAN

nafcaproic acid INN

Nafcil powder for IV or IM injection (discontinued 1998) ℞ *penicillinase-resistant penicillin antibiotic* [nafcillin sodium] 0.5, 1, 2, 10 g

nafcillin INN *penicillinase-resistant penicillin antibiotic* [also: nafcillin sodium]

nafcillin sodium USAN, USP *penicillinase-resistant penicillin antibiotic* [also: nafcillin]

nafenodone INN

nafenopin USAN, INN *antihyperlipoproteinemic*

nafetolol INN

nafimidone INN *anticonvulsant* [also: nafimidone HCl]

nafimidone HCl USAN *anticonvulsant* [also: nafimidone]

nafiverine INN

naflocort USAN, INN *topical adrenocortical steroid*

nafomine INN *muscle relaxant* [also: nafomine malate]

nafomine malate USAN *muscle relaxant* [also: nafomine]

nafoxadol INN

nafoxidine HCl USAN, INN *antiestrogen*

nafronyl oxalate USAN *vasodilator* [also: naftidrofuryl]

naftalofos USAN, INN *veterinary anthelmintic*

naftazone INN, BAN

naftidrofuryl INN *vasodilator* [also: nafronyl oxalate]

naftifine INN, BAN *broad-spectrum antifungal* [also: naftifine HCl]

naftifine HCl USAN *broad-spectrum antifungal* [also: naftifine]

Naftin cream, gel ℞ *topical antifungal* [naftifine HCl] 1%

naftopidil INN

naftoxate INN

naftypramide INN *antibacterial*

Naganol (available only from the Centers for Disease Control) ℞ *antiparasitic for African trypanosomiasis and onchocerciasis* [suramin sodium]

naganol [see: suramin sodium]

NaGHB (sodium gamma hydroxybutyrate) [see: gamma hydroxybutyrate (GHB); sodium oxybate]

nagrestipen USAN *stem cell inhibitory protein*

nalazosulfamide [see: salazosulfamide]

nalbuphine INN, BAN *narcotic agonist-antagonist analgesic; narcotic antagonist* [also: nalbuphine HCl]

nalbuphine HCl USAN *narcotic agonist-antagonist analgesic; narcotic antagonist* [also: nalbuphine] 10, 20 mg/mL injection

Naldecon sustained-release tablets, syrup, pediatric syrup, pediatric drops ℞ *decongestant; antihistamine* [phenylpropanolamine HCl; phenylephrine HCl; chlorpheniramine maleate; phenyltoloxamine citrate] 40•10•5•15 mg; 20•5•2.5•7.5 mg/5 mL; 5•1.25•0.5•2 mg/5 mL; 5•1.25•0.5•2 mg/mL ⦿ Nalfon

Naldecon CX Adult liquid ℞ *narcotic antitussive; decongestant; expectorant* [codeine phosphate; phenylpropanolamine HCl; guaifenesin] 10•12.5•200 mg/5 mL

Naldecon DX children's syrup, pediatric drops OTC *pediatric antitussive, decongestant, and expectorant* [dextromethorphan hydrobromide; phenylpropanolamine HCl; guaifenesin] 5•6.25•100 mg/5 mL; 5•6.25•50 mg/mL

Naldecon DX Adult liquid OTC *antitussive; decongestant; expectorant*

[dextromethorphan hydrobromide; phenylpropanolamine HCl; guaifenesin] 10•12.5•200 mg/5 mL

Naldecon EX children's syrup, pediatric drops OTC *pediatric decongestant and expectorant* [phenylpropanolamine HCl; guaifenesin] 6.25•100 mg/5 mL; 6.25•50 mg/mL

Naldecon Senior DX liquid OTC *antitussive; expectorant* [dextromethorphan hydrobromide; guaifenesin] 10•200 mg/5 mL

Naldecon Senior EX liquid OTC *expectorant* [guaifenesin] 200 mg/5 mL

Naldelate syrup, pediatric syrup ℞ *decongestant; antihistamine* [phenylpropanolamine HCl; phenylephrine HCl; chlorpheniramine maleate; phenyltoloxamine citrate] 20•5•2.5•7.5 mg/5 mL; 5•1.25•0.5•2 mg/5 mL

Naldelate DX Adult liquid OTC *antitussive; decongestant; expectorant* [dextromethorphan hydrobromide; phenylpropanolamine HCl; guaifenesin] 10•12.5•200 mg/5 mL

Nalfon Pulvules (capsules) ℞ *analgesic; antiarthritic; nonsteroidal anti-inflammatory drug (NSAID)* [fenoprofen calcium] 200, 300 mg ⓓ Naldecon

Nalgest sustained-release tablets, syrup, pediatric syrup, pediatric drops ℞ *decongestant; antihistamine* [phenylpropanolamine HCl; phenylephrine HCl; chlorpheniramine maleate; phenyltoloxamine citrate] 40•10•5•15 mg; 20•5•2.5•7.5 mg/5 mL; 5•1.25•0.5•2 mg/5 mL; 5•1.25•0.5•2 mg/mL

nalidixane [see: nalidixic acid]

nalidixate sodium USAN *antibacterial*

nalidixic acid USAN, USP, INN *urinary antibiotic*

Nallpen powder for IV or IM injection ℞ *penicillinase-resistant penicillin antibiotic* [nafcillin sodium] 0.5, 1, 2, 10 g

nalmefene USAN, INN, BAN *narcotic antagonist*

nalmefene HCl *narcotic antagonist*

nalmetrene [now: nalmefene]

nalmexone INN *analgesic; narcotic antagonist* [also: nalmexone HCl]

nalmexone HCl USAN *analgesic; narcotic antagonist* [also: nalmexone]

nalorphine INN [also: nalorphine HCl]

nalorphine HCl USP [also: nalorphine]

naloxiphane tartrate [see: levallorphan tartrate]

naloxone INN, BAN *narcotic antagonist* [also: naloxone HCl]

naloxone HCl USAN, USP, JAN *narcotic antagonist* [also: naloxone] 0.02, 0.4, 1 mg/mL injection

naloxone HCl & buprenorphine HCl *investigational (orphan) for opiate addictions*

naloxone HCl & pentazocine *narcotic agonist-antagonist analgesic* 0.5•50 mg oral

naltrexone USAN, INN, BAN *narcotic antagonist*

naltrexone HCl *opiate blockage and maintenance in formerly opiate-dependent individuals (orphan)* 50 mg oral

naminterol INN

[^{13}N]ammonia [see: ammonia N 13]

namoxyrate USAN, INN *analgesic*

namuron [see: cyclobarbitone]

nanafrocin INN

nandrolone BAN *anabolic* [also: nandrolone cyclotate]

nandrolone cyclotate USAN *anabolic* [also: nandrolone]

nandrolone decanoate USAN, USP *androgen/anabolic steroid for anemia of renal insufficiency; sometimes abused as a street drug*

nandrolone phenpropionate USP *androgen/anabolic steroid for metastatic breast cancer in women; sometimes abused as a street drug*

naniopine [see: nanofin]

nanofin INN

nanterinone INN, BAN

nantradol INN *analgesic* [also: nantradol HCl]

nantradol HCl USAN *analgesic* [also: nantradol]

NAPA (N-acetyl-*p*-aminophenol) [see: acetaminophen]

NAPA (N-acetyl-procainamide) [q.v.]
napactadine INN *antidepressant* [also: napactadine HCl]
napactadine HCl USAN *antidepressant* [also: napactadine]
napadisilate INN *combining name for radicals or groups* [also: napadisylate]
napadisylate BAN *combining name for radicals or groups* [also: napadisilate]
napamezole INN *antidepressant* [also: napamezole HCl]
napamezole HCl USAN *antidepressant* [also: napamezole]
naphazoline INN, BAN *topical ophthalmic decongestant and vasoconstrictor; nasal decongestant* [also: naphazoline HCl; naphazoline nitrate]
naphazoline HCl USP *topical ophthalmic decongestant and vasoconstrictor; nasal decongestant* [also: naphazoline; naphazoline nitrate] 0.1% eye drops
naphazoline HCl & antazoline phosphate *topical ocular decongestant and antihistamine* 0.05%•0.5%
naphazoline HCl & pheniramine maleate *topical ocular decongestant and antihistamine* 0.025%•0.3% eye drops
naphazoline nitrate JAN *topical ocular vasoconstrictor; nasal decongestant* [also: naphazoline HCl; naphazoline]
Naphazoline Plus eye drops OTC *topical ophthalmic decongestant and antihistamine* [naphazoline HCl; pheniramine maleate] 0.025%•0.3%
Naphcon eye drops OTC *topical ophthalmic decongestant and vasoconstrictor* [naphazoline HCl] 0.012%
Naphcon Forte Drop-Tainers (eye drops) ℞ *topical ophthalmic decongestant and vasoconstrictor* [naphazoline HCl] 0.1%
Naphcon-A Drop-Tainers (eye drops) OTC *topical ophthalmic decongestant and antihistamine* [naphazoline HCl; pheniramine maleate] 0.025%•0.3%
Naphoptic-A eye drops ℞ *topical ophthalmic decongestant and antihistamine* [naphazoline HCl; pheniramine maleate] 0.025%•0.3%
2-naphthol [see: betanaphthol]
naphthonone INN
naphthypramide [see: naftypramide]
Naphuride (available only from the Centers for Disease Control) ℞ *antiparasitic for African trypanosomiasis and onchocerciasis* [suramin sodium]
napirimus INN
napitane mesylate USAN *antidepressant; α-adrenergic blocker; norepinephrine uptake antagonist*
Naprelan controlled-release tablets ℞ *once-daily analgesic and antiarthritic; nonsteroidal anti-inflammatory drug (NSAID)* [naproxen (from naproxen sodium)] 375 (412.5), 500 (550) mg
naprodoxime INN
Napron X tablets (discontinued 2000) ℞ *analgesic; antiarthritic; nonsteroidal anti-inflammatory drug (NSAID)* [naproxen] 500 mg ⑨ Lupron; Mepron
Naprosyn tablets, oral suspension ℞ *analgesic; antiarthritic; nonsteroidal anti-inflammatory drug (NSAID)* [naproxen] 250, 375, 500 mg; 125 mg/5 mL ⑨ Meprospan; Natacyn
Naprosyn EC [see: EC-Naprosyn]
naproxen USAN, USP, INN, BAN, JAN *analgesic; antiarthritic; nonsteroidal anti-inflammatory drug (NSAID)* 250, 375, 500 mg oral; 125 mg/5 mL oral
naproxen sodium USAN, USP *analgesic; antiarthritic; antipyretic; nonsteroidal anti-inflammatory drug (NSAID)* 220, 275, 550 mg oral
naproxol USAN, INN *anti-inflammatory; analgesic; antipyretic*
napsagatran USAN, INN *antithrombotic*
napsilate INN *combining name for radicals or groups* [also: napsylate]
napsylate USAN, BAN *combining name for radicals or groups* [also: napsilate]
Naqua tablets ℞ *diuretic; antihypertensive* [trichlormethiazide] 2, 4 mg
naranol INN *antipsychotic* [also: naranol HCl]
naranol HCl USAN *antipsychotic* [also: naranol]
narasin USAN, INN, BAN *coccidiostat; veterinary growth stimulant*

naratriptan INN, BAN *vascular serotonin 5-HT$_1$ receptor agonist for migraine headache* [also: naratriptan HCl]
naratriptan HCl USAN *vascular serotonin 5-HT$_1$ receptor agonist for migraine headache* [also: naratriptan]
Narcan IV, IM, or subcu injection, neonatal injection ℞ *narcotic antagonist for opiate dependence or overdose; hypotension treatment* [naloxone HCl] 0.4, 1 mg/mL; 0.02 mg/mL ⊡ Marcaine
narcotic agonist-antagonists *a class of opioid or morphine-like analgesics with lower abuse potential than pure narcotic agonist analgesics*
narcotic agonists; narcotics *a class of opioid or morphine-like analgesics that relieve pain and induce sleep*
narcotine [see: noscapine]
narcotine HCl [see: noscapine HCl]
nard *medicinal herb* [see: spikenard]
Nardil sugar-coated tablets ℞ *antipsychotic; monoamine oxidase inhibitor (MAOI) for treatment-resistant atypical depression* [phenelzine sulfate] 15 mg ⊡ Norinyl
Naropin injection ℞ *long-acting local anesthetic* [ropivacaine HCl] 2, 5, 7.5, 10 mg/mL
narrow dock *medicinal herb* [see: yellow dock]
Nasabid prolonged-action capsules ℞ *decongestant; expectorant* [pseudoephedrine HCl; guaifenesin] 90•250 mg
Nasabid SR long-acting tablets ℞ *decongestant; expectorant* [pseudoephedrine HCl; guaifenesin] 90•500 mg
Nasacort nasal spray ℞ *corticosteroidal anti-inflammatory for seasonal or perennial rhinitis* [triamcinolone acetonide] 55 μg/spray
Nasacort AQ metered-dose aerosol ℞ *corticosteroidal anti-inflammatory for seasonal or perennial rhinitis* [triamcinolone acetonide] 55 μg/spray
Nasahist B subcu or IM injection (discontinued 1997) ℞ *antihistamine; anaphylaxis* [brompheniramine maleate] 10 mg/mL
NāSal nasal spray, nose drops OTC *nasal moisturizer* [sodium chloride (saline solution)] 0.65%
Nasal Decongestant spray OTC *nasal decongestant* [oxymetazoline HCl] 0.05%
Nasal Jelly ointment OTC *nasal moisturizer* [phenol; camphor; menthol; eucalyptus oil; oil of lavender]
Nasal Moist nasal spray OTC *nasal moisturizer* [sodium chloride (saline solution)] 0.65%
Nasal Relief nasal spray OTC *nasal decongestant* [oxymetazoline HCl] 0.05%
NasalCrom; Children's NasalCrom nasal spray OTC *anti-inflammatory/mast cell stabilizer for the prophylaxis of allergic rhinitis* [cromolyn sodium] 4% (5.2 mg/dose)
NasalCrom A nasal spray + tablets OTC *anti-inflammatory/mast cell stabilizer for the prophylaxis of allergic rhinitis; antihistamine* [cromolyn sodium; chlorpheniramine maleate] 4% (5.2 mg/dose); 4 mg
NasalCrom CA nasal spray + tablets OTC *anti-inflammatory/mast cell stabilizer for the prophylaxis of allergic rhinitis; decongestant; analgesic* [cromolyn sodium; pseudoephedrine HCl; acetaminophen] 4% (5.2 mg/dose); 30 mg•500 mg
Nasal-Ease with Zinc nasal gel OTC *nasal anti-infective, moisturizer, and emollient* [zinc acetate; aloe vera; calendula extract; alpha tocopheryl acetate]
Nasal-Ease with Zinc Gluconate nasal spray OTC *nasal moisturizer and anti-infective* [zinc gluconate]
Nasalide nasal spray ℞ *corticosteroidal anti-inflammatory for seasonal or perennial rhinitis* [flunisolide] 25 μg/dose
Nasarel metered dose nasal spray ℞ *corticosteroidal anti-inflammatory for seasonal or perennial rhinitis* [flunisolide] 25 μg/dose

Nasatab LA long-acting film-coated tablets ℞ *decongestant; expectorant* [pseudoephedrine HCl; guaifenesin] 120•500 mg

Nascobal nasal gel in metered-dose applicator ℞ *maintenance administration following intramuscular vitamin B_{12} therapy* [cyanocobalamin] 500 µg/0.1 mL dose

Nashville rabbit antithymocyte serum [see: lymphocyte immune globulin, antithymocyte]

Nashville Rabbit Antithymocyte Serum ℞ *investigational (orphan) passive immunizing agent to prevent allograft rejection in organ and bone marrow transplants* [lymphocyte immune globulin, antithymocyte (rabbit)]

Nasonex nasal spray ℞ *corticosteroid for the prophylaxis and treatment of seasonal and perennial allergic rhinitis* [mometasone furoate] 50 µg/spray

Nasturtium officinale *medicinal herb* [see: watercress]

NataChew chewable tablets ℞ *prenatal vitamin/mineral supplement* [multiple vitamins & minerals; ferrous fumarate; folic acid] ≛•29•1 mg

Natacyn eye drop suspension ℞ *ophthalmic antifungal agent* [natamycin] 5% Ⓓ Naprosyn

NataFort film-coated tablets ℞ *prenatal vitamin/iron supplement* [multiple vitamins; ferrous sulfate; folic acid] ≛•60•1 mg

NatalCare Plus film-coated tablets ℞ *vitamin/mineral/calcium/iron supplement* [multiple vitamins & minerals; calcium; iron; folic acid] ≛•200•27•1 mg

Natalins tablets (name changed to Enfamil Natalins Rx in 2001)

Natalins Rx tablets (discontinued 2001) ℞ *vitamin/calcium/iron supplement* [multiple vitamins; calcium; iron; folic acid; biotin] ≛•200•60•1•0.03 mg

natalizumab *investigational (Phase II) humanized monoclonal antibody for treatment of multiple sclerosis and Crohn disease*

natamycin USAN, USP, INN, BAN *ophthalmic fungicidal antibiotic* [also: pimaricin]

Natarex Prenatal tablets ℞ *vitamin/calcium/iron supplement* [multiple vitamins; calcium; iron; folic acid; biotin] ≛•200•60•1•0.03 mg

NataTab CFe; NataTab FA film-coated tablets ℞ *prenatal vitamin/mineral supplement* [multiple vitamins & minerals] ≛

nateglinide USAN *amino acid–derivative; oral antidiabetic agent for type 2 diabetes*

Natrecor powder for IV injection ℞ *human B-type natriuretic peptide (hBNP); vasodilator for acute congestive heart failure* [nesiritide citrate] 1.5 mg/vial

natriuretic peptide, human B-type (hBNP) [see: nesiritide; nesiritide citrate]

Natural Fiber Laxative powder OTC *bulk laxative* [psyllium hydrophilic mucilloid] 3.4 g/dose

natural killer cell stimulatory factor [see: edodekin alfa]

Natural Vegetable powder (discontinued 1999) OTC *bulk laxative* [psyllium hydrophilic mucilloid] 3.4 g/tsp.

Naturalyte oral solution OTC *electrolyte replacement* [sodium, potassium, and chloride electrolytes] 240 mL, 1 L

Nature's Choice (CAN) powder for oral solution OTC *vitamin/mineral/calcium/iron supplement* [multiple vitamins & minerals; calcium; iron; folic acid; biotin] ≛•500•4•0.08•0.06 mg

Nature's Remedy tablets OTC *stimulant laxative* [cascara sagrada; aloe] 150•100 mg

Nature's Tears eye drops OTC *ophthalmic moisturizer/lubricant* [hydroxypropyl methylcellulose] 0.4%

Naturetin tablets ℞ *antihypertensive; diuretic* [bendroflumethiazide] 5, 10 mg

Naturvus *hydrophilic contact lens material* [hefilcon B]

Naus-A-Way solution (discontinued 1997) OTC *antinauseant; antiemetic* [phosphorated carbohydrate solution (fructose, dextrose, and orthophosphoric acid)]

Nausea Relief oral solution OTC *antiemetic for nausea associated with influenza, morning sickness, motion sickness, inhalation anesthesia, or food and drink indiscretions* [phosphorated carbohydrate solution (dextrose, fructose, and phosphoric acid)] 1.87 g•1.87 g•21.5 mg per dose

Nausetrol oral solution OTC *antiemetic for nausea associated with influenza, morning sickness, motion sickness, inhalation anesthesia, or food and drink indiscretions* [phosphorated carbohydrate solution (fructose, dextrose, and orthophosphoric acid)]

Navane capsules ℞ *conventional (typical) antipsychotic* [thiothixene] 1, 2, 5, 10, 20 mg

Navane IM solution (discontinued 1997) ℞ *conventional (typical) antipsychotic* [thiothixene HCl] 2 mg/mL

Navane oral concentrate ℞ *conventional (typical) antipsychotic* [thiothixene HCl] 5 mg/mL

Navane powder for IM injection (discontinued 1998) ℞ *conventional (typical) antipsychotic* [thiothixene HCl] 5 mg/mL

Navelbine IV injection ℞ *antineoplastic for non–small cell lung cancer (NSCLC)* [vinorelbine tartrate] 10 mg/mL

naxagolide INN *antiparkinsonian; dopamine agonist* [also: naxagolide HCl]

naxagolide HCl USAN *antiparkinsonian; dopamine agonist* [also: naxagolide]

naxaprostene INN

NBI-3001 *investigational (Phase I/II, orphan) for glioblastoma or astrocytic glioma* [also: interleukin-4 Pseudomonas toxin fusion protein]

9-NC (9-nitrocamptothecin) [see: rubitecan]

ND Clear sustained-release capsules ℞ *decongestant; antihistamine* [pseudoephedrine HCl; chlorpheniramine maleate] 120•8 mg

ND Stat subcu or IM injection (discontinued 1997) ℞ *antihistamine for anaphylaxis* [brompheniramine maleate] 10 mg/mL

ND-Gesic tablets OTC *decongestant; antihistamine; analgesic* [phenylephrine HCl; chlorpheniramine maleate; pyrilamine maleate; acetaminophen] 5•2•12.5•300 mg

NE-1530 *investigational (Phase II) agent for the prevention of otitis media (clinical trials discontinued 1999)*

nealbarbital INN [also: nealbarbitone]

nealbarbitone BAN [also: nealbarbital]

nebacumab USAN, INN, BAN *antiendotoxin monoclonal antibody; investigational (orphan) for gram-negative bacteremia in endotoxin shock*

Nebcin IV or IM injection, pediatric injection, powder for injection ℞ *aminoglycoside antibiotic* [tobramycin sulfate] 10, 40 mg/mL; 10 mg/mL; 1.2 g

nebidrazine INN

nebivolol USAN, INN *antihypertensive (β-blocker)*

nebracetam INN

nebramycin USAN, INN *antibacterial*

nebramycin factor 6 [see: tobramycin]

NebuPent inhalation aerosol ℞ *antiprotozoal; treatment and prophylaxis of Pneumocystis carinii pneumonia (orphan)* [pentamidine isethionate] 300 mg

Necon 0.5/35; Necon 1/35 tablets (in packs of 21 or 28) ℞ *monophasic oral contraceptive* [norethindrone; ethinyl estradiol] 0.5 mg•35 µg; 1 mg•35 µg

Necon 1/50 tablets (in packs of 21 or 28) ℞ *monophasic oral contraceptive* [norethindrone; mestranol] 1 mg•50 µg

Necon 10/11 tablets (in packs of 28) ℞ *biphasic oral contraceptive* [norethindrone; ethinyl estradiol]
Phase 1 (10 days): 0.5 mg•35 µg;
Phase 2 (11 days): 1 mg•35 µg

nedocromil USAN, INN, BAN *anti-inflammatory; prophylactic antiallergic; mast cell stabilizer*

nedocromil calcium USAN *anti-inflammatory; prophylactic antiallergic; mast cell stabilizer*

nedocromil sodium USAN *anti-inflammatory; antiasthmatic; prophylactic antiallergic; mast cell stabilizer*

N.E.E. 1/35 tablets (discontinued 1999) ℞ *monophasic oral contraceptive* [norethindrone; ethinyl estradiol] 1 mg•35 µg

neem tree *(Azadirachta indica)* fruit, leaves, root, and oil *medicinal herb for contraception, diabetes, heart disease, malaria, skin diseases, ulcers, and worms; also used as a pesticide and insect repellent; not generally regarded as safe for infants, as it may cause death*

nefazodone INN *antidepressant; serotonin and norepinephrine uptake inhibitor* [also: nefazodone HCl]

nefazodone HCl USAN *antidepressant; serotonin and norepinephrine uptake inhibitor* [also: nefazodone]

neflumozide INN *antipsychotic* [also: neflumozide HCl]

neflumozide HCl USAN *antipsychotic* [also: neflumozide]

nefocon A USAN *hydrophobic contact lens material*

nefopam INN *analgesic* [also: nefopam HCl]

nefopam HCl USAN *analgesic* [also: nefopam]

nefrolan [see: clorexolone]

NegGram caplets, oral suspension ℞ *urinary antibiotic* [nalidixic acid] 250, 500, 1000 mg; 250 mg/5 mL

nelarabine USAN *antineoplastic for T-cell and B-cell lymphomas*

neldazosin INN

nelezaprine INN *muscle relaxant* [also: nelezaprine maleate]

nelezaprine maleate USAN *muscle relaxant* [also: nelezaprine]

nelfilcon A USAN *hydrophilic contact lens material*

nelfinavir mesylate USAN *antiretroviral HIV-1 protease inhibitor*

nelfinavir mesylate & amprenavir *investigational (Phase II) protease inhibitor combination for AIDS*

Nelova 0.5/35E; Nelova 1/35E tablets (in packs of 21 or 28) ℞ *monophasic oral contraceptive* [norethindrone; ethinyl estradiol] 0.5 mg•35 µg; 1 mg•35 µg

Nelova 1/50M tablets (in packs of 21 or 28) ℞ *monophasic oral contraceptive* [norethindrone; mestranol] 1 mg•50 µg

Nelova 10/11 tablets (in packs of 21 and 28) ℞ *biphasic oral contraceptive* [norethindrone; ethinyl estradiol] Phase 1 (10 days): 0.5 mg•35 µg; Phase 2 (11 days): 1 mg•35 µg

nemadectin USAN, INN *veterinary antiparasitic*

nemazoline INN *nasal decongestant* [also: nemazoline HCl]

nemazoline HCl USAN *nasal decongestant* [also: nemazoline]

Nembutal elixir ℞ *sedative; hypnotic; also abused as a street drug* [pentobarbital] 20 mg/5 mL ⓢ Myambutal

Nembutal Sodium capsules, IV or IM injection, suppositories ℞ *sedative; hypnotic; also abused as a street drug* [pentobarbital sodium] 50, 100 mg; 50 mg/mL; 30, 60, 120, 200 mg

neoarsphenamine NF, INN

Neocaf ℞ *investigational (orphan) for apnea of prematurity* [caffeine]

Neo-Calglucon syrup OTC *calcium supplement* [calcium glubionate] 1.8 g/5 mL

neocarzinostatin [now: zinostatin]

Neocate One + ready-to-use liquid OTC *pediatric enteral nutritional therapy* [lactose-free formula] 237 mL

Neocera (trademarked ingredient) *suppository base* [polyethylent glycol 400, 1450, and 8000; polysorbate 60]

neocid [see: chlorophenothane]

neocinchophen NF, INN

NeoCitran DM Coughs & Colds (CAN) powder for oral solution (discontinued 1999) OTC *antitussive; decongestant; antihistamine* [dextromethorphan hydrobromide; phenylephrine HCl; pheniramine maleate] 30•10•20 mg/dose

Neo-Cortef ointment (discontinued 1997) ℞ *topical corticosteroidal anti-inflammatory; antibiotic* [hydrocortisone; neomycin sulfate] 0.5%•0.5%, 1%•0.5%

Neo-Cultol jelly (discontinued 1999) OTC *emollient laxative* [mineral oil]

NeoDecadron cream (discontinued 1998) ℞ *topical corticosteroidal anti-inflammatory; antibiotic* [dexamethasone sodium phosphate; neomycin sulfate] 0.1%•0.5%

NeoDecadron Ocumeter (eye drops), ophthalmic ointment ℞ *topical ophthalmic corticosteroidal anti-inflammatory; antibiotic* [dexamethasone sodium phosphate; neomycin sulfate] 0.1%•0.35%; 0.05%•0.35%

Neo-Dexair eye drops ℞ *topical ophthalmic corticosteroidal anti-inflammatory; antibiotic* [dexamethasone sodium phosphate; neomycin sulfate] 0.1%•0.35%

Neo-Dexameth eye drops ℞ *topical ophthalmic corticosteroidal anti-inflammatory; antibiotic* [dexamethasone sodium phosphate; neomycin sulfate] 0.1%•0.35%

Neo-Diaral capsules OTC *antidiarrheal* [loperamide] 2 mg

Neo-Durabolic IM injection (discontinued 2000) ℞ *anabolic steroid for anemia of renal insufficiency* [nandrolone decanoate (in oil)] 50, 200 mg/mL

neodymium *element (Nd)*

Neo-fradin oral solution ℞ *aminoglycoside antibiotic* [neomycin sulfate] 125 mg/5 mL

Neoloid oral emulsion OTC *stimulant laxative* [castor oil] 36.4%

Neomark ℞ *investigational (NDA filed, orphan) radiosensitizer for breast and brain tumors* [broxuridine]

neo-mercazole [see: carbimazole]

Neomixin ointment OTC *topical antibiotic* [polymyxin B sulfate; neomycin sulfate; bacitracin zinc] 5000 U•3.5 mg•400 U per g 👂 neomycin

neomycin INN, BAN *antibacterial* [also: neomycin palmitate] 👂 Neomixin

neomycin B [see: framycetin]

neomycin palmitate USAN *antibacterial* [also: neomycin]

neomycin sulfate USP *aminoglycoside antibiotic* 500 mg oral; 3.5 mg/g topical

neomycin sulfate & polymyxin B sulfate & bacitracin zinc *topical antibiotic* 5 mg•10 000 U•400 U per g ophthalmic

neomycin sulfate & polymyxin B sulfate & dexamethasone *topical ophthalmic antibiotic and corticosteroidal anti-inflammatory* 0.35%•10 000 U•0.1% per mL eye drops

neomycin sulfate & polymyxin B sulfate & gramicidin *topical antibiotic* 1.75 mg•10 000 U•0.025 mg per mL eye drops

neomycin undecenoate [see: neomycin undecylenate]

neomycin undecylenate USAN *antibacterial; antifungal*

neon *element (Ne)*

Neopap suppositories OTC *analgesic; antipyretic* [acetaminophen] 125 mg

neopenyl [see: clemizole penicillin]

neoquate [see: nequinate]

Neoral soft gels, oral solution ℞ *immunosuppressant for allogenic kidney, liver, and heart transplants, rheumatoid arthritis, and psoriasis* [cyclosporine for microemulsion] 25, 100 mg (10, 50 mg available in Canada); 100 mg/mL

Neosar powder for IV injection ℞ *nitrogen mustard-type alkylating antineoplastic for multiple leukemias, lymphomas, blastomas, sarcomas and organ cancers* [cyclophosphamide] 100 mg

Neosporin cream OTC *topical antibiotic* [polymyxin B sulfate; neomycin sulfate] 10 000 U•3.5 mg per g

Neosporin Drop Dose (eye drops) ℞ *topical ophthalmic antibiotic* [polymyxin B sulfate; neomycin sulfate; gramicidin] 10 000 U•1.75 mg• 0.025 mg per mL

Neosporin ointment OTC *topical antibiotic* [polymyxin B sulfate; neomycin sulfate; bacitracin] 5000 U•3.5 mg• 400 U, 10 000 U•3.5 mg•500 U /g

Neosporin ophthalmic ointment ℞ *topical ophthalmic antibiotic* [polymyxin B sulfate; neomycin sulfate; bacitracin zinc] 10 000 U•5 mg• 400 U per g

Neosporin G.U. Irrigant solution ℞ *bactericidal* [neomycin sulfate; polymyxin B sulfate] 40 mg•200 000 U per mL

Neosporin Plus cream OTC *topical antibiotic; anesthetic* [polymyxin B sulfate; neomycin; lidocaine] 10 000 U•3.5 mg•40 mg per g

Neosporin Plus ointment OTC *topical antibiotic; anesthetic* [polymyxin B sulfate; bacitracin zinc; neomycin; lidocaine] 10 000 U•500 U•3.5 mg•40 mg per g

Neosten timed-release tablets ℞ *investigational (NDA filed) agent for osteoporosis* [sodium fluoride]

neostigmine BAN *cholinergic/anticholinesterase muscle stimulant* [also: neostigmine bromide]

neostigmine bromide USP, INN, BAN *cholinergic/anticholinesterase muscle stimulant* [also: neostigmine] 15 mg oral

neostigmine methylsulfate USP *cholinergic/anticholinesterase muscle stimulant; urinary stimulant* 1:1000 (1 mg/mL), 1:2000 (0.5 mg/mL) injection

Neostrata AHA for Age Spots and Skin Lightening gel (discontinued 1997) OTC *hyperpigmentation bleaching agent; sunscreen* [hydroquinone; glycolic acid] 2%•10%

Neo-Synephrine eye drops, viscous solution ℞ *topical ophthalmic decongestant and vasoconstrictor; mydriatic* [phenylephrine HCl] 2.5%, 10%; 10%

Neo-Synephrine nasal spray, nose drops OTC *nasal decongestant* [phenylephrine HCl] 0.25%, 0.5%, 1%; 0.125%, 0.25%, 0.5%, 1%

Neo-Synephrine 12 Hour nasal spray OTC *nasal decongestant* [oxymetazoline HCl] 0.05%

Neo-Synephrine IV, IM, or subcu injection ℞ *vasopressor for hypotensive or cardiac shock* [phenylephrine HCl] 1% (10 mg/mL)

Neo-Tabs tablets ℞ *aminoglycoside antibiotic* [neomycin sulfate] 500 mg

NeoTect kit for injection preparation ℞ *radiopharmaceutical imaging agent for lung cancer; investigational (NDA filed) for malignant melanoma and neuroendocrine disorders* [depreotide]

Neotrace-4 IV injection ℞ *intravenous nutritional therapy* [multiple trace elements (metals)]

Neotricin HC ophthalmic ointment ℞ *topical ophthalmic corticosteroidal anti-inflammatory; antibiotic* [hydrocortisone acetate; neomycin sulfate; bacitracin zinc; polymyxin B sulfate] 1%•3.5%•400 U/g•10 000 U/g

Neotrofin ℞ *investigational (Phase II/III) nerve growth factor for Alzheimer disease, spinal cord injuries, and stroke* [leteprinim potassium]

Neovastat ℞ *investigational (Phase III) shark cartilage–based antineoplastic/angiogenesis inhibitor for lung, prostate, renal, and breast cancers* [AE-941 (code name—generic name not yet assigned)] ⓢ Novastan

nepafenac USAN *topical ophthalmic anti-inflammatory and analgesic*

Nepeta cataria *medicinal herb* [see: catnip]

Nephplex Rx tablets ℞ *vitamin supplement* [multiple B vitamins; ascorbic acid; folic acid; biotin] ≛•60• 1•0.3 mg

NephrAmine 5.4% IV infusion ℞ *nutritional therapy for renal failure* [multiple essential amino acids; electrolytes]

nephritics *a class of agents that affect the kidney (a term used in folk medicine)*

Nephro-Calci tablets OTC *calcium supplement* [calcium carbonate] 1.5 g

Nephrocaps capsules ℞ *vitamin supplement* [multiple B vitamins; vitamin C; folic acid; biotin] ≛•100 mg•1 mg•150 µg

Nephro-Fer tablets OTC *hematinic* [ferrous fumarate (source of iron)] 350 mg (115 mg)

Nephro-Fer Rx film-coated tablets ℞ *hematinic* [ferrous fumarate; folic acid] 106.9•1 mg

Nephron solution for inhalation OTC *sympathomimetic bronchodilator* [racepinephrine HCl] 2.25%

Nephron FA tablets ℞ *hematinic* [ferrous fumarate; multiple B vitamins; ascorbic acid; folic acid; biotin; docusate sodium] 66.6•≛•40•1•0.3•75 mg

Nephro-Vite Rx film-coated tablets ℞ *vitamin supplement* [multiple B vitamins; vitamin C; folic acid; biotin] ≛•60 mg•1 mg•300 µg

Nephro-Vite Rx + Fe film-coated tablets ℞ *hematinic* [ferrous fumarate; multiple B vitamins; ascorbic acid; folic acid; biotin] 100•≛•60•1•0.3 mg

Nephro-Vite Vitamin B Complex and C Supplement tablets OTC *vitamin supplement* [multiple B vitamins; vitamin C; folic acid; biotin] ≛•60•0.8•0.3 mg

Nephrox oral suspension OTC *antacid; laxative* [aluminum hydroxide; mineral oil 10%] 320 mg/5 mL

nepicastat HCl USAN *dopamine β-hydroxylase inhibitor for congestive heart failure*

Nepro oral liquid OTC *enteral nutritional therapy for acute or chronic renal failure* [lactose-free formula] 240 mL

neptamustine INN *antineoplastic* [also: pentamustine]

Neptazane tablets ℞ *carbonic anhydrase inhibitor for glaucoma* [methazolamide] 25, 50 mg

neptunium *element (Np)*

nequinate USAN, INN *coccidiostat for poultry* [also: methyl benzoquate]

neraminol INN

nerbacadol INN

nerelimomab USAN *monoclonal antibody; investigational (Phase III) cytokine modulator for septic shock*

neridronic acid INN

Nerium indicum; N. oleander *medicinal herb* [see: oleander]

nervines *a class of agents that have a calming or soothing effect on the nerves (a term used in folk medicine)*

Nervocaine 1% injection ℞ *injectable local anesthetic* [lidocaine HCl] 1%

Nesacaine; Nesacaine MPF injection ℞ *injectable local anesthetic* [chloroprocaine HCl] 1%, 2%; 2%, 3%

nesapidil INN

nesiritide USAN *human B-type natriuretic peptide (hBNP); vasodilator for acute congestive heart failure*

nesiritide citrate USAN *human B-type natriuretic peptide (hBNP); vasodilator for acute congestive heart failure*

nesosteine INN

Nestabs tablets (name changed to Vitelle Nestabs OTC in 2000)

Nestabs CFB; Nestabs FA tablets ℞ *vitamin/calcium/iron supplement for pregnancy and lactation* [multiple vitamins; calcium; iron; folic acid] ≛•200•50•1 mg; ≛•200•29•1 mg

Nestrex tablets (name changed to Vitelle Nestrex in 2001)

nethalide [see: pronetalol]

netilmicin INN, BAN *aminoglycoside antibiotic* [also: netilmicin sulfate]

netilmicin sulfate USAN, USP *aminoglycoside antibiotic* [also: netilmicin]

netobimin USAN, INN, BAN *veterinary anthelmintic*

netrafilcon A USAN *hydrophilic contact lens material*

Netromicina (Mexican name for U.S. product Netromycin)

Netromycin IV or IM injection ℞ *aminoglycoside antibiotic* [netilmicin sulfate] 100 mg/mL

nettle *(Urtica dioica; U. urens)* leaves and root *medicinal herb for blood cleansing, bronchitis, diarrhea, edema, hypertension, internal and external bleeding, and rheumatism; also being investigated for hay fever and urinary tract irrigation*

nettle, hemp; bee nettle; dog nettle; hemp dead nettle *medicinal herb* [see: hemp nettle]

nettle flowers; dead nettle; stingless nettle; white nettle *medicinal herb* [see: blind nettle]

Neumega subcu injection ℞ *platelet growth factor for prevention of thrombocytopenia following chemotherapy or radiation (orphan)* [oprelvekin] 5 mg

Neupogen IV or subcu injection ℞ *hematopoietic stimulant for severe chronic neutropenia and myelodysplastic syndrome (orphan); investigational (Phase III, orphan) cytokine for CMV retinitis of AIDS* [filgrastim] 300 µg/mL

Neuprex injection ℞ *investigational (Phase III, orphan) agent for gram-negative sepsis, hemorrhagic shock, and meningococcemia; investigational agent for lung infection in cystic fibrosis* [bactericidal and permeability-increasing protein, recombinant (rBPI-21)]

neural dopaminergic cells (or precursors), porcine fetal *investigational (orphan) intracerebral implant for stage 4 and 5 Parkinson disease*

neural gabaergic cells (or precursors), porcine fetal *investigational (orphan) intracerebral implant for Huntington disease*

Neuramate tablets (discontinued 2001) ℞ *anxiolytic* [meprobamate] 400 mg

NeuRecover-DA; NeuRecover-LT; NeuRecover-SA capsules OTC *dietary supplement* [multiple vitamins & minerals; multiple amino acids; folic acid] ≛ •0.067 mg; ≛ •0.03 mg; ≛ • 0.067 mg

Neurelan *investigational (orphan) for multiple sclerosis and spinal cord injury* [fampridine]

Neurobloc (name changed to Myobloc upon marketing release in 2001)

NeuroCell-HD ℞ *investigational (orphan) intracerebral implant for patients with Huntington disease* [neural gabaergic cells, porcine fetal]

NeuroCell-PD ℞ *investigational (Phase II/III, orphan) intracerebral implant for patients with advanced Parkinson disease* [neural dopaminergic cells, porcine fetal]

Neurodep injection ℞ *parenteral vitamin therapy* [multiple B vitamins; vitamin C] ≛ •50 mg/mL

Neurodep-Caps capsules OTC *vitamin supplement* [vitamins B_1, B_6, and B_{12}] 125•125•1 mg

Neurolite injection ℞ *imaging aid for SPECT brain scans* [technetium Tc 99m bicisate]

Neurontin capsules, film-coated tablets, oral solution ℞ *anticonvulsant for partial-onset seizures; investigational (orphan) for amyotrophic lateral sclerosis* [gabapentin] 100, 300, 400 mg; 600, 800 mg; 250 mg/5 mL

neurosin [see: calcium glycerophosphate]

NeuroSlim capsules OTC *dietary supplement* [multiple vitamins & minerals; multiple amino acids; folic acid; biotin] ≛ •0.066•0.05 mg

neurotrophic growth factor [see: methionyl neurotrophic factor]

neurotrophin-1 *investigational (orphan) for motor neuron disease and amyotrophic lateral sclerosis*

neurotrophin-3 (NT-3) *investigational agent for treating peripheral neuropathies; investigational for constipation*

neustab [see: thioacetazone; thiacetazone]

Neut IV or subcu injection ℞ *pH buffer for metabolic acidosis; urinary alkalinizer* [sodium bicarbonate] 4% (0.48 mEq/mL)

neutral acriflavine [see: acriflavine]

Neutral C (CAN) capsules OTC *vitamin C supplement* [calcium polyascorbate;

lemon bioflavonoids; echinacea] 600•≛•≛ mg

Neutral C + CoEnzyme Q10 (CAN) capsules OTC *vitamin/mineral supplement* [multiple vitamins; multiple minerals; calcium ascorbate; coenzyme Q_{10}; folic acid] ≛•≛•320•10•0.5 mg

neutral insulin INN, BAN, JAN *antidiabetic* [also: insulin, neutral]

Neutralase *investigational (Phase III) agent for the reversal of heparin-induced anticoagulation for bypass surgery* [heparinase 1]

Neutralca-S (CAN) oral suspension OTC *antacid* [aluminum hydroxide; magnesium hydroxide] 200•200 mg/5 mL

neutramycin USAN, INN *antibacterial*

Neutra-Phos powder OTC *phosphorus supplement* [monobasic sodium phosphate; monobasic potassium phosphate; dibasic sodium phosphate; dibasic potassium phosphate] 250 mg/packet (P)

Neutra-Phos-K powder OTC *phosphorus supplement* [monobasic potassium phosphate; dibasic potassium phosphate] 250 mg/packet (P)

NeuTrexin powder for IV injection ℞ *antiprotozoal for AIDS-related Pneumocystis carinii pneumonia (orphan); investigational (orphan) antineoplastic for multiple cancers* [trimetrexate glucuronate] 25 mg

neutroflavine [see: acriflavine]

Neutrogena Acne Mask OTC *topical keratolytic cleansing mask for acne* [benzoyl peroxide] 5%

Neutrogena Antiseptic Cleanser for Acne-Prone Skin liquid OTC *topical cleanser for acne* [benzethonium chloride]

Neutrogena Body lotion, oil OTC *moisturizer; emollient*

Neutrogena Drying gel OTC *topical astringent and antiseptic for acne* [hamamelis water; isopropyl alcohol]

Neutrogena Moisture lotion OTC *moisturizer; emollient*

Neutrogena Non-Drying Cleansing lotion OTC *soap-free therapeutic skin cleanser*

Neutrogena Norwegian Formula Hand cream OTC *moisturizer; emollient*

Neutrogena Oil-Free Acne Wash liquid OTC *topical keratolytic cleanser for acne* [salicylic acid] 2%

Neutrogena Soap; Neutrogena Cleansing for Acne-Prone Skin; Neutrogena Baby Cleansing Formula Soap; Neutrogena Dry Skin Soap; Neutrogena Oily Skin Soap bar OTC *therapeutic skin cleanser*

Neutrogena T/Derm oil OTC *topical antipsoriatic; antiseborrheic* [coal tar] 5%

Neutrogena T/Gel shampoo, conditioner OTC *antiseborrheic; antipsoriatic; antipruritic; antibacterial* [coal tar] 2%; 1.5%

Neutrogena T/Sal shampoo OTC *antiseborrheic; antipsoriatic; antipruritic; antibacterial* [salicylic acid; coal tar] 2%•2%

nevirapine USAN, INN *antiviral nonnucleoside reverse transcriptase inhibitor (NNRTI) for HIV-1*

nevirapine & zidovudine & didanosine *investigational (Phase III) antiviral combination for HIV infection*

New Jersey tea *(Ceanothus americanus)* root bark *medicinal herb used as an astringent, expectorant, and sedative*

New Zealand green-lipped mussel *(Perna canaliculus)* freeze-dried body or gonads *natural treatment for osteoarthritis and rheumatoid arthritis*

new-estranol 1 [see: diethylstilbestrol]

new-oestranol 1 [see: diethylstilbestrol]

new-oestranol 11 [see: diethylstilbestrol dipropionate]

NewPaks (trademarked delivery form) *ready-to-use closed system containers*

New-Skin liquid, spray OTC *skin protectant; antiseptic* [hydroxyquinoline]

nexeridine INN *analgesic* [also: nexeridine HCl]

nexeridine HCl USAN *analgesic* [also: nexeridine]

Nexium enteric-coated delayed-release pellets in capsules ℞ *proton pump inhibitor for gastric and duodenal ulcers, erosive esophagitis, GERD, and other gastroesophageal disorders* [esomeprazole magnesium] 20, 40 mg

NFL (Novantrone, fluorouracil, leucovorin [rescue]) *chemotherapy protocol for breast cancer*

NG-29 *investigational (orphan) diagnostic aid for pituitary release of growth hormone*

N-Graft ℞ *investigational (orphan) intracerebral implant for patients with advanced Parkinson disease (for co-implantation with fetal neural cells)* [Sertoli cells, porcine]

N.G.T. cream ℞ *topical corticosteroidal anti-inflammatory; antifungal* [triamcinolone acetonide; nystatin] 0.1%• 100 000 U per g

Nia-Bid sustained-action capsules (discontinued 1999) OTC *vitamin B_3 supplement; antihyperlipidemic* [niacin] 400 mg

Niacels timed-release capsules (discontinued 1997) OTC *vitamin B_3 supplement; antihyperlipidemic* [niacin] 400 mg

niacin (vitamin B_3) USP *water-soluble vitamin; peripheral vasodilator; antihyperlipidemic for hypertriglyceridemia (types IV and V hyperlipidemia)* [also: nicotinic acid] 50, 100, 125, 250, 400, 500 mg oral ⓢ Minocin

niacinamide (vitamin B_3) USP *water-soluble vitamin; enzyme cofactor* [also: nicotinamide] 100, 500 mg oral

niacinamide hydroiodide *expectorant*

Niacor immediate-release tablets ℞ *vitamin B_3 therapy; peripheral vasodilator; antihyperlipidemic for hypertriglyceridemia (types IV and V hyperlipidemia)* [niacin] 500 mg

nialamide NF, INN

niaprazine INN

Niaspan extended-release tablets ℞ *vitamin B_3 therapy; peripheral vasodilator; antihyperlipidemic for hypertriglyceridemia (types IV and V hyperlipidemia)* [niacin] 500, 750, 1000 mg

NiaStase (CAN) powder for IV injection ℞ *recombinant coagulation factor VII for hemophilia A and B* [eptacog alfa (activated)] 1.2, 2.4, 4.8 mg/vial

nibroxane USAN, INN *topical antimicrobial*

Nicabate (European name for U.S. product Nicoderm)

nicafenine INN

nicainoprol INN

nicametate INN, BAN

nicaraven INN

nicarbazin BAN

nicardipine INN, BAN *vasodilator; calcium channel blocker* [also: nicardipine HCl]

nicardipine HCl USAN *antianginal; antihypertensive; vasodilator; calcium channel blocker* [also: nicardipine] 20, 30 mg oral

NicCheck I reagent strips *in vitro diagnostic aid for urine nicotine, used to determine the smoking status of the subject*

NicCheck II reagent strips *investigational in vitro diagnostic aid for urine nicotine, used to determine exposure to passive cigarette smoke*

N'Ice throat spray OTC *topical analgesic; counterirritant; mild local anesthetic* [menthol] 0.12%

N'Ice; N'Ice 'n Clear lozenges OTC *topical oral analgesic; counterirritant; mild local anesthetic* [menthol] 5 mg

N'Ice Vitamin C Drops (lozenges) OTC *vitamin C supplement* [ascorbic acid; menthol] 60•? mg

NicErase-SL ℞ *investigational (Phase III) treatment for nicotine withdrawal; clinical trials discontinued 1997* [lobeline sulfate]

nicergoline USAN, INN *vasodilator*

niceritrol INN, BAN

nicethamide BAN [also: nikethamide]

niceverine INN

nickel *element (Ni)*

niclofolan INN, BAN

niclosamide USAN, INN *anthelmintic for cestodiasis (tapeworm)*

Nico-400 timed-release capsules (discontinued 1999) OTC *vitamin B_3 supplement; antihyperlipidemic* [niacin] 400 mg

Nicobid Tempules (timed-release capsules) (discontinued 1999) OTC *vitamin B_3 supplement; antihyperlipidemic* [niacin] 125, 250, 500 mg ⓓ Nitro-Bid

nicoboxil INN

nicoclonate INN

nicocodine INN, BAN

nicocortonide INN

Nicoderm CQ transdermal patch (regular or clear) OTC *smoking deterrent; nicotine withdrawal aid* [nicotine] 7, 14, 21 mg/day

nicodicodine INN, BAN

nicoduozide (isoniazid + nicothiazone)

nicofibrate INN

nicofuranose INN

nicofurate INN

nicogrelate INN

Nicolar tablets (discontinued 1999) ℞ *vitamin B_3 therapy; antihyperlipidemic; peripheral vasodilator* [niacin] 500 mg

nicomol INN

nicomorphine INN, BAN

nicopholine INN

nicorandil USAN, INN *coronary vasodilator*

Nicorette chewing pieces OTC *smoking deterrent; nicotine withdrawal aid* [nicotine polacrilex] 2, 4 mg

Nicorette DS chewing pieces (discontinued 1997) ℞ *smoking deterrent; nicotine withdrawal aid* [nicotine polacrilex] 4 mg

Nicorette Plus (CAN) chewing pieces OTC *smoking deterrent; nicotine withdrawal aid* [nicotine polacrilex] 4 mg

nicothiazone INN

nicotinaldehyde thiosemicarbazone [see: nicothiazone]

nicotinamide (vitamin B_3) INN, BAN, JAN *water-soluble vitamin; enzyme cofactor* [also: niacinamide]

nicotinamide-adenine dinucleotide (NAD) [now: nadide]

nicotine *a very poisonous alkaloid used as an insecticide and external parasiticide; the active principle in tobacco; smoking cessation aid* [also see: tobacco] 7, 14, 21 mg/day transdermal

nicotine bitartrate USAN *smoking cessation aid*

nicotine & mecamylamine HCl *investigational (Phase III) transdermal patch for smoking cessation*

nicotine OT *investigational (Phase II) oral transmucosal form for smoking cessation*

nicotine polacrilex USAN *smoking deterrent; nicotine withdrawal aid* 2, 4 mg oral

nicotine resin complex [see: nicotine polacrilex]

Nicotinex elixir OTC *vitamin B_3 supplement; antihyperlipidemic* [niacin] 50 mg/5 mL

nicotinic acid (vitamin B_3) INN, BAN, JAN *water-soluble vitamin; peripheral vasodilator; antihyperlipidemic* [also: niacin]

nicotinic acid amide [see: niacinamide]

nicotinic acid 1-oxide [see: oxiniacic acid]

nicotinohydroxamic acid [see: nicoxamat]

6-nicotinoyl dihydrocodeine [see: nicodicodine]

6-nicotinoylcodeine [see: nicocodine]

4-nicotinoylmorpholine [see: nicopholine]

nicotinyl alcohol USAN, BAN *peripheral vasodilator*

nicotinyl tartrate

Nicotrol oral inhaler ℞ *smoking deterrent; nicotine withdrawal aid* [nicotine] 4 mg

Nicotrol transdermal patch OTC *smoking deterrent; nicotine withdrawal aid* [nicotine] 15 mg/16 hours

Nicotrol NS nasal spray ℞ *smoking deterrent; nicotine withdrawal aid* [nicotine] 0.5 mg/spray

nicotylamide [see: niacinamide]

nicoumalone BAN [also: acenocoumarol]
nicoxamat INN
nictiazem INN
nictindole INN
Nidagel (CAN) vaginal gel ℞ *antibacterial for bacterial vaginosis* [metronidazole] 0.75%
nidroxyzone INN
Nifedical XL film-coated sustained-release tablets ℞ *antianginal; antihypertensive; calcium channel blocker* [nifedipine] 30, 60 mg
nifedipine USAN, USP, INN, BAN *antianginal; antihypertensive; coronary vasodilator; calcium channel blocker; investigational (orphan) for interstitial cystitis* 10, 20, 30, 60, 90 mg oral
nifenalol INN
nifenazone INN, BAN
Niferex tablets, elixir OTC *hematinic; iron supplement* [polysaccharide-iron complex] 50 mg; 100 mg/5 mL
Niferex with Vitamin C chewable tablets (discontinued 1998) OTC *hematinic* [polysaccharide-iron complex; ascorbic acid; sodium ascorbate] 50•100•169 mg
Niferex-150 capsules OTC *hematinic; iron supplement* [polysaccharide-iron complex] 150 mg
Niferex-150 Forte capsules ℞ *hematinic* [polysaccharide-iron complex; cyanocobalamin; folic acid] 150 mg•25 µg•1 mg
Niferex-PN film-coated tablets ℞ *prenatal vitamin/iron supplement* [polysaccharide-iron complex; multiple vitamins & minerals; folic acid] 60•≛•1 mg
Niferex-PN Forte film-coated tablets ℞ *prenatal vitamin/mineral/calcium/iron supplement* [multiple vitamins & minerals; calcium; polysaccharide-iron complex; folic acid] ≛•250•60•1 mg
niflumic acid INN
nifluridide USAN *ectoparasiticide*
nifungin USAN, INN
nifuradene USAN, INN *antibacterial*
nifuralazine [see: furalazine]
nifuraldezone USAN, INN *antibacterial*
nifuralide INN
nifuramizone [see: nifurethazone]
nifuratel USAN, INN *antibacterial; antifungal; antiprotozoal (Trichomonas)*
nifuratrone USAN, INN *antibacterial*
nifurazolidone [see: furazolidone]
nifurdazil USAN, INN *antibacterial*
nifurethazone INN
nifurfoline INN
nifurhydrazone [see: nihydrazone]
nifurimide USAN, INN *antibacterial*
nifurizone INN
nifurmazole INN
nifurmerone USAN, INN *antifungal*
nifuroquine INN
nifuroxazide INN
nifuroxime NF, INN
nifurpipone (NP) INN
nifurpirinol USAN, INN *antibacterial*
nifurprazine INN
nifurquinazol USAN, INN *antibacterial*
nifursemizone USAN, INN *antiprotozoal for poultry (Histomonas)*
nifursol USAN, INN *antiprotozoal for poultry (Histomonas)*
nifurthiazole USAN, INN *antibacterial*
nifurthiline [see: thiofuradene]
nifurtimox INN, BAN *investigational anti-infective for Chagas disease (available only from Centers for Disease Control and Prevention)*
nifurtoinol INN
nifurvidine INN
nifurzide INN
Night Time Cold/Flu Relief oral liquid OTC *antitussive; decongestant; antihistamine; analgesic* [dextromethorphan hydrobromide; pseudoephedrine HCl; doxylamine succinate; acetaminophen; alcohol 10%] 30•60•12.5•1000 mg/30 mL
nightshade; nightshade vine *medicinal herb* [see: bittersweet nightshade]
nightshade, American *medicinal herb* [see: pokeweed]
nightshade, deadly *medicinal herb* [see: belladonna]

nightshade, fetid; stinking nightshade *medicinal herb* [see: henbane]
nightshade, three-leaved *medicinal herb* [see: birthroot]
Night-Time Effervescent Cold tablets for oral solution OTC *decongestant; antihistamine; analgesic; antipyretic* [phenylpropanolamine HCl; diphenhydramine citrate; aspirin] 15•38.33•325 mg
Nighttime Sleep Aid tablets OTC *antihistaminic sleep aid* [diphenhydramine HCl] 50 mg
niguldipine INN
nihydrazone INN
nikethamide NF, INN [also: nicethamide]
Nilandron tablets ℞ *antiandrogen antineoplastic for metastatic prostate cancer* [nilutamide] 50, 150 mg
nileprost INN
nilestriol INN *estrogen* [also: nylestriol]
nilprazole INN
Nilstat cream, ointment ℞ *topical antifungal* [nystatin] 100 000 U/g ⑨ Nitrostat; nystatin
Nilstat film-coated tablets (discontinued 2000) ℞ *systemic antifungal* [nystatin] 500 000 U
Nilstat oral suspension, powder for oral suspension ℞ *antifungal; oral candidiasis treatment* [nystatin] 100 000 U/mL; 150 million, 500 million, 1 billion, 2 billion U
niludipine INN
nilutamide USAN, INN, BAN *antiandrogen antineoplastic for metastatic prostate cancer*
nilvadipine USAN, INN, JAN *calcium channel antagonist*
nimazone USAN, INN *anti-inflammatory*
Nimbex IV infusion ℞ *nondepolarizing neuromuscular blocking agent for anesthesia* [cisatracurium besylate] 2, 10 mg/mL
Nimbus; Nimbus Quick Strip test kit for home use *in vitro diagnostic aid; urine pregnancy test* [monoclonal antibody-based enzyme immunoassay]
Nimbus Plus test kit for professional use *in vitro diagnostic aid; urine pregnancy test*
nimesulide INN, BAN
nimetazepam INN
nimidane USAN, INN *veterinary acaricide*
nimodipine USAN, INN, BAN *vasodilator; calcium channel blocker; investigational Alzheimer treatment*
nimorazole INN, BAN
nimustine INN
niobium *element (Nb)*
niometacin INN
Nion B Plus C caplets OTC *vitamin supplement* [multiple B vitamins; vitamin C] ≛•300 mg
Nipent powder for IV injection ℞ *antibiotic antineoplastic for hairy cell leukemia (orphan); investigational (orphan) for chronic lymphocytic leukemia and cutaneous T-cell lymphoma; investigational (Phase II) for AIDS-related non-Hodgkin lymphoma* [pentostatin] 10 mg
niperotidine INN
nipradilol INN
Nipride *brand discontinued 1992* [see: sodium nitroprusside]
niprofazone INN
niridazole USAN, INN *antischistosomal*
nisbuterol INN *bronchodilator* [also: nisbuterol mesylate]
nisbuterol mesylate USAN *bronchodilator* [also: nisbuterol]
nisin *investigational agent for severe colonic bacterial infections*
nisobamate USAN, INN *minor tranquilizer*
nisoldipine USAN, INN, BAN, JAN *coronary vasodilator; calcium channel blocker for hypertension*
nisoxetine USAN, INN *antidepressant*
nisterime INN *androgen* [also: nisterime acetate]
nisterime acetate USAN *androgen* [also: nisterime]
nitarsone USAN, INN *antiprotozoal (Histomonas)*
nitazoxanide (NTZ) INN *investigational (NDA filed, orphan) anti-infec-*

tive for AIDS-related cryptosporidial diarrhea (NDA withdrawn 1998)

Nite Time Cold Formula liquid OTC *antitussive; decongestant; antihistamine; analgesic* [dextromethorphan hydrobromide; pseudoephedrine HCl; doxylamine succinate; acetaminophen; alcohol 25%] 5•10•1.25•167 mg/5 mL

nithiamide USAN *veterinary antibacterial* [also: aminitrozole; acinitrazole]

nitracrine INN

nitrafudam INN *antidepressant* [also: nitrafudam HCl]

nitrafudam HCl USAN *antidepressant* [also: nitrafudam]

nitralamine HCl USAN *antifungal*

nitramisole INN *anthelmintic* [also: nitramisole HCl]

nitramisole HCl USAN *anthelmintic* [also: nitramisole]

nitraquazone INN

nitrates *a class of antianginal agents that cause the relaxation of vascular smooth muscles*

nitratophenylmercury [see: phenylmercuric nitrate]

nitrazepam USAN, INN, BAN, JAN *anticonvulsant; hypnotic*

Nitrazine paper for professional use *in vitro diagnostic aid for urine pH determination*

nitre, sweet spirit of [see: ethyl nitrite]

nitrefazole INN, BAN

Nitrek transdermal patch ℞ *antianginal; vasodilator* [nitroglycerin] 22.4, 44.8, 67.2 mg (0.2, 0.4, 0.6 mg/hr.)

nitrendipine USAN, INN, BAN, JAN *antihypertensive; calcium channel blocker*

nitric acid NF *acidifying agent*

nitric oxide USAN *vasodilator; inhalation gas for neonatal hypoxic respiratory failure due to persistent pulmonary hypertension (orphan); investigational (orphan) for acute adult respiratory distress syndrome; investigational to prevent reperfusion injury following lung transplants*

nitricholine perchlorate INN

***p*-nitrobenzenearsonic acid** [see: nitarsone]

Nitro-Bid ointment ℞ *antianginal; vasodilator* [nitroglycerin] 2% (15 mg/inch) ⓢ Nicobid

Nitro-Bid IV infusion ℞ *antianginal; vasodilator; perioperative antihypertensive; for congestive heart failure with myocardial infarction* [nitroglycerin] 5 mg/mL

9-nitrocamptothecin (9-NC) [now: rubitecan]

nitroclofene INN

nitrocycline USAN, INN *antibacterial*

nitrodan USAN, INN *anthelmintic*

Nitro-Derm transdermal patch (discontinued 2000) ℞ *antianginal; vasodilator* [nitroglycerin] 160 mg (0.8 mg/hr.)

Nitrodisc transdermal patch ℞ *antianginal; vasodilator* [nitroglycerin] 16, 24, 32 mg (0.2, 0.3, 0.4 mg/hr.)

Nitro-Dur transdermal patch ℞ *antianginal; vasodilator* [nitroglycerin] 20, 40, 60, 80, 120, 160 mg (0.1, 0.2, 0.3, 0.4, 0.6, 0.8 mg/hr.)

nitroethanolamine [see: aminoethyl nitrate]

nitrofuradoxadone [see: furmethoxadone]

nitrofural INN *broad-spectrum bactericidal; adjunct to burn treatment* [also: nitrofurazone]

nitrofurantoin USP, INN *urinary antibiotic* 50, 100 mg oral

nitrofurantoin sodium *urinary antibiotic*

nitrofurazone USP, BAN *broad-spectrum bactericidal; adjunct to burn treatment and skin grafting* [also: nitrofural] 0.2% topical

nitrofurmethone [see: furaltadone]

nitrofuroxizone [see: nidroxyzone]

Nitrogard transmucosal extended-release tablets ℞ *antianginal; vasodilator* [nitroglycerin] 2, 3 mg

nitrogen (N_2) NF *air displacement agent; element (N)*

nitrogen monoxide [see: nitrous oxide]

nitrogen mustard N-oxide HCl JAN *alkylating antineoplastic* [also: mechlorethamine HCl; chlormethine; mustine]

nitrogen mustards *a class of alkylating antineoplastics*

nitrogen oxide (N_2O) [see: nitrous oxide]

nitroglycerin USP *coronary vasodilator; antianginal; antihypertensive* [also: glyceryl trinitrate] 2.5, 6.5, 9 mg oral; 5 mg/mL injection; 0.2, 0.4, 0.6 mg/hr. transdermal; 2% topical ⊡ Nitroglyn

Nitroglyn extended-release capsules ℞ *antianginal; vasodilator* [nitroglycerin] 2.5, 6.5, 9, 13 mg ⊡ nitroglycerin

nitrohydroxyquinoline [see: nitroxoline]

Nitrol ointment, Appli-Kit (ointment & adhesive dosage covers) ℞ *antianginal; vasodilator* [nitroglycerin] 2% (15 mg/inch)

Nitrolan liquid OTC *enteral nutritional therapy* [lactose-free formula]

Nitrolingual Pumpspray CFC-free translingual aerosol ℞ *antianginal; vasodilator* [nitroglycerin] 0.4 mg/spray

nitromannitol [see: mannitol hexanitrate]

nitromersol USP *topical anti-infective*

nitromide USAN *coccidiostat for poultry; antibacterial*

nitromifene INN

nitromifene citrate USAN *antiestrogen*

Nitrong sustained-release tablets ℞ *antianginal; vasodilator* [nitroglycerin] 2.6, 6.5, 9 mg

Nitropress powder for IV injection, flip-top vials ℞ *vasodilator for hypertensive emergency* [sodium nitroprusside] 50 mg/dose

nitroprusside sodium [see: sodium nitroprusside]

NitroQuick sublingual tablets ℞ *antianginal; vasodilator* [nitroglycerin] 0.3, 0.4, 0.6 mg (1/200, 1/150, 1/100 gr.)

nitroscanate USAN, INN *veterinary anthelmintic*

nitrosoureas *a class of alkylating antineoplastics*

Nitrostat sublingual tablets ℞ *antianginal; vasodilator* [nitroglycerin] 0.3, 0.4, 0.6 mg (1/200, 1/150, 1/100 gr.)

nitrosulfathiazole INN [also: paranitrosulfathiazole]

NitroTab sublingual tablets ℞ *antianginal; vasodilator* [nitroglycerin] 0.3, 0.4, 0.6 mg (1/200, 1/150, 1/100 gr.)

Nitro-Time extended-release capsules ℞ *antianginal; vasodilator* [nitroglycerin] 2.5, 6.5, 9 mg

nitrous acid, sodium salt [see: sodium nitrite]

nitrous oxide (N_2O) USP *a weak inhalation general anesthetic; sometimes abused as a street drug to create a dreamy or floating sensation*

nitroxinil INN

nitroxoline INN, BAN

nivacortol INN *corticosteroid; anti-inflammatory* [also: nivazol]

nivadipine [see: nilvadipine]

nivaquine [see: chloroquine phosphate]

nivazol USAN *corticosteroid; anti-inflammatory* [also: nivacortol]

Nivea After Tan; Nivea Moisturizing; Nivea Moisturizing Extra Enriched lotion OTC *moisturizer; emollient*

Nivea Moisturizing; Nivea Skin oil OTC *moisturizer; emollient*

Nivea Moisturizing Creme Soap bar OTC *therapeutic skin cleanser*

Nivea Ultra Moisturizing Creme OTC *moisturizer; emollient*

nivimedone sodium USAN *antiallergic*

nixylic acid INN

nizatidine USAN, USP, INN, BAN, JAN *histamine H_2 antagonist for gastric and duodenal ulcers*

nizofenone INN

Nizoral cream, shampoo ℞ *topical antifungal* [ketoconazole] 2%

Nizoral tablets ℞ *systemic imidazole antifungal* [ketoconazole] 200 mg

Nizoral A-D shampoo OTC *topical antifungal for dandruff* [ketoconazole] 1%

NMP-22 *investigational (NDA filed) bladder cancer test kit*

N-Multistix; N-Multistix SG reagent strips *in vitro diagnostic aid for multiple urine products*

NNRTIs (non-nucleoside reverse transcriptase inhibitors) [see: reverse transcriptase inhibitors]

No Pain-HP roll-on OTC *topical analgesic* [capsaicin] 0.075%

nobelium *element (No)*

noberastine USAN, INN, BAN *antihistamine*

noble yarrow *medicinal herb* [see: yarrow]

nocloprost INN

nocodazole USAN, INN *antineoplastic*

nodding wakerobin *medicinal herb* [see: birthroot]

NōDōz chewable tablets (discontinued 2001) OTC *CNS stimulant; analeptic* [caffeine] 100 mg

NōDōz coated caplets OTC *CNS stimulant; analeptic* [caffeine] 200 mg

nofecainide INN

nofetumomab merpentan *monoclonal antibody imaging agent for small cell lung cancer*

nogalamycin USAN, INN *antineoplastic*

No-Hist capsules ℞ *nasal decongestant* [phenylephrine HCl; phenylpropanolamine HCl; pseudoephedrine HCl] 5•40•40 mg

Nolahist tablets OTC *piperidine antihistamine for allergic rhinitis* [phenindamine tartrate] 25 mg

Nolamine timed-release tablets ℞ *decongestant; antihistamine* [phenylpropanolamine HCl; chlorpheniramine maleate; phenindamine tartrate] 50•4•24 mg

nolatrexed dihydrochloride *investigational (Phase III) antineoplastic*

nolinium bromide USAN, INN *antisecretory; antiulcerative*

Nolvadex tablets ℞ *antiestrogen antineoplastic for advanced postmenopausal breast cancer; breast cancer prevention for high-risk patients* [tamoxifen citrate] 10, 20 mg

nomegestrol INN

nomelidine INN

nomifensine INN *antidepressant* [also: nomifensine maleate]

nomifensine maleate USAN *antidepressant* [also: nomifensine]

nonabine INN, BAN

nonabsorbable surgical suture [see: suture, nonabsorbable surgical]

nonachlazine [now: azaclorzine HCl]

nonacog alfa USAN, INN *synthetic human blood coagulation factor IX; antihemophilic for hemophilia B and Christmas disease (orphan)*

nonanedioic acid [see: azelaic acid]

nonaperone INN

nonapyrimine INN

nonathymulin INN

nondestearinated cod liver oil [see: cod liver oil, nondestearinated]

Non-Habit Forming Stool Softener capsules OTC *laxative; stool softener* [docusate sodium] 100 mg

noni ***(Morinda citrifolia)*** berries *medicinal herb for arthritis, bacterial infections, diabetes, drug addiction, headache, hypertension, liver and skin disorders, pain, and slowing aging; also used as an antioxidant*

nonionic contrast media *a class of newer radiopaque agents that, in general, have a low osmolar concentration of iodine (the contrast agent), which corresponds to a lower incidence of adverse reactions* [also called: low osmolar contrast media (LOCM)]

nonivamide INN

non-nucleoside reverse transcriptase inhibitors (NNRTIs) [see: reverse transcriptase inhibitors]

nonoxinol 4 INN *surfactant* [also: nonoxynol 4]

nonoxinol 9 INN *wetting and solubilizing agent; spermaticide* [also: nonoxynol 9]

nonoxinol 15 INN *surfactant* [also: nonoxynol 15]

nonoxinol 30 INN *surfactant* [also: nonoxynol 30]

nonoxynol 4 USAN *surfactant* [also: nonoxinol 4]

nonoxynol 9 USAN, USP *wetting and solubilizing agent; spermicide* [also: nonoxinol 9]
nonoxynol 10 NF *surfactant*
nonoxynol 15 USAN *surfactant* [also: nonoxinol 15]
nonoxynol 30 USAN *surfactant* [also: nonoxinol 30]
nonsteroidal anti-inflammatory drugs (NSAIDs) *a class of anti-inflammatory drugs that have analgesic and antipyretic effects*
nonylphenoxypolyethoxyethanol [see: nonoxynol 4, 9, 15, & 30]
Nootropil ℞ *cognition adjuvant; investigational (orphan) for myoclonus* [piracetam]
nopal plant *medicinal herb for cleansing the lymphatic system, diabetes, digestion, obesity, neutralizing toxins, and preventing arteriosclerosis*
noracymethadol INN *analgesic* [also: noracymethadol HCl]
noracymethadol HCl USAN *analgesic* [also: noracymethadol]
noradrenaline bitartrate [see: norepinephrine bitartrate]
noramidopyrine methanesulfonate sodium [see: dipyrone]
norandrostenolone phenylpropionate [see: nandrolone phenpropionate]
norastemizole *investigational (Phase III) third generation, nonsedating antihistamine for allergy*
norbolethone USAN *anabolic* [also: norboletone]
norboletone INN *anabolic* [also: norbolethone]
norbudrine INN [also: norbutrine]
norbutrine BAN [also: norbudrine]
norclostebol INN
Norco tablets ℞ *narcotic analgesic* [hydrocodone bitartrate; acetaminophen] 5•325, 7.5•325, 10•325 mg
norcodeine INN, BAN
Norcuron powder for IV injection ℞ *nondepolarizing neuromuscular blocker; adjunct to anesthesia* [vecuronium bromide] 10, 20 mg/vial
norcycline [see: sancycline]
nordazepam INN
nordefrin HCl NF
Nordette tablets (in Pilpaks of 21 or 28) ℞ *monophasic oral contraceptive; emergency postcoital contraceptive* [levonorgestrel; ethinyl estradiol] 0.15 mg•30 µg
nordinone INN
NordiPen (trademarked device) *subcu self-injector for Norditropin*
Norditropin powder for subcu injection, prefilled cartridges for NordiPen (self-injection device) ℞ *growth hormone for adults or children with congenital or endogenous growth hormone deficiency and children with growth failure due to Turner syndrome or chronic renal insufficiency* [somatropin] 4, 8 mg (12, 24 IU) per vial; 5, 10, 15 mg (15, 30, 45 IU) per 1.5 mL cartridge
Norditropin SimpleXx subcu injection ℞ *investigational (NDA filed) growth hormone for adults or children with congenital or endogenous growth hormone deficiency, children with Turner syndrome or renal-induced growth failure, or AIDS-wasting syndrome (orphan)* [somatropin]
Norel capsules ℞ *decongestant; expectorant* [phenylephrine HCl; phenylpropanolamine HCl; guaifenesin] 5•45•200 mg
Norel Plus capsules ℞ *decongestant; antihistamine; analgesic* [phenylpropanolamine HCl; chlorpheniramine maleate; phenyltoloxamine dihydrogen citrate; acetaminophen] 25•4•25•325 mg
norelgestromin USAN *investigational progestin-type contraceptive*
norephedrine HCl [see: phenylpropanolamine HCl]
norepinephrine INN *adrenergic; vasoconstrictor; vasopressor for shock* [also: norepinephrine bitartrate]
norepinephrine bitartrate USAN, USP *adrenergic; vasoconstrictor; vasopressor*

for acute hypotensive shock [also: norepinephrine]

norethandrolone NF, INN

Norethin 1/35E tablets (discontinued 1999) ℞ *monophasic oral contraceptive* [norethindrone; ethinyl estradiol] 1 mg•35 µg

Norethin 1/50M tablets (discontinued 1999) ℞ *monophasic oral contraceptive* [norethindrone; mestranol] 1 mg•50 µg

norethindrone USP *progestin for amenorrhea, abnormal uterine bleeding, and endometriosis* [also: norethisterone]

norethindrone acetate USP *progestin for amenorrhea, abnormal uterine bleeding, and endometriosis* 5 mg oral

norethisterone INN, BAN, JAN *progestin* [also: norethindrone]

norethynodrel USAN, USP *progestin* [also: noretynodrel]

noretynodrel INN *progestin* [also: norethynodrel]

noreximide INN

norfenefrine INN

Norflex sustained-release tablets, IV or IM injection ℞ *skeletal muscle relaxant* [orphenadrine citrate] 100 mg; 30 mg/mL

norfloxacin USAN, USP, INN, BAN, JAN *broad-spectrum fluoroquinolone antibiotic*

norfloxacin succinil INN

norflurane USAN, INN *inhalation anesthetic*

Norforms powder (discontinued 1998) OTC *absorbs vaginal moisture; astringent* [cornstarch; zinc oxide]

Norforms vaginal suppositories OTC *feminine deodorant* [polyethylene glycol]

Norgesic; Norgesic Forte tablets ℞ *skeletal muscle relaxant; analgesic* [orphenadrine citrate; aspirin; caffeine] 25•385•30 mg; 50•770•60 mg

norgesterone INN

norgestimate USAN, INN, BAN *progestin*

norgestomet USAN, INN *progestin*

norgestrel USAN, USP, INN *progestin*

d-norgestrel *(incorrect enantiomer designation)* [now: levonorgestrel]

D-norgestrel [see: levonorgestrel]

norgestrienone INN

Norinyl 1 + 35 tablets (in packs of 21 or 28) ℞ *monophasic oral contraceptive* [norethindrone; ethinyl estradiol] 1 mg•35 µg ⑨ Nardil

Norinyl 1 + 50 tablets (in packs of 21 or 28) ℞ *monophasic oral contraceptive* [norethindrone; mestranol] 1 mg•50 µg

Norisodrine with Calcium Iodide syrup ℞ *bronchodilator; expectorant* [isoproterenol sulfate; calcium iodide; alcohol 6%] 3•150 mg

Noritate cream ℞ *antibacterial for inflammatory lesions and acne rosacea* [metronidazole (in an emollient base)] 1%

norletimol INN

norleusactide INN [also: pentacosactride]

norlevorphanol INN, BAN

norlupinanes *a class of antibiotics* [also called: quinolizidines]

½ normal saline (½ NS; 0.45% sodium chloride) *electrolyte replacement*

normal saline (NS; 0.9% sodium chloride) *electrolyte replacement* [also: saline solution]

normal serum albumin [see: albumin, human]

Normaline tablets OTC *sodium chloride replacement; dehydration preventative* [sodium chloride] 250 mg

normethadone INN, BAN

normethandrolone [see: normethandrone]

normethandrone

normethisterone [see: normethandrone]

Normiflo deep subcu injection in prefilled syringes (discontinued 2000) ℞ *a low molecular weight heparin–type anticoagulant for the prevention of deep vein thrombosis (DVT) following knee replacement surgery* [ardeparin sodium] 5000, 10 000 U/0.5 mL

Normix ℞ *investigational (orphan) antibacterial for hepatic encephalopathy* [rifaximin]

Normodyne film-coated tablets, IV infusion ℞ *antihypertensive; α- and β-blocker* [labetalol HCl] 100, 200, 300 mg; 5 mg/mL

normorphine INN, BAN

Normosang ℞ *investigational (orphan) for acute symptomatic porphyria and myelodysplastic syndrome* [heme arginate]

Normosol-M and 5% Dextrose; Normosol-R and 5% Dextrose IV infusion ℞ *intravenous nutritional/electrolyte therapy* [combined electrolyte solution; dextrose]

Normosol-R; Normosol-R pH 7.4 IV infusion ℞ *intravenous electrolyte therapy* [combined electrolyte solution]

Noroxin film-coated tablets ℞ *broad-spectrum fluoroquinolone antibiotic* [norfloxacin] 400 mg

Norpace capsules ℞ *antiarrhythmic* [disopyramide phosphate] 100, 150 mg

Norpace CR controlled-release capsules ℞ *antiarrhythmic* [disopyramide phosphate] 100, 500 mg

norpipanone INN, BAN

Norplant implantable Silastic capsules ℞ *long-term (5 year) contraceptive system* [levonorgestrel] 216 mg (6 × 36 mg)

Norpramin film-coated tablets ℞ *tricyclic antidepressant* [desipramine HCl] 10, 25, 50, 75, 100, 150 mg ⑨ imipramine

norpseudoephedrine [see: cathine]

Nor-Q.D. tablets (in packs of 28) ℞ *oral contraceptive (progestin only)* [norethindrone] 0.35 mg

nortestosterone phenylpropionate [see: nandrolone phenpropionate]

Nor-Tet capsules ℞ *broad-spectrum antibiotic* [tetracycline HCl] 250, 500 mg

nortetrazepam INN

Nortrel tablets ℞ *monophasic oral contraceptive* [norethindrone; ethinyl estradiol] 0.5 mg•35 μg, 1 mg•35 μg

nortriptyline HCl USAN, USP, INN *tricyclic antidepressant* 10, 25, 50, 75 mg oral; 10 mg/5 mL oral ⑨ amitriptyline

Norvasc tablets ℞ *antianginal; antihypertensive; calcium channel blocker* [amlodipine] 2.5, 5, 10 mg

norvinisterone INN

norvinodrel [see: norgesterone]

Norvir soft capsules, oral solution ℞ *antiviral protease inhibitor for HIV infection* [ritonavir] 100 mg; 80 mg/mL

Norway pine; Norway spruce *medicinal herb* [see: spruce]

Norwich tablets OTC *analgesic; antipyretic; anti-inflammatory; antirheumatic* [aspirin] 325, 500 mg

Norzine IM injection, suppositories, tablets ℞ *antiemetic* [thiethylperazine maleate] 5 mg/mL; 10 mg; 10 mg

NoSalt; NoSalt Seasoned (discontinued 1997) OTC *salt substitute* [potassium chloride] 64 mEq/5 g; 34 mEq/5 g

nosantine INN, BAN

noscapine USP, INN *antitussive*

noscapine HCl NF

nosebleed *medicinal herb* [see: yarrow]

nosiheptide USAN, INN *veterinary growth stimulant*

Nōstril; Children's Nōstril nasal spray OTC *nasal decongestant* [phenylephrine HCl] 0.5%; 0.25%

Nōstrilla nasal spray OTC *nasal decongestant* [oxymetazoline HCl] 0.05%

notensil maleate [see: acepromazine]

Novacet lotion ℞ *topical acne treatment* [sulfacetamide sodium; sulfur] 10%•5%

Nova-Dec tablets OTC *vitamin/mineral/iron supplement* [multiple vitamins & minerals; iron; folic acid; biotin] ≛•30 mg•0.4 mg•30 μg

Novafed A sustained-release capsules ℞ *decongestant; antihistamine* [pseudoephedrine HCl; chlorpheniramine maleate] 120•8 mg

Novagest Expectorant with Codeine liquid ℞ *narcotic antitussive; decongestant; expectorant* [codeine phosphate; pseudoephedrine HCl; guaifenesin; alcohol 1.4%] 10•30•100 mg/5 mL

Novahistine elixir (discontinued 1997) OTC *decongestant; antihistamine* [phenylephrine HCl; chlorpheniramine maleate] 5•2 mg/5 mL

Novahistine DH syrup ℞ *narcotic antitussive; decongestant; antihistamine* [codeine phosphate; pseudoephedrine HCl; chlorpheniramine maleate; alcohol 5%] 10•30•2 mg/5 mL

Novahistine DMX oral liquid OTC *antitussive; decongestant; expectorant* [dextromethorphan hydrobromide; pseudoephedrine HCl; guaifenesin; alcohol 5%] 10•30•100 mg/5 mL

Novahistine Expectorant liquid (discontinued 1997) ℞ *narcotic antitussive; decongestant; expectorant* [codeine phosphate; pseudoephedrine HCl; guaifenesin; alcohol 7.5%] 10•30•100 mg/5 mL

novamidon [see: aminopyrine]

Novamine; Novamine 15% IV infusion ℞ *total parenteral nutrition; peripheral parenteral nutrition* [multiple essential and nonessential amino acids]

Novamoxin (CAN) capsules, chewable tablets, oral suspension ℞ *aminopenicillin antibiotic* [amoxicillin trihydrate] 250, 500 mg; 125, 250 mg; 125, 250 mg/5 mL

Novantrone IV infusion ℞ *antibiotic antineoplastic for prostate cancer or acute nonlymphocytic leukemia (ANL) (orphan); treatment for progressive and relapsing-remitting multiple sclerosis* [mitoxantrone HCl] 2 mg/mL

Novapren ℞ *investigational (Phase I) antiviral for HIV*

Novarel powder for IM injection ℞ *hormone for prepubertal cryptorchidism and hypogonadism; ovulation stimulant; testosterone stimulant* [chorionic gonadotropin] 1000 U/mL

Novasen (CAN) enteric-coated tablets OTC *analgesic; antipyretic; anti-inflammatory; antirheumatic* [aspirin] 325, 650 mg

NovaSource Renal oral liquid in Brik Paks OTC *enteral nutritional therapy for renal failure* 237 mL

Novastan (name changed to Acova upon marketing release in 2000) ⓓ Neovastat; Ovastat

novel (atypical) antipsychotics *a class of agents with a high affinity to the serotonin receptors and varying degrees of affinity to other neurotransmitter receptors; "atypical" due to the low incidence of extrapyramidal side effects (EPS)* [compare to: conventional (typical) antipsychotics]

Novo-Amiodarone (CAN) tablets ℞ *antiarrhythmic* [amiodarone HCl] 200 mg

novobiocin INN, BAN *bacteriostatic antibiotic* [also: novobiocin calcium]

novobiocin calcium USP *bacteriostatic antibiotic* [also: novobiocin]

novobiocin sodium USP *bacteriostatic antibiotic*

Novocain injection ℞ *injectable local anesthetic* [procaine HCl] 1%, 2%, 10%

Novo-Cefaclor (CAN) capsules ℞ *cephalosporin antibiotic* [cefaclor] 250, 500 mg

Novo-Cefadroxil (CAN) capsules ℞ *cephalosporin antibiotic* [cefadroxil] 500 mg

Novo-Clonazepam (CAN) tablets ℞ *anticonvulsant* [clonazepam] 0.5, 2 mg

Novo-Cyproterone (CAN) tablets ℞ *antiandrogen antineoplastic for advanced prostatic carcinoma* [cyproterone acetate] 50 mg

Novo-Difenac-K (CAN) tablets ℞ *analgesic; antiarthritic; nonsteroidal anti-inflammatory drug (NSAID)* [diclofenac potassium] 50 mg

Novo-Diltiazem CD (CAN) (once daily) controlled-delivery capsules ℞ *antihypertensive; antianginal; antiarrhythmic; calcium channel blocker* [diltiazem HCl] 120, 180, 240, 300 mg

Novo-Divalproex (CAN) enteric-coated tablets ℞ *anticonvulsant* [divalproex sodium] 125, 250, 500 mg

Novo-Domperidone (CAN) film-coated tablets ℞ *antiemetic for diabetic gas-*

troparesis and chronic gastritis [domperidone maleate] 10 mg

Novo-Fluvoxamine (CAN) tablets ℞ *selective serotonin reuptake inhibitor (SSRI) for depression and obsessive-compulsive disorder (OCD)* [fluvoxamine maleate] 50, 100 mg

Novo-Gemfibrozil (CAN) capsules, tablets ℞ *antihyperlipidemic for hypertriglyceridemia and coronary heart disease* [gemfibrozil] 300 mg; 600 mg

Novo-Glyburide (CAN) tablets ℞ *sulfonylurea antidiabetic* [glyburide] 2.5, 5 mg

Novo-Hydrazide (CAN) tablets ℞ *antihypertensive; diuretic* [hydrochlorothiazide] 25, 50 mg

Novo-Ketoconazole (CAN) tablets ℞ *broad-spectrum antifungal* [ketoconazole] 200 mg

Novolin 70/30 vials for subcu injection, Penfill (prefilled cartridges for NovoPen), prefilled syringes OTC *antidiabetic* [isophane human insulin (rDNA); human insulin (rDNA)] 100 U/mL; 1.5, 3 mL; 1.5 mL

Novolin 85/15 Penfill (prefilled cartridges for NovoPen) OTC *investigational (NDA filed) antidiabetic* [isophane human insulin (rDNA); human insulin (rDNA)]

Novolin ge 10/90 (CAN) Penfill (prefilled cartridges for NovoPen) OTC *antidiabetic* [human insulin (rDNA); isophane human insulin (rDNA)] 3 mL

Novolin ge 20/80 (CAN) Penfill (prefilled cartridges for NovoPen) OTC *antidiabetic* [human insulin (rDNA); isophane human insulin (rDNA)] 3 mL

Novolin ge 30/70 (CAN) vials for subcu injection, Penfill (prefilled cartridges for NovoPen) OTC *antidiabetic* [human insulin (rDNA); isophane human insulin (rDNA)] 100 U/mL; 1.5, 3 mL

Novolin ge 40/60 (CAN) Penfill (prefilled cartridges for NovoPen) OTC *antidiabetic* [human insulin (rDNA); isophane human insulin (rDNA)] 3 mL

Novolin ge 50/50 (CAN) Penfill (prefilled cartridges for NovoPen) OTC *antidiabetic* [human insulin (rDNA); isophane human insulin (rDNA)] 3 mL

Novolin ge Lente (CAN) vials for subcu injection OTC *antidiabetic* [human insulin zinc (rDNA)] 100 U/mL

Novolin ge NPH (CAN) vials for subcu injection, Penfill (prefilled cartridges for NovoPen) OTC *antidiabetic* [isophane human insulin (rDNA)] 100 U/mL; 1.5, 3 mL

Novolin ge Toronto (CAN) vials for subcu injection, Penfill (prefilled cartridges for NovoPen) OTC *antidiabetic* [human insulin (rDNA)] 100 U/mL; 1.5, 3 mL

Novolin ge Ultralente (CAN) vials for subcu injection OTC *antidiabetic* [human insulin zinc (rDNA)] 100 U/mL

Novolin L vials for subcu injection OTC *antidiabetic* [human insulin zinc (rDNA)] 100 U/mL

Novolin N vials for subcu injection, Penfill (prefilled cartridges for NovoPen), prefilled syringes OTC *antidiabetic* [isophane human insulin (rDNA)] 100 U/mL; 1.5, 3 mL; 1.5 mL

Novolin R vials for subcu injection, Penfill (prefilled cartridges for NovoPen), prefilled syringes OTC *antidiabetic* [human insulin (rDNA)] 100 U/mL; 1.5, 3 mL; 1.5 mL

NovoLog vials for subcu injection, Penfill (prefilled cartridges for NovoPen) ℞ *rapid-acting insulin analogue for diabetes* [human insulin aspart (rDNA)] 100 U/mL; 3 mL

Novo-Lorazem (CAN) tablets ℞ *benzodiazepine anxiolytic* [lorazepam] 0.5, 1, 2 mg

Novo-Medrone (CAN) tablets ℞ *progestin for secondary amenorrhea, abnormal uterine bleeding, and endometrial hyperplasia* [medroxyprogesterone acetate] 2.5, 5, 10 mg

Novo-Metformin (CAN) film-coated tablets ℞ *biguanide antidiabetic* [metformin HCl] 500, 850 mg

Novo-Metoprol (CAN) tablets, film-coated caplets ℞ *antihypertensive;*

antianginal; antiadrenergic (β-blocker) [metoprolol tartrate] 50, 100 mg

Novo-Moclobemide (CAN) tablets ℞ *antidepressant* [moclobemide] 100, 150, 300 mg

Novo-Naprox (CAN) tablets ℞ *analgesic; antiarthritic; nonsteroidal anti-inflammatory drug (NSAID)* [naproxen] 125, 250, 375, 500 mg

Novo-Naprox-EC (CAN) enteric-coated tablets ℞ *analgesic; antiarthritic; nonsteroidal anti-inflammatory drug (NSAID)* [naproxen] 250, 375, 500 mg

Novo-Naprox SR (CAN) sustained-release tablets ℞ *analgesic; antiarthritic; nonsteroidal anti-inflammatory drug (NSAID)* [naproxen] 750 mg

Novo-Nizatidine (CAN) capsules ℞ *histamine H_2 antagonist for treatment of gastric and duodenal ulcers* [nizatidine] 150, 300 mg

Novo-Norfloxacin (CAN) tablets ℞ *broad-spectrum fluoroquinolone antibiotic* [norfloxacin] 400 mg

NovoNorm (European name for U.S. product Prandin)

Novopaque oral/rectal suspension ℞ *radiopaque contrast medium for gastrointestinal imaging* [barium sulfate] 60%

NovoPen 1.5 prefilled reusable syringe *uses Novolin PenFill cartridges and NovoFine 30-gauge disposable needles* [insulin (several types available)] 1–40 U/injection

Novo-Ranidine (CAN) film-coated tablets ℞ *histamine H_2 antagonist for gastric and duodenal ulcers* [ranitidine HCl] 150, 300 mg

NovoRapid (European name for U.S. product NovoLog)

Novo-Salmol (CAN) tablets ℞ *sympathomimetic bronchodilator* [salbutamol sulfate] 2, 4 mg

Novo-Semide (CAN) tablets ℞ *antihypertensive; loop diuretic* [furosemide] 20, 40, 80 mg

Novo-Sertraline (CAN) capsules ℞ *selective serotonin reuptake inhibitor (SSRI) for depression* [sertraline HCl] 25, 50, 100 mg

NovoSeven powder for IV injection ℞ *coagulant for hemophilia A and B (orphan); investigational (orphan) for von Willebrand disease* [factor VIIa, recombinant] 1.2, 4.8 mg/vial

Novo-Terazosin (CAN) tablets ℞ *antihypertensive (α-blocker); treatment for benign prostatic hyperplasia (BPH)* [terazosin HCl] 1, 2, 5, 10 mg

Novo-Timol (CAN) eye drops (discontinued 2001) ℞ *topical antiglaucoma agent (β-blocker)* [timolol maleate] 0.25%, 0.5%

Novo-Triptyn (CAN) tablets ℞ *tricyclic antidepressant* [amitriptyline HCl] 10, 25, 50 mg

NovoVac ℞ *investigational (Phase I/II) antibody vaccine for melanoma*

Novoxapam (CAN) tablets ℞ *benzodiazepine anxiolytic* [oxazepam] 10, 15, 30 mg

NOVP (Novantrone, Oncovin, vinblastine, prednisone) *chemotherapy protocol for Hodgkin lymphoma*

noxiptiline INN [also: noxiptyline]

noxiptyline BAN [also: noxiptiline]

noxythiolin BAN [also: noxytiolin]

noxytiolin INN [also: noxythiolin]

NP (nifurpipone) [q.v.]

NP-27 solution, powder, spray powder, cream (discontinued 1998) OTC *topical antifungal* [tolnaftate] 1%

NPH (neutral protamine Hagedorn) insulin [see: insulin, isophane]

NPH Iletin I subcu injection (discontinued 1999) OTC *antidiabetic* [isophane insulin (beef-pork)] 100 U/mL

NPH Iletin II subcu injection OTC *antidiabetic* [isophane insulin (pork)] 100 U/mL

NPH Insulin subcu injection (discontinued 1997) OTC *antidiabetic* [isophane insulin (beef)] 100 U/mL

NPH-N subcu injection (discontinued 2000) OTC *antidiabetic* [isophane insulin (pork)] 100 U/mL

NRTIs (nucleoside reverse transcriptase inhibitors) [see: reverse transcriptase inhibitors]

NS (normal saline) [q.v.]

NS-2710 *investigational (Phase II) anxiolytic*

NSAIDs (nonsteroidal anti-inflammatory drugs) [q.v.] ⑨ InFeD

NTBC *investigational (orphan) for tyrosinemia type I*

NTZ (nitazoxanide) [q.v.]

NTZ Long Acting nasal spray, nose drops OTC *nasal decongestant* [oxymetazoline HCl] 0.05%

Nubain IV, subcu or IM injection ℞ *narcotic agonist-antagonist analgesic* [nalbuphine HCl] 10, 20 mg/mL

Nu-Beclomethasone (CAN) nasal spray ℞ *corticosteroidal anti-inflammatory for chronic asthma and rhinitis* [beclomethasone dipropionate] 50 μg/metered dose

nucleoside reverse transcriptase inhibitors (NRTIs) [see: reverse transcriptase inhibitors]

nuclomedone INN

nuclotixene INN

Nucofed capsules, syrup ℞ *narcotic antitussive; decongestant* [codeine phosphate; pseudoephedrine HCl] 20•60 mg; 20•60 mg/5 mL

Nucofed Expectorant; Nucofed Pediatric Expectorant syrup ℞ *narcotic antitussive; decongestant; expectorant* [codeine phosphate; pseudoephedrine HCl; guaifenesin; alcohol 12.5%-6%] 20•60•200 mg/5 mL; 10•30•100 mg/5 mL

Nucotuss Expectorant; Nucotuss Pediatric Expectorant liquid *narcotic antitussive; decongestant; expectorant* [codeine phosphate; pseudoephedrine HCl; guaifenesin; alcohol 12.5%-6%] 20•60•200 mg/5 mL; 10•30•100 mg/5 mL

Nu-Diltiaz-CD (CAN) capsules ℞ *antihypertensive; antianginal* [diltiazem HCl] 120, 180, 240 mg

Nu-Divalproex (CAN) tablets ℞ *anticonvulsant* [divalproex sodium] 125, 250, 500 mg

Nu-Enalapril (CAN) tablets ℞ *antihypertensive; angiotensin-converting enzyme (ACE) inhibitor* [enalapril maleate]

nufenoxole USAN, INN *antiperistaltic*

Nu-Fluvoxamine (CAN) tablets ℞ *selective serotonin reuptake inhibitor (SSRI) for depression and obsessive-compulsive disorder (OCD)* [fluvoxamine maleate]

Nu-Iron elixir OTC *hematinic; iron supplement* [polysaccharide-iron complex] 100 mg/5 mL

Nu-Iron 150 capsules OTC *hematinic; iron supplement* [polysaccharide-iron complex] 150 mg

Nu-Iron Plus elixir ℞ *hematinic* [polysaccharide-iron complex; cyanocobalamin; folic acid] 300 mg•75 μg•3 mg per 15 mL

Nu-Iron V film-coated tablets ℞ *vitamin/iron supplement* [polysaccharide-iron complex; multiple vitamins; folic acid] 60•≛•1 mg

Nu-knit (trademarked form) *oxidized cellulose hemostatic pad*

NuLev orally disintegrating tablets ℞ *GI/GU antispasmodic; antiparkinsonian; anticholinergic "drying agent" for allergic rhinitis* [hyoscyamine sulfate] 0.125 mg

NuLytely powder for oral solution ℞ *pre-procedure bowel evacuant* [polyethylene glycol–electrolyte solution (PEG 3350)] 60, 105 g/L

Nu-Moclobemide (CAN) tablets ℞ *antidepressant* [moclobemide] 100, 150 mg

Numorphan IV, IM, or subcu injection, suppositories ℞ *narcotic analgesic; preoperative support of anesthesia; investigational (orphan) for intractable pain in narcotic-tolerant patients* [oxymorphone HCl] 1, 1.5 mg/mL; 5 mg

Numzident gel OTC *topical oral anesthetic* [benzocaine] 10%

Numzit Teething gel OTC *topical oral anesthetic* [benzocaine] 7.5%

Numzit Teething lotion OTC *topical oral anesthetic* [benzocaine; alcohol 12.1%] 0.2%

Nupercainal ointment, cream OTC *topical local anesthetic* [dibucaine] 1%; 0.5%

Nupercainal rectal suppositories OTC *emollient; astringent* [cocoa butter; zinc oxide] 2.1•0.25 g

Nuprin tablets, caplets OTC *analgesic; antiarthritic; antipyretic; nonsteroidal anti-inflammatory drug (NSAID)* [ibuprofen] 200 mg

Nuprin Backache caplets OTC *analgesic; antipyretic; anti-inflammatory* [magnesium salicylate] 580 mg

Nu-Prochlor (CAN) film-coated tablets ℞ *conventional (typical) antipsychotic; antiemetic* [prochlorperazine bimaleate] 5, 10 mg

Nuquin HP cream, gel ℞ *hyperpigmentation bleaching agent; sunscreen* [hydroquinone; dioxybenzone] 4%•30 mg

Nuromax IV injection ℞ *nondepolarizing neuromuscular blocker; adjunct to anesthesia* [doxacurium chloride] 1 mg/mL

Nursette (trademarked form) *prefilled disposable bottle*

Nu-Salt OTC *salt substitute* [potassium chloride] 68 mEq/5 g

nut, oil *medicinal herb* [see: butternut]

Nu-Tears eye drops OTC *ophthalmic moisturizer/lubricant* [polyvinyl alcohol] 1.4%

Nu-Tears II eye drops OTC *ophthalmic moisturizer/lubricant* [polyvinyl alcohol; polyethylene glycol 400] 1%•1%

Nu-Timolol (CAN) tablets ℞ *antihypertensive; antiadrenergic (β-blocker); migraine prophylaxis* [timolol maleate] 5, 10, 20 mg

nutmeg *(Myristica fragrans)* seed and aril *medicinal herb for diarrhea, flatulence, inducing expectoration, insomnia, mouth sores, rheumatism, salivary stimulation, and stimulating menstruation*

nutmeg oil NF

Nutracort cream ℞ *topical corticosteroidal anti-inflammatory* [hydrocortisone] 1%

Nutracort lotion (discontinued 1997) ℞ *topical corticosteroidal anti-inflammatory* [hydrocortisone] 1%

Nutraderm cream, lotion OTC *moisturizer; emollient*

Nutraderm OTC *lotion base*

Nutraderm Bath Oil OTC *bath emollient*

Nutraloric powder OTC *enteral nutritional therapy* [milk-based formula]

Nutramigen liquid, powder OTC *hypoallergenic infant food* [enzymatically hydrolyzed protein formula]

Nutraplus cream, lotion OTC *moisturizer; emollient; keratolytic* [urea] 10%

Nutra-Soothe bath oil OTC *bath emollient* [colloidal oatmeal; light mineral oil]

Nutren 1.0 liquid OTC *enteral nutritional therapy* [lactose-free formula]

Nutren 1.5 liquid OTC *enteral nutritional therapy* [lactose-free formula]

Nutren 2.0 ready-to-use liquid OTC *enteral nutritional therapy* [lactose-free formula]

Nutricon tablets OTC *vitamin/mineral/calcium/iron supplement* [multiple vitamins & minerals; calcium; iron; folic acid; biotin] ≛•200•20•0.4•0.15 mg

Nutrilan ready-to-use liquid OTC *enteral nutritional therapy* [lactose-free formula]

Nutrilyte; Nutrilyte II IV admixture ℞ *intravenous electrolyte therapy* [combined electrolyte solution]

Nutrineal Peritoneal Dialysis Solution with 1.1% Amino Acid ℞ *investigational (orphan) nutritional supplement for continuous ambulatory peritoneal dialysis patients*

Nutropin powder for subcu injection ℞ *growth hormone for adults or children with congenital or endogenous growth hormone deficiency, children with Turner syndrome or renal-induced growth failure* [somatropin] 5, 10 mg (15, 30 IU) per vial

Nutropin AQ subcu injection ℞ *growth hormone for congenital or renal-induced growth failure and Turner syndrome (orphan); investigational (orphan) for severe burns* [somatropin] 10 mg (30 IU) per vial

Nutropin Depot sustained-release subcu injection ℞ *once- or twice-monthly doseform of Nutropin* [somatropin] 13.5, 18, 22.5 mg

Nutrox capsules OTC *dietary supplement* [multiple vitamins & minerals; multiple amino acids] ≛

Nu-Valproic (CAN) capsules ℞ *anticonvulsant* [valproic acid] 250 mg

Nuvance ℞ *investigational (Phase II) treatment for allergy, asthma, transplant rejection, and infectious diseases* [interleukin-4 receptor]

nuvenzepine INN

Nuvion ℞ *investigational monoclonal antibody for organ transplants, autoimmune diseases, and other T-lymphocyte disorders* [visilizumab]

nyctal [see: carbromal]

nydrane [see: benzchlorpropamid]

Nydrazid IM injection ℞ *tuberculostatic* [isoniazid] 100 mg/mL

nylestriol USAN *estrogen* [also: nilestriol]

nylidrin HCl USP *peripheral vasodilator* [also: buphenine]

Nymphaea odorata *medicinal herb* [see: white pond lilly]

Nyotran ℞ *investigational (NDA filed) systemic antifungal for Aspergillus fumigatus infections; investigational (Phase III) for cryptococcal meningitis* [nystatin, liposomal]

NyQuil Hot Therapy powder for oral solution OTC *antitussive; decongestant; antihistamine; analgesic* [dextromethorphan hydrobromide; pseudoephedrine HCl; doxylamine succinate; acetaminophen] 30•60•12.5•1000 mg/packet

NyQuil LiquiCaps (liquid-filled capsules) OTC *antitussive; decongestant; antihistamine; analgesic* [dextromethorphan hydrobromide; pseudoephedrine HCl; doxylamine succinate; acetaminophen] 10•30•6.25•250 mg

NyQuil Multisymptom Cold Flu Relief; NyQuil Nighttime Cold/Flu Medicine liquid OTC *antitussive; decongestant; antihistamine; analgesic* [dextromethorphan hydrobromide; pseudoephedrine HCl; doxylamine succinate; acetaminophen; alcohol 10%-25%] 5•10•2.1•167 mg/5 mL; 5•10•1.25•167 mg/5 mL

NyQuil Nighttime Cough/Cold, Children's liquid OTC *pediatric antitussive, decongestant, and antihistamine* [dextromethorphan hydrobromide; pseudoephedrine HCl; chlorpheniramine maleate] 5•10•0.67 mg/5 mL

nystatin USP, INN, BAN, JAN *polyene antifungal* 500 000 U oral; 100 000 U vaginal; 100 000 U/g topical ⑨ Nilstat; Nitrostat

Nystatin-LF (liposomal formulation) IV injection ℞ *investigational (NDA filed) systemic therapy for fungal infections; investigational (Phase II) antiviral for HIV* [nystatin]

Nystex cream, ointment ℞ *topical antifungal* [nystatin] 100 000 U/g

Nystex oral suspension ℞ *antifungal; oral candidiasis treatment* [nystatin] 100 000 U/mL

Nytcold Medicine liquid OTC *antitussive; decongestant; antihistamine; analgesic* [dextromethorphan hydrobromide; pseudoephedrine HCl; doxylamine succinate; acetaminophen; alcohol 25%] 5•10•1.25•167 mg/5 mL

Nytol tablets OTC *antihistaminic sleep aid* [diphenhydramine HCl] 25, 50 mg

NZ-1001 *investigational (orphan) phosphorylated enzyme replacement therapy for Pompe disease*

NZGLM (New Zealand green-lipped mussel) [q.v.]

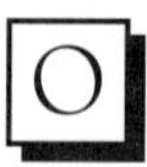

O_2 (oxygen) [q.v.]
oak *medicinal herb* [see: white oak]
OAP (Oncovin, ara-C, prednisone) *chemotherapy protocol*
oatmeal, colloidal *demulcent*
oats (*Avena sativa*) grain and straw *medicinal herb for dry itchy skin, hyperlipidemia, indigestion, insomnia, nervousness, opium addiction, reducing the desire to smoke, and strengthening the heart*
obecalp *placebo (spelled backward)*
Obenix capsules ℞ *anorexiant; CNS stimulant* [phentermine HCl] 37.5 mg
Obephen capsules (discontinued 1997) ℞ *anorexiant; CNS stimulant* [phentermine HCl] 30 mg
obidoxime chloride USAN, INN *cholinesterase reactivator*
Oby-Cap capsules (discontinued 1998) ℞ *anorexiant; CNS stimulant* [phentermine HCl] 30 mg
O-Cal f.a. tablets ℞ *vitamin/mineral/calcium/iron supplement and dental caries preventative* [multiple vitamins & minerals; calcium; iron; folic acid; sodium fluoride] ≛ •200•66•1•1.1 mg
ocaperidone USAN, INN, BAN *antipsychotic*
Occlusal-HP liquid OTC *topical keratolytic* [salicylic acid in polyacrylic vehicle] 17%
Occucoat ophthalmic solution ℞ *ophthalmic surgical aid* [hydroxypropyl methylcellulose] 2%
Ocean Mist nasal spray OTC *nasal moisturizer* [sodium chloride (saline solution)] 0.65%
ocfentanil INN *narcotic analgesic* [also: ocfentanil HCl]
ocfentanil HCl USAN *narcotic analgesic* [also: ocfentanil]
ociltide INN
Ocimum basilicum *medicinal herb* [see: basil]
ocinaplon USAN *anxiolytic*
OCL oral solution ℞ *pre-procedure bowel evacuant* [polyethylene glycol–electrolyte solution (PEG 3350)] 60 g/L
ocrase INN
ocrilate INN *tissue adhesive* [also: ocrylate]
ocrylate USAN *tissue adhesive* [also: ocrilate]
OCT (22-oxacalcitriol) [see: maxacalcitol]
octabenzone USAN, INN *ultraviolet screen*
octacaine INN
octacosactrin BAN [also: tosactide]
octacosanol (wheat germ oil) *natural supplement for increasing muscle endurance*
octadecafluorodecehydronaphthalene [see: perflunafene]
octadecanoic acid, calcium salt [see: calcium stearate]
octadecanoic acid, sodium salt [see: sodium stearate]
octadecanoic acid, zinc salt [see: zinc stearate]
1-octadecanol [see: stearyl alcohol]
9-octadecenylamine hydrofluoride [see: dectaflur]
octafonium chloride INN
Octamide PFS IV or IM injection ℞ *antiemetic for chemotherapy; GI stimulant; peristaltic* [metoclopramide HCl] 5 mg/mL
octamoxin INN
octamylamine INN
octanoic acid USAN, INN *antifungal*
octapinol INN
octastine INN
octatropine methylbromide INN, BAN *anticholinergic; peptic ulcer adjunct* [also: anisotropine methylbromide]
octatropone bromide [see: anisotropine methylbromide]
octaverine INN, BAN
octazamide USAN, INN *analgesic*
octenidine INN, BAN *topical anti-infective* [also: octenidine HCl]

octenidine HCl USAN *topical anti-infective* [also: octenidine]
octenidine saccharin USAN *dental plaque inhibitor*
Octicare ear drops, ear drop suspension ℞ *topical corticosteroidal anti-inflammatory; antibiotic* [hydrocortisone; neomycin sulfate; polymyxin B sulfate] 1%•5 mg•10 000 U per mL
octicizer USAN *plasticizer*
octil INN *combining name for radicals or groups*
octimibate INN
octinoxate USAN *ultraviolet B sunscreen*
octisalate USAN *ultraviolet sunscreen*
octisamyl [see: octamylamine]
Octocaine HCl injection ℞ *injectable local anesthetic* [lidocaine HCl; epinephrine] 2%•1:50 000, 2%•1:100 000
octoclothepine [see: clorotepine]
octocrilene INN *ultraviolet screen* [also: octocrylene]
octocrylene USAN *ultraviolet screen* [also: octocrilene]
octodecactide [see: codactide]
octodrine USAN, INN *adrenergic; vasoconstrictor; local anesthetic*
octopamine INN
octotiamine INN
octoxinol INN *surfactant/wetting agent* [also: octoxynol 9]
octoxynol 9 USAN, NF *surfactant/wetting agent; spermicide* [also: octoxinol]
OctreoScan powder for injection ℞ *radiopaque contrast medium* [oxidronate sodium] 2 mg
OctreoScan 111 ℞ *investigational radioactive imaging agent for SPECT scans of neuroendocrine tumors* [indium In 111 pentetreotide]
octreotide USAN, INN, BAN *gastric antisecretory*
octreotide acetate USAN *gastric antisecretory for acromegaly and severe diarrhea due to VIPomas and other tumors (orphan)*
octreotide pamoate USAN *antineoplastic*
octriptyline INN *antidepressant* [also: octriptyline phosphate]
octriptyline phosphate USAN *antidepressant* [also: octriptyline]
octrizole USAN, INN *ultraviolet screen*
octyl methoxycinnamate [see: octinoxate]
octyl salicylate [see: octisalate]
***S*-octyl thiobenzoate** [see: tioctilate]
octyl-2-cyanoacrylate [see: ocrylate]
octyldodecanol NF *oleaginous vehicle*
OcuCaps caplets OTC *vitamin/mineral supplement* [vitamins A, C, and E; multiple minerals] 5000 IU•400 mg•182 mg•≛
OcuClear eye drops OTC *topical ophthalmic decongestant and vasoconstrictor* [oxymetazoline HCl] 0.025%
OcuCoat prefilled syringe OTC *ophthalmic surgical aid* [hydroxypropyl methylcellulose] 2%
OcuCoat; OcuCoat PF eye drops OTC *ophthalmic moisturizer/lubricant* [hydroxypropyl methylcellulose] 0.8%
Ocudose (trademarked delivery device) *single-use eye drop dispenser*
Ocufen eye drops ℞ *topical ophthalmic nonsteroidal anti-inflammatory drug (NSAID); intraoperative miosis inhibitor* [flurbiprofen sodium] 0.03%
ocufilcon A USAN *hydrophilic contact lens material*
ocufilcon B USAN *hydrophilic contact lens material*
ocufilcon C USAN *hydrophilic contact lens material*
ocufilcon D USAN *hydrophilic contact lens material*
ocufilcon F USAN *hydrophilic contact lens material*
Ocuflox eye drops ℞ *topical fluoroquinolone antibiotic for bacterial conjunctivitis and corneal ulcers (orphan)* [ofloxacin] 0.3%
Ocumeter (trademarked delivery device) *prefilled eye drop dispenser*
Ocupress eye drops ℞ *topical antiglaucoma agent (β-blocker)* [carteolol HCl] 1%
Ocusert Pilo-20; Ocusert Pilo-40 continuous-release ocular wafer ℞ *topical antiglaucoma agent; direct-act-*

ing miotic [pilocarpine] 20 μg/hr.; 40 μg/hr.

OCuSOFT solution, pads OTC *eyelid cleanser for blepharitis or contact lenses*

OCuSoft VMS film-coated tablets OTC *vitamin/mineral supplement* [vitamins A, C, and E; multiple minerals] 5000 IU•60 mg•30 mg•≛

Ocusulf-10 eye drops ℞ *topical ophthalmic antibiotic* [sulfacetamide sodium] 10%

Ocutears (CAN) eye drops (discontinued 1998) OTC *ophthalmic moisturizer/lubricant* [hydroxypropyl methylcellulose] 0.5%

Ocutricin ophthalmic ointment ℞ *topical ophthalmic antibiotic* [polymyxin B sulfate; neomycin sulfate; bacitracin zinc] 10 000 U•3.5 mg•400 U per g

Ocuvite film-coated tablets OTC *vitamin/mineral supplement* [vitamins A, C, and E; multiple minerals] 5000 IU•60 mg•30 IU•≛

Ocuvite Extra tablets OTC *vitamin/mineral supplement* [vitamins A, C, and E; multiple minerals] 6000 IU•200 mg•50 IU•≛

Odor Free ArthriCare [see: ArthriCare, Odor Free]

Oenothera biennis *medicinal herb* [see: evening primrose]

OEP (oil of evening primrose) [see: evening primrose]

Oesclim (CAN) transdermal patch ℞ *estrogen replacement therapy for postmenopausal symptoms* [estradiol-17β hemihydrate] 25, 50 μg/day

Oesto-Mins powder OTC *vitamin/mineral supplement* [vitamins C and D; calcium; magnesium; potassium] 500 mg•100 IU•250 mg•250 mg•45 mg per 4.5 g

oestradiol BAN *estrogen replacement therapy for postmenopausal disorders; palliative therapy for prostatic and breast cancers* [also: estradiol]

oestradiol benzoate BAN [also: estradiol benzoate]

oestradiol valerate BAN *estrogen* [also: estradiol valerate]

oestriol succinate BAN *estrogen* [also: estriol; estriol succinate]

oestrogenine [see: diethylstilbestrol]

oestromenin [see: diethylstilbestrol]

oestrone BAN *estrogen replacement therapy for postmenopausal disorders; palliative therapy for prostatic and breast cancers* [also: estrone]

Off-Ezy Corn & Callus Remover kit (liquid + cushion pads) OTC *topical keratolytic* [salicylic acid in a collodion-like vehicle] 17%

Off-Ezy Wart Remover liquid OTC *topical keratolytic* [salicylic acid in a collodion-like vehicle] 17%

ofloxacin USAN, INN, BAN, JAN *broad-spectrum fluoroquinolone antibiotic; topical corneal ulcer treatment (orphan)*

ofornine USAN, INN *antihypertensive*

oftasceine INN

Ogen tablets ℞ *estrogen replacement therapy for postmenopausal symptoms* [estrone (from estropipate)] 0.625 (0.75), 1.25 (1.5), 2.5 (3) mg

Ogen vaginal cream ℞ *estrogen replacement for postmenopausal atrophic vaginitis* [estropipate] 1.5 mg/g

Ogestrel tablets ℞ *monophasic oral contraceptive; emergency postcoital contraceptive* [norgestrel; ethinyl estradiol] 0.5 mg•50 μg

OGT-918 *investigational (orphan) glucosidase inhibitor for Gaucher disease and Fabry disease*

oidiomycin *diagnostic aid for cell-mediated immunity; extract of the Oidiomycetes fungus family*

oil nut *medicinal herb* [see: butternut]

oil of evening primrose (OEP) [see: evening primrose]

oil of mustard [see: allyl isothiocyanate]

Oil of Olay Foaming Face Wash liquid OTC *topical cleanser for acne*

oil ricini [see: castor oil]

Oilatum Soap bar OTC *therapeutic skin cleanser*

ointment, hydrophilic USP *ointment base; oil-in-water emulsion*
ointment, white USP *oleaginous ointment base*
ointment, yellow USP *ointment base*
olaflur USAN, INN, BAN *dental caries prophylactic*
olamine USAN, INN *combining name for radicals or groups*
olanexidine HCl USAN *topical antibiotic for nosocomial or wound infections*
olanzapine USAN, INN *thienobenzodiazepine antipsychotic; antimanic for bipolar disorder*
olaquindox INN, BAN
old man's beard *medicinal herb* [see: fringe tree; woodbine]
old tuberculin (OT) [see: tuberculin]
Olea europaea *medicinal herb* [see: olive]
oleander *(Nerium indicum; N. oleander)* plant *medicinal herb for asthma, cancer, corns, epilepsy, and heart disease; not generally regarded as safe in any form, as it is extremely toxic*
oleandomycin INN [also: oleandomycin phosphate]
oleandomycin, triacetate ester [see: troleandomycin]
oleandomycin phosphate NF [also: oleandomycin]
oleic acid NF *emulsion adjunct*
oleic acid I 125 USAN *radioactive agent*
oleic acid I 131 USAN *radioactive agent*
oleovitamin A [now: vitamin A]
oleovitamin A & D USP *source of vitamins A and D*
oleovitamin D, synthetic [now: ergocalciferol]
olethytan 20 [see: polysorbate 80]
oletimol INN
oleum caryophylii [see: clove oil]
oleum gossypii seminis [see: cottonseed oil]
oleum maydis [see: corn oil]
oleum ricini [see: castor oil]
oleyl alcohol NF *emulsifying agent; emollient*
oligomycin D [see: rutamycin]
olive *(Olea europaea)* leaves, bark, and fruit *medicinal herb used as an antiseptic, astringent, cholagogue, demulcent, emollient, febrifuge, hypoglycemic, laxative, and tranquilizer*
olive, spurge; spurge laurel *medicinal herb* [see: mezereon]
olive oil NF *pharmaceutic aid*
olivomycin INN
olizumab *investigational (Phase III) recombinant humanized monoclonal antibody for asthma*
olmesartan *investigational (Phase III) oral angiotensin II receptor antagonist and antihypertensive*
olmidine INN
olopatadine INN *antiallergic; antiasthmatic*
olopatadine HCl USAN *antiallergic; antiasthmatic; ophthalmic antihistamine and mast cell stabilizer*
olpimedone INN
olsalazine INN, BAN *GI anti-inflammatory* [also: olsalazine sodium]
olsalazine sodium USAN *GI anti-inflammatory; treatment of ulcerative colitis* [also: olsalazine]
oltipraz INN
Olux foam ℞ *topical corticosteroidal anti-inflammatory for scalp dermatoses* [clobetasol propionate; ethanol 60%] 0.05%
olvanil USAN, INN *analgesic*
OM 401 *investigational (orphan) for sickle cell disease*
omaciclovir USAN *antiviral DNA polymerase inhibitor for herpes zoster*
OMAD (Oncovin, methotrexate/citrovorum factor, Adriamycin, dactinomycin) *chemotherapy protocol*
omalizumab *investigational (NDA filed) recombinant humanized monoclonal antibody (rhuMAb) to immunoglobulin E (anti-IgE) for treatment of asthma and allergic rhinitis*
omapatrilat *vasopeptidase inhibitor (VPI); investigational (NDA filed) endopeptidase and angiotensin-converting enzyme (ACE) inhibitor for hypertension and congestive heart failure*

omega-3 fatty acids [see: doconexent; icosapent; omega-3 marine triglycerides]

omega-3 fatty acids with all double bonds in the *cis* configuration *investigational (orphan) preventative for organ graft rejection*

omega-3 marine triglycerides BAN [12% doconexent (q.v.) + 18% icosapent (q.v.)]

omeprazole USAN, INN, BAN, JAN *proton pump inhibitor for gastric and duodenal ulcers, erosive esophagitis, GERD, and other gastroesophageal disorders*

omeprazole sodium USAN *gastric antisecretory*

omidoline INN

Omnicef capsules, oral suspension ℞ *cephalosporin antibiotic* [cefdinir] 300 mg; 125 mg/5 mL

Omniferon ℞ *investigational (Phase I) for genital herpes, multiple sclerosis, and AIDS* [interferon alfa]

OmniHIB powder for IM injection, prefilled syringes ℞ *Haemophilus influenzae type b (HIB) vaccine* [Hemophilus b conjugate vaccine; tetanus toxoid] 10•24 µg/0.5 mL

OMNIhist L.A. long-acting tablets ℞ *decongestant; antihistamine; anticholinergic* [phenylephrine HCl; chlorpheniramine maleate; methscopolamine nitrate] 20•8•2.5 mg

Omnipaque injection ℞ *radiopaque contrast medium* [iohexol (46.36% iodine)] 302, 388, 453, 518, 647, 755 mg/mL (140, 180, 210, 240, 300, 350 mg/mL)

Omnipen capsules, powder for oral suspension ℞ *aminopenicillin antibiotic* [ampicillin] 250, 500 mg; 125, 250 mg/5 mL ⊠ Unipen

Omnipen-N powder for IV or IM injection ℞ *aminopenicillin antibiotic* [ampicillin sodium] 125, 250, 500 mg, 1, 2, 10 g

Omniscan IV injection ℞ *MRI contrast medium* [gadodiamide] 287 mg/mL

omoconazole INN *antifungal*

omoconazole nitrate USAN *antifungal*

omonasteine INN

OMS Concentrate drops ℞ *narcotic analgesic* [morphine sulfate] 20 mg/mL

onapristone INN *investigational antineoplastic for hormone-dependent cancers*

Oncaspar IV or IM injection ℞ *antineoplastic for acute lymphocytic leukemia (orphan) and acute lymphoblastic leukemia* [pegaspargase] 750 IU/mL

Oncet capsules ℞ *narcotic antitussive; analgesic* [hydrocodone bitartrate; acetaminophen] 5•500 mg

Oncocine-HspE7 ℞ *investigational (Phase I) agent for cervical cancer*

Oncolym ℞ *investigational (Phase III, orphan) treatment for non-Hodgkin B-cell lymphoma (clinical trials discontinued 1999)* [iodine I 131 Lym-1 MAb]

Oncolysin B ℞ *investigational (Phase III) antineoplastic for B-cell lymphoma, leukemia, AIDS lymphoma, and myeloma; clinical trials discontinued 1997* [anti-B4-blocked ricin MAb]

Onconase ℞ *investigational (Phase III) treatment for pancreatic, breast, colorectal, prostate, and small cell lung cancers* [p30 protein]

OncoPhage ℞ *investigational (Phase III) antineoplastic for renal cell carcinoma*

OncoRad OV103 ℞ *investigational (orphan) antineoplastic for ovarian cancer* [CYT-103-Y-90 (code name —generic name not yet assigned)]

OncoScint CR/OV ℞ *radiodiagnostic imaging aid for ovarian (orphan) and colorectal cancer* [indium In 111 satumomab pendetide]

Oncostate ℞ *investigational (orphan) for renal cell carcinoma* [coumarin]

Onco-TCS *investigational (Phase II/III) antineoplastic for advanced non-Hodgkin lymphoma* [vincristine liposomal]

OncoTICE (CAN) powder for intravesical instillation ℞ *antineoplastic for urinary bladder cancer* [BCG vaccine, Tice strain] 50 mg (1–8 × 10^8 CFU)

OncoTrac imaging kit ℞ *investigational (orphan) for diagnostic imaging agent for metastasis of malignant melanoma*

[technetium Tc 99m antimelanoma murine MAb]

OncoVax-CL ℞ *investigational (Phase I/II) therapeutic vaccine for colorectal cancer*

OncoVax-Pr ℞ *investigational (Phase II) therapeutic vaccine for prostate cancer*

Oncovin IV injection, Hyporets (prefilled syringes) ℞ *antineoplastic for lung and breast cancers, various leukemias, lymphomas, and sarcomas* [vincristine sulfate] 1 mg/mL ⊡ Ancobon

Oncovite tablets OTC *vitamin supplement* [multiple vitamins] ≛

ondansetron INN, BAN *serotonin 5-HT_3 receptor antagonist; antiemetic for nausea following chemotherapy, radiation, or surgery* [also: ondansetron HCl]

ondansetron HCl USAN *serotonin 5-HT_3 receptor antagonist; antiemetic for nausea following chemotherapy, radiation, or surgery* [also: ondansetron]

Ondrox sustained-release tablets OTC *vitamin/mineral/calcium/iron supplement* [multiple vitamins & minerals; multiple amino acids; calcium; iron; folic acid; biotin] ≛ •25•3•0.67• 0.005 mg

1+1-F Creme ℞ *topical corticosteroidal anti-inflammatory; antifungal; antibacterial; local anesthetic* [hydrocortisone; clioquinol; pramoxine] 1%•3%•1%

1% HC ointment ℞ *topical corticosteroidal anti-inflammatory* [hydrocortisone] 1%

One Step Midstream Pregnancy Test stick for home use (discontinued 1998) *in vitro diagnostic aid; urine pregnancy test*

One Touch reagent strips for home use *in vitro diagnostic aid for blood glucose*

15AU81 *investigational (orphan) for primary pulmonary hypertension*

One-A-Day 55 Plus tablets OTC *geriatric vitamin/mineral supplement* [multiple vitamins & minerals; folic acid; biotin] ≛ •400•30 μg

One-A-Day Essential tablets OTC *vitamin supplement* [multiple vitamins; folic acid] ≛ •0.4 mg

One-A-Day Extras Antioxidant softgel capsules OTC *vitamin/mineral supplement* [vitamins A, C, and E; multiple minerals] 5000 IU•250 mg• 200 IU• ≛

One-A-Day Extras Vitamin C tablets (discontinued 1999) OTC *vitamin supplement* [vitamin C] 500 mg

One-A-Day Extras Vitamin E softgels (discontinued 1999) OTC *vitamin supplement* [vitamin E] 400 IU

One-A-Day Maximum Formula tablets OTC *vitamin/mineral/iron supplement* [multiple vitamins & minerals; iron; folic acid; biotin] ≛ •18 mg•0.4 mg•30 μg

One-A-Day Men's Vitamins tablets OTC *vitamin supplement* [multiple vitamins; folic acid] ≛ •0.4 mg

One-A-Day Women's Formula tablets OTC *vitamin/calcium/iron supplement* [multiple vitamins; calcium; iron; folic acid] ≛ •450•27•0.4 mg

One-Alpha (CAN) capsules, oral solution, IV injection ℞ *vitamin D therapy; calcium regulator for hypocalcemia and osteodystrophy of chronic renal dialysis and hyperparathyroidism of chronic renal failure* [alfacalcidol] 0.25, 0.5, 1 μg; 0.2 μg/mL; 2 μg/mL

1-alpha-D2 *investigational (Phase III) for secondary hyperparathyroidism in hemodialysis patients*

1DMTX/6-MP (methotrexate [with leucovorin rescue], mercaptopurine) *chemotherapy protocol for acute lymphocytic leukemia (ALL); a 1-day dosing protocol* [also: MTX/6-MP (a daily and weekly dosing protocol)]

One-Tablet-Daily OTC *vitamin supplement* [multiple vitamins; folic acid] ≛ •0.4 mg

One-Tablet-Daily with Iron OTC *vitamin/iron supplement* [multiple vitamins; iron; folic acid] ≛ •18•0.4 mg

One-Tablet-Daily with Minerals OTC *vitamin/mineral/iron supplement* [multiple vitamins & minerals; iron; folic acid; biotin] ≛ •18 mg•0.4 mg•30 μg

onion (*Allium cepa*) bulb *medicinal herb used as an anthelmintic, antiseptic, antispasmodic, carminative, diuretic, expectorant, and stomachic*

Onkolox ℞ *investigational (orphan) for renal cell carcinoma* [coumarin]

Ontak frozen solution for IV injection ℞ *antineoplastic for recurrent or persistent cutaneous T-cell lymphoma (orphan); investigational (Phase II) for non-Hodgkin lymphoma* [denileukin diftitox] 150 µg/mL

ontazolast USAN *antiasthmatic; leukotriene biosynthesis inhibitor*

ontianil INN

Onxol IV infusion ℞ *antineoplastic for ovarian and breast cancers, and non–small cell lung cancer (NSCLC), and AIDS-related Kaposi sarcoma (orphan)* [paclitaxel] 6 mg/mL

Ony-Clear solution OTC *topical antifungal* [benzalkonium chloride] 1%

ONYX-015 *investigational (Phase III) adenovirus E1B, in combination with cisplatin and 5-FU, for recurrent head and neck cancer; investigational (Phase I) for Barrett esophageal metaplasia; investigational for primary liver tumors*

OP-1 (osteogenic protein-1) [q.v.]

OPA (Oncovin, prednisone, Adriamycin) *chemotherapy protocol for pediatric Hodgkin lymphoma*

OPAL (Oncovin, prednisone, L-asparaginase) *chemotherapy protocol*

Opcon-A eye drops OTC *topical ophthalmic decongestant, antihistamine, and lubricant* [naphazoline HCl; pheniramine maleate; hydroxypropyl methylcellulose] 0.027%•0.315%•0.5%

OPEN (Oncovin, prednisone, etoposide, Novantrone) *chemotherapy protocol*

Operand solution, prep pads, swab sticks, surgical scrub, perineal wash concentrate, aerosol, Iofoam skin cleanser, ointment OTC *broad-spectrum antimicrobial* [povidone-iodine] 1%; 1%; 1%; 7.5%; 1%; 0.5%; 1%; 1%

Operand Douche concentrate OTC *antiseptic/germicidal; vaginal cleanser and deodorizer* [povidone-iodine]

Ophthaine eye drops (discontinued 1997) ℞ *topical ophthalmic anesthetic* [proparacaine HCl] 0.5%

Ophthalgan eye drops ℞ *corneal edema-reducing and clearing agent* [glycerin]

Ophthetic eye drops ℞ *topical ophthalmic anesthetic* [proparacaine HCl] 0.5%

Ophthifluor antecubital venous injection ℞ *ophthalmic diagnostic agent* [fluorescein sodium] 10%

opiniazide INN

opipramol INN *antidepressant; antipsychotic* [also: opipramol HCl]

opipramol HCl USAN *antidepressant; antipsychotic* [also: opipramol]

opium USP *narcotic analgesic; widely abused as a street drug, which is highly addictive* 10% oral

opium, powdered USP *narcotic analgesic*

Oplopanax horridus *medicinal herb* [see: devil's club]

OPP (Oncovin, procarbazine, prednisone) *chemotherapy protocol*

OPPA (Oncovin, prednisone, procarbazine, Adriamycin) *chemotherapy protocol for pediatric Hodgkin lymphoma*

oprelvekin USAN *platelet growth factor for prevention of thrombocytopenia following chemotherapy or radiation (orphan)* [also: interleukin 11, recombinant human]

Opticare PMS tablets OTC *vitamin/mineral supplement; digestive enzymes* [multiple vitamins & minerals; iron; folic acid; biotin; amylase; protease; lipase] ≛•2.5 mg•0.033 mg•10.4 µg•2500 U•2500 U•200 U

Opti-Clean solution OTC *cleaning solution for hard, soft, or rigid gas permeable contact lenses*

Opti-Clean II solution OTC *cleaning solution for hard or soft contact lenses*

Opti-Clean II Especially for Sensitive Eyes solution OTC *cleaning solution for rigid gas permeable contact lenses*

Opticrom 4% eye drops ℞ *topical ophthalmic antiallergic for vernal keratoconjunctivitis (orphan)* [cromolyn sodium]

Opticyl eye drops ℞ *cycloplegic; mydriatic* [tropicamide] 0.5%, 1%

Opti-Free solution OTC *chemical disinfecting solution for soft contact lenses* [note: one of four different products with the same name]

Opti-Free solution OTC *rewetting solution for soft contact lenses* [note: one of four different products with the same name]

Opti-Free solution OTC *surfactant cleaning solution for soft contact lenses* [note: one of four different products with the same name]

Opti-Free tablets OTC *enzymatic cleaner for soft contact lenses* [pork pancreatin] [note: one of four different products with the same name]

Optigene ophthalmic solution OTC *extraocular irrigating solution* [sterile isotonic solution]

Optigene 3 eye drops OTC *topical ophthalmic decongestant and vasoconstrictor* [tetrahydrozoline HCl] 0.05%

Optilets-500 Filmtabs (film-coated tablets) OTC *vitamin supplement* [multiple vitamins] ≛

Optilets-M-500 Filmtabs (film-coated tablets) OTC *vitamin/mineral/iron supplement* [multiple vitamins & minerals; iron] ≛•20 mg

Optimark IV injection ℞ *MRI contrast medium for imaging of the brain, head, and spine and liver structure and vascularity* [gadoversetamide]

Optimental liquid OTC *enteral nutritional therapy* 237 mL

Optimine tablets ℞ *piperidine antihistamine for allergic rhinitis and chronic urticaria* [azatadine maleate] 1 mg

Optimmune ℞ *investigational (orphan) for severe keratoconjunctivitis sicca in Sjögren syndrome* [cyclosporine]

Optimoist oral spray OTC *saliva substitute* [hydroxyethyl cellulose]

Optimox Prenatal tablets OTC *vitamin/mineral/calcium/iron supplement* [multiple vitamins & minerals; calcium; iron; folic acid] ≛•100•5•0.133 mg

Opti-One solution OTC *rewetting solution for soft contact lenses*

Opti-One Multi-Purpose solution OTC *chemical disinfecting solution for soft contact lenses*

OptiPen One (trademarked insulin delivery device) *cartridge-type subcu injector*

OptiPranolol eye drops ℞ *topical antiglaucoma agent (β-blocker)* [metipranolol HCl] 0.3%

Optiray 160; Optiray 240; Optiray 300; Optiray 320; Optiray 350 injection ℞ *radiopaque contrast medium* [ioversol (47.3% iodine)] 339 mg/mL (160 mg/mL); 509 mg/mL (240 mg/mL); 636 mg/mL (300 mg/mL); 678 mg/mL (320 mg/mL); 741 mg/mL (350 mg/mL)

Opti-Soft Especially for Sensitive Eyes solution OTC *rinsing/storage solution for soft contact lenses* [sodium chloride (preserved saline solution)]

Optison injectable suspension *ultrasound contrast medium for cardiac imaging; investigational (Phase III) diagnostic aid for infertility due to obstructed fallopian tubes* [perflutren] 3 mL

Opti-Tears solution OTC *rewetting solution for hard or soft contact lenses*

Optivar eye drops ℞ *antihistamine and mast cell stabilizer for allergic conjunctivitis* [azelastine HCl] 0.05%

Optivite P.M.T. tablets OTC *geriatric vitamin/mineral supplement* [multiple vitamins & minerals; folic acid; biotin] ≛•30•≟ μg

Opti-Zyme Enzymatic Cleaner Especially for Sensitive Eyes tablets OTC *enzymatic cleaner for soft or rigid gas permeable contact lenses* [pork pancreatin]

Optrin ℞ *investigational (Phase I/II) photodynamic therapy for age-related macular degeneration* [motexafin lutetium]

Optro ℞ *investigational agent for chronic anemia* [human hemoglobin, recombinant]

OPV (oral poliovirus vaccine) [see: poliovirus vaccine, live oral]

ORA5 liquid OTC *oral anti-infective* [copper sulfate; iodine; potassium iodide]

Orabase gel OTC *mucous membrane anesthetic* [benzocaine] 15%

Orabase Baby gel OTC *topical oral anesthetic* [benzocaine] 7.5%

Orabase HCA oral paste ℞ *topical corticosteroidal anti-inflammatory* [hydrocortisone acetate] 0.5%

Orabase Lip Healer cream OTC *topical oral anesthetic; antipruritic/counterirritant; vulnerary* [benzocaine; menthol; allantoin] 5%•0.5%•1.5%

Orabase-B oral paste OTC *topical oral anesthetic* [benzocaine] 20% ⊡ Orinase

Orabase-Plain oral paste OTC *relief from minor oral irritations* [plasticized hydrocarbon gel]

Oracit solution ℞ *urinary alkalinizing agent* [sodium citrate; citric acid] 490•640 mg/5 mL

OraDisc ℞ *investigational (Phase III) agent for canker sores* [amlexanox]

Oragrafin Calcium granules for oral suspension (discontinued 1999) ℞ *radiopaque contrast medium for cholecystography* [ipodate calcium (61.7% iodine)] 3 g/packet

Oragrafin Sodium capsules (discontinued 2001) ℞ *radiopaque contrast medium for cholecystography* [ipodate sodium (61.4% iodine)] 500 mg (307 mg)

Orajel liquid OTC *topical oral anesthetic* [benzocaine; alcohol 44.2%] 20%

Orajel; Orajel Brace-aid; Orajel/d; Denture Orajel; Baby Orajel; Baby Orajel Nighttime Formula gel OTC *topical oral anesthetic* [benzocaine] 20%; 20%; 10%; 10%; 7.5%; 10%

Orajel Mouth-Aid liquid, gel OTC *mucous membrane anesthetic* [benzocaine] 20%

Orajel Perioseptic liquid OTC *topical oral anti-inflammatory and anti-infective for braces* [carbamide peroxide] 15%

Orajel Tooth & Gum Cleanser, Baby gel OTC *removes plaque-like film* [poloxamer 407; simethicone] 2%•0.12%

Oralease ℞ *investigational (Phase III) analgesic for pain due to oral ulcers*

Oralet (trademarked dosage form) *oral lozenge/lollipop*

Oralgen; Oralin ℞ *investigational (Phase II/III) oral insulin formulation*

Oralone Dental paste ℞ *topical corticosteroidal anti-inflammatory* [triamcinolone acetonide] 0.1%

Oraminic II subcu or IM injection (discontinued 1997) ℞ *antihistamine for anaphylaxis* [brompheniramine maleate] 10 mg/mL

Oramorph SR sustained-release tablets ℞ *narcotic analgesic* [morphine sulfate] 15, 30, 60, 100 mg

orange flower oil NF *flavoring agent; perfume*

orange flower water NF

orange oil NF

orange peel tincture, sweet NF

orange root *medicinal herb* [see: goldenseal]

orange spirit, compound NF

orange swallow wort *medicinal herb* [see: pleurisy root]

orange syrup NF

Orap tablets ℞ *antidyskinetic for Tourette syndrome* [pimozide] 1, 2 mg (4 mg available in Canada)

Oraphen-PD elixir OTC *analgesic; antipyretic* [acetaminophen] 120 mg/5 mL

Orapred oral solution ℞ *corticosteroid; anti-inflammatory* [prednisolone sodium phosphate] 15 mg/5 mL

Orarinse ℞ *investigational (Phase II) mucositis treatment*

orarsan [see: acetarsone] ⊡ Oracin; Orasone

Orasept liquid OTC *oral astringent; antiseptic* [tannic acid; methylbenzethonium chloride; alcohol 53.31%] 12.16%•1.53%

Orasept throat spray OTC *topical oral anesthetic; antiseptic* [benzocaine; methylbenzethonium chloride] 0.996%•1.037%

Orasol liquid OTC *topical oral anesthetic; antipruritic/counterirritant; antiseptic* [benzocaine; phenol; alcohol 70%] 6.3%•0.5%

OraSolv (trademarked delivery system) *investigational (NDA filed)*

Orasone tablets ℞ *corticosteroid; anti-inflammatory; immunosuppressant* [prednisone] 1, 5, 10, 20, 50 mg ⓓ Oracin; orarsan

OraSure reagent kit for home use *in vitro diagnostic aid for HIV antibodies*

OraSure HIV-1 reagent kit for professional use *in vitro diagnostic aid for HIV antibodies using oral mucosal transudate* [single-sample, three-test kit: two ELISA assays + Western Blot assay]

orazamide INN

Orazinc capsules, tablets OTC *zinc supplement* [zinc sulfate] 220 mg; 110 mg

orbofiban acetate USAN *platelet aggregation inhibitor; fibrinogen receptor antagonist*

orbutopril INN

orchanet *medicinal herb* [see: henna *(Alkanna)*]

orciprenaline INN, BAN *bronchodilator* [also: metaproterenol polistirex]

orciprenaline polistirex [see: metaproterenol polistirex]

orciprenaline sulfate [see: metaproterenol sulfate]

orconazole INN *antifungal* [also: orconazole nitrate]

orconazole nitrate USAN *antifungal* [also: orconazole]

Ordrine AT extended-release capsules ℞ *antitussive; decongestant* [caramiphen edisylate; phenylpropanolamine HCl] 40•75 mg

oregano *medicinal herb* [see: marjoram]

Oregon grape *(Mahonia aquifolium)* rhizome and root *medicinal herb for acne, blood disorders, eczema, jaundice, liver disorders, promoting digestion, psoriasis, and staphylococcal infections*

orestrate INN

orestrol [see: diethylstilbestrol dipropionate]

Oretic tablets ℞ *antihypertensive; diuretic* [hydrochlorothiazide] 25, 50 mg ⓓ Oreton

Oreton Methyl tablets, buccal tablets (discontinued 2001) ℞ *androgen replacement for hypogonadism or testosterone deficiency in men, delayed puberty in boys, and metastatic breast cancer in women; also abused as a street drug* [methyltestosterone] 10 mg ⓓ Oretic

Orexin chewable tablets OTC *vitamin supplement* [vitamins B_1, B_6, and B_{12}] 8.1 mg•4.1 mg•25 μg

ORG 33062 *investigational (Phase III) antidepressant*

Organidin NR tablets, oral liquid ℞ *expectorant* [guaifenesin] 200 mg; 100 mg/5 mL

organoclay [see: bentoquatam]

Orgaran deep subcu injection ℞ *anticoagulant/antithrombotic for prevention of deep vein thrombosis (DVT) following hip replacement surgery* [danaparoid sodium] 750 anti-Xa U/0.6 mL

orgotein USAN, INN, BAN *anti-inflammatory; antirheumatic; investigational (orphan) for amyotrophic lateral sclerosis and to prevent donor organ reperfusion injury* [previously known as superoxide dismutase (SOD)]

orgotein, recombinant human *investigational (orphan) for bronchopulmonary dysplasia of premature neonates*

orienticine A; orienticine D [see: orientiparcin]

orientiparcin INN [a mixture of orienticine A and orienticine D]

Origanum vulgare *medicinal herb* [see: marjoram]

Orimune oral suspension ℞ *poliomyelitis vaccine* [poliovirus vaccine, live oral trivalent] 0.5 mL

Orinase tablets ℞ *sulfonylurea antidiabetic* [tolbutamide] 500 mg ⊡ Orabase; Ornade; Ornex; Tolinase

Orinase Diagnostic powder for IV injection ℞ *in vivo diagnostic aid for pancreatic islet cell adenoma (insulinoma)* [tolbutamide sodium] 1 g/vial

oritavancin diphosphate USAN *antibiotic; peptidoglycan synthesis inhibitor*

Orlaam IV injection ℞ *narcotic analgesic for management of opiate addiction (orphan)* [levomethadyl acetate HCl] 10 mg/mL

orlipastat [see: orlistat]

orlistat USAN, INN *lipase inhibitor to suppress the absorption of dietary fats, leading to weight loss*

ormaplatin USAN *antineoplastic*

Ormazine IV or IM injection (discontinued 1998) ℞ *conventional (typical) antipsychotic* [chlorpromazine HCl] 25 mg/mL

ormetoprim USAN, INN *antibacterial*

Ornade Spansules (sustained-release capsules) ℞ *decongestant; antihistamine* [phenylpropanolamine HCl; chlorpheniramine maleate] 75•12 mg ⊡ Orinase; Ornex

Ornex No Drowsiness caplets OTC *decongestant; analgesic; antipyretic* [pseudoephedrine HCl; acetaminophen] 30•325 mg ⊡ Orex; Orinase; Ornade

ornidazole USAN, INN *anti-infective*

Ornidyl IV injection concentrate ℞ *antiprotozoal for Trypanosoma brucei gambiense (sleeping sickness) infection (orphan)* [eflornithine HCl] 200 mg/mL

ornipressin INN

ornithine (L-ornithine) INN

ornithine vasopressin [see: ornipressin]

ornoprostil INN

Oros (trademarked delivery system) *patterned-release tablets*

orotic acid INN

orotirelin INN

orpanoxin USAN, INN *anti-inflammatory*

orphenadine citrate [see: orphenadrine citrate]

orphenadrine INN, BAN *skeletal muscle relaxant; antihistamine* [also: orphenadrine citrate]

orphenadrine citrate USP *skeletal muscle relaxant; antihistamine* [also: orphenadrine] 100 mg oral; 30 mg/mL injection

orphenadrine HCl *anticholinergic; antiparkinsonian*

Orphengesic; Orphengesic Forte tablets ℞ *skeletal muscle relaxant; analgesic* [orphenadrine citrate; aspirin; caffeine] 25•385•30 mg; 50•770•60 mg

orpressin [see: ornipressin]

orris root *(Iris florentina)* *medicinal herb used as a diuretic and stomachic*

ortetamine INN

orthesin [see: benzocaine]

Ortho 0.5/35; Ortho 1/35 (CAN) tablets (in packs of 21 or 28) ℞ *monophasic oral contraceptive* [norethindrone; ethinyl estradiol] 0.5 mg•35 µg; 1 mg•35 µg

Ortho 7/7/7 (CAN) tablets (in packs of 21 or 28) ℞ *triphasic oral contraceptive* [norethindrone; ethinyl estradiol]
Phase 1 (7 days): 0.5 mg•35 µg;
Phase 2 (7 days): 0.75 mg•35 µg;
Phase 3 (7 days): 1 mg•35 µg

Ortho Dienestrol vaginal cream ℞ *estrogen replacement for postmenopausal atrophic vaginitis* [dienestrol] 0.01%

Ortho Evra ℞ *investigational progestin-type contraceptive* [norelgestromin]

Ortho Tri-Cyclen tablets (in Dialpaks and Veridates of 21 or 28) ℞ *triphasic oral contraceptive; treatment for acne vulgaris in females* [norgestimate; ethinyl estradiol]
Phase 1 (7 days): 0.18 mg•35 µg;
Phase 2 (7 days): 0.215 mg•35 µg;
Phase 3 (7 days): 0.25 mg•35 µg

Ortho-Cept tablets (in Dialpaks and Veridates of 21 or 28) ℞ *monophasic oral contraceptive* [desogestrel; ethinyl estradiol] 0.15 mg•30 µg

Orthoclone OKT3 IV injection ℞ *immunosuppressant for renal, cardiac,* *and hepatic transplants* [muromonab-CD3] 5 mg/5 mL [2] Ortho-Creme

orthocresol NF

Ortho-Cyclen tablets (in Dialpaks and Veridates of 21 or 28) ℞ *monophasic oral contraceptive* [norgestimate; ethinyl estradiol] 0.25 mg•35 μg

Ortho-Est tablets ℞ *estrogen replacement therapy for postmenopausal symptoms* [estrone (from estropipate)] 0.625 (0.75), 1.25 (1.5) mg

Ortho-Gynol vaginal gel OTC *spermicidal contraceptive (for use with a diaphragm)* [octoxynol 9] 1%

Ortholinum ℞ *investigational (orphan) for spasmodic torticollis* [botulinum toxin, type F]

Ortho-Novum 1/35 tablets (in Dialpaks and Veridates of 21 or 28) ℞ *monophasic oral contraceptive* [norethindrone; ethinyl estradiol] 1 mg•35 μg

Ortho-Novum 1/50 tablets (in Dialpaks of 21 or 28) ℞ *monophasic oral contraceptive* [norethindrone; mestranol] 1 mg•50 μg

Ortho-Novum 7/7/7 tablets (in Dialpaks and Veridates of 21 or 28) ℞ *triphasic oral contraceptive* [norethindrone; ethinyl estradiol]
Phase 1 (7 days): 0.5 mg•35 μg;
Phase 2 (7 days): 0.75 mg•35 μg;
Phase 3 (7 days): 1 mg•35 μg

Ortho-Novum 10/11 tablets (in Dialpaks of 21 or 28; in Veridates of 28) ℞ *biphasic oral contraceptive* [norethindrone; ethinyl estradiol]
Phase 1 (10 days): 0.5 mg•35 μg;
Phase 2 (11 days): 1 mg•35 μg

Ortho-Prefest tablets (in packs of 30) ℞ *hormone replacement therapy for postmenopausal symptoms* [estradiol-17β; norgestimate] 1•0 mg×3 days; 1•0.09 mg×3 days; repeat without interruption

orthotolidine

Orthovisc (European name for U.S. products Hyalgan, Supartz)

Orthoxicol Cough syrup OTC *antitussive; decongestant; antihistamine* [dextromethorphan hydrobromide; phenylpropanolamine HCl; chlorpheniramine maleate; alcohol 8%] 6.7•8.3•1.3 mg/5 mL

Orudis capsules ℞ *analgesic; antiarthritic; nonsteroidal anti-inflammatory drug (NSAID)* [ketoprofen] 25, 50, 75 mg

Orudis KT tablets OTC *analgesic; antiarthritic; antipyretic; nonsteroidal anti-inflammatory drug (NSAID)* [ketoprofen] 12.5 mg

Oruvail sustained-release pellets in capsules ℞ *once-daily antiarthritic; nonsteroidal anti-inflammatory drug (NSAID)* [ketoprofen] 100, 150, 200 mg

oryzanol A, B, and C *medicinal herb* [see: rice bran oil]

Orzel tablets ℞ *investigational (NDA filed) oral agent for colorectal cancer* [uracil; tegafur; leucovorin calcium]

osalmid INN

osarsal [see: acetarsone]

Os-Cal 250+D; Os-Cal 500+D film-coated tablets OTC *dietary supplement* [calcium carbonate; vitamin D] 250 mg•125 IU; 500 mg•200 IU

Os-Cal 500 tablets, chewable tablets OTC *calcium supplement* [calcium carbonate] 1.25 g

Os-Cal Fortified tablets OTC *vitamin/calcium/iron supplement* [multiple vitamins; calcium carbonate; iron] ≛•250•5 mg

Os-Cal Fortified Multivitamin & Minerals tablets OTC *vitamin/mineral/calcium/iron supplement* [multiple vitamins & minerals; calcium carbonate; iron] ≛•250•5 mg

oseltamivir phosphate USAN *antiviral; neuraminidase inhibitor for prophylaxis and treatment of influenza A and B infections*

osmadizone INN

Osmitrol IV infusion ℞ *antihypertensive; osmotic diuretic* [mannitol] 5%, 10%, 15%, 20%

osmium *element (Os)*

Osmoglyn solution ℞ *osmotic diuretic* [glycerin] 50%

Osmolite; Osmolite HN liquid OTC *enteral nutritional therapy* [lactose-free formula]

Osmorhiza longistylis *medicinal herb* [see: sweet cicely]

osmotic diuretics *a class of diuretics that increase excretion of sodium and chloride and decrease tubular absorption of water*

Osmunda cinnamomea; O. regalis *medicinal herb* [see: buckhorn brake]

OspA [see: lipoprotein OspA, recombinant]

Ossigel ℞ *investigational (Phase I) agent to accelerate healing of bone fractures* [ersofermin; hyaluronate sodium]

OST-577 *investigational human anti-hepatitis B antibody*

Ostac (CAN) capsules, IV infusion ℞ *bisphosphonate bone resorption inhibitor for hypercalcemia of malignancy and osteolysis due to bone metastasis of malignant tumors* [clodronate disodium] 400 mg; 30 mg/mL

Ostavir ℞ *investigational (Phase II) anti-hepatitis B monoclonal antibody* [tuvirumab]

Osteocalcin subcu or IM injection ℞ *calcium regulator for hypercalcemia, Paget disease, and postmenopausal osteoporosis* [calcitonin (salmon)] 200 IU/mL

Osteo-D ℞ *calcium regulator; investigational (orphan) for familial hypophosphatemic rickets* [secalciferol]

osteogenic protein-1 (OP-1) *investigational (NDA filed) morphogenic protein that enhances motor function following stroke*

Osteomark *investigational enzyme-linked immunoassay for monitoring bone resorption; investigational agent for primary hyperparathyroidism and metastatic bone tumors* [monoclonal antibodies]

OsteoMax effervescent powder for oral solution OTC *dietary supplement* [calcium citrate; vitamin D; magnesium] 500 mg•200 IU•200 mg

Osteo-Mins powder OTC *dietary supplement* [multiple minerals; vitamins C and D] * •500 mg•100 IU

Ostiderm lotion OTC *for hyperhidrosis and bromhidrosis* [aluminum sulfate; zinc oxide] 14.5•? mg/g

Ostiderm roll-on OTC *for hyperhidrosis and bromhidrosis* [aluminum chlorohydrate; camphor; alcohol] ?•?•?

ostreogrycin INN, BAN

osvarsan [see: acetarsone]

Oswego tea *(Monarda didyma)* leaves and flowers *medicinal herb used as a calmative, rubefacient, and stimulant*

OT (old tuberculin) [see: tuberculin]

Otic Domeboro ear drops ℞ *antibacterial; antifungal* [acetic acid; aluminum acetate] 2%•?

Otic-Care ear drops, otic suspension ℞ *topical corticosteroidal anti-inflammatory; antibiotic* [hydrocortisone; neomycin sulfate; polymyxin B sulfate] 1%•5 mg•10 000 U per mL

otilonium bromide INN, BAN

Oti-Med ear drops ℞ *topical corticosteroidal anti-inflammatory; antibacterial; topical local anesthetic* [hydrocortisone; chloroxylenol; pramoxine HCl] 10•1•10 mg/mL

otimerate sodium INN

OtiTricin otic suspension ℞ *topical corticosteroidal anti-inflammatory; antibiotic* [hydrocortisone; neomycin sulfate; polymyxin B sulfate] 1%•5 mg•10 000 U per mL

Otobiotic Otic ear drops ℞ *topical corticosteroidal anti-inflammatory; antibiotic* [hydrocortisone; polymyxin B sulfate] 0.5%•10 000 U per mL ⊠ Urobiotic

Otocain ear drops ℞ *topical local anesthetic* [benzocaine] 20%

Otocalm ear drops ℞ *topical local anesthetic; analgesic* [benzocaine; antipyrine] 1.4%•5.4%

Otocort ear drops, otic suspension ℞ *topical corticosteroidal anti-inflammatory; antibiotic* [hydrocortisone; neomycin sulfate; polymyxin B sulfate] 1%•5 mg•10 000 U per mL

Otomar-HC ear drops ℞ *topical corticosteroidal anti-inflammatory; local anesthetic; antibacterial* [hydrocortisone; pramoxine HCl; chloroxylenol] 10•10•1 mg/mL

Otomycet-HC ear drops ℞ *topical corticosteroidal anti-inflammatory; antibacterial; antifungal* [hydrocortisone; acetic acid] 1%•2%

Otomycin-HPN Otic ear drops ℞ *topical corticosteroidal anti-inflammatory; antibiotic* [hydrocortisone; neomycin sulfate; polymyxin B sulfate] 1%•5 mg•10 000 U per mL

Otosporin ear drops ℞ *topical corticosteroidal anti-inflammatory; antibiotic* [hydrocortisone; neomycin sulfate; polymyxin B sulfate] 1%•5 mg•10 000 U per mL

Otrivin nasal spray, nose drops, pediatric drops OTC *nasal decongestant* [xylometazoline HCl] 0.1%; 0.1%; 0.05% ⊡ Lotrimin

ouabain USP

Our Lady's mint *medicinal herb* [see: spearmint]

Outgro solution OTC *pain relief for ingrown toenails* [tannic acid; chlorobutanol; isopropyl alcohol 83%] 25%•5%

ovandrotone albumin INN, BAN

OvaRex ℞ *investigational (Phase II, orphan) therapeutic vaccine for epithelial ovarian cancer* [monoclonal antibody B43.13] ⊡ O-Vax

Ovastat ℞ *investigational (orphan) for ovarian cancer* [treosulfan] ⊡ Novastan

O-Vax ℞ *investigational (Phase III, orphan) therapeutic vaccine for adjuvant treatment of ovarian cancer* [autologous cell (AC) vaccine] ⊡ Ovarex

Ovcon-35 tablets (in packs of 21 or 28) ℞ *monophasic oral contraceptive* [norethindrone; ethinyl estradiol] 0.4 mg•35 µg

Ovcon-50 tablets (in packs of 28) ℞ *monophasic oral contraceptive* [norethindrone; ethinyl estradiol] 1 mg•50 µg

Overtime tablets OTC *CNS stimulant; analeptic* [caffeine] 200 mg

Ovide lotion ℞ *pediculicide* [malathion; isopropyl alcohol 78%] 0.5%

Ovidrel powder for subcu injection ℞ *fertility stimulant for anovulatory women; adjuvant therapy for cryptorchidism* [choriogonadotropin alfa] 250 µg

ovine corticotropin-releasing hormone [see: corticorelin ovine triflutate]

Ovoid (trademarked dosage form) *sugar-coated tablet*

Ovral tablets (in Pilpaks of 28) ℞ *monophasic oral contraceptive; emergency postcoital contraceptive* [norgestrel; ethinyl estradiol] 0.5 mg•50 µg

Ovrette tablets (in packs of 28) ℞ *oral contraceptive (progestin only); emergency postcoital contraceptive* [norgestrel] 0.075 mg

OvuGen test kit *in vitro diagnostic aid to predict ovulation time*

OvuKIT Self-Test kit for home use *in vitro diagnostic aid to predict ovulation time*

OvuQuick Self-Test kit for home use *in vitro diagnostic aid to predict ovulation time*

[^{15}O]water [see: water O 15]

ox bile extract [see: bile salts]

oxabolone cipionate INN

oxabrexine INN

22-oxacalcitriol (OCT) [see: maxacalcitol]

oxaceprol INN

oxacillin INN *penicillinase-resistant penicillin antibiotic* [also: oxacillin sodium]

oxacillin sodium USAN, USP *penicillinase-resistant penicillin antibiotic* [also: oxacillin] 250, 500 mg oral; 250 mg/5 mL oral; 0.25, 0.5, 1, 2, 4, 10 g injection

oxadimedine INN

oxadimedine HCl [see: oxadimedine]

oxadoddy *medicinal herb* [see: Culver root]

oxaflozane INN

oxaflumazine INN

oxafuradene [see: nifuradene]

oxagrelate USAN, INN *platelet antiaggregatory agent*

oxalinast INN
oxaliplatin USAN, INN *investigational (orphan) alkylating antineoplastic for ovarian and colorectal cancers*
Oxalis acetosella *medicinal herb* [see: wood sorrel]
oxamarin INN *hemostatic* [also: oxamarin HCl]
oxamarin HCl USAN *hemostatic* [also: oxamarin]
oxametacin INN
oxamisole INN *immunoregulator* [also: oxamisole HCl]
oxamisole HCl USAN *immunoregulator* [also: oxamisole]
oxamniquine USAN, USP, INN *antischistosomal; anthelmintic for schistosomiasis (flukes)*
oxamphetamine hydrobromide [see: hydroxyamphetamine hydrobromide]
oxamycin [see: cycloserine]
oxanamide INN
Oxandrin gel ℞ *investigational (Phase II) steroid for AIDS-wasting syndrome* [oxandrolone]
Oxandrin tablets ℞ *anabolic steroid; investigational (orphan) for muscular dystrophy, AIDS-wasting syndrome, and alcoholic hepatitis; also abused as a street drug to increase muscle mass* [oxandrolone] 2.5 mg
oxandrolone USAN, USP, INN, BAN, JAN *anabolic steroid; investigational (Phase III, orphan) for AIDS-wasting syndrome; investigational (orphan) for muscular dystrophy and alcoholic hepatitis; also abused as a street drug to increase muscle mass*
oxantel INN *anthelmintic* [also: oxantel pamoate]
oxantel pamoate USAN *anthelmintic* [also: oxantel]
oxantrazole HCl [see: piroxantrone HCl]
oxapadol INN
oxapium iodide INN
oxaprazine
oxapropanium iodide INN
oxaprotiline INN *antidepressant* [also: oxaprotiline HCl]
oxaprotiline HCl USAN *antidepressant* [also: oxaprotiline]
oxaprozin USAN, INN, BAN *antiarthritic; nonsteroidal anti-inflammatory drug (NSAID)* 600 mg oral
oxarbazole USAN, INN *antiasthmatic*
oxarutine [see: ethoxazorutoside]
oxatomide USAN, INN *antiallergic; antiasthmatic*
oxazafone INN
oxazepam USAN, USP, INN *benzodiazepine anxiolytic; minor tranquilizer; alcohol withdrawal therapy* 10, 15, 30 mg oral
oxazidione INN
oxazolam INN
oxazolidin [see: oxyphenbutazone]
oxazolidinediones *a class of anticonvulsants*
oxazorone INN
oxcarbazepine INN *anticonvulsant for partial seizures in adults or children*
oxdralazine INN
oxeladin INN, BAN
oxendolone USAN, INN *antiandrogen for benign prostatic hypertrophy*
oxepinac INN
oxerutins BAN
oxetacaine INN *topical anesthetic* [also: oxethazaine]
oxetacillin INN
2-oxetanone [see: propiolactone]
oxethazaine USAN, BAN *topical anesthetic* [also: oxetacaine]
oxetorone INN *migraine-specific analgesic* [also: oxetorone fumarate]
oxetorone fumarate USAN *migraine-specific analgesic* [also: oxetorone]
Oxeze (CAN) Turbuhaler (dry powder in a metered-dose inhaler) ℞ *twice-daily bronchodilator for asthma* [formoterol fumarate] 6, 12 μg/dose
oxfenamide [see: oxiramide]
oxfendazole USAN, INN *anthelmintic*
oxfenicine USAN, INN, BAN *vasodilator*
oxibendazole USAN, INN *anthelmintic*
oxibetaine INN
oxibuprocaine chloride [see: benoxinate HCl]

oxichlorochine sulfate [see: hydroxychloroquine sulfate]
oxicinchophen [see: oxycinchophen]
oxiconazole INN, BAN *broad-spectrum topical antifungal* [also: oxiconazole nitrate]
oxiconazole nitrate USAN *broad-spectrum topical antifungal* [also: oxiconazole]
oxicone [see: oxycodone]
oxidized cellulose [see: cellulose, oxidized]
oxidized cholic acid [see: dehydrocholic acid]
oxidized regenerated cellulose [see: cellulose, oxidized regenerated]
oxidopamine USAN, INN *ophthalmic adrenergic*
oxidronate sodium *parenteral radiopaque contrast medium*
oxidronic acid USAN, INN, BAN *calcium regulator*
oxifenamate [see: hydroxyphenamate]
oxifentorex INN
Oxi-Freeda tablets OTC *dietary supplement* [multiple vitamins & minerals; multiple amino acids]
oxifungin INN *antifungal* [also: oxifungin HCl]
oxifungin HCl USAN *antifungal* [also: oxifungin]
oxilorphan USAN, INN *narcotic antagonist*
oximetazoline HCl [see: oxymetazoline HCl]
oximetholone [see: oxymetholone]
oximonam USAN, INN *antibacterial*
oximonam sodium USAN *antibacterial*
oxindanac INN
oxiniacic acid INN
oxiperomide USAN, INN *antipsychotic*
oxipertine [see: oxypertine]
oxipethidine [see: hydroxypethidine]
oxiphenbutazone [see: oxyphenbutazone]
oxiphencyclimine chloride [see: oxyphencyclimine HCl]
Oxipor VHC lotion OTC *topical antipsoriatic; antiseborrheic; keratolytic* [coal tar solution; alcohol 79%] 25%
oxiprocaine [see: hydroxyprocaine]
oxiprogesterone caproate [see: hydroxyprogesterone caproate]
oxipurinol INN *xanthine oxidase inhibitor* [also: oxypurinol]
oxiracetam INN, BAN *investigational treatment for Alzheimer disease*
oxiramide USAN, INN *antiarrhythmic*
oxisopred INN
Oxistat cream, lotion ℞ *broad-spectrum topical antifungal* [oxiconazole nitrate] 1%
oxistilbamidine isethionate [see: hydroxystilbamidine isethionate]
oxisuran USAN, INN *antineoplastic*
oxitefonium bromide INN
oxitetracaine [see: hydroxytetracaine]
oxitetracycline [see: oxytetracycline]
oxitriptan INN
oxitriptyline INN
oxitropium bromide INN, BAN
Oxizole (CAN) cream, lotion ℞ *broad-spectrum topical antifungal* [oxiconazole nitrate] 1%
oxmetidine INN, BAN *antagonist to histamine H_2 receptors* [also: oxmetidine HCl]
oxmetidine HCl USAN *antagonist to histamine H_2 receptors* [also: oxmetidine]
oxmetidine mesylate USAN *antagonist to histamine H_2 receptors*
oxodipine INN
oxogestone INN *progestin* [also: oxogestone phenpropionate]
oxogestone phenpropionate USAN *progestin* [also: oxogestone]
oxoglurate INN *combining name for radicals or groups*
oxolamine INN
oxolinic acid USAN, INN *antibacterial*
oxomemazine INN
oxonazine INN
4-oxopentanoic acid, calcium salt [see: calcium levulinate]
oxophenarsine INN [also: oxophenarsine HCl]
oxophenarsine HCl USP [also: oxophenarsine]
5-oxoproline [see: pidolic acid]
oxoprostol INN, BAN

oxothiazolidine carboxylate (L-2-oxothiazolidine-4-carboxylic acid) *investigational (Phase II) immunomodulator for AIDS; investigational (orphan) for adult respiratory distress syndrome and amyotrophic lateral sclerosis (ARDS trials discontinued 1998)*

oxozepam [see: oxazepam]

oxpentifylline BAN *peripheral vasodilator; hemorheologic agent* [also: pentoxifylline]

oxpheneridine INN

oxprenoate potassium INN

oxprenolol INN *coronary vasodilator* [also: oxprenolol HCl]

oxprenolol HCl USAN, USP *coronary vasodilator* [also: oxprenolol]

OxSODrol ℞ *investigational (Phase III) anti-inflammatory and antirheumatic; investigational (Phase III) for the prevention of bronchopulmonary dysplasia* [orgotein (previously known as superoxide dismutase, or SOD)]

Oxsoralen lotion ℞ *topical psoralens for repigmentation of idiopathic vitiligo* [methoxsalen] 1%

Oxsoralen-Ultra capsules ℞ *systemic psoralens for the treatment of severe recalcitrant psoriasis* [methoxsalen] 10 mg

oxtriphylline USP *bronchodilator* [also: choline theophyllinate] 100, 200 mg oral; 50, 100 mg/5 mL oral

Oxy 5 for Sensitive Skin, Advanced Formula; Oxy for Sensitive Skin, Advanced Formula gel OTC *topical keratolytic for acne* [benzoyl peroxide] 5%; 2.5%

Oxy 5 Tinted lotion OTC *topical keratolytic for acne* [benzoyl peroxide] 5%

Oxy 10 Advanced Formula gel OTC *topical keratolytic for acne* [benzoyl peroxide] 10%

Oxy 10 Wash liquid OTC *topical keratolytic for acne* [benzoyl peroxide] 10%

Oxy Medicated Cleanser & Pads OTC *topical keratolytic cleanser for acne* [salicylic acid; alcohol] 0.5%•22%, 0.5%•40%, 2%•50%

Oxy Medicated Soap bar OTC *medicated cleanser for acne* [triclosan] 1%

Oxy Night Watch; Oxy Night Watch for Sensitive Skin lotion OTC *topical keratolytic for acne* [salicylic acid] 2%; 1%

Oxy ResiDon't Medicated Face Wash liquid (discontinued 1997) OTC *medicated cleanser for acne* [triclosan] 0.6%

oxybenzone USAN, USP, INN *ultraviolet screen*

oxybuprocaine INN, BAN *topical anesthetic* [also: benoxinate HCl; oxybuprocaine HCl]

oxybuprocaine HCl JAN *topical anesthetic* [also: benoxinate HCl; oxybuprocaine]

oxybutynin INN, BAN *anticholinergic; urinary antispasmodic* [also: oxybutynin chloride]

oxybutynin chloride USAN, USP *anticholinergic; urinary antispasmodic for urge urinary incontinence and frequency* [also: oxybutynin] 5 mg oral; 5 mg/5 mL oral

Oxycel pads, pledgets, strips ℞ *topical local hemostat for surgery* [cellulose, oxidized]

oxychlorosene USAN *topical anti-infective*

oxychlorosene sodium USAN *topical anti-infective*

oxycinchophen INN, BAN

oxyclipine INN *anticholinergic* [also: propenzolate HCl]

oxyclipine HCl [see: propenzolate HCl]

oxyclozanide INN, BAN

Oxycocet (CAN) tablets ℞ *narcotic analgesic* [oxycodone HCl; acetaminophen] 5•325 mg

oxycodone USAN, INN, BAN *narcotic analgesic; also abused as a street drug*

oxycodone HCl USAN, USP *narcotic analgesic; also abused as a street drug* 5 mg oral

oxycodone terephthalate USP *narcotic analgesic; also abused as a street drug*

OxyContin controlled-release tablets ℞ *narcotic analgesic; also abused as a* *street drug* [oxycodone HCl] 10, 20, 40, 80, 160 mg

Oxydess II tablets ℞ *CNS stimulant; amphetamine* [dextroamphetamine sulfate] 10 mg

oxydimethylquinazine [see: antipyrine]

oxydipentonium chloride INN

oxyethyltheophylline [see: etofylline]

OxyFast oral drops ℞ *narcotic analgesic* [oxycodone HCl] 20 mg/mL

oxyfedrine INN, BAN

oxyfenamate INN *minor tranquilizer* [also: hydroxyphenamate]

oxyfilcon A USAN *hydrophilic contact lens material*

oxygen (O_2) USP *medicinal gas; element (O)*

oxygen, polymeric *investigational (orphan) for sickle cell anemia*

oxygen 93 percent USP *medicinal gas*

Oxygent emulsion ℞ *investigational (Phase III) intravascular oxygen carrier to reduce need for blood transfusions in surgical patients* [perflubron]

OxyIR immediate-release capsules ℞ *narcotic analgesic* [oxycodone HCl] 5 mg

oxymesterone INN, BAN

oxymetazoline INN, BAN *topical ocular vasoconstrictor; nasal decongestant* [also: oxymetazoline HCl] ⑨ oxymetholone

oxymetazoline HCl USAN, USP *topical ocular vasoconstrictor; nasal decongestant* [also: oxymetazoline] 0.05% nasal

oxymetholone USAN, USP, INN, BAN *androgen; anabolic steroid; also abused as a street drug* ⑨ oxymetazoline; oxymorphone

oxymethylene urea [see: polynoxylin]

oxymorphone INN, BAN *narcotic analgesic* [also: oxymorphone HCl] ⑨ oxymetholone

oxymorphone HCl USP *narcotic analgesic; investigational (orphan) for intractable pain in narcotic-tolerant patients* [also: oxymorphone]

oxypendyl INN

oxypertine USAN, INN *antidepressant*

oxyphenbutazone USP, INN *anti-inflammatory; antirheumatic; antipyretic; analgesic*

oxyphencyclimine INN *anticholinergic* [also: oxyphencyclimine HCl]

oxyphencyclimine HCl USP *peptic ulcer adjunct* [also: oxyphencyclimine]

oxyphenhydrazine [see: carsalam]

oxyphenisatin BAN *laxative* [also: oxyphenisatin acetate; oxyphenisatine]

oxyphenisatin acetate USAN *laxative* [also: oxyphenisatine; oxyphenisatin]

oxyphenisatine INN *laxative* [also: oxyphenisatin acetate; oxyphenisatin]

oxyphenonium bromide

oxyphylline [see: etofylline]

oxypurinol USAN *xanthine oxidase inhibitor* [also: oxipurinol]

oxypyrronium bromide INN

oxyquinoline USAN *disinfectant/antiseptic*

oxyquinoline benzoate [see: benzoxiquine]

oxyquinoline sulfate USAN, NF *complexing agent*

oxyridazine INN

Oxysept solution + tablets OTC *two-step chemical disinfecting system for soft contact lenses* [hydrogen peroxide-based] 3%

Oxysept 2 solution OTC *rinsing/storage solution for soft contact lenses* [sodium chloride (saline solution)]

oxysonium iodide INN

oxytetracycline USP, INN *bacteriostatic antibiotic; antirickettsial*

oxytetracycline calcium USP *antibacterial*

oxytetracycline HCl USP *bacteriostatic antibiotic; antirickettsial* 250 mg oral

oxytocics *a class of posterior pituitary hormones that stimulate contraction of the myometrium (uterine muscle)*

oxytocin USP, INN *posterior pituitary hormone; oxytocic for induction of labor* 10 U/mL injection

Oxyzal Wet Dressing liquid OTC *antiseptic dressing for minor infections* [oxyquinoline sulfate; benzalkonium chloride]

Oysco 500 chewable tablets OTC *calcium supplement* [calcium carbonate] 1.25 g

Oyst-Cal 500 film-coated tablets OTC *calcium supplement* [calcium carbonate] 1.25 g

Oyst-Cal-D film-coated tablets OTC *dietary supplement* [calcium carbonate; vitamin D] 250 mg•125 IU

Oyster Calcium tablets OTC *dietary supplement* [calcium carbonate; vitamins A and D] 375 mg•800 IU•200 IU

Oyster Calcium 500 + D tablets OTC *dietary supplement* [calcium carbonate; vitamin D] 500 mg•125 IU

Oyster Calcium with Vitamin D tablets OTC *dietary supplement* [calcium carbonate; vitamin D] 250 mg•125 IU

Oyster Shell Calcium with Vitamin D tablets OTC *calcium supplement* [calcium carbonate; vitamin D] 250 mg•125 IU

Oyster Shell Calcium-500 tablets OTC *calcium supplement* [calcium carbonate] 1.25 g

Oystercal 500 tablets OTC *calcium supplement* [calcium carbonate] 1.25 g

Oystercal-D 250 tablets OTC *dietary supplement* [calcium carbonate; vitamin D] 250 mg•125 IU

oz; gamma-oz *medicinal herb* [see: rice bran oil]

ozagrel INN *investigational antiasthmatic* [also: ozagrel sodium]

ozagrel sodium JAN *investigational antiasthmatic* [also: ozagrel]

ozolinone USAN, INN *diuretic*

P

P & S liquid OTC *antimicrobial hair dressing* [phenol]

P & S shampoo OTC *antiseborrheic; keratolytic* [salicylic acid] 2%

P & S Plus gel OTC *topical antipsoriatic; antiseborrheic; keratolytic* [coal tar solution; salicylic acid] 8%•2%

p30 protein *investigational (Phase III) adjunct to chemotherapy for pancreatic, breast, colorectal, prostate, and small cell lung cancers*

^{32}P [see: chromic phosphate P 32]

^{32}P [see: polymetaphosphate P 32]

^{32}P [see: sodium phosphate P 32]

P-53 *investigational (Phase II) antipsoriatic*

p53 adenoviral gene *investigational (Phase II) gene therapy for cancer* [also: adenoviral p53 gene]

P-54 *investigational (Phase II) COX-2 inhibitor for osteoarthritis*

P-081 *investigational isoflavone that increases HDL cholesterol in menopausal women*

P_1E_1; P_2E_1; P_4E_1; P_6E_1 Drop-Tainers (eye drops) ℞ *topical antiglaucoma agent* [pilocarpine HCl; epinephrine bitartrate] 1%•1%; 2%•1%; 4%•1%; 6%•1%

P_3E_1 Drop-Tainers (eye drops) (discontinued 1998) ℞ *topical antiglaucoma agent* [pilocarpine HCl; epinephrine bitartrate] 3%•1%

P-414 *investigational (Phase II) oral heparin for deep vein thrombosis*

P-748 *investigational (Phase II) imaging agent for pulmonary emboli*

PAB (para-aminobenzoate) [see: aminobenzoic acid]

PABA (para-aminobenzoic acid) [now: aminobenzoic acid]

PABA sodium [see: aminobenzoate sodium]

Pabalate enteric-coated tablets (discontinued 2000) OTC *analgesic; antipyretic; anti-inflammatory* [sodium salicylate; aminobenzoate sodium] 300•300 mg

PAB-Esc-C (Platinol, Adriamycin, bleomycin, escalating doses of

cyclophosphamide) *chemotherapy protocol*

pabestrol D [see: diethylstilbestrol dipropionate]

PAC; PAC-I (Platinol, Adriamycin, cyclophosphamide) *chemotherapy protocol for ovarian and endometrial cancer; "I" stands for "Indiana protocol," used for ovarian cancer only*

P-A-C Analgesic tablets OTC *analgesic; antipyretic; anti-inflammatory* [aspirin; caffeine] 400•32 mg

PACE (Platinol, Adriamycin, cyclophosphamide, etoposide) *chemotherapy protocol*

Pacerone tablets ℞ *antiarrhythmic for acute ventricular tachycardia and fibrillation (orphan)* [amiodarone HCl] 200, 400 mg

PA-CI (Adriamycin, cisplatin) *chemotherapy protocol for pediatric hepatoblastoma*

Pacis powder for intravesical instillation ℞ *antineoplastic for urinary bladder cancer* [BCG vaccine, Montreal strain] 120 mg (2.4–12 × 10^8 CFU)

Packer's Pine Tar shampoo, soap OTC *antiseborrheic; antipsoriatic; antipruritic; antibacterial* [pine tar]

paclitaxel USAN, INN, BAN *antineoplastic for ovarian and breast cancers, non–small cell lung cancer (NSCLC), and AIDS-related Kaposi sarcoma (orphan); investigational (Phase I/II) micellular formulation for multiple sclerosis* 6 mg/mL injection

paclitaxel & carboplatin & etoposide *chemotherapy protocol for primary adenocarcinoma and small cell lung cancer*

paclitaxel & trastuzumab *chemotherapy protocol for breast cancer*

paclitaxel & vinorelbine tartrate *chemotherapy protocol for breast cancer*

pacrinolol INN

padimate INN *ultraviolet screen* [also: padimate A]

padimate A USAN *ultraviolet screen* [also: padimate]

padimate O USAN *ultraviolet screen*

Paeonia officinalis *medicinal herb* [see: peony]

PAF-AH (platelet-activating factor acetylhydrolase) [see: platelet-activating factor acetylhydrolast, recombinant]

Pafase ℞ *investigational (Phase II/III) platelet-activating factor for acute respiratory distress syndrome* [acetylhydrolase]

pafenolol INN

paflufocon A USAN *hydrophobic contact lens material*

paflufocon B USAN *hydrophobic contact lens material*

paflufocon C USAN *hydrophobic contact lens material*

paflufocon D USAN *hydrophobic contact lens material*

paflufocon E USAN *hydrophobic contact lens material*

Pagoclone ℞ *investigational (Phase II) treatment for panic disorders*

pagoclone USAN *anxiolytic*

PAH (para-aminohippurate) [see: aminohippuric acid]

PAHA (para-aminohippuric acid) [see: aminohippuric acid]

Pain Bust-R II cream OTC *topical analgesic; counterirritant* [methyl salicylate; menthol] 17%•12%

Pain Doctor cream OTC *topical analgesic; topical anesthetic; antipruritic* [capsaicin; methyl salicylate; menthol] 0.025%•25%•10%

Pain Gel Plus OTC *topical analgesic; counterirritant* [menthol] 4%

Pain Reliever tablets (discontinued 2000) OTC *analgesic; antipyretic; anti-inflammatory* [acetaminophen; aspirin; caffeine] 250•250•65 mg

paint, Indian *medicinal herb* [see: bloodroot]

paint, yellow Indian *medicinal herb* [see: goldenseal]

paint root, red *medicinal herb* [see: bloodroot]

Pain-X gel OTC *topical analgesic; counterirritant* [capsaicin; menthol; camphor] 0.05%•5%•4%

PALA disodium [see: sparfosate sodium]
palatrigine INN, BAN
paldimycin USAN, INN *antibacterial*
paldimycin A [see: paldimycin]
paldimycin B [see: paldimycin]
pale gentian *medicinal herb* [see: gentian]
palestrol [see: diethylstilbestrol]
Palgic-D extended-release tablets ℞ *decongestant; antihistamine* [pseudoephedrine HCl; carbinoxamine maleate] 90•8 mg
Palgic-DS syrup ℞ *decongestant; antihistamine* [pseudoephedrine HCl; carbinoxamine maleate] 30•2 mg/5 mL
palinavir USAN *antiviral; HIV-1 protease inhibitor*
palinum [see: cyclobarbitone]
palivizumab *monoclonal antibody for prophylaxis of respiratory syncytial virus (RSV) in infants*
palladium *element (Pd)*
palladium Pd 103 *investigational radioactive "seeds" for ultrasound-guided brachytherapy for adenocarcinoma of the prostate*
palm, dwarf; dwarf palmetto; pan palm *medicinal herb* [see: saw palmetto]
palmidrol INN
Palmitate-A 5000 tablets OTC *vitamin supplement* [vitamin A palmitate] 5000 IU
palmitic acid USAN *ultrasound contrast medium for echocardiography*
palmoxirate sodium USAN *antidiabetic* [also: palmoxiric acid]
palmoxiric acid INN *antidiabetic* [also: palmoxirate sodium]
palonosetron HCl USAN *antiemetic; antinauseant; serotonin 5-HT$_3$ antagonist; investigational (Phase III) for chemotherapy-induced nausea and vomiting*
PALS coated tablets OTC *systemic deodorant for ostomy, breath, and body odors* [chlorophyllin copper complex] 100 mg
PAM; L-PAM (phenylalanine mustard) [see: melphalan]
2-PAM (2-pyridine aldoxime methylchloride) [see: pralidoxime chloride]
pamabrom USAN *nonprescription diuretic*
pamaqueside USAN *hypocholesterolemic; cholesterol absorption inhibitor; antiatherosclerotic*
pamaquine naphthoate NF
pamatolol INN *antiadrenergic (β-receptor)* [also: pamatolol sulfate]
pamatolol sulfate USAN *antiadrenergic (β-receptor)* [also: pamatolol]
Pamelor capsules, oral solution ℞ *tricyclic antidepressant* [nortriptyline HCl] 10, 25, 50, 75 mg; 10 mg/5 mL ⑨ Dymelor; Panlor
pamidronate disodium USAN *bisphosphonate bone resorption inhibitor for Paget disease, hypercalcemia of malignancy, breast cancer, and multiple myeloma*
pamidronic acid INN, BAN
Pamine tablets ℞ *GI antispasmodic; anticholinergic; peptic ulcer treatment* [methscopolamine bromide] 2.5 mg
Pamisyl ℞ *investigational (orphan) for ulcerative colitis* [aminosalicylic acid]
pamoate USAN, USP *combining name for radicals or groups* [also: embonate]
Pamprin, Nighttime powder OTC *antihistaminic sleep aid; analgesic* [diphenhydramine HCl; acetaminophen] 50•650 mg
Pamprin Maximum Pain Relief caplets OTC *analgesic; antipyretic; diuretic* [acetaminophen; magnesium salicylate; pamabrom] 250•250•25 mg
Pamprin Multi-Symptom caplets, tablets OTC *analgesic; antipyretic; diuretic; antihistaminic sleep aid* [acetaminophen; pamabrom; pyrilamine maleate] 500•25•15 mg
Pan C Ascorbate; Pan C-500 tablets OTC *vitamin C supplement with multiple bioflavonoids* [vitamin C; citrus bioflavonoids; hesperidin] 200•100•100 mg; 500•100•100 mg

Panacet 5/500 tablets ℞ *narcotic analgesic* [hydrocodone bitartrate; acetaminophen] 5•500 mg

panadiplon USAN, INN *anxiolytic*

Panadol tablets, caplets OTC *analgesic; antipyretic* [acetaminophen] 500 mg

Panadol, Children's chewable tablets, liquid OTC *analgesic; antipyretic* [acetaminophen] 80 mg; 160 mg/5 mL

Panadol, Infants' drops OTC *analgesic; antipyretic* [acetaminophen] 100 mg/mL

Panadol, Junior caplets OTC *analgesic; antipyretic* [acetaminophen] 160 mg

Panafil ointment ℞ *topical enzyme for wound debridement; vulnerary; wound deodorant* [papain; urea; chlorophyllin copper complex] 521 700 IU/g•10%•0.5%

Panafil White ointment ℞ *topical enzyme for wound debridement; vulnerary* [papain; urea] 10%•10%

Panalgesic cream OTC *topical analgesic; counterirritant* [methyl salicylate; menthol] 35%•4%

Panalgesic Gold liniment OTC *topical analgesic; counterirritant; antiseptic* [methyl salicylate; camphor; menthol; alcohol 22%] 55%•3.1%•1.25%

Panasal 5/500 tablets ℞ *narcotic analgesic* [hydrocodone bitartrate; aspirin] 5•500 mg

Panasol-S tablets ℞ *corticosteroid; anti-inflammatory; immunosuppressant* [prednisone] 1 mg ⑨ Panscol

Panavir ℞ *investigational (Phase II) antiviral for HIV and AIDS* [probucol]

Panax ginseng; P. shin-seng **(Korean ginseng)** *medicinal herb* [see: ginseng]

Panax horridum *medicinal herb* [see: devil's club]

Panax pseudoginseng **(Chikusetsu ginseng; Himalayan ginseng; Sanchi ginseng; Zhuzishen)** *medicinal herb* [see: ginseng]

Panax quinquefolia **(American ginseng)** *medicinal herb* [see: ginseng]

Panax **spp.** *medicinal herb* [see: ginseng]

Panax trifolius **(dwarf ginseng)** *medicinal herb* [see: ginseng]

Pancof-HC oral liquid ℞ *narcotic antitussive; decongestant; antihistamine* [hydrocodone bitartrate; pseudoephedrine HCl; chlorpheniramine maleate; alcohol 5%] 3•15•2 mg/5 mL

Pancof-XL; Pancof XP liquid ℞ *narcotic antitussive; decongestant; expectorant* [hydrocodone bitartrate; pseudoephedrine HCl; guaifenesin] 3•15•100 mg/5 mL; 2.5•15•100 mg/5 mL

pancopride USAN, INN *antiemetic; anxiolytic; peristaltic stimulant*

Pancrease; Pancrease MT 4; Pancrease MT 10; Pancrease MT 16; Pancrease MT 20 capsules containing enteric-coated microtablets ℞ *digestive enzymes* [lipase; protease; amylase] 4.5•25•20; 4.5•12•12; 10•30•30; 16•48•48; 20•44•56 thousand USP units

pancreatin USP *digestive enzyme*

Pancreatin, 4X; Pancreatin, 8X tablets OTC *digestive enzymes* [pancreatin; lipase; protease; amylase] 2400 mg•12 000 U•60 000 U•60 000 U; 7200 mg•22 500 U•180 000 U•180 000 U

Pancrecarb MS-8 delayed-release capsules ℞ *digestive enzymes for exocrine pancreatic insufficiency in cystic fibrosis and chronic pancreatitis* [lipase; protease; amylase] 8•45•40 thousand USP units

pancrelipase USAN, USP *digestive enzyme* 8000 lipase U•30 000 protease U•30 000 amylase U

Pancrezyme 4X tablets OTC *digestive enzymes* [pancreatin; lipase; protease; amylase] 2400 mg•12 000 U•60 000 U•60 000 U

pancuronium bromide USAN, INN *nondepolarizing neuromuscular blocker; muscle relaxant; adjunct to anesthesia* 1, 2 mg/mL injection

Pandel cream ℞ *topical corticosteroidal anti-inflammatory* [hydrocortisone probutate] 0.1%

Panex; Panex 500 tablets (discontinued 1997) OTC *analgesic; antipyretic* [acetaminophen] 325 mg; 500 mg

Panfil G capsules, syrup ℞ *antiasthmatic; bronchodilator; expectorant* [dyphylline; guaifenesin] 200•100 mg; 100•50 mg/5 mL

Panglobulin powder for IV infusion ℞ *passive immunizing agent for HIV and idiopathic thrombocytopenic purpura (ITP)* [immune globulin] 1, 3, 6, 12 g

Panhematin powder for IV injection ℞ *enzyme inhibitor for recurring attacks of acute intermittent porphyria (AIP)* [hemin] 301 mg/dose

panidazole INN, BAN

Panitone-500 tablets OTC *analgesic; antipyretic* [acetaminophen] 500 mg

Panlor DC capsules ℞ *narcotic analgesic* [dihydrocodeine bitartrate; acetaminophen; caffeine] 16•356.4•30 mg ⊠ Pamelor

Panmist JR long-acting tablets ℞ *decongestant; expectorant* [pseudoephedrine HCl; guaifenesin] 45•600 mg

PanMist-DM extended-release caplets ℞ *antitussive; decongestant; expectorant* [dextromethorphan hydrobromide; pseudoephedrine HCl; guaifenesin] 30•45•600 mg

Panmycin capsules ℞ *broad-spectrum antibiotic* [tetracycline HCl] 250 mg

Pannaz tablets ℞ *decongestant; antihistamine; anticholinergic* [pseudoephedrine HCl; chlorpheniramine maleate; methscopolamine nitrate] 90•8•2.5 mg

panomifene INN

Panorex ℞ *antineoplastic adjunct (orphan status withdrawn 1997)* [edrecolomab] ⊠ Panarex

Panoxyl cleansing bar ℞ *topical keratolytic for acne* [benzoyl peroxide] 5%, 10% ⊠ Benoxyl

Panoxyl AQ 2½; Panoxyl 5; Panoxyl AQ 5; Panoxyl 10; Panoxyl AQ 10 gel ℞ *topical keratolytic for acne* [benzoyl peroxide] 2.5%; 5%; 5%; 10%; 10%

Panretin capsules ℞ *investigational (Phase III, orphan) treatment for Kaposi sarcoma, psoriasis, myelodysplastic syndrome (MDS), and acute promyelocytic leukemia (APL)* [alitretinoin]

Panretin gel ℞ *topical treatment for cutaneous lesions of AIDS-related Kaposi sarcoma (orphan)* [alitretinoin] 0.1%

Panscol lotion, ointment OTC *topical keratolytic* [salicylic acid] 3% ⊠ Panasol

pansy (*Viola tricolor*) plant *medicinal herb used as an anodyne, demulcent, diaphoretic, diuretic, expectorant, laxative, and vulnerary*

pantenicate INN

panthenol USAN, USP, INN *B complex vitamin*

D-panthenol [see: dexpanthenol]

Panthoderm cream OTC *antipruritic; vulnerary; emollient* [dexpanthenol] 2%

Panto IV (CAN) powder for IV injection ℞ *proton pump inhibitor for erosive esophagitis associated with gastroesophageal reflux disease (GERD)* [pantoprazole sodium] 40 mg/vial

Panto IV (CAN) powder for IV injection ℞ *proton pump inhibitor for gastroesophageal reflux disease (GERD) and eradication of H. pylori infection* [pantoprazole sodium]

Pantoloc (CAN) enteric-coated tablets ℞ *proton pump inhibitor for erosive esophagitis associated with gastroesophageal reflux disease (GERD)* [pantoprazole sodium] 40 mg

pantoprazole USAN, INN, BAN *proton pump inhibitor for erosive esophagitis associated with gastroesophageal reflux disease (GERD)*

pantoprazole sodium USAN *proton pump inhibitor for erosive esophagitis associated with gastroesophageal reflux disease (GERD)*

pantothenic acid (vitamin B_5) BAN *water-soluble vitamin; enzyme cofactor* [also: calcium pantothenate]

DL-pantothenic acid [see: calcium pantothenate, racemic]

pantothenol [see: dexpanthenol]

pantothenyl alcohol [see: panthenol]

D-pantothenyl alcohol [see: dexpanthenol]

Pantozol ℞ *investigational proton pump inhibitor for gastroesophageal reflux disease (GERD)* [pantoprazole]

panuramine INN, BAN

papain USP *topical proteolytic enzyme for necrotic tissue debridement*

Papain Urea Chlorophyllin ointment ℞ *topical enzyme for wound debridement; vulnerary; wound deodorant* [papain; urea; chlorophyllin copper complex] 521 700 IU/g•10%•0.5%

Papain Urea Debriding ointment ℞ *topical enzyme for wound debridement; vulnerary* [papain; urea] 1 100 000 IU/g•10%

papaverine BAN *peripheral vasodilator; smooth muscle relaxant; orphan status withdrawn 1996* [also: papaverine HCl]

papaverine HCl USP *peripheral vasodilator; smooth muscle relaxant for cerebral, myocardial, and peripheral ischemias* [also: papaverine] 150 mg oral; 30 mg/mL

papaveroline INN, BAN

papaya *(Carica papaya)* leaves, fruit, juice, and seeds *medicinal herb for aiding digestion, gas, insect bites, and intestinal worms*

Papaya Enzyme chewable tablets OTC *digestive enzymes* [papain; amylase] 60•60 mg

Papirine ℞ *investigational antiviral*

Paplex Ultra solution ℞ *topical keratolytic* [salicylic acid in flexible collodion] 26%

papoose root *medicinal herb* [see: blue cohosh]

Par Glycerol elixir ℞ *expectorant* [iodinated glycerol] 60 mg/5 mL

Para Special Lice and Nits (CAN) spray, shampoo OTC *pediculicide* [piperonyl butoxide; bioallethrin] 2.64%•0.66%; 4.4%•1.1%

para-aminobenzoate (PAB) [see: aminobenzoic acid]

Para-Aminobenzoic Acid tablets, powder OTC *"possibly effective" for scleroderma and other skin diseases and Peyronie disease* [aminobenzoic acid] 100, 500 mg; 120 g

para-aminobenzoic acid (PABA) [now: aminobenzoic acid]

para-aminohippurate (PAH) [see: aminohippuric acid]

para-aminohippurate sodium [see: aminohippurate sodium]

para-aminohippuric acid (PAHA) [see: aminohippuric acid]

para-aminosalicylate (PAS) [see: aminosalicylic acid]

para-aminosalicylic acid (PASA) [see: aminosalicylic acid]

Parabolan *brand name for trenbolone hexahydrobenzylcarbonate, a European veterinary anabolic steroid abused as a street drug*

parabromdylamine maleate [see: brompheniramine maleate]

paracetaldehyde [see: paraldehyde]

paracetamol INN, BAN *analgesic; antipyretic* [also: acetaminophen]

parachlorometaxylenol (PCMX) *topical antiseptic; broad-spectrum antibacterial*

parachlorophenol (PCP) USP *topical antibacterial*

parachlorophenol, camphorated USP *topical dental anti-infective*

paracodin [see: dihydrocodeine]

paraffin NF *stiffening agent*

paraffin, liquid [see: mineral oil]

paraffin, synthetic NF *stiffening agent*

Paraflex caplets ℞ *skeletal muscle relaxant* [chlorzoxazone] 250 mg

paraflutizide INN

Parafon Forte DSC caplets ℞ *skeletal muscle relaxant* [chlorzoxazone] 500 mg ⑨ Pantopon

paraformaldehyde USP

Paraguay tea *medicinal herb* [see: yerba maté]

Para-Hist HD liquid ℞ *narcotic antitussive; decongestant; antihistamine* [hydrocodone bitartrate; phenylephrine HCl; chlorpheniramine maleate] 1.67•5•2 mg/5 mL

parahydrecin [now: isomerol]

Paral oral liquid, rectal liquid ℞ *sedative; hypnotic* [paraldehyde]
paraldehyde USP *hypnotic; sedative; anticonvulsant* 1 g/mL oral or rectal
paramethadione USP, INN, BAN *anticonvulsant* ⚠ paramethasone
paramethasone INN *corticosteroid; anti-inflammatory* [also: paramethasone acetate] ⚠ paramethadione
paramethasone acetate USAN, USP *corticosteroid; anti-inflammatory* [also: paramethasone]
para-nitrosulfathiazole NF [also: nitrosulfathiazole]
paranyline HCl USAN *anti-inflammatory* [also: renytoline]
parapenzolate bromide USAN, INN *anticholinergic*
Paraplatin powder for IV injection ℞ *alkylating antineoplastic for ovarian and other cancers* [carboplatin] 50, 150, 450 mg
parapropamol INN
pararosaniline embonate INN *antischistosomal* [also: pararosaniline pamoate]
pararosaniline pamoate USAN *antischistosomal* [also: pararosaniline embonate]
parasympathomimetics *a class of agents that produce effects similar to those of the parasympathetic nervous system* [also called: cholinergic agonists]
Parathar powder for IV injection ℞ *in vivo diagnostic aid for parathyroid-induced hypocalcemia (orphan)* [teriparatide acetate] 200 U
parathesin [see: benzocaine]
parathiazine INN
parathyroid USP *hormone*
parathyroid hormone (1-34), biosynthetic human [see: teriparatide]
parathyroid hormone (1-84), recombinant human *investigational (Phase III) agent to increase bone mineral content and density in postmenopausal osteoporosis*
paraxazone INN
parbendazole USAN, INN *anthelmintic*
parconazole INN *antifungal* [also: parconazole HCl]
parconazole HCl USAN *antifungal* [also: parconazole]
parecoxib USAN *COX-2 inhibitor; anti-inflammatory; analgesic*
parecoxib sodium USAN *COX-2 inhibitor; anti-inflammatory; analgesic*
Paredrine eye drops ℞ *mydriatic* [hydroxyamphetamine hydrobromide] 1%
paregoric (PG) USP (a preparation of opium, anise oil, benzoic acid, camphor, alcohol, and glycerin) *antiperistaltic; narcotic analgesic; sometimes abused as a street drug* 2 mg/5 mL oral
Paremyd eye drops ℞ *mydriatic; weak cycloplegic* [hydroxyamphetamine hydrobromide; tropicamide] 1%•0.25%
parenabol [see: boldenone undecylenate]
Parepectolin concentrated liquid OTC *GI adsorbent; antidiarrheal* [attapulgite] 600 mg/15 mL
pareptide INN *antiparkinsonian* [also: pareptide sulfate]
pareptide sulfate USAN *antiparkinsonian* [also: pareptide]
parethoxycaine INN
parethoxycaine HCl [see: parethoxycaine]
Par-F tablets ℞ *vitamin/mineral/calcium/iron supplement* [multiple vitamins & minerals; calcium; iron; folic acid] ≛•250•60•1 mg
pargeverine INN
pargolol INN
pargyline INN *antihypertensive* [also: pargyline HCl]
pargyline HCl USAN, USP *antihypertensive* [also: pargyline]
paricalcitol USAN *synthetic vitamin D analogue for osteodystrophy and hyperparathyroidism secondary to chronic renal failure*
paridocaine INN
Parlodel SnapTabs (scored tablets), capsules ℞ *dopamine agonist for Parkinson disease; lactation inhibitor; treats acro-*

megaly, infertility, and hypogonadism [bromocriptine mesylate] 2.5 mg; 5 mg

Par-Natal Plus 1 Improved tablets ℞ *vitamin/calcium/iron supplement* [multiple vitamins; calcium; iron; folic acid] ≛•200•65•1 mg

Parnate film-coated tablets ℞ *monoamine oxidase inhibitor (MAOI) for reactive depression (a major depressive episode without melancholia)* [tranylcypromine sulfate] 10 mg

parodilol INN

parodyne [see: antipyrine]

paroleine [see: mineral oil]

paromomycin INN, BAN *aminoglycoside antibiotic; amebicide* [also: paromomycin sulfate]

Paromomycin ℞ *investigational (orphan) for tuberculosis,* Mycobacterium avium *complex, and visceral leishmaniasis* [aminosidine]

paromomycin sulfate USP *aminoglycoside antibiotic; amebicide* [also: paromomycin]

paroxetine USAN, INN, BAN *selective serotonin reuptake inhibitor (SSRI) for depression, obsessive-compulsive disorder, and panic disorder*

paroxetine HCl *selective serotonin reuptake inhibitor (SSRI) for depression, obsessive-compulsive disorder, panic disorder, social anxiety disorder, and generalized anxiety disorder*

paroxyl [see: acetarsone]

paroxypropione INN

parpanit HCl [see: caramiphen HCl]

parsalmide INN

Parsidol tablets (discontinued 1997) ℞ *anticholinergic; antiparkinsonian* [ethopropazine HCl] 10, 50 mg

parsley ***(Petroselinum sativum)*** leaves and root *medicinal herb for amenorrhea, bladder infections, blood building and cleansing, body lice, colic, dysmenorrhea, flatulence, gallstones, inducing abortion, jaundice, nephritis, prostate disorders, and urinary retention*

parsley fern *medicinal herb* [see: tansy]

parsnip, cow; wooly parsnip *medicinal herb* [see: masterwort]

Parthenocissus quinquefolia *medicinal herb* [see: American ivy]

partricin USAN, INN *antifungal; antiprotozoal*

partridge berry *medicinal herb* [see: squaw vine; wintergreen]

Partuss LA long-acting tablets ℞ *decongestant; expectorant* [phenylpropanolamine HCl; guaifenesin] 75•400 mg

parvaquone INN, BAN ge

Parvlex tablets OTC *hematinic* [ferrous fumarate; multiple B vitamins & minerals; vitamin C; folic acid] 100•≛•50•0.1 mg

PAS (para-aminosalicylate) [see: aminosalicylic acid]

PASA (para-aminosalicylic acid) [see: aminosalicylic acid]

Paser delayed-release granules ℞ *treatment for multidrug-resistant tuberculosis (MDR-TB) (orphan)* [aminosalicylic acid] 4 g/packet

pasiniazid INN

pasque flower ***(Anemone patens)*** plant *medicinal herb used as a diaphoretic, diuretic, and rubefacient; not generally regarded as safe due to toxicity*

passion flower ***(Passiflora incarnata)*** plant *medicinal herb for asthma, bronchitis, eye infections, fever, inflamed hemorrhoids, insomnia, menopause, nervousness, pain related to neurasthenia, and attention-deficit disorder, nervousness, and excitability in children*

Pastilles (dosage form) *troches*

Patanol Drop-Tainer (eye drops) ℞ *topical ophthalmic antihistamine and mast cell stabilizer for allergic conjunctivitis* [olopatadine HCl] 0.1%

PATCO (prednisone, ara-C, thioguanine, cyclophosphamide, Oncovin) *chemotherapy protocol*

Pathilon film-coated tablets (discontinued 2001) ℞ *peptic ulcer treatment adjunct* [tridihexethyl chloride] 25 mg ⑨ Pathocil

Pathocil capsules, powder for oral suspension ℞ *penicillinase-resistant penicillin antibiotic* [dicloxacillin sodium]

250, 500 mg; 62.5 mg/5 mL ⊡ Bactocill; Pathilon; Placidyl

patience, garden *medicinal herb* [see: yellow dock]

patience dock *medicinal herb* [see: bistort]

pau d'arco *(Lapacho colorado; L. morado)* inner bark *medicinal herb for boils, blood cleansing, cancer, Candida albicans infections, chlorosis, diabetes, leukemia, pain, skin wounds, and syphilis*

Paullinia cupana; P. sorbilis *medicinal herb* [see: guarana]

paulomycin USAN, INN *antibacterial*

Pausinystalia johimbe *medicinal herb* [see: yohimbe]

pauson *medicinal herb* [see: bloodroot]

Pavabid Plateau Caps (controlled-release capsules) ℞ *peripheral vasodilator; smooth muscle relaxant for cerebral, myocardial, and peripheral ischemias* [papaverine HCl] 150 mg ⊡ Pavased

Pavagen TD timed-release capsules ℞ *peripheral vasodilator; smooth muscle relaxant for cerebral, myocardial, and peripheral ischemias* [papaverine HCl] 150 mg

Pavarine Spancaps (timed-release capsules) (discontinued 1997) ℞ *peripheral vasodilator; smooth muscle relaxant for cerebral, myocardial, and peripheral ischemias* [papaverine HCl] 150 mg

Pavatine timed-release capsules (discontinued 1997) ℞ *peripheral vasodilator; smooth muscle relaxant for cerebral, myocardial, and peripheral ischemias* [papaverine HCl] 150 mg ⊡ Pavatym

PAVe (procarbazine, Alkeran, Velban) *chemotherapy protocol*

Paverolan Lanacaps (timed-release capsules) (discontinued 1997) ℞ *peripheral vasodilator; smooth muscle relaxant for cerebral, myocardial, and peripheral ischemias* [papaverine HCl] 150 mg ⊡ Pavulon

Pavulon IM injection ℞ *nondepolarizing neuromuscular blocker; adjunct to anesthesia* [pancuronium bromide] 1, 2 mg/mL ⊡ Paverolan

pawpaw *(Asimina triloba)* fruit *medicinal herb used as an antimicrobial and antineoplastic*

paxamate INN

Paxarel tablets ℞ *anxiolytic; sedative* [acecarbromal] 250 mg

Paxene ℞ *antineoplastic for ovarian and breast cancers, non–small cell lung cancer (NSCLC), and AIDS-related Kaposi sarcoma (orphan)* [paclitaxel]

Paxil film-coated tablets, oral suspension ℞ *selective serotonin reuptake inhibitor (SSRI) for depression, obsessive-compulsive disorder (OCD), panic disorder, social anxiety disorder, and generalized anxiety disorder (GAD)* [paroxetine HCl] 10, 20, 30, 40 mg; 10 mg/5 mL

Paxil CR film-coated controlled-release tablets (discontinued 2000) ℞ *selective serotonin reuptake inhibitor (SSRI) for depression* [paroxetine HCl] 12.5, 25 mg

pazelliptine INN

pazinaclone USAN *anxiolytic*

Pazo Hemorrhoid ointment OTC *temporary relief of hemorrhoidal symptoms; topical vasoconstrictor; counterirritant; astringent* [ephedrine sulfate; camphor; zinc oxide] 0.2%•2%•5%

Pazo Hemorrhoid suppositories OTC *temporary relief of hemorrhoidal symptoms; topical vasoconstrictor; astringent* [ephedrine sulfate; zinc oxide] 3.8•96.5 mg

pazoxide USAN, INN *antihypertensive*

PBV (Platinol, bleomycin, vinblastine) *chemotherapy protocol*

PBZ elixir (discontinued 1997) ℞ *antihistamine* [tripelennamine HCl] 37.5 mg/5 mL

PBZ tablets ℞ *antihistamine* [tripelennamine HCl] 25, 50 mg

PBZ (pyribenzamine) [see: tripelennamine]

PBZ-SR extended-release tablets ℞ *antihistamine* [tripelennamine HCl] 100 mg

PC (paclitaxel, carboplatin) *chemotherapy protocol for bladder and non–small cell lung cancer (NSCLC)*
PC (paclitaxel, cisplatin) *chemotherapy protocol for non–small cell lung cancer (NSCLC)*
PC (phosphatidylcholine) [see: lecithin]
PCE Dispertabs (delayed-release tablets) ℞ *macrolide antibiotic* [erythromycin] 333, 500 mg
PCE (Platinol, cyclophosphamide, etoposide) *chemotherapy protocol*
PCE (polymer-coated erythromycin) [see: erythromycin]
PCMX (parachlorometaxylenol) [q.v.]
PCOs (procyanidolic oligomers) [q.v.]
PCP (parachlorophenol) [q.v.]
PCP (phenylcyclohexyl piperidine) *a powerful veterinary analgesic/anesthetic widely abused as a hallucinogenic street drug* [medically known as phencyclidine HCl]
PCV (procarbazine, CCNU, vincristine) *chemotherapy protocol for brain tumors*
PDE-3 (phosphodiesterase-3) inhibitors *a class of platelet aggregation inhibitors*
PDGA (pteroyldiglutamic acid)
PDLA (phosphinicodilactic acid) [see: foscolic acid]
PDP Liquid Protein OTC *dietary supplement* [hydrolyzed protein; L-tryptophan] 15•?̲ g/30 mL
PE (paclitaxel, estramustine) *chemotherapy protocol for prostate cancer*
PE (phenylephrine) [q.v.]
PE (polyethylene) [q.v.]
pea, ground squirrel *medicinal herb* [see: twin leaf]
pea, turkey; wild turkey pea *medicinal herb* [see: turkey corn]
peach *(Prunus persica)* bark and leaves *medicinal herb for bladder disorders, chest congestion, chronic bronchitis, nausea, and water retention*
peanut oil NF *solvent*
PEB (Platinol, etoposide, bleomycin) *chemotherapy protocol*
pecazine INN, BAN
pecazine acetate [see: pecazine]
pecilocin INN, BAN
pecocycline INN
pectin USP *suspending agent; protectant; GI adsorbent*
pectorals *a class of agents that relieve disorders of the respiratory tract, such as expectorants*
Pedameth capsules, liquid ℞ *urinary acidifier to control ammonia production* [racemethionine] 200 mg; 75 mg/5 mL
PediaCare Allergy Formula liquid OTC *antihistamine* [chlorpheniramine maleate] 1 mg/5 mL
PediaCare Cold-Allergy chewable tablets OTC *pediatric decongestant and antihistamine* [pseudoephedrine HCl; chlorpheniramine maleate] 15•1 mg
PediaCare Cough-Cold Formula chewable tablets, liquid OTC *pediatric antitussive, decongestant, and antihistamine* [dextromethorphan hydrobromide; pseudoephedrine HCl; chlorpheniramine maleate] 5•15•1 mg; 5•15•1 mg/5 mL
PediaCare Fever oral suspension, oral drops OTC *analgesic; antiarthritic; antipyretic; nonsteroidal anti-inflammatory drug (NSAID)* [ibuprofen] 100 mg/5 mL; 40 mg/mL
PediaCare Infant's Decongestant drops OTC *nasal decongestant* [pseudoephedrine HCl] 7.5 mg/0.8 mL
PediaCare NightRest Cough-Cold liquid OTC *pediatric antitussive, decongestant, and antihistamine* [dextromethorphan hydrobromide; pseudoephedrine HCl; chlorpheniramine maleate] 7.5•15•1 mg/5 mL
Pediacof syrup ℞ *pediatric narcotic antitussive, decongestant, antihistamine, and expectorant* [codeine phosphate; phenylephrine HCl; chlorpheniramine maleate; potassium iodide; alcohol 5%] 5•2.5•0.75•75 mg/5 mL
Pediacon DX children's syrup, pediatric drops OTC *pediatric antitussive, decon-*

gestant, and expectorant [dextromethorphan hydrobromide; phenylpropanolamine HCl; guaifenesin] 5•6.25•100 mg/5 mL; 5•6.25•50 mg/mL

Pediacon EX pediatric drops OTC *pediatric decongestant and expectorant* [phenylpropanolamine HCl; guaifenesin] 6.25•50 mg/mL

Pediaflor drops ℞ *dental caries preventative* [sodium fluoride] 1.1 mg/mL

Pedialyte oral solution, freezer pops OTC *electrolyte replacement* [sodium, potassium, and chloride electrolytes]

Pediamist low-pressure nasal spray OTC *nasal moisturizer for children* [sodium chloride (saline solution)]

Pediapred oral solution ℞ *corticosteroid; anti-inflammatory* [prednisolone sodium phosphate] 5 mg/5 mL

PediaSure; PediaSure with Fiber ready-to-use liquid OTC *total or supplementary infant feeding*

Pediatric Electrolyte oral solution OTC *electrolyte replacement* [dextrose; multiple electrolytes] 1 L

Pediazole oral suspension ℞ *antibiotic* [erythromycin ethylsuccinate; sulfisoxazole acetyl] 200•600 mg/5 mL

Pedi-Bath Salts (discontinued 2000) OTC *bath emollient*

Pedi-Boro Soak Paks powder packets OTC *astringent wet dressing (modified Burow solution)* [aluminum sulfate; calcium acetate]

Pedi-Cort V Creme (discontinued 2000) ℞ *topical corticosteroidal anti-inflammatory; antifungal; antibacterial* [hydrocortisone; clioquinol] 1%•3%

pediculicides *a class of agents effective against head and pubic lice*

Pedi-Dri powder ℞ *topical antifungal* [nystatin] 100 000 U/g

Pediotic ear drop suspension ℞ *topical corticosteroidal anti-inflammatory; antibiotic* [hydrocortisone; neomycin sulfate; polymyxin B sulfate] 1%•5 mg•10 000 U per mL

Pedi-Pro foot powder OTC *topical antifungal; anhidrotic* [zinc undecylenate; aluminum chlorohydrate; menthol; chloroxylenol]

Pedituss Cough syrup ℞ *pediatric narcotic antitussive, decongestant, antihistamine, and expectorant* [codeine phosphate; phenylephrine HCl; chlorpheniramine maleate; potassium iodide] 5•2.5•0.75•75 mg/5 mL

Pedi-Vit-A Creme OTC *moisturizer; emollient* [vitamin A] 100 000 U/30 g

Pedotic otic suspension ℞ *topical corticosteroidal anti-inflammatory; antibiotic* [hydrocortisone; neomycin sulfate; polymyxin B sulfate] 1%•5 mg•10 000 U per mL

PedTE-Pak-4 IV injection ℞ *intravenous nutritional therapy* [multiple trace elements (metals)] ≛

Pedtrace-4 IV injection ℞ *intravenous nutritional therapy* [multiple trace elements (metals)]

PedvaxHIB IM injection ℞ *pediatric (2–71 months) vaccine for Haemophilus influenzae type b (HIB)* [Hemophilus b conjugate vaccine; *Neisseria meningitidis* OMPC] 7.5•125 μg/0.5 mL

pefloxacin USAN, INN, BAN *antibacterial*

pefloxacin mesylate USAN *antibacterial*

PEG (polyethylene glycol) [q.v.]

PEG-ADA (polyethylene glycol-adenosine deaminase) [see: pegademase bovine]

pegademase INN *adenosine deaminase (ADA) replacement* [also: pegademase bovine]

pegademase bovine USAN *adenosine deaminase (ADA) replacement for severe combined immunodeficiency disease (orphan)* [also: pegademase]

PEG-adenosine deaminase (PEG-ADA) [see: pegademase bovine]

Peganone tablets ℞ *hydantoin anticonvulsant* [ethotoin] 250, 500 mg

PEG-L-asparaginase [see: pegaspargase]

pegaspargase (PEG-L-asparaginase) USAN, INN *antineoplastic for acute lymphocytic leukemia (orphan) and acute lymphoblastic leukemia*

Pegasys ℞ *investigational (orphan) agent for renal call carcinoma; investi-*

gational (NDA filed) for chronic hepatitis C [PEG-interferon alfa-2a]

PEG-camptothecin *investigational prodrug form of camptothecin, a hormonal antineoplastic topoisomerase I inhibitor*

PEG-ES (polyethylene glycol–electrolyte solution) [q.v.]

PEG-glucocerebrosidase *investigational (orphan) chronic enzyme replacement therapy for Gaucher disease*

PEG-hemoglobin *investigational blood replacement*

PEG-interferon alfa-2a *investigational (orphan) agent for renal cell carcinoma; investigational (NDA filed) for hepatitis C*

peginterferon alfa-2b *antiviral for chronic hepatitis C*

PEG-interleukin-2 *investigational (Phase II) cytokine for AIDS; investigational (orphan) for primary immunodeficiencies associated with T-cell defects*

PEG-Intron powder for subcu injection *antiviral; long-acting formulation of Intron A for chronic hepatitis C; investigational (Phase III) for malignant melanoma and chronic myelogenous leukemia* [peginterferon alfa-2b] 100, 160, 240, 300 µg/mL

peglicol 5 oleate USAN *emulsifying agent*

pegnartograstim USAN *immunostimulant adjunct to cancer chemotherapy*

pegorgotein USAN, INN *free-radical scavenger; investigational to prevent irreversible brain damage after head trauma*

pegoterate USAN, INN *suspending agent*

pegoxol 7 stearate USAN *emulsifying agent*

PEG-SOD (polyethylene glycol-superoxide dismutase) [see: pegorgotein]

PEG-uricase (polyethylene glycol-urate oxidase) *investigational*

pegvisomant USAN *investigational (Phase III, orphan) growth hormone receptor antagonist for acromegaly*

pegylated megakaryocyte growth factor [see: megakaryocyte growth and development factor, pegylated, recombinant human]

Pelamine tablets (discontinued 1997) ℞ *antihistamine* [tripelennamine HCl] 50 mg

pelanserin INN *antihypertensive; vasodilator; serotonin adrenergic blocker* [also: pelanserin HCl]

pelanserin HCl USAN *antihypertensive; vasodilator; serotonin adrenergic blocker* [also: pelanserin]

peldesine USAN *purine nucleoside phosphorylase inhibitor for psoriasis; investigational (orphan) for cutaneous T-cell lymphoma; investigational (Phase III) for HIV*

peliomycin USAN, INN *antineoplastic*

pellants *a class of agents that purify or cleanse the system, particularly the blood* [also called: depurants; depuratives]

pelretin USAN, INN *antikeratinizing agent*

pelrinone INN *cardiotonic* [also: pelrinone HCl]

pelrinone HCl USAN *cardiotonic* [also: pelrinone]

PemADD tablets ℞ *CNS stimulant for attention-deficit hyperactivity disorder (ADHD)* [pemoline] 18.75, 37.5, 75 mg

PemADD CT chewable tablets ℞ *CNS stimulant for attention-deficit hyperactivity disorder (ADHD)* [pemoline] 37.5 mg

pemedolac USAN, INN *analgesic*

pemerid INN *antitussive* [also: pemerid nitrate]

pemerid nitrate USAN *antitussive* [also: pemerid]

pemetrexed disodium USAN *antineoplastic; thymidylate synthase inhibitor; dihydrofolate reductase inhibitor; glycinamide ribonucleotide formyl transferase inhibitor*

pemirolast INN *ophthalmic antiallergic; mast cell stabilizer* [also: pemirolast potassium]

pemirolast potassium USAN *ophthalmic antiallergic; mast cell stabilizer* [also: pemirolast]

pemoline USAN, INN, BAN, JAN *CNS stimulant for attention-deficit hyperac-*

tivity disorder (ADHD) and narcolepsy 18.75, 37.5, 75 mg oral
pempidine INN, BAN
penamecillin USAN, INN, BAN *antibacterial*
penbutolol INN, BAN *antihypertensive; antiadrenergic (β-blocker)* [also: penbutolol sulfate]
penbutolol sulfate USAN *antihypertensive; antiadrenergic (β-blocker)* [also: penbutolol]
penciclovir USAN, INN, BAN *topical antiviral for herpes infections*
penciclovir sodium USAN *antiviral for herpes infections*
pendecamaine INN, BAN
pendiomide [see: azamethonium bromide]
Penecare cream, lotion OTC *moisturizer; emollient* [lactic acid]
Penecort cream, solution ℞ *topical corticosteroidal anti-inflammatory* [hydrocortisone] 1%
penems *a class of broad-spectrum antibiotics*
Penetrex film-coated tablets ℞ *broad-spectrum fluoroquinolone antibiotic* [enoxacin] 200, 400 mg
PenFill (trademarked form) *insulin injector refill cartridge*
penfluridol USAN, INN *antipsychotic*
penflutizide INN
pengitoxin INN
penicillamine USAN, USP, INN *metal chelating agent; antirheumatic* ⌧ penicillin
penicillin aluminum
penicillin benzathine phenoxymethyl [now: penicillin V benzathine]
penicillin calcium USP
penicillin G benzathine USP *natural penicillin antibiotic* [also: benzathine benzylpenicillin; benzathine penicillin; benzylpenicillin benzathine]
penicillin G hydrabamine *natural penicillin antibiotic*
penicillin G potassium USP *natural penicillin antibiotic* [also: benzylpenicillin potassium] 1, 2, 3 million U injection
penicillin G procaine USP *natural penicillin antibiotic* [also: procaine penicillin]
penicillin G redox [see: redox-penicillin G]
penicillin G sodium USP *natural penicillin antibiotic* [also: benzylpenicillin sodium]
penicillin hydrabamine phenoxymethyl [now: penicillin V hydrabamine]
penicillin N [see: adicillin]
penicillin O [see: almecillin]
penicillin O chloroprocaine
penicillin O potassium
penicillin O sodium
penicillin phenoxymethyl [now: penicillin V]
penicillin potassium G [see: penicillin G potassium]
penicillin potassium phenoxymethyl [now: penicillin V potassium]
penicillin V USAN, USP *natural penicillin antibiotic* [also: phenoxymethylpenicillin]
penicillin V benzathine USAN, USP *natural penicillin antibiotic*
penicillin V hydrabamine USAN, USP *natural penicillin antibiotic*
penicillin V potassium USAN, USP *natural penicillin antibiotic*
Penicillin VK tablets, oral solution ℞ *natural penicillin antibiotic* [penicillin V potassium] 250, 500 mg; 125, 250 mg/5 mL
penicillin-152 potassium [see: phenethicillin potassium] ⌧ penicillamine; Polycillin
penicillinase INN, BAN
penicillinase-resistant penicillins *a subclass of penicillins (q.v.)*
penicillinphenyrazine [see: phenyracillin]
penicillins *a class of bactericidal antibiotics effective against both gram-positive and gram-negative bacteria; divided into natural, penicillinase-resistant,*

aminopenicillin, and extended-spectrum penicillins

penidural [see: benzathine penicillin]

penimepicycline INN

penimocycline INN

penirolol INN

Pen-Kera cream OTC *moisturizer; emollient*

Penlac nail lacquer ℞ *topical antifungal for onychomycosis* [ciclopirox] 8%

penmesterol INN

Pennsaid ℞ *investigational (NDA filed) topical NSAID for rheumatoid arthritis and osteoarthritis pain* [diclofenac potassium]

pennyroyal *(Hedeoma pulegeoides; Mentha pulegium)* plant *medicinal herb for childbirth pain, colds, colic, fever, gas, inducing abortion and menstruation, mouth sores, respiratory illnesses, and venomous bites; also used as an insect repellent; not generally regarded as safe for ingestion, as it is toxic*

penoctonium bromide INN

penprostene INN

penta tea *medicinal herb* [see: jiaogulan]

pentabamate USAN, INN *minor tranquilizer*

Pentacarinat IV or IM injection ℞ *antiprotozoal; treatment and prophylaxis of Pneumocystis carinii pneumonia (orphan)* [pentamidine isethionate] 300 mg

Pentacea ℞ *investigational (orphan) antineoplastic for small cell lung cancer*

pentacosactride BAN [also: norleusactide]

pentacynium chloride INN

pentacyone chloride [see: pentacynium chloride]

pentaerithritol tetranicotinate [see: niceritrol]

pentaerithrityl tetranitrate INN *vasodilator* [also: pentaerythritol tetranitrate]

pentaerythritol tetranitrate (PETN) USP *coronary vasodilator; antianginal* [also: pentaerithrityl tetranitrate]

pentaerythritol trinitrate [see: pentrinitrol]

pentafilcon A USAN *hydrophilic contact lens material*

pentafluranol INN, BAN

pentafuside *investigational (Phase II) antiviral fusion inhibitor for HIV and AIDS*

pentagastrin USAN, INN, JAN *gastric secretion indicator*

pentagestrone INN

pentalamide INN, BAN

pentalyte USAN, USP, NF *electrolyte combination*

Pentam 300 IV or IM injection ℞ *antiprotozoal; treatment and prophylaxis of Pneumocystis carinii pneumonia (orphan)* [pentamidine isethionate] 300 mg

pentamethazene [see: azamethonium bromide]

pentamethonium bromide INN, BAN

pentamethylenetetrazol [see: pentylenetetrazol]

pentamidine INN, BAN

pentamidine isethionate *antiprotozoal; treatment and prophylaxis of Pneumocystis carinii pneumonia (orphan)* 300 mg injection

pentamin [see: azamethonium bromide]

pentamorphone USAN, INN *narcotic analgesic*

pentamoxane INN

pentamoxane HCl [see: pentamoxane]

pentamustine USAN *antineoplastic* [also: neptamustine]

pentanedial [see: glutaral]

pentanitrol [see: pentaerythritol tetranitrate]

pentaphonate

pentapiperide INN

pentapiperium methylsulfate USAN *anticholinergic* [also: pentapiperium metilsulfate]

pentapiperium metilsulfate INN *anticholinergic* [also: pentapiperium methylsulfate]

pentaquine INN [also: pentaquine phosphate]

pentaquine phosphate USP [also: pentaquine]

Pentasa controlled-release capsules ℞ *anti-inflammatory for ulcerative colitis, proctosigmoiditis, and proctitis* [mesalamine] 250 mg

pentasodium colistinmethanesulfonate [see: colistimethate sodium]

Pentaspan ℞ *leukapheresis adjunct to improve leukocyte yield (orphan)* [pentastarch]

pentastarch USAN, BAN *leukapheresis adjunct; red cell sedimenting agent; centrifugal leukocyte harvesting aid (orphan)*

pentavalent gas gangrene antitoxin

Pentazine injection (discontinued 1997) ℞ *antihistamine; sedative; antiemetic; motion sickness relief* [promethazine HCl] 50 mg/mL ⑨ Phenazine

Pentazine VC with Codeine liquid ℞ *narcotic antitussive; antihistamine* [codeine phosphate; promethazine HCl] 10•6.25 mg/5 mL

pentazocine USAN, USP, INN, BAN *narcotic agonist-antagonist analgesic; also abused as a street drug*

pentazocine HCl USAN, USP *narcotic agonist-antagonist analgesic; also abused as a street drug*

pentazocine HCl & acetaminophen *narcotic analgesic* 25•650 mg oral

pentazocine lactate USAN, USP *analgesic*

pentazocine & naloxone HCl *narcotic agonist-antagonist analgesic; also abused as a street drug* 50•0.5 mg oral

pentetate calcium trisodium USAN *plutonium chelating agent* [also: calcium trisodium pentetate]

pentetate calcium trisodium Yb 169 USAN *radioactive agent*

pentetate disodium [see: pentetic acid, sodium salts]

pentetate indium disodium In 111 USAN *diagnostic aid; radioactive agent*

pentetate monosodium [see: pentetic acid, sodium salts]

pentetate pentasodium [see: pentetic acid, sodium salts]

pentetate tetrasodium [see: pentetic acid, sodium salts]

pentetate trisodium [see: pentetic acid, sodium salts]

pentetate trisodium calcium [see: pentetate calcium trisodium]

pentethylcyclanone [see: cyclexanone]

pentetic acid USAN, BAN *diagnostic aid*

pentetic acid, sodium salts *diagnostic aid*

pentetrazol INN [also: pentylenetetrazol]

penthanil diethylenetriamine pentaacetic acid (DTPA) [see: pentetic acid]

penthienate bromide NF

Penthrane liquid for vaporization ℞ *inhalation general anesthetic* [methoxyflurane]

penthrichloral INN, BAN

pentiapine INN *antipsychotic* [also: pentiapine maleate]

pentiapine maleate USAN *antipsychotic* [also: pentiapine]

penticide [see: chlorophenothane]

pentifylline INN, BAN

pentigetide USAN, INN *antiallergic*

pentisomicin USAN, INN *anti-infective*

pentisomide INN

pentizidone INN *antibacterial* [also: pentizidone sodium]

pentizidone sodium USAN *antibacterial* [also: pentizidone]

pentobarbital USP, INN *sedative; hypnotic; also abused as a street drug* [also: pentobarbitone; pentobarbital calcium] ⑨ phenobarbital

pentobarbital calcium JAN *sedative; hypnotic; also abused as a street drug* [also: pentobarbital; pentobarbitone]

pentobarbital sodium USP, JAN *sedative; hypnotic; also abused as a street drug* [also: pentobarbitone sodium] 100 mg oral; 50 mg/mL injection

pentobarbitone BAN *sedative; hypnotic; also abused as a street drug* [also: pentobarbital]

pentobarbitone sodium BAN *sedative; hypnotic; also abused as a street drug* [also: pentobarbital sodium]

Pentolair eye drops ℞ *mydriatic; cycloplegic* [cyclopentolate HCl] 1%

pentolinium tartrate NF [also: pentolonium tartrate]

pentolonium tartrate INN [also: pentolinium tartrate]

pentolonum bitartrate [see: pentolinium tartrate]

pentomone USAN, INN *prostate growth inhibitor*

pentopril USAN, INN *angiotensin-converting enzyme (ACE) inhibitor*

pentorex INN

pentosalen BAN

pentosan polysulfate sodium USAN, INN *urinary tract anti-inflammatory and analgesic for interstitial cystitis (orphan)* [also: pentosan polysulphate sodium]

pentosan polysulphate sodium BAN *urinary tract anti-inflammatory and analgesic* [also: pentosan polysulfate sodium]

Pentostam (available only from the Centers for Disease Control) ℞ *investigational anti-infective for leishmaniasis* [sodium stibogluconate]

pentostatin USAN, INN *potentiator; antibiotic antineoplastic for hairy cell leukemia (orphan); investigational (orphan) for chronic lymphocytic leukemia and cutaneous T-cell lymphoma; investigational (Phase II) for AIDS-related non-Hodgkin lymphoma*

Pentothal powder for IV injection ℞ *barbiturate general anesthetic* [thiopental sodium] 2%, 2.5% (20, 25 mg/mL) ⑨ pentrinitrol

Pentothal rectal suspension (discontinued 1997) ℞ *barbiturate general anesthetic* [thiopental sodium] 400 mg/g ⑨ pentrinitrol;

pentoxifylline USAN, INN *peripheral vasodilator; hemorheologic agent* [also: oxpentifylline] 400 mg oral

pentoxiverine citrate [see: carbetapentane citrate]

pentoxyverine INN [also: carbetapentane citrate]

pentoxyverine citrate [see: carbetapentane citrate]

Pentrax; Pentrax Gold shampoo OTC *antiseborrheic; antipsoriatic; antipruritic; antibacterial* [coal tar] 4.3%; 4%

pentrinitrol USAN, INN *coronary vasodilator* ⑨ Pentothal

***tert*-pentyl alcohol** [see: amylene hydrate]

6-pentyl-*m*-cresol [see: amylmetacresol]

pentylenetetrazol NF [also: pentetrazol]

pentymal [see: amobarbital]

Pen-V tablets (discontinued 1998) ℞ *natural penicillin antibiotic* [penicillin V potassium] 250, 500 mg

Pen-Vee K tablets, powder for oral solution ℞ *natural penicillin antibiotic* [penicillin V potassium] 250, 500 mg; 125, 250 mg/5 mL

peony *(Paeonia officinalis)* root (other parts are poisonous) *medicinal herb used as an antispasmodic, diuretic, and sedative*

Pepcid film-coated tablets, powder for oral suspension, IV injection, preloaded syringes for IV ℞ *histamine H_2 antagonist for gastric and duodenal ulcers* [famotidine] 20, 40 mg; 40 mg/5 mL; 10 mg/mL; 20 mg

Pepcid AC ("acid controller") tablets, chewable tablets, gelcaps OTC *histamine H_2 antagonist for heartburn and acid indigestion* [famotidine] 10 mg

Pepcid Complete chewable tablets OTC *combination antacid and histamine H_2 antagonist for heartburn and acid indigestion* [calcium carbonate; magnesium hydroxide; famotidine] 800•165•10 mg

Pepcid RPD rapidly disintegrating tablets ℞ *histamine H_2 antagonist for gastric and duodenal ulcers* [famotidine] 20, 40 mg

pepleomycin [see: peplomycin sulfate]

peplomycin INN *antineoplastic* [also: peplomycin sulfate]

peplomycin sulfate USAN *antineoplastic* [also: peplomycin]

pepper, African red; American red pepper; bird pepper; cayenne pepper; chili pepper; cockspur pepper; garden pepper; red pep-

per; **Spanish pepper** *medicinal herb* [see: cayenne]

pepper, Jamaica *medicinal herb* [see: allspice]

pepper, java; tailed pepper *medicinal herb* [see: cubeb]

pepper, water *medicinal herb* [see: knotweed]

pepper, wild *medicinal herb* [see: mezereon]

pepperidge bush *medicinal herb* [see: barberry]

peppermint NF *flavoring agent; perfume*

peppermint *(Mentha piperita)* leaves *medicinal herb for appetite stimulation, colds, colic, indigestion, fever, gas and heartburn, headache, shock, sore throat, and toothache*

peppermint oil NF *flavoring agent*

peppermint spirit USP *flavoring agent; perfume*

peppermint water NF *flavored vehicle*

pepsin *digestive aid*

pepstatin USAN, INN *pepsin enzyme inhibitor*

Peptamen ready-to-use liquid OTC *enteral nutritional therapy for GI impairment*

Peptavlon subcu injection ℞ *in vivo diagnostic aid for gastrointestinal function* [pentagastrin] 250 µg/mL

Peptic Relief chewable tablets, liquid OTC *antidiarrheal; antinauseant* [bismuth subsalicylate] 262 mg; 87.3 mg/5 mL

Pepto Diarrhea Control oral solution OTC *antidiarrheal* [loperamide HCl] 1 mg/5 mL

Pepto-Bismol chewable tablets, caplets, liquid OTC *antidiarrheal; antinauseant* [bismuth subsalicylate] 262 mg; 262 mg; 262, 524 mg/15 mL

peraclopone INN

peradoxime INN

perafensine INN

peralopride INN

peraquinsin INN

perastine INN

peratizole INN, BAN

perbufylline INN

Perchloracap capsules ℞ *radioimaging adjunct* [potassium perchlorate] 200 mg

Percocet tablets ℞ *narcotic analgesic* [oxycodone HCl; acetaminophen] 2.5•325, 5•325, 7.5•500, 10•650 mg

Percodan; Percodan-Demi tablets ℞ *narcotic analgesic; also abused as a street drug* [oxycodone HCl; oxycodone terephthalate; aspirin] 4.5•0.38•325 mg; 2.25•0.19•325 mg ⓢ Decadron

Percogesic tablets OTC *antihistamine; analgesic* [phenyltoloxamine citrate; acetaminophen] 30•325 mg

Percolone tablets ℞ *narcotic analgesic* [oxycodone HCl] 5 mg

Perdiem granules OTC *bulk laxative* [psyllium] 4.03 g/tsp. ⓢ Pyridium

Perdiem Overnight Relief granules OTC *bulk laxative; stimulant laxative* [psyllium; senna] 3.25•0.74 g/tsp.

Perfect Image (CAN) capsules OTC *chromium supplement* [chromium chloride] 200 µg

Perfectoderm gel OTC *topical keratolytic for acne* [benzoyl peroxide] 5%

perfilcon A USAN *hydrophilic contact lens material*

perflenapent USAN *ultrasound contrast medium*

perflexane USAN *investigational (NDA filed) ultrasound contrast medium for cardiac imaging*

perflisopent USAN *ultrasound contrast medium*

perfluamine INN, BAN

perflubron USAN, INN *blood substitute; oral MRI contrast medium; investigational (Phase III) agent for pediatric acute respiratory distress syndrome (ARDS); investigational (Phase III) intravascular oxygen carrier to reduce need for blood transfusions in surgery patients*

perflunafene INN, BAN

perflutren USAN *ultrasound contrast medium for cardiac imaging; investigational (Phase III) for gynecologic imaging*

perfomedil INN

perfosfamide USAN *antineoplastic; orphan status withdrawn 1996*
pergolide INN, BAN *dopamine agonist; antiparkinsonian* [also: pergolide mesylate]
pergolide mesylate USAN *dopamine agonist; antiparkinsonian; investigational (orphan) for Tourette syndrome* [also: pergolide]
Pergonal powder for IM injection ℞ *ovulation stimulant for women; spermatogenesis stimulant for men* [menotropins] 75, 150 IU/ampule
perhexiline INN *coronary vasodilator* [also: perhexiline maleate]
perhexiline maleate USAN *coronary vasodilator* [also: perhexiline]
Periactin syrup (discontinued 2001) ℞ *piperidine antihistamine* [cyproheptadine HCl] 2 mg/5 mL ⑨ Taractan
Periactin tablets ℞ *piperidine antihistamine* [cyproheptadine HCl] 4 mg ⑨ Taractan
periciazine INN *phenothiazine antipsychotic* [also: pericyazine]
Peri-Colace capsules, syrup OTC *stimulant laxative; stool softener* [casanthranol; docusate sodium] 30•100 mg; 30•60 mg/15 mL
pericyazine BAN *phenothiazine antipsychotic* [also: periciazine]
Peridex mouth rinse ℞ *antimicrobial; gingivitis treatment; investigational (orphan) for oral mucositis in bone marrow transplant patients* [chlorhexidine gluconate; alcohol 11.6%] 0.12%
Peridin-C tablets OTC *vitamin C supplement with bioflavonoids* [ascorbic acid; hesperidin] 200•200 mg
Peri-Dos softgels OTC *stimulant laxative; stool softener* [casanthranol; docusate sodium] 30•100 mg
perilla *(Perilla frutescens)* plant *medicinal herb for asthma, inducing sweating, nausea, gastrointestinal spasms, and sunstroke*
perillyl alcohol (POH) *investigational (Phase II) monoterpene antineoplastic for advanced colorectal carcinoma and pancreatic cancer*
perimetazine INN
perindopril USAN, INN, BAN *antihypertensive; angiotensin-converting enzyme (ACE) inhibitor*
perindopril erbumine USAN *angiotensin-converting enzyme (ACE) inhibitor for essential hypertension*
perindoprilat INN, BAN
PerioChip biodegradable polymer implant ℞ *antimicrobial adjunct to scaling and root planing procedures in periodontitis* [chlorhexidine gluconate] 2.5 mg
PerioGard mouth rinse ℞ *antimicrobial; gingivitis treatment* [chlorhexidine gluconate; alcohol 11.6%] 0.12%
Periostat capsules (discontinued 2001) ℞ *antibiotic for periodontal disease* [doxycycline hyclate] 20 mg
Periostat tablets ℞ *antibiotic for periodontal disease* [doxycycline hyclate] 20 mg
peripheral vasodilators *a class of cardiovascular drugs that cause dilation of the blood vessels*
Periploca sylvestris *medicinal herb* [see: gymnema]
perisoxal INN
periwinkle *(Catharanthus roseus)* plant *medicinal herb for cancer, diabetes, diarrhea, insect stings, nervousness, ocular inflammation, and ulcers; not generally regarded as safe for ingestion because of toxicity*
perlapine USAN, INN *hypnotic*
Perles (dosage form) *soft gelatin capsule*
permanganic acid, potassium salt [see: potassium permanganate]
Permapen Isoject (unit dose syringe) for deep IM injection ℞ *natural penicillin antibiotic* [penicillin G benzathine] 1 200 000 U
Permax tablets ℞ *dopamine agonist; antiparkinsonian; investigational (orphan) for Tourette syndrome* [pergolide mesylate] 0.05, 0.25, 1 mg
permethrin USAN, INN, BAN *ectoparasiticide*
Permitil tablets, oral concentrate ℞ *conventional (typical) antipsychotic*

[fluphenazine HCl] 2.5, 5, 10 mg; 5 mg/mL

Perna canaliculus *natural remedy* [see: New Zealand green-lipped mussel]

Pernox Scrub; Pernox Lathering Lotion OTC *abrasive cleanser for acne* [sulfur; salicylic acid]

peroxide, dibenzoyl [see: benzoyl peroxide]

Peroxin A 5; Peroxin A 10 gel ℞ *topical keratolytic for acne* [benzoyl peroxide] 5%; 10%

Peroxyl mouth rinse, oral gel OTC *cleansing of oral wounds* [hydrogen peroxide] 1.5%

perphenazine USP, INN *phenothiazine antipsychotic; antiemetic; intractable hiccough relief* 2, 4, 8, 16 mg oral; 16 mg/5 mL

Persa-Gel; Persa-Gel W 5%; Persa-Gel W 10% gel ℞ *topical keratolytic for acne* [benzoyl peroxide] 5%, 10%; 5%; 10%

Persantine sugar-coated tablets ℞ *platelet aggregation inhibitor* [dipyridamole] 25, 50, 75 mg ⓢ Pertofrane

Persantine IV injection ℞ *diagnostic aid for coronary artery function* [dipyridamole] 10 mg

Persea americana; P. gratissima *medicinal herb* [see: avocado]

Persian bark; Persian berries *medicinal herb* [see: buckthorn]

Persian walnut *medicinal herb* [see: English walnut]

persic oil NF *vehicle*

persilic acid INN

Pertropin capsules OTC *dietary lipotropic agent* [linolenic acid; multiple essential fatty acids] 7 mins.

Pertussin CS; Pertussin ES syrup OTC *antitussive* [dextromethorphan hydrobromide] 3.5 mg/5 mL; 15 mg/5 mL

pertussis immune globulin USP *passive immunizing agent*

pertussis immune human globulin [now: pertussis immune globulin]

pertussis vaccine USP *active immunizing agent*

pertussis vaccine, acellular [see: diphtheria & tetanus toxoids & acellular pertussis (DTaP) vaccine, adsorbed]

pertussis vaccine, adsorbed USP *active immunizing agent*

pertussis vaccine, component (alternate name for acellular pertussis vacine) [see: diphtheria & tetanus toxoids & acellular pertussis (DTaP) vaccine, adsorbed]

pertussis vaccine, whole-cell [see: diphtheria & tetanus toxoids & whole-cell pertussis (DTwP) vaccine, adsorbed]

Peruvian balsam NF *topical local protectant; rubefacient*

Peruvian balsam *(Myroxylon balsamum; M. pereirae)* oil *medicinal herb for edema, expelling worms, hemostasis, topical infections, and wound healing*

Peruvian bark; yellow Peruvian bark *medicinal herb* [see: quinine]

Peruvian ginseng *medicinal herb* [see: maca]

Petasites hybridus *medicinal herb* [see: butterbur]

pethidine INN, BAN *narcotic analgesic; also abused as a street drug* [also: meperidine HCl]

pethidine HCl [see: meperidine HCl]

PETN (pentaerythritol tetranitrate) [q.v.]

petrichloral INN

petrolatum USP *ointment base; emollient/protectant* [also: yellow petrolatum]

petrolatum, hydrophilic USP *absorbent ointment base; topical protectant*

petrolatum, liquid [see: mineral oil]

petrolatum, liquid emulsion [see: mineral oil emulsion]

petrolatum, white USP, JAN *oleaginous ointment base; topical protectant*

petrolatum gauze [see: gauze, petrolatum]

petroleum benzin [see: benzin, petroleum]

petroleum distillate inhalants *vapors from butane, toluene, acetone, ben-*

zene, gasoline, etc. which produce psychoactive effects, abused as street drugs [see also: nitrous oxide; volatile nitrites]

petroleum jelly [see: petrolatum]

Petroselinum sativum *medicinal herb* [see: parsley]

Peumus boldus *medicinal herb* [see: boldo]

pexantel INN

pexiganan acetate USAN *investigational (NDA filed) broad-spectrum topical antibiotic for impetigo and diabetic foot ulcers*

PFA (phosphonoformic acid) [see: foscarnet sodium]

Pfaffia paniculata *medicinal herb* [see: suma]

Pfeiffer's Allergy tablets (discontinued 1997) OTC *antihistamine* [chlorpheniramine maleate] 4 mg

Pfeiffer's Cold Sore lotion OTC *topical oral anesthetic; analgesic; counterirritant* [gum benzoin; camphor; menthol; eucalyptol; alcohol 85%] 7%•?•?•?

Pfizerpen powder for injection ℞ *natural penicillin antibiotic* [penicillin G potassium] 1, 5, 20 million U

Pfizerpen-AS IM injection (discontinued 1997) ℞ *bactericidal antibiotic* [penicillin G procaine] 300 000 U/mL

PFL (Platinol, fluorouracil, leucovorin [rescue]) *chemotherapy protocol for head, neck, and gastric cancer*

PFT (L-phenylalanine mustard, fluorouracil, tamoxifen) *chemotherapy protocol*

PG (paregoric) [q.v.]

PG (prostaglandin) [q.v.]

PGA (pteroylglutamic acid) [see: folic acid]

PGE_1 (prostaglandin E_1) [now: alprostadil]

PGE_2 (prostaglandin E_2) [now: dinoprostone]

$PGF_{2\alpha}$ (prostaglandin $F_{2\alpha}$) [see: dinoprost]

$PGF_{2\alpha}$ (prostaglandin $F_{2\alpha}$) THAM [see: dinoprost tromethamine]

PGG glucan *investigational (Phase III) immunotherapeutic to prevent postsurgical infections following non-colorectal GI surgery (clinical trials discontinued 1999)*

PGI_2 (prostaglandin I_2) [now: epoprostenol]

PGX (prostaglandin X) [now: epoprostenol]

Phaenicia sericata *natural treatment* [see: maggots]

Phanadex Cough syrup OTC *antitussive; decongestant; antihistamine; expectorant* [dextromethorphan hydrobromide; phenylpropanolamine HCl; pyrilamine maleate; guaifenesin] 15•25•40•100 mg/5 mL

Phanatuss Cough syrup OTC *antitussive; expectorant* [dextromethorphan hydrobromide; guaifenesin] 10•85 mg/5 mL

phanchinone [see: phanquinone; phanquone]

phanquinone INN [also: phanquone]

phanquone BAN [also: phanquinone]

pharmaceutical glaze [see: glaze, pharmaceutical]

Pharmaflur; Pharmaflur df; Pharmaflur 1.1 chewable tablets ℞ *dental caries preventative* [sodium fluoride] 2.2 mg; 2.2 mg; 1.1 mg

Pharmalgen subcu or IM injection ℞ *venom sensitivity testing (subcu); venom desensitization therapy (IM)* [extracts of honeybee, yellow jacket, yellow hornet, white-faced hornet, mixed vespid, and wasp venom]

Pharmia regina *natural treatment* [see: maggots]

Pharmorubicin PFS; Pharmorubicin RDF (CAN) IV injection ℞ *antibiotic antineoplastic* [epirubicin HCl] 2 mg/mL; 10, 50 mg/vial

Phazyme tablets, drops OTC *antiflatulent* [simethicone] 60 mg; 40 mg/0.6 mL ⓢ Pherazine

Phazyme (CAN) oral liquid OTC *antiflatulent* [simethicone] 125 mg/5 mL

Phazyme 95 tablets OTC *antiflatulent* [simethicone] 95 mg

Phazyme 125 softgels OTC *antiflatulent* [simethicone] 125 mg

phebutazine [see: febuverine]
phebutyrazine [see: febuverine]
phemfilcon A USAN *hydrophilic contact lens material*
phenacaine INN [also: phenacaine HCl]
phenacaine HCl USP [also: phenacaine]
phenacemide USP, INN, BAN *anticonvulsant*
phenacetin USP, INN *(withdrawn from market)* ⊠ phenazocine
phenacon [see: fenaclon]
phenactropinium chloride INN, BAN
phenacyl 4-morpholineacetate [see: mobecarb]
N-phenacylhomatropinium chloride [see: phenactropinium chloride]
phenacylpivalate [see: pibecarb]
Phenadex Children's Cough/Cold syrup (discontinued 1998) OTC *pediatric antitussive, decongestant, and expectorant* [dextromethorphan hydrobromide; phenylpropanolamine HCl; guaifenesin; alcohol 5%] 5•6.25•100 mg/5 mL
Phenadex Pediatric Cough/Cold drops (discontinued 1998) OTC *pediatric antitussive, decongestant, and expectorant* [dextromethorphan hydrobromide; phenylpropanolamine HCl; guaifenesin] 5•6.25•50 mg/mL
Phenadex Senior liquid (discontinued 1998) OTC *antitussive; expectorant* [dextromethorphan hydrobromide; guaifenesin] 10•200 mg/5 mL
phenadoxone INN, BAN
phenaglycodol INN
Phenahist-TR sustained-release tablets ℞ *decongestant; antihistamine; anticholinergic* [phenylpropanolamine HCl; phenylephrine HCl; chlorpheniramine maleate; hyoscyamine sulfate; atropine sulfate; scopolamine hydrobromide] 50•25•8•0.19•0.04•0.01 mg
phenamazoline INN
phenamazoline HCl [see: phenamazoline]
Phenameth tablets (discontinued 1997) ℞ *antihistamine; sedative; antiemetic; motion sickness relief* [promethazine HCl] 25 mg
Phenameth DM syrup ℞ *antitussive; antihistamine* [dextromethorphan hydrobromide; promethazine HCl; alcohol] 15•6.25 mg/5 mL
phenampromide INN
Phenapap tablets OTC *decongestant; analgesic* [pseudoephedrine HCl; acetaminophen] 30•325 mg
Phenapap Sinus Headache & Congestion tablets OTC *decongestant; antihistamine; analgesic* [pseudoephedrine HCl; chlorpheniramine maleate; acetaminophen] 30•2•325 mg
Phenaphen with Codeine No. 3 & No. 4 capsules ℞ *narcotic analgesic* [codeine phosphate; acetaminophen] 30•325 mg; 60•325 mg
phenaphthazine
phenarbutal [see: phetharbital]
phenarsone sulfoxylate INN
Phenaseptic throat spray OTC *topical antipruritic/counterirritant; mild local anesthetic* [phenol] 1.4%
Phenate timed-release tablets ℞ *decongestant; antihistamine; analgesic* [phenylpropanolamine HCl; chlorpheniramine maleate; acetaminophen] 40•4•325 mg
Phenazine 50 injection (discontinued 1997) ℞ *antihistamine; sedative; antiemetic; motion sickness relief* [promethazine HCl] 50 mg/mL ⊠ Pentazine; phenelzine; Phenoxine; Pherazine
Phenazo (CAN) tablets ℞ *urinary analgesic* [phenazopyridine HCl] 100, 200 mg
phenazocine INN ⊠ phenacetin
phenazocine hydrobromide [see: phenazocine]
phenazone INN, BAN *analgesic* [also: antipyrine]
phenazopyridine INN, BAN *urinary tract analgesic* [also: phenazopyridine HCl]
phenazopyridine HCl USAN, USP *urinary tract analgesic* [also: phenazopyridine] 100, 200 mg oral
phenbenicillin BAN [also: fenbenicillin]

phenbutazone sodium glycerate USAN *anti-inflammatory*
phenbutrazate BAN [also: fenbutrazate]
phencarbamide USAN *anticholinergic* [also: fencarbamide]
Phenchlor S.H.A. sustained-release tablets ℞ *decongestant; antihistamine; anticholinergic* [phenylpropanolamine HCl; phenylephrine HCl; chlorpheniramine maleate; hyoscyamine sulfate; atropine sulfate; scopolamine hydrobromide] 50•25•8•0.19•0.04•0.01 mg
phencyclidine INN *anesthetic* [also: phencyclidine HCl]
phencyclidine HCl USAN *anesthetic* [also: phencyclidine]
phendimetrazine INN *anorexiant* [also: phendimetrazine tartrate]
phendimetrazine tartrate USP *anorexiant; CNS stimulant* [also: phendimetrazine] 35, 105 mg oral
Phendryl; Phendryl Children's Allergy Medicine elixir (discontinued 1997) OTC *antihistamine* [diphenhydramine HCl] 12.5 mg/5 mL
phenelzine INN, BAN *antidepressant; MAO inhibitor* [also: phenelzine sulfate] ⓓ Phenazine; Phenylzin
phenelzine sulfate USP *antidepressant; MAO inhibitor* [also: phenelzine]
phenemal [see: phenobarbital]
Phenerbel-S tablets ℞ *GI anticholinergic; sedative; analgesic* [belladonna alkaloids; phenobarbital; ergotamine tartrate] 0.2•40•0.6 mg
Phenergan tablets, suppositories, injection ℞ *antihistamine; sedative; antiemetic; motion sickness relief* [promethazine HCl] 12.5, 25, 50 mg; 12.5, 25, 50 mg; 25, 50 mg/mL ⓓ Phenaphen; Theragran
Phenergan Fortis syrup ℞ *antihistamine; sedative; antiemetic; motion sickness relief* [promethazine HCl; alcohol 1.5%] 25 mg/5 mL
Phenergan Plain syrup ℞ *antihistamine; sedative; antiemetic; motion sickness relief* [promethazine HCl] 6.25 mg/5 mL
Phenergan VC syrup ℞ *decongestant; antihistamine* [phenylephrine HCl; promethazine HCl; alcohol 7%] 5•6.25 mg/5 mL
Phenergan VC with Codeine syrup ℞ *narcotic antitussive; decongestant; antihistamine* [codeine phosphate; phenylephrine HCl; promethazine HCl; alcohol 7%] 10•5•6.25 mg/5 mL
Phenergan with Codeine syrup ℞ *narcotic antitussive; antihistamine* [codeine phosphate; promethazine HCl; alcohol 7%] 10•6.25 mg/5 mL
Phenergan with Dextromethorphan syrup ℞ *antitussive; antihistamine* [dextromethorphan hydrobromide; promethazine HCl; alcohol 7%] 15•6.25 mg/5 mL
pheneridine INN
phenethanol [see: phenylethyl alcohol]
phenethazine [see: fenethazine]
phenethicillin potassium USP [also: pheneticillin]
phenethyl alcohol BAN *antimicrobial agent* [also: phenylethyl alcohol]
N-phenethylanthranilic acid [see: enfenamic acid]
phenethylazocine bromide [see: phenazocine hydrobromide]
phenethylhydrazine sulfate [see: phenelzine sulfate]
pheneticillin INN [also: phenethicillin potassium]
pheneticillin potassium [see: phenethicillin potassium]
Phenetron tablets, syrup (discontinued 1997) ℞ *antihistamine; antitussive* [chlorpheniramine maleate] 4 mg; 2 mg/5 mL
phenetsal [see: acetaminosalol]
pheneturide INN, BAN [also: acetylpheneturide]
Phenex-1 powder OTC *formula for infants with phenylketonuria*
Phenex-2 powder OTC *enteral nutritional therapy for phenylketonuria (PKU)*
phenformin INN, BAN *biguanide hypoglycemic agent* [also: phenformin HCl]
phenformin HCl USP *hypoglycemic agent (removed from market by FDA*

in 1977, now available as an investigational drug) [also: phenformin]
phenglutarimide INN, BAN
Phenhist DH with Codeine liquid ℞ *narcotic antitussive; decongestant; antihistamine* [codeine phosphate; pseudoephedrine HCl; chlorpheniramine maleate; alcohol 5%] 10•30•2 mg/5 mL
Phenhist Expectorant liquid ℞ *narcotic antitussive; decongestant; expectorant* [codeine phosphate; pseudoephedrine HCl; guaifenesin; alcohol 7.5%] 10•30•100 mg/5 mL
phenicarbazide INN
phenidiemal [see: phetharbital]
phenindamine INN *piperidine antihistamine* [also: phenindamine tartrate]
phenindamine tartrate USAN *piperidine antihistamine for allergic rhinitis* [also: phenindamine]
phenindione USP, INN *anticoagulant*
pheniodol sodium INN [also: iodoalphionic acid]
pheniprazine INN, BAN
pheniprazine HCl [see: pheniprazine]
pheniramine INN [also: pheniramine maleate]
pheniramine maleate USAN *antihistamine* [also: pheniramine]
pheniramine maleate & naphazoline HCl *topical ocular antihistamine and decongestant* 0.3%•0.025% eye drops
phenisonone hydrobromide
phenmetraline HCl [see: phenmetrazine HCl]
phenmetrazine INN, BAN *anorexiant; CNS stimulant; also abused as a street drug* [also: phenmetrazine HCl]
phenmetrazine HCl USP *anorexiant; CNS stimulant; also abused as a street drug* [also: phenmetrazine]
phenobamate [see: febarbamate]
phenobarbital USP, INN, JAN *anticonvulsant; hypnotic; sedative; also abused as a street drug* [also: phenobarbitone] 15, 30, 60, 100 mg oral; 15, 20 mg/5 mL oral ⊠ pentobarbital
phenobarbital sodium USP, INN, JAN *anticonvulsant; hypnotic; sedative; also abused as a street drug* 30, 60, 65, 130 mg/mL injection
phenobarbitone BAN *anticonvulsant; hypnotic; sedative; also abused as a street drug* [also: phenobarbital]
phenobutiodil INN
phenododecinium bromide [see: domiphen bromide]
Phenoject-50 injection (discontinued 1997) ℞ *antihistamine; motion sickness relief; sleep aid; antiemetic; sedative* [promethazine HCl] 50 mg/mL
phenol USP *topical antiseptic/antipruritic; local anesthetic; preservative*
phenol, liquefied USP *topical antipruritic*
phenol, sodium salt [see: phenolate sodium]
phenol red [see: phenolsulfonphthalein]
phenolate sodium USAN *disinfectant*
Phenolated Calamine lotion OTC *topical poison ivy treatment* [calamine; zinc oxide; phenol] 8%•8%•1%
Phenolax wafers (discontinued 1998) OTC *stimulant laxative* [phenolphthalein] 64.8 mg
phenolphthalein USP, INN *stimulant laxative* [banned in all OTC laxatives in 1999]
phenolphthalein, white [see: phenolphthalein]
phenolphthalein, yellow USP *stimulant laxative* [banned in all OTC laxatives in 1999]
phenolsulfonphthalein USP
phenolsulphonate sodium USP
phenomorphan INN, BAN
phenomycilline [see: penicillin V]
phenoperidine INN, BAN
phenopryldiasulfone sodium [see: solasulfone]
Phenoptic eye drops ℞ *topical ophthalmic decongestant and vasoconstrictor; mydriatic* [phenylephrine HCl] 2.5%
phenosulfophthalein [see: phenolsulfonphthalein]
phenothiazine NF, INN *antipsychotic*
phenothiazines *a class of dopamine receptor antagonists with antipsychotic, hypotensive, antiemetic, antispasmodic, and antihistaminic activity*

phenothrin INN, BAN
phenoxazoline HCl [see: fenoxazoline HCl]
Phenoxine tablets OTC *diet aid* [phenylpropanolamine HCl] 25 mg ⓢ Phenazine
phenoxybenzamine INN *antihypertensive* [also: phenoxybenzamine HCl]
phenoxybenzamine HCl USP *antihypertensive; pheochromocytomic agent* [also: phenoxybenzamine]
phenoxymethylpenicillin INN *natural penicillin antibiotic* [also: penicillin V]
phenoxypropazine BAN [also: fenoxypropazine]
phenoxypropylpenicillin [see: propicillin]
phenozolone [see: fenozolone]
phenprobamate INN, BAN
phenprocoumon USAN, USP, INN *anticoagulant*
phenprocumone [see: phenprocoumon]
phenpromethadrine [see: phenpromethamine]
phenpromethamine INN
phenpropamine citrate [see: alverine citrate]
phensuximide USP, INN, BAN *succinimide anticonvulsant*
phentermine USAN, INN *anorexiant; CNS stimulant; an adrenergic isomer of amphetamine* ⓢ phentolamine
phentermine HCl USP *anorexiant; CNS stimulant; the water-soluble form of phentermine for oral administration* 8, 15, 18.75, 30, 37.5 mg oral
phenthiazine [see: phenothiazine]
phentolamine INN, BAN *antihypertensive; pheochromocytomic agent* [also: phentolamine HCl] ⓢ phentermine; Ventolin
phentolamine HCl USP *antihypertensive; pheochromocytomic agent* [also: phentolamine]
phentolamine mesilate INN, JAN *antiadrenergic; antihypertensive; pheochromocytomic agent* [also: phentolamine mesylate]
phentolamine mesylate USP *antihypertensive; α-adrenergic blocker; pheochromocytomic agent; investigational (Phase III) oral treatment for erectile dysfunction* [also: phentolamine mesilate] 5 mg injection
phentolamine methanesulfonate [now: phentolamine mesylate]
Phentrol 2; Phentrol 4; Phentrol 5 capsules ℞ *anorexiant; CNS stimulant* [phentermine HCl] 30 mg
phentydrone
Phenurone tablets (discontinued 1997) ℞ *anticonvulsant* [phenacemide] 500 mg
phenyl aminosalicylate USAN, BAN *antibacterial; tuberculostatic* [also: fenamisal]
phenyl salicylate NF *analgesic; not generally regarded as safe and effective as an antidiarrheal*
phenylalanine (L-phenylalanine) USAN, USP, INN *essential amino acid; symbols: Phe, F*
phenylalanine ammonia-lyase *investigational (orphan) for hyperphenylalaninemia*
phenylalanine mustard (PAM) [see: melphalan]
L-phenylalanine mustard (L-PAM) [see: melphalan]
Phenylase *investigational (orphan) for hyperphenylalaninemia* [phenylalanine ammonia-lyase]
phenylazo diamino pyridine HCl [see: phenazopyridine HCl]
phenylbenzyl atropine [see: xenytropium bromide]
phenylbutazone USP, INN *antirheumatic; anti-inflammatory; antipyretic; analgesic*
phenylbutylpiperadines *a class of dopamine receptor antagonists with conventional (typical) antipsychotic activity* [also called: butyrophenones]
phenylbutyrate sodium [see: sodium phenylbutyrate]
2-phenylbutyrylurea [see: pheneturide; acetylpheneturide]
phenylcarbinol [see: benzyl alcohol]

phenylcinchoninic acid [now: cinchophen]

α-phenyl-*p*-cresol carbamate [see: diphenan]

phenylcyclohexyl piperidine (PCP) [see: PCP; phencyclidine HCl]

2-phenylcyclopentylamine HCl [see: cypenamine HCl]

phenyldimazone [see: normethadone]

Phenyldrine timed-release tablets OTC *diet aid* [phenylpropanolamine HCl] 75 mg

phenylephrine (PE) INN, BAN *nasal decongestant; ocular vasoconstrictor; vasopressor for hypotensive or cardiac shock* [also: phenylephrine HCl]

phenylephrine bitartrate *bronchodilator; vasoconstrictor*

phenylephrine HCl USP *nasal decongestant; ocular vasoconstrictor; vasopressor for hypotensive or cardiac shock* [also: phenylephrine] 0.25%, 0.5%, 1% nose drops or spray; 2.5%, 10% eye drops; 1% injection

phenylephrine HCl & phenylpropanolamine HCl & guaifenesin *nasal decongestant; expectorant* 5•45•200 mg oral

phenylephrine tannate *nasal decongestant*

phenylephrine tannate, chlorpheniramine tannate, and pyrilamine tannate *decongestant; antihistamine* 25•8•25 mg oral

phenylethanol [see: phenylethyl alcohol]

phenylethyl alcohol USP *antimicrobial agent; preservative* [also: phenethyl alcohol]

phenylethylmalonylurea [see: phenobarbital]

Phenylfenesin L.A. extended-action tablets ℞ *decongestant; expectorant* [phenylpropanolamine HCl; guaifenesin] 75•400 mg

Phenylfenesin L.A. long-acting tablets ℞ *decongestant; expectorant* [phenylpropanolamine HCl; guaifenesin] 75•400 mg

Phenyl-Free liquid OTC *special diet for infants with phenylketonuria (PKU)*

Phenylgesic tablets OTC *antihistamine; analgesic* [phenyltoloxamine citrate; acetaminophen] 30•325 mg

phenylhydrazone *investigational (Phase I) antiviral for AIDS-related Kaposi sarcoma*

phenylindanedione [see: phenindione]

phenylmercuric acetate NF *antimicrobial agent; preservative*

phenylmercuric borate INN

phenylmercuric chloride NF

phenylmercuric nitrate NF *antimicrobial agent; preservative; topical antiseptic*

phenylone [see: antipyrine]

phenylpropanolamine (PPA) INN, BAN *vasoconstrictor; nasal decongestant; nonprescription diet aid* [also: phenylpropanolamine HCl]

phenylpropanolamine HCl USP *vasoconstrictor; nasal decongestant; nonprescription diet aid* [also: phenylpropanolamine] 25, 50, 75 mg oral

phenylpropanolamine HCl & chlorpheniramine maleate *decongestant; antihistamine* 75•12 mg

phenylpropanolamine HCl & phenylephrine HCl & guaifenesin *nasal decongestant; expectorant* 45•5•200 mg oral

phenylpropanolamine polistirex USAN *adrenergic; vasoconstrictor*

1-phenylsemicarbazide [see: phenicarbazide]

phenylthilone [see: phenythilone]

phenyltoloxamine INN *antihistamine; sleep aid*

phenyltoloxamine citrate *antihistamine; sleep aid*

phenyltriazines *a class of anticonvulsants*

phenyracillin INN

phenyramidol HCl USAN *analgesic; skeletal muscle relaxant* [also: fenyramidol]

phenythilone INN

phenytoin USAN, USP, INN, BAN *hydantoin anticonvulsant* 125 mg/5 mL oral

phenytoin redox [see: redox-phenytoin]

phenytoin sodium USP *hydantoin anticonvulsant* 100 mg oral; 50 mg/mL injection

Pherazine DM syrup ℞ *antitussive; antihistamine* [dextromethorphan hydrobromide; promethazine HCl; alcohol 7%] 15•6.25 mg/5 mL

Pherazine VC with Codeine syrup ℞ *narcotic antitussive; decongestant; antihistamine* [codeine phosphate; phenylephrine HCl; promethazine HCl; alcohol 7%] 10•5•6.25 mg/5 mL

Pherazine with Codeine syrup ℞ *narcotic antitussive; antihistamine* [codeine phosphate; promethazine HCl; alcohol 7%] 10•6.25 mg/5 mL

phetharbital INN

phezathion [see: fezatione]

Phicon cream OTC *topical anesthetic; emollient* [pramoxine HCl; vitamins A and E] 0.5%•7500 IU•2000 IU

Phicon F cream OTC *topical anesthetic; antifungal* [pramoxine HCl; undecylenic acid] 0.05%•8%

Phillips' Chewable tablets OTC *antacid* [magnesium hydroxide] 311 mg

Phillips' Laxative gelcaps (discontinued 1998) OTC *stimulant laxative; stool softener* [phenolphthalein; docusate sodium] 90•83 mg

Phillips' LaxCaps capsules (discontinued 1998) OTC *stimulant laxative; stool softener* [phenolphthalein; docusate sodium] 90•83 mg

Phillips' Liqui-Gels OTC *laxative; stool softener* [docusate sodium] 100 mg

Phillips' Milk of Magnesia; Concentrated Phillips' Milk of Magnesia liquid OTC *antacid; saline laxative* [magnesium hydroxide] 400 mg/5 mL; 800 mg/5 mL

pHisoDerm; pHisoDerm for Baby liquid OTC *soap-free therapeutic skin cleanser*

pHisoDerm Cleansing Bar OTC *therapeutic skin cleanser*

pHisoHex liquid ℞ *bacteriostatic skin cleanser* [hexachlorophene] 3% 🄬 Fostex

phloropropiophenone [see: flopropione]

pholcodine INN

pholedrine INN, BAN

pholescutol [see: folescutol]

Phoradendron flavescens; P. serotinum; P. tomentosum *medicinal herb* [see: mistletoe]

PhosChol softgels, liquid concentrate OTC *neurotransmitter; lipotropic* [phosphatidylcholine] 565, 900 mg; 3 g/5 mL

phoscolic acid [see: foscolic acid]

Phos-Flur oral rinse ℞ *topical dental caries preventative* [acidulated phosphate fluoride] 0.44 mg/mL

PhosLo tablets, capsules, gelcaps ℞ *buffering agent for hyperphosphatemia in end-stage renal disease (orphan)* [calcium acetate] 667 mg; 333.3, 667 mg; 667 mg

phosphate salt of tricyclic nucleoside [now: triciribine phosphate]

phosphatidylcholine (PC) [see: lecithin]

phosphatidylglycerol *investigational (orphan) for neonatal respiratory distress syndrome*

phosphinic acid [see: hypophosphorous acid]

2,2′-phosphinicodilactic acid (PDLA) [see: foscolic acid]

Phosphocol P 32 suspension for intracavitary instillation, interstitial injection ℞ *radiopharmaceutical antineoplastic* [chromic phosphate P 32] 10, 15 mCi

phosphocysteamine *investigational (orphan) for cystinosis*

phosphodiesterase-3 (PDE-3) inhibitors *a class of platelet aggregation inhibitors*

Phospholine Iodide powder for eye drops ℞ *topical antiglaucoma agent; irreversible cholinesterase inhibitor miotic* [echothiophate iodide] 0.03%, 0.125%

phosphonoformic acid (PFA) [see: foscarnet sodium]

phosphonomethoxypropyladenine (PMPA) [see: tenofovir]

phosphorated carbohydrate solution (hyperosmolar solution with phosphoric acid) *antiemetic for nausea associated with influenza, morning sickness, motion sickness, inhalation anesthesia, or food and drink indiscretions*

phosphoric acid NF *solvent; acidifying agent*

phosphoric acid, aluminum salt [see: aluminum phosphate gel]

phosphoric acid, calcium salt [see: calcium phosphate, dibasic]

phosphoric acid, chromium salt [see: chromic phosphate Cr 51 & P 32]

phosphoric acid, diammonium salt [see: ammonium phosphate]

phosphoric acid, dipotassium salt [see: potassium phosphate, dibasic]

phosphoric acid, disodium salt heptahydrate [see: sodium phosphate, dibasic]

phosphoric acid, disodium salt hydrate [see: sodium phosphate, dibasic]

phosphoric acid, magnesium salt [see: magnesium phosphate]

phosphoric acid, monopotassium salt [see: potassium phosphate, monobasic]

phosphoric acid, monosodium salt dihydrate [see: sodium phosphate, monobasic]

phosphoric acid, monosodium salt monohydrate [see: sodium phosphate, monobasic]

phosphorofluoridic acid, disodium salt [see: sodium monofluorophosphate]

phosphorus *element (P)*

Phospho-Soda [see: Fleet Phospho-Soda]

phosphothiamine [see: monophosphothiamine]

Photofrin powder for IV injection ℞ *laser light–activated antineoplastic for photodynamic therapy of esophageal (orphan) and non–small cell lung cancers (NSCLC); investigational (orphan) for bladder cancer* [porfimer sodium] 75 mg

PhotoPoint ℞ *investigational (Phase III) photosensitizer for wet age-related macular degeneration (AMD)* [rostaporfin]

phoxim INN, BAN

Phrenilin tablets ℞ *analgesic; barbiturate sedative* [acetaminophen; butalbital] 325•50 mg

Phrenilin Forte capsules ℞ *analgesic; barbiturate sedative* [acetaminophen; butalbital] 650•50 mg

PHRT (procarbazine, hydroxyurea, radiotherapy) *chemotherapy protocol*

phthalofyne USAN *veterinary anthelmintic* [also: ftalofyne]

phthalylsulfacetamide NF

phthalylsulfamethizole INN

phthalylsulfathiazole USP, INN

phylcardin [see: aminophylline]

phyllindon [see: aminophylline]

Phyllocontin controlled-release tablets ℞ *antiasthmatic; bronchodilator* [aminophylline] 225 mg

phylloquinone [see: phytonadione]

Phylorinol liquid OTC *topical antipruritic/counterirritant; mild local anesthetic; antiseptic; astringent; oral deodorant* [phenol; boric acid; strong iodine solution; chlorophyllin copper complex] 0.6%•?•?•?

Phylorinol mouthwash/gargle OTC *topical antipruritic/counterirritant; mild local anesthetic* [phenol] 0.6%

physic root *medicinal herb* [see: Culver root]

physiological irrigating solution *for general irrigating, washing and rinsing; not for injection*

Physiolyte liquid ℞ *sterile irrigant* [physiological irrigating solution]

PhysioSol liquid ℞ *sterile irrigant* [physiological irrigating solution]

Physiotens ℞ *investigational centrally acting sympatholytic for hypertension, congestive heart failure, and type 2 diabetes* [moxonidine]

physostigmine USP, BAN *reversible cholinesterase inhibitor miotic for glaucoma; investigational (NDA filed) for*

Alzheimer disease ⓓ pyridostigmine; Prostigmin
physostigmine salicylate USP *cholinergic to reverse anticholinergic overdose; investigational (orphan) for Friedreich and other inherited ataxias*
physostigmine sulfate USP *ophthalmic cholinergic for glaucoma; miotic*
phytate persodium USAN *pharmaceutic aid*
phytate sodium USAN *calcium-chelating agent*
phytic acid [see: fytic acid]
Phytolacca americana; P. decandra; P. rigida *medicinal herb* [see: pokeweed]
phytomenadione (vitamin K_1) INN, BAN *fat-soluble vitamin; prothrombogenic* [also: phytonadione]
phytonadiol sodium diphosphate INN
phytonadione (vitamin K_1) USP, JAN *fat-soluble vitamin; prothrombogenic* [also: phytomenadione] 2 mg/mL injection
PIA (Platinol, ifosfamide, Adriamycin) *chemotherapy protocol*
pibecarb INN
piberaline INN
piboserod HCl USAN *selective serotonin 5-HT_4 receptor antagonist for irritable bowel syndrome*
pibrozelesin hydrobromide USAN *antineoplastic*
picafibrate INN
picartamide INN
Picea excelsa; P. mariana *medicinal herb* [see: spruce tree]
picenadol INN *analgesic* [also: picenadol HCl]
picenadol HCl USAN *analgesic* [also: picenadol]
picilorex INN
pick purse; pickpocket *medicinal herb* [see: shepherd's purse]
piclamilast USAN *phosphodiesterase IV inhibitor for asthma*
piclonidine INN
piclopastine INN
picloxydine INN, BAN
picobenzide INN
picodralazine INN
picolamine INN
piconol INN
picoperine INN
picoprazole INN
picotrin INN *keratolytic* [also: picotrin diolamine]
picotrin diolamine USAN *keratolytic* [also: picotrin]
Picovir ℞ *investigational (Phase III) viral replication inhibitor for viral respiratory infections, including the common cold* [pleconaril]
Picrasma excelsa *medicinal herb* [see: quassia]
picric acid [see: trinitrophenol]
picrotoxin NF
picumast INN, BAN
picumeterol INN, BAN *bronchodilator* [also: picumeterol fumarate]
picumeterol fumarate USAN *bronchodilator* [also: picumeterol]
pidolacetamol INN
pidolic acid INN
pifarnine USAN, INN *gastric antiulcerative*
pifenate INN, BAN
pifexole INN
piflutixol INN
pifoxime INN
pigeonberry *medicinal herb* [see: pokeweed]
piketoprofen INN
Pilagan eye drops ℞ *topical antiglaucoma agent; direct-acting miotic* [pilocarpine nitrate] 1%, 2%, 4%
pildralazine INN
pilewort *(Erechtites hieracifolia)* plant *medicinal herb used as an astringent and emetic*
Pilocar eye drops ℞ *topical antiglaucoma agent; direct-acting miotic* [pilocarpine HCl] 0.5%, 1%, 2%, 3%, 4%, 6%
pilocarpine USP, BAN *antiglaucoma agent; ophthalmic cholinergic*
pilocarpine HCl USP *ophthalmic cholinergic; antiglaucoma; miotic; treatment of xerostomia and keratoconjunctivitis sicca due to radiotherapy or Sjögren syndrome (orphan); also for dry mouth* 0.5%, 1%, 2%, 4%, 6%, 8% eye drops

pilocarpine nitrate USP *ophthalmic cholinergic; antiglaucoma; miotic*

Pilopine HS ophthalmic gel ℞ *topical antiglaucoma agent; direct-acting miotic* [pilocarpine HCl] 4%

Piloptic-½; Piloptic-1; Piloptic-2; Piloptic-3; Piloptic-4; Piloptic-6 eye drops ℞ *topical antiglaucoma agent; direct-acting miotic* [pilocarpine HCl] 0.5%; 1%; 2%; 3%; 4%; 6%

Pilopto-Carpine eye drops ℞ *topical antiglaucoma agent; direct-acting miotic* [pilocarpine HCl] 4%

Pilostat eye drops ℞ *topical antiglaucoma agent; direct-acting miotic* [pilocarpine HCl] 0.5%, 1%, 2%, 3%, 4%, 6%

Pilpak (trademarked packaging form) *patient compliance package*

Pima syrup ℞ *expectorant* [potassium iodide] 325 mg/5 mL

pimagedine HCl USAN *advanced glycosylation inhibitor for type 1 diabetes; investigational (Phase III) for diabetics in end-stage renal disease*

pimaricin JAN *ophthalmic antibacterial/antifungal antibiotic* [also: natamycin]

pimeclone INN

pimecrolimus USAN *immunosuppressant for atopic dermatitis*

pimefylline INN

pimelautide INN

Pimenta dioica; P. officinalis *medicinal herb* [see: allspice]

pimetacin INN

pimethixene INN

pimetine INN *antihyperlipoproteinemic* [also: pimetine HCl]

pimetine HCl USAN *antihyperlipoproteinemic* [also: pimetine]

pimetixene [see: pimethixene]

pimetremide INN

pimeverine [see: pimetremide]

piminodine INN [also: piminodine esylate]

piminodine esylate NF [also: piminodine]

piminodine ethanesulfonate [see: piminodine esylate]

pimobendan USAN, INN *cardiotonic*

pimonidazole INN, BAN

pimozide USAN, USP, INN, BAN, JAN *antidyskinetic for Tourette syndrome; diphenylbutylpiperidine antipsychotic; neuroleptic*

pimpernel; small pimpernel *medicinal herb* [see: burnet]

pimpernel, blue *medicinal herb* [see: skullcap]

pimpernel, water *medicinal herb* [see: brooklime]

Pimpinella anisum *medicinal herb* [see: anise]

Pimpinella magna; P. saxifrage *medicinal herb* [see: burnet]

pinacidil USAN, INN *antihypertensive*

pinadoline USAN, INN *analgesic*

pinafide INN

pinaverium bromide INN *GI antispasmodic*

pinazepam INN

pincainide INN

Pindac (approved but not currently being marketed) ℞ *antihypertensive* [pinacidil]

pindolol USAN, USP, INN, BAN *antihypertensive; antiadrenergic (β-blocker)* 5, 10 mg oral

pine, Norway *medicinal herb* [see: spruce]

pine, prince's *medicinal herb* [see: pipsissewa]

pine bark extract *natural free radical scavenger for inflammatory collagen disease and peripheral vascular disease; contains 80%–85% procyanidolic oligomers (PCOs)*

pine needle oil NF

pine tar USP

pineapple *(Ananas comosus)* fruit *medicinal herb for constipation, jaundice, soft tissue inflammation, and topical wound debridement*

Pink Bismuth liquid OTC *antidiarrheal; antinauseant* [bismuth subsalicylate] 130, 262 mg/15 mL

pinolcaine INN

pinoxepin INN *antipsychotic* [also: pinoxepin HCl]

pinoxepin HCl USAN *antipsychotic* [also: pinoxepin]

Pin-Rid soft gel capsules, liquid OTC *anthelmintic for ascariasis (roundworm) and enterobiasis (pinworm)* [pyrantel pamoate] 180 mg; 50 mg/mL
Pinus palustris *natural remedy* [see: turpentine]
Pinus strobus *medicinal herb* [see: white pine]
Pin-X liquid OTC *anthelmintic for ascariasis (roundworm) and enterobiasis (pinworm)* [pyrantel pamoate] 50 mg/mL
pioglitazone INN *thiazolidinedione antidiabetic; increases cellular response to insulin without increasing insulin secretion* [also: pioglitazone HCl]
pioglitazone HCl USAN *thiazolidinedione antidiabetic; increases cellular response to insulin without increasing insulin secretion* [also: pioglitazone]
pipacycline INN
pipamazine INN
pipamperone USAN, INN *antipsychotic*
pipaneperone [see: pipamperone]
pipazetate INN *antitussive* [also: pipazethate]
pipazethate USAN *antitussive* [also: pipazetate]
pipe plant; Dutchman's pipe; Indian pipe *medicinal herb* [see: fit root]
pipebuzone INN
pipecuronium bromide USAN, INN, BAN *muscle relaxant; nondepolarizing neuromuscular blocker; adjunct to anesthesia*
pipemidic acid INN
pipenzolate bromide INN
pipenzolate methylbromide [see: pipenzolate bromide]
pipenzolone bromide [see: pipenzolate bromide]
pipequaline INN
Piper cubeba *medicinal herb* [see: cubeb]
Piper methysticum *medicinal herb* [see: kava kava]
piperacetazine USAN, USP, INN *antipsychotic* ⑨ piperazine
piperacillin INN, BAN *extended-spectrum penicillin antibiotic* [also: piperacillin sodium]
piperacillin sodium USAN, USP, JAN *extended-spectrum penicillin antibiotic* [also: piperacillin]
piperamide INN *anthelmintic* [also: piperamide maleate]
piperamide maleate USAN *anthelmintic* [also: piperamide]
piperamine [see: bamipine]
piperazine USP *anthelmintic for enterobiasis (pinworm) and ascariasis (roundworm)* ⑨ piperacetazine
piperazine calcium edetate INN *anthelmintic* [also: piperazine edetate calcium]
piperazine citrate USP *anthelmintic* 250 mg oral; 500 mg/mL oral
piperazine citrate hydrate [see: piperazine citrate]
piperazine edetate calcium USAN *anthelmintic* [also: piperazine calcium edetate]
piperazine estrone sulfate [now: estropipate]
piperazine hexahydrate [see: piperazine citrate]
piperazine phosphate
piperazine phosphate monohydrate [see: piperazine phosphate]
piperazine theophylline ethanoate [see: acefylline piperazine]
piperidine phosphate
piperidines *a class of antihistamines*
piperidolate INN [also: piperidolate HCl]
piperidolate HCl USP [also: piperidolate]
piperilate [see: pipethanate]
piperine USP
piperocaine INN [also: piperocaine HCl]
piperocaine HCl USP [also: piperocaine]
piperonyl butoxide *pediculicide for lice*
piperoxan INN
piperphenidol HCl
piperylone INN
pipethanate INN
pipobroman USAN, USP, INN *alkylating antineoplastic*
pipoctanone INN
pipofezine INN
piposulfan USAN, INN *antineoplastic*

pipotiazine INN *phenothiazine antipsychotic* [also: pipotiazine palmitate]
pipotiazine palmitate USAN *phenothiazine antipsychotic* [also: pipotiazine]
pipoxizine INN
pipoxolan INN *muscle relaxant* [also: pipoxolan HCl]
pipoxolan HCl USAN *muscle relaxant* [also: pipoxolan]
Pipracil powder for IV or IM injection ℞ *extended-spectrum penicillin antibiotic* [piperacillin sodium] 2, 3, 4, 40 g/vial
pipradimadol INN
pipradrol INN [also: pipradrol HCl]
pipradrol HCl NF [also: pipradrol]
pipramadol INN
pipratecol INN
piprinhydrinate INN, BAN
piprocurarium iodide INN
piprofurol INN
piprozolin USAN, INN *choleretic*
pipsissewa *(Chimaphila umbellata)* plant *medicinal herb used as an astringent, diaphoretic, and diuretic*
piquindone INN *antipsychotic* [also: piquindone HCl]
piquindone HCl USAN *antipsychotic* [also: piquindone]
piquizil INN *bronchodilator* [also: piquizil HCl]
piquizil HCl USAN *bronchodilator* [also: piquizil]
piracetam USAN, INN, BAN *cognition adjuvant; investigational (orphan) for myoclonus* ⑨ piroxicam
pirandamine INN *antidepressant* [also: pirandamine HCl]
pirandamine HCl USAN *antidepressant* [also: pirandamine]
pirarubicin INN
piraxelate INN
pirazmonam INN *antimicrobial* [also: pirazmonam sodium]
pirazmonam sodium USAN *antimicrobial* [also: pirazmonam]
pirazofurin INN *antineoplastic* [also: pyrazofurin]
pirazolac USAN, INN, BAN *antirheumatic*
pirbenicillin INN *antibacterial* [also: pirbenicillin sodium]
pirbenicillin sodium USAN *antibacterial* [also: pirbenicillin]
pirbuterol INN *sympathomimetic bronchodilator* [also: pirbuterol acetate]
pirbuterol acetate USAN *sympathomimetic bronchodilator* [also: pirbuterol]
pirbuterol HCl USAN *bronchodilator*
pirdonium bromide INN
pirenoxine INN
pirenperone USAN, INN, BAN *tranquilizer*
pirenzepine INN, BAN *treatment for peptic ulcers* [also: pirenzepine HCl]
pirenzepine HCl USAN, JAN *treatment for peptic ulcers* [also: pirenzepine]
pirepolol INN
piretanide USAN, INN *diuretic*
pirfenidone USAN, INN *analgesic; anti-inflammatory; antipyretic*
piribedil INN
piribenzyl methylsulfate [see: bevonium metilsulfate]
piridicillin INN *antibacterial* [also: piridicillin sodium]
piridicillin sodium USAN *antibacterial* [also: piridicillin]
piridocaine INN
piridocaine HCl [see: piridocaine]
piridoxilate INN, BAN
piridronate sodium USAN *calcium regulator*
piridronic acid INN
pirifibrate INN
pirinidazole INN
pirinitramide [see: piritramide]
pirinixic acid INN
pirinixil INN
piriprost USAN *antiasthmatic*
piriprost potassium USAN *antiasthmatic*
piriqualone INN
pirisudanol INN
piritramide INN, BAN
piritrexim INN *antiproliferative agent* [also: piritrexim isethionate]
piritrexim isethionate USAN *antiproliferative; orphan status withdrawn 1996* [also: piritrexim]
pirlimycin HCl USAN *antibacterial*
pirlindole INN
pirmagrel USAN, INN *thromboxane synthetase inhibitor*

pirmenol INN *antiarrhythmic* [also: pirmenol HCl]
pirmenol HCl USAN *antiarrhythmic* [also: pirmenol]
pirnabin INN *antiglaucoma agent* [also: pirnabine]
pirnabine USAN *antiglaucoma agent* [also: pirnabin]
piroctone USAN, INN *antiseborrheic*
piroctone olamine USAN *antiseborrheic*
pirodavir USAN, INN, BAN *antiviral*
piroglirine INN *antidiabetic* [also: piroglirine tartrate]
piroglirine tartrate USAN *antidiabetic* [also: piroglirine]
piroheptine INN
pirolate USAN, INN *antiasthmatic*
pirolazamide USAN, INN *antiarrhythmic*
piromidic acid INN
piroxantrone INN *antineoplastic* [also: piroxantrone HCl]
piroxantrone HCl USAN *antineoplastic* [also: piroxantrone]
piroxicam USAN, USP, INN, BAN, JAN *antiarthritic; nonsteroidal anti-inflammatory drug (NSAID)* 10, 20 mg oral 🔊 piracetam
piroxicam β-cyclodextrin [see: piroxicam betadex]
piroxicam betadex USAN *analgesic; antirheumatic; nonsteroidal anti-inflammatory drug (NSAID)*
piroxicam cinnamate USAN *anti-inflammatory*
piroxicam olamine USAN *analgesic; anti-inflammatory*
piroxicillin INN
piroximone USAN, INN, BAN *cardiotonic*
pirozadil INN
pirprofen USAN, INN, BAN *anti-inflammatory*
pirquinozol USAN, INN *antiallergic*
pirralkonium bromide INN
pirroksan [now: proroxan HCl]
pirsidomine USAN, INN *vasodilator*
pirtenidine INN
pistachio *medicinal herb* [see: witch hazel]
pitch tree, Canada; hemlock pitch tree *medicinal herb* [see: hemlock]
pitcher plant ***(Sarracenia purpurea)*** root *medicinal herb used as an astringent, diuretic, and stimulant*
pitenodil INN
Pitocin IV, IM injection ℞ *oxytocic for induction of labor, postpartum bleeding, and incomplete abortion* [oxytocin] 10 U/mL 🔊 Pitressin
pitofenone INN
Pitressin IM or subcu injection ℞ *pituitary antidiuretic hormone for diabetes insipidus or prevention of abdominal distention* [vasopressin] 20 U/mL 🔊 Pitocin
Pitrex (CAN) cream OTC *topical antifungal* [tolnaftate] 1%
pituitary, anterior
pituitary, posterior USP *antidiuretic hormone*
pituxate INN
pivalate USAN, INN, BAN *combining name for radicals or groups*
pivampicillin INN *aminopenicillin antibiotic* [also: pivampicillin HCl]
pivampicillin HCl USAN *aminopenicillin antibiotic* [also: pivampicillin]
pivampicillin pamoate USAN *antibacterial*
pivampicillin probenate USAN *antibacterial*
Pivanex ℞ *investigational (Phase II) small-molecule antineoplastic for stage III and IV non–small cell lung cancer (NSCLC)*
pivenfrine INN
pivmecillinam INN, BAN *aminopenicillin antibiotic* [also: amdinocillin pivoxil; pivmecillinam HCl]
pivmecillinam HCl JAN *aminopenicillin antibiotic* [also: amdinocillin pivoxil; pivmecillinam]
pivopril USAN *antihypertensive*
pivoxazepam INN
pivoxetil USAN, INN *combining name for radicals or groups*
pivoxil USAN, INN *combining name for radicals or groups*
pivsulbactam BAN *β-lactamase inhibitor; penicillin/cephalosporin synergist* [also: sulbactam pivoxil]

pix pini [see: pine tar]

Pixykine ℞ *investigational second-generation colony stimulating factor for neutropenia and thrombocytopenia* [milodistim]

pizotifen INN, BAN *anabolic; antidepressant; serotonin inhibitor (migraine specific)* [also: pizotyline]

pizotyline USAN *anabolic; antidepressant; serotonin inhibitor (migraine specific)* [also: pizotifen]

placebo *no medicinal value* [also: obecalp]

Placidyl capsules ℞ *hypnotic* [ethchlorvynol] 200, 500, 750 mg ⓢ Pathocil

plafibride INN

plague vaccine USP *active bacterin for plague (Yersinia pestis)* 1.8–2.2 × 10^8 bacilli/mL IM injection

Plan B tablets (in packs of 2) ℞ *emergency postcoital contraceptive (progestin only)* [levonorgestrel] 0.75 mg

planadalin [see: carbromal]

Plantago lanceolata; P. major **and other species** *medicinal herb* [see: plantain]

Plantago ovata **(psyllium)** *medicinal herb* [see: plantain]

plantago seed USP *laxative*

plantain (*Plantago lanceolata; P. major* and other species) leaves and seeds *medicinal herb for bed-wetting, bladder infections, blood poisoning, constipation, diarrhea, diverticulitis, edema, hyperlipidemia, kidney disorders, neuralgia, snake bites, sores, and topical inflammation*

Plaquase powder for injection ℞ *investigational (orphan) for Peyronie disease* [collagenase]

Plaquenil Sulfate film-coated tablets ℞ *antimalarial; antirheumatic* [hydroxychloroquine sulfate] 200 mg

Plasbumin-5; Plasbumin-25 IV infusion ℞ *blood volume expander for shock, burns, and hypoproteinemia* [human albumin] 5%; 25%

plasma, antihemophilic human USP

plasma concentrate factor IX [see: factor IX complex]

plasma expanders *a class of therapeutic blood modifiers used to increase the volume of circulating blood* [also called: blood volume expanders]

plasma protein fraction USP *blood volume supporter*

plasma protein fraction, human [now: plasma protein fraction]

plasma protein fractions *a class of therapeutic blood modifiers used to regulate the volume of circulating blood*

plasma thromboplastin component (PTC) [see: factor IX]

Plasma-Lyte A pH 7.4; Plasma-Lyte R; Plasma-Lyte 56; Plasma-Lyte 148 IV infusion ℞ *intravenous electrolyte therapy* [combined electrolyte solution]

Plasma-Lyte M (R; 56; 148) and 5% Dextrose IV infusion ℞ *intravenous nutritional/electrolyte therapy* [combined electrolyte solution; dextrose]

Plasmanate IV infusion ℞ *blood volume expander for shock due to burns, trauma and surgery* [plasma protein fraction] 5%

Plasma-Plex IV infusion ℞ *blood volume expander for shock due to burns, trauma and surgery* [plasma protein fraction] 5%

Plasmatein IV infusion ℞ *blood volume expander for shock due to burns, trauma and surgery* [plasma protein fraction] 5%

plasmin BAN [also: fibrinolysin, human]

Plateau Cap (trademarked dosage form) *controlled-release capsule*

platelet cofactor II [see: factor IX]

platelet concentrate USP *platelet replenisher*

platelet-activating factor acetylhydrolase, recombinant (rPAF-AH) *investigational (Phase II) for asthma; investigational (Phase II) for endoscopic retrograde cholangiopancreatography (ERCP)*

Platinol powder for IV injection (discontinued 1997) ℞ *alkylating antineoplastic for testicular, ovarian, blad-*

der, lung, head, neck, and esophageal cancers [cisplatin] 10, 50 mg
Platinol-AQ IV injection ℞ *alkylating antineoplastic for metastatic testicular tumors, metastatic ovarian tumors, and advanced bladder cancer* [cisplatin] 1 mg/mL
platinum *element (Pt)*
***cis*-platinum** [now: cisplatin]
***cis*-platinum II** [now: cisplatin]
platinum diamminodichloride [see: cisplatin]
plaunotol INN
plauracin USAN, INN *veterinary growth stimulant*
Plavix coated tablets ℞ *platelet aggregation inhibitor for stroke, myocardial infarction, and peripheral artery disease* [clopidogrel bisulfate] 75 mg
Plax, Advanced Formula mouthwash/gargle OTC [sodium pyrophosphate]
pleconaril USAN *investigational (Phase III) viral replication inhibitor for treatment of viral respiratory infection and viral meningitis; investigational for polio myelitis*
Plegisol solution ℞ *cardioplegic solution* [calcium chloride; magnesium chloride; potassium chloride; sodium chloride] 17.6•325.3•119.3•643 mg/100 mL
Plendil extended-release tablets ℞ *antihypertensive; calcium channel blocker* [felodipine] 2.5, 5, 10 mg ⓢ Prinivil
Pletal tablets ℞ *vasodilator and platelet aggregation inhibitor for intermittent claudication* [cilostazol] 50, 100 mg
pleurisy root *(Asclepias tuberosa)* *medicinal herb for asthma, bronchitis, dysentery, emphysema, fever, pleurisy, and pneumonia*
pleuromulin INN
Pliagel solution OTC *surfactant cleaning solution for soft contact lenses*
plicamycin USAN, USP, INN *antibiotic antineoplastic*
plomestane USAN *antineoplastic; aromatase inhibitor*
plum *(Prunus americana; P. domestica; P. spinosa)* fruit and bark *medicinal herb used as an anthelmintic, astringent, and laxative*
Plus Sinus (CAN) extended-release caplets (discontinued 2001) OTC *nasal decongestant* [pseudoephedrine HCl] 120 mg
plutonium *element (Pu)*
PM Caps (CAN) OTC *vitamin supplement* [multiple vitamins; folic acid] ≛•0.2 mg
PMB 200; PMB 400 tablets (discontinued 1998) ℞ *estrogen replacement therapy for postmenopausal symptoms; anxiolytic* [conjugated estrogens; meprobamate] 0.45•200 mg; 0.45•400 mg
pMDI (dosage form) *pressurized metered-dose inhaler*
PMEA *investigational (Phase I/II) antiviral nucleoside analogue for HIV and various herpesvirus types* [also: GS 393]
PMMA (polymethyl methacrylate) [q.v.]
PMPA (phosphonomethoxypropyladenine) [see: tenofovir]
PMPA (phosphonomethoxypropyladenine) prodrug [see: tenofovir disoproxil fumarate]
PMS-Bethanechol Chloride (CAN) tablets (discontinued 1998) ℞ *cholinergic urinary stimulant for postsurgical and postpartum urinary retention* [bethanechol chloride] 10, 25, 50 mg
PMS-Bezafibrate (CAN) tablets ℞ *antihyperlipidemic* [bezafibrate] 200 mg
PMS-Bromocriptine (CAN) tablets, capsules ℞ *dopamine agonist for Parkinson disease; lactation inhibitor; growth hormone suppressant for acromegaly* [bromocriptine mesylate] 2.5 mg; 5 mg
PMS-Captopril (CAN) tablets ℞ *antihypertensive; angiotensin-converting enzyme (ACE) inhibitor* [captopril] 12.5, 25, 50, 100 mg
PMS-Carbamazepine CR (CAN) controlled-release tablets ℞ *anticonvulsant; analgesic for trigeminal neuralgia; antimanic* [carbamazepine] 200, 400 mg

PMS-Conjugated Estrogens (CAN) tablets ℞ *estrogen replacement therapy for postmenopausal symptoms* [conjugated estrogens] 0.3, 0.625, 0.9, 1.25 mg

PMS-Desferoxamine (CAN) powder for IM, IV, or subcu injection ℞ *adjunct treatment for iron intoxication or overload* [deferoxamine mesylate] 500 mg

PMS-Dexamethasone (CAN) injection ℞ *corticosteroidal anti-inflammatory* [dexamethasone sodium phosphate] 4, 10 mg/mL

PMS-Dexamethasone (CAN) tablets, elixir, eye drops, ear drops ℞ *corticosteroidal anti-inflammatory* [dexamethasone] 0.5, 0.75, 4 mg; 0.5 mg/5 mL; 0.1%; 0.1%

PMS-Dicitrate (CAN) oral solution ℞ *urinary alkalinizing agent* [sodium citrate; citric acid] 500•334 mg/5 mL

PMS-Diclofenac (CAN) tablets, suppositories ℞ *analgesic; antiarthritic; nonsteroidal anti-inflammatory drug (NSAID)* [diclofenac sodium] 25, 50 mg; 25, 50 mg

PMS-Diclofenac SR (CAN) slow-release tablets ℞ *analgesic; antiarthritic; nonsteroidal anti-inflammatory drug (NSAID)* [diclofenac sodium] 75, 100 mg

PMS-Dipivefrin (CAN) eye drops ℞ *topical antiglaucoma agent* [dipivefrin HCl] 0.1%

PMS-Fenofibrate Micro (CAN) capsules ℞ *antihyperlipidemic* [fenofibrate, micronized] 200 mg

PMS-Fluorometholone (CAN) eye drops ℞ *topical ophthalmic corticosteroidal anti-inflammatory* [fluorometholone] 0.1%

PMS-Fluphenazine (CAN) tablets, elixir (discontinued 1998) ℞ *conventional (typical) antipsychotic* [fluphenazine decanoate] 1, 2, 5 mg; 2.5 mg/5 mL

PMS-Fluphenazine Decanoate (CAN) subcu or IM injection ℞ *conventional (typical) antipsychotic* [fluphenazine decanoate] 25, 100 mg/mL

PMS-Fluvoxamine (CAN) film-coated tablets ℞ *selective serotonin reuptake inhibitor (SSRI) for depression and obsessive-compulsive disorder (OCD)* [fluvoxamine maleate] 50, 100 mg

PMS-Gabapentin (CAN) capsules ℞ *anticonvulsant for partial-onset seizures* [gabapentin] 100, 300, 400 mg

PMS-Haloperidol (CAN) IM injection (discontinued 1998) ℞ *conventional (typical) antipsychotic; antidyskinetic for Tourette syndrome* [haloperidol lactate] 2 mg/mL

PMS-Haloperidol LA (CAN) IM injection ℞ *conventional (typical) antipsychotic; antidyskinetic for Tourette syndrome* [haloperidol decanoate] 50, 100 mg/mL

PMS-Indapamide (CAN) tablets ℞ *antihypertensive; diuretic* [indapamide] 1.25, 2.5 mg

PMS-Levobunolol (CAN) eye drops ℞ *topical antiglaucoma agent* [levobunolol HCl] 5 mg/mL

PMS-Lithium Carbonate (CAN) capsules ℞ *antipsychotic for manic episodes of a bipolar disorder* [lithium carbonate] 150, 300, 600 mg

PMS-Lithium Citrate (CAN) syrup ℞ *antipsychotic for manic episodes of a bipolar disorder* [lithium citrate] 300 mg/5 mL

PMS-Minocycline (CAN) capsules ℞ *tetracycline antibiotic* [minocycline HCl] 50, 100 mg

PMS-Moclobemide (CAN) tablets ℞ *antidepressant* [moclobemide] 100, 150 mg

PMS-Nizatidine (CAN) capsules ℞ *histamine H_2 antagonist for treatment of gastric and duodenal ulcers* [nizatidine] 150, 300 mg

PMS-Oxybutynin (CAN) tablets, syrup ℞ *urinary antispasmodic* [oxybutynin chloride] 2.5, 5 mg; 5 mg/5 mL

PMS-Pindolol (CAN) tablets ℞ *antihypertensive; antianginal* [pindolol] 5, 10, 15, 80, 160 mg

PMS-Polytrimethoprim (CAN) eye drops ℞ *topical ophthalmic antibiotic* [polymyxin B sulfate; trimethoprim sulfate] 10 000 U•1 mg per mL

PMS-Ranitidine (CAN) film-coated tablets ℞ *histamine H_2 antagonist for gas-*

tric and duodenal ulcers [ranitidine HCl] 150, 300 mg

PMS-Sotalol (CAN) tablets ℞ *antiarrhythmic* [sotalol HCl] 80, 160 mg

PMS-Sucralfate (CAN) tablets ℞ *cytoprotective agent for gastric ulcers* [sucralfate]

PMS-Tamoxifen (CAN) tablets ℞ *antiestrogen antineoplastic for breast cancer* [tamoxifen citrate] 10, 20 mg

PMS-Terazosin (CAN) tablets ℞ *antihypertensive (α-blocker); treatment for benign prostatic hyperplasia (BPH)* [terazosin HCl] 1, 2, 5, 10 mg

PMS-Terbinafine (CAN) tablets ℞ *systemic allylamine antifungal* [terbinafine HCl] 250 mg

PMS-Ticlopidine (CAN) film-coated tablets ℞ *platelet aggregation inhibitor for stroke* [ticlopidine HCl] 250 mg

PMS-Tobramycin (CAN) eye drops ℞ *topical antibiotic* [tobramycin] 0.3%

P-MVAC (Platinol, methotrexate, vinblastine, Adriamycin, carboplatin) *chemotherapy protocol*

PNCRM7 *investigational pneumococcal conjugate vaccine for otitis media*

Pneumo 23 (CAN) subcu or IM injection ℞ *active immunization against 23 strains of Streptococcus pneumoniae* [pneumococcal vaccine, polyvalent] 0.5 mL

pneumococcal vaccine, 7-valent *active bacterin for pneumococcal pneumonia (polysaccharide isolates of 7 strains of Streptococcus pneumoniae: 4, 6B, 9V, 14, 18C, 19F, and 23F)*

pneumococcal vaccine, polyvalent *active bacterin for pneumococcal pneumonia (polysaccharide isolates of 23 strains of Streptococcus pneumoniae)*

Pneumomist sustained-release tablets ℞ *expectorant* [guaifenesin] 600 mg

Pneumopent for inhalation ℞ *investigational (orphan) prophylaxis of Pneumocystis carinii pneumonia* [pentamidine isethionate]

Pneumotussin tablets ℞ *narcotic antitussive; expectorant* [hydrocodone bitartrate; guaifenesin] 2.5•300 mg

Pneumotussin HC syrup ℞ *narcotic antitussive; expectorant* [hydrocodone bitartrate; guaifenesin] 5•100 mg/5 mL

Pneumovax 23 subcu or IM injection ℞ *active immunization against 23 strains of Streptococcus pneumoniae* [pneumococcal vaccine, polyvalent] 25 µg of each strain per 0.5 mL dose

Pnu-Imune 23 subcu or IM injection ℞ *active immunization against 23 strains of Streptococcus pneumoniae* [pneumococcal vaccine, polyvalent] 25 µg of each strain per 0.5 mL dose

pobilukast edamine USAN *antiasthmatic*

POC (procarbazine, Oncovin, CCNU) *chemotherapy protocol for pediatric brain tumors*

POCA (prednisone, Oncovin, cytarabine, Adriamycin) *chemotherapy protocol*

POCC (procarbazine, Oncovin, cyclophosphamide, CCNU) *chemotherapy protocol*

Pockethaler (trademarked delivery device) *nasal inhalation aerosol*

pod pepper *medicinal herb* [see: cayenne]

podilfen INN

Podocon-25 liquid ℞ *topical keratolytic for genital warts* [podophyllum resin] 25%

podofilox USAN *topical antimitotic for genital warts* [also: podophyllotoxin]

Podofin liquid ℞ *topical keratolytic for genital warts* [podophyllum resin] 25% ⊡ podophyllin

podophyllin [see: podophyllum resin] ⊡ Podofin

podophyllotoxin BAN *topical antimitotic* [also: podofilox]

podophyllotoxins *a class of mitotic-inhibiting antineoplastics derived from podophyllotoxin*

podophyllum USP *caustic; cytotoxic agent for genital warts*

Podophyllum peltatum *medicinal herb* [see: mandrake]

podophyllum resin USP *caustic; cytotoxic agent for genital warts*

POH (perillyl alcohol) [q.v.]

poinsettia *(Euphorbia pulcherrima; E. poinsettia; Poinsettia pulcher-*

rima) plant and sap *medicinal herb for fever, pain relief, stimulating lactation, toothache, and warts; also used as an antibacterial and depilatory*

Point-Two oral rinse ℞ *topical dental caries preventative* [sodium fluoride; alcohol 6%] 0.2%

poison, dog *medicinal herb* [see: dog poison]

Poison Antidote Kit OTC *emergency treatment for various poisons* [syrup of ipecac; charcoal suspension] 30•60 mL

poison ash *medicinal herb* [see: fringe tree]

poison flag *medicinal herb* [see: blue flag]

poison hemlock *(Conium maculatum)* plant *medicinal herb that has been used for analgesia and sedation and as a method of execution; it is extremely poisonous*

poison ivy extract, alum precipitated USAN *ivy poisoning counteractant*

poison oak *(Tocicodendron diversilobum)* extract *medicinal herb used in homeopathic remedies for osteoarthritis*

poison oak extract USAN *antiallergic*

Poison Oak-N-Ivy Armor lotion OTC *topical poison ivy protectant*

poke root *(Phytolacca decandra)* *medicinal herb* [see: pokeweed]

pokeweed *(Phytolacca americana; P. decandra; P. rigida)* root and young shoots *medicinal herb for arthritis, blood cleansing, bowel evacuation, dysmenorrhea, mucous membrane inflammation and discharge, mumps, pain, rheumatism, ringworm, scabies, syphilis, and tonsillitis; not generally regarded as safe and effective*

polacrilin USAN, INN *pharmaceutic aid*

polacrilin potassium USAN, NF *tablet disintegrant*

Poladex timed-release tablets (discontinued 1997) ℞ *antihistamine* [dexchlorpheniramine maleate] 4, 6 mg

Polaramine tablets, Repetabs (repeat-action tablets), syrup ℞ *antihistamine* [dexchlorpheniramine maleate] 2 mg; 4, 6 mg; 2 mg/5 mL

Polaramine Expectorant liquid ℞ *decongestant; antihistamine; expectorant* [pseudoephedrine sulfate; dexchlorpheniramine maleate; guaifenesin; alcohol 7.2%] 20•2•100 mg/5 mL

poldine methylsulfate USAN, USP *anticholinergic* [also: poldine metilsulfate]

poldine metilsulfate INN *anticholinergic* [also: poldine methylsulfate]

polecat weed *medicinal herb* [see: skunk cabbage]

policapram USAN, INN *tablet binder*

policresulen INN

polidexide sulfate INN

polidocanol

polifeprosan INN *pharmaceutic aid; implantable, biodegradable drug carrier* [also: polifeprosan 20]

polifeprosan 20 USAN *pharmaceutic aid; implantable, biodegradable drug carrier* [also: polifeprosan]

poligeenan USAN, INN *dispersing agent*

poliglecaprone 25 USAN *absorbable surgical suture material*

poliglecaprone 90 USAN *absorbable surgical suture coating*

poliglusam USAN *antihemorrhagic*

polignate sodium USAN *pepsin enzyme inhibitor*

polihexanide INN [also: polyhexanide]

poliomyelitis vaccine [now: poliovirus vaccine, inactivated]

poliovirus vaccine, enhanced inactivated (eIPV) *active immunizing agent for poliomyelitis*

poliovirus vaccine, inactivated (IPV) USP *active immunizing agent for poliomyelitis*

poliovirus vaccine, live oral (OPV) USP *active immunizing agent for poliomyelitis*

polipropene 25 USAN *tablet excipient*

polisaponin INN

politef INN *prosthetic aid* [also: polytef]

polixetonium chloride USAN, INN *preservative*

Polocaine injection ℞ *injectable local anesthetic* [mepivacaine HCl] 1%, 2%, 3%

Polocaine injection ℞ *injectable local anesthetic* [mepivacaine HCl; levonordefrin] 2%•1:20 000
Polocaine MPF injection ℞ *injectable local anesthetic* [mepivacaine HCl] 1%, 1.5%, 2%
polonium *element (Po)*
poloxalene USAN, INN, BAN *surfactant*
poloxamer USAN, NF, INN, BAN *ointment and suppository base; tablet binder*
poloxamer 124 USAN *surfactant; emulsifier; solubilizer; stabilizer*
poloxamer 188 USAN *surfactant; emulsifier; solubilizer; investigational (Phase III, orphan) for sickle cell crisis; investigational (orphan) for severe burns and vasospasm following cerebral aneurysm repair*
poloxamer 237 USAN *surfactant; emulsifier; solubilizer; stabilizer*
poloxamer 331 *investigational (orphan) for toxoplasmosis of AIDS*
poloxamer 338 USAN *surfactant; emulsifier; solubilizer; stabilizer*
poloxamer 407 USAN *surfactant; emulsifier; solubilizer; stabilizer*
poly I: poly C12U *investigational (Phase III, orphan) antiviral/immunomodulator for HIV, renal cell carcinoma, metastatic melanoma, and chronic fatigue syndrome*
polyamine-methylene resin
polyanhydroglucose [see: dextran]
polyanhydroglucuronic acid [see: dextran]
polybenzarsol INN
polybutester USAN *surgical suture material*
polybutilate USAN *surgical suture coating*
polycarbokane [see: polycarbophil]
polycarbophil USP, INN, BAN *bulk laxative; antidiarrheal*
Polycillin capsules, powder for oral suspension, pediatric drops (discontinued 1998) ℞ *aminopenicillin antibiotic* [ampicillin] 250, 500 mg; 125, 250, 500 mg/5 mL; 100 mg/mL ⑨ penicillin
Polycillin-N powder for IV or IM injection (discontinued 1998) ℞ *aminopenicillin antibiotic* [ampicillin sodium] 0.125, 0.25, 0.5, 1, 2, 10 g
Polycillin-PRB powder for oral suspension (discontinued 1998) ℞ *antibiotic for Neisseria gonorrhoeae* [ampicillin; probenecid] 3.5•1 g
Polycitra syrup ℞ *urinary alkalinizing agent* [potassium citrate; sodium citrate; citric acid] 550•500•334 mg/5 mL
Polycitra-K oral solution, crystals for oral solution ℞ *urinary alkalizing agent* [potassium citrate; citric acid] 1100•334 mg/5 mL; 3300•1002 mg/packet
Polycitra-LC solution ℞ *urinary alkalizing agent* [potassium citrate; sodium citrate; citric acid] 550•500•334 mg/5 mL
Polycose liquid, powder OTC *carbohydrate caloric supplement* [glucose polymers]
polydextrose USAN *food additive*
polydimethylsiloxane *surgical aid (retinal tamponade) for retinal detachment*
Polydine ointment, scrub, solution OTC *broad-spectrum antimicrobial* [povidone-iodine]
polydioxanone USAN *absorbable surgical suture material*
polyelectrolyte 211 [see: sodium alginate]
polyenes *a class of antifungals produced by a species of Streptomyces that damage fungal cell membranes*
polyestradiol phosphate INN, BAN *antineoplastic; estrogen*
polyetadene INN *antacid* [also: polyethadene]
polyethadene USAN *antacid* [also: polyetadene]
polyethylene excipient NF *stiffening agent*
polyethylene glycol (PEG) NF *ophthalmic moisturizer; ointment and suppository base; solvent; hyperosmotic laxative; pre-procedure bowel evacuant*
polyethylene glycol *n* (*n* refers to the molecular weight: 300, 400, 1000, etc.)

polyethylene glycol *n* dioleate (*n* refers to the molecular weight: 300, 400, 1000, etc.)

polyethylene glycol 8 monostearate [see: polyoxyl 8 stearate]

polyethylene glycol 1000 monocetyl ether [see: cetomacrogol 1000]

polyethylene glycol 1540 NF

polyethylene glycol 4000 USP [also: macrogol 4000]

polyethylene glycol 6000 USP

polyethylene glycol–electrolyte solution (PEG-ES) *pre-procedure bowel evacuant* [contains PEG 3350]

polyethylene glycol monoleyl ether [see: polyoxyl 10 oleyl ether]

polyethylene glycol monomethyl ether NF *excipient*

polyethylene glycol monostearate [see: polyoxyl 40 & 50 stearate]

polyethylene glycol-superoxide dismutase (PEG-SOD) [see: pegorgotein]

polyethylene oxide NF *suspending and viscosity agent; tablet binder*

polyferose USAN *hematinic*

Polygala senega *medicinal herb* [see: senega]

Polygam powder for IV infusion (discontinued 2001; replaced by Polygam S/D) ℞ *passive immunizing agent for HIV* [immune globulin] 50 mg/mL

Polygam S/D freeze-dried powder for IV infusion ℞ *passive immunizing agent for HIV, idiopathic thrombocytopenic purpura (ITP), and B-cell chronic lymphocytic leukemia* [immune globulin, solvent/detergent treated] 50 mg/mL

polygeline INN, BAN

polyglactin 370 USAN *absorbable surgical suture coating*

polyglactin 910 USAN *absorbable surgical suture material*

polyglycolic acid USAN, INN *surgical suture material*

polyglyconate USAN, BAN *absorbable surgical suture material*

Polygonatum multiflorum; P. odoratum *medicinal herb* [see: Solomon's seal]

Polygonum aviculare; P. hydropiper; P. persicaria; P. punctatum *medicinal herb* [see: knotweed]

Polygonum bistorta *medicinal herb* [see: bistort]

Polygonum multiflorum *medicinal herb* [see: fo-ti; ho-shou-wu]

PolyHeme ℞ *investigational (Phase III) blood substitute* [human hemoglobin cross-linked with glutaral]

polyhexanide BAN [also: polihexanide]

Poly-Histine elixir (discontinued 2001) ℞ *antihistamine* [pheniramine maleate; pyrilamine maleate; phenyltoloxamine citrate] 4•4•4 mg/5 mL

Poly-Histine CS syrup ℞ *narcotic antitussive; decongestant; antihistamine* [codeine phosphate; phenylpropanolamine HCl; brompheniramine maleate] 10•12.5•2 mg/5 mL

Poly-Histine DM syrup ℞ *antitussive; decongestant; antihistamine* [dextromethorphan hydrobromide; phenylpropanolamine HCl; brompheniramine maleate] 10•12.5•2 mg/5 mL

Poly-Histine-D sustained-release capsules, elixir ℞ *decongestant; antihistamine* [phenylpropanolamine HCl; phenyltoloxamine citrate; pyrilamine maleate; pheniramine maleate] 50•16•16•16 mg; 12.5•4•4•4 mg/5 mL

Poly-Histine-D Ped Caps sustained-release capsules ℞ *pediatric decongestant and antihistamine* [phenylpropanolamine HCl; phenyltoloxamine citrate; pyrilamine maleate; pheniramine maleate] 25•8•8•8 mg

poly-ICLC *investigational (orphan) for primary brain tumors*

polyloxyl 8 stearate USAN *surfactant*

polymacon USAN *hydrophilic contact lens material*

polymanoacetate [now: acemannan]

polymeric oxygen [see: oxygen, polymeric]

polymetaphosphate P 32 USAN *radioactive agent*

polymethyl methacrylate (PMMA) *rigid hydrophobic polymer used for hard contact lenses*

polymixin E [see: colistin sulfate]
polymonine
Polymox capsules, powder for oral suspension, pediatric drops (discontinued 1998) ℞ *aminopenicillin antibiotic* [amoxicillin] 250, 500 mg; 125, 250 mg/5 mL; 50 mg/mL
polymyxin BAN *bactericidal antibiotic* [also: polymyxin B sulfate; polymyxin B]
polymyxin B INN *bactericidal antibiotic* [also: polymyxin B sulfate; polymyxin]
polymyxin B sulfate USP *bactericidal antibiotic* [also: polymyxin B; polymyxin] 500 000 U/vial eye drops or injection
polymyxin B sulfate & bacitracin zinc *topical antibiotic* 10 000•500 U/g ophthalmic
polymyxin B sulfate & bacitracin zinc & neomycin sulfate *topical antibiotic* 10 000 U•400 U•5 mg per g ophthalmic
polymyxin B sulfate & gramicidin & neomycin sulfate *topical antibiotic* 10 000 U•0.025 mg•1.75 mg per mL eye drops
polymyxin B sulfate & neomycin sulfate & dexamethasone *topical ophthalmic antibiotic and corticosteroidal anti-inflammatory* 10 000 U•0.35%•0.1% per mL eye drops
polymyxin B sulfate & trimethoprim sulfate [CG] *topical ophthalmic antibiotic* 10 000 U•1 mg per mL
polymyxin B_1 [see: polymyxin B]
polymyxin B_2 [see: polymyxin B]
polymyxin B_3 [see: polymyxin B]
polymyxin E [see: colistin sulfate]
polynoxylin INN, BAN
polyolprepolymer *topical base for creams and gels*
polyoxyethylene 20 sorbitan monolaurate [see: polysorbate 20]
polyoxyethylene 20 sorbitan monooleate [see: polysorbate 80]
polyoxyethylene 20 sorbitan monopalmitate [see: polysorbate 40]
polyoxyethylene 20 sorbitan monostearate [see: polysorbate 60]
polyoxyethylene 20 sorbitan trioleate [see: polysorbate 85]
polyoxyethylene 20 sorbitan tristearate [see: polysorbate 65]
polyoxyethylene 50 stearate [now: polyoxyl 50 stearate]
polyoxyethylene glycol 1000 monocetyl ether [see: cetomacrogol 1000]
polyoxyethylene nonyl phenol *surfactant/wetting agent*
polyoxyl 10 oleyl ether NF *surfactant*
polyoxyl 20 cetostearyl ether NF *surfactant*
polyoxyl 35 castor oil NF *emulsifying agent; surfactant*
polyoxyl 40 hydrogenated castor oil NF *emulsifying agent; surfactant*
polyoxyl 40 stearate USAN, NF *surfactant*
polyoxyl 50 stearate NF *surfactant; emulsifying agent*
polyoxypropylene 15 stearyl ether USAN *solvent*
polyphosphoric acid, sodium salt [see: sodium polyphosphate]
Polypodium vulgare *medicinal herb* [see: female fern]
Poly-Pred eye drop suspension ℞ *topical ophthalmic corticosteroidal anti-inflammatory; antibiotic* [prednisolone acetate; neomycin sulfate; polymyxin B sulfate] 0.5%•0.35%•10 000 U per mL
polypropylene glycol NF
polyribonucleotide [see: poly I: poly C12U]
polysaccharide-iron complex *hematinic; iron supplement* 150 mg oral
Polysorb Hydrate cream OTC *moisturizer; emollient*
polysorbate 20 USAN, NF, INN *surfactant/wetting agent*
polysorbate 40 USAN, NF, INN *surfactant*
polysorbate 60 USAN, NF, INN *surfactant*
polysorbate 65 USAN, INN *surfactant*
polysorbate 80 USAN, NF, INN *surfactant/wetting agent; viscosity-increasing agent*
polysorbate 85 USAN, INN *surfactant*

Polysporin ointment, powder OTC *topical antibiotic* [polymyxin B sulfate; bacitracin zinc] 10 000•500 U/g

Polysporin ophthalmic ointment OTC *topical ophthalmic antibiotic* [polymyxin B sulfate; bacitracin zinc] 10 000•500 U/g

Polytabs-F chewable tablets ℞ *pediatric vitamin supplement and dental caries preventative* [multiple vitamins; fluoride; folic acid] ≛•1•0.3 mg

Polytar shampoo, soap OTC *antiseborrheic; antipsoriatic; antipruritic; antibacterial* [coal tar, pine tar, and juniper tar solution] 2.5%; 1%

Polytar Bath oil OTC *antipsoriatic; antiseborrheic; antipruritic; emollient* [coal tar, pine tar, and juniper tar solution] 25%

polytef USAN *prosthetic aid* [also: politef]

polytetrafluoroethylene (PTFE) [see: polytef]

polythiazide USAN, USP, INN *diuretic; antihypertensive*

Polytrim eye drops ℞ *topical ophthalmic antibiotic* [polymyxin B sulfate; trimethoprim] 10 000 U•1 mg per mL

polyurethane foam USAN *internal bone splint*

polyvalent Crotaline antivenin [see: antivenin (Crotalidae) polyvalent]

polyvalent gas gangrene antitoxin [see: gas gangrene antitoxin, pentavalent]

polyvidone INN *dispersing, suspending and viscosity-increasing agent* [also: povidone]

Poly-Vi-Flor chewable tablets ℞ *pediatric vitamin supplement and dental caries preventative* [multiple vitamins; sodium fluoride; folic acid] ≛•0.25•0.3, ≛•0.5•0.3, ≛•1•0.3 mg

Poly-Vi-Flor drops ℞ *pediatric vitamin supplement and dental caries preventative* [multiple vitamins; sodium fluoride] ≛•0.25, ≛•0.5 mg/mL

Poly-Vi-Flor with Iron chewable tablets ℞ *pediatric vitamin/iron supplement and dental caries preventative* [multiple vitamins & minerals; sodium fluoride; iron; folic acid] ≛•0.25•12•0.3, ≛•0.5•12•0.3, ≛•1•12•0.3 mg

Poly-Vi-Flor with Iron drops ℞ *pediatric vitamin/iron supplement and dental caries preventative* [multiple vitamins & minerals; sodium fluoride; iron] ≛•0.25•10, ≛•0.5•10 mg/mL

polyvinyl acetate phthalate NF *coating agent*

polyvinyl alcohol (PVA) USP *ophthalmic moisturizer; viscosity-increasing agent*

polyvinyl chloride, radiopaque *oral radiopaque contrast medium for severe constipation*

polyvinylpyrrolidone [now: povidone]

Poly-Vi-Sol chewable tablets OTC *vitamin supplement* [multiple vitamins; folic acid] ≛•0.3 mg

Poly-Vi-Sol drops OTC *vitamin supplement* [multiple vitamins] ≛

Poly-Vi-Sol with Iron chewable tablets OTC *vitamin/iron supplement* [multiple vitamins; iron; folic acid] ≛•12•0.3 mg

Poly-Vi-Sol with Iron drops OTC *vitamin/iron supplement* [multiple vitamins; iron] ≛•10 mg/mL

Poly-Vitamin drops OTC *vitamin supplement* [multiple vitamins] ≛

Polyvitamin Fluoride chewable tablets ℞ *pediatric vitamin supplement and dental caries preventative* [multiple vitamins; fluoride; folic acid] ≛•0.5•0.3, ≛•1•0.3 mg

Polyvitamin Fluoride drops ℞ *pediatric vitamin supplement and dental caries preventative* [multiple vitamins; fluoride] ≛•0.25, ≛•0.5 mg/mL

Polyvitamin Fluoride with Iron chewable tablets ℞ *pediatric vitamin/iron supplement and dental caries preventative* [multiple vitamins & minerals; fluoride; iron; folic acid] ≛•1•12•0.3 mg

Poly-Vitamin with Iron drops OTC *vitamin/iron supplement* [multiple vitamins; iron] ≛•10 mg/mL

Polyvitamin with Iron and Fluoride drops ℞ *pediatric vitamin/iron*

supplement and dental caries preventative [multiple vitamins; iron; fluoride] ≛•10•0.25 mg/mL

Polyvitamins with Fluoride and Iron chewable tablets ℞ *pediatric vitamin/iron supplement and dental caries preventative* [multiple vitamins; fluoride; iron; folic acid] ≛•0.5•12•0.3 mg

pomegranate *(Punica granatum)* seeds and fruit rind *medicinal herb used as an anthelmintic and astringent*

POMP (prednisone, Oncovin, methotrexate, Purinethol) *chemotherapy protocol*

ponalrestat USAN, INN, BAN *aldose reductase inhibitor*

Pondimin tablets (discontinued 1997) ℞ *anorexiant; CNS depressant* [fenfluramine HCl] 20 mg

ponfibrate INN

Ponstel capsules ℞ *analgesic; nonsteroidal anti-inflammatory drug (NSAID)* [mefenamic acid] 250 mg 🔊 Pronestyl

Pontocaine cream OTC *topical local anesthetic* [tetracaine HCl] 1%

Pontocaine ointment OTC *topical local anesthetic* [tetracaine; menthol] 0.5%•0.5%

Pontocaine HCl Mono-Drop (eye drops) ℞ *topical ophthalmic anesthetic* [tetracaine HCl] 0.5%

Pontocaine HCl solution ℞ *nose/throat anesthetic to abolish laryngeal and esophageal reflex* [tetracaine HCl; chlorobutanol] 2%•0.4%

Pontocaine HCl spinal injection, powder for reconstitution ℞ *injectable local anesthetic* [tetracaine HCl] 0.2%, 0.3%, 1%

poplar *(Populus tremuloides)* bark and buds *medicinal herb used as an antiperiodic, balsamic, febrifuge, and stomachic*

poplar, balsam *medicinal herb* [see: balm of Gilead]

poplar, black *medicinal herb* [see: black poplar]

Po-Pon-S sugar-coated tablets OTC *vitamin/mineral supplement* [multiple vitamins & minerals] ≛

Populus balsamifera; P. candicans *medicinal herb* [see: balm of Gilead]

Populus nigra; P. tremula *medicinal herb* [see: black poplar]

Populus tremuloides *medicinal herb* [see: poplar]

poractant alfa BAN *porcine lung extract containing 90% phospholipids for emergency rescue and treatment of respiratory distress syndrome (RDS) in premature infants (orphan)*

Porcelana cream OTC *hyperpigmentation bleaching agent* [hydroquinone] 2%

Porcelana with Sunscreen cream OTC *hyperpigmentation bleaching agent; sunscreen* [hydroquinone; padimate O] 2%•2.5%

porcine islet preparation, encapsulated *investigational (orphan) antidiabetic for type 1 patients on immunosuppression*

porfimer sodium USAN, INN *laser light–activated antineoplastic for photodynamic therapy (PDT) of esophageal (orphan) and non–small cell lung cancers (NSCLC); investigational (orphan) for bladder cancer*

porfiromycin USAN, INN, BAN *antibacterial; investigational (Phase III, orphan) antineoplastic for head, neck, and cervical cancers*

***Porites* spp.** *natural material* [see: coral]

porofocon A USAN *hydrophobic contact lens material*

porofocon B USAN *hydrophobic contact lens material*

Portagen powder OTC *enteral nutritional therapy* [lactose-free formula]

porton asparaginase [see: Erwinia L-asparaginase]

posaconazole USAN *antifungal*

posatirelin INN

posedrine [see: benzchlorpropamid]

Posicor tablets (discontinued 1998) ℞ *vasodilator and calcium channel blocker for hypertension and chronic stable* *angina* [mibefradil dihydrochloride] 50, 100 mg ⊡ Proscar

poskine INN, BAN

posterior pituitary [see: pituitary, posterior]

Posture tablets OTC *calcium supplement* [calcium phosphate, tribasic] 1565.2 mg

Posture-D film-coated tablets OTC *dietary supplement* [calcium phosphate, tribasic; vitamin D] 600 mg•125 IU

Potaba tablets, capsules, Envules (powder for reconstitution) ℞ *water-soluble vitamin; "possibly effective" for scleroderma and other skin diseases and Peyronie disease* [aminobenzoate potassium] 500 mg; 500 mg; 2 g

Potable Aqua tablets OTC *emergency disinfectant for drinking water* [tetraglycine hydroperiodide (source of iodine)] 16.7% (6.68%)

Potasalan liquid ℞ *potassium supplement* [potassium chloride; alcohol 4%] 20 mEq/15 mL

potash, sulfurated USP *source of sulfides*

potassic saline, lactated NF

potassium *element (K)*

potassium acetate USP *electrolyte replenisher* 2, 4 mEq/mL injection

potassium acid phosphate *urinary acidifier*

potassium alpha-phenoxyethyl penicillin [see: phenethicillin potassium]

potassium alum [see: alum, potassium]

potassium aminobenzoate [see: aminobenzoate potassium]

potassium aspartate [see: L-aspartate potassium]

potassium aspartate & magnesium aspartate USAN *nutrient*

potassium benzoate NF *preservative*

potassium benzyl penicillin [see: penicillin G potassium]

potassium bicarbonate USP *pH buffer; electrolyte replacement*

potassium bitartrate USAN

potassium borate *pH buffer*

potassium canrenoate JAN *aldosterone antagonist* [also: canrenoate potassium; canrenoic acid]

potassium carbonate USP *alkalizing agent*

potassium chloride (KCl) USP *electrolyte replenisher* 600, 750 mg oral; 20, 40 mEq/15 mL oral; 20 mEq/pkt oral; 2, 10, 20, 30, 40, 60, 90 mEq/mL injection

potassium chloride K 42 USAN *radioactive agent*

potassium citrate USP *electrolyte replacement; urinary alkalizer for nephrolithiasis and hypocitruria prevention (orphan)*

potassium clavulanate & amoxicillin [see: amoxicillin]

potassium clavulanate & ticarcillin [see: ticarcillin disodium]

potassium dichloroisocyanurate [see: troclosene potassium]

potassium gamma hydroxybutyrate (KGHB) [see: gamma hydroxybutyrate (GHB)]

potassium glucaldrate USAN, INN *antacid*

potassium gluconate USP *electrolyte replenisher* 500, 595 mg oral; 20 mEq/15 mL oral

potassium guaiacolsulfonate USP *expectorant* [also: sulfogaiacol]

potassium hydroxide (KOH) NF *alkalizing agent*

potassium hydroxymethoxybenzenesulfonate hemihydrate [see: potassium guaiacolsulfonate]

potassium iodide USP *antifungal; expectorant; iodine supplement; thyroid agent* 1 g/mL oral

potassium mercuric iodide NF

potassium metabisulfite NF *antioxidant*

potassium metaphosphate NF *buffering agent*

potassium nitrate *tooth desensitizer*

potassium nitrazepate INN

potassium para-aminobenzoate (PAB) [see: aminobenzoate potassium]

potassium penicillin G [see: penicillin G potassium]

potassium perchlorate *radioimaging adjunct*

potassium permanganate USP *topical anti-infective*

potassium phosphate, dibasic USP *calcium regulator; phosphorus replacement; pH buffer*

potassium phosphate, monobasic NF *pH buffer; phosphorus replacement*

potassium sodium tartrate USP *laxative*

potassium sorbate NF *antimicrobial agent*

potassium tetraborate *pH buffer*

potassium thiocyanate NF

potassium-sparing diuretics *a class of diuretic agents that interfere with sodium reabsorption, thus decreasing potassium secretion*

potato, wild; wild sweet potato vine *medicinal herb* [see: wild jalap]

Potentilla anserina; P. canadensis; P. reptans *medicinal herb* [see: cinquefoil]

Potentilla tormentilla *medicinal herb* [see: tormentil]

Povidine ointment, scrub, solution OTC *broad-spectrum antimicrobial* [povidone-iodine] 10%, 5%, 10%

povidone USAN, USP *dispersing, suspending and viscosity-increasing agent* [also: polyvidone]

povidone I 125 USAN *radioactive agent*

povidone I 131 USAN *radioactive agent*

povidone-iodine USP, BAN *broad-spectrum antimicrobial* 10% topical

powdered cellulose [see: cellulose, powdered]

powdered ipecac [see: ipecac, powdered]

powdered opium [see: opium, powdered]

PowderJect (trademarked device) ℞ *investigational device for the needleless injection of drugs in powder form*

PowerMate tablets OTC *vitamin/mineral supplement* [multiple vitamins & minerals] ≛

PowerVites tablets OTC *vitamin/mineral supplement* [multiple vitamins & minerals; folic acid; biotin] ≛ •150•25 µg

PPA (phenylpropanolamine) [q.v.]

PPD (purified protein derivative [of tuberculin]) [see: tuberculin]

PPG-15 stearyl ether [now: polyoxypropylene 15 stearyl ether]

PPRT-321 *investigational (Phase II) saw palmetto derivative for benign prostatic hyperplasia*

practolol USAN, INN *antiadrenergic (β-receptor)*

prajmalium bitartrate INN, BAN

pralidoxime chloride USAN, USP *cholinesterase reactivator for organophosphate poisoning and anticholinesterase overdose* 600 mg injection ⑨ pyridoxine; pramoxine

pralidoxime iodide USAN, INN *cholinesterase reactivator* ⑨ pyridoxine; pramoxine

pralidoxime mesylate USAN *cholinesterase reactivator* ⑨ pyridoxine; pramoxine

pralmorelin dihydrochloride USAN *growth hormone secretagogue*

PrameGel gel OTC *topical local anesthetic* [pramoxine HCl; menthol] 1%•0.5%

Pramidin nasal spray (commercially available in Italy) ℞ *investigational antiemetic for chemotherapy* [metoclopramide HCl]

Pramilet FA Filmtabs (film-coated tablets) ℞ *prenatal vitamin/mineral/calcium/iron supplement* [multiple vitamins & minerals; calcium; iron; folic acid] ≛ •250•40•1 mg

pramipexole USAN, INN *dopamine agonist; antiparkinsonian; investigational for depression and schizophrenia*

pramipexole dihydrochloride USAN *dopamine agonist; antiparkinsonian; investigational for depression and schizophrenia*

pramiracetam INN *cognition adjuvant* [also: pramiracetam HCl]

pramiracetam HCl USAN *cognition adjuvant* [also: pramiracetam]

pramiracetam sulfate USAN *cognition adjuvant; orphan status withdrawn 1996*

pramiverine INN, BAN

pramlintide USAN *synthetic amylin analogue to slow gastric emptying; investi-*

gational (Phase III) antidiabetic for type 1 and type 2 diabetes

pramlintide acetate USAN *synthetic amylin analogue to slow gastric emptying; investigational (Phase III) antidiabetic for type 1 and type 2 diabetes*

pramocaine INN *topical anesthetic* [also: pramoxine HCl; pramoxine]

pramocaine HCl [see: pramoxine HCl]

Pramosone cream, lotion, ointment ℞ *topical corticosteroidal anti-inflammatory; local anesthetic* [hydrocortisone acetate; pramoxine] 1%•1%, 2.5%•1%; 2.5%•1%; 2.5%•1% ⑨ pramoxine

pramoxine BAN *topical local anesthetic* [also: pramoxine HCl; pramocaine] ⑨ pralidoxime; Pramosone

Pramoxine HC anorectal aerosol foam ℞ *topical corticosteroidal anti-inflammatory; local anesthetic* [hydrocortisone acetate; pramoxine HCl] 1%•1%

pramoxine HCl USP *topical local anesthetic* [also: pramocaine; pramoxine]

prampine INN, BAN

Prandase (CAN) tablets ℞ *alpha-glucosidase inhibitor for type 2 diabetes* [acarbose] 50, 100 mg

Prandin tablets ℞ *oral antidiabetic agent that stimulates release of insulin from the pancreas for type 2 diabetes* [repaglinide] 0.5, 1, 2 mg

pranidipine INN

pranlukast INN, BAN *investigational treatment for asthma*

pranolium chloride USAN, INN *antiarrhythmic*

pranoprofen INN

pranosal INN

praseodymium *element (Pr)*

prasterone INN

Pravachol tablets ℞ *HMG-CoA reductase inhibitor for hyperlipidemia, hypertriglyceridemia, atherosclerosis, coronary procedures, and recurrent myocardial infarctions* [pravastatin sodium] 10, 20, 40 mg ⑨ Primacor

pravadoline INN *analgesic* [also: pravadoline maleate]

pravadoline maleate USAN *analgesic* [also: pravadoline]

pravastatin INN, BAN *HMG-CoA reductase inhibitor for hyperlipidemia, hypertriglyceridemia, atherosclerosis, coronary procedures, and recurrent myocardial infarctions* [also: pravastatin sodium]

pravastatin sodium USAN, JAN *HMG-CoA reductase inhibitor for hyperlipidemia, hypertriglyceridemia, atherosclerosis, coronary procedures, and recurrent myocardial infarctions* [also: pravastatin]

Prax lotion, cream OTC *topical local anesthetic* [pramoxine HCl] 1%

praxadine INN

prazepam USAN, USP, INN *sedative; anxiolytic* 5 mg oral ⑨ prazepine; prazosin

prazepine INN ⑨ prazepam

praziquantel USAN, USP, INN, BAN *anthelmintic for schistosomiasis (flukes)*

prazitone INN, BAN

prazocillin INN

prazosin INN, BAN *antihypertensive; α_1-adrenergic blocker* [also: prazosin HCl] ⑨ prazepam

prazosin HCl USAN, USP, JAN *antihypertensive; α_1-adrenergic blocker* [also: prazosin] 1, 2, 5 mg oral

Pre-Attain liquid OTC *enteral nutritional therapy* [lactose-free formula]

PreCare Conceive film-coated tablets ℞ *pre-conception vitamin/mineral/calcium/iron supplement* [multiple vitamins & minerals; calcium; iron; folic acid] ≛•200•30•1 mg

PreCare Prenatal film-coated caplet ℞ *vitamin/mineral/calcium/iron supplement for pregnancy and lactation* [multiple vitamins & minerals; calcium; iron; folic acid] ≛•250•40•1 mg

precatory bean (*Abrus precatorius*) plant *medicinal herb for eye inflammation, hastening labor, and stimulating abortion; not generally regarded as safe, as it is highly toxic and ingestion may be fatal*

Precedex IV infusion ℞ *sedative for intubated and ventilated patients in an* *intensive care setting; premedication to anesthesia* [dexmedetomidine HCl] 100 µg/mL

precipitated calcium carbonate JAN *antacid; calcium replenisher* [also: calcium carbonate]

precipitated chalk [see: calcium carbonate]

precipitated sulfur [see: sulfur, precipitated]

Precision High Nitrogen Diet powder OTC *enteral nutritional therapy* [lactose-free formula]

Precision LR Diet powder OTC *enteral nutritional therapy* [lactose-free formula]

preclamol INN

Precose tablets ℞ *alpha-glucosidase inhibitor for type 2 diabetes* [acarbose] 25, 50, 100 mg

Pred Mild; Pred Forte eye drop suspension ℞ *topical ophthalmic corticosteroidal anti-inflammatory* [prednisolone acetate] 0.12%; 1%

Predalone 50 IM injection ℞ *corticosteroid; anti-inflammatory* [prednisolone acetate] 50 mg/mL

Predcor-50 IM injection ℞ *corticosteroid; anti-inflammatory* [prednisolone acetate] 50 mg/mL

Pred-G eye drop suspension ℞ *topical ophthalmic corticosteroidal anti-inflammatory; antibiotic* [prednisolone acetate; gentamicin sulfate] 1%•0.3%

Pred-G S.O.P. ophthalmic ointment ℞ *ophthalmic topical corticosteroidal anti-inflammatory; antibiotic* [prednisolone acetate; gentamicin sulfate; chlorobutanol] 0.6%•0.3%•0.5%

prednazate USAN, INN *anti-inflammatory*

prednazoline INN

prednicarbate USAN, INN *corticosteroid; anti-inflammatory*

Prednicen-M tablets ℞ *corticosteroid; anti-inflammatory; immunosuppressant* [prednisone] 5 mg

prednimustine USAN, INN *antineoplastic; investigational for malignant non-Hodgkin lymphomas; orphan status withdrawn 1998*

Prednisol TBA intra-articular, intralesional, or soft tissue injection ℞ *corticosteroid; anti-inflammatory* [prednisolone tebutate] 20 mg/mL

prednisolamate INN, BAN

prednisolone USP, INN *corticosteroidal anti-inflammatory* 5 mg oral; 15 mg/5 mL oral ⑨ prednisone

prednisolone acetate USP, BAN *corticosteroidal anti-inflammatory* 1% eye drops; 25, 50 mg/mL injection

prednisolone hemisuccinate USP *corticosteroidal anti-inflammatory*

prednisolone sodium phosphate USP *corticosteroidal anti-inflammatory* 0.125%, 1% eye drops

prednisolone sodium succinate USP *corticosteroidal anti-inflammatory*

prednisolone steaglate INN, BAN *corticosteroidal anti-inflammatory*

prednisolone tebutate USP *corticosteroidal anti-inflammatory* 20 mg/mL injection

prednisone USP, INN *corticosteroid; anti-inflammatory; immunosuppressant* 1, 5, 20 mg oral ⑨ prednisolone

prednival USAN *corticosteroid; anti-inflammatory*

prednylidene INN, BAN

prefenamate INN

Prefest [see: Ortho-Prefest]

Prefill (dosage form) *prefilled applicator*

Preflex Daily Cleaner Especially for Sensitive Eyes solution OTC *surfactant cleaning solution for soft contact lenses*

Prefrin Liquifilm eye drops OTC *topical ophthalmic decongestant* [phenylephrine HCl] 0.12%

pregabalin USAN *gabamimetic anticonvulsant*

pregelatinized starch [see: starch, pregelatinized]

Pregestimil powder OTC *hypoallergenic infant food for severe malabsorption disorders* [enzymatically hydrolyzed protein formula]

pregnandiol JAN

pregneninolone [see: ethisterone]

pregnenolone INN *non-hormonal sterol derivative* [also: pregnenolone succinate]

pregnenolone succinate USAN *non-hormonal sterol derivative* [also: pregnenolone]

Pregnosis slide test for home use *in vitro diagnostic aid; urine pregnancy test* [latex agglutination test]

Pregnyl powder for IM injection ℞ *hormone for prepubertal cryptorchidism and hypogonadism; ovulation stimulant* [chorionic gonadotropin] 1000 U/mL

Prehist sustained-release capsules ℞ *decongestant; antihistamine* [phenylephrine HCl; chlorpheniramine maleate] 20•8 mg

Prehist D sustained-release tablets, sustained-release capsules ℞ *decongestant; antihistamine; anticholinergic* [phenylephrine HCl; chlorpheniramine maleate; methscopolamine nitrate] 20•8•2.5 mg

Prelone syrup ℞ *corticosteroid; anti-inflammatory* [prednisolone; alcohol 5%] 5, 15 mg/5 mL

Prelu-2 timed-release capsules ℞ *anorexiant; CNS stimulant* [phendimetrazine tartrate] 105 mg

premafloxacin USAN, INN *veterinary antibacterial*

Premarin tablets ℞ *estrogen replacement therapy for postmenopausal symptoms; palliative therapy for prostate and breast cancer; investigational (Phase III) for Alzheimer disease* [conjugated estrogens] 0.3, 0.625, 0.9, 1.25, 2.5 mg

Premarin vaginal cream ℞ *estrogen replacement for postmenopausal atrophic vaginitis* [conjugated estrogens] 0.625 mg/g

Premarin Intravenous IV or IM injection ℞ *treatment of abnormal uterine bleeding due to hormonal imbalance* [conjugated estrogens] 25 mg

Premarin with Methyltestosterone tablets (discontinued 1999) ℞ *hormone replacement therapy for postmenopausal symptoms* [conjugated estrogens; methyltestosterone] 0.625•5, 1.25•10 mg

premazepam INN, BAN

PremesisRx tablets ℞ *prenatal vitamin/mineral supplement* [vitamin B_6; vitamin B_{12}; folic acid; calcium carbonate] 75 mg•12 µg•1 mg•200 mg

Premphase tablets (in packs of 28) ℞ *hormone replacement therapy for postmenopausal symptoms* [Phase 1: conjugated estrogens; Phase 2: conjugated estrogens; medroxyprogesterone acetate] 0.625 mg; 0.625•5 mg

Prempro tablets ℞ *hormone replacement therapy for postmenopausal symptoms* [conjugated estrogens; medroxyprogesterone acetate] 0.625•2.5, 0.625•5 mg

Prēmsyn PMS caplets OTC *analgesic; antipyretic; diuretic; antihistaminic sleep aid* [acetaminophen; pamabrom; pyrilamine maleate] 500•25•15 mg

prenalterol INN, BAN *adrenergic* [also: prenalterol HCl]

prenalterol HCl USAN *adrenergic* [also: prenalterol]

Prenatal H.P. tablets ℞ *vitamin/calcium/iron supplement* [multiple vitamins; calcium; iron; folic acid] ≛•50•30•0.8 mg

Prenatal Maternal tablets ℞ *vitamin/mineral/calcium/iron supplement* [multiple vitamins & minerals; calcium; iron; folic acid; biotin] ≛•250•60•1•0.03 mg

Prenatal MR 90 delayed-release film-coated tablets ℞ *vitamin/calcium/iron supplement* [multiple vitamins; calcium; iron; folic acid] ≛•250•90•1 mg

Prenatal Plus; Prenatal Plus Improved tablets ℞ *vitamin/calcium/iron supplement* [multiple vitamins; calcium; iron; folic acid] ≛•200•65•1 mg

Prenatal Plus Iron tablets ℞ *vitamin/calcium/iron supplement* [multiple vitamins; calcium; iron; folic acid] ≛•200•27•1 mg

Prenatal Plus with Betacarotene tablets ℞ *vitamin/calcium/iron supplement* [multiple vitamins; calcium; iron; folic acid] ≛ •200•65•1 mg

Prenatal Rx tablets ℞ *vitamin/calcium/iron supplement* [multiple vitamins; calcium; iron; folic acid] ≛ •175•29.5•1 mg

Prenatal Rx with Betacarotene tablets ℞ *vitamin/calcium/iron supplement* [multiple vitamins; calcium; iron; folic acid; biotin] ≛ •200•60•1•0.03 mg

Prenatal with Folic Acid tablets OTC *vitamin/calcium/iron supplement* [multiple vitamins; calcium; iron; folic acid] ≛ •200•60•0.8 mg

Prenatal Z delayed-release film-coated tablets ℞ *vitamin/calcium/iron supplement* [multiple vitamins; calcium; iron; folic acid] ≛ •300•65•1 mg

Prenatal-1 + Iron tablets ℞ *vitamin/calcium/iron supplement* [multiple vitamins; calcium; iron; folic acid] ≛ •200•65•1 mg

Prenatal-S tablets OTC *vitamin/calcium/iron supplement* [multiple vitamins; calcium; iron; folic acid] ≛ •200•60•0.8 mg

Prenate Advance; Prenate 90 delayed-release film-coated tablets ℞ *prenatal vitamin/calcium/iron supplement* [multiple vitamins; calcium; iron; folic acid] ≛ •200•90•1 mg; ≛ •250•90•1 mg

Prenate Ultra delayed-release film-coated tablets (discontinued 2000) ℞ *prenatal vitamin/calcium/iron supplement* [multiple vitamins; calcium; iron; folic acid] ≛ •200•90•1 mg

Prenavite tablets OTC *vitamin/calcium/iron supplement* [multiple vitamins; calcium; iron; folic acid] ≛ •200•60•0.8 mg

prenisteine INN

prenoverine INN

prenoxdiazine INN

prenylamine USAN, INN *coronary vasodilator*

Preparation H anorectal cream, anorectal ointment OTC *temporary relief of hemorrhoidal symptoms* [shark liver oil; phenylephrine HCl] 3%•0.25%

Preparation H cleansing tissues OTC *moisturizer and cleanser for external rectal/vaginal areas* [propylene glycol]

Preparation H rectal suppositories OTC *temporary relief of hemorrhoidal symptoms* [shark liver oil] 3%

Preparation H Cooling Gel OTC *temporary relief of hemorrhoidal symptoms* [phenylephrine HCl; hamamelis water; alcohol 7.5%] 0.25%•50%

prepared chalk [see: calcium carbonate]

Prepcat oral suspension ℞ *radiopaque contrast medium for gastrointestinal imaging* [barium sulfate] 1.5%

Pre-Pen solution for dermal scratch test ℞ *diagnostic aid for penicillin hypersensitivity* [benzylpenicilloyl polylysine] 0.25 mL

Pre-Pen/MDM solution for dermal scratch test ℞ *investigational (orphan) for penicillin hypersensitivity assessment* [benzylpenicillin]

Prepidil gel ℞ *prostaglandin for cervical ripening at term* [dinoprostone] 0.5 mg

Prepulsid (CAN) tablets, oral suspension (discontinued 2001) ℞ *treatment for nocturnal heartburn due to gastroesophageal reflux disease (GERD)* [cisapride] 5, 10, 20 mg; 1 mg/mL

pretamazium iodide INN, BAN

prethcamide

prethrombin [see: prothrombin complex, activated]

pretiadil INN

Pretts Diet-Aid chewable tablets OTC *diet aid* [sodium carboxymethylcellulose; alginic acid; sodium bicarbonate] 100•200•70 mg

Pretty Feet & Hands cream OTC *moisturizer; emollient*

Pretz solution OTC *nasal moisturizer* [sodium chloride (saline solution)] 0.6%

Pretz Irrigating solution OTC *for postoperative irrigation* [sodium chloride (saline solution); glycerin; eriodictyon] 0.75%

Pretz Moisturizing nose drops OTC *nasal moisturizer* [sodium chloride (saline solution); glycerin; eriodictyon] 0.75%

Pretz-D nasal spray OTC *nasal decongestant and moisturizer* [ephedrine sulfate] 0.25%

PretzPak ointment OTC *antimicrobial postoperative nasal pack* [benzyl alcohol; polyethylene glycol; carboxymethylcellulose; urea; allantoin]

Prevacid delayed-release capsules ℞ *proton pump inhibitor for gastric and duodenal ulcers, erosive esophagitis, GERD, and other gastroesophageal disorders* [lansoprazole] 15, 30 mg

Prevalite powder for oral suspension ℞ *cholesterol-lowering antihyperlipidemic; also used for biliary obstruction* [cholestyramine resin] 4 g/dose

Prevatac ℞ *investigational (Phase III) agent to prevent recurrence of prostate cancer* [exisulind]

Preven kit (4 film-coated tablets + pregnancy test) ℞ *emergency postcoital contraceptive* [levonorgestrel; ethinyl estradiol] 0.25•0.05 mg ⓢ Preveon

Prevent-X powder for oral solution OTC *dietary supplement* [multiple vitamins & minerals; multiple amino acids] ≛

Preveon ℞ *investigational (Phase III) nucleotide reverse transcriptase inhibitor (NRTI) for advanced HIV and AIDS (clinical trials discontinued 1999); investigational (Phase III) treatment for chronic hepatitis B virus (HBV) infections* [adefovir dipivoxil] ⓢ Preven

PreviDent gel (for self-application) ℞ *topical dental caries preventative* [sodium fluoride] 1.1%

PreviDent 5000 Plus cream (for self-application) ℞ *topical dental caries preventative* [sodium fluoride] 1.1%

PreviDent Rinse oral solution ℞ *topical dental caries preventative* [sodium fluoride] 0.2%

Prevnar IM injection ℞ *active immunization against 7 strains of Streptococcus pneumoniae in infants and toddlers* [pneumococcal vaccine, 7-valent] 2–4 µg of each strain per 0.5 mL dose

Prevpac three-drug daily pack ℞ *triple therapy for H. pylori: an antisecretory and two antibiotics* [lansoprazole; clarithromycin; amoxicillin] 2×30 mg; 2×500 mg; 4×500 mg

PreVue *B. burgdorferi* Antibody Detection Assay reagent kit for professional use *in vitro diagnostic aid for Lyme disease*

prezatide copper acetate USAN, INN *immunomodulator; investigational (Phase II) wound-healing gel for venous leg ulcers*

Prezios ℞ *investigational vitamin D_3 analogue for the topical treatment of psoriasis* [maxacalcitol]

pribecaine INN

prickly ash *(Xanthoxylum americanum; X. fraxineum)* bark *medicinal herb for fever, mouth sores, poor circulation, ulcers, and wounds*

prickly juniper *(Juniperus oxycedrus)* *medicinal herb* [see: juniper]

prickly pear *medicinal herb* [see: nopal]

pride of China *(Melia azedarach)* root bark and fruit *medicinal herb used as an anthelmintic, astringent, bitter tonic, emetic, emmenagogue, and purgative*

pride weed *medicinal herb* [see: fleabane; horseweed]

pridefine INN *antidepressant* [also: pridefine HCl]

pridefine HCl USAN *antidepressant* [also: pridefine]

prideperone INN

pridinol INN

priest's crown *medicinal herb* [see: dandelion]

prifelone USAN, INN *dermatologic anti-inflammatory*

prifinium bromide INN

Priftin film-coated tablets ℞ *antibacterial for tuberculosis (orphan); investigational (orphan) for AIDS-related*

Mycobacterium avium complex (MAC) [rifapentine] 150 mg

prifuroline INN

priliximab USAN, INN *monoclonal antibody to treat autoimmune lymphoproliferative diseases and in organ transplants*

prilocaine USAN, INN, BAN *topical local anesthetic*

prilocaine HCl USAN, USP *topical local anesthetic* [also: propitocaine HCl]

Prilosec delayed-release capsules ℞ *proton pump inhibitor for gastric and duodenal ulcers, erosive esophagitis, GERD, and other gastroesophageal disorders* [omeprazole] 10, 20, 40 mg ⊡ Prozac

primachine phosphate [see: primaquine phosphate]

Primacor IV infusion ℞ *vasodilator for congestive heart failure* [milrinone lactate] 0.2, 1 mg/mL ⊡ Pravachol

Primacor in 5% Dextrose IV infusion ℞ *vasodilator for congestive heart failure* [milrinone lactate; dextrose] 200 μg/mL; 5% ⊡ Pravachol

primaperone INN

primaquine INN *antimalarial* [also: primaquine phosphate]

primaquine phosphate USP *antimalarial; prevention of malarial relapse* [also: primaquine] 26.3 mg oral

primaquine phosphate & clindamycin HCl *investigational (orphan) for AIDS-associated Pneumocystis carinii pneumonia*

Primatene tablets OTC *bronchodilator; decongestant; expectorant* [ephedrine HCl; guaifenesin] 12.5•200 mg

Primatene tablets (discontinued 1998) OTC *antiasthmatic; bronchodilator; decongestant; sedative* [theophylline; ephedrine HCl; phenobarbital] 130•24•7.5 mg

Primatene Dual Action tablets (discontinued 2000) OTC *antiasthmatic; bronchodilator; decongestant; expectorant* [theophylline; ephedrine HCl; guaifenesin] 60•12.5•100 mg

Primatene Mist inhalation aerosol OTC *sympathomimetic bronchodilator* [epinephrine] 0.2 mg/dose

Primatene Mist Suspension inhalation aerosol (discontinued 1999) OTC *sympathomimetic bronchodilator* [epinephrine bitartrate] 0.3 mg/dose

Primatuss Cough Mixture 4 liquid OTC *antitussive; antihistamine* [dextromethorphan hydrobromide; chlorpheniramine maleate; alcohol 10%] 15•2 mg/5 mL

Primatuss Cough Mixture 4D liquid OTC *antitussive; decongestant; expectorant* [dextromethorphan hydrobromide; pseudoephedrine HCl; guaifenesin; alcohol 10%] 10•20•67 mg/5 mL

Primaxin I.M. powder for injection ℞ *carbapenem antibiotic* [imipenem; cilastatin sodium] 500•500, 750•750 mg

Primaxin I.V. powder for injection ℞ *carbapenem antibiotic* [imipenem; cilastatin sodium] 250•250, 500•500 mg

primidolol USAN, INN *antihypertensive; antianginal; antiarrhythmic*

primidone USP, INN, BAN *anticonvulsant for grand mal, psychomotor, or focal epileptic seizures* 50, 250 mg oral

Primobolan *brand name for methenolone acetate, a European anabolic steroid abused as a street drug*

Primobolan Depot *brand name for methenolone enanthate, a European anabolic steroid abused as a street drug*

Primsol oral solution ℞ *antibiotic for otitis media in children and urinary tract infections in adults* [trimethoprim HCl] 50 mg/5 mL

primycin INN

prince's pine *medicinal herb* [see: pipsissewa]

Principen capsules, powder for oral suspension ℞ *aminopenicillin antibiotic* [ampicillin] 250, 500 mg; 125, 250 mg/5 mL

Prinivil tablets ℞ *antihypertensive; angiotensin-converting enzyme (ACE) inhibitor* [lisinopril] 2.5, 5, 10, 20, 40 mg ⊡ Plendil

prinodolol [see: pindolol]

prinomastat USAN *investigational (Phase III) matrix metalloprotease inhibitor for advanced non–small cell* *lung cancer (NSCLC) and prostate cancer (clinical trials discontinued 2000); investigational (Phase II) for age-related macular degeneration*

prinomide INN *antirheumatic* [also: prinomide tromethamine]

prinomide tromethamine USAN *antirheumatic* [also: prinomide]

prinoxodan USAN, INN *cardiotonic*

Prinzide tablets ℞ *antihypertensive; angiotensin-converting enzyme (ACE) inhibitor; diuretic* [hydrochlorothiazide; lisinopril] 12.5•10 mg

Prinzide 12.5; Prinzide 25 tablets ℞ *antihypertensive; angiotensin-converting enzyme (ACE) inhibitor; diuretic* [hydrochlorothiazide; lisinopril] 12.5•20 mg; 25•20 mg

Priorix (CAN) injection ℞ *active immunizing agent* [measles, mumps, and rubella virus vaccine, live attenuated] 0.5 mL

Priscoline HCl IV injection ℞ *peripheral vasodilator for neonatal persistent pulmonary hypertension* [tolazoline HCl] 25 mg/mL ⊡ Apresoline

pristinamycin INN, BAN

privet, Egyptian *medicinal herb* [see: henna *(Lawsonia)*]

Privine nasal spray, nose drops OTC *nasal decongestant* [naphazoline HCl] 0.05%

prizidilol INN, BAN *antihypertensive* [also: prizidilol HCl]

prizidilol HCl USAN *antihypertensive* [also: prizidilol]

PRO 367 *investigational (Phase I/II) radiolabeled antigen-binding agent for HIV infection*

PRO 542 *investigational (Phase I/II) recombinant fusion protein, antigen-binding agent, and HIV attachment inhibitor for HIV infection*

PRO 2000 *investigational (Phase I) antiviral and microbicide gel for HIV infection*

Pro Skin capsules OTC *vitamin/zinc supplement* [vitamins A, B_5, C, and E; zinc] 6250 IU•10 mg•100 mg•100 IU•10 mg

PRO-2000 gel ℞ *investigational (Phase I) topical microbicide that functions as a chemical barrier to prevent HIV infection and sexually transmitted diseases*

Pro-50 injection (discontinued 1997) ℞ *antihistamine; sedative; antiemetic; motion sickness relief* [promethazine HCl] 50 mg/mL

proadifen INN *non-specific synergist* [also: proadifen HCl]

proadifen HCl USAN *non-specific synergist* [also: proadifen]

ProAmatine tablets ℞ *vasopressor for orthostatic hypotension (orphan)* [midodrine HCl] 2.5, 5 mg

proanthocyanidins *natural free radical scavenger found in grape seed extract and pine bark extract* [also: procyanidolic oligomers (PCOs); procyanidins]

Probalan tablets (discontinued 1997) ℞ *uricosuric for gout* [probenecid] 500 mg

Probampacin powder for oral suspension (discontinued 1998) ℞ *antibiotic for Neisseria gonorrhoeae* [ampicillin; probenecid] 3.5•1 g

Pro-Banthīne tablets ℞ *peptic ulcer treatment adjunct; antispasmodic; antisecretory* [propantheline bromide] 7.5, 15 mg

probarbital sodium NF, INN

Probax gel OTC *relief from minor oral irritations* [propolis] 2%

Probec-T tablets OTC *vitamin supplement* [multiple B vitamins; vitamin C] ≛•600 mg

Proben-C tablets (discontinued 1997) ℞ *treatment for frequent, recurrent attacks of gouty arthritis* [probenecid; colchicine] 500•0.5 mg

probenecid USP, INN, BAN *uricosuric for gout* 500 mg oral

probenecid & colchicine *treatment for frequent, recurrent attacks of gouty arthritis* 500•0.5 mg oral

Probeta ℞ *investigational antihypertensive (β-blocker)* [bisoprolol]

probicromil calcium USAN *prophylactic antiallergic* [also: ambicromil]

Pro-Bionate capsules, powder OTC *dietary supplement; fever blister treat-*

ment; not generally regarded as safe and effective as an antidiarrheal [*Lactobacillus acidophilus*] 2 billion U; 2 billion U/g

probucol USAN, USP, INN *antihyperlipidemic; investigational (Phase II) antiviral for HIV and AIDS*

probutate USAN *combining name for radicals or groups* [also: buteprate]

procainamide INN *antiarrhythmic* [also: procainamide HCl]

procainamide HCl USP *antiarrhythmic* [also: procainamide] 250, 375, 500, 750 mg oral; 100, 500 mg/mL injection

procaine INN *local anesthetic* [also: procaine borate] ⓢ Procan

procaine borate NF *local anesthetic* [also: procaine] ⓢ Procan

procaine HCl USP *injectable local anesthetic; investigational (Phase II) for HIV infection; sometimes used as a treatment for the overall effects of aging such as alopecia, arthritis, cerebral atherosclerosis, hypertension, progressive dementia, and sexual dysfunction* 1%, 2% ⓢ Procan

procaine penicillin BAN *bactericidal antibiotic* [also: penicillin G procaine] ⓢ Procan

ProcalAmine IV infusion ℞ *peripheral parenteral nutrition* [multiple essential and nonessential amino acids; electrolytes]

Pro-Cal-Sof capsules (discontinued 1999) OTC *laxative; stool softener* [docusate calcium] 240 mg

Procanbid extended-release film-coated tablets ℞ *twice-daily antiarrhythmic* [procainamide HCl] 500, 1000 mg

procarbazine INN *antineoplastic* [also: procarbazine HCl] ⓢ dacarbazine

procarbazine HCl USAN, USP *antineoplastic for Hodgkin disease* [also: procarbazine]

Procardia capsules ℞ *antianginal; antihypertensive; calcium channel blocker* [nifedipine] 10, 20 mg

Procardia XL film-coated sustained-release tablets ℞ *antianginal; antihypertensive; calcium channel blocker* [nifedipine] 30, 60, 90 mg

procaterol INN, BAN *bronchodilator* [also: procaterol HCl]

procaterol HCl USAN *bronchodilator* [also: procaterol]

prochlorperazine USP, INN *phenothiazine antipsychotic; antiemetic*

prochlorperazine bimaleate *phenothiazine antipsychotic; antiemetic*

prochlorperazine edisylate USP *phenothiazine antipsychotic; antiemetic* 5 mg/mL injection

prochlorperazine ethanedisulfonate [see: prochlorperazine edisylate]

prochlorperazine maleate USP *phenothiazine antipsychotic; antiemetic* 5, 10, 25 mg oral

prochlorperazine mesylate *phenothiazine antipsychotic; antiemetic*

procinolol INN

procinonide USAN, INN *adrenocortical steroid*

Proclim (CAN) tablets (discontinued 2001) ℞ *progestin* [medroxyprogesterone acetate] 2.5, 5, 10 mg

proclonol USAN, INN *anthelmintic; antifungal*

procodazole INN

proconvertin [see: factor VII]

Procort cream, spray OTC *topical corticosteroidal anti-inflammatory* [hydrocortisone] 1%

Procrit IV or subcu injection ℞ *stimulates RBC production; for anemia of chronic renal failure, HIV, or chemotherapy (orphan)* [epoetin alfa] 2000, 3000, 4000, 10 000, 20 000 U/mL

Proctocort anorectal cream, suppositories ℞ *topical corticosteroidal anti-inflammatory* [hydrocortisone] 1%; 30 mg

ProctoCream-HC anorectal cream (discontinued 2000) ℞ *topical corticosteroidal anti-inflammatory; local anesthetic* [hydrocortisone acetate; pramoxine HCl] 1%•1%

ProctoCream-HC 2.5% anorectal cream ℞ *topical corticosteroidal anti-*

inflammatory [hydrocortisone acetate] 2.5%

Proctodan-HC (CAN) anorectal ointment, suppositories ℞ *topical corticosteroidal anti-inflammatory, local anesthetic, and astringent* [hydrocortisone acetate; pramoxine HCl; zinc sulfate] 0.5%•1%•0.5%; 10•20•10 mg

ProctoFoam NS anorectal aerosol foam OTC *topical local anesthetic* [pramoxine HCl] 1%

Proctofoam-HC anorectal aerosol foam ℞ *topical corticosteroidal anti-inflammatory; local anesthetic* [hydrocortisone acetate; pramoxine HCl] 1%•1%

Pro-Cute lotion OTC *moisturizer; emollient*

procyanidolic oligomers (PCOs) *natural free radical scavenger found in grape seed extract and pine bark extract* [also: proanthocyanidins; procyanidins]

ProCycle Gold tablets OTC *vitamin/mineral/iron supplement* [multiple vitamins & minerals; iron; folic acid; biotin] ≛•3•0.067•≟ mg

procyclidine HCl USP *anticholinergic; antiparkinsonian; skeletal muscle relaxant* [also: procyclidine]

procymate INN

Procysteine ℞ *investigational (Phase II) immunomodulator for AIDS; investigational (orphan) for amyotrophic lateral sclerosis; investigational (Phase III, orphan) for adult respiratory distress syndrome (ARDS trials discontinued 1998)* [oxothiazolidine carboxylate]

prodeconium bromide INN

Proderm aerosol OTC *topical wound spray for decubitus ulcers* [castor oil; peruvian balsam] 650•72.5 mg/0.82 mL

prodilidine INN *analgesic* [also: prodilidine HCl]

prodilidine HCl USAN *analgesic* [also: prodilidine]

prodipine INN

Prodium tablets OTC *urinary analgesic* [phenazopyridine HCl] 95 mg

prodolic acid USAN, INN *anti-inflammatory*

pro-drugs *a class of agents which metabolize into a therapeutic or more potent form in the body*

profadol INN *analgesic* [also: profadol HCl]

profadol HCl USAN *analgesic* [also: profadol]

Profasi powder for IM injection ℞ *hormone for prepubertal cryptorchidism and hypogonadism; ovulation stimulant* [chorionic gonadotropin] 500, 1000 U/mL

Profen II; Profen LA timed-release tablets ℞ *decongestant; expectorant* [phenylpropanolamine HCl; guaifenesin] 37.5•600 mg; 75•600 mg

Profen II DM extended-release tablets ℞ *decongestant; expectorant; antitussive* [pseudoephedrine HCl; guaifenesin; dextromethorphan hydrobromide] 45•800•30 mg

Profen Forte DM extended-release tablets ℞ *decongestant; expectorant; antitussive* [pseudoephedrine HCl; guaifenesin; dextromethorphan hydrobromide] 90•800•60 mg

Profenal Drop-Tainers (eye drops) ℞ *ocular nonsteroidal anti-inflammatory drug (NSAID); intraoperative miosis inhibitor* [suprofen] 1%

profenamine INN *antiparkinsonian* [also: ethopropazine HCl; ethopropazine]

profenamine HCl [see: ethopropazine HCl]

profexalone INN

Profiber liquid OTC *enteral nutritional therapy* [lactose-free formula]

Profilate HP IV injection (discontinued 1997) ℞ *antihemophilic to correct coagulation deficiency* [antihemophilic factor VIII:C in heptane]

Profilnine SD powder for IV injection ℞ *anticoagulant to correct factor IX deficiency (hemophilia B; Christmas disease)* [coagulation factors II, VII, IX, and X, solvent/detergent treated]

Proflavanol C (CAN) tablets OTC *vitamin C supplement* [vitamin C as mixed ascorbates] 100 mg

proflavine INN [also: proflavine dihydrochloride]

proflavine dihydrochloride NF [also: proflavine]

proflavine sulfate NF

proflazepam INN

ProFree/GP Weekly Enzymatic Cleaner tablets OTC *enzymatic cleaner for rigid gas permeable contact lenses* [papain]

progabide USAN, INN *anticonvulsant; muscle relaxant*

Progestasert intrauterine device (IUD) ℞ *long-term (1 year) contraceptive insert* [progesterone] 38 mg

progesterone USP, INN *progestin; intrauterine contraceptive; investigational (orphan) for in vitro fertilization and embryo transfer* 50 mg/mL injection

progestins *a class of sex hormones that cause a sloughing of the endometrial lining, also used as a hormonal antineoplastic*

proglumetacin INN

proglumide USAN, INN, BAN, JAN *anticholinergic*

Proglycem capsules, oral suspension ℞ *emergency antihypertensive; vasodilator; glucose-elevating agent* [diazoxide] 50 mg; 50 mg/mL

Prograf capsules, IV infusion ℞ *immunosuppressant for liver transplants; investigational for other organ transplants* [tacrolimus] 1, 5 mg; 5 mg/mL

proguanil INN, BAN, DCF *antimalarial; dihydrofolate reductase inhibitor* [also: chloroguanide HCl]

proguanil HCl [see: chloroguanide HCl]

ProHance injection ℞ *MRI contrast media for brain and spine imaging* [gadoteridol] 279.3 mg/mL

proheptazine INN

ProHIBiT IM injection (discontinued 2000) ℞ *pediatric (1½–5 years) vaccine for Haemophilus influenzae type b (HIB)* [Hemophilus b conjugate vaccine (with a diphtheria conjugate carrier)] 25•(18) µg/0.5 mL

proinsulin human USAN *antidiabetic*

Prolastin inhalation aerosol ℞ *investigational (Phase II) delivery form* [$alpha_1$-proteinase inhibitor]

Prolastin IV injection ℞ *chronic replacement therapy for hereditary $alpha_1$-proteinase inhibitor deficiency, which leads to progressive panacinar emphysema (orphan)* [$alpha_1$-proteinase inhibitor] 20 mg/mL

ProLease (trademarked delivery system) *sustained-release injection*

Proleukin powder for IV infusion ℞ *antineoplastic for metastatic melanoma and renal cell carcinoma (orphan); investigational (Phase III, orphan) agent for immunodeficiency diseases and acute myelogenous leukemia (AML); investigational (Phase II) for Hodgkin lymphoma* [aldesleukin] 18 million IU/mL

proligestone INN

proline (L-proline) USAN, USP, INN *nonessential amino acid; symbols: Pro, P* ⊡ Prolene

prolintane INN *antidepressant* [also: prolintane HCl]

prolintane HCl USAN *antidepressant* [also: prolintane]

Prolixin tablets, elixir, oral concentrate, IM injection ℞ *conventional (typical) antipsychotic* [fluphenazine HCl] 1, 2.5, 5, 10 mg; 2.5 mg/5 mL; 5 mg/mL; 2.5 mg/mL

Prolixin Decanoate subcu or IM injection, Unimatic (prefilled) syringe ℞ *conventional (typical) antipsychotic* [fluphenazine decanoate] 25 mg/mL

Prolixin Enanthate subcu or IM injection ℞ *conventional (typical) antipsychotic* [fluphenazine enanthate] 25 mg/mL

prolonium iodide INN

Proloprim tablets ℞ *anti-infective; antibacterial* [trimethoprim] 100, 200 mg

ProMACE (prednisone, methotrexate [with leucovorin rescue], Adriamycin, cyclophosphamide, etoposide) *chemotherapy protocol for non-Hodgkin lymphoma*

ProMACE/cytaBOM (ProMACE [above], cytarabine, bleomycin, Oncovin, mitoxantrone) *chemotherapy protocol for non-Hodgkin lymphoma*

ProMACE/MOPP (full course of ProMACE, followed by MOPP) *chemotherapy protocol for non-Hodgkin lymphoma*

ProMaxx-100 extended release ℞ *investigational LH-RH analogue for prostate cancer*

promazine INN *phenothiazine antipsychotic* [also: promazine HCl] ⊠ Promethazine

promazine HCl USP *phenothiazine antipsychotic* [also: promazine] 25, 50 mg/mL injection

Promega Pearls (softgels) OTC *dietary supplement* [omega-3 fatty acids; multiple vitamins & minerals] 600•≛, 1000•≛ mg

promegestone INN

promelase INN

ProMem ℞ *investigational (NDA filed) acetylcholinesterase (AChE) inhibitor for Alzheimer dementia* [metrifonate]

promestriene INN

Prometh VC Plain liquid ℞ *decongestant; antihistamine* [phenylephrine HCl; promethazine HCl] 5•6.25 mg/5 mL

Prometh VC with Codeine syrup ℞ *narcotic antitussive; decongestant; antihistamine* [codeine phosphate; phenylephrine HCl; promethazine HCl; alcohol] 10•5•6.25 mg/5 mL

Prometh with Codeine syrup ℞ *narcotic antitussive; antihistamine* [codeine phosphate; promethazine HCl] 10•6.25 mg/5 mL

Prometh with Dextromethorphan syrup ℞ *antitussive; antihistamine* [dextromethorphan hydrobromide; promethazine HCl; alcohol 7%] 15•6.25 mg/5 mL

Prometh-50 injection (discontinued 1997) ℞ *antihistamine; sedative; antiemetic; motion sickness relief* [promethazine HCl] 50 mg/mL

promethazine INN *phenothiazine antihistamine; antiemetic; antidopaminergic; motion sickness relief* [also: promethazine HCl]

Promethazine DM syrup ℞ *antitussive; antihistamine* [dextromethorphan hydrobromide; promethazine HCl; alcohol] 15•6.25 mg/5 mL

promethazine HCl USP *phenothiazine antihistamine; antiemetic; antidopaminergic; motion sickness relief* [also: promethazine] 25, 50 mg oral; 6.25 mg/5 mL oral; 50 mg suppositories; 25, 50 mg/mL injection

promethazine teoclate INN *phenothiazine antihistamine*

Promethazine VC syrup ℞ *decongestant; antihistamine* [phenylephrine HCl; promethazine HCl] 5•6.25 mg/5 mL

Promethazine VC Plain syrup ℞ *decongestant; antihistamine* [phenylephrine HCl; promethazine HCl; alcohol 7%] 5•6.25 mg/5 mL

Promethazine VC with Codeine syrup ℞ *narcotic antitussive; decongestant; antihistamine* [codeine phosphate; phenylephrine HCl; promethazine HCl; alcohol] 10•5•6.25 mg/5 mL

promethestrol [see: methestrol]

Promethist with Codeine syrup ℞ *narcotic antitussive; decongestant; antihistamine* [codeine phosphate; phenylephrine HCl; promethazine HCl; alcohol] 10•5•6.25 mg/5 mL

promethium *element (Pm)*

Prometrium capsules ℞ *progestin for secondary amenorrhea and to prevent endometrial hyperplasia* [progesterone, micronized] 100, 200 mg

Prominol tablets ℞ *analgesic; antipyretic; sedative* [acetaminophen; butalbital] 650•50 mg

Promit IV injection ℞ *monovalent hapten for prophylaxis of dextran-induced anaphylactic reactions* [dextran 1] 150 mg/mL

ProMod powder OTC *oral protein supplement* [D-whey protein concentrate; soy lecithin]

promolate INN
promoxolane INN
prompt insulin zinc [see: insulin zinc, prompt]
Promycin *investigational (Phase III, orphan) antineoplastic for head, neck, and cervical cancers* [porfiromycin]
Pronemia Hematinic capsules ℞ *hematinic* [ferrous fumarate; cyanocobalamin; ascorbic acid; intrinsic factor concentrate; folic acid] 115 mg•15 µg•150 mg•75 mg•1 mg
Pronestyl capsules, tablets, IV or IM injection ℞ *antiarrhythmic* [procainamide HCl] 250, 375, 500 mg; 250, 375, 500 mg; 100, 500 mg/mL ⓓ Ponstel
Pronestyl-SR sustained-release tablets ℞ *antiarrhythmic* [procainamide HCl] 500 mg
pronetalol INN [also: pronethalol]
pronethalol BAN [also: pronetalol]
Pronto shampoo + creme rinse OTC *pediculicide for lice* [pyrethrins; piperonyl butoxide] 0.33%•4%
Propac powder OTC *oral protein supplement* [whey protein; lactose]
Propacet 100 film-coated tablets ℞ *narcotic analgesic* [propoxyphene napsylate; acetaminophen] 100•650 mg
propacetamol INN
propafenone INN, BAN *antiarrhythmic* [also: propafenone HCl]
propafenone HCl USAN *antiarrhythmic* [also: propafenone] 150, 225 mg oral
Propagest tablets OTC *nasal decongestant* [phenylpropanolamine HCl] 25 mg
propamidine INN, BAN, DCF
propamidine isethionate *investigational (orphan) eye drops for Acanthamoeba keratitis*
propaminodiphen [see: pramiverine]
propane NF *aerosol propellant*
1,2-propanediol [see: propylene glycol]
propanidid USAN, INN *intravenous anesthetic*
propanocaine INN
propanoic acid, sodium salt hydrate [see: sodium propionate]
2-propanol [see: isopropyl alcohol]
2-propanone [see: acetone]
propantheline bromide USP, INN *GI antispasmodic; peptic ulcer adjunct* 15 mg oral
PROPApH Acne cream OTC *topical keratolytic for acne* [salicylic acid] 2%
PROPApH Cleansing; PROPApH Cleansing for Sensitive Skin; PROPApH Cleansing Maximum Strength pads OTC *topical keratolytic for acne* [salicylic acid] 0.5%; 0.5%; 2%
PROPApH Cleansing for Normal/Combination Skin; PROPApH Cleansing for Oily Skin lotion OTC *topical keratolytic for acne* [salicylic acid] 0.5%
PROPApH Foaming Face Wash liquid ℞ *topical keratolytic cleanser for acne* [salicylic acid] 2%
PROPApH Peel-Off Acne Mask OTC *topical keratolytic for acne* [salicylic acid] 2%
proparacaine HCl USP *topical ophthalmic anesthetic* [also: proxymetacaine] 0.5% eye drops
proparacaine HCl & fluorescein sodium *topical ophthalmic anesthetic; corneal disclosing agent* 0.5%•0.25%
propatyl nitrate USAN *coronary vasodilator* [also: propatylnitrate]
propatylnitrate INN *coronary vasodilator* [also: propatyl nitrate]
propazolamide INN
Propecia film-coated tablets ℞ *androgen hormone inhibitor for androgenic alopecia in men* [finasteride] 1 mg
1-propene homopolymer [see: polipropene 25]
propenidazole INN
propentofylline INN
***p*-propenylanisole** [see: anethole]
propenzolate HCl USAN *anticholinergic* [also: oxyclipine]
propericiazine [see: periciazine]
properidine INN, BAN
propetamide INN
propetandrol INN
prophenamine HCl [see: ethopropazine HCl]

Pro-Phree powder OTC *supplement to breast milk* [protein-free formula with vitamins & minerals]

Prophyllin ointment OTC *topical antifungal; vulnerary; wound deodorant* [sodium propionate; chlorophyll derivatives] 5%•0.0125%

propicillin INN, BAN

propikacin USAN, INN *antibacterial*

Propimex-1 powder OTC *formula for infants with propionic or methylmalonicacidemia*

Propimex-2 powder OTC *enteral nutritional therapy for propionic or methylmalonic acidemia*

Propine eye drops ℞ *topical antiglaucoma agent* [dipivefrin HCl] 0.1%

propinetidine INN

propiodal [see: prolonium iodide]

propiolactone (β-propiolactone) USAN, INN *disinfectant*

propiomazine USAN, INN *preanesthetic sedative*

propiomazine HCl USP *sedative; analgesic adjunct*

propionic acid NF *antimicrobial; acidifying agent*

propionyl erythromycin lauryl sulfate [see: erythromycin estolate]

propipocaine INN

propiram INN, BAN *narcotic agonist-antagonist analgesic* [also: propiram fumarate]

propiram fumarate USAN *investigational (Phase III) narcotic agonist-antagonist analgesic* [also: propiram]

propisergide INN

propitocaine HCl JAN *topical local anesthetic* [also: prilocaine HCl]

propiverine INN

propizepine INN

Proplex T IV infusion ℞ *antihemophilic to correct factor VII, VIII (hemophilia A), and IX (hemophilia B; Christmas disease) deficiencies* [coagulation factors II, VII, IX, and X, heat treated] 30 mL

propofol USAN, INN, BAN *general anesthetic* 1% injection

propolis *natural resin collected from the buds of certain trees by bees and used as an antibiotic, anti-inflammatory, antioxidant, antineoplastic, fungicide, immune system stimulant, and vulnerary*

propoxate INN

propoxycaine INN *local anesthetic* [also: propoxycaine HCl]

propoxycaine HCl USP *local anesthetic* [also: propoxycaine]

propoxyphene HCl USAN, USP *narcotic analgesic* [also: dextropropoxyphene HCl] 65 mg oral

propoxyphene napsylate USAN, USP *narcotic analgesic*

propranolol INN, BAN *antiarrhythmic; antihypertensive; antianginal; antiadrenergic (β-blocker); migraine prophylaxis* [also: propranolol HCl]

propranolol HCl USAN, USP *antiarrhythmic; antihypertensive; antianginal; antiadrenergic (β-blocker); migraine prophylaxis* [also: propranolol] 10, 20, 40, 60, 80, 90, 120, 160 mg oral; 4, 8, 80 mg/mL oral; 1 mg/mL injection

Propulsid tablets, oral suspension (discontinued 2000) ℞ *treatment for nocturnal heartburn due to gastroesophageal reflux disease (GERD)* [cisapride] 10, 20 mg; 1 mg/mL

propyl *p*-aminobenzoate [see: risocaine]

propyl docetrizoate INN, BAN

propyl gallate NF *antioxidant*

propyl *p*-hydroxybenzoate [see: propylparaben]

propyl *p*-hydroxybenzoate, sodium salt [see: propylparaben sodium]

N-propylajmalinium tartrate [see: prajmalinum bitartrate]

propylene carbonate NF *gelling agent*

propylene glycol USP *humectant; solvent; suspending and viscosity-increasing agent*

propylene glycol alginate NF *suspending agent; viscosity-increasing agent*

propylene glycol diacetate NF *solvent*

propylene glycol ether of methylcellulose [see: hydroxypropyl methylcellulose]
propylene glycol monostearate NF *emulsifying agent*
propylhexedrine USP, INN, BAN *vasoconstrictor; nasal decongestant*
propyliodone USP, INN *radiopaque contrast medium (56.7% iodine)*
propylorvinol [see: etorphine]
propylparaben USAN, NF *antifungal agent; preservative*
propylparaben sodium USAN, NF *antimicrobial preservative*
2-propylpentanoic acid [see: valproic acid]
propylthiouracil (PTU) USP, INN *thyroid inhibitor*
2-propylvaleramide [see: valpromide]
propylvaleric acid [see: valproic acid]
propyperone INN
propyphenazone INN, BAN
propyromazine bromide INN
proquamezine BAN [also: aminopromazine]
proquazone USAN, INN *anti-inflammatory*
proquinolate USAN, INN *coccidiostat for poultry*
prorenoate potassium USAN, INN *aldosterone antagonist*
Prorex-25; Prorex-50 injection (discontinued 1997) ℞ *antihistamine; sedative; antiemetic; motion sickness relief* [promethazine HCl] 25 mg/mL; 50 mg/mL
proroxan INN *antiadrenergic (α-receptor)* [also: proroxan HCl]
proroxan HCl USAN *antiadrenergic (α-receptor)* [also: proroxan]
Proscar film-coated tablets ℞ *androgen hormone inhibitor for benign prostatic hyperplasia (BPH)* [finasteride] 5 mg ⑨ Posicor
proscillaridin USAN, INN *cardiotonic*
proscillaridin A [see: proscillaridin]
Prosed/DS sugar-coated tablets ℞ *urinary antibiotic; antiseptic; analgesic; antispasmodic* [methenamine; phenyl salicylate; methylene blue; benzoic acid; atropine sulfate; hyoscyamine sulfate] 81.6•36.2•10.8•9•0.06•0.06 mg
ProSobee liquid, powder OTC *hypoallergenic infant food* [soy protein formula]
Pro-Sof Plus capsules (discontinued 1999) OTC *stimulant laxative; stool softener* [casanthranol; docusate sodium] 30•100 mg
ProSol 20% IV infusion ℞ *total parenteral nutrition* [multiple essential and nonessential amino acids] 20 g
ProSom tablets ℞ *sedative; hypnotic* [estazolam] 1, 2 mg
Prosorba Column for dialysis ℞ *treatment for rheumatoid arthritis* [protein A]
prospidium chloride INN
prostacyclin [now: epoprostenol]
prostaglandin agonists *a class of antiglaucoma agents that reduce intraocular pressure (IOP) by increasing the outflow of aqueous humor*
prostaglandin E_1 (PGE_1) [now: alprostadil]
prostaglandin E_1 enol ester *investigational (orphan) for advanced chronic critical limb ischemia*
prostaglandin E_2 (PGE_2) [see: dinoprostone]
prostaglandin $F_{2\alpha}$ ($PGF_{2\alpha}$) [see: dinoprost]
prostaglandin I_2 (PGI_2) [now: epoprostenol]
prostaglandin X (PGX) [now: epoprostenol]
prostaglandins *a class of agents that stimulate uterine contractions, used for abortions, cervical ripening, and postpartum hemorrhage*
prostalene USAN, INN *prostaglandin*
Prostaphlin capsules, powder for oral solution, powder for IV or IM injection (discontinued 1998) ℞ *penicillinase-resistant penicillin antibiotic* [oxacillin sodium] 250, 500 mg; 250 mg/5 mL; 0.5, 1, 2, 4, 10 g
ProstaScint *imaging agent for prostate cancer and its metastases* [capromab pendetide]

ProStep transdermal patch (discontinued 2001) ℞ *smoking deterrent; nicotine withdrawal aid* [nicotine] 11, 22 mg/day

Prostigmin subcu or IM injection ℞ *cholinergic urinary stimulant for postsurgical urinary retention* [neostigmine methylsulfate] 1:1000 (1 mg/mL), 1:2000 (0.5 mg/mL), 1:4000 (0.25 mg/mL) (1:400 [2.5 mg/mL] available in Canada) ⑨ physostigmine

Prostigmin tablets ℞ *myasthenia gravis treatment; antidote for neuromuscular blockers* [neostigmine bromide] 15 mg

Prostin E2 vaginal suppository ℞ *prostaglandin-type abortifacient* [dinoprostone] 20 mg

Prostin VR Pediatric IV injection ℞ *vasodilator; platelet aggregation inhibitor* [alprostadil] 500 µg/mL

prosulpride INN

prosultiamine INN

protactinium *element (Pa)*

protamine sulfate USP, INN *antidote to heparin overdose* [also: protamine sulphate] 10 mg/mL injection

protamine sulphate BAN *antidote to heparin overdose* [also: protamine sulfate]

protamine zinc insulin (PZI) INN *antidiabetic* [also: insulin, protamine zinc; insulin zinc protamine]

Protar Protein shampoo (discontinued 1998) OTC *antiseborrheic; antipsoriatic; antipruritic; antibacterial* [coal tar] 5%

protargin, mild [see: silver protein, mild]

protease *digestive enzyme* [100 IU/mg in pancrelipase; 25 IU/mg in pancreatin]

protease inhibitors *a class of antivirals that block HIV replication*

ProTech First Aid Stick liquid OTC *topical antiseptic; analgesic* [lidocaine; povidone-iodine] 2.5%•10%

Protectol Medicated powder OTC *topical antifungal* [calcium undecylenate] 15%

Protegra softgels OTC *vitamin/mineral supplement* [multiple vitamins & minerals] ≛

Protegrin mouthwash ℞ *investigational (Phase III) rinse for oral mucositis* [IB-367 (code name—generic name not yet assigned)]

protein A *treatment for rheumatoid arthritis*

protein C concentrate *investigational (orphan) anticoagulant for protein C deficiency*

protein hydrolysate USP *fluid and nutrient replenisher*

α_1-proteinase inhibitor [see: alpha$_1$-proteinase inhibitor]

Protenate IV infusion ℞ *blood volume expander for shock due to burns, trauma and surgery* [plasma protein fraction] 5%

proterguride INN

Prothazine subcu or IM injection (discontinued 1997) ℞ *antihistamine; sedative; antiemetic; motion sickness relief* [promethazine HCl] 25, 50 mg/mL

Prothazine Plain syrup (discontinued 1997) ℞ *antihistamine; sedative; antiemetic; motion sickness relief* [promethazine HCl] 6.25 mg/5 mL

Prothecan ℞ *investigational hormonal antineoplastic for solid tumors* [PEG-camptothecin]

protheobromine INN

Prothiaden ℞ *investigational (NDA filed) tricyclic antidepressant* [dothiepin HCl]

prothionamide BAN [also: protionamide]

prothipendyl INN

prothipendyl HCl [see: prothipendyl]

prothixene INN

prothrombin complex, activated BAN

Protilase capsules containing enteric-coated spheres ℞ *digestive enzymes* [lipase; protease; amylase] 4000•25 000•20 000 U

ProTime test kit for home use *in vitro diagnostic aid for the management of anticoagulation therapy*

protiofate INN

protionamide INN [also: prothionamide]

protirelin USAN, INN, BAN *prothyrotropin; diagnostic aid for thyroid function;*

investigational (orphan) for infant respiratory distress syndrome of prematurity

protizinic acid INN

protokylol HCl

proton pump inhibitors *a class of gastric antisecretory agents that inhibit the ATPase "proton pump" within the gastric parietal cell* [also called: ATPase inhibitors; substituted benzimidazoles]

Protonix enteric-coated delayed-release tablets ℞ *proton pump inhibitor for erosive esophagitis associated with gastroesophageal reflux disease (GERD)* [pantoprazole sodium] 20, 40 mg

Protonix I.V. powder for infusion ℞ *proton pump inhibitor for erosive esophagitis associated with gastroesophageal reflux disease (GERD)* [pantoprazole sodium] 40 mg/vial

Protopam Chloride IV injection ℞ *antidote for organophosphate poisoning and anticholinesterase overdose* [pralidoxime chloride] 1 g ⓢ Protamine

Protopic ointment ℞ *topical immunosuppressant for eczema* [tacrolimus] 0.03%, 0.1%

Protostat tablets ℞ *antibiotic; antiprotozoal; amebicide* [metronidazole] 250, 500 mg

protoveratrine A

Protovir ℞ *investigational (Phase I) antiviral for AIDS-related cytomegalovirus* [sevirumab]

Protox ℞ *investigational (orphan) for toxoplasmosis of AIDS; investigational (Phase II) for treatment of bacterial and viral infections* [poloxamer 331]

protriptyline INN *tricyclic antidepressant* [also: protriptyline HCl]

protriptyline HCl USAN, USP *tricyclic antidepressant* [also: protriptyline] 5, 10 mg oral

Protropin powder for IM or subcu injection ℞ *growth hormone for congenital growth failure due to lack of endogenous growth hormone (orphan)* [somatrem] 5, 10 mg (15, 30 IU) per vial

Protropin II ℞ *growth hormone for adults or children with congenital or endogenous growth hormone deficiency, children with Turner syndrome or renal-induced growth failure, or AIDS-wasting syndrome (orphan); investigational (orphan) for severe burns* [somatropin]

Protuss liquid ℞ *narcotic antitussive; expectorant* [hydrocodone bitartrate; potassium guaiacolsulfonate] 5•300 mg/5 mL

Protuss DM film-coated tablets ℞ *antitussive; decongestant; expectorant* [dextromethorphan hydrobromide; pseudoephedrine HCl; guaifenesin] 30•60•600 mg

Protuss-D liquid ℞ *narcotic antitussive; decongestant; expectorant* [hydrocodone bitartrate; pseudoephedrine HCl; potassium guaiacolsulfonate] 5•30•300 mg/5 mL

prourokinase [see: saruplase]

Proventil inhalation aerosol ℞ *sympathomimetic bronchodilator* [albuterol] 90 µg/dose

Proventil tablets, Repetabs (extended-release tablets), syrup, solution for inhalation ℞ *sympathomimetic bronchodilator* [albuterol sulfate] 2, 4 mg; 4 mg; 2 mg/5 mL; 0.083%, 0.5%

Proventil HFA CFC-free inhalation aerosol ℞ *sympathomimetic bronchodilator* [albuterol sulfate] 90 µg/dose

Provera tablets ℞ *progestin for secondary amenorrhea, abnormal uterine bleeding, and endometrial hyperplasia* [medroxyprogesterone acetate] 2.5, 5, 10 mg ⓢ Covera; Provir; Trovert

Provigil caplets ℞ *analeptic for excessive daytime sleepiness of narcolepsy (orphan); investigational for fatigue associated with multiple sclerosis* [modafinil] 100, 200 mg

Provir ℞ *investigational (Phase III) treatment for AIDS-related diarrhea* [crofelemer] ⓢ Provera; Trovert

Proviron *brand name for mesterolone, an androgen abused with anabolic steroid street drugs*

provitamin A [see: beta carotene]

Provocholine powder for reconstitution for inhalation ℞ *bronchocon-*

strictor for in vivo pulmonary function challenge test [methacholine chloride] 100 mg/5 mL

proxazole USAN, INN *smooth muscle relaxant; analgesic; anti-inflammatory*

proxazole citrate USAN *smooth muscle relaxant; analgesic; anti-inflammatory*

proxetil INN *combining name for radicals or groups*

proxibarbal INN

proxibutene INN

proxicromil USAN, INN *antiallergic*

proxifezone INN

Proxigel OTC *topical oral anti-inflammatory and anti-infective for braces* [carbamide peroxide] 10%

proxorphan INN *analgesic; antitussive* [also: proxorphan tartrate]

proxorphan tartrate USAN *analgesic; antitussive* [also: proxorphan]

proxymetacaine INN, BAN *topical ophthalmic anesthetic* [also: proparacaine HCl]

proxymetacaine HCl [see: proparacaine HCl]

proxyphylline INN, BAN

Prozac Pulvules (capsules), tablets, oral solution ℞ *selective serotonin reuptake inhibitor (SSRI) for depression, obsessive-compulsive disorder (OCD), and bulimia nervosa* [fluoxetine HCl] 10, 20, 40 mg; 10 mg; 20 mg/5 mL ⊠ Prilosec

Prozac Weekly enteric-coated delayed-release pellets in capsules ℞ *selective serotonin reuptake inhibitor (SSRI) for depression; once-weekly dosing for maintenance therapy* [fluoxetine HCl] 90 mg

prozapine INN

Prozine-50 IM injection ℞ *conventional (typical) antipsychotic* [promazine HCl] 50 mg/mL

prucalopride HCl USAN *investigational (Phase III) prokinetic agent for post-ileus and opioid-induced constipation*

prucalopride succinate USAN *investigational (Phase III) prokinetic agent for post-ileus and opioid-induced constipation*

Prulet tablets (discontinued 1998) OTC *stimulant laxative* [white phenolphthalein] 60 mg

Prunella vulgaris *medicinal herb* [see: woundwort]

Prunus africana *medicinal herb* [see: pygeum]

Prunus americana; P. domestica; P. spinosa *medicinal herb* [see: plum]

Prunus amygdalus *medicinal herb* [see: almond]

Prunus armeniaca *medicinal herb* [see: apricot]

Prunus persica *medicinal herb* [see: peach]

Prunus serotina *medicinal herb* [see: wild black cherry]

Prunus virginiana *medicinal herb* [see: wild cherry]

Pryme (name changed to LYMErix upon release in 1999)

PSE (pseudoephedrine HCl) [q.v.]

Pseudo liquid OTC *nasal decongestant* [pseudoephedrine HCl] 30 mg/5 mL

Pseudo-Car DM syrup ℞ *antitussive; decongestant; antihistamine* [dextromethorphan hydrobromide; pseudoephedrine HCl; carbinoxamine maleate] 15•60•4 mg/5 mL

Pseudo-Chlor sustained-release capsules ℞ *decongestant; antihistamine* [pseudoephedrine HCl; chlorpheniramine maleate] 120•8 mg

pseudoephedrine INN, BAN *vasoconstrictor; nasal decongestant* [also: pseudoephedrine HCl]

pseudoephedrine HCl USAN, USP *vasoconstrictor; nasal decongestant* [also: pseudoephedrine] 30, 60 mg oral; 30 mg/5 mL oral

pseudoephedrine HCl & carbinoxamine maleate *decongestant; antihistamine* 60•4 mg/5 mL oral; 25•2 mg/mL oral

pseudoephedrine HCl & dextromethorphan hydrobromide & brompheniramine maleate *nasal decongestant; antitussive; antihistamine* 80•15•4 mg/5 mL oral

pseudoephedrine polistirex USAN *nasal decongestant*

pseudoephedrine sulfate USAN, USP *bronchodilator; nasal decongestant*

pseudoephedrine tannate *bronchodilator; nasal decongestant*

Pseudofrin (CAN) tablets OTC *decongestant* [pseudoephedrine HCl] 60 mg

Pseudo-Gest tablets OTC *nasal decongestant* [pseudoephedrine HCl] 30, 60 mg

Pseudo-Gest Plus tablets OTC *decongestant; antihistamine* [pseudoephedrine HCl; chlorpheniramine maleate] 60•4 mg

***Pseudomonas aeruginosa* purified extract** *investigational (orphan) agent to increase platelet count in immune thrombocytopenic purpura*

***Pseudomonas* immune globulin** [see: mucoid exopolysaccharide *Pseudomonas* hyperimmune globulin]

pseudomonic acid A [see: mupirocin]

Pseudostat ℞ *investigational (Phase II) theraccine for chronic bronchitis*

psilocin *a hallucinogenic street drug closely related to psilocybin*

psilocybin BAN *a hallucinogenic street drug derived from the Psilocybe mexicana mushroom* [also: psilocybine]

psilocybine INN, DCF *a hallucinogenic street drug derived from the Psilocybe mexicana mushroom* [also: psilocybin]

psoralens *a class of oral or topical skin photosensitizing agents used with ultraviolet A light (320–400 nm wavelength) for the treatment of severe recalcitrant psoriasis*

Psor-a-set bar OTC *therapeutic skin cleanser; topical keratolytic* [salicylic acid] 2%

Psorcon cream, ointment (name changed to Psorcon E in 2000)

Psorcon E cream, ointment ℞ *topical corticosteroidal anti-inflammatory* [diflorasone diacetate] 0.05%

PsoriGel OTC *topical antipsoriatic; antiseborrheic; antiseptic* [coal tar solution; alcohol 33%] 7.5%

Psovascar *investigational (Phase I/II) angiogenesis inhibitor for psoriasis*

psyllium *(Plantago ovata)* *medicinal herb* [see: plantain]

psyllium husk USP *bulk laxative*

psyllium hydrocolloid *bulk laxative*

psyllium hydrophilic mucilloid *bulk laxative*

psyllium seed [see: plantago seed]

PT-14 *investigational peptide analogue for erectile dysfunction*

PTC (plasma thromboplastin component) [see: factor IX]

P.T.E.-4; P.T.E.-5 IV injection ℞ *intravenous nutritional therapy* [multiple trace elements (metals)]

pterins *a class of investigational antineoplastics*

pteroyldiglutamic acid (PDGA)

pteroylglutamic acid (PGA) [see: folic acid]

PTFE (polytetrafluoroethylene) [see: polytef]

PTU (propylthiouracil) [q.v.]

Pt/VM (Platinol, VM-26) *chemotherapy protocol for pediatric neuroblastoma*

ptyalagogues *a class of agents that stimulate the secretion of saliva* [also called: sialagogues]

puccoon, yellow *medicinal herb* [see: goldenseal]

Pueraria lobata; P. thunbergiana *medicinal herb* [see: kudzu]

puffball *medicinal herb* [see: dandelion]

Pulmicort Respules (single-dose ampule for inhalation) ℞ *corticosteroidal anti-inflammatory for chronic asthma in children* [budesonide] 0.25, 0.5 mg

Pulmicort Turbuhaler (dry powder in a metered-dose inhaler) ℞ *corticosteroidal anti-inflammatory for chronic asthma* [budesonide] 160 µg/dose

Pulmocare ready-to-use liquid OTC *enteral nutritional therapy for pulmonary problems*

Pulmonaria officinalis *medicinal herb* [see: lungwort]

pulmonary surfactant replacement, porcine [now: poractant alfa]

Pulmozyme solution for nebulization ℞ *reduces respiratory viscoelasticity of* *sputum in cystic fibrosis (orphan)* [dornase alfa] 1 mg/mL

pulse VAC *chemotherapy protocol for sarcomas* [see: VAC pulse]

pulse VAC (vincristine, Adriamycin, cyclophosphamide) *chemotherapy protocol* [also: VAC]

PulsePak (trademarked dosage form) *one-week dosage pack*

Pulvule (trademarked dosage form) *bullet-shaped capsule*

pumice USP *dental abrasive*

pumitepa INN

Punctum Plug ℞ *blocks the puncta and canaliculus to eliminate tear loss in keratitis sicca* [silicone plug]

Punica granatum *medicinal herb* [see: pomegranate]

Puralube ophthalmic ointment OTC *ocular moisturizer/lubricant* [white petrolatum; mineral oil]

Puralube Tears eye drops OTC *ophthalmic moisturizer/lubricant* [polyvinyl alcohol; polyethylene glycol 400] 1%•1%

Puregon (CAN) subcu or IM injection ℞ *recombinant follicle-stimulating hormone (FSH) for the induction of ovulation and development of multiple follicles for assisted reproductive technology (ART)* [follitropin beta] 50, 100 IU

purgatives *a class of agents that cause vigorous evacuation of the bowels by increasing bulk, stimulating peristaltic action, etc.* [also called: cathartics]

Purge oral liquid OTC *stimulant laxative* [castor oil] 95%

purified cotton [see: cotton, purified]

purified protein derivative (PPD) of tuberculin [see: tuberculin]

purified rayon [see: rayon, purified]

purified siliceous earth [see: siliceous earth, purified]

purified water [see: water, purified]

***H*-purin-6-amine** [see: adenine]

purine nucleoside phosphorylase *investigational (Phase III) treatment for psoriasis*

Purinethol tablets ℞ *antimetabolite antineoplastic for multiple leukemias* [mercaptopurine] 50 mg

Purinol (CAN) tablets (discontinued 1998) ℞ *xanthine oxidase inhibitor for gout and hyperuricemia* [allopurinol] 100, 300 mg

Purlytin *investigational (Phase III) PhotoPoint photodynamic therapy for advanced metastatic breast cancer involving the skin and age-related macular degeneration* [rostaporfin]

puromycin USAN, INN *antineoplastic; antiprotozoal (Trypanosoma)*

puromycin HCl USAN *antineoplastic; antiprotozoal (Trypanosoma)*

purple angelica *medicinal herb* [see: angelica]

purple boneset *medicinal herb* [see: boneset]

purple cone flower *medicinal herb* [see: echinacea]

purple leptandra *medicinal herb* [see: Culver root]

Purpose Alpha Hydroxy Moisture lotion, cream OTC *moisturizer; emollient; exfoliant* [glycolic acid] 8%

Purpose Dry Skin cream OTC *moisturizer; emollient*

Purpose Soap bar OTC *therapeutic skin cleanser*

purshiana bark *medicinal herb* [see: cascara sagrada]

purslain, water *medicinal herb* [see: brooklime]

purvain *medicinal herb* [see: blue vervain]

pussywillow *medicinal herb* [see: willow]

PUVA *an acronym for psoralens (P) and ultraviolet A (UVA) light, used as a treatment for severe recalcitrant psoriasis* [see: psoralens; methoxsalen]

PVA (polyvinyl alcohol) [q.v.]

PVA (prednisone, vincristine, asparaginase) *chemotherapy protocol for acute lymphocytic leukemia (ALL)*

PVB (Platinol, vinblastine, bleomycin) *chemotherapy protocol for testicular cancer and adenocarcinoma*

PVC (polyvinyl chloride) [see: polyvinyl chloride, radiopaque]
PVDA (prednisone, vincristine, daunorubicin, asparaginase) *chemotherapy protocol for acute lymphocytic leukemia (ALL)*
PVP; PVP-16 (Platinol, VP-16) *chemotherapy protocol*
PVS Basics ℞ *hydrophobic contact lens material* [paflufocon E]
P-V-Tussin syrup ℞ *narcotic antitussive; decongestant; antihistamine* [hydrocodone bitartrate; pseudoephedrine HCl; chlorpheniramine maleate; alcohol 5%] 2.5•30•2 mg/5 mL
P-V-Tussin tablets ℞ *narcotic antitussive; antihistamine; expectorant* [hydrocodone bitartrate; phenindamine tartrate; guaifenesin] 5•25•200 mg
Pycnanthemum virginianum *medicinal herb* [see: wild hyssop]
Pycnogenol *natural free radical scavenger; a registered trade name for pine bark extract* [see: pine bark extract]
pygeum *(Prunus africana; Pygeum africanum)* bark *medicinal herb for prostate gland enlargement and urinary disorders*
Pylori-Check test kit for professional use *in vivo diagnostic aid for H. pylori in the breath*
Pylorid (CAN) film-coated tablets (discontinued 2001) ℞ *histamine H_2 antagonist for duodenal ulcers with H. pylori infection* [ranitidine bismuth citrate] 400 mg
Pyloriset reagent kit for professional use *in vitro diagnostic aid for GI disorders*
pyrabrom USAN *antihistamine*
pyradone [see: aminopyrine]
pyrantel INN *anthelmintic for ascariasis (roundworm) and enterobiasis (pinworm)* [also: pyrantel pamoate]
pyrantel pamoate USAN, USP *anthelmintic for ascariasis (roundworm) and enterobiasis (pinworm)* [also: pyrantel]
pyrantel tartrate USAN *anthelmintic*
pyrathiazine HCl [see: parathiazine]
pyrazinamide (PZA) USP, INN, BAN *bactericidal; primary tuberculostatic* 500 mg oral
pyrazinecarboxamide [see: pyrazinamide]
pyrazofurin USAN *antineoplastic* [also: pirazofurin]
pyrazoline [see: antipyrine]
pyrazolopyrimidines *a class of sedatives and hypnotics with rapid onset and short duration of action, used in the short-term treatment of insomnia*
pyrbenzindole [see: benzindopyrine HCl]
pyrbuterol HCl [see: pirbuterol HCl]
pyrethrins *a class of natural pesticides derived from pyrethrum flowers, especially Chrysanthemum cinerariaefolium and C. coccineum*
Pyrethrum parthenium *medicinal herb* [see: feverfew]
pyribenzamine (PBZ) [see: tripelennamine]
pyricarbate INN
pyridarone INN
Pyridiate; Pyridate No. 2 tablets ℞ *urinary analgesic* [phenazopyridine HCl] 100 mg; 200 mg
4-pyridinamine [see: fampridine]
2-pyridine aldoxime methylchloride (2-PAM) [see: pralidoxime chloride]
3-pyridinecarboxamide [see: niacinamide]
3-pyridinecarboxylic acid [see: niacin]
4-pyridinecarboxylic acid hydrazide [see: isoniazid]
3-pyridinecarboxylic acid methyl ester [see: methyl nicotinate]
3-pyridinemethanol [see: nicotinyl alcohol]
2-pyridinemethanol [see: piconol]
3-pyridinemethanol tartrate [see: nicotinyl tartrate]
Pyridium tablets ℞ *urinary analgesic* [phenazopyridine HCl] 100, 200 mg ⓓ Dyrenium; pyridoxine; pyrithione; pyritidium
Pyridium Plus tablets ℞ *urinary analgesic; antispasmodic; sedative*

[phenazopyridine HCl; hyoscyamine hydrobromide; butabarbital] 150•0.3•15 mg

pyridofylline INN

pyridostigmine bromide USP, INN *cholinergic/anticholinesterase muscle stimulant* ⊡ physostigmine

pyridoxal-5′-phosphate [see: pyridoxine HCl]

pyridoxamine [see: pyridoxine HCl]

pyridoxine (vitamin B_6) INN *water-soluble vitamin; enzyme cofactor* [also: pyridoxine HCl] ⊡ pralidoxime; Pyridium

pyridoxine HCl (vitamin B_6) USP *water-soluble vitamin; enzyme cofactor* [also: pyridoxine] 50, 100, 250, 500 mg oral; 100 mg/mL injection ⊡ pralidoxime; Pyridium

β-pyridylcarbinol [see: nicotinyl alcohol]

pyridylmethanol *me+* [see: nicotinyl alcohol]

9-[3-pyridylmethyl]-9-deazaguanine *investigational for cutaneous T-cell lymphoma; orphan status withdrawn 1998*

pyrilamine maleate USP *anticholinergic; antihistamine; sleep aid* [also: mepyramine]

pyrilamine tannate, phenylephrine tannate, and chlorpheniramine tannate *antihistamine; decongestant* 25•25•8 mg oral

pyrimethamine USP, INN *folic acid antagonist for malaria suppression and transmission control; toxoplasmosis treatment adjunct*

pyrimethamine & sulfadiazine *Toxoplasma gondii encephalitis treatment (orphan)*

pyrimidinedione [see: uracil]

pyrimitate INN, BAN

Pyrinex Pediculicide shampoo OTC *pediculicide for lice* [pyrethrins; piperonyl butoxide; deodorized kerosene] 0.2%•2%•0.8%

pyrinoline USAN, INN *antiarrhythmic*

Pyrinyl liquid OTC *pediculicide for lice* [pyrethrins; piperonyl butoxide; deodorized kerosene] 0.2%•2%•0.8%

Pyrinyl II liquid OTC *pediculicide for lice* [pyrethrins; piperonyl butoxide] 0.3%•3%

Pyrinyl Plus shampoo OTC *pediculicide for lice* [pyrethrins; piperonyl butoxide] 0.3%•3%

pyrithen [see: chlorothen citrate]

pyrithione sodium USAN *topical antimicrobial* ⊡ Pyridium

pyrithione zinc USAN, INN, BAN *antibacterial; antifungal; antiseborrheic*

pyrithyldione INN

pyritidium bromide INN ⊡ Pyridium

pyritinol INN, BAN

pyrodifenium bromide [see: prifinium bromide]

pyrogallic acid [see: pyrogallol]

pyrogallol NF

pyrophendane INN

pyrophenindane [see: pyrophendane]

pyrovalerone INN *CNS stimulant* [also: pyrovalerone HCl]

pyrovalerone HCl USAN *CNS stimulant* [also: pyrovalerone]

pyroxamine INN *antihistamine* [also: pyroxamine maleate]

pyroxamine maleate USAN *antihistamine* [also: pyroxamine]

pyroxylin USP, INN *pharmaceutic necessity for collodion*

pyrrobutamine phosphate USP

pyrrocaine USAN, INN *local anesthetic*

pyrrocaine HCl NF

pyrrolifene INN *analgesic* [also: pyrroliphene HCl]

pyrrolifene HCl [see: pyrroliphene HCl]

pyrroliphene HCl USAN *analgesic* [also: pyrrolifene]

pyrrolnitrin USAN, INN *antifungal*

pyrroxane [now: proroxan HCl]

Pyrroxate capsules OTC *decongestant; antihistamine; analgesic* [phenylpropanolamine HCl; chlorpheniramine maleate; acetaminophen] 25•4•650 mg

Pyrus malus *medicinal herb* [see: apple]

pyrvinium chloride INN
pyrvinium embonate [see: pyrvinium pamoate]
pyrvinium pamoate USP *anthelmintic* [also: viprynium embonate]
pytamine INN
PYtest reagent kit for professional use *in vitro diagnostic aid for H. pylori in the breath* [carbon C 14 urea] 1 mCi
PZA (pyrazinamide) [q.v.]
PZI (protamine zinc insulin) [q.v.]

QS-21 *investigational (Phase II) immune system stimulant for AIDS vaccines*
QTest test stick for home use *in vitro diagnostic aid; urine pregnancy test*
QTest Ovulation test kit for professional use *in vitro diagnostic aid to predict ovulation time*
quadazocine INN, BAN *opioid antagonist* [also: quadazocine mesylate]
quadazocine mesylate USAN *opioid antagonist* [also: quadazocine]
Quadramet IV injection ℞ *radiopharmaceutical for treatment of bone pain from osteoblastic metastatic tumors* [samarium Sm 153 lexidronam] 1850 MBq/mL (50 mCi/mL)
Quadrinal tablets ℞ *antiasthmatic; bronchodilator; decongestant; expectorant; sedative* [theophylline; ephedrine HCl; potassium iodide; phenobarbital] 65•24•320•24 mg
quadrosilan INN
quaking aspen *medicinal herb* [see: poplar]
Quantaffirm reagent kit for professional use *in vitro diagnostic aid for mononucleosis*
Quarzan capsules ℞ *anticholinergic; peptic ulcer treatment* [clidinium bromide] 2.5, 5 mg ⊡ Questran
quassia *(Picrasma excelsa; Quassia amara)* bark *medicinal herb used as an anthelmintic, antimalarial, appetizer, digestive aid, febrifuge, insecticide, pediculicide, and tonic*
quatacaine INN
quaternium-18 bentonite [see: bentoquatam]
quazepam USAN, INN *sedative; hypnotic*
quazinone USAN, INN *cardiotonic*
quazodine USAN, INN *cardiotonic; bronchodilator*
quazolast USAN, INN *antiasthmatic; mediator release inhibitor*
Queen Anne's lace *medicinal herb* [see: carrot]
queen of the meadow *medicinal herb* [see: boneset; meadowsweet]
queen of the meadow *(Eupatorium purpureum)* leaves *medicinal herb for bursitis, gallstones, kidney infections and stones, neuralgias, rheumatism, ringworm, urinary disorders, and water retention*
Quelicin IV or IM injection ℞ *neuromuscular blocker* [succinylcholine chloride] 20, 50, 100 mg/mL
Quelidrine Cough syrup OTC *antitussive; decongestant; antihistamine; expectorant* [dextromethorphan hydrobromide; ephedrine HCl; phenylephrine HCl; chlorpheniramine maleate; ammonium chloride; ipecac; alcohol 2%] 10 mg•5 mg•5 mg•2 mg•40 mg•0.005 mL per 5 mL
Quercetin tablets OTC *dietary supplement* [eucalyptus bioflavonoids] 50, 250 mg
Quercus alba *medicinal herb* [see: white oak]
Questran; Questran Light powder for oral suspension ℞ *cholesterol-lowering antihyperlipidemic; also used for biliary obstruction* [cholestyramine resin] 4 g/dose
quetiapine fumarate USAN *dibenzothiazepine antipsychotic*

Quibron; Quibron-300 capsules ℞ *antiasthmatic; bronchodilator; expectorant* [theophylline; guaifenesin] 150•90 mg; 300•180 mg

Quibron-T Dividose (multiple-scored tablets) ℞ *antiasthmatic; bronchodilator* [theophylline] 300 mg

Quibron-T/SR sustained-release Dividose (multiple-scored tablets) ℞ *antiasthmatic; bronchodilator* [theophylline] 300 mg

Quick AC Enema Kit concentrated rectal suspension ℞ *radiopaque contrast medium for gastrointestinal imaging* [barium sulfate] 150%

Quick Care solutions OTC *two-step chemical disinfecting system for soft contact lenses* [hydrogen peroxide-based]

Quick Pep tablets (discontinued 2001) OTC *CNS stimulant; analeptic* [caffeine] 150 mg

Quicklets (trademarked dosage form) *quickly dissolving tablets*

Quickscreen test kit for home use *in vitro diagnostic aid for detection of multiple illicit drugs in the urine*

quick-set *medicinal herb* [see: hawthorn]

QuickVue *H. pylori* gII test kit for professional use *in vitro diagnostic aid for H. pylori in serum or plasma*

QuickVue Influenza Test for professional use *in vitro diagnostic aid for detection of influenza A and B from nasal excretions*

QuickVue Pregnancy Test cassettes for professional use *in vitro diagnostic aid; urine pregnancy test*

Quiess IM injection (discontinued 1998) ℞ *anxiolytic; antiemetic* [hydroxyzine HCl] 50 mg/mL

quifenadine INN

quiflapon sodium USAN *leukotriene biosynthesis inhibitor for asthma and inflammatory bowel disease*

Quilimmune-M ℞ *investigational (Phase II) vaccine against malaria*

Quilimmune-P ℞ *investigational (Phase II) vaccine against pneumonia in elderly patients*

quillaia *(Quillaja saponaria)* bark *medicinal herb for bronchitis and cough; also used topically for dandruff and scalp itchiness*

quillifoline INN

quilostigmine USAN *cholinesterase inhibitor for Alzheimer disease*

quinacainol INN

quinacillin INN, BAN

quinacrine HCl USP *antimalarial; anthelmintic for giardiasis and cestodiasis (tapeworm)* [also: mepacrine] ⊡ quinidine

Quinaglute Dura-Tabs (sustained-release tablets) ℞ *antiarrhythmic* [quinidine gluconate] 324 mg

Quinalan sustained-release tablets (discontinued 2000) ℞ *antiarrhythmic* [quinidine gluconate] 324 mg

quinalbarbitone sodium BAN *hypnotic; sedative* [also: secobarbital sodium]

quinaldine blue USAN *obstetric diagnostic aid*

quinambicide [see: clioquinol]

quinapril INN, BAN *angiotensin-converting enzyme (ACE) inhibitor; antihypertensive; adjunct to CHF therapy* [also: quinapril HCl]

quinapril HCl USAN *angiotensin-converting enzyme (ACE) inhibitor; antihypertensive; adjunct to CHF therapy* [also: quinapril]

quinaprilat USAN, INN *antihypertensive; angiotensin-converting enzyme (ACE) inhibitor*

quinazosin INN *antihypertensive* [also: quinazosin HCl]

quinazosin HCl USAN *antihypertensive* [also: quinazosin]

quinbolone USAN, INN *anabolic*

quincarbate INN

quindecamine INN *antibacterial* [also: quindecamine acetate]

quindecamine acetate USAN *antibacterial* [also: quindecamine]

quindonium bromide USAN, INN *antiarrhythmic*

quindoxin INN, BAN

quinelorane INN *antihypertensive; antiparkinsonian* [also: quinelorane HCl]

quinelorane HCl USAN *antihypertensive; antiparkinsonian* [also: quinelorane]
quinestradol INN, BAN
quinestrol USAN, USP, INN, BAN *estrogen replacement therapy for postmenopausal disorders*
quinetalate INN *smooth muscle relaxant* [also: quinetolate]
quinethazone USP, INN *diuretic; antihypertensive*
quinetolate USAN *smooth muscle relaxant* [also: quinetalate]
quinezamide INN
quinfamide USAN, INN *antiamebic*
quingestanol INN *progestin* [also: quingestanol acetate]
quingestanol acetate USAN *progestin* [also: quingestanol]
quingestrone USAN, INN *progestin*
Quinidex Extentabs (extended-release tablets) ℞ *antiarrhythmic* [quinidine sulfate] 300 mg
quinidine NF, BAN *antiarrhythmic* ⓢ clonidine; quinacrine; Quinatime; quinine
quinidine gluconate USP *antiarrhythmic; antimalarial* 324 mg oral; 80 mg/mL injection
quinidine polygalacturonate *antiarrhythmic*
quinidine sulfate USP *antiarrhythmic* 300 mg oral
quinine (*Cinchona calisaya; C. ledgeriana; C. succirubra*) NF, BAN bark *medicinal herb for cancer, fever, hemorrhoids, indigestion, inducing abortion, jaundice, malaria, mouth and throat diseases, parasites, stimulation of hair growth, and varicose veins* ⓢ quinidine
quinine ascorbate USAN *smoking deterrent*
quinine biascorbate [now: quinine ascorbate]
quinine bisulfate NF
quinine dihydrochloride NF *investigational anti-infective for pernicious malaria*
quinine ethylcarbonate NF
quinine glycerophosphate NF
quinine HCl NF
quinine hydrobromide NF
quinine hypophosphite NF
quinine monohydrobromide [see: quinine hydrobromide]
quinine monohydrochloride [see: quinine HCl]
quinine monosalicylate [see: quinine salicylate]
quinine phosphate NF
quinine phosphinate [see: quinine hypophosphite]
quinine salicylate NF
quinine sulfate USP *antimalarial cinchona alkaloid; treatment of nocturnal leg cramps* 200, 260, 325 mg oral
quinine sulfate dihydrate [see: quinine sulfate]
quinine tannate USP
Quinine-Odan (CAN) capsules OTC *antimalarial* [quinine sulfate] 200, 300 mg
quinisocaine INN [also: dimethisoquin HCl; dimethisoquin]
quinocide INN
8-quinolinol [see: oxyquinoline]
8-quinolinol benzoate [see: benzoxiquine]
quinolizidines *a class of antibiotics based on the quinolizidine (norlupinane) structure* [also called: norlupinanes]
quinolones [see: fluoroquinolones]
Quinora tablets ℞ *antiarrhythmic* [quinidine sulfate] 300 mg
quinoxyl [see: chiniofon]
quinpirole INN *antihypertensive* [also: quinpirole HCl]
quinpirole HCl USAN *antihypertensive* [also: quinpirole]
quinprenaline INN *bronchodilator* [also: quinterenol sulfate]
quinprenaline sulfate [see: quinterenol sulfate]
Quinsana Plus powder OTC *topical antifungal* [tolnaftate] 1%
quinsy berry *medicinal herb* [see: currant]
Quintabs tablets OTC *vitamin supplement* [multiple vitamins; folic acid] ≛•0.1 mg
Quintabs-M tablets OTC *vitamin/mineral/iron supplement* [multiple vita-

mins & minerals; iron; folic acid] ≛ •18•0.4 mg

quinterenol sulfate USAN *bronchodilator* [also: quinprenaline]

quintiofos INN, BAN

3-quinuclidinol benzoate [see: benzoclidine]

quinuclium bromide USAN, INN *antihypertensive*

quinupramine INN

quinupristin USAN, INN *streptogramin antibiotic; bacteriostatic to gram-positive infections*

quinupristin & dalfopristin *two streptogramin antibiotics that are synergistically bactericidal to gram-positive infections; investigational (NDA filed) for pneumonia*

quipazine INN *antidepressant; oxytocic* [also: quipazine maleate]

quipazine maleate USAN *antidepressant; oxytocic* [also: quipazine]

quisultazine INN

quisultidine [see: quisultazine]

Quixin eye drops ℞ *topical fluoroquinolone antibiotic for bacterial conjunctivitis* [levofloxacin] 0.5%

QVAR CFC-free oral pMDI (pressurized metered-dose inhaler) ℞ *corticosteroidal anti-inflammatory for chronic asthma* [beclomethasone dipropionate] 40, 80 µg/puff

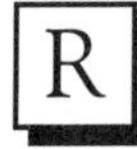

R & C shampoo OTC *pediculicide for lice* [pyrethrins; piperonyl butoxide] 0.3%•3%

R & D Calcium Carbonate/600 ℞ *investigational (orphan) for hyperphosphatemia of end-stage renal disease* [calcium carbonate]

R-121919 *investigational (Phase I) agent for anxiety and depression*

RA Lotion OTC *topical acne treatment* [resorcinol; alcohol 43%] 3%

RabAvert IM injection ℞ *rabies vaccine for pre-exposure vaccination or post-exposure prophylaxis* [rabies vaccine, chick embryo cell] 2.5 IU

rabeprazole INN *proton pump inhibitor for duodenal ulcers, erosive or ulcerative gastroesophageal reflux disease (GERD), and other gastroesophageal disorders* [also: rabeprazole sodium]

rabeprazole sodium USAN *proton pump inhibitor for duodenal ulcers, erosive or ulcerative gastroesophageal reflux disease (GERD), and other gastroesophageal disorders* [also: rabeprazole]

rabies immune globulin (RIG) USP *passive immunizing agent for rabies prophylaxis and treatment*

rabies vaccine USP *active immunizing agent* Challenge Virus Standard (CVS)

rabies vaccine, adsorbed (RVA) [see: rabies vaccine]

rabies vaccine, DCO (diploid cell origin) [see: rabies vaccine]

rabies vaccine, HDCV (human diploid cell vaccine) [see: rabies vaccine]

race ginger *medicinal herb* [see: ginger]

racecadotril [see: acetorphan]

racefemine INN

racefenicol INN *antibacterial* [also: racephenicol]

racemethadol [see: dimepheptanol]

racemethionine USAN, USP *urinary acidifier* [also: methionine (the DL- form)]

racemethorphan INN, BAN

racemetirosine INN

racemic amphetamine phosphate

racemic amphetamine sulfate [see: amphetamine sulfate]

racemic calcium pantothenate [see: calcium pantothenate, racemic]

racemoramide INN, BAN

racemorphan INN

racephedrine HCl USAN

racephenicol USAN *antibacterial* [also: racefenicol]
racepinefrine INN *sympathomimetic bronchodilator* [also: racepinephrine]
racepinephrine USP *sympathomimetic bronchodilator* [also: racepinefrine]
racepinephrine HCl USP *sympathomimetic bronchodilator*
raclopride INN, BAN
raclopride C 11 USAN *radiopharmaceutical*
racoonberry *medicinal herb* [see: mandrake]
ractopamine INN *veterinary growth stimulant* [also: ractopamine HCl]
ractopamine HCl USAN *veterinary growth stimulant* [also: ractopamine]
radio-chromated serum albumin [see: albumin, chromated]
radio-iodinated I 125 serum albumin [see: albumin, iodinated]
radio-iodinated I 131 serum albumin [see: albumin, iodinated]
radiomerisoprol ^{197}Hg [see: merisoprol Hg 197]
radioselenomethionine ^{75}Se [see: selenomethionine Se 75]
radiotolpovidone I 131 INN *hypoalbuminemia test; radioactive agent* [also: tolpovidone I 131]
radish *(Raphanus sativus)* root *medicinal herb used as an antispasmodic, astringent, cholagogue, and diuretic*
radium *element (Ra)*
radon *element (Rn)*
rAd/p53 gene therapy *investigational (Phase I) therapy for cancer*
rafoxanide USAN, INN *anthelmintic*
ragged cup *(Silphium perfoliatum)* root and gum *medicinal herb used as an antispasmodic, diaphoretic, and stimulant*
ragwort *medicinal herb* [see: life root]
ralitoline USAN, INN *anticonvulsant*
raloxifene INN *antiestrogen; selective estrogen receptor modulator (SERM) for the prevention and treatment of postmenopausal osteoporosis* [also: raloxifene HCl]
raloxifene HCl USAN *antiestrogen; selective estrogen receptor modulator (SERM) for the prevention and treatment of postmenopausal osteoporosis* [also: raloxifene]
raltitrexed USAN *antimetabolite antineoplastic; investigational (Phase III) thymidylate synthase inhibitor for advanced colorectal cancer*
raluridine USAN *antiviral*
rambufaside [see: meproscillarin]
ramciclane INN
ramifenazone INN
ramipril USAN, INN, BAN *antihypertensive; angiotensin-converting enzyme (ACE) inhibitor*
ramiprilat INN
ramixotidine INN
ramnodigin INN
ramoplanin USAN, INN *investigational (Phase III) antibiotic for vancomycin-resistant Enterococcus faecium (VREF)*
Ramses vaginal jelly OTC *spermicidal contraceptive* [nonoxynol 9] 5%
Ramses Extra premedicated condom OTC *spermicidal/barrier contraceptive* [nonoxynol 9] 15%
ranimustine INN
ranimycin USAN, INN *antibacterial*
ranitidine USAN, INN, BAN *histamine H_2 antagonist for gastric ulcers* 150, 300 mg oral
ranitidine bismuth citrate USAN *histamine H_2 antagonist for gastric ulcers with H. pylori infection* [also: ranitidine bismutrex]
ranitidine bismutrex BAN *histamine H_2 antagonist for gastric ulcers with H. pylori infection* [also: ranitidine bismuth citrate]
ranitidine HCl USP, JAN *histamine H_2 antagonist for gastric ulcers* 75 mg oral; 15 mg/mL oral
ranolazine INN *antianginal* [also: ranolazine HCl]
ranolazine HCl USAN *investigational (Phase III) antianginal for chronic stable angina* [also: ranolazine]

Ranunculus acris; R. bulbosus; R. scleratus *medicinal herb* [see: buttercup]

rapacuronium bromide USAN *neuromuscular blocker; adjunct to general anesthesia*

Rapamune tablets, oral solution ℞ *immunosuppressant for renal transplantation* [sirolimus] 1 mg; 1 mg/mL

rapamycin [now: sirolimus]

Raphanus sativus *medicinal herb* [see: radish]

RapidVue test kit for home use *in vitro diagnostic aid; urine pregnancy test*

Rapimine (name changed to Emadine upon marketing release in 1998)

Raplon IV injection (discontinued 2001) ℞ *rapid-onset, short-acting neuromuscular blocker for skeletal muscle relaxation as an adjunct to general anesthesia* [rapacuronium bromide] 100, 200 mg

rasagiline INN

rasagiline mesylate USAN *antiparkinsonian; monoamine oxidase B (MAO-B) inhibitor; investigational (Phase III) for Parkinson disease*

raspberry, ground *medicinal herb* [see: goldenseal]

raspberry, red; wild red raspberry *medicinal herb* [see: red raspberry]

raspberry [syrup] USP

rathyronine INN

rattleroot *medicinal herb* [see: black cohosh]

rattlesnake antivenin [see: antivenin (Crotalidae) polyvalent]

rattlesnake root *medicinal herb* [see: birthroot; black cohosh; senega]

rattleweed *medicinal herb* [see: black cohosh]

rauwolfia serpentina USP *antihypertensive; peripheral antiadrenergic; antipsychotic*

Rauzide tablets ℞ *antihypertensive; diuretic* [bendroflumethiazide; rauwolfia serpentina] 4•50 mg

Ravocaine & Novocaine with Levophed injection ℞ *injectable local anesthetic for dental procedures* [propoxycaine HCl; procaine; norepinephrine bitartrate] 7.2•36•0.12 mg/1.8 mL

Raxar film-coated tablets; Rax-Pack (10 tablets) (discontinued 1999) ℞ *broad-spectrum fluoroquinolone antibiotic* [grepafloxacin HCl] 200, 400, 600 mg

rayon, purified USAN, USP *surgical aid*

razinodil INN

razobazam INN

razoxane INN, BAN

^{86}**Rb** [see: rubidium chloride Rb 86]

RBC-CD4 *investigational (Phase I/II) antiviral for HIV*

rBPI (bactericidal and permeability-increasing protein, recombinant) [q.v.]

rCD4 (recombinant soluble human CD4) [see: CD4, recombinant soluble human]

RCF liquid OTC *hypoallergenic infant formula* [soy protein formula, carbohydrate free]

Reabilan; Reabilan HN ready-to-use liquid OTC *enteral nutritional therapy* [lactose-free formula]

Reactine (CAN) film-coated tablets, syrup ℞ *once-daily antihistamine* [cetirizine HCl] 5, 10 mg; 5 mg/5 mL

reactrol [see: clemizole HCl]

rebamipide INN

Rebetol capsules ℞ *nucleoside antiviral* [ribavirin] 200 mg

Rebetron capsules + subcu or IM injection ℞ *combination treatment for chronic hepatitis* C [Rebetol (ribavirin capsules); Intron A (interferon alfa-2b injection)] 200 mg•3 million IU

Rebif (CAN) powder for injection, prefilled syringe ℞ *immunomodulator for relapsing remitting multiple sclerosis (orphan) and condylomata acuminata; investigational (orphan) for malignant melanoma, metastatic renal cell carcinoma, T-cell lymphoma, and Kaposi sarcoma* [interferon beta-1a] 3, 12 MIU/vial; 6, 12 MIU/0.5 mL

reboxetine INN *investigational (NDA filed) fast-acting selective norepinephrine reuptake inhibitor for depression*

reboxetine mesylate USAN *investigational (NDA filed) fast-acting selective norepinephrine reuptake inhibitor for depression*

recainam INN, BAN *antiarrhythmic* [also: recainam HCl]

recainam HCl USAN *antiarrhythmic* [also: recainam]

recainam tosylate USAN *antiarrhythmic*

recanescin [see: deserpidine]

Receptin ℞ *investigational (Phase II) antiviral for AIDS; orphan status withdrawn 1997* [CD4, recombinant soluble human]

reclazepam USAN, INN *sedative*

Reclomide tablets ℞ *antidopaminergic; antiemetic for chemotherapy; peristaltic* [metoclopramide HCl] 10 mg

Recombigen HIV-1 LA Test reagent kit for professional use *in vitro diagnostic aid for HIV-1 antibodies in blood, serum, or plasma* [latex agglutination test]

recombinant alpha$_1$ antitrypsin [see: alpha$_1$ antitrypsin, recombinant]

recombinant antihemophilic factor [see: antihemophilic factor, recombinant]

recombinant factor VIIa [see: factor VIIa, recombinant]

recombinant factor VIII [see: antihemophilic factor, recombinant]

recombinant human activated protein C (rhAPC) [see: drotrecogin alfa]

recombinant human CD4 immunoglobulin G [CD4 immunoglobulin G, recombinant human]

recombinant human deoxyribonuclease (rhDNase) [see: dornase alfa]

recombinant human erythropoietin [see: erythropoietin, recombinant human]

recombinant human growth hormone (rhGH) [see: somatropin]

recombinant human interferon beta [see: interferon beta, recombinant human]

recombinant human interleukin-1 receptor (rhIL-1R; rhu IL-1R) [see: interleukin-1 receptor]

recombinant human superoxide dismutase (SOD) [see: superoxide dismutase, recombinant human]

recombinant interferon alfa-2a [see: interferon alfa-2a, recombinant]

recombinant interferon alfa-2b [see: interferon alfa-2b, recombinant]

recombinant interferon beta [see: interferon beta, recombinant]

recombinant interleukin-2 [see: interleukin-2, recombinant]

recombinant methionyl granulocyte CSF [see: methionyl granulocyte CSF, recombinant]

recombinant methionyl human granulocyte CSF [see: methionyl human granulocyte CSF, recombinant]

recombinant soluble human CD4 (rCD4) [see: CD4, recombinant soluble human]

recombinant tissue plasminogen activator (rtPA; rt-PA) [see: alteplase]

Recombinate powder for IV injection ℞ *antihemophilic to correct coagulation deficiency* [antihemophilic factor VIII, recombinant] 250, 500, 1000 IU

Recombivax HB adult IM injection, pediatric/adolescent IM injection, dialysis formulation ℞ *active immunizing agent for hepatitis B and D* [hepatitis B virus vaccine, recombinant] 10 µg/mL; 5 µg/0.5 mL; 40 µg/mL

Rectacort rectal suppositories ℞ *corticosteroidal anti-inflammatory* [hydrocortisone acetate] 10%

Rectagene rectal suppositories OTC *temporary relief of hemorrhoidal symptoms* [live yeast cell derivative; shark liver oil] 2000 SRF U/oz.

Rectagene II rectal suppositories (discontinued 1997) OTC *temporary relief of hemorrhoidal symptoms* [bismuth subgallate; bismuth resorcin compound; benzyl benzoate; peruvian balsam; zinc oxide] 2.25%•1.75%•1.2%•1.8%•11%

Rectagene Medicated Rectal Balm ointment OTC *temporary relief of hemorrhoidal symptoms* [shark liver oil; phenyl mercuric nitrate; live yeast cell derivative] 3%•1:10 000•66.67 U/g

Rectolax suppositories OTC *stimulant laxative* [bisacodyl] 10 mg

red bay; red laurel *medicinal herb* [see: magnolia]

red bearberry *medicinal herb* [see: uva ursi]

red blood cells [see: blood cells, red]

red bush tea *(Aspalathus contaminata; A. linearis; Borbonia pinifolia)* leaves and stems *medicinal herb used as a free radical scavenger; investigational antineoplastic; investigational for preventing brain damage caused by aging*

red clover *(Trifolium pratense)* flower *medicinal herb for blood cleansing, bronchitis, cancer, clearing toxins, nervous disorders, and spasms*

Red Cross Toothache liquid OTC *topical oral analgesic* [eugenol] 85%

red currant *(Ribes rubrum)* *medicinal herb* [see: currant]

red elm *medicinal herb* [see: slippery elm]

red ferric oxide [see: ferric oxide, red]

red ink berries; red ink plant *medicinal herb* [see: pokeweed]

red laurel; red bay *medicinal herb* [see: magnolia]

red legs *medicinal herb* [see: bistort]

red mulberry *(Morus rubra)* *medicinal herb* [see: mulberry]

red oak *(Quercus rubra)* *medicinal herb* [see: white oak]

red paint root *medicinal herb* [see: bloodroot]

red pepper; African red pepper; American red pepper *medicinal herb* [see: cayenne]

red pimpernel *(Anagallis arvensis)* plant *medicinal herb used as a cholagogue, diaphoretic, diuretic, expectorant, nervine, purgative, and stimulant*

red puccoon *medicinal herb* [see: bloodroot]

red raspberry *(Rubus idaeus; R. strigosus)* leaves *medicinal herb for childbirth afterpains, diarrhea and other bowel disorders, fever, flu, morning sickness, menstrual disorders, mouth sores, nausea, and vomiting*

red root *medicinal herb* [see: bloodroot; danshen; New Jersey tea]

red sarsaparilla *medicinal herb* [see: sarsaparilla]

red veterinarian petrolatum (RVP) [see: petrolatum]

red weed *medicinal herb* [see: pokeweed]

redberry *medicinal herb* [see: ginseng]

Redi Vial (trademarked packaging form) *dual-compartment vial*

Rediject (trademarked delivery system) *prefilled disposable syringe*

Redipak (trademarked packaging form) *unit dose or unit-of-issue package*

RediTabs (trademarked dosage form) *rapidly disintegrating tablets*

redmond clay (montmorillonite) *natural remedy for bug bites and stings and other skin problems*

Reducin ℞ *investigational (orphan) for nonoperative management of cutaneous fistulas of the GI tract and bleeding esophageal varices* [somatostatin]

Redutemp tablets OTC *analgesic; antipyretic* [acetaminophen] 500 mg

Redux capsules (discontinued 1997) ℞ *anorexiant and appetite suppressant for long-term dieting* [dexfenfluramine HCl] 15 mg

Reese's Pinworm soft gel capsules, liquid OTC *anthelmintic for ascariasis (roundworm) and enterobiasis (pinworm)* [pyrantel pamoate] 180 mg; 50 mg/mL

ReFacto powder for IV injection *long-term treatment for hemophilia A (orphan); short-term bleeding prophylaxis for surgical procedures* [antihemophilic factor, recombinant] 250, 500, 1000 IU/vial

Refludan powder for IV injection *anticoagulant for heparin-induced thrombocytopenia (orphan)* [lepirudin] 50 mg

Refresh eye drops OTC *ophthalmic moisturizer/lubricant* [polyvinyl alcohol] 1.4%

Refresh Plus; Refresh Tears eye drops OTC *ophthalmic moisturizer/lubricant* [carboxymethylcellulose] 0.5%

Refresh P.M. ophthalmic ointment OTC *ocular moisturizer/lubricant* [white petrolatum; mineral oil; lanolin]

refrigerants *a class of agents that lower abnormal body heat (a term used in folk medicine)*

Rēgain snack bar OTC *enteral nutritional therapy for impaired renal function* [multiple essential amino acids] ⓢ Rogaine

Regitine IV or IM injection ℞ *antihypertensive for pheochromocytoma; α-blocker* [phentolamine mesylate] 5 mg/mL

Reglan tablets, syrup, IV infusion ℞ *antidopaminergic; antiemetic for chemotherapy; peristaltic* [metoclopramide HCl] 5, 10 mg; 5 mg/5 mL; 5 mg/mL ⓢ Regonol

Regonol IM or IV injection ℞ *cholinergic/anticholinesterase muscle stimulant; muscle relaxant reversal* [pyridostigmine bromide] 5 mg/mL ⓢ Reglan

regramostim USAN, INN *antineutropenic; hematopoietic stimulant; biologic response modifier; bone marrow stimulant*

Regranex gel ℞ *recombinant platelet-derived growth factor B for chronic diabetic foot ulcers* [becaplermin] 0.01%

Regressin ℞ *investigational tumor growth inhibitor and apoptosis inducer for bladder cancer*

Regroton tablets ℞ *antihypertensive; diuretic* [chlorthalidone; reserpine] 50•0.25 mg ⓢ Hygroton

Regulace capsules (discontinued 1999) OTC *stimulant laxative; stool softener* [casanthranol; docusate sodium] 30•100 mg

Regular Iletin I subcu injection (discontinued 1999) OTC *antidiabetic* [insulin (beef-pork)] 100 U/mL

Regular Iletin II subcu injection OTC *antidiabetic* [insulin (pork)] 100 U/mL

Regular Iletin II U-500 (concentrated) subcu or IM injection (discontinued 2000) ℞ *antidiabetic* [insulin (pork)] 500 U/mL

Regular Insulin subcu injection (discontinued 1997) OTC *antidiabetic* [insulin (pork)] 100 U/mL

Regular Purified Pork Insulin subcu injection (discontinued 2000) OTC *antidiabetic* [insulin] 100 U/mL

regulator, female *medicinal herb* [see: life root]

Regulax SS capsules OTC *laxative; stool softener* [docusate sodium] 100 mg

Reguloid powder OTC *bulk laxative* [psyllium hydrophilic mucilloid] 3.4 g/tsp.

Reguloid Sugar Free powder (discontinued 1999) OTC *bulk laxative* [psyllium hydrophilic mucilloid] 3.4 g/tbsp.

Regutol tablets (discontinued 1997) OTC *stool softener* [docusate sodium] 100 mg

Rehydralyte oral solution OTC *electrolyte replacement* [sodium, potassium, and chloride electrolytes]

reishi mushrooms body and stem *medicinal herb for AIDS, allergies, fatigue, heart problems, and insomnia*

Rejuva-A (CAN) cream ℞ *treatment for photodamaged skin* [tretinoin] 0.025%

Relafen film-coated tablets ℞ *antiarthritic; nonsteroidal anti-inflammatory drug (NSAID)* [nabumetone] 500, 750 mg

relaxin *investigational (orphan) for progressive systemic sclerosis; investigational (Phase II/III) for scleroderma*

Release+ (CAN) capsules OTC *vitamin C/manganese supplement* [calcium ascorbate; manganese citrate] 30•1.25 mg

Release-Tabs (dosage form) *timed-release tablets*

Relenza Rotadisks (powder for oral inhalation, for use with Diskhaler device) *antiviral for the treatment of acute influenza A and B infections* [zanamivir] 5 mg

Reliable Gentle Laxative delayed-release enteric-coated tablets, suppositories OTC *stimulant laxative* [bisacodyl] 5 mg; 10 mg

Relief eye drops OTC *topical ophthalmic decongestant* [phenylephrine HCl] 0.12%

relomycin USAN, INN *antibacterial*

Relpax ℞ *investigational (NDA filed) serotonin 5-HT_{1D}-receptor agonist for migraine* [eletriptan hydrobromide]

remacemide INN *neuroprotective anticonvulsant* [also: remacemide HCl]

remacemide HCl USAN *neuroprotective anticonvulsant* [also: remacemide]

Remeron coated tablets, SolTabs (orally disintegrating tablets) ℞ *tetracyclic antidepressant* [mirtazapine] 15, 30, 45 mg ⑫ Femiron

Remicade powder for IV infusion ℞ *anti-inflammatory; anti-TNFα (tumor necrosis factor alpha) monoclonal antibody for severe and fistulizing Crohn disease (orphan) and rheumatoid arthritis (with methotrexate)* [infliximab] 100 mg/vial

Remifemin Menopause tablets OTC *natural remedy for postmenopausal symptoms* [black cohosh (standardized extract)] ≈20 mg (1 mg triterpene glycosides)

remifentanil INN, BAN *short-acting narcotic analgesic for general anesthesia* [also: remifentanil HCl]

remifentanil HCl USAN *short-acting narcotic analgesic for general anesthesia* [also: remifentanil]

remikiren INN

Reminyl film-coated tablets ℞ *acetylcholinesterase inhibitor to increase cognition in Alzheimer disease* [galantamine hydrobromide] 4, 8, 12 mg

remiprostol USAN, INN *antiulcerative*

Remodulin continuous subcu infusion ℞ *investigational (NDA filed) prostacyclin analogue for pulmonary arterial hypertension (PAH) and peripheral vascular disease (PVD); investigational (Phase II) for critical limb ischemia (CLI)* [treprostinil sodium]

remoxipride USAN, INN, BAN *antipsychotic*

remoxipride HCl USAN *antipsychotic*

Remular-S tablets ℞ *skeletal muscle relaxant* [chlorzoxazone] 250 mg

Remune ℞ *investigational (Phase III) immunostimulant theraccine adjunct for HIV* [HIV-1 immunogen, gp120-depleted, inactivated]

Renacidin powder for solution ℞ *bladder and catheter irrigant for apatite or struvite calculi (orphan)* [citric acid; D-gluconic acid lactone; magnesium hydroxycarbonate] 6.602•0.198•3.177 g/100 mL

Renacidin Irrigation solution ℞ *bladder and catheter irrigant for apatite or struvite calculi (orphan)* [citric acid; glucono-delta-lactone; magnesium carbonate]

Renagel capsules, film-coated tablets ℞ *phosphate-binding polymer for hyperphosphatemia of end-stage renal disease* [sevelamer HCl] 403 mg; 400, 800 mg

RenAmin IV infusion ℞ *nutritional therapy for renal failure* [multiple essential and nonessential amino acids; electrolytes]

renanolone INN

Renese tablets ℞ *diuretic; antihypertensive* [polythiazide] 1, 2, 4 mg

Renese-R tablets ℞ *antihypertensive; diuretic* [polythiazide; reserpine] 2•0.25 mg

rennet, cheese *medicinal herb* [see: bedstraw]

Reno-30 intracavitary instillation ℞ *radiopaque contrast medium for urological imaging* [diatrizoate meglumine (46.67% iodine)] 300 mg/mL (141 mg/mL)

RenoCal-76 injection ℞ *radiopaque contrast medium* [diatrizoate meglumine; diatrizoate sodium (48.7% total iodine)] 660•100 mg/mL (370 mg/mL)

Reno-Dip; Reno-60 injection ℞ *radiopaque contrast medium* [diatrizoate meglumine (46.67% iodine)] 300 mg/mL (141 mg/mL); 600 mg/mL (282 mg/mL)

Renografin-60 injection ℞ *radiopaque contrast medium* [diatrizoate meglumine; diatrizoate sodium (48.75% total iodine)] 520•80 mg/mL (292.5 mg/mL)

Renografin-76 injection (discontinued 1999) ℞ *radiopaque contrast medium* [diatrizoate meglumine; diatrizoate sodium (48.75% total iodine)] 66%•10% (37%)

Reno-M-Dip; Reno-M-30; Reno-M-60 injection (name changed to Reno-Dip, Reno-30, and Reno-60 in 1999)

Renoquid tablets ℞ *broad-spectrum bacteriostatic* [sulfacytine] 250 mg

Renova cream ℞ *retinoid for photodamage, fine wrinkles, mottled hyperpigmentation, and roughness of facial skin* [tretinoin] 0.02%, 0.05%

Renovist; Renovist II injection (discontinued 1999) ℞ *radiopaque contrast medium* [diatrizoate meglumine; diatrizoate sodium (53.8% total iodine)] 34.3%•35% (37%); 28.5%•29.1% (31%)

Renovue-Dip; Renovue-65 injection (discontinued 1999) ℞ *radiopaque contrast medium* [iodamide meglumine (46% iodine)] 24%; 65%

Rentamine Pediatric oral suspension ℞ *pediatric antitussive, decongestant, and antihistamine* [carbetapentane tannate; phenylephrine tannate; ephedrine tannate; chlorpheniramine tannate] 30•5•5•4 mg/5 mL

rentiapril INN

ReNu solution OTC *rinsing/storage solution for soft contact lenses* [sodium chloride (preserved saline solution)]

ReNu Effervescent Enzymatic Cleaner; ReNu Thermal Enzymatic Cleaner tablets OTC *enzymatic cleaner for soft contact lenses* [subtilisin]

ReNu Multi-Purpose solution OTC *chemical disinfecting solution for soft contact lenses*

renytoline INN *anti-inflammatory* [also: paranyline HCl]

renytoline HCl [see: paranyline HCl]

renzapride INN, BAN

ReoPro IV injection ℞ *platelet aggregation inhibitor for PTCA and acute arterial occlusive disorders* [abciximab] 2 mg/mL

Reosyn ℞ *investigational antineoplastic* [reovirus]

reovirus *investigational antineoplastic*

repaglinide USAN *oral antidiabetic agent that stimulates release of insulin from the pancreas for type 2 diabetes*

Repan capsules (discontinued 2000) ℞ *analgesic; barbiturate sedative* [acetaminophen; caffeine; butalbital] 325•40•50 mg ⊡ Riopan

Repan tablets ℞ *analgesic; barbiturate sedative* [acetaminophen; caffeine; butalbital] 325•40•50 mg ⊡ Riopan

Repan CF caplets ℞ *analgesic; barbiturate sedative* [acetaminophen; butalbital] 650•50 mg

Repetab (trademarked dosage form) *extended-release tablet*

repirinast USAN, INN *antiallergic; antiasthmatic*

Replagal ℞ *investigational (NDA filed) enzyme replacement therapy for Fabry disease* [agalsidase alfa]

Replens vaginal gel OTC *lubricant* [glycerin; mineral oil]

Replete ready-to-use liquid OTC *enteral nutritional therapy* [lactose-free formula]

rEPO (recombinant erythropoietin) [see: epoetin alfa; epoetin beta]

Reposans-10 capsules ℞ *benzodiazepine anxiolytic* [chlordiazepoxide HCl] 10 mg

repository corticotropin [see: corticotropin, repository]

repromicin USAN, INN *antibacterial*

Repronex powder for IM or subcu injection ℞ *ovulation stimulant for women; spermatogenesis stimulant for men* [menotropins] 75, 150 IU/ampule

reproterol INN, BAN *bronchodilator* [also: reproterol HCl]

reproterol HCl USAN *bronchodilator* [also: reproterol]

Requip film-coated tablets ℞ *dopamine agonist; antiparkinsonian; investigational* *for restless leg syndrome (RLS)* [ropinirole HCl] 0.25, 0.5, 1, 2, 4, 5 mg

Resaid sustained-release capsules ℞ *decongestant; antihistamine* [phenylpropanolamine HCl; chlorpheniramine maleate] 75•12 mg

Rescaps-D S.R. sustained-release capsules ℞ *antitussive; decongestant* [caramiphen edisylate; phenylpropanolamine HCl] 40•75 mg

rescimetol INN

rescinnamine NF, INN, BAN *antihypertensive; rauwolfia derivative*

Rescon liquid OTC *decongestant; antihistamine* [phenylpropanolamine HCl; chlorpheniramine maleate] 12.5•2 mg/5 mL

Rescon sustained-release capsules ℞ *decongestant; antihistamine* [pseudoephedrine HCl; chlorpheniramine maleate] 120•12 mg

Rescon JR controlled-release capsules ℞ *pediatric decongestant and antihistamine* [pseudoephedrine HCl; chlorpheniramine maleate] 60•4 mg

Rescon-DM liquid OTC *antitussive; decongestant; antihistamine* [dextromethorphan hydrobromide; pseudoephedrine HCl; chlorpheniramine maleate] 10•30•2 mg/5 mL

Rescon-ED controlled-release capsules ℞ *decongestant; antihistamine* [pseudoephedrine HCl; chlorpheniramine maleate] 120•8 mg

Rescon-GG liquid OTC *decongestant; expectorant* [phenylephrine HCl; guaifenesin] 5•100 mg/5 mL

Rescriptor tablets ℞ *antiretroviral; non-nucleoside reverse transcriptase inhibitor (NNRTI) for HIV-1* [delavirdine mesylate] 100, 200 mg

Rescue Pak (trademarked dosage form) *unit dose package*

Rescula eye drops ℞ *prostaglandin* $F_{2\alpha}$ *analogue for glaucoma and ocular hypertension* [unoprostone isopropyl] 0.15%

Resectisol solution ℞ *genitourinary irrigant* [mannitol] 5 g/100 mL

reserpine USP, INN *antihypertensive; peripheral antiadrenergic; rauwolfia derivative* 0.1, 0.25 mg oral

resibufogenin [see: bufogenin]

resiniferatoxin (RTX) *investigational (Phase II) neuronal desensitizing agent for urge incontinence*

Resinol ointment OTC *topical poison ivy treatment* [calamine; zinc oxide; resorcinol] 6%•12%•2%

resocortol butyrate USAN *topical anti-inflammatory*

Resol oral solution OTC *electrolyte replacement* [sodium, potassium, chloride, calcium, magnesium, and phosphate electrolytes]

Resolve/GP solution OTC *cleaning solution for hard or rigid gas permeable contact lenses*

resorantel INN

resorcin [see: resorcinol]

resorcin acetate [see: resorcinol monoacetate]

resorcin brown NF

resorcinol USP *keratolytic; antifungal*

resorcinol monoacetate USP *antiseborrheic; keratolytic*

Resource; Resource Plus ready-to-use liquid OTC *enteral nutritional therapy* [lactose-free formula]

ReSource Diabetic; ReSource Fruit Beverage; ReSource Just for Kids ready-to-use liquid in Brik Paks OTC *enteral nutritional therapy* [lactose-free formula] 237 mL

Resovist ℞ *investigational superparamagnetic diagnostic aid* [ferucarbotran]

Respa-1st sustained-release tablets ℞ *decongestant; expectorant* [pseudoephedrine HCl; guaifenesin] 58•600 mg

Respa-DM sustained-release tablets ℞ *antitussive; expectorant* [dextromethorphan hydrobromide; guaifenesin] 28•600 mg

Respa-GF sustained-release tablets ℞ *expectorant* [guaifenesin] 600 mg

Respahist sustained-release capsules ℞ *decongestant; antihistamine* [pseudoephedrine HCl; brompheniramine maleate] 60•6 mg

Respaire-60; Respaire-120 extended-release capsules ℞ *decongestant; expectorant* [pseudoephedrine HCl; guaifenesin] 60•200 mg; 120•250 mg

Respalor ready-to-use liquid OTC *enteral nutritional therapy for pulmonary problems*

Respbid sustained-release tablets ℞ *antiasthmatic; bronchodilator* [theophylline] 250, 500 mg

RespiGam IV infusion ℞ *preventative for respiratory syncytial virus (RSV) infections in high-risk infants (orphan); investigational (orphan) treatment for RSV* [respiratory syncytial virus immune globulin, solvent/detergent treated] 50 mg/mL

Respihaler (trademarked delivery system) *oral inhalation aerosol*

RespiPak (trademarked packaging form) *tablets in daily compliance packaging*

Respiracult-Strep culture paddles for professional use *in vitro diagnostic test for Group A streptococci from throat and nasopharyngeal sources*

respiratory syncytial virus immune globulin (RSV-IG) *preventative for respiratory syncytial virus (RSV) infections in high-risk infants (orphan); investigational (orphan) treatment for RSV*

Respirgard II (trademarked delivery system) *nebulizer*

Respules (trademarked delivery system) *single-dose ampule for inhalation*

Restasis eye drops ℞ *investigational (NDA filed, orphan) emulsion for Sjögren keratoconjunctivitis sicca* [cyclosporine] 0.05%

restoratives *a class of agents that promote a restoration of strength and vigor (a term used in folk medicine)*

Restore powder (discontinued 1999) OTC *bulk laxative* [psyllium hydrophilic mucilloid] 3.4 g/dose

Restoril capsules ℞ *benzodiazepine sedative; hypnotic* [temazepam] 7.5, 15, 30 mg ⊡ Risperdal; Vistaril; Zestril

Retavase powder for IV infusion ℞ *thrombolytic; tissue plasminogen activator (tPA) for acute myocardial infarction* [reteplase] 18.8 mg (10.8 IU)

retelliptine INN

reteplase USAN, INN *thrombolytic; tissue plasminogen activator (tPA) for acute myocardial infarction*

reticulose *investigational (Phase III) viral replication inhibitor for HIV and HPV (human papilloma virus)*

Retin-A cream, gel, liquid ℞ *topical keratolytic for acne* [tretinoin] 0.025%, 0.05%, 0.1% (0.01% available in Canada); 0.025%, 0.1%; 0.05%

Retin-A Micro gel ℞ *topical keratolytic for acne* [tretinoin] 0.1%

retinal pigmented epithelial cells, human, on collagen microcarriers *investigational (orphan) for stage 3 and 4 Parkinson disease*

retinamide R-II *investigational (orphan) for myelodysplastic syndrome*

retinoic acid (all-*trans*-retinoic acid) [see: tretinoin]

9-*cis*-retinoic acid [see: alitretinoin]

13-*cis*-retinoic acid [see: isotretinoin]

retinoids *a class of antineoplastics chemically related to vitamin A*

Retinol cream OTC *moisturizer; emollient* [vitamin A] 100 000 IU

retinol INN, BAN *vitamin* A_1

Retinol-A cream OTC *moisturizer; emollient* [vitamin A palmitate] 10 000 IU/g

Retrovir film-coated tablets, capsules, syrup, IV injection ℞ *nucleoside reverse transcriptase inhibitor (NRTI) antiviral for HIV, AIDS, and AIDS-related complex (orphan)* [zidovudine] 300 mg; 100 mg; 50 mg/5 mL; 10 mg/mL

Revasc ℞ *investigational thrombin inhibitor* [desirudin]

revenast INN

Reversa UV with Cosmederm-7 (CAN) cream, lip balm OTC *moisturizer; emollient; exfoliant; anti-irritant* [glycolic acid; strontium chloride] 4%•?, 8%•?; 2%•?

reverse transcriptase (RT) inhibitors *a class of antiretroviral drugs that inhibit the activity of reverse transcriptase in viral cells, preventing cell replication; subdivided into nucleoside (purine- or pyrimidine-based) and nonnucleoside types* [reverse transcriptase is also known as DNA polymerase]

reversible proton pump inhibitors [see: proton pump inhibitors]

Reversol IV or IM injection ℞ *myasthenia gravis treatment; antidote to curare overdose* [edrophonium chloride] 10 mg/mL

Revex IV, IM, or subcu injection ℞ *opioid antagonist for narcotic overdose* [nalmefene] 100 µg/mL, 1 mg/mL

Rēv-Eyes powder for eye drops ℞ *miotic to reverse iatrogenic mydriasis* [dapiprazole HCl] 0.5%

ReVia tablets ℞ *narcotic antagonist for opiate dependence or overdose (orphan) and alcoholism* [naltrexone HCl] 50 mg

revospirone INN, BAN

Rexigen Forte sustained-release capsules ℞ *anorexiant; CNS stimulant* [phendimetrazine tartrate] 105 mg

Rexolate IM injection ℞ *analgesic; antipyretic; anti-inflammatory; antirheumatic* [sodium thiosalicylate] 50 mg/mL

Rezamid lotion OTC *topical acne treatment* [sulfur; resorcinol; alcohol] 5%•2%•28%

Rezipas ℞ *investigational (orphan) for ulcerative colitis* [aminosalicylic acid]

Rezulin film-coated tablets (discontinued 2000) ℞ *thiazolidinedione antidiabetic; increases cellular response to insulin without increasing insulin secretion* [troglitazone] 200, 300, 400 mg

R-Frone ℞ *investigational (orphan) for metastatic renal cell carcinoma, malignant melanoma, and Kaposi sarcoma* [interferon beta-1a, recombinant]

rGCR (recombinant glucocerebrosidase) [see: glucocerebrosidase, recombinant retroviral vector]

rG-CSF (recombinant granulocyte colony-stimulating factor) [see: lenograstim]

R-Gel OTC *topical analgesic* [capsaicin] 0.025%

R-Gen elixir ℞ *expectorant* [iodinated glycerol] 60 mg/5 mL

R-gene 10 IV injection ℞ *diagnostic aid for pituitary (growth hormone) function* [arginine HCl] 10% (950 mOsm/L)

RGG0853, E1A lipid complex *investigational (orphan) for advanced ovarian cancer*

rGM-CSF; rhGM-CSF; rhuGM-CSF (granulocyte-macrophage colony-stimulating factor) [q.v.]

rgp160; rgp160 IIIB; rgp160 MN (recombinant glycoprotein) *investigational (Phase I–III) antiviral (treatment) and vaccine (preventative) for HIV* [also: AIDS vaccine]

Rh_0(D) immune globulin USP *passive immunizing agent; obstetric Rh factor immunity suppressant; treatment for immune thrombocytopenic purpura (ITP) (orphan)*

Rh_0(D) immune human globulin [now: Rh_0(D) immune globulin]

Rhamnus cathartica; R. frangula *medicinal herb* [see: buckthorn]

Rhamnus purshiana *medicinal herb* [see: cascara sagrada]

rhAPC (recombinant human activated protein C) [see: drotrecogin alfa]

rhATIII (recombinant human antithrombin III) [see: antithrombin III]

rHb1.1 (recombinant hemoglobin) [see: hemoglobin, recombinant human]

rhDNase (recombinant human deoxyribonuclease) [see: dornase alfa]

Rheaban caplets OTC *antidiarrheal; GI adsorbent* [activated attapulgite] 750 mg

rhenium *element (Re)*

Rheomacrodex IV infusion ℞ *plasma volume expander for shock due to hemorrhage, burns, or surgery* [dextran 40] 10%

RheothRx Copolymer (name changed to Flocor in 1998)

rheotran (45) [see: dextran 45]
rhetinic acid [see: enoxolone]
Rheum palmatum *medicinal herb* [see: rhubarb]
Rheumatex slide tests for professional use *in vitro diagnostic aid for rheumatoid factor in the blood* ⊠ Rheumatrex
rheumatism root *medicinal herb* [see: twin leaf; wild yam]
rheumatism weed *medicinal herb* [see: pipsissewa]
Rheumaton slide tests for professional use *in vitro diagnostic aid for rheumatoid factor in serum or synovial fluid*
Rheumatrex Dose Pack (tablets) ℞ *antimetabolite antineoplastic for leukemia; systemic antipsoriatic; antirheumatic; investigational (orphan) for juvenile rheumatoid arthritis* [methotrexate sodium] 2.5 mg ⊠ Rheumatex
rhFSH (recombinant human follicle-stimulating hormone) [see: menotropins]
rhGH (recombinant human growth hormone) [see: somatropin]
rhIGF-1 (recombinant human insulin-like growth factor-1) [now: mecasermin]
rhIL-1R; rhu IL-1R (recombinant human interleukin-1 receptor) [see: interleukin-1 receptor]
rhIL-11 (recombinant human interleukin-11) [see: interleukin-11, recombinant human]
rhIL-12 (recombinant human interleukin-12) [see: interleukin-12]
Rhinall nasal spray, nose drops OTC *nasal decongestant* [phenylephrine HCl] 0.25%
Rhinatate tablets ℞ *decongestant; antihistamine* [phenylephrine tannate; chlorpheniramine tannate; pyrilamine tannate] 25•8•25 mg
Rhinocaps capsules OTC *decongestant; analgesic; antipyretic* [phenylpropanolamine HCl; acetaminophen; aspirin] 20•162•162 mg
Rhinocort nasal inhalation aerosol ℞ *corticosteroidal anti-inflammatory for seasonal or perennial rhinitis* [budesonide] 32 µg/dose
Rhinocort (CAN) Turbuhaler (dry powder in a metered-dose inhaler) ℞ *intranasal steroidal anti-inflammatory* [budesonide] 100 µg/dose
Rhinocort Aqua nasal spray ℞ *intranasal steroidal anti-inflammatory* [budesonide] 32 µg/spray
Rhinolar-EX; Rhinolar-EX 12 sustained-release capsules ℞ *decongestant; antihistamine* [phenylpropanolamine HCl; chlorpheniramine maleate] 75•8 mg; 75•12 mg
Rhinosyn; Rhinosyn-PD liquid OTC *decongestant; antihistamine* [pseudoephedrine HCl; chlorpheniramine maleate; alcohol] 60•4 mg/5 mL; 30•2 mg/5 mL
Rhinosyn-DM liquid OTC *antitussive; decongestant; antihistamine* [dextromethorphan hydrobromide; pseudoephedrine HCl; chlorpheniramine maleate; alcohol 1.4%] 15•30•2 mg/5 mL
Rhinosyn-DMX syrup OTC *antitussive; expectorant* [dextromethorphan hydrobromide; guaifenesin] 15•100 mg/5 mL
Rhinosyn-X liquid OTC *antitussive; decongestant; expectorant* [dextromethorphan hydrobromide; pseudoephedrine HCl; guaifenesin; alcohol 7.5%] 10•30•100 mg/5 mL
rhodine [see: aspirin]
rhodium *element (Rh)*
Rho-Fluphenazine Decanoate (CAN) subcu or IM injection ℞ *conventional (typical) antipsychotic* [fluphenazine decanoate] 25, 100 mg/mL
RhoGAM IM injection ℞ *obstetric Rh factor immunity suppressant* [Rh_0(D) immune globulin] 300 µg
Rhoxal-amiodarone (CAN) tablets ℞ *antiarrhythmic for acute ventricular tachycardia and fibrillation (orphan)* [amiodarone HCl] 200 mg
Rhoxal-diltiazem CD (CAN) (once daily) sustained-release capsules ℞ *antihypertensive; antianginal; antiarrhythmic;*

calcium channel blocker [diltiazem HCl] 120, 180, 240, 300 mg

Rhoxal-famotidine (CAN) film-coated tablets ℞ *histamine H_2 antagonist for gastric and duodenal ulcers* [famotidine] 20, 40 mg

Rhoxal-fluoxetine (CAN) capsules ℞ *selective serotonin reuptake inhibitor (SSRI) for depression, obsessive-compulsive disorder (OCD), and bulimia nervosa* [fluoxetine HCl] 10, 20 mg

Rhoxal-minocycline (CAN) capsules ℞ *tetracycline antibiotic* [minocycline HCl] 50, 100 mg

Rhoxal-orphenadrine (CAN) sustained-release tablets ℞ *skeletal muscle relaxant* [orphenadrine citrate] 100 mg

Rhoxal-oxaprozin (CAN) film-coated caplets ℞ *antiarthritic; nonsteroidal anti-inflammatory drug (NSAID)* [oxaprozin] 600 mg

Rhoxal-ranitidine (CAN) film-coated tablets ℞ *histamine H_2 antagonist for gastric and duodenal ulcers* [ranitidine HCl] 150, 300 mg

Rhoxal-ticlopidine (CAN) film-coated tablets ℞ *platelet aggregation inhibitor for stroke* [ticlopidine HCl] 250 mg

Rhoxal-timolol (CAN) eye drops ℞ *topical antiglaucoma agent (β-blocker)* [timolol maleate] 0.25%, 0.5%

Rhoxal-valproic (CAN) capsules, enteric-coated capsules ℞ *anticonvulsant* [valproic acid] 250 mg; 500 mg

rhubarb *(Rheum palmatum)* root *medicinal herb for colon and liver disorders*

Rhuli gel OTC *topical poison ivy treatment* [benzyl alcohol; menthol; camphor] 2%•0.3%•0.3%

Rhuli spray OTC *topical poison ivy treatment* [benzocaine; calamine; camphor] 5%•13.8%•0.7%

rhuMAb-E25 [now: omalizumab]

rhuMAb-VEGF *investigational (Phase III) recombinant humanized monoclonal antibody to vascular endothelial growth factor used in combination with chemotherapy to treat colorectal and non–small cell lung cancer (NSCLC)*

Rhus glabra *medicinal herb* [see: sumach]

Riba 3.0 SIA reagent kit for professional use *in vitro diagnostic aid for hepatitis* C [strip immunoblot assay (SIA)]

ribaminol USAN, INN *memory adjuvant*

ribavirin USP, INN *antiviral for severe lower respiratory tract infections; investigational (Phase II/III) for HIV; investigational (orphan) for hemorrhagic fever with renal syndrome* [also: tribavirin]

Ribes nigrum; R. rubrum *medicinal herb* [see: currant]

ribgrass; ribwort *medicinal herb* [see: plantain]

riboflavin (vitamin B_2) USP, INN *water-soluble vitamin; enzyme cofactor* 50, 100 mg oral

riboflavin 5′-phosphate sodium USP *vitamin*

riboflavine [see: riboflavin]

riboprine USAN, INN *antineoplastic*

ribostamycin INN, BAN

riboxamide [see: tiazofurin]

ricainide [see: indecainide HCl]

rice bran oil (gamma oryzanol) extract *medicinal herb used as a hypolipidemic and to treat gastrointestinal and menopausal symptoms*

richweed *medicinal herb* [see: black cohosh; stone root]

ricin (blocked) conjugated murine MAb (anti-B4) *investigational (orphan) for B-cell lymphoma, leukemia, and treatment of bone marrow in non-T-cell ALL; clinical trials discontinued 1997*

ricin (blocked) conjugated murine MAb (anti-MY9) *investigational (orphan) for myeloid leukemia (including AML), ex vivo treatment of autologous bone marrow in AML, and blast crisis in CML*

ricin (blocked) conjugated murine MAb (CD6) *investigational (orphan) for T-cell leukemias, lymphomas, and other mature T-cell malignancies*

ricin (blocked) conjugated murine MAb (N901) *investigational (orphan) for small cell lung cancer*

RID liquid OTC *pediculicide for lice* [pyrethrins; piperonyl butoxide; petroleum distillate] 0.3%•3%•1.2%

RID mousse (aerosol foam) OTC *pediculicide for lice* [pyrethrins; piperonyl butoxide] 0.33%•4%

Rid-A-Pain gel OTC *topical oral anesthetic* [benzocaine] 10%

Rid-a-Pain-HP cream OTC *topical analgesic* [capsaicin] 0.075%

Ridaura capsules ℞ *antirheumatic* [auranofin] 3 mg

ridazolol INN

RIDD (recombinant interleukin-2, dacarbazine, DDP) *chemotherapy protocol*

Ridenol elixir OTC *analgesic; antipyretic* [acetaminophen] 80 mg/5 mL

ridogrel USAN, INN, BAN *thromboxane synthetase inhibitor*

rifabutin USAN, INN *antiviral; antibacterial; for prevention of* Mycobacterium avium *complex (MAC) in advanced HIV patients (orphan)*

Rifadin capsules, powder for IV injection ℞ *tuberculostatic (orphan)* [rifampin] 150, 300 mg; 600 mg ⑨ Ritalin

rifalazil USAN *investigational (Phase II) rifampin derivative for* Mycobacterium avium *complex (MAC) and* Mycobacterium tuberculosis

Rifamate capsules ℞ *tuberculostatic* [rifampin; isoniazid] 300•150 mg

rifametane USAN, INN *antibacterial*

rifamexil USAN *antibacterial*

rifamide USAN, INN *antibacterial*

rifampicin INN, BAN, JAN *antibacterial* [also: rifampin]

rifampin USAN, USP *antibacterial; antituberculosis agent (orphan)* [also: rifampicin] 150, 300 mg oral

rifampin & isoniazid & pyrazinamide *short-course treatment of tuberculosis (orphan)*

rifamycin INN, BAN

rifamycin diethylamide [see: rifamide]

rifamycin M-14 [see: rifamide]

rifapentine USAN, INN, BAN *antibacterial for tuberculosis (orphan); investigational (orphan) for AIDS-related* Mycobacterium avium *complex (MAC)*

Rifater tablets ℞ *short-course treatment for tuberculosis (orphan)* [rifampin; isoniazid; pyrazinamide] 120•50•300 mg

rifaxidin [see: rifaximin]

Rifaximin ℞ *investigational (Phase III) antibiotic for bacterial infectious diarrhea (BID)* [ritamycin]

rifaximin USAN, INN *antibacterial; investigational (orphan) for hepatic encephalopathy*

rIFN-A (recombinant interferon alfa) [see: interferon alfa-2a, recombinant]

rIFN-α2 (recombinant interferon alfa-2) [see: interferon alfa-2b, recombinant]

rIFN-B (recombinant interferon beta) [see: interferon beta-1b, recombinant]

rIFN-beta ℞ *investigational (orphan) for malignant melanoma, metastatic renal cell carcinoma, T-cell lymphoma, and Kaposi sarcoma* [interferon beta, recombinant]

rifomycin [see: rifamycin]

RIG (rabies immune globulin) [q.v.]

RIGScan *investigational imaging agent*

rilapine INN

rilmazafone INN

rilmenidine INN

rilopirox INN

rilozarone INN

Rilutek film-coated tablets ℞ *amyotrophic lateral sclerosis (ALS) treatment (orphan); investigational (orphan) for Huntington disease; investigational (Phase III) for Parkinson disease* [riluzole] 50 mg

riluzole USAN, INN *amyotrophic lateral sclerosis (ALS) treatment (orphan); investigational (orphan) for Huntington disease; investigational (Phase III) for Parkinson disease*

Rimactane capsules ℞ *tuberculostatic* [rifampin] 300 mg

Rimadyl (approved but not currently being marketed) ℞ *nonsteroidal anti-*

inflammatory drug (NSAID); analgesic; antipyretic [carprofen]

rimantadine INN *antiviral for prophylaxis and treatment of influenza A infections* [also: rimantadine HCl]

rimantadine HCl USAN *antiviral for prophylaxis and treatment of influenza A infections* [also: rimantadine]

rimazolium metilsulfate INN

rimcazole INN *antipsychotic* [also: rimcazole HCl]

rimcazole HCl USAN *antipsychotic* [also: rimcazole]

rimexolone USAN, INN, BAN *ophthalmic corticosteroidal anti-inflammatory*

rimiterol INN *bronchodilator* [also: rimiterol hydrobromide]

rimiterol hydrobromide USAN *bronchodilator* [also: rimiterol]

rimoprogin INN

Rimso-50 solution for bladder instillation ℞ *anti-inflammatory for symptomatic relief of interstitial cystitis* [dimethyl sulfoxide (DMSO)] 50%

Rinade B.I.D. sustained-release capsules ℞ *decongestant; antihistamine* [pseudoephedrine HCl; chlorpheniramine maleate] 120•8 mg

Ringer injection USP *fluid and electrolyte replenisher* [also: compound solution of sodium chloride]

Ringer injection, lactated USP *fluid and electrolyte replenisher; systemic alkalizer* [also: compound solution of sodium lactate]

Ringer irrigation USP *irrigation solution*

Ringer solution [now: Ringer's irrigation]

riodipine INN

Riopan suspension OTC *antacid* [magaldrate] 540 mg/5 mL

Riopan Plus chewable tablets, oral suspension OTC *antacid; antiflatulent* [magaldrate; simethicone] 480•20, 1080•20 mg; 540•40, 1080•40 mg/5 mL

rioprostil USAN, INN *gastric antisecretory*

ripazepam USAN, INN *minor tranquilizer*

ripple grass *medicinal herb* [see: plantain]

risedronate sodium USAN *bisphosphonate bone resorption inhibitor for Paget disease and treatment or prevention of postmenopausal and glucocorticoid-induced osteoporosis*

rismorelin porcine USAN *growth stimulant for growth hormone deficiencies*

risocaine USAN, INN *local anesthetic*

risotilide HCl USAN *antiarrhythmic*

Risperdal long-acting injection ℞ *investigational (NDA filed) delivery form* [risperidone (encapsulated in polymer microspheres)] ⊡ Restoril

Risperdal tablets, oral drops ℞ *novel (atypical) antipsychotic* [risperidone] 0.25, 0.5, 1, 2, 3, 4 mg; 1 mg/mL ⊡ Restoril

risperidone USAN, INN, BAN *benzisoxazole antipsychotic; neuroleptic*

ristianol INN, BAN *immunoregulator* [also: ristianol phosphate]

ristianol phosphate USAN *immunoregulator* [also: ristianol]

ristocetin USP, INN, BAN

Ritadex ℞ *investigational (NDA filed) CNS stimulant for attention-deficit hyperactivity disorder (ADHD) and narcolepsy* [dexmethylphenidate HCl]

Ritalin tablets ℞ *CNS stimulant for attention-deficit hyperactivity disorder (ADHD) and narcolepsy; also abused as a street drug* [methylphenidate HCl] 5, 10, 20 mg ⊡ Ismelin; Rifadin

Ritalin-SR sustained-release tablets ℞ *CNS stimulant for attention-deficit hyperactivity disorder (ADHD) and narcolepsy* [methylphenidate HCl] 20 mg

ritamycin *investigational (Phase III) antibiotic for bacterial infectious diarrhea (BID)*

ritanserin USAN, INN, BAN *serotonin S_2 antagonist; investigational agent for various psychiatric illnesses and substance abuse* 10 mg oral

ritiometan INN

ritodrine USAN, INN *smooth muscle relaxant*

ritodrine HCl USAN, USP *smooth muscle relaxant; uterine relaxant to arrest preterm labor* 0.3, 10, 15 mg/mL injection

ritolukast USAN, INN *antiasthmatic; leukotriene antagonist*

ritonavir USAN, INN *antiviral protease inhibitor for HIV infection*

ritonavir & lamivudine & saquinavir mesylate *investigational (Phase II) protease inhibitor and nucleoside reverse transcriptase inhibitor combination for HIV infection*

ritonavir & zidovudine & saquinavir mesylate *investigational (Phase II) protease inhibitor combination for HIV infection*

ritropirronium bromide INN

ritrosulfan INN

Rituxan IV infusion ℞ *monoclonal antibody for non-Hodgkin B-cell lymphoma (orphan)* [rituximab] 10 mg/mL

rituximab USAN *monoclonal antibody for non-Hodgkin B-cell lymphoma (orphan)*

Riva-Diclofenac (CAN) enteric-coated tablets ℞ *analgesic; antiarthritic; nonsteroidal anti-inflammatory drug (NSAID)* [diclofenac sodium] 50 mg

Riva-Diclofenac-K (CAN) film-coated slow-release tablets ℞ *analgesic; antiarthritic; nonsteroidal anti-inflammatory drug (NSAID)* [diclofenac potassium] 75 mg

Riva-Loperamide (CAN) caplets OTC *antidiarrheal* [loperamide HCl] 2 mg

Riva-Lorazepam (CAN) tablets ℞ *benzodiazepine anxiolytic* [lorazepam] 0.5, 1, 2 mg

Riva-Naproxen (CAN) tablets ℞ *analgesic; antiarthritic; nonsteroidal anti-inflammatory drug (NSAID)* [naproxen] 250, 375, 500 mg

Riva-Norfloxacin (CAN) film-coated tablets ℞ *broad-spectrum fluoroquinolone antibiotic* [norfloxacin] 400 mg

rivastigmine USAN *acetylcholinesterase inhibitor to increase cognition in Alzheimer disease*

rivastigmine tartrate *acetylcholinesterase inhibitor to increase cognition in Alzheimer disease*

rivoglitazone USAN *antidiabetic for type 2 diabetes*

rizatriptan benzoate USAN *vascular serotonin 5-HT_1 receptor agonist for migraine headache*

rizatriptan sulfate USAN *vascular serotonin 5-HT_1 receptor agonist for migraine headache*

rizolipase INN

r-metHuLeptin [see: metreleptin]

RMP-7 (receptor-mediated permeabilizer) [see: lobradimil]

RMS suppositories ℞ *narcotic analgesic* [morphine sulfate] 5, 10, 20, 30 mg

rNPA (recombinant novel plasminogen activator) [see: novel plasminogen activator]

rob elder *medicinal herb* [see: elderberry]

Robafen AC Cough syrup ℞ *narcotic antitussive; expectorant* [codeine phosphate; guaifenesin; alcohol 3.5%] 10•100 mg/5 mL

Robafen CF liquid OTC *antitussive; decongestant; expectorant* [dextromethorphan hydrobromide; phenylpropanolamine HCl; guaifenesin] 10•12.5•100 mg/5 mL

Robafen DAC syrup ℞ *narcotic antitussive; decongestant; expectorant* [codeine phosphate; pseudoephedrine HCl; guaifenesin; alcohol 1.4%] 10•30•100 mg/5 mL

Robafen DM syrup OTC *antitussive; expectorant* [dextromethorphan hydrobromide; guaifenesin; alcohol 1.4%] 10•100 mg/5 mL

RoBathol Bath Oil OTC *bath emollient*

Robaxin tablets, IV or IM injection ℞ *skeletal muscle relaxant* [methocarbamol] 500, 750 mg; 100 mg/mL

Robaxisal tablets ℞ *skeletal muscle relaxant; analgesic* [methocarbamol; aspirin] 400•325 mg ⊡ Robaxacet

robenidine INN *coccidiostat for poultry* [also: robenidine HCl]

robenidine HCl USAN *coccidiostat for poultry* [also: robenidine]

Robicap (trademarked dosage form) *capsule*

Robicillin VK tablets (discontinued 1998) ℞ *natural penicillin antibiotic* [penicillin V potassium] 250, 500 mg

Robimycin Robitabs (enteric-coated tablets) (discontinued 1998) ℞ *macrolide antibiotic* [erythromycin] 250 mg

Robinul tablets, IV or IM injection ℞ *GI antispasmodic; anticholinergic; peptic ulcer treatment adjunct; antisecretory* [glycopyrrolate] 1 mg; 0.2 mg/5 mL

Robinul Forte tablets ℞ *GI antispasmodic; anticholinergic; peptic ulcer treatment adjunct; antisecretory* [glycopyrrolate] 2 mg

Robitab (trademarked dosage form) *tablet*

Robitet Robicaps (capsules) (discontinued 1997) ℞ *broad-spectrum antibiotic* [tetracycline HCl] 250, 500 mg

Robitussin syrup OTC *expectorant* [guaifenesin; alcohol 3.5%] 100 mg/5 mL

Robitussin A-C syrup ℞ *narcotic antitussive; expectorant* [codeine phosphate; guaifenesin; alcohol 3.5%] 10•100 mg/5 mL

Robitussin Cold & Cough Liqui-Gels (capsules) OTC *antitussive; decongestant; expectorant* [dextromethorphan hydrobromide; pseudoephedrine HCl; guaifenesin] 10•30•200 mg

Robitussin Cough Calmers lozenge OTC *antitussive* [dextromethorphan hydrobromide] 5 mg

Robitussin Cough & Cold; Robitussin Pediatric Cough & Cold liquid OTC *antitussive; decongestant* [dextromethorphan hydrobromide; pseudoephedrine HCl] 15•30 mg/5 mL; 7.5•15 mg/5 mL

Robitussin Cough Drops lozenge OTC *topical analgesic; mild anesthetic* [menthol] 7.4, 10 mg

Robitussin Honey Cough DM (CAN) honey-based syrup OTC *antitussive* [dextromethorphan hydrobromide] 10 mg/5 mL

Robitussin Liquid Center Cough Drops lozenges OTC *topical analgesic; counterirritant; mild local anesthetic* [menthol] 10 mg

Robitussin Night Relief liquid OTC *antitussive; decongestant; antihistamine; analgesic* [dextromethorphan hydrobromide; pseudoephedrine HCl; pyrilamine maleate; acetaminophen] 5•10•8.3•108.3 mg/5 mL

Robitussin Pediatric liquid OTC *antitussive* [dextromethorphan hydrobromide] 7.5 mg/5 mL

Robitussin Severe Congestion Liqui-Gels (capsules) OTC *decongestant; expectorant* [pseudoephedrine HCl; guaifenesin] 30•200 mg

Robitussin-CF liquid OTC *antitussive; decongestant; expectorant* [dextromethorphan hydrobromide; phenylpropanolamine HCl; guaifenesin; alcohol 4.75%] 10•12.5•100 mg/5 mL

Robitussin-DAC syrup ℞ *narcotic antitussive; decongestant; expectorant* [codeine phosphate; pseudoephedrine HCl; guaifenesin; alcohol 1.9%] 10•30•100 mg/5 mL

Robitussin-DM liquid OTC *antitussive; expectorant* [dextromethorphan hydrobromide; guaifenesin] 10•100 mg/5 mL

Robitussin-PE syrup OTC *decongestant; expectorant* [pseudoephedrine HCl; guaifenesin; alcohol 1.4%] 30•100 mg/5 mL

Rocaltrol capsules, oral solution ℞ *vitamin D therapy for hypoparathyroidism and hypocalcemia of chronic renal dialysis; decreases severity of psoriatic lesions* [calcitriol] 0.25, 0.5 μg; 1 μg/mL

rocastine INN *antihistamine* [also: rocastine HCl]

rocastine HCl USAN *antihistamine* [also: rocastine]

Rocephin powder or frozen premix for IV or IM injection ℞ *cephalosporin antibiotic* [ceftriaxone sodium] 0.25, 0.5, 1, 2, 10 g

rochelle salt [see: potassium sodium tartrate]

rociverine INN

rock brake; rock polypod *medicinal herb* [see: female fern]

rock elm *medicinal herb* [see: slippery elm]

rock parsley *medicinal herb* [see: parsley]

rock rose *(Helianthemum canadense)* plant *medicinal herb used as an astringent and tonic*

Rocky Mountain grape *medicinal herb* [see: Oregon grape]

Rocky Mountain spotted fever vaccine USP

rocuronium bromide USAN, INN, BAN *neuromuscular blocking agent*

R.O.-Dexsone (CAN) eye drops (discontinued 1998) ℞ *topical ophthalmic corticosteroidal anti-inflammatory* [dexamethasone sodium phosphate] 0.1%

rodocaine USAN, INN *local anesthetic*

rodorubicin INN

rofecoxib *analgesic; antiarthritic; antipyretic; COX-2 inhibitor; nonsteroidal anti-inflammatory drug (NSAID)*

rofelodine INN

Roferon-A subcu or IM injection, prefilled syringes ℞ *antineoplastic/antiviral for hairy cell leukemia, Kaposi sarcoma (orphan), and chronic myelogenous leukemia (orphan); investigational (orphan) for renal cell carcinoma* [interferon alfa-2a] 3, 6, 9, 36 million IU/mL; 6, 9 million IU/0.5 mL

roflurane USAN, INN *inhalation anesthetic*

Rogaine for Men; Rogaine for Women; Rogaine Extra Strength for Men topical solution OTC *hair growth stimulant* [minoxidil] 2%; 2%; 5% 🔊 Rēgain

rogletimide USAN, INN, BAN *antineoplastic; aromatase inhibitor*

Rohypnol (not approved for use in the U.S.) ℞ *sedative and hypnotic; smuggled into the U.S. as a street drug, commonly called "roofies" or "the date rape drug"* [flunitrazepam]

rokitamycin INN

Rolaids, Calcium Rich chewable tablets OTC *antacid* [magnesium hydroxide; calcium carbonate] 80•412 mg

Rolatuss Expectorant liquid ℞ *narcotic antitussive; decongestant; antihistamine; expectorant* [codeine phosphate; phenylephrine HCl; chlorpheniramine maleate; ammonium chloride; alcohol 5%] 9.85•5•2•33.3 mg/5 mL

Rolatuss Plain liquid OTC *decongestant; antihistamine* [phenylephrine HCl; chlorpheniramine maleate; alcohol 5%] 5•2 mg/5 mL

Rolatuss with Hydrocodone liquid ℞ *narcotic antitussive; decongestant; antihistamine* [hydrocodone bitartrate; phenylpropanolamine HCl; phenylephrine HCl; pyrilamine maleate; pheniramine maleate] 1.7•3.3•5•3.3•3.3 mg/5 mL

Rolazar ℞ *investigational antineoplastic* [pemetrexed disodium]

roletamide USAN, INN *hypnotic*

rolgamidine USAN, INN, BAN *antidiarrheal*

rolicton [see: amisometradine]

rolicyclidine INN

rolicypram BAN *antidepressant* [also: rolicyprine]

rolicyprine USAN, INN *antidepressant* [also: rolicypram]

rolipram USAN, INN *tranquilizer*

rolitetracycline USAN, USP, INN *antibacterial*

rolitetracycline nitrate USAN *antibacterial*

rolodine USAN, INN *skeletal muscle relaxant*

rolziracetam INN, BAN

Roman camomile *medicinal herb* [see: chamomile]

Roman laurel *medicinal herb* [see: laurel]

romazarit USAN, INN, BAN *anti-inflammatory; antirheumatic*

Romazicon IV injection ℞ *benzodiazepine antagonist to reverse anesthesia or treat overdose* [flumazenil] 0.1 mg/mL

rometin [see: clioquinol]

romifenone INN

romifidine INN

Romilar AC oral liquid ℞ *narcotic antitussive; expectorant* [codeine phosphate; guaifenesin] 10•100 mg/5 mL

romurtide INN

ronactolol INN

Rondamine-DM pediatric drops ℞ *pediatric antitussive, decongestant, and antihistamine* [dextromethorphan hydrobromide; pseudoephedrine

HCl; carbinoxamine maleate] 4•25•2 mg/5 mL

Rondec chewable tablets ℞ *decongestant; antihistamine* [pseudoephedrine HCl; brompheniramine maleate] 60•4 mg

Rondec film-coated tablets, syrup, pediatric drops ℞ *decongestant; antihistamine* [pseudoephedrine HCl; carbinoxamine maleate] 60•4 mg; 60•4 mg/5 mL; 25•2 mg/mL

Rondec-DM syrup, pediatric drops ℞ *antitussive; decongestant; antihistamine* [dextromethorphan hydrobromide; pseudoephedrine HCl; carbinoxamine maleate] 15•60•4 mg/5 mL; 4•25•2 mg/mL

Rondec-TR timed-release Filmtabs (film-coated tablets) ℞ *decongestant; antihistamine* [pseudoephedrine HCl; carbinoxamine maleate] 120•8 mg

ronidazole USAN, INN *antiprotozoal*

ronifibrate INN

ronipamil INN

ronnel USAN *systemic insecticide* [also: fenclofos; fenchlorphos]

ropinirole INN, BAN *dopamine agonist; antiparkinsonian* [also: ropinirole HCl]

ropinirole HCl USAN *dopamine agonist; antiparkinsonian* [also: ropinirole]

ropitoin INN *antiarrhythmic* [also: ropitoin HCl]

ropitoin HCl USAN *antiarrhythmic* [also: ropitoin]

ropivacaine INN *long-acting local anesthetic*

ropivacaine HCl *long-acting local anesthetic*

ropizine USAN, INN *anticonvulsant*

roquinimex USAN, INN *investigational (Phase II) immunomodulator for HIV; investigational for bone marrow transplant for leukemia; clinical trials for MS discontinued 1997; orphan status withdrawn 1998*

***Rosa acicularis; R. canina; R. rugosa* and other species** *medicinal herb* [see: rose]

rosamicin [now: rosaramicin]

rosamicin butyrate [now: rosaramicin butyrate]

rosamicin propionate [now: rosaramicin propionate]

rosamicin sodium phosphate [now: rosaramicin sodium phosphate]

rosamicin stearate [now: rosaramicin stearate]

rosaprostol INN

rosaramicin USAN, INN *antibacterial*

rosaramicin butyrate USAN *antibacterial*

rosaramicin propionate USAN *antibacterial*

rosaramicin sodium phosphate USAN *antibacterial*

rosaramicin stearate USAN *antibacterial*

rosary pea *medicinal herb* [see: precatory bean]

rose (*Rosa acicularis; R. canina; R. rugosa* and other species) flowers and hips *medicinal herb for blood cleansing, cancer, colds, flu, infections, and sore throat; also used as a diuretic, mild laxative, and source of vitamin C*

rose, sun *medicinal herb* [see: rock rose]

rose bengal *diagnostic aid for corneal injury and pathology* 1.3 mg/strip

rose bengal sodium (^{131}I) INN *hepatic function test; radioactive agent* [also: rose bengal sodium I 131]

rose bengal sodium I 125 USAN *radioactive agent*

rose bengal sodium I 131 USAN, USP *hepatic function test; radioactive agent* [also: rose bengal sodium (^{131}I)]

rose laurel *medicinal herb* [see: mountain laurel]

rose oil NF *perfume*

rose petal aqueous infusion *ocular emollient*

rose water, stronger NF *perfume*

rose water ointment USP *emollient; ointment base*

rosemary *(Rosmarinus officinalis)* leaves *medicinal herb for flatulence, gastrointestinal spasm, halitosis, heart tonic, inducing diaphoresis, migraine headache, promoting menstrual flow, stimulating abortion, and stomach disorders*

Rosets ophthalmic strips OTC *corneal disclosing agent* [rose bengal] 1.3 mg
rosiglitazone maleate USAN *thiazolidinedione antidiabetic; increases cellular response to insulin without increasing insulin secretion*
rosin USP
rosoxacin USAN, INN *antibacterial* [also: acrosoxacin]
rostaporfin USAN *investigational (Phase III) photosensitizer for wet age-related macular degeneration (AMD); investigational (Phase III) treatment for various cancers by photodynamic therapy*
rosterolone INN
rosuvastatin calcium USAN *investigational (NDA filed) HMG-CoA reductase inhibitor for hyperlipidemia*
Rotacaps (trademarked form) *encapsulated powder for inhalation*
Rotadisk (trademarked dosage form) *powder for inhalation* [used in a Diskhaler]
rotamicillin INN
Rotamune ℞ *investigational oral rotavirus vaccine*
RotaShield powder for oral liquid (discontinued 1999) ℞ *immunization against gastroenteritis in infants* [rotavirus vaccine, live] 2.5 mL
rotavirus vaccine *live oral immunization against gastroenteritis in infants*
rotoxamine USAN, INN *antihistamine*
rotoxamine tartrate NF
rotraxate INN
round-leaved plantain *medicinal herb* [see: plantain]
rovelizumab USAN *immunomodulator; immunoglobulin G4 monoclonal antibody; investigational (Phase III) cell adhesion inhibitor for acute ischemic stroke*
Rowasa suppositories, rectal suspension enema ℞ *anti-inflammatory for active ulcerative colitis, proctosigmoiditis and proctitis* [mesalamine] 500 mg; 4 g/60 mL
roxadimate USAN, INN *sunscreen*
Roxanol suppositories ℞ *narcotic analgesic* [morphine sulfate] 5, 10, 20, 30 mg
Roxanol; Roxanol 100; Roxanol Rescudose; Roxanol T; Roxanol UD oral solution ℞ *narcotic analgesic* [morphine sulfate] 20 mg/mL; 100 mg/5 mL; 10 mg/2.5 mL; 20 mg/mL; 10 mg/2.5 mL, 20 mg/5 mL, 30 mg/1.5 mL
roxarsone USAN, INN *antibacterial*
roxatidine INN, BAN *histamine H_2 antagonist for gastric and duodenal ulcers* [also: roxatidine acetate HCl]
roxatidine acetate HCl USAN *histamine H_2 antagonist for gastric and duodenal ulcers* [also: roxatidine]
roxibolone INN
Roxicet tablets, oral solution ℞ *narcotic analgesic* [oxycodone HCl; acetaminophen] 5•325 mg; 5•325 mg/5 mL
Roxicet 5/500 caplets ℞ *narcotic analgesic* [oxycodone HCl; acetaminophen] 5•500 mg
Roxicodone tablets, oral solution, Intensol (concentrated oral solution) ℞ *narcotic analgesic* [oxycodone HCl] 5, 15, 30 mg; 5 mg/5 mL; 20 mg/mL
roxifiban acetate USAN *antithrombotic; fibrinogen receptor antagonist*
Roxilox capsules ℞ *narcotic analgesic* [oxycodone HCl; acetaminophen] 5•500 mg
Roxin ℞ *investigational (NDA filed) histamine H_2 antagonist for duodenal and gastric ulcers* [roxatidine acetate HCl]
roxindole INN
Roxiprin tablets ℞ *narcotic analgesic* [oxycodone HCl; oxycodone terephthalate; aspirin] 4.5•0.38•325 mg
roxithromycin USAN, INN *antibacterial*
roxolonium metilsulfate INN
roxoperone INN
royal jelly *natural remedy for improving fertility and increasing longevity*
rp24 *investigational antiviral for AIDS* [also: AIDS vaccine]
rPA; r-PA (recombinant plasminogen activator) *more properly called "recombinant tissue plasminogen activator" (rtPA)* [see: alteplase; anistreplase; lanoteplase; monteplase; reteplase; saruplase; tenecteplase]

rPAF-AH (recombinant platelet-activating factor acetylhydrolase) [see: platelet-activating factor acetylhydrolase, recombinant]

RPI-4610 *investigational anticancer agent*

r-ProUK ℞ *investigational (Phase III) prourokinase clot-dissolving agent for stroke* [saruplase, recombinant]

R/S lotion OTC *topical acne treatment* [sulfur; resorcinol; alcohol] 5%•2%•28%

RSD-921 *investigational (Phase II) local anesthetic and antiarrhythmic*

RSV-IG (respiratory syncytial virus immune globulin) [q.v.]

RT (reverse transcriptase) inhibitors [q.v.]

R-Tanna 12 oral suspension ℞ *decongestant; antihistamine* [phenylephrine tannate; pyrilamine tannate] 5•30 mg/5 mL

R-Tannamine tablets, pediatric oral suspension ℞ *decongestant; antihistamine* [phenylephrine tannate; chlorpheniramine tannate; pyrilamine tannate] 25•8•25 mg; 5•2•12.5 mg/5 mL

R-Tannate tablets, pediatric oral suspension ℞ *decongestant; antihistamine* [phenylephrine tannate; chlorpheniramine tannate; pyrilamine tannate] 25•8•25 mg; 5•2•12.5 mg/5 mL

R-Tannic-S A/D oral suspension ℞ *decongestant; antihistamine* [phenylephrine tannate; pyrilamine tannate] 5•30 mg/5 mL

rtPA; rt-PA (recombinant tissue plasminogen activator) [see: alteplase; anistreplase; lanoteplase; monteplase; reteplase; saruplase; tenecteplase]

RTX (resiniferatoxin) [q.v.]

Rubazyme reagent kit for professional use *in vitro diagnostic aid for rubella virus IgG antibodies in serum* [enzyme immunoassay (EIA)]

rubbing alcohol [see: alcohol, rubbing]

rubbing isopropyl alcohol [see: isopropyl alcohol, rubbing]

rubefacients *a class of gentle local irritants that redden the skin by producing active or passive hyperemia*

rubella & mumps virus vaccine, live *active immunizing agent for rubella and mumps*

rubella virus vaccine, live USP *active immunizing agent for rubella*

rubeola vaccine [see: measles virus vaccine, live]

Rubex powder for IV injection ℞ *anthracycline antibiotic antineoplastic* [doxorubicin HCl] 50, 100 mg

rubidium *element (Rb)*

rubidium chloride Rb 82 USAN *radioactive diagnostic aid for cardiac disease*

rubidium chloride Rb 86 USAN *radioactive agent*

rubitecan USAN *investigational (Phase III) topoisomerase I inhibitor antineoplastic for pancreatic cancer*

Rubramin PC IM or subcu injection ℞ *antianemic; vitamin B_{12} supplement* [cyanocobalamin] 100, 1000 µg/mL

Rubus fructicosus; R. villosus *medicinal herb* [see: blackberry]

Rubus idaeus; R. strigosus *medicinal herb* [see: red raspberry]

rue (*Ruta bracteosa; R. graveolens; R. montana*) plant *medicinal herb for cramps, hypertension, hysteria, muscle strains, neuralgia, nervous disorders, sciatica, stimulation of abortion and menstruation, tendon strains, and trauma*

rufinamide USAN *anticonvulsant*

rufloxacin INN

rufocromomycin INN, BAN *antineoplastic* [also: streptonigrin]

Ru-lets M 500 film-coated tablets OTC *vitamin/mineral supplement* [multiple vitamins & minerals] ≛

RuLox oral suspension OTC *antacid* [aluminum hydroxide; magnesium hydroxide] 225•200 mg/5 mL

RuLox #1; RuLox #2 chewable tablets OTC *antacid* [aluminum hydroxide; magnesium hydroxide] 200•200 mg; 400•400 mg

RuLox Plus chewable tablets, oral suspension OTC *antacid; antiflatulent* [aluminum hydroxide; magnesium hydroxide; simethicone] 200•200•25 mg; 500•450•40 mg/5 mL

rum cherry *medicinal herb* [see: wild black cherry]

Rumex acetosa *medicinal herb* [see: sorrel]

Rumex crispus *medicinal herb* [see: yellow dock]

Rumex hymenosepalus *medicinal herb* [see: canaigre]

Rum-K liquid ℞ *potassium supplement* [potassium chloride] 30 mEq/15 mL

Ruscus aculeatus *medicinal herb* [see: butcher's broom]

rush, sweet *medicinal herb* [see: calamus]

Ruta bracteosa; R. graveolens; R. montana *medicinal herb* [see: rue]

rutamycin USAN, INN *antifungal*

ruthenium *element (Ru)*

rutin NF *a bioflavonoid* [also: rutoside]

rutoside INN [also: rutin]

Ru-Tuss liquid (discontinued 2000) OTC *decongestant; antihistamine* [phenylephrine HCl; chlorpheniramine maleate; alcohol 5%] 5•2 mg/5 mL

Ru-Tuss DE prolonged-action film-coated tablets (discontinued 2000) ℞ *decongestant; expectorant* [pseudoephedrine HCl; guaifenesin] 120•600 mg

Ru-Tuss Expectorant liquid (discontinued 2000) OTC *antitussive; decongestant; expectorant* [dextromethorphan hydrobromide; pseudoephedrine HCl; guaifenesin; alcohol 10%] 10•30•100 mg/5 mL

Ru-Tuss with Hydrocodone liquid (discontinued 2000) ℞ *narcotic antitussive; decongestant; antihistamine* [hydrocodone bitartrate; phenylpropanolamine HCl; phenylephrine HCl; pyrilamine maleate; pheniramine maleate; alcohol 5%] 1.7•3.3•5•3.3•3.3 mg/5 mL

ruvazone INN

Ru-Vert-M film-coated tablets (discontinued 1998) ℞ *anticholinergic; antivertigo agent; motion sickness preventative* [meclizine HCl] 25 mg

RVA (rabies vaccine, adsorbed) [see: rabies vaccine]

RVP (red veterinarian petrolatum) [see: petrolatum]

RxPak; ℞Pak (trademarked form) *prescription package*

Rymed capsules ℞ *decongestant; expectorant* [pseudoephedrine HCl; guaifenesin] 30•250 mg

Rymed liquid OTC *decongestant; expectorant* [pseudoephedrine HCl; guaifenesin; alcohol 1.4%] 30•100 mg/5 mL

Rymed-TR long-acting caplets ℞ *decongestant; expectorant* [phenylpropanolamine HCl; guaifenesin] 75•400 mg

Ryna liquid OTC *decongestant; antihistamine* [pseudoephedrine HCl; chlorpheniramine maleate] 30•2 mg/5 mL

Ryna-C liquid ℞ *narcotic antitussive; decongestant; antihistamine* [codeine phosphate; pseudoephedrine HCl; chlorpheniramine maleate] 10•30•2 mg/5 mL

Ryna-CX liquid ℞ *narcotic antitussive; decongestant; expectorant* [codeine phosphate; pseudoephedrine HCl; guaifenesin] 10•30•100 mg/5 mL

Rynatan pediatric oral suspension ℞ *decongestant; antihistamine* [phenylephrine tannate; chlorpheniramine tannate; pyrilamine tannate] 5•2•12.5 mg/5 mL

Rynatan tablets ℞ *decongestant; antihistamine* [pseudoephedrine sulfate; azatadine maleate] 120•1 mg

Rynatan-12 S oral suspension ℞ *pediatric decongestant and antihistamine* [phenylephrine tannate; pyrilamine tannate] 5•30 mg/5 mL

Rynatan-S oral suspension ℞ *pediatric decongestant and antihistamine* [phenylephrine tannate; chlorpheniramine tannate; pyrilamine tannate] 5•2•12.5 mg/5 mL

Rynatuss tablets, pediatric suspension ℞ *antitussive; decongestant; antihistamine* [carbetapentane tannate; phenylephrine tannate; ephedrine tannate; chlorpheniramine tannate] 60•10•10•5 mg; 30•5•5•4 mg/5 mL

Rythmol film-coated tablets ℞ *antiarrhythmic* [propafenone HCl] 150, 225, 300 mg

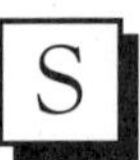

S-2 solution for inhalation OTC *sympathomimetic bronchodilator* [racepinephrine HCl] 2.25%
^{35}S [see: sodium sulfate S 35]
SA (salicylic acid) [q.v.]
SA (serum albumin) [see: albumin, human]
Sabatia angularis *medicinal herb* [see: American centaury]
Sab-Betaxolol (CAN) eye drops ℞ *topical antiglaucoma agent (β-blocker)* [betaxolol HCl] 0.5%
sabcomeline HCl USAN *muscarinic receptor agonist for Alzheimer disease*
Sab-Cortimyxin (CAN) ophthalmic ointment ℞ *topical ophthalmic corticosteroidal anti-inflammatory; antibiotic* [hydrocortisone; neomycin sulfate; polymyxin B sulfate] 1%•0.35%•10 000 U per mL
sabeluzole USAN, INN, BAN *anticonvulsant; antihypoxic*
Sabin vaccine [see: poliovirus vaccine, live oral]
Sabril (commercially available in 40 foreign countries) ℞ *investigational anticonvulsant* [vigabatrin]
Sacarasa (name changed to Sucraid in 1997)
saccharated ferric oxide JAN *hematinic* [also: iron sucrose]
saccharated iron; saccharated iron oxide [see: iron sucrose; saccharated ferric oxide]
saccharin NF *flavoring agent*
saccharin calcium USP *non-nutritive sweetener*
saccharin sodium USP *non-nutritive sweetener*
sacred bark *medicinal herb* [see: cascara sagrada]
sacrosidase USAN *enzyme replacement therapy for congenital sucrase-isomaltase deficiency (orphan)*
Saf-Clens spray OTC *wound cleanser*
Safe Tussin 30 liquid OTC *antitussive; expectorant* [dextromethorphan hydrobromide; guaifenesin] 15•100 mg/5 mL
safflower *(Carthamus tinctorius)* flowers *medicinal herb for delirium, digestive disorders, fever, gout, inducing sweating, jaundice, liver disorders, lowering cholesterol, promoting expectoration, uric acid build-up, and urinary disorders*
safflower oil USP *oleaginous vehicle; essential fatty acid supplement*
saffron *(Crocus sativus)* flowers *medicinal herb for fever, gout, inducing sweating, measles, rheumatism, scarlet fever, and sedation; also used as an aphrodisiac and expectorant*
saffron, American; bastard saffron *medicinal herb* [see: safflower]
safingol USAN *antipsoriatic; antineoplastic adjunct*
safingol HCl USAN *antipsoriatic; antineoplastic adjunct*
safrole USP
sagackhomi *medicinal herb* [see: uva ursi]
sage *(Salvia lavandulaefolia; S. lyrata; S. officinalis)* leaves *medicinal herb for cough, diarrhea, dysmenorrhea, fever, gastritis, gum and mouth sores, memory improvement, nausea, nervous disorders, and sore throat*
sailor's tobacco *medicinal herb* [see: mugwort]
St. Benedict thistle *medicinal herb* [see: blessed thistle]
St. James' weed; St. James' wort *medicinal herb* [see: shepherd's purse]
St. John's wort *(Hypericum perforatum)* plant *medicinal herb for AIDS, antiviral therapy, anxiety, bronchitis, cancer, childbirth afterpains, depression, gastritis, insomnia, and skin disorders* 300 mg oral (CAN)
St. Joseph Adult Chewable Aspirin chewable tablets OTC *analgesic; antipyretic; anti-inflammatory* [aspirin] 81 mg
St. Joseph Aspirin-Free Fever Reducer for Children liquid (dis-

continued 1997) OTC *analgesic; antipyretic* [acetaminophen] 160 mg/5 mL

St. Joseph Aspirin-Free for Children chewable tablets (discontinued 1997) OTC *analgesic; antipyretic* [acetaminophen] 80 mg

St. Joseph Aspirin-Free Infant Drops (discontinued 1997) OTC *analgesic; antipyretic* [acetaminophen] 100 mg/mL

St. Joseph Cold Tablets for Children chewable tablets OTC *pediatric decongestant and analgesic* [phenylpropanolamine HCl; acetaminophen] 3.125•80 mg

St. Joseph Cough Suppressant syrup OTC *antitussive* [dextromethorphan hydrobromide] 7.5 mg/5 mL

St. Josephwort *medicinal herb* [see: basil]

Saizen powder for subcu or IM injection, cool.click (needle-free subcu injector) ℞ *growth hormone for adults or children with congenital or endogenous growth hormone deficiency, children with Turner syndrome or renal-induced growth failure* [somatropin] 5 mg (15 IU) per vial

SalAc liquid OTC *topical keratolytic cleanser for acne* [salicylic acid] 2%

salacetamide INN

salacetin [see: aspirin]

Sal-Acid plaster OTC *topical keratolytic* [salicylic acid in a collodion-like vehicle] 40%

Salactic Film liquid OTC *topical keratolytic* [salicylic acid in a collodion-like vehicle] 17%

salafibrate INN

Salagen film-coated tablets ℞ *treatment of xerostomia and keratoconjunctivitis sicca due to radiotherapy or Sjögren syndrome (orphan); also for dry mouth* [pilocarpine HCl] 5 mg

salantel USAN, INN *veterinary anthelmintic*

salazodine INN

Salazopyrin (European name for U.S. product Azulfidine)

salazosulfadimidine INN [also: salazosulphadimidine]

salazosulfamide INN

salazosulfapyridine JAN *broad-spectrum bacteriostatic; anti-inflammatory for ulcerative colitis; antirheumatic* [also: sulfasalazine; sulphasalazine]

salazosulfathiazole INN

salazosulphadimidine BAN [also: salazosulfadimidine]

salbutamol INN, BAN *sympathomimetic bronchodilator* [also: albuterol]

Salbutamol Nebuamp (CAN) solution for nebulization ℞ *sympathomimetic bronchodilator* [salbutamol sulfate] 2.5 mL/ampule

salbutamol sulfate JAN *sympathomimetic bronchodilator* [also: albuterol sulfate]

salcatonin BAN *synthetic analogue of calcitonin (salmon); calcium regulator; investigational osteoporosis treatment* [also: calcitonin salmon (synthesis)]

salcetogen [see: aspirin]

Sal-Clens Acne Cleanser gel OTC *topical keratolytic for acne* [salicylic acid] 2%

salcolex USAN, INN *analgesic; anti-inflammatory; antipyretic*

SalEst test kit for professional use *in vitro diagnostic aid for estriol levels in saliva, used to predict spontaneous preterm labor and delivery*

saletamide INN *analgesic* [also: salethamide maleate]

saletamide maleate [see: salethamide maleate]

salethamide maleate USAN *analgesic* [also: saletamide]

saletin [see: aspirin]

Saleto tablets OTC *analgesic; antipyretic; anti-inflammatory* [acetaminophen; aspirin; salicylamide; caffeine] 115•210•65•16 mg

Saleto CF tablets OTC *antitussive; decongestant; analgesic* [dextromethorphan hydrobromide; phenylpropanolamine; acetaminophen] 10•12.5•325 mg

Saleto-200 tablets (discontinued 2000) OTC *analgesic; antiarthritic; antipyretic; nonsteroidal anti-inflammatory drug (NSAID)* [ibuprofen] 200 mg

Saleto-400; Saleto-600; Saleto-800 tablets (discontinued 2000) ℞ *analgesic; antiarthritic; antipyretic; nonsteroidal anti-inflammatory drug (NSAID)* [ibuprofen] 400 mg; 600 mg; 800 mg
Saleto-D capsules OTC *decongestant; analgesic; antipyretic* [phenylpropanolamine HCl; acetaminophen; salicylamide; caffeine] 18•240•120•16 mg
Salflex film-coated tablets OTC *analgesic; antipyretic; anti-inflammatory; antirheumatic* [salsalate] 500, 750 mg
salfluverine INN
salicain [now: salicyl alcohol]
salicin USP
salicin willow *medicinal herb* [see: willow]
salicyl alcohol USAN *local anesthetic*
salicylamide USP *analgesic*
salicylanilide NF
salicylate meglumine USAN *antirheumatic; analgesic*
salicylates *a class of drugs that have analgesic, antipyretic, and anti-inflammatory effects*
salicylazosulfapyridine [now: sulfasalazine]
salicylic acid (SA) USP *keratolytic; antiseborrheic; antipsoriatic*
salicylic acid, bimolecular ester [see: salsalate]
salicylic acid acetate [see: aspirin]
Salicylic Acid and Sulfur Soap bar OTC *medicated cleanser for acne* [salicylic acid; precipitated sulfur] 3%•10%
Salicylic Acid Cleansing bar OTC *medicated cleanser for acne* [salicylic acid] 2%
salicylic acid dihydrogen phosphate [see: fosfosal]
salicylsalicylic acid [see: salsalate]
saligenin [now: salicyl alcohol]
saligenol [now: salicyl alcohol]
salinazid INN, BAN
saline, lactated potassic [see: potassic saline, lactated]
saline laxatives *a subclass of laxatives that work by attracting and retaining water in the intestines to increase intraluminal pressure and cholecystokinin release* [see also: laxatives]
saline solution (SS) [also: normal saline]
SalineX nasal mist, nose drops OTC *nasal moisturizer* [sodium chloride (saline solution)] 0.4%
saliniazid [see: salinazid]
salinomycin INN, BAN
Saliva Substitute oral solution OTC *saliva substitute* [carboxymethylcellulose sodium]
Salivart oral spray OTC *saliva substitute* [carboxymethylcellulose sodium] 1%
Salix lozenges OTC *saliva substitute* [carboxymethylcellulose]
Salix alba; S. caprea; S. nigra; S. purpurea *medicinal herb* [see: willow]
salmaterol [see: salmeterol]
salmefamol INN, BAN
salmeterol USAN, INN, BAN *sympathomimetic bronchodilator*
salmeterol xinafoate USAN *adrenergic; sympathomimetic bronchodilator*
salmisteine INN
salmon calcitonin [see: salcatonin]
Salmonella typhi **vaccine** [see: typhoid vaccine]
Salmonine subcu or IM injection ℞ *calcium regulator for hypercalcemia, Paget disease, and postmenopausal osteoporosis* [calcitonin (salmon)] 200 IU/mL
salmotin [see: adicillin]
salnacedin USAN *topical anti-inflammatory*
Salofalk (CAN) enteric-coated tablets ℞ *for acute ulcerative colitis and the prevention of Crohn disease relapse following bowel resection* [mesalamine (5-aminosalicylic acid)] 250, 500 mg
Salofalk (CAN) suppositories, rectal suspension enema ℞ *anti-inflammatory for distal ulcerative colitis (DUC) and ulcerative proctitis* [mesalamine (5-aminosalicylic acid)] 250, 500 mg; 2, 4 g/58 mL
Sal-Oil-T hair dressing ℞ *antipsoriatic; antiseborrheic; keratolytic* [coal tar; salicylic acid] 10%•6%

salol [see: phenyl salicylate]
Sal-Plant gel OTC *topical keratolytic* [salicylic acid in a collodion-like vehicle] 17%
Salprofen IV injection ℞ *investigational (orphan) for patent ductus arteriosus* [ibuprofen]
salprotoside INN
salsalate USAN, USP, INN, BAN *analgesic; antipyretic; anti-inflammatory; antirheumatic* 500, 750 mg oral
Salsitab film-coated tablets ℞ *analgesic; antipyretic; anti-inflammatory; antirheumatic* [salsalate] 500, 750 mg
Sal-Tropine tablets ℞ *GI/GU antispasmodic; antiparkinsonian; anticholinergic "drying agent" for the respiratory tract; antidote to insecticide poisoning* [atropine sulfate] 0.4 mg
Saluron tablets ℞ *diuretic; antihypertensive* [hydroflumethiazide] 50 mg
Salutensin; Salutensin-Demi tablets ℞ *antihypertensive* [hydroflumethiazide; reserpine] 50•0.125 mg; 25•0.125 mg ⓢ Diutensen
saluzide [see: opiniazide]
salvarsan [see: arsphenamine]
salverine INN
Salvia lavandulaefolia; S. lyrata; S. officinalis *medicinal herb* [see: sage]
Salvia miltiorrhiza *medicinal herb* [see: danshen]
samarium *element (Sm)*
samarium Sm 153 EDTMP (ethylenediaminetetramethylenephosphoric acid) [see: samarium Sm 153 lexidronam]
samarium Sm 153 lexidronam USAN *radiopharmaceutical for treatment of bone pain from osteoblastic metastatic tumors*
Sambucus canadensis; S. ebulus; S. nigra; S. racemosa *medicinal herb* [see: elder flower; elderberry]
Sanchi ginseng *(Panax pseudoginseng)* *medicinal herb* [see: ginseng]
sancycline USAN, INN *antibacterial*
sandalwood *(Santalum album)* oil *medicinal herb for headache, stomach ache, and urogenital disorders; also used topically as an antiseptic and astringent*
Sandimmune gel capsules, oral solution, IV infusion ℞ *immunosuppressant for allogenic kidney, liver, and heart transplants; investigational for many other uses* [cyclosporine] 25, 50, 100 mg; 100 mg/mL; 50 mg/mL
Sandimmune ophthalmic ointment ℞ *investigational (orphan) for keratoconjunctivitis sicca, keratoplasty graft rejection, and corneal melting syndrome* [cyclosporine] 2%
Sandimmune Neoral (CAN) soft gels, oral solution [see: Neoral]
Sandoglobulin powder for IV infusion ℞ *passive immunizing agent for HIV and idiopathic thrombocytopenic purpura (ITP)* [immune globulin] 1, 3, 6, 12 g
SandoPak (trademarked packaging form) *unit dose blister package*
Sandostatin subcu or IV injection ℞ *gastric antisecretory for acromegaly and severe diarrhea due to VIPomas and other tumors (orphan)* [octreotide acetate] 0.05, 0.1, 0.2, 0.5, 1 mg/mL ⓢ simvastatin; zinostatin
Sandostatin LAR Depot suspension for IM injection ℞ *gastric antisecretory for acromegaly and severe diarrhea due to VIPomas and other tumors (orphan)* [octreotide acetate]
sanfetrinem INN, BAN *antibacterial* [also: sanfetrinem sodium]
sanfetrinem cilexetil USAN *antibacterial*
sanfetrinem sodium USAN *antibacterial* [also: sanfetrinem]
SangCya oral solution ℞ *immunosuppressive to prevent solid organ transplant rejection* [cyclosporine; alcohol 10.5%] 100 mg/mL
Sanguinaria canadensis *medicinal herb* [see: bloodroot]
sanguinarine chloride [now: sanguinarium chloride]
sanguinarium chloride USAN, INN *antifungal; antimicrobial; anti-inflammatory*
sanicle *(Sanicula europea; S. marilandica)* root *medicinal herb used as*

an astringent, expectorant, discutient, depurative, nervine, and vulnerary

Sani-Pak (trademarked packaging form) *sanitary dispensing box*

Sani-Supp suppositories OTC *hyperosmolar laxative* [glycerin]

Sanorex tablets ℞ *anorexiant; CNS stimulant; investigational (orphan) treatment for Duchenne muscular dystrophy* [mazindol] 1, 2 mg

Sansert tablets ℞ *agent for migraine and vascular headaches* [methysergide maleate] 2 mg

Santalum album *medicinal herb* [see: sandalwood]

santonin NF

Santyl ointment ℞ *topical enzyme for biochemical debridement* [collagenase] 250 U/g

saperconazole USAN, INN, BAN *antifungal*

Saponaria officinalis *medicinal herb* [see: soapwort]

saprisartan INN, BAN *antihypertensive; angiotensin II antagonist* [also: saprisartan potassium]

saprisartan potassium USAN *antihypertensive; angiotensin II antagonist* [also: saprisartan]

sapropterin INN

saquinavir USAN, INN, BAN *antiretroviral protease inhibitor for HIV infection* [also: saquinavir mesylate]

saquinavir & amprenavir *investigational (Phase II) protease inhibitor combination for AIDS*

saquinavir mesylate USAN *antiretroviral protease inhibitor for HIV infection* [also: saquinavir]

saquinavir mesylate & ritonavir & lamivudine *investigational (Phase II) protease inhibitor and nucleoside reverse transcriptase inhibitor combination for HIV infection*

saquinavir mesylate & ritonavir & zidovudine *investigational (Phase II) protease inhibitor combination for HIV infection*

Sarafem capsules ℞ *selective serotonin reuptake inhibitor (SSRI) for premenstrual dysphoric disorder (PMDD)* [fluoxetine HCl] 10, 20 mg

sarafloxacin INN, BAN *anti-infective; DNA gyrase inhibitor* [also: sarafloxacin HCl]

sarafloxacin HCl USAN *anti-infective; DNA gyrase inhibitor* [also: sarafloxacin]

saralasin INN *antihypertensive* [also: saralasin acetate]

saralasin acetate USAN *antihypertensive; investigational (Phase I/II) mouthwash for oral candidiasis* [also: saralasin]

Saratoga ointment OTC *astringent; antiseptic; wound protectant* [zinc oxide; boric acid; eucalyptol]

sarcolysin INN

L-sarcolysin [see: melphalan]

Sardo Bath & Shower oil OTC *bath emollient*

Sardoettes towelettes OTC *moisturizer; emollient*

sargramostim USAN, INN, BAN *antineutropenic for bone marrow transplant and graft delay (orphan); investigational (Phase III) for malignant melanoma; investigational (Phase III) cytokine for HIV infection; investigational (Phase II) cytokine for HIV infection*

sargramostim & HGP-30 *investigational (Phase I) combination for HIV infection*

sarmazenil INN

sarmoxicillin USAN, INN *antibacterial*

Sarna Anti-Itch foam, lotion OTC *topical analgesic; counterirritant* [camphor; menthol] 0.5%•0.5%

saroten [see: amitriptyline]

Sarothamnus scoparius *medicinal herb* [see: broom]

sarpicillin USAN, INN *antibacterial*

Sarracenia purpurea *medicinal herb* [see: pitcher plant]

sarsaparilla (*Smilax* spp.) root *medicinal herb for blood cleansing (binding and expulsion of endotoxins), joint aches including arthritis and rheumatism, hormonal disorders, skin diseases* *including leprosy and psoriasis, and syphilis*

saruplase INN *investigational (Phase III) prourokinase clot-dissolving agent for stroke*

sassafras *(Sassafras albidum; S. officinale)* root and bark *medicinal herb for acne, blood cleansing, insect bites and stings, obesity, psoriasis, skin diseases, and water retention; not generally regarded as safe because of serious side effects; banned by the FDA as a carcinogen*

sassafras, swamp *medicinal herb* [see: magnolia]

SAStid Soap bar OTC *medicated cleanser for acne* [precipitated sulfur] 10%

saterinone INN

satinflower *medicinal herb* [see: chickweed]

satranidazole INN

satraplatin USAN *antineoplastic*

satumomab INN, BAN *radiodiagnostic monoclonal antibody for ovarian and colorectal carcinoma* [also: indium In 111 satumomab pendetide]

satumomab pendetide [see: indium In 111 satumomab pendetide]

Satureja hortensis *medicinal herb* [see: summer savory]

Satureja montana; S. obovata *medicinal herb* [see: winter savory]

savory *medicinal herb* [see: summer savory; winter savory]

savoxepin INN

Savvy vaginal gel ℞ *investigational (Phase I/II) microbicide and spermicide for HIV infection*

saw palmetto *(Serenoa repens; S. serrulata)* berries *medicinal herb for benign prostatic hypertrophy and genitourinary, glandular, and reproductive disorders; also used to enlarge breasts, increase sperm production, promote weight gain, and enhance sexual vigor*

saxifrage, burnet; European burnet saxifrage; small burnet saxifrage; small saxifrage *medicinal herb* [see: burnet]

saxifrax *medicinal herb* [see: sassafras]

SB-210396 *investigational (Phase III) anti-CD4 antibody for rheumatoid arthritis* [also: IDEC-CE9.1]

SB-217969 *investigational (Phase I/II) anti-CD4 antibody for the treatment of rheumatoid arthritis*

SC (succinylcholine) [see: succinylcholine chlorine]

SCA proteins (single-chain antigen-binding proteins) *a class of investigational antineoplastics*

Scabene lotion, shampoo (discontinued 1998) ℞ *pediculicide for lice; scabicide* [lindane] 1%

scabicides *a class of agents effective against scabies*

scabwort *medicinal herb* [see: elecampane]

Scadan scalp lotion OTC *antiseptic; antiseborrheic* [myristyltrimethylammonium bromide; stearyl dimethyl benzyl ammonium chloride] 1%•0.1%

Scalpicin liquid OTC *topical antiseborrheic* [salicylic acid] 3%

Scalpicin liquid (discontinued 1999) OTC *topical corticosteroidal anti-inflammatory* [hydrocortisone] 1%

scaly dragon's claw *medicinal herb* [see: coral root]

scammony, wild *medicinal herb* [see: wild jalap]

scandium *element (Sc)*

scarlet bergamot *medicinal herb* [see: Oswego tea]

scarlet berry *medicinal herb* [see: bittersweet nightshade]

scarlet fever streptococcus toxin

scarlet red NF *promotes wound healing*

Scarlet Red Ointment Dressings medication-impregnated gauze ℞ *wound dressing; vulnerary* [scarlet red] 5%

scarlet sumach *medicinal herb* [see: sumach]

SCCS (simethicone-coated cellulose suspension) [see: SonoRx]

sCD4-PE40 [see: alvircept sudotox]

SCF (stem cell factor) [q.v.]

SCH-58500 *investigational (Phase II) gene therapy for liver and colorectal tumors*

Schamberg lotion OTC *topical analgesic; antiseptic; astringent; antifungal; counterirritant* [zinc oxide; menthol; phenol] 8.25%•0.25%•1.5%

Scheinpharm Tobramycin (CAN) IV or IM injection (discontinued 2000) ℞ *aminoglycoside antibiotic* [tobramycin sulfate] 10, 40 mg/mL

Schick test [see: diphtheria toxin for Schick test]

Schick test control USP *dermal reactivity indicator*

Schirmer Tear Test ophthalmic strips *diagnostic tear flow test aid*

schizandra (*Schisandra arisanensis; S. chinensis; S. rubriflora; S. sphenanthera*) berries *medicinal herb for cough, gastrointestinal disorders, increasing energy and mental alertness, nervous disorders, respiratory illnesses, and stress; also used as a liver protectant*

Scleromate IV injection ℞ *sclerosing agent for varicose veins* [morrhuate sodium] 50 mg/mL

Sclerosol aerosol ℞ *investigational (NDA filed, orphan) treatment for malignant pleural effusion and pneumothorax via intrapleural thoracoscopy administration* [talc, sterile]

scoke *medicinal herb* [see: pokeweed]

Scopace tablets ℞ *GI antispasmodic; anticholinergic CNS depressant; motion sickness preventative* [scopolamine hydrobromine] 0.4 mg

scopafungin USAN *antibacterial; antifungal*

Scope mouthwash OTC *oral antiseptic* [cetylpyridinium chloride]

scopolamine *oral/transdermal motion sickness preventative*

scopolamine hydrobromide USP *GI antispasmodic; anticholinergic CNS depressant; motion sickness preventative; cycloplegic; mydriatic* [also: hyoscine hydrobromide] 0.3, 0.4, 0.86, 1 mg/mL injection

scopolamine methyl nitrate [see: methscopolamine nitrate]

scopolamine methylbromide [see: methscopolamine bromide]

Scott's Emulsion OTC *vitamin supplement* [vitamins A and D] 1250•100 IU/5 mL

Scot-Tussin Allergy; Scot-Tussin Allergy Relief Formula Clear oral liquid OTC *antihistamine* [diphenhydramine HCl] 12.5 mg/5 mL

Scot-Tussin DM liquid OTC *antitussive; antihistamine* [dextromethorphan hydrobromide; chlorpheniramine maleate] 15•2 mg/5 mL

Scot-Tussin DM Cough Chasers lozenges OTC *antitussive* [dextromethorphan hydrobromide] 2.5 mg

Scot-k$>Tussin Expectorant sugar-free liquid OTC *expectorant* [guaifenesin] 100 mg/5 mL

Scot-Tussin Original 5-Action Cold Formula syrup, sugar-free liquid OTC *decongestant; antihistamine; analgesic* [phenylephrine HCl; pheniramine maleate; sodium citrate; sodium salicylate; caffeine citrate] 4.2•13.3•83.3•83.3•25 mg

Scot-Tussin Senior Clear liquid OTC *antitussive; expectorant* [dextromethorphan hydrobromide; guaifenesin] 15•200 mg/5 mL

sCR1 (soluble complement receptor 1) *investigational (Phase I/II) complement inhibitor for severe burns, adult respiratory distress syndrome, and reperfusion injury* [also: TP-10]

Scriptene ℞ *investigational (Phase II) heterodimer antiviral for AIDS* [zidovudine; didanosine]

scrofula plant *medicinal herb* [see: figwort]

Scrophularia nodosa *medicinal herb* [see: figwort]

scullcap *medicinal herb* [see: skullcap]

scuroforme [see: butyl aminobenzoate]

Scutellaria lateriflora *medicinal herb* [see: skullcap]

SD (streptodornase) [q.v.]

^{75}Se [see: selenomethionine Se 75]

sea girdles *medicinal herb* [see: kelp *(Laminaria)*]

Sea Mist nasal spray OTC *nasal moisturizer* [sodium chloride (saline solution)] 0.65%

Seale's Lotion Modified OTC *topical acne treatment* [sulfur] 6.4%

sealroot; sealwort *medicinal herb* [see: Solomon's seal]

Sea-Omega 30; Sea-Omega 50 softgels OTC *dietary supplement* [omega-3 fatty acids] 1200 mg; 1000 mg

seawrack *medicinal herb* [see: kelp *(Fucus)*]

Seba-Nil Cleansing Mask scrub OTC *abrasive cleanser for acne*

Seba-Nil Oily Skin Cleanser liquid OTC *topical cleanser for acne* [alcohol; acetone]

Sebasorb lotion OTC *topical keratolytic for acne* [salicylic acid; attapulgite] 2%•10%

Sebex shampoo OTC *antiseborrheic; keratolytic* [sulfur; salicylic acid] 2%•2%

Sebex-T shampoo OTC *antiseborrheic; antipsoriatic; keratolytic* [sulfur; salicylic acid; coal tar] 2%•2%•5%

Sebizon lotion ℞ *bacteriostatic; antiseborrheic* [sulfacetamide sodium] 10%

Sebucare hair lotion OTC *antiseborrheic; keratolytic* [salicylic acid; alcohol 61%] 1.8%

Sebulex shampoo (discontinued 1997) OTC *antiseborrheic; keratolytic* [sulfur; salicylic acid] 2%•2%

Sebulex with Conditioners shampoo OTC *antiseborrheic; keratolytic* [sulfur; salicylic acid] 2%•2%

Sebulon shampoo (discontinued 1997) OTC *antiseborrheic; antibacterial; antifungal* [pyrithione zinc] 2%

Sebutone cream shampoo, liquid shampoo (discontinued 1997) OTC *antiseborrheic; antipsoriatic; keratolytic* [coal tar; sulfur; salicylic acid] 0.5%•2%•2%

secalciferol USAN, INN, BAN *calcium regulator; investigational (orphan) for familial hypophosphatemic rickets*

secbutabarbital sodium INN *sedative; hypnotic* [also: butabarbital sodium]

secbutobarbitone BAN *sedative; hypnotic* [also: butabarbital]

seclazone USAN, INN *anti-inflammatory; uricosuric*

secnidazole INN, BAN

secobarbital USP, INN *hypnotic; sedative*

secobarbital sodium USP, JAN *hypnotic; sedative; also abused as a street drug* [also: quinalbarbitone sodium] 100 mg oral; 50 mg/mL injection

Seconal Sodium Pulvules (capsules) ℞ *sedative; hypnotic; also abused as a street drug* [secobarbital sodium] 100 mg

secoverine INN

Secran liquid OTC *vitamin supplement* [vitamins B_1, B_3, and B_{12}; alcohol 17%] 10 mg•10 mg•25 µg per 5 mL

secretin INN, BAN *diagnostic aid for pancreatic function*

Secretin Ferring powder for IV injection ℞ *diagnostic aid for pancreatic function* [secretin] 10 CU/mL

secretory leukocyte protease inhibitor *investigational (orphan) for congenital alpha$_1$-antitrypsin deficiency, cystic fibrosis, and bronchopulmonary dysplasia*

Sectral capsules ℞ *antihypertensive; antiarrhythmic; antiadrenergic (β-blocker)* [acebutolol HCl] 200, 400 mg

Secule (trademarked packaging form) *single-dose vial*

securinine INN

sedaform [see: chlorobutanol]

Sedapap caplets ℞ *analgesic; barbiturate sedative* [acetaminophen; butalbital] 650•50 mg

sedatine [see: antipyrine]

sedatives *a class of soothing agents that reduce excitement, nervousness, distress, or irritation* [also called: calmatives]

sedecamycin USAN, INN *veterinary antibacterial*

sedeval [see: barbital]

sedge, sweet *medicinal herb* [see: calamus]

sedoxantrone trihydrochloride [now: ledoxantrone trihydrochloride]

seganserin INN, BAN

seglitide INN *antidiabetic* [also: seglitide acetate]

seglitide acetate USAN *antidiabetic* [also: seglitide]

SelCID ℞ *investigational (Phase I) selective cytokine inhibitory drug*

Seldane tablets (discontinued 1998) ℞ *nonsedating antihistamine* [terfenadine] 60 mg

Seldane-D sustained-release tablets (discontinued 1998) ℞ *decongestant; antihistamine* [pseudoephedrine HCl; terfenadine] 120•60 mg

Selecor tablets ℞ *investigational (NDA filed) antihypertensive; antianginal; β-blocker* [celiprolol HCl]

Select-A-Jet (trademarked delivery system) *syringe system*

selective estrogen receptor modulators (SERMs) *a class of osteoporosis prevention agents that reduce bone resorption and decrease overall bone turnover in postmenopausal women*

selective serotonin 5-HT$_3$ (hydroxytryptamine) blockers *a class of antiemetic and antinauseant agents used primarily after emetogenic cancer chemotherapy* [also called: 5-HT$_3$ receptor antagonists]

selective serotonin reuptake inhibitors (SSRIs) *a class of oral antidepressants that inhibit neuronal uptake of serotonin (5-HT), a CNS neurotransmitter*

selegiline INN, BAN *dopaminergic antiparkinsonian; investigational (Phase III) transdermal treatment for depression* [also: selegiline HCl]

selegiline HCl USAN *dopaminergic antiparkinsonian (orphan)* [also: selegiline] 5 mg oral

selenious acid USP *dietary selenium supplement* 65.4 µg/mL injection

selenium *element (Se)*

selenium dioxide, monohydrated [see: selenious acid]

selenium sulfide USP *antifungal; antiseborrheic* 1%, 2.5% topical

selenomethionine (^{75}Se) INN *pancreas function test; radioactive agent* [also: selenomethionine Se 75]

selenomethionine Se 75 USAN, USP *pancreas function test; radioactive agent* [also: selenomethionine (^{75}Se)]

Sele-Pak IV injection ℞ *intravenous nutritional therapy* [selenious acid] 65.4 µg/mL

Selepen IV injection ℞ *intravenous nutritional therapy* [selenious acid] 65.4 µg/mL

selfotel USAN *N-methyl-D-aspartate (NMDA) antagonist for treatment of stroke-induced impairment*

Seloken (foreign name for U.S. product Lopressor)

Seloken ZOC (foreign name for U.S. product Toprol XL)

selprazine INN

Selsun lotion/shampoo ℞ *antiseborrheic; antifungal* [selenium sulfide] 2.5%

Selsun Blue; Selsun Gold for Women lotion/shampoo OTC *antiseborrheic* [selenium sulfide] 1%

sematilide INN *antiarrhythmic* [also: sematilide HCl]

sematilide HCl USAN *antiarrhythmic* [also: sematilide]

semduramicin USAN, INN *coccidiostat*

semduramicin sodium USAN *coccidiostat*

Semicid vaginal suppositories OTC *spermicidal contraceptive* [nonoxynol 9] 100 mg

semisodium valproate BAN *anticonvulsant; antipsychotic for manic episodes; migraine prophylaxis* [also: divalproex sodium; valproate semisodium]

semparatide acetate USAN *parathyroid hormone analogue to enhance fracture healing*

Semprex-D capsules ℞ *decongestant; antihistamine* [pseudoephedrine HCl; acrivastine] 60•8 mg

semustine USAN, INN *antineoplastic*

senecio, golden *medicinal herb* [see: life root]

Senecio aureus; S. jacoboea; S. vulgaris *medicinal herb* [see: life root]

senega (*Polygala senega*) root *medicinal herb used as an antitussive for asthma, chronic bronchitis, croup, lung congestion, and pneumonia*

Senexon tablets OTC *stimulant laxative* [sennosides] 8.6 mg

Senilezol elixir ℞ *vitamin/iron supplement* [multiple B vitamins; ferric pyrophosphate] ≛•3.3 mg

senna USP *stimulant laxative*

senna (*Cassia acutifolia; C. angustifolia; C. senna*) leaves *medicinal herb for bowel evacuation before gastrointestinal procedures, constipation, edema, and expelling worms*

Senna-Gen tablets OTC *stimulant laxative* [sennosides] 8.6 mg

sennosides USP *stimulant laxative*

Senokot suppositories (discontinued 1999) OTC *stimulant laxative* [senna concentrate] 652 mg

Senokot tablets, granules, syrup OTC *stimulant laxative* [sennosides] 8.6 mg; 15 mg/5 mL; 8.8 mg/5 mL

Senokot-S tablets OTC *stimulant laxative; stool softener* [sennosides; docusate sodium] 8.6•50 mg

SenokotXtra tablets OTC *stimulant laxative* [sennosides] 17 mg

Senolax tablets (discontinued 1997) OTC *stimulant laxative* [senna concentrate] 187 mg

Sensability kit OTC *breast self-examination aid*

Sensamide ℞ *investigational (Phase II/III) radiosensitizer for inoperable non–small cell lung cancer (NSCLC)* [metoclopramide HCl]

Sensitive Eyes; Sensitive Eyes Plus solution OTC *rinsing/storage solution for soft contact lenses* [sodium chloride (preserved saline solution)]

Sensitive Eyes Daily Cleaner; Sensitive Eyes Saline/Cleaning Solution OTC *surfactant cleaning solution for soft contact lenses*

Sensitive Eyes Drops OTC *rewetting solution for soft contact lenses*

Sensitivity Protection Crest toothpaste OTC *tooth desensitizer; topical dental caries preventative* [potassium nitrate; sodium fluoride]

Sensodyne Cool Gel toothpaste OTC *tooth desensitizer; topical dental caries preventative* [potassium nitrate; sodium fluoride]

Sensodyne Fresh Mint toothpaste OTC *tooth desensitizer; dental caries preventative* [potassium nitrate; sodium monofluorophosphate]

Sensodyne-SC toothpaste OTC *tooth desensitizer* [strontium chloride hexahydrate] 10%

SensoGARD gel OTC *topical oral anesthetic* [benzocaine] 20%

Sensorcaine injection ℞ *injectable local anesthetic* [bupivacaine HCl] 0.25%, 0.5%

Sensorcaine injection ℞ *injectable local anesthetic* [bupivacaine HCl; epinephrine] 0.25%•1:200 000; 0.5%•1:200 000

Sensorcaine MPF injection ℞ *injectable local anesthetic* [bupivacaine HCl] 0.25%, 0.5%, 0.75%

Sensorcaine MPF injection ℞ *injectable local anesthetic* [bupivacaine HCl; epinephrine] 0.25%•1:200 000, 0.5%•1:200 000, 0.75%•1:200 000

Sensorcaine MPF Spinal injection ℞ *injectable local anesthetic* [bupivacaine HCl] 0.75%

Sentinel test kit for professional use *urine test for HIV-1 antibodies* ⊡ fentanyl

sepazonium chloride USAN, INN *topical anti-infective*

seperidol HCl USAN *antipsychotic* [also: clofluperol]

Seprafilm hydrated gel film *to reduce the incidence, extent, and severity of postoperative adhesions* [hyaluronate sodium; carboxymethylcellulose]

seprilose USAN *antirheumatic*

seproxetine HCl USAN *antidepressant*

Septa ointment OTC *topical antibiotic* [polymyxin B sulfate; neomycin sulfate; bacitracin] 5000 U•3.5 mg•400 U per g ⊡ Cipro; Septra

Septi-Soft solution ℞ *antiseptic; disinfectant* [triclosan] 0.25%

Septisol foam ℞ *bacteriostatic skin cleanser* [hexachlorophene; alcohol 56%] 0.23%

Septisol solution ℞ *antiseptic; disinfectant* [triclosan] 0.25%

Septocaine intraoral injection ℞ *local anesthetic for dentistry* [articaine HCl; epinephrine] 4%•1:100 000

septomonab [see: nebacumab]

Septopal polymethyl methacrylate (PMMA) beads on surgical wire ℞ *investigational (orphan) for chronic osteomyelitis* [gentamicin sulfate]

Septra tablets, oral suspension ℞ *anti-infective; antibacterial* [trimethoprim; sulfamethoxazole] 80•400 mg; 40•200 mg/5 mL ⊠ Cipro; Septa

Septra DS tablets ℞ *anti-infective; antibacterial* [trimethoprim; sulfamethoxazole] 160•800 mg

Septra IV infusion ℞ *anti-infective; antibacterial* [trimethoprim; sulfamethoxazole] 80•400 mg/5 mL

Sequels (trademarked dosage form) *sustained-release capsule or tablet*

sequifenadine INN

seractide INN *adrenocorticotropic hormone* [also: seractide acetate]

seractide acetate USAN *adrenocorticotropic hormone* [also: seractide]

Ser-Ap-Es tablets ℞ *antihypertensive; vasodilator; diuretic* [hydrochlorothiazide; reserpine; hydralazine HCl] 15•0.1•25 mg ⊠ Catapres

seratrodast USAN, INN *anti-inflammatory; antiasthmatic; thromboxane receptor antagonist*

Serax capsules, tablets ℞ *benzodiazepine anxiolytic* [oxazepam] 10, 15, 30 mg; 15 mg ⊠ Eurax; Urex; Xerac

serazapine HCl USAN *anxiolytic*

Sereine solution OTC *cleaning solution for hard contact lenses* [note: one of three different products with the same name]

Sereine solution OTC *wetting solution for hard contact lenses* [note: one of three different products with the same name]

Sereine solution OTC *wetting/soaking solution for hard contact lenses* [note: one of three different products with the same name]

Serenoa repens; S. serrulata *medicinal herb* [see: saw palmetto]

Serentil tablets, oral concentrate, IM injection ℞ *conventional (typical) antipsychotic* [mesoridazine besylate] 10, 25, 50, 100 mg; 25 mg/mL; 25 mg/mL ⊠ Surital

Serevent oral metered dose inhaler, Diskus (oral inhalation powder device) ℞ *twice-daily sympathomimetic bronchodilator for asthma and bronchospasm* [salmeterol xinafoate] 25 μg/dose; 50 μg/dose

serfibrate INN

sergolexole INN *antimigraine* [also: sergolexole maleate]

sergolexole maleate USAN *antimigraine* [also: sergolexole]

serine (L-serine) USAN, USP, INN *nonessential amino acid; symbols: Ser, S*

L-serine diazoacetate [see: azaserine]

84-L-serineplasminogen activator [see: monteplase]

sermetacin USAN, INN *anti-inflammatory*

sermorelin INN, BAN *growth hormone deficiency diagnosis and treatment* [also: sermorelin acetate]

sermorelin acetate USAN *diagnostic aid for pituitary function; treatment for growth hormone deficiency (orphan), anovulation, and AIDS-related weight loss* [also: sermorelin]

SERMs (selective estrogen receptor modulators) *a class of osteoporosis prevention agents that reduce bone resorption and decrease overall bone turnover in postmenopausal women*

Seromycin Pulvules (capsules) ℞ *bacteriostatic; tuberculostatic; treatment for acute urinary tract infections* [cycloserine] 250 mg

Serophene tablets ℞ *ovulation stimulant* [clomiphene citrate] 50 mg

Seroquel tablets ℞ *novel (atypical) antipsychotic* [quetiapine fumarate] 25, 100, 200, 300 mg

Serostim powder for subcu injection ℞ *growth hormone for adults or children with congenital or endogenous growth hormone deficiency, children with Turner syndrome or renal-induced growth failure, or AIDS-wasting syndrome (orphan)* [somatropin] 4, 5, 6 mg (12, 15, 18 IU) per vial

serotonin (5-hydroxytriptamine$_1$; 5-HT$_1$) [see: selective serotonin reuptake inhibitors; vascular serotonin receptor antagonists]

Seroxat (European name for U.S. product Paxil)

SERPACWA (Skin Exposure Reduction Paste Against Chemical Warfare Agents) cream ℞ *to delay absorption of chemical warfare agents through the skin when applied before exposure; used in conjunction with MOPP (Mission Oriented Protective Posture) gear* [polytef; perfluoroalkylpolyether]

serrapeptase INN

Serratia marcescens **extract (polyribosomes)** *investigational (orphan) for primary brain malignancies*

sertaconazole INN

sertindole USAN, INN *antipsychotic; neuroleptic*

Sertoli cells, porcine *investigational (orphan) intracerebral implant for stage 4 and 5 Parkinson disease (for co-implantation with fetal neural cells)*

sertraline INN, BAN *selective serotonin reuptake inhibitor (SSRI) for depression, obsessive-compulsive disorder (OCD), panic disorder, and post-traumatic stress disorder* [also: sertraline HCl]

sertraline HCl USAN *selective serotonin reuptake inhibitor (SSRI) for depression, obsessive-compulsive disorder (OCD), panic disorder, and post-traumatic stress disorder (PTSD)* [also: sertraline]

serum albumin (SA) [see: albumin, human]

serum albumin, iodinated (^{125}I) human [see: albumin, iodinated I 125 serum]

serum albumin, iodinated (^{131}I) human [see: albumin, iodinated I 131 serum]

serum fibrinogen (SF) [see: fibrinogen, human]

serum globulin (SG) [see: globulin, immune]

serum gonadotrophin [see: gonadotrophin, serum]

serum gonadotropin [see: gonadotrophin, serum]

serum prothrombin conversion accelerator (SPCA) factor [see: factor VII]

Serutan granules OTC *bulk laxative* [psyllium] 2.5 g/tsp.

Serutan powder (discontinued 1999) OTC *bulk laxative* [psyllium] 3.4 g/tsp.

Serzone tablets ℞ *antidepressant* [nefazodone HCl] 50, 100, 150, 200, 250 mg

Serzone-5HT$_2$ (CAN) tablets ℞ *antidepressant* [nefazodone HCl] 50, 100, 150, 200 mg

sesame oil NF *solvent; oleaginous vehicle*

Sesame Street Complete chewable tablets OTC *vitamin/mineral/calcium/iron supplement* [multiple vitamins & minerals; calcium; iron; folic acid; biotin] ≛•80•10•0.2•0.015 mg

Sesame Street Plus Extra C chewable tablets OTC *vitamin supplement* [multiple vitamins; folic acid] ≛•0.2 mg

Sesame Street Plus Iron chewable tablets OTC *vitamin/iron supplement* [multiple vitamins; iron; folic acid] ≛•10•0.2 mg

setastine INN

setazindol INN

setiptiline INN

setoperone USAN, INN *antipsychotic*

setwall *medicinal herb* [see: valerian]

Seudotabs tablets OTC *nasal decongestant* [pseudoephedrine HCl] 30 mg

sevelamer HCl USAN *phosphate-binding polymer for hyperphosphatemia of end-stage renal disease*

7 + 3 protocol (cytarabine, daunorubicin) *chemotherapy protocol for acute myelocytic leukemia (AML)*

7 + 3 protocol (cytarabine, idarubicin) *chemotherapy protocol for acute myelocytic leukemia (AML)*

7 + 3 protocol (cytarabine, mitoxantrone) *chemotherapy protocol for acute myelocytic leukemia (AML)*

seven barks *medicinal herb* [see: hydrangea]

7E3 MAb [see: abciximab]

sevirumab USAN, INN *investigational (Phase I) antiviral for AIDS; orphan status withdrawn 1996*

sevitropium mesilate INN

sevoflurane USAN, INN *inhalation general anesthetic*

sevopramide INN

sezolamide HCl USAN *carbonic anhydrase inhibitor*

SF (serum fibrinogen) [see: fibrinogen, human]

SFC lotion OTC *soap-free therapeutic skin cleanser*

sfericase INN

SG (serum globulin) [see: globulin, immune]

SG (soluble gelatin) [see: gelatin]

shamrock, Indian *medicinal herb* [see: birthroot]

shamrock, water *medicinal herb* [see: buckbean]

shark cartilage (derived from *Sphyrna lewini, Squalus acanthias,* and other species) *natural remedy for cancer* [also: squalamine]

shark liver oil *emollient/protectant*

shavegrass *medicinal herb* [see: horsetail]

sheep laurel *medicinal herb* [see: mountain laurel]

Sheik Elite premedicated condom OTC *spermicidal/barrier contraceptive* [nonoxynol 9] 8%

shell flower *medicinal herb* [see: turtlebloom]

shellac NF *tablet coating agent*

Shepard's Cream Lotion; Shepard's Skin Cream OTC *moisturizer; emollient*

shepherd's club *medicinal herb* [see: mullein]

shepherd's heart *medicinal herb* [see: shepherd's purse]

shepherd's purse *(Capsella bursa-pastoris)* plant *medicinal herb for bleeding, ear disease, hypertension, painful menstruation, and urinary bleeding*

shigoka *medicinal herb* [see: Siberian ginseng]

shiitake mushrooms *(Lentinula edodes; Tricholomopsis edodes)* stem and cap *medicinal herb for boosting the immune system, cancer, lowering cholesterol, and viral illnesses*

Shohl solution, modified (sodium citrate & citric acid) *urinary alkalizer; compounding agent*

short chain fatty acids *investigational (orphan) for left-sided ulcerative colitis and chronic radiation proctitis*

short-leaved buchu *medicinal herb* [see: buchu]

Shur-Clens solution OTC *wound cleanser* [poloxamer 188] 20%

Shur-Seal vaginal gel OTC *spermicidal contraceptive (for use with a diaphragm)* [nonoxynol 9] 2%

siagoside INN

sialagogues *a class of agents that stimulate the secretion of saliva* [also called: ptyalagogues]

Sibelium ℞ *investigational (orphan) vasodilator for alternating hemiplegia* [flunarizine HCl]

Siberian ginseng *(Acanthopanax senticosus; Eleutherococcus senticosus)* root *medicinal herb for age spots, blood diseases, depression, hemorrhage, immune system stimulation, increasing endurance and longevity, normalizing blood pressure, platelet aggregation inhibition, sexual stimulation, and stress* [also see: ginseng]

Siblin granules (discontinued 1997) OTC *bulk laxative* [blond psyllium seed coatings] 2.5 g/tsp.

sibopirdine USAN *cognition enhancer for Alzheimer disease; nootropic*

sibrafiban USAN *platelet inhibitor; fibrinogen receptor antagonist; investigational (Phase III) oral glycoprotein IIb/IIIa receptor antagonist for acute coronary syndrome*

sibutramine INN, BAN *anorexiant for the treatment of obesity; monoamine reuptake inhibitor antidepressant* [also: sibutramine HCl]

sibutramine HCl USAN *anorexiant for the treatment of obesity; monoamine reuptake inhibitor antidepressant* [also: sibutramine]

siccanin INN

Sickledex test kit for professional use *in vitro diagnostic aid for hemoglobin S (sickle cell)*

sicklewort *medicinal herb* [see: woundwort]

side-flowering skullcap *medicinal herb* [see: skullcap]

SigPak (trademarked packaging form) *unit-of-use package*

Sigtab tablets OTC *vitamin supplement* [multiple vitamins; folic acid] ≛ • 0.4 mg

Sigtab-M tablets OTC *vitamin/mineral/calcium/iron supplement* [multiple vitamins & minerals; calcium; iron; folic acid; biotin] ≛ • 200 • 18 • 0.4 • 0.045 mg

siguazodan INN, BAN

Silace syrup OTC *laxative; stool softener* [docusate sodium] 60 mg/15 mL

Silace-C syrup OTC *stimulant laxative; stool softener* [casanthranol; docusate sodium; alcohol 10%] 30 • 60 mg/15 mL

Siladryl elixir OTC *antihistamine* [diphenhydramine HCl] 12.5 mg/5 mL

Silafed syrup OTC *decongestant; antihistamine* [pseudoephedrine HCl; triprolidine HCl] 30 • 1.25 mg/5 mL

silafilcon A USAN *hydrophilic contact lens material*

silafocon A USAN *hydrophobic contact lens material*

Silaminic Cold syrup OTC *decongestant; antihistamine* [phenylpropanolamine HCl; chlorpheniramine maleate] 12.5 • 2 mg/5 mL

Silaminic Expectorant syrup OTC *decongestant; expectorant* [phenylpropanolamine HCl; guaifenesin; alcohol 5%] 12.5 • 100 mg/5 mL

silandrone USAN, INN *androgen*

Silapap, Children's liquid OTC *analgesic; antipyretic* [acetaminophen] 80 mg/2.5 mL

Silapap, Infant's drops OTC *analgesic; antipyretic* [acetaminophen] 100 mg/mL

Sildec-DM syrup, pediatric drops ℞ *antitussive; decongestant; antihistamine* [dextromethorphan hydrobromide; pseudoephedrine HCl; carbinoxamine maleate] 15 • 60 • 4 mg/5 mL; 4 • 25 • 2 mg/mL

sildenafil citrate USAN *selective vasodilator for erectile dysfunction*

Sildicon-E pediatric drops OTC *pediatric decongestant and expectorant* [phenylpropanolamine HCl; guaifenesin] 6.25 • 30 mg/mL

Silfedrine, Children's liquid OTC *nasal decongestant* [pseudoephedrine HCl] 30 mg/5 mL

silibinin INN

silica, dental-type NF *pharmaceutic aid*

silica gel [now: silicon dioxide]

siliceous earth, purified NF *filtering medium*

silicic acid, magnesium salt [see: magnesium trisilicate]

silicon *element (Si)*

silicon dioxide NF *dispersing and suspending agent*

silicon dioxide, colloidal NF *suspending agent; tablet and capsule diluent*

silicone

Silicone No. 2 ointment OTC *skin protectant* [silicone; hydrophobic starch derivative] 10% • ≟

silicone oil [see: polydimethylsiloxane]

silicristin INN

silidianin INN

silkweed *medicinal herb* [see: milkweed; pleurisy root]

silky swallow wort; Virginia silk *medicinal herb* [see: milkweed]

silodrate USAN *antacid* [also: simaldrate]

Silphen Cough syrup OTC *antihistamine; antitussive* [diphenhydramine HCl; alcohol 5%] 12.5 mg/5 mL

Silphen DM syrup OTC *antitussive* [dextromethorphan hydrobromide; alcohol 5%] 10 mg/5 mL

Silphium perfoliatum *medicinal herb* [see: ragged cup]

Siltapp with Dextromethorphan HBr Cold & Cough elixir ℞ *antitussive; decongestant; antihistamine* [dextromethorphan hydrobromide; phenylpropanolamine HCl; brompheniramine maleate] 10•12.5•2 mg/5 mL

Sil-Tex liquid ℞ *decongestant; expectorant* [phenylpropanolamine HCl; phenylephrine HCl; guaifenesin; alcohol 5%] 20•5•100 mg/5 mL

Siltussin syrup OTC *expectorant* [guaifenesin; alcohol 3.5%] 100 mg/5 mL

Siltussin DM syrup OTC *antitussive; expectorant* [dextromethorphan hydrobromide; guaifenesin] 10•100 mg/5 mL

Siltussin-CF liquid OTC *antitussive; decongestant; expectorant* [dextromethorphan hydrobromide; phenylpropanolamine HCl; guaifenesin; alcohol 4.75%] 10•12.5•100 mg/5 mL

Silvadene cream ℞ *broad-spectrum bactericidal for adjunctive burn treatment* [silver sulfadiazine] 10 mg/g ⑨ Azulfidine

silver *element (Ag)*

silver nitrate USP *ophthalmic neonatal anti-infective; strong caustic* 1% eye drops; 10%, 25%, 50%, 75% topical

silver nitrate, toughened USP *caustic*

silver protein, mild NF *ophthalmic antiseptic; ophthalmic surgical aid*

silver sulfadiazine (SSD) USAN, USP *broad-spectrum bactericidal; adjunct to burn therapy* [also: sulfadiazine silver]

silverweed; silver cinquefoil *medicinal herb* [see: cinquefoil]

Silybum marianum *medicinal herb* [see: milk thistle]

Simaal Gel; Simaal Gel 2 liquid (discontinued 2000) OTC *antacid; antiflatulent* [aluminum hydroxide; magnesium hydroxide; simethicone] 200•200•20 mg/5 mL; 500•400•40 mg/5 mL

simaldrate INN *antacid* [also: silodrate]

Simdax *investigational cardiotonic and vasodilator for congestive heart failure* [levosimendan]

simethicone USAN, USP *antiflatulent; adjunct to gastrointestinal imaging* 80 mg oral; 40 mg/0.6 mL oral

simethicone-coated cellulose suspension (SCCS) [see: SonoRx]

simetride INN

simfibrate INN

Similac Human Milk Fortifier powder OTC *supplementary infant feeding (add to breast milk)* 900 mg packets

Similac Low Iron liquid, powder OTC *total or supplementary infant feeding*

Similac PM 60/40 Low-Iron liquid OTC *formula for infants predisposed to hypocalcemia* [whey formula with lowered mineral levels]

Similac with Iron liquid, powder OTC *total or supplementary infant feeding*

simple syrup [see: syrup]

Simpler's joy *medicinal herb* [see: blue vervain]

Simplet tablets OTC *decongestant; antihistamine; analgesic* [pseudoephedrine HCl; chlorpheniramine maleate; acetaminophen] 60•4•650 mg ⑨ Singlet

Simron soft gelatin capsules (discontinued 1998) OTC *hematinic* [ferrous gluconate (source of iron)] 86 mg (10 mg)

Simron Plus capsules OTC *vitamin/iron supplement* [multiple vitamins; ferrous gluconate; folic acid] ≛•10•0.1 mg

simtrazene USAN, INN *antineoplastic*

Simulect powder for IV infusion *immunosuppressant; IL-2 receptor antagonist for the prevention of acute rejection of renal transplants (orphan)* [basiliximab] 20 mg

simvastatin USAN, INN, BAN *HMG-CoA reductase inhibitor for hyperlipidemia, hypertriglyceridemia, and coro-*

nary heart disease ⓢ Sandostatin; zinostatin

Sinapils tablets OTC *decongestant; antihistamine; analgesic* [phenylpropanolamine HCl; chlorpheniramine maleate; acetaminophen; caffeine] 12.5•2•325•32.5 mg

Sinapis alba *medicinal herb* [see: mustard]

sinapultide USAN *pulmonary surfactant for respiratory distress syndrome*

Sinarest; Sinarest Sinus tablets OTC *decongestant; antihistamine; analgesic* [pseudoephedrine HCl; chlorpheniramine maleate; acetaminophen] 30•2•500 mg; 30•2•325 mg

Sinarest, No Drowsiness tablets OTC *decongestant; analgesic; antipyretic* [pseudoephedrine HCl; acetaminophen] 30•500 mg

Sinarest 12 Hour nasal spray OTC *nasal decongestant* [oxymetazoline HCl] 0.05%

sincalide USAN, INN *choleretic; diagnostic aid for gallbladder function*

Sine-Aid tablets, caplets, gelcaps OTC *decongestant; analgesic; antipyretic* [pseudoephedrine HCl; acetaminophen] 30•500 mg

Sine-Aid IB caplets OTC *decongestant; analgesic* [pseudoephedrine HCl; ibuprofen] 30•200 mg

sinefungin USAN, INN *antifungal*

Sinemet 10/100; Sinemet 25/100; Sinemet 25/250 tablets ℞ *antiparkinsonian; dopamine precursor; decarboxylase inhibitor* [carbidopa; levodopa] 10•100 mg; 25•100 mg; 25•250 mg

Sinemet CR sustained-release tablets ℞ *antiparkinsonian; dopamine precursor; decarboxylase inhibitor* [carbidopa; levodopa] 25•100, 50•200 mg

Sine-Off No Drowsiness Formula caplets OTC *decongestant; analgesic; antipyretic* [pseudoephedrine HCl; acetaminophen] 30•500 mg

Sine-Off Sinus Medicine caplets OTC *decongestant; antihistamine; analgesic* [pseudoephedrine HCl; chlorpheniramine maleate; acetaminophen] 30•2•500 mg

Sinequan capsules, oral concentrate ℞ *tricyclic antidepressant and anxiolytic* [doxepin HCl] 10, 25, 50, 75, 100, 150 mg; 10 mg/mL

Sinex nasal spray OTC *nasal decongestant* [phenylephrine HCl] 0.5%

Sinex 12-Hour nasal spray OTC *nasal decongestant* [oxymetazoline HCl] 0.05%

single-chain antigen-binding proteins (SCA proteins) *a class of investigational antineoplastics*

SingleJect (trademarked dosage form) *prefilled syringe*

Singlet for Adults tablets OTC *decongestant; antihistamine; analgesic* [pseudoephedrine HCl; chlorpheniramine maleate; acetaminophen] 60•4•650 mg ⓢ Simplet

Singulair chewable tablets, film-coated tablets ℞ *leukotriene receptor inhibitor for prophylaxis and chronic treatment of asthma* [montelukast sodium] 4, 5 mg; 10 mg

Sinografin intracavitary instillation ℞ *radiopaque contrast medium for gynecological imaging* [diatrizoate meglumine; iodipamide meglumine (47.8% total iodine)] 727•268 mg/mL (380 mg/mL)

sinorphan [now: ecadotril]

sintropium bromide INN

Sinufed Timecelles (sustained-release capsules) ℞ *decongestant; expectorant* [pseudoephedrine HCl; guaifenesin] 60•300 mg

Sinulin tablets OTC *decongestant; antihistamine; analgesic* [phenylpropanolamine HCl; chlorpheniramine maleate; acetaminophen] 25•4•650 mg

Sinumist-SR sustained-release Capsulets (capsule-shaped tablet) ℞ *expectorant* [guaifenesin] 600 mg

Sinupan controlled-release capsules ℞ *decongestant; expectorant* [phenylephrine HCl; guaifenesin] 40•200 mg

Sinus Headache & Congestion tablets OTC *decongestant; antihistamine; analgesic* [pseudoephedrine HCl;

chlorpheniramine maleate; acetaminophen] 30•2•500 mg

Sinus Relief tablets OTC *decongestant; analgesic* [pseudoephedrine HCl; acetaminophen] 30•325 mg

Sinusol-B subcu or IM injection (discontinued 1997) ℞ *antihistamine for anaphylaxis* [brompheniramine maleate] 10 mg/mL

Sinustop Pro capsules OTC *nasal decongestant* [pseudoephedrine HCl] 60 mg

Sinutab Non-Drying liquid capsules OTC *decongestant; expectorant* [pseudoephedrine HCl; guaifenesin] 30•200 mg

Sinutab Sinus Allergy caplets, tablets OTC *decongestant; antihistamine; analgesic* [pseudoephedrine HCl; chlorpheniramine maleate; acetaminophen] 30•2•500 mg

Sinutab Without Drowsiness caplets OTC *decongestant; analgesic; antipyretic* [pseudoephedrine HCl; acetaminophen] 30•500 mg

Sinutab Without Drowsiness tablets OTC *decongestant; analgesic; antipyretic* [pseudoephedrine HCl; acetaminophen] 30•325 mg; 30•500 mg

SinuVent long-acting tablets ℞ *decongestant; expectorant* [phenylpropanolamine HCl; guaifenesin] 75•600 mg

Sirdalud (foreign name for U.S. product Zanaflex)

sirolimus USAN *immunosuppressant for renal transplantation*

sisomicin USAN, INN *antibacterial* [also: sissomicin]

sisomicin sulfate USAN, USP *antibacterial*

sissomicin BAN *antibacterial* [also: sisomicin]

sitafloxacin USAN *antibacterial; DNA-gyrase inhibitor*

sitalidone INN

sitofibrate INN

sitogluside USAN, INN *antiprostatic hypertrophy*

sitosterols NF

Sitzmarks capsules ℞ *radiopaque contrast medium for severe constipation* [polyvinyl chloride, radiopaque] 24 rings/capsule

sizofiran INN

SK (streptokinase) [q.v.]

Skeeter Stik liquid OTC *topical local anesthetic; counterirritant* [lidocaine; menthol] 4%•1%

Skelaxin tablets ℞ *skeletal muscle relaxant* [metaxalone] 400 mg

Skelid tablets ℞ *bisphosphonate bone resorption inhibitor for Paget disease* [tiludronate disodium] 240 mg

skin respiratory factor (SRF) *claimed to promote wound healing*

Skin Shield liquid OTC *skin protectant; topical local anesthetic* [dyclonine HCl; benzethonium chloride] 0.75%•0.2%

Skinoren (German name for U.S. product Azelex)

skullcap *(Scutellaria lateriflora)* plant *medicinal herb for convulsions, epilepsy, fever, hypertension, infertility, insomnia, nervous disorders, rabies, and restlessness*

skunk cabbage *(Symplocarpus foetidus)* root *medicinal herb used as an antispasmodic, diuretic, emetic, expectorant, pectoral, stimulant, and sudorific*

skunk weed *medicinal herb* [see: skunk cabbage]

SL (sodium lactate) [q.v.]

Sleep-Eze 3 tablets OTC *antihistaminic sleep aid* [diphenhydramine HCl] 25 mg

Sleepinal capsules, soft gels OTC *antihistaminic sleep aid* [diphenhydramine HCl] 50 mg

Sleepwell 2-nite tablets OTC *antihistaminic sleep aid* [diphenhydramine HCl] 25 mg

Slim-Mint gum OTC *decrease taste perception of sweetness* [benzocaine] 6 mg

slippery elm *(Ulmus fulva; U. rubra)* inner bark *medicinal herb for asthma, blackened or bruised eyes, boils, bronchitis, burns, cold sores, colitis, cough, diaper rash, diarrhea, indigestion, lung disorders, sore throat, and urinary tract inflammation*

slippery root *medicinal herb* [see: comfrey]

Slo-bid Gyrocaps (extended-release capsules) ℞ *antiasthmatic; bronchodilator* [theophylline] 50, 75, 100, 125, 200, 300 mg

Slocaps (trademarked form) *sustained-release capsules*

Slo-Niacin controlled-release tablets OTC *vitamin B_3 supplement; antihyperlipidemic* [niacin] 250, 500, 750 mg

Slonnon (Japanese name for U.S. product Acova)

Slo-phyllin tablets, syrup, Gyrocaps (extended-release capsules) ℞ *antiasthmatic; bronchodilator* [theophylline] 100, 200 mg; 80 mg/15 mL; 60, 125, 250 mg

Slo-phyllin GG capsules, syrup ℞ *antiasthmatic; bronchodilator; expectorant* [theophylline; guaifenesin] 150•90 mg; 150•90 mg/15 mL

Slo-Salt-K slow-release tablets OTC *sodium chloride/potassium replacement; dehydration preventative* [sodium chloride; potassium chloride] 410•150 mg

slow channel blockers *a class of coronary vasodilators that inhibit cardiac muscle contraction and slow cardiac electrical conduction velocity* [also called: calcium channel blockers; calcium antagonists]

Slow Fe slow-release tablets OTC *hematinic* [ferrous sulfate, dried (source of iron)] 160 mg (50 mg)

Slow Fe with Folic Acid slow-release tablets OTC *hematinic* [ferrous sulfate; folic acid] 50•0.4 mg

Slow Fluoride slow-release tablets ℞ *investigational agent for postmenopausal osteoporosis* [sodium fluoride]

Slow-K controlled-release tablets ℞ *potassium supplement* [potassium chloride] 600 mg (8 mEq)

Slow-Mag delayed-release enteric-coated tablets OTC *magnesium supplement* [magnesium chloride] 535 mg ⊡ Flomax; Zomig

SLT hair lotion OTC *antiseborrheic; antipsoriatic; keratolytic; antiseptic* [coal tar; salicylic acid; lactic acid; alcohol 65%] 2%•3%•5%

small burnet saxifrage *medicinal herb* [see: burnet]

small pimpernel *medicinal herb* [see: burnet]

small saxifrage *medicinal herb* [see: burnet]

smallpox vaccine USP *active immunizing agent*

SMART anti-CD3 antibody *investigational (Phase I) immunosuppressant*

SMART anti-gpIIb/IIIa monoclonal antibody *investigational cardiovascular antiplatelet agent*

SMART anti-tac; humanized anti-tac [now: daclizimab]

SMART M195 antibody *investigational (Phase III) agent for acute myelogenous leukemia*

SmartMist (trademarked form) *hand-held inhalation device*

smartweed; water smartweed *medicinal herb* [see: knotweed]

SMF (streptozocin, mitomycin, fluorouracil) *chemotherapy protocol for pancreatic cancer*

***Smilax* spp.** *medicinal herb* [see: sarsaparilla]

smooth sumach *medicinal herb* [see: sumach]

SMX; SMZ (sulfamethoxazole) [q.v.]

SMZ-TMP (sulfamethoxazole & trimethoprim) [q.v.]

SN (streptonigrin) [q.v.]

snake bite *medicinal herb* [see: birthroot]

snake head *medicinal herb* [see: turtlebloom]

snake lily *medicinal herb* [see: blue flag]

snake weed *medicinal herb* [see: bistort; plantain]

snakebite antivenin [see: antivenin, Crotalidae & Micrurus fulvius]

snakeroot *medicinal herb* [see: echinacea]

snakeroot, black *medicinal herb* [see: black cohosh; sanicle]

Snaplets-DM granules OTC *pediatric antitussive and decongestant* [dextromethorphan hydrobromide; phenylpropanolamine HCl] 5•6.25 mg/packet

Snaplets-EX granules OTC *pediatric decongestant and expectorant* [phenylpropanolamine HCl; guaifenesin] 6.25•50 mg/packet

Snaplets-FR granules (discontinued 1997) OTC *analgesic; antipyretic* [acetaminophen] 80 mg/packet

Snaplets-Multi granules OTC *pediatric antitussive, decongestant, and antihistamine* [dextromethorphan hydrobromide; phenylpropanolamine HCl; chlorpheniramine maleate] 5•6.25•1 mg/packet

snapping hazel *medicinal herb* [see: witch hazel]

SnapTab (trademarked dosage form) *scored tablet*

SnET2 (tin ethyl etiopurpurin) [now: rostaporfin]

Snooze Fast tablets OTC *antihistaminic sleep aid* [diphenhydramine HCl] 50 mg

Sno-Strips ophthalmic strips *diagnostic tear flow test aid*

snout, swine *medicinal herb* [see: dandelion]

snowball, wild *medicinal herb* [see: New Jersey tea]

snowdrop tree; snowflower *medicinal herb* [see: fringe tree]

SNX-482 *investigational selective R-type calcium channel blocker for treatment of brain and neurological disorders*

Soac-Lens solution OTC *wetting/soaking solution for hard contact lenses*

soap, green USP *detergent*

soapwort ***(Saponaria officinalis)*** plant and roots *medicinal herb for acne, boils, eczema, poison ivy rash and psoriasis; also used in skin disinfectants and soaps*

SOD (superoxide dismutase) [see: orgotein]

soda lime NF *carbon dioxide absorbent*

sodium *element (Na)*

sodium acetate USP *dialysis aid; electrolyte replenisher; pH buffer* 2, 4 mEq/mL (16.4%, 32.8%) injection

sodium acetate trihydrate [see: sodium acetate]

sodium acetrizoate INN, BAN [also: acetrizoate sodium]

sodium acetylsalicylate *analgesic*

sodium acid phosphate *urinary acidifier*

sodium acid pyrophosphate *urinary acidifier*

sodium alginate NF *suspending agent*

sodium amidotrizoate INN *oral/rectal/parenteral radiopaque contrast medium (59.87% iodine)* [also: diatrizoate sodium; sodium diatrizoate]

sodium aminobenzoate [see: aminobenzoate sodium]

sodium amylopectin sulfate [see: sodium amylosulfate]

sodium amylosulfate USAN *enzyme inhibitor*

sodium anoxynaphthonate BAN *blood volume and cardiac output test* [also: anazolene sodium]

sodium antimony gluconate [see: sodium stibogluconate]

sodium antimonylgluconate BAN

sodium apolate INN, BAN *anticoagulant* [also: lyapolate sodium]

sodium arsenate, exsiccated NF

sodium arsenate As 74 USAN *radioactive agent*

sodium ascorbate (vitamin C) USP, INN *water-soluble vitamin; antiscorbutic*

sodium aurothiomalate INN *antirheumatic* [also: gold sodium thiomalate]

sodium aurotiosulfate INN [also: gold sodium thiosulfate]

sodium azodisalicylate [now: olsalazine sodium]

sodium benzoate USAN, NF, JAN *antihyperammonemic; antifungal agent; preservative*

sodium benzoate & caffeine *stimulant for respiratory depression due to an overdose of CNS depressants* 250 mg/mL injection

sodium benzoate & sodium phenylacetate *to prevent and treat hyperammonemia of urea cycle enzymopathy (orphan)*

sodium benzyl penicillin [see: penicillin G sodium]

sodium bicarbonate USP *electrolyte replenisher; systemic alkalizer; antacid* 325, 600, 650 mg oral; 0.5, 0.6, 0.9, 1 mEq/mL (4.2%, 5%, 7.5%, 8.4%) injection

sodium biphosphate *urinary acidifier; pH buffer*

sodium bisulfite NF *antioxidant*

sodium bitionolate INN *topical anti-infective* [also: bithionolate sodium]

sodium borate NF *alkalizing agent; antipruritic; bacteriostatic agent in cold creams, eye washes, and mouth rinses*

sodium borocaptate (^{10}B) INN *antineoplastic; radioactive agent* [also: borocaptate sodium B 10]

sodium cacodylate NF

sodium calcium edetate INN *heavy metal chelating agent* [also: edetate calcium disodium; sodium calciumedetate; calcium disodium edetate]

sodium calciumedetate BAN *heavy metal chelating agent* [also: edetate calcium disodium; sodium calcium edetate; calcium disodium edetate]

sodium caprylate *antifungal*

sodium carbonate NF *alkalizing agent*

sodium chloride (NaCl) USP *ophthalmic hypertonic; electrolyte replacement; abortifacient; diluent* [sterile isotonic solution] 650, 1000, 2250 mg oral; 0.45%, 0.9%, 3%, 5%, 14.6%, 23.4% injection/diluent

0.45% sodium chloride (½ normal saline; ½ NS) *electrolyte replacement*

0.9% sodium chloride (normal saline; NS) *electrolyte replacement* [also: saline solution]

sodium chloride, compound solution of INN *fluid and electrolyte replenisher* [also: Ringer injection]

sodium chloride Na 22 USAN *radioactive agent*

sodium chondroitin sulfate [see: chondroitin sulfate sodium]

sodium chromate (^{51}Cr) INN *blood volume test; radioactive agent* [also: sodium chromate Cr 51]

sodium chromate Cr 51 USAN *blood volume test; radioactive agent* [also: sodium chromate (^{51}Cr)]

sodium citrate USP *systemic alkalizer; pH buffer; antacid; investigational (orphan) adjunct to leukapheresis procedures*

sodium colistin methanesulfonate [see: colistimethate sodium]

sodium cromoglycate [see: cromolyn sodium]

sodium cyclamate NF, INN

sodium cyclohexanesulfamate [see: sodium cyclamate]

sodium dehydroacetate NF *antimicrobial preservative*

sodium dehydrocholate INN [also: dehydrocholate sodium]

sodium denyl [see: phenytoin sodium]

sodium diatrizoate BAN *oral/rectal/parenteral radiopaque contrast medium (59.87% iodine)* [also: diatrizoate sodium; sodium amidotrizoate]

sodium dibunate INN, BAN

sodium dicloroacetate (sodium DCA) USAN *pyruvate dehydrogenase activator; investigational (orphan) for acute head trauma and neurologic injury; investigational (orphan) for lactic acidosis and homozygous familial hypercholesterolemia*

sodium diethyldithiocarbamate [see: ditiocarb sodium]

sodium diiodomethanesulfonate [see: dimethiodal sodium]

sodium dioctyl sulfosuccinate INN *stool softener; surfactant* [also: docusate sodium]

sodium diphenylhydantoin [see: phenytoin sodium]

sodium diprotrizoate INN, BAN [also: diprotrizoate sodium]

Sodium Diuril powder for IV injection ℞ *diuretic* [chlorothiazide] 500 mg

sodium edetate [see: edetate sodium]

sodium estrone sulfate *estrogen replacement therapy for postmenopausal disorders* 0.625, 1.25, 2.5, 5 mg oral

sodium etasulfate INN *detergent* [also: sodium ethasulfate]

sodium ethasulfate USAN *detergent* [also: sodium etasulfate]

sodium feredetate INN [also: sodium ironedetate]

sodium ferric gluconate *hematinic for iron deficiency of chronic hemodialysis with erythropoietin therapy*

sodium fluoride USP *fluoride replacement therapy; dental caries preventative; investigational agent for treatment of postmenopausal osteoporosis* 1.1, 2.2 mg oral; 0.125 mg/drop oral

sodium fluoride F 18 USP

sodium fluoride & phosphoric acid USP *dental caries prophylactic*

sodium formaldehyde sulfoxylate NF *preservative*

sodium gamma hydroxybutyrate (NaGHB) [see: gamma hydroxybutyrate (GHB); sodium oxybate]

sodium gammahydroxyburate [see: sodium oxybate]

sodium gentisate INN

sodium glucaspaldrate INN, BAN

sodium gluconate USP *electrolyte replenisher*

sodium glucosulfone USP

sodium glutamate

sodium glycerophosphate NF

sodium glycocholate [see: bile salts]

sodium gualenate INN [also: azulene sulfonate sodium]

sodium hyaluronate [see: hyaluronate sodium]

sodium hydroxide NF *alkalizing agent*

sodium hydroxybenzenesulfonate [see: phenolsulphonate sodium]

sodium 4-hydroxybutyrate [see: sodium oxybate]

sodium hypochlorite USP, JAN *disinfectant and bleach used for utensils and equipment; topical dissolution of dental caries*

sodium hypochlorite, diluted NF [also: antiformin, dental]

sodium hypophosphite NF

sodium iodide USP *dietary iodine supplement*

sodium iodide (^{123}I) JAN *thyroid function test; radioactive agent* [also: sodium iodide I 123]

sodium iodide (^{125}I) INN *thyroid function test; radioactive agent* [also: sodium iodide I 125]

sodium iodide (^{131}I) JAN *antineoplastic for thyroid carcinoma; radioactive agent for hyperthyroidism* [also: sodium iodide I 131]

sodium iodide I 123 USP *radioactive agent; diagnostic aid for thyroid function* [also: sodium iodide (^{123}I)] 3.7, 7.4 MBq oral

sodium iodide I 125 USAN, USP *thyroid function test; radioactive agent* [also: sodium iodide (^{125}I)]

sodium iodide I 131 USAN, USP, INN *antineoplastic for thyroid carcinoma; radioactive agent for hyperthyroidism* [also: sodium iodide (^{131}I)] 0.75–100 mCi, 3.5–150 mCi oral

sodium iodohippurate (^{131}I) INN, JAN *renal function test; radioactive agent* [also: iodohippurate sodium I 131]

sodium iodomethanesulfonate [see: methiodal sodium]

sodium iopodate JAN *oral radiopaque contrast medium for cholecystography (61.4% iodine)* [also: ipodate sodium; sodium ipodate]

sodium iotalamate (^{125}I) INN *radioactive agent* [also: iothalamate sodium I 125]

sodium iotalamate (^{131}I) INN *radioactive agent* [also: iothalamate sodium I 131]

sodium iothalamate BAN *parenteral radiopaque contrast medium (59.9% iodine)* [also: iothalamate sodium]

sodium ioxaglate BAN *radiopaque contrast medium* [also: ioxaglate sodium]

sodium ipodate INN, BAN *oral radiopaque contrast medium for cholecystography (61.4% iodine)* [also: ipodate sodium; sodium iopodate]

sodium ironedetate BAN [also: sodium feredetate]

sodium lactate (SL) USP *electrolyte replenisher* 167 mEq/L (1/6 molar) injection

sodium lactate, compound solution of INN *electrolyte and fluid replenisher; systemic alkalizer* [also: Ringer injection, lactated]

sodium lauryl sulfate NF *surfactant/wetting agent* [also: laurilsulfate]

sodium lignosulfonate [see: polignate sodium]

sodium metabisulfite NF *antioxidant*

sodium metrizoate INN *radiopaque contrast medium* [also: metrizoate sodium]

sodium monododecyl sulfate [see: sodium lauryl sulfate]

sodium monofluorophosphate USP *dental caries prophylactic*

sodium monomercaptoundecahydro-closo-dodecaborate *investigational (orphan) for boron neutron capture therapy (BNCT) for glioblastoma multiforme*

sodium morrhuate INN *sclerosing agent* [also: morrhuate sodium]

sodium nitrite USP *antidote to cyanide poisoning*

sodium nitroferricyanide [see: sodium nitroprusside]

sodium nitroferricyanide dihydrate [see: sodium nitroprusside]

sodium nitroprusside USP *emergency antihypertensive; vasodilator* 50 mg/dose injection

sodium noramidopyrine methanesulfonate [see: dipyrone]

sodium oxybate USAN *adjunct to anesthesia; investigational (NDA filed, orphan) for narcolepsy, cataplexy, sleep paralysis, and hypnagogic hallucinations*

sodium oxychlorosene [see: oxychlorosene sodium]

sodium paratoluenesulfan chloramide [see: chloramine-T]

sodium penicillin G [see: penicillin G sodium]

sodium pentosan polysulfate [see: pentosan polysulfate sodium]

sodium perborate *topical antiseptic/germicidal*

sodium perborate monohydrate USAN

sodium pertechnetate Tc 99m USAN, USP *radioactive agent*

sodium phenolate [see: phenolate sodium]

sodium phenylacetate USAN *antihyperammonemic*

sodium phenylacetate & sodium benzoate *to prevent and treat hyperammonemia of urea cycle enzymopathy (orphan)*

sodium phenylbutyrate USAN *antihyperammonemic for urea cycle disorders (orphan); investigational (orphan) for various sickling disorders*

sodium phosphate (^{32}P) INN *antineoplastic; antipolycythemic; neoplasm test* [also: sodium phosphate P 32]

sodium phosphate, dibasic USP *saline laxative; phosphorus replacement; pH buffer*

sodium phosphate, monobasic USP *saline laxative; phosphorus replacement; pH buffer*

sodium phosphate P 32 USAN, USP *antipolycythemic; radiopharmaceutical antineoplastic for various leukemias and skeletal metastases* [also: sodium phosphate (^{32}P)] 0.67 mCi/mL

sodium picofosfate INN

sodium picosulfate INN

sodium polyphosphate USAN *pharmaceutic aid*

sodium polystyrene sulfonate USP *potassium-removing ion-exchange resin for hyperkalemia* 15 g/60 mL oral

sodium propionate NF *preservative; antifungal*

sodium propionate hydrate [see: sodium propionate]

sodium 2-propylvalerate [see: valproate sodium]

sodium psylliate NF

sodium pyrophosphate USAN *pharmaceutic aid*

sodium radiochromate [see: sodium chromate Cr 51]

sodium rhodanate [see: thiocyanate sodium]

sodium salicylate (SS) USP *analgesic; antipyretic; anti-inflammatory; antirheumatic* 325, 650 mg oral

sodium starch glycolate NF *tablet excipient*

sodium stearate NF *emulsifying and stiffening agent*

sodium stearyl fumarate NF *tablet and capsule lubricant*

sodium stibocaptate INN [also: stibocaptate]

sodium stibogluconate INN, BAN, DCF *investigational antiparasitic for leishmaniasis and trypanosomiasis*

Sodium Sulamyd eye drops, ophthalmic ointment ℞ *topical ophthalmic antibiotic* [sulfacetamide sodium] 10%, 30%; 10%

sodium sulfacetamide [see: sulfacetamide sodium]

sodium sulfate USP *calcium regulator*

sodium sulfate S 35 USAN *radioactive agent*

sodium sulfocyanate [see: thiocyanate sodium]

sodium taurocholate [see: bile salts]

sodium tetradecyl (STD) sulfate INN *sclerosing agent; investigational (orphan) for bleeding esophageal varices*

sodium thiomalate, gold [see: gold sodium thiomalate]

sodium thiosalicylate *analgesic; antipyretic; anti-inflammatory; antirheumatic* 50 mg/mL injection

sodium thiosulfate USP *antidote to cyanide poisoning; antiseptic; antifungal* 25% (250 mg/mL) IV injection

sodium thiosulfate, gold [see: gold sodium thiosulfate]

sodium thiosulfate & hydroxocobalamin *investigational (orphan) for severe acute cyanide poisoning*

sodium timerfonate INN *topical anti-infective* [also: thimerfonate sodium]

sodium trimetaphosphate USAN *pharmaceutic aid*

sodium tyropanoate INN *oral radiopaque contrast medium for cholecystography (57.4% iodine)* [also: tyropanoate sodium]

sodium valproate [see: valproate sodium]

Sodol Compound tablets ℞ *skeletal muscle relaxant; analgesic* [carisoprodol; aspirin] 200•325 mg

sofalcone INN

Sofenol 5 lotion OTC *moisturizer; emollient*

Soft Mate Comfort Drops for Sensitive Eyes OTC *rewetting solution for soft contact lenses*

Soft Mate Consept solution + aerosol spray OTC *two-step chemical disinfecting system for soft contact lenses* [hydrogen peroxide based] 3%

Soft Mate Disinfecting for Sensitive Eyes solution OTC *chemical disinfecting solution for soft contact lenses*

Soft Mate Hands Off Daily Cleaner solution OTC *surfactant cleaning solution for soft contact lenses*

soft pine *medicinal herb* [see: white pine]

Soft Sense lotion OTC *moisturizer; emollient*

Softabs (trademarked dosage form) *chewable tablets*

softgels (dosage form) *soft gelatin capsules*

SoftWear solution OTC *rinsing/storage solution for soft contact lenses* [sodium chloride (preserved saline solution)]

Solage topical solution ℞ *keratolytic and bleaching agent for solar lentigines* [mequinol; tretinoin] 2%•0.01%

Solanum dulcamara *medicinal herb* [see: bittersweet nightshade]

solapsone BAN [also: solasulfone]

Solaquin cream OTC *hyperpigmentation bleaching agent in a sunscreen base* [hydroquinone] 2%

Solaquin Forte cream, gel ℞ *hyperpigmentation bleaching agent; sunscreen* [hydroquinone; ethyl dihydroxypropyl PABA; dioxybenzone; oxybenzone] 4%•5%•3%•2%

Solaraze gel ℞ *topical treatment for actinic keratoses (AK)* [diclofenac potassium] 3%

Solarcaine aerosol spray, lotion OTC *topical local anesthetic; antiseptic* [benzocaine; triclosan] 20%•0.13%

Solarcaine Aloe Extra Burn Relief spray, gel, cream OTC *topical local anesthetic* [lidocaine] 0.5%

solasulfone INN [also: solapsone]

soldier's woundwort *medicinal herb* [see: yarrow]

Solfoton tablets, capsules ℞ *long-acting barbiturate sedative, hypnotic, and anticonvulsant* [phenobarbital] 16 mg

Solganal IM injection ℞ *antirheumatic* [aurothioglucose] 50 mg/mL

Solidago nemoralis; S. odora; S. virgaurea *medicinal herb* [see: goldenrod]

Solomon's seal *(Polygonatum multiflorum; P. odoratum)* root *medicinal herb used as an astringent, demulcent, emetic, and expectorant*

solpecainol INN

SolTabs (trademarked dosage form) *orally disintegrating tablets*

Soltice Quick-Rub OTC *topical analgesic; counterirritant* [methyl salicylate; camphor; menthol; eucalyptus oil]

soluble complement receptor [see: complement receptor type I, soluble recombinant human]

soluble ferric pyrophosphate [see: ferric pyrophosphate, soluble]

soluble gelatin (SG) [see: gelatin]

Solu-Cortef powder for IV or IM injection ℞ *corticosteroid; anti-inflammatory* [hydrocortisone sodium succinate] 100, 250, 500, 1000 mg/vial

Solu-Medrol powder for IV or IM injection ℞ *corticosteroid; anti-inflammatory; immunosuppressant* [methylprednisolone sodium succinate] 40, 125, 500, 1000, 2000 mg/vial

Solumol OTC *ointment base*

Solurex intra-articular, intralesional, soft tissue, or IM injection ℞ *corticosteroid; anti-inflammatory* [dexamethasone sodium phosphate] 4 mg/mL

Solurex LA intralesional, intra-articular, soft tissue, or IM injection ℞ *corticosteroid; anti-inflammatory* [dexamethasone acetate] 8 mg/mL

Soluspan (trademarked form) *injectable suspension*

Soluvite C.T. chewable tablets ℞ *pediatric vitamin supplement and dental caries preventative* [multiple vitamins; fluoride; folic acid] ≛•1•0.3 mg

Soluvite-f drops ℞ *pediatric vitamin supplement and dental caries preventative* [vitamins A, C, and D; fluoride] 1500 IU•35 mg•400 IU•0.25 mg per 0.6 mL

Solvent-G OTC *liquid base*

Solvet (trademarked dosage form) *soluble tablet*

solypertine INN *antiadrenergic* [also: solypertine tartrate]

solypertine tartrate USAN *antiadrenergic* [also: solypertine]

Soma tablets ℞ *skeletal muscle relaxant* [carisoprodol] 350 mg

Soma Compound tablets ℞ *skeletal muscle relaxant; analgesic* [carisoprodol; aspirin] 200•325 mg

Soma Compound with Codeine tablets ℞ *skeletal muscle relaxant; analgesic* [carisoprodol; aspirin; codeine phosphate] 200•325•16 mg

Somagard ℞ *investigational (orphan) LH-RH agonist for central precocious puberty* [deslorelin]

somagrebove USAN *veterinary galactopoietic agent*

somalapor USAN, INN, BAN *porcine growth hormone*

somantadine INN *antiviral* [also: somantadine HCl]

somantadine HCl USAN *antiviral* [also: somantadine]

SomatoKine ℞ *investigational (Phase II, orphan) agent for treatment of muscle degradation following severe burns and hip fracture surgery; investigational (Phase II) for type 1 diabetes* [IGF-BP3 complex]

somatomedin-C [see: mecasermin]

somatorelin INN *growth hormone-releasing factor (GH-RF)*

somatostatin (SS) INN, BAN *growth hormone-release inhibiting factor; investigational (orphan) for cutaneous gastrointestinal fistulas and bleeding esophageal varices*

somatotropin, human [see: somatropin]

Somatrel ℞ *investigational (orphan) diagnostic aid for pituitary release of growth hormone* [NG-29 (code name —generic name not yet assigned)]

somatrem USAN, INN, BAN *growth hormone for congenital growth failure due to lack of endogenous growth hormone (orphan)*

somatropin USAN, INN, BAN, JAN *growth hormone for adults or children with congenital or endogenous growth hormone deficiency, children with Turner syndrome or renal-induced growth failure, or AIDS-wasting syndrome (orphan); investigational (orphan) for severe burns* [also: human growth hormone]

somatropin & glutamine *investigational (orphan) for GI malabsorption due to short bowel syndrome*

Somavert injection ℞ *investigational (Phase III, orphan) growth hormone receptor antagonist for acromegaly* [pegvisomant]

somavubove USAN, INN *veterinary galactopoietic agent*

somenopor USAN *porcine growth hormone*

sometribove USAN, INN, BAN *veterinary growth stimulant*

sometripor USAN, INN, BAN *veterinary growth stimulant*

somfasepor USAN *veterinary growth stimulant*

somidobove USAN, INN *synthetic bovine growth hormone*

Sominex tablets, caplets OTC *antihistaminic sleep aid* [diphenhydramine HCl] 25 mg; 50 mg

Sominex Pain Relief tablets OTC *antihistaminic sleep aid; analgesic* [diphenhydramine HCl; acetaminophen] 25•500 mg

Sonata capsules ℞ *rapid-onset, short-duration hypnotic for the short-term treatment of insomnia* [zaleplon] 5, 10 mg

Sonazoid ℞ *investigational (NDA filed) ultrasound contrast agent*

sonepiprazole mesylate USAN *dopamine D_4 antagonist; antipsychotic*

SonoRx oral suspension ℞ *ultrasound imaging agent to reduce gas shadowing* [simethicone-coated cellulose] 7.5 mg/mL

Soothaderm lotion OTC *topical anesthetic; topical antihistamine; emollient* [pyrilamine maleate; benzocaine; zinc oxide] 2.07•2.08•41.35 mg/mL

sopecainol [see: solpecainol]

sopitazine INN

sopromidine INN

soproxil USAN *combining name for radicals or groups* [also: disoproxil]

soquinolol INN

sorb apple *medicinal herb* [see: mountain ash]

sorbic acid NF *antimicrobial agent; preservative*

sorbide nitrate [see: isosorbide dinitrate]

sorbimacrogol laurate 300 [see: polysorbate 20]

sorbimacrogol oleate 300 [see: polysorbate 80]

sorbimacrogol palmitate 300 [see: polysorbate 40]

sorbimacrogol stearate [see: polysorbate 60]

sorbimacrogol tristearate 300 [see: polysorbate 65]

sorbinicate INN

sorbinil USAN, INN, BAN *aldose reductase enzyme inhibitor*

sorbitan laurate INN *surfactant* [also: sorbitan monolaurate]

sorbitan monolaurate USAN, NF *surfactant* [also: sorbitan laurate]

sorbitan monooleate USAN, NF *surfactant* [also: sorbitan oleate]

sorbitan monopalmitate USAN, NF *surfactant* [also: sorbitan palmitate]

sorbitan monostearate USAN, NF *surfactant* [also: sorbitan stearate]

sorbitan oleate INN *surfactant* [also: sorbitan monooleate]

sorbitan palmitate INN *surfactant* [also: sorbitan monopalmitate]

sorbitan sesquioleate USAN, INN *surfactant*

sorbitan stearate INN *surfactant* [also: sorbitan monostearate]
sorbitan trioleate USAN, INN *surfactant*
sorbitan tristearate USAN, INN *surfactant*
sorbitol NF *flavoring agent; tablet excipient; urologic irrigant* 3%, 3.3%
sorbitol (solution) USP *flavoring agent; tablet excipient*
Sorbitrate tablets, sublingual tablets, chewable tablets ℞ *antianginal; vasodilator* [isosorbide dinitrate] 5, 10, 20, 30, 40 mg; 2.5, 5 mg; 5, 10 mg
Sorbsan pads *absorbent dressing for wet wounds* [calcium alginate fiber]
Sorbus americana; S. aucuparia *medicinal herb* [see: mountain ash]
Soriatane capsules ℞ *systemic antipsoriatic* [acitretin] 10, 25 mg
sorivudine USAN, INN, BAN *antiviral for varicella zoster and herpes zoster in immunocompromised patients; orphan status withdrawn 1997*
sornidipine INN
sorrel *(Rumex acetosa)* plant *medicinal herb used as an antiscorbutic, astringent, diuretic, laxative, refrigerant, and vermifuge*
sorrel, common; mountain sorrel; white sorrel *medicinal herb* [see: wood sorrel]
sorrel, Jamaica *medicinal herb* [see: hibiscus]
sotalol INN, BAN *antiarrhythmic; antiadrenergic (β-blocker)* [also: sotalol HCl]
sotalol HCl USAN *antiadrenergic (β-blocker); antiarrhythmic for ventricular arrhythmias (orphan)* [also: sotalol] 80, 120, 160, 240 mg oral
soterenol INN *adrenergic; bronchodilator* [also: soterenol HCl]
soterenol HCl USAN *adrenergic; bronchodilator* [also: soterenol]
Sotradecol IV injection, Dosette (unit-of-use injection) ℞ *sclerosing agent; investigational (orphan) for bleeding esophageal varices* [sodium tetradecyl sulfate] 1%, 3%
sour dock *medicinal herb* [see: yellow dock]
sourberry; sowberry *medicinal herb* [see: barberry]
sourgrass *medicinal herb* [see: sorrel]
Southern ginseng *medicinal herb* [see: jiaogulan]
Soviet gramicidin [see: gramicidin S]
sowberry; sourberry *medicinal herb* [see: barberry]
soy; soya; soybean *(Glycine max)* *medicinal herb and food crop; isoflavone compounds provide phytoestrogens to alleviate menopausal symptoms, including osteoporosis, and provide antineoplastic, cardiovascular, and gastrointestinal benefits*
Soyalac; I-Soyalac liquid, powder OTC *hypoallergenic infant food* [soy protein formula]
soybean oil USP *pharmaceutic necessity*
spaglumic acid INN
Span C tablets OTC *vitamin C supplement with bioflavonoids* [ascorbic acid and rose hips; citrus bioflavonoids] 200•300 mg
Spancap No. 1 sustained-release capsules ℞ *CNS stimulant* [dextroamphetamine sulfate] 15 mg
Spancaps (dosage form) *timed-release capsules*
Span-FF controlled-release capsules (discontinued 1998) OTC *hematinic* [ferrous fumarate (source of iron)] 325 mg (106 mg)
Spanidin *investigational (orphan) immunosuppressant for acute renal graft rejection* [gusperimus]
Spanish chestnut *medicinal herb* [see: horse chestnut]
Spanish pepper *medicinal herb* [see: cayenne]
Spansule (trademarked dosage form) *sustained-release capsule*
sparfloxacin USAN, INN, BAN *broad-spectrum fluoroquinolone antibiotic*
sparfosate sodium USAN *antineoplastic* [also: sparfosic acid]
sparfosic acid INN *antineoplastic* [also: sparfosate sodium]

Sparine tablets (discontinued 2001) ℞ *conventional (typical) antipsychotic* [promazine HCl] 25, 50 mg

Sparine Tubex (cartridge-needle unit for IM injection) (discontinued 1998) ℞ *conventional (typical) antipsychotic* [promazine HCl] 50 mg/mL

Sparkles effervescent granules OTC *antacid; aid in endoscopic examination* [sodium bicarbonate; citric acid; simethicone] 2000•1500•?mg/dose

sparsomycin USAN, INN *antineoplastic*

Spartaject ℞ *investigational (Phase II/III) intravenous delivery device*

sparteine INN *oxytocic* [also: sparteine sulfate]

sparteine sulfate USAN *oxytocic* [also: sparteine]

Spasmolin tablets ℞ *GI antispasmodic; anticholinergic; sedative* [atropine sulfate; scopolamine hydrobromide; hyoscyamine hydrobromide; phenobarbital] 0.0194•0.0065•0.1037•16.2 mg

SPC3 *investigational (Phase I/II) treatment for HIV*

SPCA (serum prothrombin conversion accelerator) factor [see: factor VII]

spearmint NF

spearmint *(Mentha spicata)* leaves *medicinal herb for colds, colic, flu, gas, nausea, and vomiting*

spearmint oil NF

Spec-T lozenges OTC *topical oral anesthetic* [benzocaine] 10 mg

Spec-T Sore Throat/Cough Suppressant lozenges OTC *topical oral anesthetic; antitussive* [benzocaine; dextromethorphan hydrobromide] 10•10 mg

Spec-T Sore Throat/Decongestant lozenges OTC *decongestant; topical oral anesthetic* [phenylpropanolamine HCl; phenylephrine HCl; benzocaine] 10.5•5•10 mg

Spectazole cream ℞ *topical antifungal* [econazole nitrate] 1%

spectinomycin INN *antibiotic* [also: spectinomycin HCl]

spectinomycin HCl USAN, USP *antibiotic* [also: spectinomycin]

Spectracef capsules ℞ *broad-spectrum cephalosporin antibiotic* [cefditoren pivoxil] 200, 400 mg

Spectrobid film-coated tablets ℞ *aminopenicillin antibiotic* [bacampicillin HCl] 400 mg

Spectrobid powder for oral suspension (discontinued 1997) ℞ *aminopenicillin antibiotic* [bacampicillin HCl] 125 mg/5 mL

Spectrocin Plus ointment OTC *topical antibiotic; local anesthetic* [neomycin sulfate; polymyxin B sulfate; bacitracin; lidocaine] 5000 U•3.5 mg•400 U•5 mg per g

Spectro-Jel liquid OTC *soap-free therapeutic skin cleanser*

speedwell *(Veronica officinalis)* flowering plant *medicinal herb used as a diuretic, expectorant, and stomachic*

speedwell, tall *medicinal herb* [see: Culver root]

spenbolic [see: methandriol]

spermaceti, synthetic [see: cetyl esters wax]

spermicides *a class of topical contraceptive agents that kill the male sperm*

Spersadex (CAN) eye drops (discontinued 1998) ℞ *topical ophthalmic corticosteroidal anti-inflammatory* [dexamethasone sodium phosphate] 0.1%

Spexil ℞ *investigational (Phase III) broad-spectrum aminocyclitol antibiotic for respiratory, gynecologic, and abdominal infections* [trospectomycin]

Spherulin intradermal injection ℞ *diagnostic aid for coccidioidomycosis* [coccidioidin] 1:100, 1:10

spiceberry *medicinal herb* [see: wintergreen]

spiclamine INN

spiclomazine INN

spicy wintergreen *medicinal herb* [see: wintergreen]

spider bite antivenin [see: antivenin (Latrodectus mactans)]

spignet *medicinal herb* [see: spikenard]

spikenard ***(Aralia racemosa)*** root *medicinal herb for asthma, childbirth, cough, and rheumatism*

spindle tree *medicinal herb* [see: wahoo]

spiperone USAN, INN *antipsychotic*

spiradoline INN *analgesic* [also: spiradoline mesylate]

spiradoline mesylate USAN *analgesic* [also: spiradoline]

spiramide INN

spiramycin USAN, INN, BAN *macrolide antibiotic* [also: acetylspiramycin]

spirapril INN, BAN *angiotensin-converting enzyme (ACE) inhibitor* [also: spirapril HCl]

spirapril HCl USAN *angiotensin-converting enzyme (ACE) inhibitor* [also: spirapril]

spiraprilat USAN, INN *angiotensin-converting enzyme (ACE) inhibitor*

spirazine INN

spirazine HCl [see: spirazine]

spirendolol INN

spirgetine INN

spirilene INN, BAN

spirit of nitrous ether [see: ethyl nitrite]

Spiriva ℞ *investigational once-daily inhaled bronchodilator for chronic obstructive pulmonary disease (COPD)* [tiotropium]

spirobarbital sodium

spirofylline INN

spirogermanium INN, BAN *antineoplastic* [also: spirogermanium HCl]

spirogermanium HCl USAN *antineoplastic* [also: spirogermanium]

spirohydantoin mustard [now: spiromustine]

spiromustine USAN, INN *antineoplastic*

spironolactone USP, INN, BAN, JAN *antihypertensive; potassium-sparing diuretic; aldosterone antagonist* 25, 50, 100 mg oral

spiroplatin USAN, INN, BAN *antineoplastic*

spirorenone INN

Spiros (trademarked delivery system) ℞ *investigational inhaler*

spirotriazine HCl [see: spirazine]

spiroxamide [see: spiroxatrine]

spiroxasone USAN, INN *diuretic*

spiroxatrine INN

spiroxepin INN

spirulina ***(Spirulina pratensis)*** plant *medicinal herb for chronic disease, enhancing antibody production, lowering serum lipids and triglycerides, and reducing gastric secretory activity; also used as a blood builder and food supplement*

spizofurone INN

SPL (staphage lysate) [q.v.]

SPL-Serologic types I and III solution for subcu injection, nasal aerosol, nasal drop, oral, or topical irrigation (discontinued 2000) ℞ *staphylococcal or polymicrobial vaccine* [staphage lysate (*Staphylococcus aureus* vaccine; Staphylococcus bacteriophage plaque-forming units)]

spoonwood *medicinal herb* [see: linden tree]

Sporanox capsules, PulsePak (one-week dose package), IV infusion ℞ *systemic triazole antifungal* [itraconazole] 100 mg; 28×100 mg; 10 mg/mL

Sporanox oral solution ("swish and swallow") ℞ *antifungal for esophageal and oropharyngeal candidiasis in immunocompromised patients* [itraconazole] 10 mg/mL

Sporidin-G ℞ *investigational (orphan) for treatment of Cryptosporidium-induced diarrhea in immunocompromised patients* [*Cryptosporidium parvum* bovine colostrum IgG concentrate]

Sports Spray OTC *topical analgesic; counterirritant; antiseptic* [methyl salicylate; menthol; camphor; alcohol 58%] 3.5%•10%•5%

Sportscreme OTC *topical analgesic* [trolamine salicylate] 10%

Sportscreme Ice gel OTC *topical analgesic; counterirritant* [trolamine; menthol] ?•2%

spotted alder *medicinal herb* [see: witch hazel]

spotted comfrey *medicinal herb* [see: lungwort]

spotted cranesbill *medicinal herb* [see: alum root]

spotted geranium *medicinal herb* [see: alum root]

spotted hemlock; spotted cowbane; spotted parsley *medicinal herb* [see: poison hemlock]

spotted lungwort *medicinal herb* [see: lungwort]

spotted thistle *medicinal herb* [see: blessed thistle]

spp. plural of species

SPPG (sulfated polysaccharide peptidoglycan) [see: tecogalan sodium]

Spray-U-Thin oral spray OTC *diet aid* [phenylpropanolamine HCl] 6.58 mg

spring wintergreen *medicinal herb* [see: wintergreen]

Sprinkle Caps (trademarked form) *powder*

sprodiamide USAN *heart and CNS imaging aid for MRI*

spruce *(Picea excelsa; P. mariana)* young shoots *medicinal herb used as a calmative, diaphoretic, expectorant, and pectoral*

spruce, Norway *medicinal herb* [see: spruce]

spruce, weeping *medicinal herb* [see: hemlock]

SPS oral suspension ℞ *potassium-removing agent for hyperkalemia* [sodium polystyrene sulfonate] 15 g/60 mL

S-P-T "liquid" capsules (discontinued 2000) ℞ *natural thyroid replacement for hypothyroidism or thyroid cancer* [thyroid, desiccated porcine] 60, 120, 180, 300 mg

spurge laurel; spurge olive *medicinal herb* [see: mezereon]

squalamine *natural remedy; investigational (Phase III, orphan) angiogenesis inhibitor for the treatment of solid tumors; investigational (Phase II) for advanced non–small cell lung cancer (NSCLC)* [also: shark cartilage]

squalane NF *oleaginous vehicle*

square, carpenter's *medicinal herb* [see: figwort]

squaw balm; squaw mint *medicinal herb* [see: pennyroyal]

squaw root *medicinal herb* [see: black cohosh; blue cohosh]

squaw tea *medicinal herb* [see: ephedra]

squaw vine *(Mitchella repens)* plant *medicinal herb for easing childbirth, lactation, and menstruation and for uterine disorders*

squaw weed *medicinal herb* [see: life root]

squawberry *medicinal herb* [see: squaw vine]

squill *(Urginea indica; U. maritima; U. scilla)* bulb *medicinal herb for edema and inducing emesis and expectoration; also used as a rat poison*

squirrel pea, ground *medicinal herb* [see: twin leaf]

SR-57746 *investigational (Phase III) agent for Alzheimer disease*

^{85}Sr [see: strontium chloride Sr 85]

^{85}Sr [see: strontium nitrate Sr 85]

^{85}Sr [see: strontium Sr 85]

SRC Expectorant liquid ℞ *narcotic antitussive; decongestant; expectorant* [hydrocodone bitartrate; pseudoephedrine HCl; guaifenesin; alcohol 12.5%] 5•60•200 mg/5 mL

SRF (skin respiratory factor) [q.v.]

SS (saline solution)

SS (sodium salicylate) [q.v.]

SS (somatostatin) [q.v.]

SSD (silver sulfadiazine) [q.v.]

SSD; SSD AF cream ℞ *broad-spectrum bactericidal for adjunctive burn treatment* [silver sulfadiazine] 10 mg/g

SSKI oral solution ℞ *expectorant* [potassium iodide] 1 g/mL

SSRIs (selective serotonin reuptake inhibitors) [q.v.]

S.S.S. High Potency Vitamin Tablets OTC *vitamin/mineral/iron supplement* [multiple vitamins & minerals; iron; biotin] ≛•27•0.0225 mg

S.S.S. Vitamin and Mineral Complex oral liquid OTC *vitamin/mineral/iron supplement* [multiple vitamins & minerals; iron; biotin; alcohol 6.6%] ≛•3•0.1 mg

S.T. 37 solution OTC *topical antiseptic* [hexylresorcinol] 0.1%

S-T Cort lotion ℞ *topical corticosteroidal anti-inflammatory* [hydrocortisone] 0.5%

S-T Forte 2 liquid ℞ *narcotic antitussive; antihistamine* [hydrocodone bitartrate; chlorpheniramine maleate] 2.5•2 mg/5 mL

ST1-RTA immunotoxin (SR 44163) *investigational for graft vs. host disease and B-chronic lymphocytic leukemia; orphan status withdrawn 1998*

Staarvisc intraocular injection ℞ *viscoelastic agent for ophthalmic surgery* [hyaluronate sodium]

stable factor [see: factor VII]

Stachys officinalis *medicinal herb* [see: betony]

Stadol IV or IM injection ℞ *narcotic agonist-antagonist analgesic* [butorphanol tartrate] 1, 2 mg/mL

Stadol NS nasal spray ℞ *narcotic agonist-antagonist analgesic; antimigraine agent* [butorphanol tartrate] 10 mg/mL

staff vine *medicinal herb* [see: bittersweet nightshade]

Stagesic capsules ℞ *narcotic analgesic* [hydrocodone bitartrate; acetaminophen] 5•500 mg

staggerweed *medicinal herb* [see: turkey corn]

staghorn *medicinal herb* [see: club moss]

Stahist sustained-release tablets ℞ *decongestant; antihistamine; anticholinergic* [phenylephrine HCl; pseudoephedrine HCl; chlorpheniramine maleate; hyoscyamine sulfate; atropine sulfate; scopolamine hydrobromide] 25•40•8•0.19•0.04•0.01 mg

stallimycin INN *antibacterial* [also: stallimycin HCl]

stallimycin HCl USAN *antibacterial* [also: stallimycin]

Stamoist E sustained-release tablets ℞ *decongestant; expectorant* [pseudoephedrine HCl; guaifenesin] 120•500 mg

Stamoist LA sustained-release tablets ℞ *decongestant; expectorant* [phenylpropanolamine HCl; guaifenesin] 75•400 mg

Stanate ℞ *investigational bilirubin inhibitor for neonatal hyperbilirubinemia*

standard VAC *chemotherapy protocol for sarcomas* [see: VAC standard]

Stanford V (mechlorethamine, doxorubicin, vinblastine, vincristine, bleomycin, etoposide, prednisone) *chemotherapy protocol for Hodgkin lymphoma*

stannous chloride USAN *pharmaceutic aid*

stannous fluoride USP *dental caries prophylactic*

stannous pyrophosphate USAN *skeletal imaging aid*

stannous sulfur colloid USAN *bone, liver and spleen imaging aid*

stannsoporfin USAN *investigational bilirubin inhibitor for neonatal hyperbilirubinemia*

stanolone BAN *investigational (orphan) for AIDS-wasting syndrome* [also: androstanolone]

stanozolol USAN, USP, INN, BAN *androgen; anabolic steroid*

staphage lysate (SPL) *active bacterin for staphylococcal infections*

Staphcillin powder for IV or IM injection (discontinued 1998) ℞ *penicillinase-resistant penicillin antibiotic* [methicillin sodium] 1, 4, 6, 10 g

StaphVAX ℞ *investigational (Phase III) vaccine against Staphylococcus aureus infection of end-stage renal disease*

Staphylococcus aureus **vaccine** [see: staphage lysate]

star anise *(Illicium anisatum; I. verum)* seeds *medicinal herb used as a carminative, stimulant, and stomachic; also added to other herbal medications to improve digestibility and taste*

star chickweed; starweed *medicinal herb* [see: chickweed]

star grass *(Aletris farinosa)* root and rhizome *medicinal herb for diarrhea, dysmenorrhea and menstrual discomfort, gas and colonic cramps, and rheumatism*

star root *medicinal herb* [see: star grass]

starch NF *dusting powder; pharmaceutic aid*

starch, pregelatinized NF *tablet excipient*

starch, topical USP *dusting powder*

starch carboxymethyl ether, sodium salt [see: sodium starch glycolate]

starch glycerite NF

starch 2-hydroxyethyl ether [see: hetastarch; pentastarch]

Starlix tablets ℞ *amino acid–derivative; antidiabetic agent for type 2 diabetes* [nateglinide] 60, 120 mg

Starnoc (CAN) capsules ℞ *rapid-onset, short-duration hypnotic for the short-term treatment of insomnia* [zaleplon] 5, 10 mg

Star-Otic ear drops OTC *antibacterial; antifungal* [acetic acid; aluminum acetate; boric acid]

Starsis (Japanese name for U.S. product Starlix)

Starvisc [see: Staarvisc]

starwort; mealy starwort *medicinal herb* [see: chickweed; star grass]

Stat-Crit electrode device for professional use *in vitro diagnostic aid for hemoglobin/hematocrit measurement*

STATdose (trademarked device) *prefilled syringes for self-administration*

Staticin topical solution ℞ *topical antibiotic for acne* [erythromycin] 1.5%

"statins" *brief term for a class of antihyperlipidemics that include atorvastatin, cerivastatin, fluvastatin, lovastatin, pravastatin, and simvastatin* [see: HMG-CoA reductase inhibitors]

statolon USAN *antiviral* [also: vistatolon]

Stat-One gel OTC *topical antiseptic* [hydrogen peroxide] 3%

Stat-One gel OTC *topical antiseptic* [isopropyl alcohol] 70%

Stat-Pak (trademarked packaging form) *unit-dose package*

Statuss Expectorant liquid ℞ *narcotic antitussive; decongestant; expectorant* [codeine phosphate; phenylpropanolamine HCl; guaifenesin; alcohol 5%] 10•12.5•100 mg/5 mL

Statuss Green liquid ℞ *narcotic antitussive; decongestant; antihistamine* [hydrocodone bitartrate; phenylpropanolamine HCl; phenylephrine HCl; pyrilamine maleate; pheniramine maleate; alcohol 5%] 1.67•3.3•5•3.3•3.3 mg/5 mL

staunch, blood *medicinal herb* [see: fleabane; horseweed]

stavudine USAN, INN *nucleoside reverse transcriptase inhibitor (NRTI) antiviral for HIV-1 infection*

Stay Alert tablets (discontinued 2001) OTC *CNS stimulant; analeptic* [caffeine] 200 mg

Stay Awake tablets OTC *CNS stimulant; analeptic* [caffeine] 200 mg

Stay-Wet 3; Stay-Wet 4 solution OTC *disinfecting/wetting/soaking solution for rigid gas permeable contact lenses*

STD (sodium tetradecyl sulfate) [q.v.]

steaglate INN *combining name for radicals or groups*

STEAM (streptonigrin, thioguanine, cyclophosphamide, actinomycin, mitomycin) *chemotherapy protocol*

stearethate 40 [see: polyoxyl 40 stearate]

stearic acid NF *emulsion adjunct; tablet and capsule lubricant*

stearyl alcohol NF *emulsion adjunct*

stearyl dimethyl benzyl ammonium chloride

stearylsulfamide INN

Stedicor *investigational antiarrhythmic* [azimilide dihydrochloride]

steffimycin USAN, INN *antibacterial; antiviral*

Stelazine film-coated tablets, oral concentrate, IM injection ℞ *conventional (typical) antipsychotic; anxiolytic* [trifluoperazine HCl] 1, 2, 5, 10 mg; 10 mg/mL; 2 mg/mL

Stellaria media *medicinal herb* [see: chickweed]

stem cell factor (SCF) *investigational (Phase III) agent for blood-related disorders and chemotherapy "rescue"*

stem cells, hematopoietic *investigational (Phase I/II) gene therapy for HIV*

Stemetil (CAN) film-coated tablets ℞ *conventional (typical) antipsychotic; antiemetic* [prochlorperazine bimaleate] 5, 10 mg

Stemetil (CAN) oral liquid, IV or IM injection ℞ *conventional (typical) antipsychotic; antiemetic* [prochlorperazine mesylate] 5 mg/5 mL; 5 mg/mL

Stemetil (CAN) suppositories ℞ *conventional (typical) antipsychotic; antiemetic* [prochlorperazine] 10 mg

Stemgen (CAN) powder for subcu injection ℞ *recombinant human stem cell factor; hematopoietic growth factor; adjunct to myelosuppressive and myeloablative therapy (investigational [orphan] in the U.S.)* [ancestim] 187.5 mg/vial

stenbolone INN *anabolic steroid; also abused as a street drug* [also: stenbolone acetate]

stenbolone acetate USAN *anabolic steroid; also abused as a street drug* [also: stenbolone]

Step 2 creme rinse OTC *for use following a pediculicide shampoo to remove lice eggs from hair*

stepronin INN

Sterapred; Sterapred DS tablets, Unipak (dispensing pack) ℞ *corticosteroid; anti-inflammatory* [prednisone] 5 mg; 10 mg

Sterculia tragacantha; S. urens; S. villosa *medicinal herb* [see: karaya gum]

stercuronium iodide INN

Sterecyt ℞ *investigational antineoplastic for malignant non-Hodgkin lymphomas; orphan status withdrawn 1998* [prednimustine]

Steri-Dose (trademarked delivery system) *prefilled disposable syringe*

SteriNail solution OTC *topical antifungal* [undecylenic acid; tolnaftate] ?•?

Steri-Vial (trademarked packaging form) *ampule*

Sterules (trademarked dosage form) *solution for nebulization*

stevaladil INN

stevia *(Stevia rebaudiana)* leaves *medicinal herb used as a non-caloric sugar substitute; also used for diabetes, food cravings, hypertension, obesity, and tobacco cravings*

stibamine glucoside INN, BAN

stibocaptate BAN [also: sodium stibocaptate]

stibophen NF

stibosamine INN

stickwort; sticklewort *medicinal herb* [see: agrimony]

stigmata maidis (corn silk) *medicinal herb* [see: Indian corn]

stilbamidine isethionate [see: stilbamidine isetionate]

stilbamidine isetionate INN

stilbazium iodide USAN, INN *anthelmintic*

stilbestroform [see: diethylstilbestrol]

stilbestrol [see: diethylstilbestrol] ⑨ Stilphostrol

stilbestronate [see: diethylstilbestrol dipropionate]

stilboestroform [see: diethylstilbestrol]

stilboestrol BAN *estrogen* [also: diethylstilbestrol]

stilboestrol DP [see: diethylstilbestrol dipropionate]

stillingia *(Stillingia ligustina)* root *medicinal herb for acne, eczema, and other skin disorders, blood cleansing, liver disorders, respiratory illnesses, and syphilis*

Stilnoct; Stilnox (European name for U.S. product Ambien)

stilonium iodide USAN, INN *antispasmodic*

Stilphostrol tablets, IV injection (discontinued 2001) ℞ *hormonal antineoplastic for palliative therapy of advanced prostatic carcinoma* [diethylstilbestrol diphosphate] 50 mg; 250 mg ⑨ Disophrol; stilbestrol

stilronate [see: diethylstilbestrol dipropionate]

Stimate nasal spray ℞ *antidiuretic; posterior pituitary hormone for hemophilia A and von Willebrand disease (orphan)* [desmopressin acetate] 150 µg/dose

stimulant laxatives *a subclass of laxatives that work by direct action on the intestinal mucosa and nerve plexus to increase peristaltic action* [see also: laxatives]

stimulants *a class of agents that excite the activity of physiological processes*

Stimulon ℞ *investigational (Phase I/II) immune system stimulant for AIDS vaccines* [QS-21 (code name—generic name not yet assigned)]

Sting-Eze concentrate OTC *topical antihistamine; antipruritic; anesthetic; bacteriostatic* [diphenhydramine HCl; camphor; phenol; benzocaine; eucalyptol]

stinging nettle *medicinal herb* [see: nettle]

Sting-Kill swabs OTC *topical local anesthetic* [benzocaine; menthol] 20%•1%

stingless nettle *medicinal herb* [see: blind nettle]

stinking nightshade *medicinal herb* [see: henbane]

stirimazole INN, BAN

stiripentol USAN, INN *anticonvulsant*

stirocainide INN

stirofos USAN *veterinary insecticide*

stitchwort *medicinal herb* [see: chickweed]

Stoko Gard cream OTC *topical protection from the effects of poison ivy*

stomachics *a class of agents that promote the functional activity of the stomach*

stone root *(Collinsonia canadensis)* roots and leaves *medicinal herb used as a diuretic and vulnerary*

Stool Softener capsules OTC *laxative; stool softener* [docusate sodium] 100, 250 mg

Stool Softener; Stool Softener DC capsules OTC *laxative; stool softener* [docusate calcium] 240 mg

stool-softening laxatives *a subclass of laxatives that work by increasing the amount of fat and water in the stool to ease its movement through the intestines* [see also: laxatives]

Stop gel ℞ *topical dental caries preventative* [stannous fluoride] 0.4%

storax USP

storax *(Liquidambar orientalis; L. styraciflua)* leaves and gum *medicinal herb for diarrhea, inducing expectoration, parasitic infections, promoting sweating and diuresis, skin sores and wounds, and sore throat*

Storzfen eye drops ℞ *topical ophthalmic decongestant and vasoconstrictor; mydriatic* [phenylephrine HCl] 2.5%

Storzine 2 eye drops ℞ *topical antiglaucoma agent; direct-acting miotic* [pilocarpine HCl] 2%

Storz-N-D eye drops ℞ *topical ophthalmic corticosteroidal anti-inflammatory; antibiotic* [dexamethasone sodium phosphate; neomycin sulfate] 0.1%•0.35%

Storz-N-P-D eye drop suspension ℞ *topical ophthalmic corticosteroidal anti-inflammatory; antibiotic* [dexamethasone; neomycin sulfate; polymyxin B sulfate] 0.1%•0.35%•10 000 U/mL

Storz-Sulf eye drops ℞ *topical ophthalmic antibiotic* [sulfacetamide sodium] 10%

stramonium [see: jimsonweed]

strawberry *(Fragaria vesca)* leaves *medicinal herb for blood cleansing, diarrhea, eczema, intestinal disorders, preventing miscarriage, and stomach cleansing*

strawberry bush; strawberry tree *medicinal herb* [see: wahoo]

Strep Detect slide tests for professional use *in vitro diagnostic aid for streptococcal antigens in throat swabs*

Streptase powder for IV or intracoronary infusion ℞ *thrombolytic enzyme for lysis of thrombi and catheter clearance* [streptokinase] 250 000, 750 000, 1 500 000 IU ⓢ Streptonase

streptococcus immune globulin, group B *investigational for neonatal group B streptococcal infection; orphan status withdrawn 1998*

streptodornase (SD) INN, BAN

streptoduocin USP

streptogramins *a class of antibiotics, isolated from Streptomyces pristinaespirales, used for gram-positive infections*

streptokinase (SK) INN *thrombolytic enzymes for myocardial infarction, thrombosis or embolism* ⓢ Streptonase

streptomycin INN, BAN *aminoglycoside antibiotic; primary tuberculostatic* [also: streptomycin sulfate]

streptomycin sulfate USP *aminoglycoside antibiotic; primary tuberculostatic* [also: streptomycin] 1 g injection

Streptonase-B test kit for professional use *in vitro diagnostic test for DNAse-B streptococcal antigens in serum* Streptase; streptokinase

streptoniazid INN *antibacterial* [also: streptonicozid]

streptonicozid USAN *antibacterial* [also: streptoniazid]

streptonigrin (SN) USAN *antineoplastic* [also: rufocromomycin]

streptovarycin INN

streptozocin USAN, INN *nitrosourea-type alkylating antineoplastic for metastatic islet cell carcinoma of the pancreas*

streptozotocin [see: streptozocin]

Streptozyme slide tests for professional use *in vitro diagnostic test for streptococcal extracellular antigens in blood, plasma, and serum*

Stress 600 with Zinc tablets OTC *vitamin/mineral supplement* [multiple vitamins & minerals; folic acid; biotin] ≛•400•45 μg

Stress B Complex tablets OTC *vitamin/mineral supplement* [multiple vitamins & minerals; folic acid; biotin] ≛•400•45 μg

Stress B Complex with Vitamin C timed-release tablets OTC *vitamin/mineral supplement* [multiple B vitamins; vitamin C; zinc] ≛•300•15 mg

Stress Formula 600 tablets OTC *vitamin supplement* [multiple vitamins; folic acid; biotin] ≛•400•45 μg

Stress Formula Vitamins capsules, tablets OTC *vitamin supplement* [multiple vitamins; folic acid; biotin] ≛•400•45 μg

Stress Formula with Iron film-coated tablets OTC *vitamin/iron supplement* [multiple B vitamins; vitamins C and E; ferrous fumarate; folic acid; biotin] ≛•500 mg•30 IU•27 mg•0.4 mg•45 μg

Stress Formula with Zinc tablets OTC *vitamin/iron supplement* [multiple B vitamins; vitamins C and E; multiple minerals; folic acid; biotin] ≛•500 mg•30 IU•≛•0.4 mg•45 μg

StressForm "605" with Iron tablets OTC *vitamin/iron supplement* [multiple B vitamins; vitamins C and E; iron; folic acid; biotin] ≛•605 mg•30 IU•27 mg•0.4 mg•45 μg

Stresstabs tablets OTC *vitamin supplement* [multiple vitamins; folic acid; biotin] ≛•400•45 μg

Stresstabs + Iron film-coated tablets OTC *vitamin/iron supplement* [multiple B vitamins; vitamins C and E; ferrous fumarate; folic acid; biotin] ≛•500 mg•30 IU•18 mg•0.4 mg•45 μg

Stresstabs + Zinc film-coated tablets OTC *vitamin/mineral supplement* [multiple vitamins & minerals; folic acid; biotin] ≛•400•45 μg

Stresstein powder OTC *enteral nutritional therapy for moderate to severe stress or trauma* [multiple branched chain amino acids]

Stri-Dex pads OTC *topical keratolytic cleanser for acne* [salicylic acid; alcohol] 0.5%•28%, 2%•44%, 2%•54%

Stri-Dex Cleansing bar OTC *medicated cleanser for acne* [triclosan] 1%

Stri-Dex Clear gel OTC *topical acne treatment* [salicylic acid; alcohol] 2%•9.3%

Stri-Dex Face Wash solution OTC *medicated cleanser for acne* [triclosan] 1%

strinoline INN

striped alder *medicinal herb* [see: winterberry; witch hazel]

Stromectol tablets ℞ *anthelmintic for strongyloidiasis and onchocerciasis* [ivermectin] 3, 6 mg

strong ammonia solution [see: ammonia solution, strong]

Strong Iodine solution, tincture ℞ *thyroid-blocking therapy; topical antimicrobial* [iodine; potassium iodide] 5%•10%; 7%•5%

Strong Start chewable tablets, caplets ℞ *vitamin/calcium/iron supplement* [multiple vitamins; calcium; iron; folic acid] ≛•200•29•1 mg

stronger rose water [see: rose water, stronger]
strontium *element (Sr)*
strontium chloride *topical anti-irritant*
strontium chloride Sr 85 USAN *radioactive agent*
strontium chloride Sr 89 USAN *radioactive agent; analgesic for metastatic bone pain*
strontium nitrate Sr 85 USAN *radioactive agent*
strontium salicylate NF
strontium Sr 85 USP
Strovite tablets ℞ *vitamin supplement* [multiple B vitamins; vitamin C; folic acid] ≛•500•0.5 mg
Strovite Advance caplets ℞ *geriatric vitamin/mineral therapy* [multiple vitamins & minerals; folic acid; biotin; alpha lipoic acid; lutein] ≛•1•0.1•15•5 mg
Strovite Plus; Strovite Forte caplets ℞ *geriatric vitamin/mineral therapy* [multiple vitamins & minerals; folic acid; biotin] ≛•800•150 μg; ≛•1000•150 μg
structum *natural remedy* [see: chondroitin sulfate]
strychnine NF *an extremely poisonous CNS stimulant; occasionally abused as a street drug in combination with LSD*
strychnine glycerophosphate NF
strychnine nitrate NF
strychnine phosphate NF
strychnine sulfate NF
strychnine valerate NF
Stuart Formula tablets OTC *vitamin/mineral/iron supplement* [multiple vitamins & minerals; iron; folic acid] ≛•18•0.1 mg
Stuart Prenatal tablets OTC *vitamin/calcium/iron supplement* [multiple vitamins; calcium; iron; folic acid] ≛•200•60•0.8 mg
Stuartnatal Plus tablets ℞ *vitamin/calcium/iron supplement* [multiple vitamins; calcium; iron; folic acid] ≛•200•65•1 mg
stugeron [see: cinnarizine]
stutgin [see: cinnarizine]
Stye ophthalmic ointment OTC *emollient* [white petrolatum; mineral oil; boric acid]
styptics *a class of hemostatic agents that stop bleeding of the skin by astringent action* [see also: astringents; hemostatics]
Stypto-Caine solution OTC *to stop bleeding of minor cuts* [aluminum chloride; tetracaine HCl; oxyquinoline sulfate] 250•2.5•1 mg/g
styramate INN
styronate resins
SU-5416 *investigational (Phase III) angiogenesis inhibitor for colorectal and non–small cell lung cancers (NSCLC); investigational (Phase II/III) for AIDS-related Kaposi sarcoma*
subathizone INN
Subdue (CAN) oral liquid OTC *enteral nutritional therapy for patients with inflammatory bowel disease*
subendazole INN
Sublimaze IV or IM injection ℞ *narcotic analgesic; anesthetic* [fentanyl citrate] 0.05 mg/mL
sublimed sulfur [see: sulfur, sublimed]
Sublingual B Total drops OTC *vitamin supplement* [multiple B vitamins; vitamin C] ≛•60 mg/mL
substance F [see: demecolcine]
substituted benzimidazoles *a class of gastric antisecretory agents that inhibit the ATPase "proton pump" within the gastric parietal cell* [also called: proton pump inhibitors; ATPase inhibitors]
Suby G solution; Suby solution G (citric acid, magnesium oxide, sodium carbonate) *urologic irrigant to dissolve phosphatic calculi*
succimer USAN, INN, BAN *heavy metal chelating agent for lead poisoning (orphan); investigational (orphan) for mercury poisoning and cysteine kidney stones*
succinchlorimide NF
succinimides *a class of anticonvulsants*
succinylcholine chloride USP *neuromuscular blocker; muscle relaxant;*

anesthesia adjunct [also: suxamethonium chloride] 20 mg/mL injection
succinyldapsone [see: succisulfone]
succinylsulfathiazole USP
succisulfone INN
succory *medicinal herb* [see: chicory]
Succus Cineraria Maritima eye drops ℞ *treatment for optic opacity caused by cataract* [senecio compositae; hamamelis water; boric acid]
suclofenide INN, BAN
Sucraid oral solution ℞ *enzyme replacement therapy for congenital sucrase-isomaltase deficiency (orphan)* [sacrosidase] 8500 IU/mL
sucralfate USAN, INN, BAN *cytoprotective agent for gastric ulcers; investigational (orphan) for oral mucositis and stomatitis following cancer radiation or chemotherapy* 1 g oral
sucralose BAN
sucralox INN, BAN
sucrase *orphan status withdrawn 1997* ⓢ sucrose
Sucrets throat spray OTC *topical antipruritic/counterirritant; mild local anesthetic* [dyclonine HCl] 0.1%
Sucrets Children's Sore Throat; Vapor Lemon Sucrets; Sucrets Maximum Strength lozenges OTC *topical antipruritic/counterirritant; mild local anesthetic* [dyclonine HCl] 1.2 mg; 2 mg; 3 mg
Sucrets Cough Control; Sucrets 4-Hour Cough lozenges OTC *antitussive* [dextromethorphan hydrobromide] 5 mg; 15 mg
Sucrets Sore Throat lozenges OTC *oral antiseptic* [hexylresorcinol] 2.4 mg
sucrose NF *flavoring agent; tablet excipient* ⓢ sucrase
sucrose octaacetate NF *alcohol denaturant*
sucrosofate potassium USAN *antiulcerative*
Sudafed tablets OTC *nasal decongestant* [pseudoephedrine HCl] 30, 60 mg
Sudafed, Children's chewable tablets OTC *nasal decongestant* [pseudoephedrine HCl] 15 mg
Sudafed 12 Hour Caplets extended-release tablets OTC *nasal decongestant* [pseudoephedrine HCl] 120 mg
Sudafed Cold & Cough liquid caps OTC *antitussive; decongestant; expectorant; analgesic* [dextromethorphan hydrobromide; pseudoephedrine HCl; guaifenesin; acetaminophen] 10•30•100•250 mg
Sudafed Plus tablets OTC *decongestant; antihistamine* [pseudoephedrine HCl; chlorpheniramine maleate] 60•4 mg
Sudafed Severe Cold caplets, tablets OTC *antitussive; decongestant; analgesic* [dextromethorphan hydrobromide; pseudoephedrine HCl; acetaminophen] 15•30•500 mg
Sudafed Sinus tablets, caplets OTC *decongestant; analgesic; antipyretic* [pseudoephedrine HCl; acetaminophen] 30•500 mg
Sudafed Sinus Advance (CAN) caplets OTC *decongestant; analgesic; antipyretic* [pseudoephedrine HCl; ibuprofen] 30•200 mg
Sudal 60/500 film-coated sustained-release tablets ℞ *decongestant; expectorant* [pseudoephedrine HCl; guaifenesin] 60•500 mg
Sudal 120/600 film-coated sustained-release tablets (discontinued 1998) ℞ *decongestant; expectorant* [pseudoephedrine HCl; guaifenesin] 120•600 mg
Sudex tablets (discontinued 1997) OTC *decongestant* [pseudoephedrine HCl] 30 mg
sudexanox INN
sudismase INN
SudoGest Sinus tablets OTC *decongestant; analgesic; antipyretic* [pseudoephedrine HCl; acetaminophen] 30•500 mg
sudorifics *a class of agents that promote profuse perspiration* [also called: diaphoretics]
sudoxicam USAN, INN *anti-inflammatory*

Sufenta IV injection ℞ *narcotic analgesic; anesthetic* [sufentanil citrate] 50 μg/mL

sufentanil USAN, INN, BAN *narcotic analgesic*

sufentanil citrate USAN *narcotic analgesic* 50 μg/mL injection

sufosfamide INN

sufotidine USAN, INN, BAN *antagonist to histamine* H_2 *receptors*

sugar, compressible NF *flavoring agent; tablet excipient*

sugar, confectioner's NF *flavoring agent; tablet excipient*

sugar, invert (50% dextrose & 50% fructose) USP *fluid and nutrient replenisher; caloric replacement*

sugar spheres NF *solid carrier vehicle*

sulamserod HCl USAN *selective 5-*HT_4 *receptor antagonist; antiarrhythmic; treatment for urge incontinence*

Sulamyd [see: Sodium Sulamyd]

Sular extended-release tablets ℞ *calcium channel blocker for hypertension* [nisoldipine] 10, 20, 30, 40 mg

sulazepam USAN, INN *minor tranquilizer*

sulbactam INN, BAN *β-lactamase inhibitor; penicillin/cephalosporin synergist*

sulbactam benzathine USAN *β-lactamase inhibitor; penicillin/cephalosporin synergist*

sulbactam pivoxil USAN *β-lactamase inhibitor; penicillin/cephalosporin synergist* [also: pivsulbactam]

sulbactam sodium USAN, USP *β-lactamase inhibitor; penicillin/cephalosporin synergist*

sulbenicillin INN

sulbenox USAN, INN *veterinary growth stimulant*

sulbentine INN

sulbutiamine INN [also: bisibutiamine]

sulclamide INN

sulconazole INN, BAN *antifungal* [also: sulconazole nitrate]

sulconazole nitrate USAN, USP *topical antifungal* [also: sulconazole]

sulergine [see: disulergine]

sulesomab USAN *monoclonal antibody; diagnostic aid for infectious lesions* [also: technetium Tc 99m sulesomab]

Sulf-10 eye drops ℞ *topical ophthalmic antibiotic* [sulfacetamide sodium] 10% ⓩ Sulten-10

sulfabenz USAN, INN *antibacterial; coccidiostat for poultry*

sulfabenzamide USAN, USP, INN *bacteriostatic antibiotic*

sulfabromomethazine sodium NF

sulfacarbamide INN [also: sulphaurea]

sulfacecole INN

sulfacetamide USP, INN *bacteriostatic antibiotic*

sulfacetamide sodium USP *bacteriostatic antibiotic* 10%, 30% eye drops

Sulfacet-R lotion ℞ *topical antibiotic for acne* [sulfacetamide sodium; sulfur] 10%•5%

sulfachlorpyridazine INN

sulfachrysoidine INN

sulfacitine INN *antibacterial* [also: sulfacytine]

sulfaclomide INN

sulfaclorazole INN

sulfaclozine INN

sulfacombin [see: sulfadiazine]

sulfacytine USAN *broad-spectrum bacteriostatic* [also: sulfacitine]

sulfadiasulfone sodium INN *antibacterial; leprostatic* [also: acetosulfone sodium]

sulfadiazine USP, INN, JAN *broad-spectrum sulfonamide bacteriostatic* [also: sulphadiazine] 500 mg oral

sulfadiazine & pyrimethamine *Toxoplasma gondii encephalitis treatment (orphan)*

sulfadiazine silver JAN *broad-spectrum bactericidal; adjunct to burn therapy* [also: silver sulfadiazine]

sulfadiazine sodium USP, INN *antibacterial* [also: sulphadiazine sodium]

sulfadicramide INN, DCF

sulfadicrolamide [see: sulfadicramide]

sulfadimethoxine NF [also: sulphadimethoxine]

sulfadimidine INN, BAN *antibacterial* [also: sulfamethazine]

sulfadoxine USAN, USP *bacteriostatic; antimalarial adjunct*
sulfaethidole NF, INN [also: sulphaethidole]
sulfafurazole INN *broad-spectrum sulfonamide bacteriostatic* [also: sulfisoxazole; sulphafurazole]
sulfaguanidine NF, INN
sulfaguanole INN
sulfaisodimidine [see: sulfisomidine]
Sulfalax Calcium capsules (discontinued 1999) OTC *laxative; stool softener* [docusate calcium] 240 mg
sulfalene USAN, INN *antibacterial* [also: sulfametopyrazine]
sulfaloxic acid INN [also: sulphaloxic acid]
sulfamates *a class of broad-spectrum anticonvulsants*
sulfamazone INN
sulfamerazine USP, INN *broad-spectrum bacteriostatic*
sulfamerazine sodium NF, INN
sulfameter USAN *antibacterial* [also: sulfametoxydiazine; sulfamethoxydiazine]
sulfamethazine USP *broad-spectrum bacteriostatic* [also: sulfadimidine]
sulfamethizole USP, INN, JAN *broad-spectrum sulfonamide bacteriostatic* [also: sulphamethizole] ⑨ sulfamethoxazole
sulfamethoxazole (SMX; SMZ) USAN, USP, INN, JAN *broad-spectrum sulfonamide antibiotic* [also: sulphamethoxazole; acetylsulfamethoxazole; sulfamethoxazole sodium] ⑨ sulfamethizole
sulfamethoxazole sodium JAN *broad-spectrum sulfonamide antibiotic* [also: sulfamethoxazole; sulphamethoxazole; acetylsulfamethoxazole]
sulfamethoxydiazine BAN *antibacterial* [also: sulfameter; sulfametoxydiazine]
sulfamethoxypyridazine USP, INN [also: sulphamethoxypyridazine]
sulfamethoxypyridazine acetyl
sulfametin [see: sulfameter]
sulfametomidine INN
sulfametopyrazine BAN *antibacterial* [also: sulfalene]
sulfametoxydiazine INN *antibacterial* [also: sulfameter; sulfamethoxydiazine]
sulfametrole INN, BAN
sulfamidothiodiazol [see: glybuzole]
sulfamonomethoxine USAN, INN, BAN *antibacterial*
sulfamoxole USAN, INN *antibacterial* [also: sulphamoxole]
***p*-sulfamoylbenzoic acid** [see: carzenide]
4′-sulfamoylsuccinanilic acid [see: sulfasuccinamide]
Sulfamylon cream ℞ *broad-spectrum bacteriostatic for second- and third-degree burns* [mafenide acetate] 85 mg/g
Sulfamylon powder for topical solution ℞ *broad-spectrum bacteriostatic to prevent meshed autograft loss on second- and third-degree burns (orphan)* [mafenide acetate] 5%
sulfanilamide NF, INN *broad-spectrum sulfonamide antibiotic*
sulfanilanilide [see: sulfabenz]
sulfanilate zinc USAN *antibacterial*
N-sulfanilylacetamide [see: sulfacetamide]
N-sulfanilylacetamide monosodium salt monohydrate [see: sulfacetamide sodium]
N-*p*-sulfanilylphenylglycine sodium [see: acediasulfone sodium]
N-sulfanilylstearamide [see: stearylsulfamide]
4′-sulfanilylsuccinanilic acid [see: succisulfone]
sulfanilylurea [see: sulfacarbamide]
sulfanitran USAN, INN, BAN *antibacterial; coccidiostat for poultry*
sulfaperin INN
sulfaphenazole INN [also: sulphaphenazole]
sulfaphtalythiazol [see: phthalysulfathiazole]
sulfaproxyline INN [also: sulphaproxyline]
sulfapyrazole INN, BAN *antibacterial* [also: sulfazamet]
sulfapyridine USP, INN *investigational (orphan) dermatitis herpetiformis suppressant* [also: sulphapyridine]

sulfapyridine sodium NF
sulfaquinoxaline INN, BAN
sulfarsphenamine NF, INN
sulfasalazine USAN, USP, INN *broad-spectrum bacteriostatic; antirheumatic; anti-inflammatory for ulcerative colitis* [also: sulphasalazine; salazosulfapyridine] 500 mg oral
sulfasomizole USAN, INN *antibacterial* [also: sulphasomizole]
sulfastearyl [see: stearylsulfamide]
sulfasuccinamide INN
sulfasymazine INN
sulfated polysaccharide peptidoglycan (SPPG) [see: tecogalan sodium]
sulfathiazole USP, INN *bacteriostatic antibiotic* [also: sulphathiazole] ⑳ sulfisoxazole
sulfathiazole sodium NF
sulfathiocarbamide [see: sulfathiourea]
sulfathiourea INN
sulfatolamide INN
Sulfatrim oral suspension ℞ *anti-infective; antibacterial* [trimethoprim; sulfamethoxazole] 40•200 mg/5 mL
sulfatroxazole INN
sulfatrozole INN
sulfazamet USAN *antibacterial* [also: sulfapyrazole]
sulfinalol INN *antihypertensive* [also: sulfinalol HCl]
sulfinalol HCl USAN *antihypertensive* [also: sulfinalol]
sulfinpyrazone USP, INN *uricosuric for gout* [also: sulphinpyrazone] 100, 200 mg oral
sulfiram INN [also: monosulfiram]
sulfisomidine [also: sulphasomidine]
sulfisoxazole USP, JAN *broad-spectrum sulfonamide antibiotic* [also: sulfafurazole; sulphafurazole] 500 mg oral ⑳ sulfathiazole
sulfisoxazole acetyl USP *broad-spectrum sulfonamide antibiotic*
sulfisoxazole diolamine USAN, USP *broad-spectrum sulfonamide antibiotic*
Sulfoam shampoo OTC *antiseborrheic; keratolytic* [salicylic acid] 2%
sulfobenzylpenicillin [see: sulbenicillin]
sulfobromophthalein sodium USP *hepatic function test*
sulfobromphthalein sodium [see: sulfobromophthalein sodium]
sulfogaiacol INN *expectorant* [also: potassium guaiacolsulfonate]
Sulfoil liquid OTC *soap-free therapeutic skin cleanser* [sulfonated castor oil]
sulfomyxin USAN, INN *antibacterial* [also: sulphomyxin sodium]
sulfonal [see: sulfonmethane]
sulfonamides *a class of broad-spectrum bacteriostatic antibiotics effective against both gram-positive and gram-negative organisms*
sulfonated hydrogenated castor oil [see: hydroxystearin sulfate]
sulfonethylmethane NF
sulfonmethane NF
sulfonterol INN *bronchodilator* [also: sulfonterol HCl]
sulfonterol HCl USAN *bronchodilator* [also: sulfonterol]
sulfonylureas *a class of antidiabetic agents that stimulate insulin production in the pancreas*
Sulforcin lotion OTC *topical acne treatment* [sulfur; resorcinol; alcohol] 5%•2%•11.65%
sulforidazine INN
sulfosalicylic acid
sulfoxone sodium USP *antibacterial; leprostatic* [also: aldesulfone sodium]
Sulfoxyl Regular; Sulfoxyl Strong lotion ℞ *topical keratolytic for acne* [benzoyl peroxide; sulfur] 5%•2%; 10%•5%
sulfur *element (S)* [see: sulfur, precipitated; sulfur, sublimed]
sulfur, precipitated USP *scabicide; topical antibacterial; topical exfoliant*
sulfur, sublimed USP *scabicide; topical antibacterial; topical exfoliant*
sulfur dioxide NF *antioxidant*
Sulfur Soap bar OTC *medicated cleanser for acne* [precipitated sulfur] 10%
sulfurated lime solution [see: lime, sulfurated]
sulfurated potash [see: potash, sulfurated]

sulfuric acid NF *acidifying agent*
sulfuric acid, aluminum ammonium salt, dodecahydrate [see: alum, ammonium]
sulfuric acid, aluminum potassium salt, dodecahydrate [see: alum, potassium]
sulfuric acid, aluminum salt, hydrate [see: aluminum sulfate]
sulfuric acid, barium salt [see: barium sulfate]
sulfuric acid, calcium salt [see: calcium sulfate]
sulfuric acid, copper salt pentahydrate [see: cupric sulfate]
sulfuric acid, disodium salt decahydrate [see: sodium sulfate]
sulfuric acid, magnesium salt [see: magnesium sulfate]
sulfuric acid, manganese salt [see: manganese sulfate]
sulfuric acid, zinc salt hydrate [see: zinc sulfate]
sulfurous acid, monosodium salt [see: sodium bisulfite]
sulglicotide INN [also: sulglycotide]
sulglycotide BAN [also: sulglicotide]
sulicrinat INN
sulindac USAN, USP, INN, BAN *antiarthritic; nonsteroidal anti-inflammatory drug (NSAID) for ankylosing spondylitis and acute bursitis/tendinitis* 150, 200 mg oral ⑨ Zoladex
sulisatin INN
sulisobenzone USAN, INN *ultraviolet screen*
sulmarin USAN, INN *hemostatic*
Sulmasque mask OTC *antibacterial and exfoliant for acne* [sulfur] 6.4%
sulmazole INN
sulmepride INN
sulnidazole USAN, INN *antiprotozoal (Trichomonas)*
sulocarbilate INN
suloctidil USAN, INN, BAN *peripheral vasodilator*
sulodexide INN
sulofenur USAN, INN *antineoplastic*
sulopenem USAN, INN *antibacterial*
sulosemide INN
sulotroban USAN, INN, BAN *treatment for glomerulonephritis*
suloxifen INN *bronchodilator* [also: suloxifen oxalate]
suloxifen oxalate USAN *bronchodilator* [also: suloxifen]
sulphabutin [see: busulfan]
sulphadiazine BAN *broad-spectrum bacteriostatic* [also: sulfadiazine]
sulphadiazine sodium BAN *antibacterial* [also: sulfadiazine sodium]
sulphadimethoxine BAN [also: sulfadimethoxine]
sulphaethidole BAN [also: sulfaethidole]
sulphafurazole BAN *broad-spectrum sulfonamide bacteriostatic* [also: sulfisoxazole; sulfafurazole]
sulphaloxic acid BAN [also: sulfaloxic acid]
sulphamethizole BAN *broad-spectrum sulfonamide bacteriostatic* [also: sulfamethizole]
sulphamethoxazole BAN *broad-spectrum sulfonamide bacteriostatic* [also: sulfamethoxazole; acetylsulfamethoxazole; sulfamethoxazole sodium]
sulphamethoxypyridazine BAN [also: sulfamethoxypyridazine]
sulphamoxole BAN *antibacterial* [also: sulfamoxole]
sulphan blue BAN *lymphangiography aid* [also: isosulfan blue]
sulphaphenazole BAN [also: sulfaphenazole]
sulphaproxyline BAN [also: sulfaproxyline]
sulphapyridine BAN *dermatitis herpetiformis suppressant* [also: sulfapyridine]
sulphasalazine BAN *broad-spectrum bacteriostatic; antirheumatic; anti-inflammatory for ulcerative colitis* [also: sulfasalazine; salazosulfapyridine]
sulphasomidine BAN [also: sulfisomidine]
sulphasomizole BAN *antibacterial* [also: sulfasomizole]
sulphathiazole BAN *antibacterial* [also: sulfathiazole]
sulphaurea BAN [also: sulfacarbamide]

sulphinpyrazone BAN *uricosuric for gout* [also: sulfinpyrazone]

sulphocarbolate sodium [see: phenolsulphonate sodium]

Sulpho-Lac cream, soap OTC *antibacterial and exfoliant for acne* [sulfur] 5%

Sulpho-Lac Acne Medication cream OTC *antibacterial; exfoliant* [sulfur; zinc sulfate] 5%•27%

sulphomyxin sodium BAN *antibacterial* [also: sulfomyxin]

sulphonal [see: sulfonmethane]

sulpiride USAN, INN *antidepressant*

sulprosal INN

sulprostone USAN, INN *prostaglandin*

Sulster eye drops (discontinued 1998) ℞ *topical ophthalmic corticosteroidal anti-inflammatory; antibiotic* [prednisolone sodium phosphate; sulfacetamide sodium] 0.25%•1%

sultamicillin USAN, INN, BAN *antibacterial*

sulthiame USAN *anticonvulsant* [also: sultiame]

sultiame INN *anticonvulsant* [also: sulthiame]

sultopride INN

sultosilic acid INN

Sultrin Triple Sulfa vaginal inserts, vaginal cream (discontinued 2001) ℞ *broad-spectrum bacteriostatic* [sulfathiazole; sulfacetamide; sulfabenzamide] 172.5•143.75•184 mg; 3.42%•2.86%•3.7%

sultroponium INN

sulukast USAN, INN *antiasthmatic; leukotriene antagonist*

sulverapride INN

suma *(Pfaffia paniculata)* bark and root *medicinal herb for circulatory disorders, chronic disease, fatigue, hormone regulation, immune system stimulation, lowering cholesterol levels, and stress; also used as a tonic*

Sumacal powder OTC *carbohydrate caloric supplement* [glucose polymers]

sumacetamol INN, BAN

sumach *(Rhus glabra)* bark, leaves, and berries *medicinal herb used as an antiseptic, astringent, diaphoretic, diuretic, emmenagogue, febrifuge, and refrigerant*

sumarotene USAN, INN *keratolytic*

sumatriptan INN, BAN *vascular serotonin 5-HT$_1$ receptor agonist for migraine and cluster headaches* [also: sumatriptan succinate]

sumatriptan succinate USAN *vascular serotonin 5-HT$_1$ receptor agonist for migraine and cluster headaches* [also: sumatriptan]

sumetizide INN

summer savory *(Calamintha hortensis; Satureja hortensis)* leaves and stems *medicinal herb for diarrhea, nausea, promoting expectoration, relieving gas and flatulence, and stimulation of menstruation; also used as an aphrodisiac*

Summer's Eve Disposable Douche solution OTC *antifungal; vaginal cleanser and deodorizer; acidity modifier* [sodium benzoate; citric acid]

Summer's Eve Disposable Douche; Summer's Eve Disposable Douche Extra Cleansing solution OTC *vaginal cleanser and deodorizer; acidity modifier* [vinegar (acetic acid)]

Summer's Eve Feminine Bath liquid OTC *for external perivaginal cleansing*

Summer's Eve Feminine Powder OTC *absorbs vaginal moisture* [cornstarch; benzethonium chloride]

Summer's Eve Feminine Wash liquid, wipes OTC *for external perivaginal cleansing*

Summer's Eve Medicated Disposable Douche solution OTC *antiseptic/germicidal; vaginal cleanser and deodorizer* [povidone-iodine] 0.3%

Summer's Eve Post-Menstrual Disposable Douche solution OTC *vaginal cleanser and deodorizer; acidity modifier* [monosodium phosphate; disodium phosphate]

Summit Extra Strength coated caplets OTC *analgesic; antipyretic; anti-inflammatory* [acetaminophen; aspirin; caffeine] 250•250•65 mg

Sumycin syrup ℞ *broad-spectrum antibiotic* [tetracycline HCl] 125 mg/5 mL

Sumycin '250'; Sumycin '500' capsules, tablets ℞ *broad-spectrum antibiotic* [tetracycline HCl] 250 mg; 500 mg

sun rose *medicinal herb* [see: rock rose]

sunagrel INN

suncillin INN *antibacterial* [also: suncillin sodium]

suncillin sodium USAN *antibacterial* [also: suncillin]

sunepitron HCl USAN *anxiolytic; antidepressant*

SunKist Multivitamins Complete, Children's chewable tablets OTC *vitamin/mineral/iron supplement* [multiple vitamins & minerals; iron; folic acid; biotin] ≛•18 mg•400 µg•40 µg

SunKist Multi-Vitamins + Extra C chewable tablets OTC *vitamin supplement* [multiple vitamins; folic acid] ≛•0.3 mg

SunKist Multivitamins + Iron, Children's chewable tablets OTC *vitamin/iron supplement* [multiple vitamins; iron; folic acid] ≛•15•0.3 mg

SunKist Vitamin C caplets (discontinued 1999) OTC *vitamin C supplement* [ascorbic acid and sodium ascorbate] 500 mg

SunKist Vitamin C chewable tablets OTC *vitamin C supplement* [ascorbic acid and sodium ascorbate] 60, 250, 500 mg

Supac tablets (discontinued 2000) OTC *analgesic; antipyretic; anti-inflammatory* [acetaminophen; aspirin; caffeine] 160•230•32 mg

Supartz intra-articular injection ℞ *viscoelastic lubricant and "shock absorber" for osteoarthritis* [hyaluronate sodium] 25 mg/2.5 mL prefilled syringe

Super CalciCaps tablets OTC *dietary supplement* [dibasic calcium phosphate; calcium gluconate; calcium carbonate; vitamin D] 400 mg (Ca)•42 mg (P)•133 IU

Super CalciCaps M-Z tablets OTC *dietary supplement* [vitamins A and D; multiple minerals] 1667 mg•133 IU•≛

Super Calcium '1200' softgels OTC *dietary supplement* [calcium; vitamin D] 600 mg•200 IU

Super Citro Cee sustained-release tablets (discontinued 1999) OTC *vitamin C supplement with multiple bioflavonoids* [ascorbic acid; rose hips; lemon bioflavonoids; rutin] 500•500•500•50 mg

Super Complex C-500 Caplets (discontinued 1999) OTC *vitamin C supplement with multiple bioflavonoids* [ascorbic acid; citrus bioflavonoids; hesperidin; rutin] 500•100•25•50 mg

Super D Perles (capsules) OTC *vitamin supplement* [vitamins A and D] 10 000•400 IU

Super Flavons; Super Flavons-300 tablets OTC *dietary supplement* [mixed bioflavonoids] 300 mg

Super Hi Potency tablets OTC *vitamin/mineral supplement* [multiple vitamins & minerals; folic acid; biotin] ≛•0.4 mg•0.075 mg

Super Ivy-Dry lotion OTC *topical poison ivy treatment* [zinc acetate; benzyl alcohol; isopropanol] 2%•10%•35%

Super Quints-50 tablets OTC *vitamin supplement* [multiple B vitamins; folic acid; biotin] ≛•400•50 µg

Superdophilus powder OTC *dietary supplement; fever blister treatment; not generally regarded as safe and effective as an antidiarrheal* [*Lactobacillus acidophilus*] 2 billion U/g

SuperEPA 1200; SuperEPA 2000 softgels OTC *dietary supplement* [omega-3 fatty acids] 1200 mg; 1000 mg

superoxide dismutase (SOD) [see: orgotein]

Superplex-T tablets OTC *vitamin supplement* [multiple B vitamins; vitamin C] ≛•500 mg

supidimide INN

Suplena ready-to-use liquid OTC *enteral nutritional therapy for renal failure* [multiple essential amino acids]

Suppap-120; Suppap-650 suppositories (discontinued 1997) OTC *analgesic; antipyretic* [acetaminophen] 120 mg; 650 mg

Supprelin subcu injection ℞ *gonadotropin-releasing hormone for central precocious puberty (orphan)* [histrelin acetate] 120, 300, 600 µg/0.6 mL

Suppress lozenges OTC *antitussive* [dextromethorphan hydrobromide] 7.5 mg

Supprette (trademarked dosage form) *suppository*

Suprane liquid for vaporization ℞ *inhalation general anesthetic* [desflurane]

Suprax film-coated tablets, powder for oral suspension ℞ *cephalosporin antibiotic* [cefixime] 200, 400 mg; 100 mg/5 mL

Suprefact (CAN) nasal solution ℞ *LH-RH analogue; hormonal antineoplastic for prostatic cancer and endometriosis* [buserelin acetate] 1 mg/mL

Suprefact; Suprefact Depot (CAN) subcu injection ℞ *LH-RH analogue; hormonal antineoplastic for prostatic cancer and endometriosis* [buserelin acetate] 1 mg/mL; 6.6 mg/dose

suproclone USAN, INN *sedative*

suprofen USAN, INN, BAN *ocular nonsteroidal anti-inflammatory drug (NSAID); antimiotic*

Supule (trademarked dosage form) *suppository*

suramin hexasodium USAN *investigational (NDA filed, orphan) growth factor antagonist for prostate cancer*

suramin sodium USP, BAN *antiparasitic for African trypanosomiasis and onchocerciasis*

Surbex Filmtabs (film-coated tablets) OTC *vitamin supplement* [multiple B vitamins] ≛

Surbex 750 with Iron Filmtabs (film-coated tablets) OTC *vitamin/iron supplement* [multiple B vitamins; vitamins C and E; ferrous sulfate, dried; folic acid] ≛ •750 mg•30 IU•27 mg•0.4 mg

Surbex 750 with Zinc Filmtabs (film-coated tablets) OTC *vitamin/zinc supplement* [multiple vitamins; zinc sulfate; folic acid] ≛ •22.5•0.4 mg

Surbex-T; Surbex with C Filmtabs (film-coated tablets) OTC *vitamin supplement* [multiple B vitamins; vitamin C] ≛ •500 mg; ≛ •250 mg

Surbu-Gen-T film-coated tablets OTC *vitamin supplement* [multiple B vitamins; vitamin C] ≛ •500 mg

Sure Cell Chlamydia Test reagent kit for professional use *in vitro diagnostic aid for Chlamydia trachomatis* [monoclonal antibody-based enzyme-linked immunosorbent assay]

Sure Cell Herpes (HSV) Test reagent kit for professional use *in vitro diagnostic aid for herpes simplex virus in genital, rectal, oral, or dermal swabs* [monoclonal antibody-based enzyme-linked immunosorbent assay (ELISA)]

Sure Cell Pregnancy test kit for professional use *in vitro diagnostic aid; urine pregnancy test* [monoclonal/polyclonal antibody ELISA test]

Sure Cell Streptococci test kit for professional use *in vitro diagnostic aid for Group A streptococcal antigens in blood and throat swabs* [enzyme-linked immunosorbent assay (ELISA)]

SureLac chewable tablets OTC *digestive aid for lactose intolerance* [lactase enzyme] 3000 U

surface active extract of saline lavage of bovine lungs [see: beractant]

surfactant laxatives *a subclass of laxatives that work by increasing the amount of fat and water in the stool to ease its movement through the intestines* [more commonly called stool softeners]

surfactant TA [see: beractant]

surfactant TA, modified bovine lung [see: beractant]

Surfak Liquigels (capsules) OTC *laxative; stool softener* [docusate calcium] 240 mg
Surfaxin ℞ *investigational (Phase II/III, orphan) KL4 pulmonary surfactant for acute respiratory distress syndrome (ARDS) and meconium aspiration syndrome (MAS)* [lucinactant]
surfilcon A USAN *hydrophilic contact lens material*
Surfol Post-Immersion Bath Oil OTC *bath emollient*
surfomer USAN, INN *hypolipidemic*
Surgel vaginal gel OTC *lubricant* [propylene glycol; glycerin]
surgibone USAN *internal bone splint*
surgical catgut [see: suture, absorbable surgical]
surgical gut [see: suture, absorbable surgical]
Surgicel strips, Nu-knit pads ℞ *topical local hemostat for surgery* [cellulose, oxidized]
suricainide INN *antiarrhythmic* [also: suricainide maleate]
suricainide maleate USAN, INN *antiarrhythmic* [also: suricainide]
suriclone INN, BAN
Surinam wood *medicinal herb* [see: quassia]
suritozole USAN, INN *antidepressant*
Surmontil capsules ℞ *tricyclic antidepressant* [trimipramine maleate] 25, 50, 100 mg
Surodex intraocular injection ℞ *investigational (Phase II) corticosteroidal anti-inflammatory* [dexamethasone]
suronacrine INN *cholinesterase inhibitor* [also: suronacrine maleate]
suronacrine maleate USAN *cholinesterase inhibitor* [also: suronacrine]
Surpass chewing gum OTC *antacid* [calcium carbonate] 300, 450 mg
Survanta suspension for intratracheal instillation ℞ *pulmonary surfactant for neonatal respiratory distress syndrome or respiratory failure (orphan)* [beractant] 25 mg/mL
Susano elixir ℞ *GI antispasmodic; anticholinergic; sedative* [atropine sulfate; scopolamine hydrobromide; hyoscyamine hydrobromide; phenobarbital] 0.0194•0.0065•0.1037•16.2 mg/5 mL
Sus-Phrine subcu injection ℞ *sympathomimetic bronchodilator for bronchial asthma, bronchospasm and COPD; vasopressor for shock* [epinephrine] 1:200 (5 mg/mL)
Sustacal powder OTC *enteral nutritional therapy* [milk-based formula]
Sustacal pudding OTC *enteral nutritional therapy* [milk-based formula]
Sustacal ready-to-use liquid OTC *enteral nutritional therapy* [lactose-free formula]
Sustacal Basic; Sustacal Plus ready-to-use liquid OTC *enteral nutritional therapy* [lactose-free formula]
Sustagen powder OTC *enteral nutritional therapy* [milk-based formula]
Sustaire timed-release tablets ℞ *antiasthmatic; bronchodilator* [theophylline] 100, 300 mg
Sustiva capsules ℞ *antiviral non-nucleoside reverse transcriptase inhibitor (NNRTI) for HIV infection* [efavirenz] 50, 100, 200 mg
sutilains USAN, USP, INN, BAN *topical proteolytic enzymes for necrotic tissue debridement*
sutoprofen [see: suprofen]
suture, absorbable surgical USP *surgical aid*
suture, nonabsorbable surgical USP *surgical aid*
suxamethone [see: succinylcholine chloride]
suxamethonium chloride INN, BAN *neuromuscular blocking agent* [also: succinylcholine chloride]
suxemerid INN *antitussive* [also: suxemerid sulfate]
suxemerid sulfate USAN *antitussive* [also: suxemerid]
suxethonium chloride INN
suxibuzone INN
swallow wort, orange *medicinal herb* [see: pleurisy root]

swallow wort, silky *medicinal herb* [see: milkweed]

swamp cabbage *medicinal herb* [see: skunk cabbage]

swamp laurel; swamp sassafras *medicinal herb* [see: magnolia]

sweet, mountain *medicinal herb* [see: New Jersey tea]

sweet, winter *medicinal herb* [see: marjoram]

sweet anise; sweet chervil *medicinal herb* [see: sweet cicely]

sweet balm *medicinal herb* [see: lemon balm]

sweet basil *medicinal herb* [see: basil]

sweet bay *medicinal herb* [see: laurel]

sweet birch *medicinal herb* [see: birch]

sweet birch oil [see: methyl salicylate]

sweet cicely *(Osmorhiza longistylis)* root *medicinal herb used as a carminative, expectorant, and stomachic*

sweet clover *medicinal herb* [see: melilot]

sweet dock *medicinal herb* [see: bistort]

sweet elder *medicinal herb* [see: elderberry]

sweet elm *medicinal herb* [see: slippery elm]

sweet fennel *medicinal herb* [see: fennel]

sweet flag *medicinal herb* [see: calamus]

sweet grass *medicinal herb* [see: calamus]

sweet leaf *medicinal herb* [see: stevia]

sweet magnolia *medicinal herb* [see: magnolia]

sweet marjoram *medicinal herb* [see: marjoram]

sweet myrtle *medicinal herb* [see: calamus]

sweet orange peel tincture [see: orange peel tincture, sweet]

sweet potato vine, wild *medicinal herb* [see: wild jalap]

sweet root *medicinal herb* [see: calamus]

sweet rush *medicinal herb* [see: calamus]

sweet sedge *medicinal herb* [see: calamus]

sweet spirit of nitre [see: ethyl nitrite]

sweet vernal grass *(Anthoxanthum odoratum)* *natural flavoring; not generally regarded as safe; banned by the FDA*

sweet violet *medicinal herb* [see: violet]

sweet water lily; sweet-scented water lily *medicinal herb* [see: white pond lily]

sweet weed *medicinal herb* [see: marsh mallow]

sweet woodruff *(Asperula odorata; Galium odoratum)* plant *medicinal herb for diuresis, inducing expectoration, liver disorders, promoting wound healing, relieving gastrointestinal spasms, and sedation*

Sweet'n Fresh Clotrimazole-7 cream, vaginal suppositories (discontinued 2001) OTC *antifungal* [clotrimazole] 1%; 100 mg

sweet-scented pond lily; sweet-scented water lily *medicinal herb* [see: white pond lily]

sweetwood *medicinal herb* [see: licorice]

Swim-Ear ear drops OTC *antiseptic* [isopropyl alcohol] 95%

swine snout *medicinal herb* [see: dandelion]

Syllact powder OTC *bulk laxative* [psyllium husks] 3.3 g/tsp.

Syllamalt powder (discontinued 1999) OTC *bulk laxative* [barley malt soup extract; psyllium husks] 4•3 g/tsp.

Symax-SR sustained-release caplets ℞ *GI/GU antispasmodic; antiparkinsonian; anticholinergic "drying agent" for allergic rhinitis and hyperhidrosis* [hyoscyamine sulfate] 0.375 mg

symclosene USAN, INN *topical anti-infective*

symetine INN *antiamebic* [also: symetine HCl]

symetine HCl USAN *antiamebic* [also: symetine]

Symlin ℞ *synthetic amylin analogue to slow gastric emptying; investigational (Phase III) antidiabetic for type 1 and type 2 diabetes* [pramlintide acetate]

Symmetrel capsules, syrup ℞ *antiviral; dopaminergic antiparkinsonian agent* [amantadine HCl] 100 mg; 50 mg/5 mL

sympatholytics *a class of cardiovascular drugs that block the passage of impulses* *through the sympathetic nervous system* [also called: antiadrenergics]

sympathomimetics *a class of bronchodilators that relax the bronchial muscles, reducing bronchospasm; a class of cardiac agents that increase myocardial contractility, causing a vasopressor effect to counteract shock (inadequate tissue perfusion)* [also called: adrenergic agonists]

Symphytum officinale; S. tuberosum *medicinal herb* [see: comfrey]

Symplocarpus foetidus *medicinal herb* [see: skunk cabbage]

Synacol CF tablets OTC *antitussive; expectorant* [dextromethorphan hydrobromide; guaifenesin] 15•200 mg

Synacort cream ℞ *topical corticosteroidal anti-inflammatory* [hydrocortisone] 1%, 2.5%

Synagis IM injection ℞ *monoclonal antibody for prophylaxis of respiratory syncytial virus (RSV) in infants* [palivizumab] 50, 100 mg

Synalar cream, ointment, topical solution ℞ *topical corticosteroidal anti-inflammatory* [fluocinolone acetonide] 0.01, 0.25%; 0.025%; 0.01%

Synalar-HP cream ℞ *topical corticosteroidal anti-inflammatory* [fluocinolone acetonide] 0.2%

Synalgos-DC capsules ℞ *narcotic analgesic* [dihydrocodeine bitartrate; aspirin; caffeine] 16•356.4•30 mg

Synapton SR ℞ *investigational (NDA filed) sustained-release acetylcholinesterase inhibitor for Alzheimer disease* [physostigmine]

Synarel nasal spray ℞ *gonadotropin-releasing hormone for central precocious puberty (orphan) and endometriosis* [nafarelin acetate] 2 mg/mL (200 µg/spray)

Synemol cream ℞ *topical corticosteroidal anti-inflammatory* [fluocinolone acetonide] 0.025%

Synercid powder for IV infusion ℞ *semi-synthetic streptogramin antibiotic for life-threatening infections* [quinupristin; dalfopristin] 150•350 mg/10 mL

synestrin [see: diethylstilbestrol]

synnematin B [see: adicillin]

Synophylate-GG syrup ℞ *antiasthmatic; bronchodilator; expectorant* [theophylline; guaifenesin; alcohol 10%] 150•100 mg/15 mL

Synovir (name changed to Thalomid upon marketing release in 1998)

Syn-Rx controlled-release tablets (14-day, 56-tablet regimen) ℞ *decongestant; expectorant* [pseudoephedrine HCl; guaifenesin] 60•600 mg

Synsorb Cd ℞ *investigational (Phase III) antidiarrheal for AIDS-related diarrhea due to Clostridium difficile infection*

Synsorb-Pk ℞ *investigational (Phase III, orphan) E. coli neutralizer for traveler's diarrhea and hemolytic uremic syndrome (HUS)* [8-methoxycarbonyloctyl oligosaccharides]

synthestrin [see: diethylstilbestrol]

synthetic lung surfactant [see: colfosceril palmitate]

synthetic monosaccharides *a class of investigational synthetic carbohydrates with immunomodulatory and anti-inflammatory effects being evaluated for the treatment of rheumatic arthritis*

synthetic paraffin [see: paraffin, synthetic]

synthetic spermaceti [now: cetyl esters wax]

synthoestrin [see: diethylstilbestrol]

Synthroid tablets, powder for injection ℞ *synthetic thyroid T_4 hormone* [levothyroxine sodium] 25, 50, 75, 88, 100, 112, 125, 150, 175, 200, 300 µg; 200, 500 µg ⓢ Euthroid

Syntocinon IV, IM injection (discontinued 1998) ℞ *oxytocic for induction of labor, postpartum bleeding, and incomplete abortion* [oxytocin] 10 U/mL

Syntocinon nasal spray (discontinued 1998) ℞ *oxytocic for initial milk let-down* [oxytocin] 40 U/mL

synvinolin [now: simvastatin]

Synvisc intra-articular injection ℞ *viscoelastic lubricant and "shock* *absorber" for osteoarthritis* [hylan G-F 20] 16 mg/2 mL

Syprine capsules ℞ *copper chelating agent for Wilson disease (orphan)* [trientine HCl] 50 mg

Syracol CF tablets OTC *antitussive; expectorant* [dextromethorphan hydrobromide; guaifenesin] 15•200 mg

syrosingopine NF, INN, BAN

syrup NF *flavoring agent*

syrupus cerasi [see: cherry juice]

Syrvite liquid OTC *vitamin supplement* [multiple vitamins] ≛

Syzygium aromaticum *medicinal herb* [see: cloves]

(S)-zopiclone [see: esopiclone]

T-2 protocol (dactinomycin, doxorubicin, vincristine, cyclophosphamide, radiation) *chemotherapy protocol*

T_3 (liothyronine sodium) [q.v.]

T_4 (levothyroxine sodium) [q.v.]

T4, recombinant soluble human *investigational (Phase I/II) antiviral for HIV*

T4 endonuclease V (T4N5), liposome encapsulated *investigational (orphan) for prevent cutaneous neoplasms in xeroderma pigmentosum*

T-10 protocol (methotrexate, doxorubicin, cisplatin, bleomycin, cyclophosphamide, dactinomycin) *chemotherapy protocol*

T-1249 *investigational for HIV infection*

Tab-A-Vite tablets OTC *vitamin supplement* [multiple vitamins; folic acid] ≛•0.4 mg

Tab-A-Vite + Iron tablets OTC *vitamin/iron supplement* [multiple vitamins; iron; folic acid] ≛•18•0.4 mg

Tabebuia avellanedae; T. impetiginosa *medicinal herb* [see: pau d'arco]

Tabernanthe iboga *street drug* [see: iboga]

tabilautide INN

Tabloid (trademarked dosage form) *tablet with raised lettering*

Tabules (dosage form) *tablets*

Tac-3 IM, intra-articular, intrabursal, intradermal injection ℞ *corticosteroid; anti-inflammatory* [triamcinolone acetonide] 3 mg/mL

Tac-40 suspension for injection ℞ *corticosteroid; anti-inflammatory* [triamcinolone acetonide] 40 mg/mL

Tacaryl syrup (discontinued 1997) ℞ *antihistamine* [methdilazine HCl] 4 mg/5 mL

Tace capsules (discontinued 1998) ℞ *hormone for estrogen replacement therapy or inoperable prostatic carcinoma* [chlorotrianisene] 12, 25 mg

TA-CIN *investigational cancer vaccine*

taclamine INN *minor tranquilizer* [also: taclamine HCl]

taclamine HCl USAN *minor tranquilizer* [also: taclamine]

tacmahac *medicinal herb* [see: balm of Gilead]

tacrine INN, BAN *reversible cholinesterase inhibitor; cognition adjuvant for Alzheimer dementia* [also: tacrine HCl]

tacrine HCl USAN *reversible cholinesterase inhibitor; cognition adjuvant for Alzheimer dementia* [also: tacrine]

tacrolimus USAN, INN *immunosuppressant for liver transplants; topical treatment for eczema; investigational (Phase III) treatment for rheumatoid arthritis*

TAD (thioguanine, ara-C, daunorubicin) *chemotherapy protocol for acute myelocytic leukemia (AML)* [also: DAT; DCT]

tadalafil USAN *phosphodiesterase-5 (PDE-5) inhibitor; investigational (NDA filed) treatment for male erectile and female sexual dysfunction*

taeniacides *a class of agents that destroy tapeworms* [see also: anthelmintics; vermicides; vermifuges]

Tagamet film-coated tablets ℞ *histamine H_2 antagonist for gastric and duodenal ulcers and gastric hypersecretory conditions* [cimetidine] 300, 400, 800 mg ⊠ Tegopen

Tagamet liquid, IV or IM injection, premixed injection ℞ *histamine H_2 antagonist for gastric and duodenal ulcers and gastric hypersecretory conditions* [cimetidine HCl] 300 mg/5 mL; 300 mg/2 mL; 300 mg/vial

Tagamet 100 (British name for U.S. product Tagamet HB [in the 100 mg strength])

Tagamet HB film-coated tablets, oral suspension OTC *histamine H_2 antagonist for episodic heartburn and acid indigestion* [cimetidine] 100, 200 mg; 200 mg

taglutimide INN

taheebo *medicinal herb* [see: pau d'arco]

TA-HPV ℞ *investigational (orphan) for cervical cancer* [vaccinia virus vaccine for human papillomavirus (HPV), recombinant]

tail, colt's; cow's tail; horse tail; mare's tail *medicinal herb* [see: fleabane; horseweed]

tail, lion's *medicinal herb* [see: motherwort]

tailed cubebs; tailed pepper *medicinal herb* [see: cubeb]

TAK-603 *investigational (orphan) for Crohn disease*

Talacen caplets ℞ *narcotic agonist-antagonist analgesic; antipyretic* [pentazocine HCl; acetaminophen] 25•650 mg

talampicillin INN *antibacterial* [also: talampicillin HCl]

talampicillin HCl USAN *antibacterial* [also: talampicillin]

talastine INN

talbutal USP, INN *sedative; hypnotic*

talc USP, JAN *dusting powder; tablet and capsule lubricant*

talc, sterile aerosol *investigational (NDA filed, orphan) treatment for malignant pleural effusion and pneumothorax via intrapleural thoracoscopy administration*

taleranol USAN, INN *gonadotropin enzyme inhibitor*

talinolol INN

talipexole INN

talisomycin USAN, INN *antineoplastic*

tall speedwell *medicinal herb* [see: Culver root]

tall veronica *medicinal herb* [see: Culver root]

TALL-104 *investigational killer cell line derived from cells of a patient with a rare form of T-cell leukemia for metastatic cancer*

tallimustine INN *investigational antineoplastic for leukemia and solid tumors*

tallow shrub *medicinal herb* [see: bayberry]

tallysomycin A [now: talisomycin]

talmetacin USAN, INN *analgesic; anti-inflammatory; antipyretic*

talmetoprim INN

talnetant HCl USAN *NK_3 receptor antagonist for urinary frequency, urgency, and incontinence*

talniflumate USAN, INN *anti-inflammatory; analgesic*

talopram INN *catecholamine potentiator* [also: talopram HCl]

talopram HCl USAN *catecholamine potentiator* [also: talopram]

talosalate USAN, INN *analgesic; anti-inflammatory*

Taloxa (foreign name for U.S. product Felbatol)

taloximine INN, BAN

talsaclidine INN

talsaclidine fumarate USAN *muscarinic M_1 agonist for Alzheimer disease*

talsupram INN

taltibride [see: metibride]

taltrimide INN

taludipine [see: teludipine]

taludipine HCl [see: teludipine HCl]

Talwin IV, subcu or IM injection ℞ *narcotic agonist-antagonist analgesic; also abused as a street drug* [pentazocine lactate] 30 mg/mL

Talwin Compound caplets ℞ *narcotic agonist-antagonist analgesic; antipyretic; also abused as a street drug* [pentazocine HCl; aspirin] 12.5•325 mg

Talwin NX tablets ℞ *narcotic agonist-antagonist analgesic; also abused as a street drug* [pentazocine HCl; naloxone HCl] 50•0.5 mg

tamarind *(Tamarindus indica)* fruit and leaves *medicinal herb used as an anthelmintic, laxative, and refrigerant*

Tambocor tablets ℞ *antiarrhythmic* [flecainide acetate] 50, 100, 150 mg

tameridone USAN, INN, BAN *veterinary sedative*

tameticillin INN

tametraline INN *antidepressant* [also: tametraline HCl]

tametraline HCl USAN *antidepressant* [also: tametraline]

Tamiflu capsules, oral suspension ℞ *antiviral for the prophylaxis and treatment of influenza A and B infections* [oseltamivir phosphate] 75 mg; 12 mg/mL

Tamine S.R. sustained-release tablets ℞ *decongestant; antihistamine* [phenylpropanolamine HCl; phenylephrine HCl; brompheniramine maleate] 15•15•12 mg

tamitinol INN

tamoxifen INN, BAN *antiestrogen antineoplastic for breast cancer* [also: tamoxifen citrate]

tamoxifen citrate USAN, USP, JAN *antiestrogen antineoplastic for breast cancer; breast cancer prevention for high-risk patients* [also: tamoxifen] 10, 20 mg oral

tamoxifen citrate & DTIC *chemotherapy protocol for malignant melanoma*

tampramine INN *antidepressant* [also: tampramine fumarate]

tampramine fumarate USAN *antidepressant* [also: tampramine]

Tamp-R-Tel (trademarked packaging form) *tamper-evident cartridge-needle unit*

tamsulosin INN *alpha$_1$-adrenergic blocker for benign prostatic hypertrophy (BPH)* [also: tamsulosin HCl]

tamsulosin HCl USAN, JAN *alpha$_1$-adrenergic blocker for benign prostatic hypertrophy (BPH)* [also: tamsulosin]

Tanac gel OTC *topical oral anesthetic; vulnerary* [dyclonine HCl; allantoin] 1%•0.5%

Tanac liquid OTC *topical oral anesthetic; antiseptic* [benzocaine; benzalkonium chloride] 10%•0.12%

Tanac Dual Core stick OTC *topical oral anesthetic; antiseptic; astringent* [benzocaine; benzalkonium chloride; tannic acid] 7.5%•0.12%•6%

Tanacetum parthenium *medicinal herb* [see: feverfew]

Tanacetum vulgare *medicinal herb* [see: tansy]

Tanafed oral suspension ℞ *decongestant; antihistamine* [pseudoephedrine tannate; chlorpheniramine tannate] 75•4.5 mg/5 mL

tandamine INN *antidepressant* [also: tandamine HCl]

tandamine HCl USAN *antidepressant* [also: tandamine]

tandospirone INN, BAN *anxiolytic* [also: tandospirone citrate]

tandospirone citrate USAN *anxiolytic* [also: tandospirone]

taniplon INN

tannic acid USP, JAN *astringent; topical mucosal protectant*

tannic acid acetate [see: acetyltannic acid]

Tannic-12 oral suspension ℞ *pediatric antitussive, decongestant, and antihistamine* [carbetapentane tannate; phenylephrine tannate; chlorpheniramine tannate] 30•5•4 mg/5 mL

tannin [see: tannic acid]

tannyl acetate [see: acetyltannic acid]

Tanoral tablets ℞ *decongestant; antihistamine* [phenylephrine tannate; chlorpheniramine tannate; pyrilamine tannate] 25•8•25 mg

tansy *(Chrysanthemum vulgare; Tanacetum vulgare)* leaves and seeds *medicinal herb for inducing diaphoresis, promoting wound healing, relieving spasms, stimulating menstruation, and treating worm infections*

tantalum *element (Ta)*

Tantrum ℞ *investigational (orphan) radioprotectant for oral mucosa following radiation therapy for head and neck cancer* [benzydamine HCl]

Tao capsules ℞ *macrolide antibiotic* [troleandomycin] 250 mg

taoryi edisylate [see: caramiphen edisylate]

Tapanol tablets, caplets, gelcaps OTC *analgesic; antipyretic* [acetaminophen] 325, 500 mg; 500 mg; 500 mg

Tapazole tablets ℞ *antithyroid agent* [methimazole] 5, 10 mg

tape, adhesive USP *surgical aid*

taprostene INN

tar [see: coal tar]

tarweed *medicinal herb* [see: yerba santa]

Tarabine PFS subcu, intrathecal, or IV injection ℞ *antimetabolite antineoplastic for various leukemias* [cytarabine] 20 mg/mL

Taraphilic Ointment OTC *topical antipsoriatic; antiseborrheic* [coal tar] 1%

Taraxacum officinale *medicinal herb* [see: dandelion]

Targocid (commercially available in 13 foreign countries) ℞ *investigational (NDA filed) glycopeptide antibiotic* [teicoplanin]

Targretin capsules, gel ℞ *synthetic retinoid analogue antineoplastic for cutaneous T-cell lymphoma (CTCL); investigational (Phase II/III) for AIDS-related Kaposi sarcoma (clinical trials discontinued 1999)* [bexarotene] 75 mg; 1% ⊡ Tegopen; Tegrin

Targretin gel ℞ *investigational (NDA filed) synthetic retinoid analogue antineoplastic for cutaneous T-cell lymphoma* [bexarotene] 1%

Tarka film-coated combination-release tablets ℞ *once-daily antihypertensive; angiotensin-converting enzyme (ACE) inhibitor; calcium channel blocker* [trandolapril (immediate release); verapamil HCl (extended release)] 2•180, 1•240, 2•240, 4•240 mg

Tarlene hair lotion OTC *antiseborrheic; antipsoriatic; keratolytic* [salicylic acid; coal tar] 2.5%•2%

Taro-Desoximetasone (CAN) cream, gel (name changed to Desoxi in 2001)

Taro-Warfarin (CAN) tablets ℞ *coumarin-derivative anticoagulant* [warfarin sodium] 1, 2, 2.5, 3, 4, 5, 6, 7.5, 10 mg

tarragon (*Artemisia dracunculus*) flowering plant *medicinal herb used as a diuretic, emmenagogue, hypnotic, and stomachic*

Tarsum shampoo OTC *antipsoriatic; antiseborrheic; keratolytic* [coal tar; salicylic acid] 10%•5%

tartar emetic [see: antimony potassium tartrate]

tartaric acid NF *buffering agent*

Tasmar film-coated tablets ℞ COMT *inhibitor; adjunct to carbidopa and levodopa for Parkinson disease* [tolcapone] 100, 200 mg

tasosartan USAN, INN *antihypertensive; angiotensin II antagonist (NDA withdrawn 1998)*

tasuldine INN

TAT antagonist *investigational (Phase I/II) antiviral for HIV infection*

taurine INN [also: aminoethylsulfonic acid]

taurocholate sodium [see: sodium taurocholate]

taurolidine INN, BAN *investigational antitoxin for the treatment of sepsis*

tauromustine INN *investigational treatment for renal cancer and multiple sclerosis*

tauroselcholic acid INN, BAN

taurultam INN, BAN

Tavist tablets, syrup ℞ *antihistamine* [clemastine fumarate] 2.68 mg; 0.67 mg/5 mL

Tavist Allergy tablets OTC *antihistamine* [clemastine fumarate] 1.34 mg

Tavist Allergy/Sinus/Headache caplets OTC *decongestant; antihistamine; analgesic* [pseudoephedrine HCl;

clemastine fumarate; acetaminophen] 30•0.335•500 mg

Tavist-1 tablets (name changed to Tavist Allergy in 1999) OTC *antihistamine* [clemastine fumarate] 1.34 mg

Tavist-D film-coated sustained-release tablets OTC *decongestant; antihistamine* [phenylpropanolamine HCl; clemastine fumarate] 75•1.34 mg

taxanes; taxoids *a class of antineoplastics that inhibits cancer cell mitosis by disrupting the cells' microtubular network*

Taxol IV infusion ℞ *antineoplastic for ovarian and breast cancers, and non–small cell lung cancer (NSCLC), and AIDS-related Kaposi sarcoma (orphan)* [paclitaxel] 6 mg/mL

Taxotere IV infusion ℞ *antineoplastic for advanced or metastatic breast cancer and non–small cell lung cancer (NSCLC)* [docetaxel] 20, 80 mg/vial

***Taxus bacatta* and other species** *medicinal herb* [see: yew]

tazadolene INN *analgesic* [also: tazadolene succinate]

tazadolene succinate USAN *analgesic* [also: tazadolene]

tazanolast INN

tazarotene USAN, INN *retinoid prodrug; topical keratolytic for acne and psoriasis*

tazasubrate INN, BAN

tazeprofen INN

Tazicef powder or frozen premix for IV or IM injection ℞ *cephalosporin antibiotic* [ceftazidime] 1, 2, 6 g

Tazidime powder for IV or IM injection ℞ *cephalosporin antibiotic* [ceftazidime] 0.5, 1, 2, 6 g

tazifylline INN *antihistamine* [also: tazifylline HCl]

tazifylline HCl USAN *antihistamine* [also: tazifylline]

taziprinone INN

tazobactam USAN, INN, BAN *β-lactamase inhibitor; penicillin synergist*

tazobactam sodium USAN *β-lactamase inhibitor; penicillin synergist*

Tazocin (European name for U.S. product Zosyn)

tazofelone USAN *investigational (Phase II) treatment for ulcerative colitis and Crohn disease*

tazolol INN *cardiotonic* [also: tazolol HCl]

tazolol HCl USAN *cardiotonic* [also: tazolol]

tazomeline citrate USAN *cholinergic agonist for Alzheimer disease*

Tazorac cream, gel ℞ *retinoid pro-drug; topical keratolytic for acne and psoriasis* [tazarotene] 0.05%, 0.1%

TBC-3B *investigational (Phase I) vaccine for AIDS*

TBC-11251 *investigational (Phase II) endothelin-A antagonist for congestive heart failure*

TBZ (thiabendazole) [q.v.]

TC (thioguanine, cytarabine) *chemotherapy protocol*

3TC [now: lamivudine]

^{99m}Tc [see: macrosalb (^{99m}Tc)]

^{99m}Tc [see: sodium pertechnetate Tc 99m]

^{99m}Tc [see: technetium Tc 99m albumin]

^{99m}Tc [see: technetium Tc 99m albumin aggregated]

^{99m}Tc [see: technetium Tc 99m albumin colloid]

^{99m}Tc [see: technetium Tc 99m albumin microaggregated]

^{99m}Tc [see: technetium Tc 99m antimony trisulfide colloid]

^{99m}Tc [see: technetium Tc 99m biciromab]

^{99m}Tc [see: technetium Tc 99m bicisate]

^{99m}Tc [see: technetium Tc 99m disofenin]

^{99m}Tc [see: technetium Tc 99m etidronate]

^{99m}Tc [see: technetium Tc 99m exametazine]

^{99m}Tc [see: technetium Tc 99m ferpentetate]

^{99m}Tc [see: technetium Tc 99m furifosmin]

^{99m}Tc [see: technetium Tc 99m gluceptate]

^{99m}Tc [see: technetium Tc 99m lidofenin]

^{99m}Tc [see: technetium Tc 99m mebrofenin]
^{99m}Tc [see: technetium Tc 99m medronate]
^{99m}Tc [see: technetium Tc 99m medronate disodium]
^{99m}Tc [see: technetium Tc 99m mertiatide]
^{99m}Tc [see: technetium Tc 99m oxidronate]
^{99m}Tc [see: technetium Tc 99m pentetate]
^{99m}Tc [see: technetium Tc 99m pentetate calcium trisodium]
^{99m}Tc [see: technetium Tc 99m (pyro- & trimeta-) phosphates]
^{99m}Tc [see: technetium Tc 99m pyrophosphate]
^{99m}Tc [see: technetium Tc 99m red blood cells]
^{99m}Tc [see: technetium Tc 99m sestamibi]
^{99m}Tc [see: technetium Tc 99m siboroxime]
^{99m}Tc [see: technetium Tc 99m succimer]
^{99m}Tc [see: technetium Tc 99m sulfur colloid]
^{99m}Tc [see: technetium Tc 99m teboroxime]
^{99m}Tc [see: technetium Tc 99m tetrofosmin]
^{99m}Tc [see: technetium Tc 99m tiatide]
TCC (trichlorocarbanilide) [see: triclocarban]
T-cell gene therapy *investigational (Phase III) treatment for HIV infection*
T-cell receptor (TCR) peptide *investigational (Phase II) theraccine for rheumatoid arthritis*
TCF (Taxol, cisplatin, fluorouracil) *chemotherapy protocol for esophageal cancer*
TCR (T-cell receptor) peptide [q.v.]
TD; Td (tetanus & diphtheria [toxoids]) *the designation TD (or DT) denotes the pediatric vaccine; Td denotes the adult vaccine* [see: diphtheria & tetanus toxoids, adsorbed]
tea, Canada; mountain tea; redberry tea *medicinal herb* [see: wintergreen]
tea tree oil *(Melaleuca alternifolia)* *medicinal herb for acne, boils, burns, Candida infections, cold sores, joint pain, skin disorders, staphylococcal and streptococcal infections, and sunburn; also used as a douche for trichomonal cervicitis and vaginal candidiasis*
TEAB (tetraethylammonium bromide) [see: tetrylammonium bromide]
teaberry oil [see: methyl salicylate]
TEAC (tetraethylammonium chloride) [q.v.]
teamster's tea *medicinal herb* [see: ephedra]
Tear Drop eye drops (discontinued 1998) OTC *ophthalmic moisturizer/lubricant* [polyvinyl alcohol]
TearGard eye drops OTC *ocular moisturizer/lubricant* [hydroxyethylcellulose]
Teargen eye drops OTC *ophthalmic moisturizer/lubricant* [polyvinyl alcohol]
Tearisol eye drops OTC *ophthalmic moisturizer/lubricant* [hydroxypropyl methylcellulose] 0.5%
Tears Naturale; Tears Naturale II; Tears Naturale Free eye drops OTC *ophthalmic moisturizer/lubricant* [hydroxypropyl methylcellulose] 0.3%
Tears Plus eye drops OTC *ophthalmic moisturizer/lubricant* [polyvinyl alcohol] 1.4%
Tears Renewed eye drops OTC *ophthalmic moisturizer/lubricant* [hydroxypropyl methylcellulose] 0.3%
Tears Renewed ophthalmic ointment OTC *ocular moisturizer/lubricant* [white petrolatum; mineral oil]
TearSaver Punctum Plugs ℞ *blocks the puncta and canaliculus to eliminate tear loss in keratitis sicca* [silicone plug]
Tebamide suppositories, pediatric suppositories ℞ *antiemetic; anticholinergic* [trimethobenzamide HCl; benzocaine] 200 mg•2%; 100 mg•2%
tebatizole INN
tebethion [see: thioacetazone; thiacetazone]

tebufelone USAN, INN *analgesic; anti-inflammatory*
tebuquine USAN, INN *antimalarial*
tebutate USAN, INN *combining name for radicals or groups*
TEC (thiotepa, etoposide, carboplatin) *chemotherapy protocol*
teceleukin USAN, INN, BAN *immunostimulant; investigational (orphan) for metastatic renal cell carcinoma and metastatic malignant melanoma*
teceleukin & interferon alfa-2a *investigational (orphan) for metastatic renal cell carcinoma and metastatic malignant melanoma*
technetium *element (Tc)*
technetium (^{99m}Tc) dimercaptosuccinic acid JAN *diagnostic aid for renal function testing* [also: technetium Tc 99m succimer]
technetium (^{99m}Tc) human serum albumin JAN *radioactive agent*
technetium (^{99m}Tc) labeled macroaggregated human albumin JAN [also: macrosalb (^{99m}Tc)]
technetium (^{99m}Tc) methylenediphosphonate JAN *radioactive diagnostic aid for skeletal imaging* [also: technetium Tc 99m medronate]
technetium (^{99m}Tc) phytate JAN *radioactive agent*
technetium Tc 99m albumin USP *radioactive agent*
technetium Tc 99m albumin aggregated USAN, USP *radioactive diagnostic aid for lung imaging*
technetium Tc 99m albumin colloid USAN, USP *radioactive agent*
technetium Tc 99m albumin microaggregated USAN *radioactive agent*
technetium Tc 99m antimelanoma murine MAb *investigational (orphan) for diagnostic imaging agent for metastases of malignant melanoma*
technetium Tc 99m antimony trisulfide colloid USAN *radioactive agent*
technetium Tc 99m apcitide *radiopharmaceutical diagnostic aid for acute venous thrombosis*
technetium Tc 99m arcitumomab USAN *radiopharmaceutical diagnostic aid for recurrent or metastatic thyroid and colorectal cancers*
technetium Tc 99m bectumomab *monoclonal antibody; investigational (Phase III, orphan) diagnostic aid for non-Hodgkin B-cell lymphoma, AIDS-related lymphomas, and other acute and chronic B-cell leukemias* [also: bectumomab]
technetium Tc 99m biciromab *radioactive diagnostic aid for deep vein thrombosis*
technetium Tc 99m bicisate USAN, INN, BAN *radioactive diagnostic aid for brain imaging*
technetium Tc 99m depreotide [see: depreotide]
technetium Tc 99m disofenin USP *radioactive diagnostic aid for hepatobiliary function testing*
technetium Tc 99m DMSA (dimercaptosuccinic acid) [see: technetium Tc 99m succimer]
technetium Tc 99m DTPA (diethylenetriaminepentaacetic acid) [see: technetium Tc 99m pentetate]
technetium Tc 99m etidronate USP *radioactive agent*
technetium Tc 99m exametazine USAN *radioactive agent*
technetium Tc 99m ferpentetate USP *radioactive agent*
technetium Tc 99m furifosmin USAN, INN *radioactive agent; diagnostic aid for cardiac disease*
technetium Tc 99m gluceptate USP *radioactive agent*
technetium Tc 99m HSA (human serum albumin) [see: technetium Tc 99m albumin]
technetium Tc 99m iron ascorbate pentetic acid complex [now: technetium Tc 99m ferpentetate]
technetium Tc 99m lidofenin USAN, USP *radioactive agent*
technetium Tc 99m MAA (microaggregated albumin) [see: technetium Tc 99m albumin aggregated]

technetium Tc 99m MDP (methylenediphosphonate) [see: technetium Tc 99m medronate]
technetium Tc 99m mebrofenin USAN, USP *radioactive agent*
technetium Tc 99m medronate USP *radioactive diagnostic aid for skeletal imaging* [also: technetium (^{99m}Tc) methylenediphosphonate]
technetium Tc 99m medronate disodium USAN *radioactive agent*
technetium Tc 99m mertiatide USAN *radioactive diagnostic aid for renal function testing*
technetium Tc 99m murine MAb IgG$_2$a to B cell [now: technetium Tc 99m bectumomab]
technetium Tc 99m murine MAb to human alpha-fetoprotein (AFP) *investigational (orphan) diagnostic aid for AFP-producing tumors, hepatoblastoma, and hepatocellular carcinoma*
technetium Tc 99m murine MAb to human chorionic gonadotropin (hCG) *investigational (orphan) diagnostic aid for hCG-producing tumors*
technetium Tc 99m oxidronate USP *radioactive diagnostic aid for skeletal imaging*
technetium Tc 99m pentetate USP *radioactive agent* [also: human serum albumin diethylenetriaminepentaacetic acid technetium (^{99m}Tc)]
technetium Tc 99m pentetate calcium trisodium USAN *radioactive agent*
technetium Tc 99m pentetate sodium [now: technetium Tc 99m pentetate]
technetium Tc 99m (pyro- and trimeta-) phosphates USP *radioactive agent*
technetium Tc 99m pyrophosphate USP, JAN *radioactive agent*
technetium Tc 99m red blood cells USAN *radioactive agent*
technetium Tc 99m sestamibi USAN, INN, BAN *radioactive/radiopaque diagnostic aid for cardiac perfusion imaging and mammography*
technetium Tc 99m siboroxime USAN, INN *radioactive diagnostic aid for brain imaging*
technetium Tc 99m sodium gluceptate [now: technetium Tc 99m gluceptate]
technetium Tc 99m succimer USP *diagnostic aid for renal function testing* [also: technetium (^{99m}Tc) dimercaptosuccinic acid]
technetium Tc 99m sulesomab *monoclonal antibody; diagnostic aid for infectious lesions* [also: sulesomab]
technetium Tc 99m sulfur colloid (TSC) USAN, USP *radioactive agent*
technetium Tc 99m teboroxime USAN, INN, BAN *radioactive/radiopaque diagnostic aid for cardiac perfusion imaging*
technetium Tc 99m tetrofosmin *radioactive agent for cardiovascular imaging*
technetium Tc 99m tiatide BAN
technetium Tc 99m TSC (technetium sulfur colloid) [see: technetium Tc 99m sulfur colloid]
technetium Tc 99m-labeled CEA scan [see: arcitumomab]
Techtide [see: P829 Techtide]
teclothiazide INN, BAN
teclozan USAN, INN *antiamebic*
Tecnu Poison Oak-N-Ivy liquid OTC *topical poison ivy treatment* [deodorized mineral spirits]
tecogalan sodium USAN *antiangiogenic antineoplastic*
Teczem film-coated extended-release tablets ℞ *antihypertensive; angiotensin-converting enzyme (ACE) inhibitor; calcium channel blocker* [diltiazem maleate; enalapril maleate] 180•5 mg
tedisamil INN *investigational calcium channel blocker for ischemic heart disease and arrhythmias*
Tedrigen tablets OTC *antiasthmatic; bronchodilator; decongestant; sedative* [theophylline; ephedrine HCl; phenobarbital] 120•22.5•7.5 mg
tefazoline INN
tefenperate INN

tefludazine INN
teflurane USAN, INN *inhalation anesthetic*
teflutixol INN
tegafur USAN, INN, BAN *antineoplastic; prodrug of fluorouracil*
tegaserod USAN *investigational (NDA filed) selective serotonin 5-HT$_4$ receptor antagonist for irritable bowel syndrome*
Tegison capsules ℞ *systemic antipsoriatic* [etretinate] 10, 25 mg
Tegopen capsules, powder for oral solution (discontinued 1998) ℞ *penicillinase-resistant penicillin antibiotic* [cloxacillin sodium] 250, 500 mg; 125 mg/5 mL ⊠ Tagamet; Tegrin; Targretin
Tegretol chewable tablets, tablets, oral suspension ℞ *anticonvulsant; analgesic for trigeminal neuralgia; antimanic* [carbamazepine] 100 mg; 200 mg; 100 mg/5 mL ⊠ Tegrin
Tegretol-XR extended-release tablets ℞ *twice-daily anticonvulsant; antipsychotic* [carbamazepine] 100, 200, 400 mg
Tegrin for Psoriasis cream, lotion, soap OTC *topical antipsoriatic; antiseborrheic; antiseptic* [coal tar solution] 5% ⊠ Tegopen; Tegretol; Targretin
Tegrin Medicated gel shampoo, lotion shampoo OTC *antiseborrheic; antipsoriatic; antipruritic; antibacterial* [coal tar] 5%
Tegrin Medicated Extra Conditioning; Advanced Formula Tegrin shampoo OTC *antiseborrheic; antipsoriatic; antipruritic; antibacterial* [coal tar] 7%
Tegrin-HC ointment OTC *topical corticosteroidal anti-inflammatory* [hydrocortisone] 1%
Tegrin-LT shampoo/conditioner OTC *pediculicide for lice* [pyrethrins; piperonyl butoxide technical] 0.33%•3.15%
teholamine [see: aminophylline]
TEIB (triethyleneiminobenzoquinone) [see: triaziquone]
teicoplanin USAN, INN, BAN *glycopeptide antibacterial antibiotic*
teicoplanin $A_{2\text{-}1}$, $A_{2\text{-}2}$, $A_{2\text{-}3}$, $A_{2\text{-}4}$, $A_{2\text{-}5}$, $A_{3\text{-}1}$ *components of teicoplanin*
Telachlor timed-release capsules (discontinued 1997) ℞ *antihistamine* [chlorpheniramine maleate] 8, 12 mg
Teladar cream ℞ *topical corticosteroidal anti-inflammatory* [betamethasone dipropionate] 0.05%
Teldrin timed-release capsules (discontinued 1997) OTC *antihistamine* [chlorpheniramine maleate] 12 mg ⊠ Tedral
Teldrin 12-Hour Allergy Relief sustained-release capsules OTC *decongestant; antihistamine* [phenylpropanolamine HCl; chlorpheniramine maleate] 75•8 mg
Tel-E-Amp (trademarked packaging form) *unit dose ampule*
Tel-E-Dose (trademarked packaging form) *unit dose package*
Tel-E-Ject (trademarked delivery system) *prefilled disposable syringe*
telenzepine INN
Tel-E-Pack (trademarked packaging form) *packaging system*
Telepaque tablets ℞ *radiopaque contrast medium for cholecystography* [iopanoic acid (66.68% iodine)] 500 mg (333.4 mg)
Tel-E-Vial (trademarked packaging form) *unit dose vial*
telinavir USAN *antiviral; HIV protease inhibitor*
Teline; Teline-500 capsules (discontinued 1997) ℞ *broad-spectrum antibiotic* [tetracycline HCl] 250 mg; 500 mg
telithromycin *investigational (NDA filed) broad-spectrum ketolide antibiotic*
tellurium *element (Te)*
telmisartan USAN *long-acting antihypertensive; angiotensin II receptor antagonist*
teloxantrone INN *antineoplastic* [also: teloxantrone HCl]
teloxantrone HCl USAN *antineoplastic* [also: teloxantrone]
teludipine INN, BAN *antihypertensive; calcium channel antagonist* [also: teludipine HCl]

teludipine HCl USAN *antihypertensive; calcium channel antagonist* [also: teludipine]

temafloxacin INN, BAN *antibacterial; microbial DNA topoisomerase inhibitor* [also: temafloxacin HCl]

temafloxacin HCl USAN *antibacterial; microbial DNA topoisomerase inhibitor* [also: temafloxacin]

temarotene INN

tematropium methylsulfate USAN *anticholinergic* [also: tematropium metilsulfate]

tematropium metilsulfate INN *anticholinergic* [also: tematropium methylsulfate]

temazepam USAN, INN *benzodiazepine hypnotic; minor tranquilizer* 7.5, 15, 30 mg oral

Temazin Cold syrup OTC *decongestant; antihistamine* [phenylpropanolamine HCl; chlorpheniramine maleate] 12.5•2 mg/5 mL

Tembid (trademarked dosage form) *sustained-action capsule*

temefos USAN, INN *veterinary ectoparasiticide*

temelastine USAN, INN, BAN *antihistamine*

temocapril HCl USAN *antihypertensive*

temocillin USAN, INN, BAN *antibacterial*

Temodal (CAN) capsules ℞ *alkylating antineoplastic for refractory anaplastic astrocytoma and recurrent malignant glioma* [temozolomide] 5, 20, 100, 250 mg

Temodar capsules ℞ *alkylating antineoplastic for refractory anaplastic astrocytoma; investigational (NDA filed) for recurrent malignant glioma and metastatic malignant melanoma* [temozolomide] 5, 20, 100, 250 mg

temodox USAN, INN *veterinary growth stimulant*

temoporfin USAN, INN, BAN *photosensitizer for photodynamic cancer therapy; investigational (NDA filed) for head and neck cancer*

Temovate ointment, gel, cream, scalp application ℞ *topical corticosteroidal anti-inflammatory* [clobetasol propionate] 0.05%

Temovate Emollient cream ℞ *topical corticosteroidal anti-inflammatory* [clobetasol propionate in an emollient base] 0.05%

temozolomide USAN, INN, BAN *alkylating antineoplastic for refractory anaplastic astrocytoma; investigational (NDA filed) for malignant glioma and metastatic malignant melanoma*

TEMP (tamoxifen, etoposide, mitoxantrone, Platinol) *chemotherapy protocol*

Tempium ℞ *investigational treatment for Alzheimer disease* [lazabemide HCl]

Tempo chewable tablets OTC *antacid; antiflatulent* [aluminum hydroxide; magnesium hydroxide; calcium carbonate; simethicone] 133•81•414•20 mg

Tempra (CAN) FirsTabs (quick-dissolving tablets), chewable tablets, syrup, oral drops OTC *pediatric analgesic and antipyretic* [acetaminophen] 160 mg; 80 mg; 80, 160 mg/5 mL; 80 mg/mL

Tempra Quicklets (quickly dissolving tablets) OTC *analgesic; antipyretic* [acetaminophen] 80, 160 mg

Tempra 1 drops OTC *analgesic; antipyretic* [acetaminophen] 100 mg/mL

Tempra 2 syrup OTC *analgesic; antipyretic* [acetaminophen] 160 mg/5 mL

Tempra 3 chewable tablets OTC *analgesic; antipyretic* [acetaminophen] 80, 160 mg

Tempule (trademarked dosage form) *timed-release capsule or tablet*

temurtide USAN, INN, BAN *vaccine adjuvant*

10 Benzagel; 5 Benzagel gel ℞ *topical keratolytic for acne* [benzoyl peroxide] 10%; 5%

10% LMD IV injection ℞ *plasma volume expander for shock due to hemorrhage, burns, or surgery* [dextran 40] 10%

tenamfetamine INN

Tencet capsules ℞ *analgesic; antipyretic; sedative* [acetaminophen; caffeine; butalbital] 325•40•50 mg

Tencon capsules ℞ *analgesic; barbiturate sedative* [acetaminophen; butalbital] 650•50 mg

tendamistat INN

Tenecteplase ℞ *investigational (NDA filed) thrombolytic*

tenecteplase USAN *thrombolytic for acute myocardial infarction; genetically engineered mutation of tissue plasminogen activator (tPA)*

Tenex tablets ℞ *antihypertensive; antiadrenergic* [guanfacine HCl] 1, 2 mg ⑨ Xanax

tenidap USAN, INN *anti-inflammatory for osteoarthritis and rheumatoid arthritis; cytokine inhibitor*

tenidap sodium USAN *anti-inflammatory for osteoarthritis and rheumatoid arthritis*

tenilapine INN

teniloxazine INN

tenilsetam INN

teniposide USAN, INN, BAN *antineoplastic for refractory childhood acute lymphocytic leukemia (orphan)*

Ten-K controlled-release tablets ℞ *potassium supplement* [potassium chloride] 750 mg (10 mEq)

tenoate INN *combining name for radicals or groups*

tenocyclidine INN

tenofovir USAN *antiviral reverse transcriptase inhibitor*

tenofovir disoproxil fumarate (tenofovir DF) USAN *investigational (NDA filed) oral antiviral nucleotide reverse transcriptase inhibitor (NRTI) for HIV infection*

tenonitrozole INN

Tenoretic 50; Tenoretic 100 tablets ℞ *antihypertensive; β-blocker; diuretic* [chlorthalidone; atenolol] 25•50 mg; 25•100 mg

Tenormin tablets, IV injection ℞ *antihypertensive; antianginal; antiadrenergic (β-blocker)* [atenolol] 25, 50, 100 mg; 5 mg/10 mL

Tenovil ℞ *investigational (Phase I) immunomodulator for HIV infection; investigational (Phase II) for psoriasis* [interleukin-10]

tenoxicam USAN, INN, BAN *anti-inflammatory*

Tensilon IV or IM injection ℞ *myasthenia gravis treatment; antidote to curare overdose* [edrophonium chloride] 10 mg/mL

Ten-Tab (trademarked dosage form) *controlled-release tablet*

Tenuate tablets, Dospan (controlled-release tablets) ℞ *anorexiant; CNS stimulant* [diethylpropion HCl] 25 mg; 75 mg

tenylidone INN

teoclate INN *combining name for radicals or groups* [also: theoclate]

teopranitol INN

teoprolol INN

tepirindole INN

tepoxalin USAN, INN *antipsoriatic*

teprenone INN

teprosilate INN *combining name for radicals or groups*

teprotide USAN, INN *angiotensin-converting enzyme (ACE) inhibitor*

Tequin film-coated tablets, IV infusion ℞ *broad-spectrum fluoroquinolone antibiotic* [gatifloxacin] 200, 400 mg; 200, 400 mg/vial

Terak with Polymyxin B Sulfate ophthalmic ointment ℞ *topical ophthalmic antibiotic* [oxytetracycline HCl; polymyxin B sulfate] 5 mg•10 000 U per g

Terazol 3 vaginal inserts, vaginal cream ℞ *antifungal* [terconazole] 80 mg; 0.8%

Terazol 7 vaginal cream ℞ *antifungal* [terconazole] 0.4%

terazosin INN, BAN *α_1-adrenergic blocker for hypertension and benign prostatic hyperplasia* [also: terazosin HCl]

terazosin HCl USAN *α_1-adrenergic blocker for hypertension and benign prostatic hyperplasia* [also: terazosin] 1, 5, 10 mg oral

terbinafine USAN, INN, BAN *systemic allylamine antifungal* [also: terbinafine HCl]
terbinafine HCl JAN *allylamine antifungal* [also: terbinafine]
terbium *element (Tb)*
terbogrel USAN *platelet aggregation inhibitor*
terbucromil INN
terbufibrol INN
terbuficin INN
terbuprol INN
terbutaline INN, BAN *sympathomimetic bronchodilator* [also: terbutaline sulfate]
terbutaline sulfate USAN, USP *sympathomimetic bronchodilator* [also: terbutaline] 2.5, 5 mg oral
terciprazine INN
terconazole USAN, INN, BAN *topical antifungal*
terfenadine USAN, USP, INN, JAN *piperidine antihistamine*
terflavoxate INN
terfluranol INN
terguride INN *investigational dopamine agonist for central nervous system disorders*
teriparatide USAN, INN *diagnostic aid for hypocalcemia; anabolic osteoporosis treatment for women*
teriparatide acetate USAN, JAN *diagnostic aid for parathyroid-induced hypocalcemia (orphan)*
terizidone INN
terlakiren USAN *antihypertensive; renin inhibitor*
terlipressin INN, BAN *investigational (orphan) for bleeding esophageal varices*
ternidazole INN
terodiline INN, BAN, JAN *coronary vasodilator* [also: terodiline HCl]
terodiline HCl USAN *coronary vasodilator; investigational agent for urinary incontinence* [also: terodiline]
terofenamate INN
teroxalene INN *antischistosomal* [also: teroxalene HCl]
teroxalene HCl USAN *antischistosomal* [also: teroxalene]
teroxirone USAN, INN *antineoplastic*
terpin hydrate USP *(disapproved for use as an expectorant in 1991)* 85 mg/5 mL oral
terpinol [see: terpin hydrate]
Terra-Cortril eye drop suspension (discontinued 2000) ℞ *topical ophthalmic corticosteroidal anti-inflammatory; antibiotic* [hydrocortisone acetate; oxytetracycline HCl] 1.5%•0.5%
terrafungine [see: oxytetracycline]
Terramycin capsules ℞ *broad-spectrum tetracycline antibiotic* [oxytetracycline HCl] 250 mg ⊡ Garamycin; Theramycin
Terramycin IM injection ℞ *broad-spectrum tetracycline antibiotic* [oxytetracycline; lidocaine] 50 mg•2%, 125 mg•2% per mL
Terramycin with Polymyxin B ophthalmic ointment ℞ *topical ophthalmic antibiotic* [oxytetracycline HCl; polymyxin B sulfate] 5 mg•10 000 U per g
Tersaseptic shampoo/cleanser OTC *soap-free therapeutic cleanser*
tertatolol INN, BAN
tertiary amyl alcohol [see: amylene hydrate]
***tert*-pentyl alcohol** [see: amylene hydrate]
Tesamone IM injection (discontinued 2001) ℞ *androgen replacement for delayed puberty or breast cancer* [testosterone] 100 mg/mL
tesicam USAN, INN *anti-inflammatory*
tesimide USAN, INN *anti-inflammatory*
Teslac tablets ℞ *hormonal antineoplastic for palliative treatment of disseminated breast carcinoma* [testolactone] 50 mg
Teslascan IV injection ℞ *MRI contrast medium for liver imaging* [mangofodipir trisodium] 37.9 mg/mL (50 μmol/mL)
tesmilifene HCl USAN *antihistamine; chemopotentiator for adjunctive treatment of malignant tumors*
TESPA (triethylenethiophosphoramide) [see: thiotepa]
Tessalon Perles (capsules) ℞ *antitussive* [benzonatate] 100, 200 mg

Test Pack kit for professional use *in vitro diagnostic aid for Group A streptococcal antigens in throat swabs* [enzyme immunoassay]

Testandro IM injection (discontinued 2001) ℞ *androgen replacement for delayed puberty or breast cancer* [testosterone] 100 mg/mL

Test-Estro Cypionates IM injection (discontinued 1999) ℞ *hormone replacement therapy for postmenopausal symptoms* [estradiol cypionate; testosterone cypionate] 2•50 mg/mL

Testoderm; Testoderm with Adhesive transdermal patch (for scrotal area) ℞ *hormone replacement therapy for hypogonadism in men* [testosterone] 4, 6 mg/day (10, 15 mg total)

Testoderm TTS transdermal patch (for nonscrotal skin) ℞ *hormone replacement therapy for hypogonadism in men* [testosterone] 5 mg/day (328 mg total)

testolactone USAN, USP, INN *androgen; hormonal antineoplastic for palliative treatment of disseminated breast cancer* ⑨ testosterone

Testopel pellets for subcu implantation ℞ *hormone replacement therapy for hypogonadism* [testosterone] 75 mg

testosterone USP, INN, BAN *androgen replacement for hypogonadism or testosterone deficiency in men; investigational (Phase II, orphan) for AIDS-wasting syndrome and delayed puberty in boys* ⑨ testolactone

Testosterone Aqueous IM injection ℞ *androgen replacement for hypogonadism, delayed puberty, and androgen-responsive metastatic cancers* [testosterone] 25, 50, 100 mg/mL

testosterone cyclopentanepropionate [see: testosterone cypionate]

testosterone cyclopentylpropionate [see: testosterone cypionate]

testosterone cypionate USP *parenteral androgen; sometimes abused as a street drug*

testosterone enanthate USP *parenteral androgen replacement for testosterone deficiency in men, delayed puberty in boys, and metastatic breast cancer in women; sometimes abused as a street drug*

testosterone heptanoate [see: testosterone enanthate]

testosterone ketolaurate USAN, INN *androgen*

testosterone 3-oxododecanoate [see: testosterone ketolaurate]

testosterone phenylacetate USAN *androgen*

testosterone propionate USP *parenteral androgen; investigational (orphan) for vulvar dystrophies*

TestPack [see: Abbott TestPack]

Testred capsules ℞ *androgen replacement for hypogonadism or testosterone deficiency in men, delayed puberty in boys, and metastatic breast cancer in women; also abused as a street drug* [methyltestosterone] 10 mg

tetanus antitoxin USP *passive immunizing agent*

tetanus & gas gangrene antitoxins NF

tetanus & gas gangrene polyvalent antitoxin [see: tetanus & gas gangrene antitoxins]

tetanus immune globulin (TIG) USP *passive immunizing agent for post-exposure tetanus prophylaxis in patients with incomplete or uncertain pre-exposure immunization with tetanus toxoids*

tetanus immune human globulin [now: tetanus immune globulin]

tetanus toxoid USP *active immunizing agent* 4 LfU/0.5 mL

tetanus toxoid, adsorbed USP *active immunizing agent* 5 LfU/0.5 mL

tetiothalein sodium [see: iodophthalein sodium]

tetnicoran [see: nicofurate]

tetrabarbital INN

tetrabenazine INN, BAN *investigational (orphan) for Huntington disease and severe tardive dyskinesia*

TetraBriks (trademarked delivery form) *ready-to-use liquid containers*

tetracaine USP, INN *topical local anesthetic* [also: amethocaine]

tetracaine HCl USP, JAN *topical local anesthetic* [also: amethocaine HCl]
Tetracap capsules ℞ *broad-spectrum antibiotic* [tetracycline HCl] 250 mg
tetrachlorodecaoxide *investigational (Phase III) immunomodulator and growth factor for HIV and AIDS*
tetrachloroethylene USP
tetrachloromethane [see: carbon tetrachloride]
tetracosactide INN *adrenocorticotropic hormone* [also: cosyntropin; tetracosactrin]
tetracosactrin BAN *adrenocorticotropic hormone* [also: cosyntropin; tetracosactide]
tetracyclics *a class of antidepressants which enhance noradrenergic and serotonergic activity by blocking norepinephrine or serotonin uptake*
tetracycline USP, INN, BAN *bacteriostatic antibiotic; antirickettsial*
tetracycline HCl USP *bacteriostatic antibiotic; antirickettsial* 100, 250, 500 mg oral; 125 mg/5 mL oral
tetracycline phosphate complex USP, BAN *antibacterial*
tetracyclines *a class of bacteriostatic, antimicrobial antibiotics*
tetradecanoic acid, methylethyl ester [see: isopropyl myristate]
tetradonium bromide INN
tetraethylammonium bromide (TEAB) [see: tetrylammonium bromide]
tetraethylammonium chloride (TEAC)
tetraethylthiuram disulfide [see: disulfiram]
tetrafilcon A USAN *hydrophilic contact lens material*
tetraglycine hydroperiodide *source of iodine for disinfecting water*
tetrahydroacridinamine (THA) [see: tacrine HCl]
tetrahydroaminoacridine (THA) [see: tacrine HCl]
tetrahydrocannabinol (THC) [see: dronabinol]
tetrahydrolipstatin [see: orlistat]
tetrahydrozoline BAN *vasoconstrictor; nasal decongestant; topical ophthalmic decongestant* [also: tetrhydrozoline HCl; tetryzoline]
tetrahydrozoline HCl USP *vasoconstrictor; nasal decongestant; topical ophthalmic decongestant* [also: tetryzoline; tetrahydrozoline] 0.05% eye drops
tetraiodophenolphthalein sodium [see: iodophthalein sodium]
Tetralan syrup (discontinued 1997) ℞ *broad-spectrum antibiotic* [tetracycline HCl] 125 mg/5 mL
Tetralan "250"; Tetralan-500 capsules (discontinued 1997) ℞ *broad-spectrum antibiotic* [tetracycline HCl] 250 mg; 500 mg
tetrallobarbital [see: butalbital]
tetramal [see: tetrabarbital]
tetrameprozine [see: aminopromazine]
tetramethrin INN
tetramethylene dimethanesulfonate [see: busulfan]
tetramisole INN *anthelmintic* [also: tetramisole HCl]
tetramisole HCl USAN *anthelmintic* [also: tetramisole]
Tetramune IM injection (discontinued 2001) ℞ *pediatric vaccine for diphtheria, pertussis, tetanus, and Haemophilus influenzae type b* [diphtheria & tetanus toxoids & whole-cell pertussis (DTwP) vaccine; Hemophilus b conjugate vaccine] 0.5 mL
tetranitrol [see: erythrityl tetranitrate]
tetrantoin
TetraPaks (trademarked delivery form) *ready-to-use open system containers*
Tetrasine; Tetrasine Extra eye drops OTC *topical ophthalmic decongestant and vasoconstrictor* [tetrahydrozoline HCl] 0.05%
tetrasodium ethylenediaminetetraacetate [see: edetate sodium]
tetrasodium pyrophosphate [see: sodium pyrophosphate]
tetrazepam INN
tetrazolast INN *antiallergic; antiasthmatic* [also: tetrazolast meglumine]

tetrazolast meglumine USAN *antiallergic; antiasthmatic* [also: tetrazolast]
tetridamine INN *analgesic; anti-inflammatory* [also: tetrydamine]
tetriprofen INN
tetrofosmin USAN, INN, BAN *diagnostic aid*
tetronasin BAN [also: tetronasin 5930]
tetronasin 5930 INN [also: tetronasin]
tetroquinone USAN, INN *systemic keratolytic*
tetroxoprim USAN, INN *antibacterial*
tetrydamine USAN *analgesic; anti-inflammatory* [also: tetridamine]
tetrylammonium bromide INN
tetryzoline INN *vasoconstrictor; nasal decongestant; topical ocular decongestant* [also: tetrahydrozoline HCl; tetrahydrozoline]
tetryzoline HCl [see: tetrahydrozoline HCl]
tetterwort *medicinal herb* [see: bloodroot; celandine]
Teveten tablets *antihypertensive; angiotensin II receptor antagonist* [eprosartan mesylate] 400, 600 mg
Texacort solution ℞ *topical corticosteroidal anti-inflammatory* [hydrocortisone] 1%
texacromil INN
tezacitabine USAN *antineoplastic for colon and rectal cancers*
tezosentan *investigational (Phase III) parenteral antihypertensive*
6-TG (6-thioguanine) [see: thioguanine]
TG (thyroglobulin) [q.v.]
T-Gen suppositories, pediatric suppositories ℞ *antiemetic; anticholinergic* [trimethobenzamide HCl; benzocaine] 200 mg•2%; 100 mg•2%
T-Gesic capsules ℞ *narcotic analgesic* [hydrocodone bitartrate; acetaminophen] 5•500 mg
αTGI (α-triglycidyl isocyanurate) [see: teroxirone]
TH (theophylline) [q.v.]
TH (thyroid hormone) [see: levothyroxine sodium]
TH-9506 *investigational GRF 1-29 growth hormone-releasing factor analogue*
THA (tetrahydroaminoacridine or tetrahydroacridinamine) [see: tacrine HCl]
thalidomide USAN, INN, BAN *sedative; hypnotic; immunomodulator for erythema nodosum leprosum (ENL) (orphan); investigational (Phase III, orphan) cytokine inhibitor for graft vs. host disease, AIDS-wasting syndrome, lupus, and mycobacterial infections; investigational (Phase II, orphan) for various cancers*
Thalitone tablets ℞ *antihypertensive; diuretic* [chlorthalidone] 15, 25 mg
thallium *element (Tl)* ⑨ Valium
thallous chloride Tl 201 USAN, USP *radiopaque contrast medium; radioactive agent*
Thalomid capsules ℞ *immunomodulator for erythema nodosum leprosum (ENL) (orphan); investigational (Phase III, orphan) for graft vs. host disease, AIDS-wasting syndrome, lupus, and mycobacterial infections; investigational (Phase II) for various cancers; investigational for Crohn disease* [thalidomide] 50 mg
Tham IV infusion ℞ *corrects systemic acidosis associated with cardiac bypass surgery or cardiac arrest* [tromethamine] 18 g/500 mL (150 mEq/500 mL)
thaumatin BAN
THC (tetrahydrocannabinol) [see: dronabinol]
THC (thiocarbanidin)
thebacon INN, BAN
theine [see: caffeine]
thenalidine INN
thenium closilate INN *veterinary anthelmintic* [also: thenium closylate]
thenium closylate USAN *veterinary anthelmintic* [also: thenium closilate]
thenyldiamine INN
thenylpyramine HCl [see: methapyrilene HCl]
Theo-24 timed-release capsules ℞ *antiasthmatic; bronchodilator* [theophylline] 100, 200, 300 mg

Theobid Duracaps (sustained-release capsules) ℞ *antiasthmatic; bronchodilator* [theophylline] 260 mg
theobromine NF
theobromine calcium salicylate NF
theobromine sodium acetate NF
theobromine sodium salicylate NF
Theobromo cacao *medicinal herb* [see: cocoa]
Theochron extended-release tablets ℞ *antiasthmatic; bronchodilator* [theophylline] 100, 200, 300 mg
theoclate BAN *combining name for radicals or groups* [also: teoclate]
Theoclear L.A. extended-release capsules ℞ *antiasthmatic; bronchodilator* [theophylline] 130, 260 mg
Theoclear-80 oral solution ℞ *antiasthmatic; bronchodilator* [theophylline] 80 mg/15 mL ⑨ Theolair
theodrenaline INN, BAN
Theodrine tablets OTC *antiasthmatic; bronchodilator; decongestant* [theophylline; ephedrine HCl] 120•22.5 mg
Theo-Dur extended-release tablets ℞ *antiasthmatic; bronchodilator* [theophylline] 100, 200, 300, 450 mg
theofibrate USAN *antihyperlipoproteinemic* [also: etofylline clofibrate]
Theolair tablets, liquid ℞ *antiasthmatic; bronchodilator* [theophylline] 125, 250 mg; 80 mg/15 mL ⑨ Theoclear; Thyrolar
Theolair-SR sustained-release tablets ℞ *antiasthmatic; bronchodilator* [theophylline] 200, 250, 300, 500 mg
Theolate liquid ℞ *antiasthmatic; bronchodilator; expectorant* [theophylline; guaifenesin] 150•90 mg/15 mL
Theomax DF pediatric syrup ℞ *antiasthmatic; bronchodilator; decongestant; antihistamine* [theophylline; ephedrine sulfate; hydroxyzine HCl; alcohol 5%] 97.5•18.75•7.5 mg/15 mL
theophyldine [see: aminophylline]
theophyllamine [see: aminophylline]
Theophyllin KI elixir ℞ *antiasthmatic; bronchodilator; expectorant* [theophylline; potassium iodide] 80•130 mg/15 mL
theophylline (TH) USP, BAN *bronchodilator* 100, 125, 200, 300, 450 mg oral; 80 mg/15 mL oral
theophylline aminoisobutanol [see: ambuphylline]
theophylline calcium salicylate *bronchodilator*
theophylline ethylenediamine [now: aminophylline]
theophylline monohydrate [see: theophylline]
theophylline olamine USP
theophylline sodium acetate NF
theophylline sodium glycinate USP *smooth muscle relaxant*
Theo-Sav controlled-release tablets ℞ *antiasthmatic; bronchodilator* [theophylline] 100, 200, 300 mg
Theospan-SR timed-release capsules ℞ *antiasthmatic; bronchodilator* [theophylline] 130, 260 mg
Theostat 80 syrup ℞ *antiasthmatic; bronchodilator* [theophylline; alcohol 1%] 80 mg/15 mL
Theovent timed-release capsules ℞ *antiasthmatic; bronchodilator* [theophylline] 125, 250 mg
Theo-X controlled-release tablets ℞ *antiasthmatic; bronchodilator* [theophylline] 100, 200, 300 mg
Thera Hematinic tablets OTC *hematinic; vitamin supplement* [ferrous fumarate; multiple vitamins; folic acid] 66.7•≛•0.33 mg
Thera Multi-Vitamin liquid OTC *vitamin supplement* [multiple vitamins] ≛
Therabid tablets OTC *vitamin supplement* [multiple vitamins] ≛
Therac lotion OTC *topical acne treatment* [colloidal sulfur] 10%
theraccines *a class of vaccines with therapeutic action, usually used to help prevent the spread of cancer*
TheraCys powder for intravesical instillation ℞ *antineoplastic for urinary bladder cancer* [BCG vaccine, live] 81 mg (1.8–19.2 $\times 10^8$ CFU)
TheraDerm transdermal patch ℞ *investigational (orphan) for AIDS-wasting syndrome* [testosterone]

TheraDerm-MTX transdermal patch ℞ *investigational hormone replacement for female testosterone deficiency* [estradiol; testosterone]

Therafectin ℞ *investigational (NDA filed) synthetic monosaccharide anti-inflammatory for rheumatoid arthritis* [amiprilose HCl]

TheraFlu Flu, Cold & Cough; NightTime TheraFlu powder for oral solution OTC *antitussive; decongestant; antihistamine; analgesic* [dextromethorphan hydrobromide; pseudoephedrine HCl; chlorpheniramine maleate; acetaminophen] 20•60•4•650 mg/packet; 30•60•4•1000 mg/packet ⊡ Thera-Flur

TheraFlu Flu & Cold Medicine powder for oral solution OTC *decongestant; antihistamine; analgesic* [pseudoephedrine HCl; chlorpheniramine maleate; acetaminophen] 60•4•650 mg/packet

TheraFlu Non-Drowsy Flu, Cold & Cough powder for oral solution OTC *antitussive; decongestant; analgesic* [dextromethorphan hydrobromide; pseudoephedrine HCl; acetaminophen] 30•60•100 mg/packet

TheraFlu Non-Drowsy Formula caplets OTC *antitussive; decongestant; analgesic* [dextromethorphan hydrobromide; pseudoephedrine HCl; acetaminophen] 15•30•500 mg

Thera-Flur; Thera-Flur-N gel (for self-application) ℞ *topical dental caries preventative* [sodium fluoride] 1.1% ⊡ TheraFlu

Thera-Gesic cream OTC *topical analgesic; counterirritant* [methyl salicylate; menthol] 15%•≟

Theragran caplets OTC *vitamin supplement* [multiple vitamins; folic acid; biotin] ≛•400•30 μg ⊡ Theragyn

Theragran liquid OTC *vitamin supplement* [multiple vitamins] ≛ ⊡ Phenergan

Theragran AntiOxidant softgels OTC *vitamin/mineral supplement* [vitamins A, C, and E; multiple minerals] 5000 IU•250 mg•200 IU•≛

Theragran Hematinic tablets ℞ *hematinic; vitamin/mineral supplement* [ferrous fumarate; multiple vitamins & minerals; folic acid] 66.7•≛•0.33 mg

Theragran Stress Formula tablets OTC *vitamin/iron supplement* [multiple B vitamins; vitamins C and E; ferrous fumarate; folic acid; biotin] ≛•600 mg•30 IU•27 mg•0.4 mg•45 μg

Theragran-M caplets OTC *vitamin/mineral/calcium/iron supplement* [multiple vitamins & minerals; calcium; iron; folic acid; biotin] ≛•40•27•0.4•0.03 mg

Theragyn ℞ *investigational (Phase III, orphan) adjuvant treatment for ovarian cancer* ⊡ Theragran

Thera-Hist syrup OTC *decongestant; antihistamine* [phenylpropanolamine HCl; chlorpheniramine maleate] 12.5•2 mg/5 mL

Thera-Ject (trademarked delivery system) *prefilled disposable syringe*

Thera-M tablets OTC *vitamin/mineral/iron supplement* [multiple vitamins & minerals; iron; folic acid; biotin] ≛•27 mg•0.4 mg•35 μg

Theramine Expectorant liquid OTC *decongestant; expectorant* [phenylpropanolamine HCl; guaifenesin] 12.5•100 mg/5 mL

Theramycin Z topical solution ℞ *topical antibiotic for acne* [erythromycin] 2% ⊡ Garamycin; Terramycin

TheraPatch transdermal patch OTC *external analgesic* [methyl salicylate; menthol; camphor]

TheraPatch Cold Sore patch OTC *topical local anesthetic and antipruritic* [lidocaine; camphor; aloe vera; eucalyptus oil] 4%•0.5%•≟•≟

Therapeutic tablets OTC *vitamin supplement* [multiple vitamins; folic acid; biotin] ≛•400•30 μg

Therapeutic B with C capsules OTC *vitamin supplement* [multiple B vitamins; vitamin C] ≛•300 mg

Therapeutic Bath lotion, oil OTC *moisturizer; emollient*

Therapeutic Mineral Ice; Therapeutic Mineral Ice Exercise Formula gel OTC *topical analgesic; counterirritant* [menthol] 2%; 4%

Therapeutic-H tablets OTC *hematinic; vitamin supplement* [ferrous fumarate; multiple vitamins; folic acid] 66.7•≛•0.33 mg

Therapeutic-M tablets OTC *vitamin/mineral/iron supplement* [multiple vitamins & minerals; iron; folic acid; biotin] ≛•27 mg•0.4 mg•30 µg

Theraplex T shampoo OTC *antiseborrheic; antipsoriatic; antipruritic; antibacterial* [coal tar] 1%

Theraplex Z shampoo OTC *antiseborrheic; antibacterial; antifungal* [pyrithione zinc] 2%

Theraseed ℞ *investigational radioactive "seeds" for ultrasound-guided brachytherapy for adenocarcinoma of the prostate* [palladium Pd 103] 0.665 Gy (66.5 rads)

Theratope-STn ℞ *investigational (Phase III) theraccine for recurrent or metastatic breast and colorectal cancer*

Theravee tablets OTC *vitamin supplement* [multiple vitamins; folic acid; biotin] ≛•400•15 µg

Theravee Hematinic tablets OTC *hematinic; vitamin supplement* [ferrous fumarate; multiple vitamins; folic acid] 66.7•≛•0.33 mg

Theravee-M tablets OTC *vitamin/mineral/iron supplement* [multiple vitamins & minerals; iron; folic acid; biotin] ≛•27 mg•0.4 mg•15 µg

Theravim tablets OTC *vitamin supplement* [multiple vitamins; folic acid; biotin] ≛•400•35 µg

Theravim-M tablets OTC *vitamin/mineral/iron supplement* [multiple vitamins & minerals; iron; folic acid; biotin] ≛•27 mg•0.4 mg•30 µg

Theravite liquid OTC *vitamin supplement* [multiple vitamins] ≛ 🔊 Therevac

Therems tablets OTC *vitamin supplement* [multiple vitamins; folic acid; biotin] ≛•400•15 µg

Therems-M tablets OTC *vitamin/mineral/iron supplement* [multiple vitamins & minerals; iron; folic acid; biotin] ≛•27 mg•0.4 mg•30 µg

Therevac-Plus disposable enema OTC *hyperosmotic laxative; stool softener; local anesthetic* [glycerin; docusate sodium; benzocaine] 275•283•20 mg 🔊 Theravite

Therevac-SB disposable enema OTC *hyperosmotic laxative; stool softener* [glycerin; docusate sodium] 275•283 mg

Thermazene cream ℞ *broad-spectrum bactericidal for adjunctive burn treatment* [silver sulfadiazine] 10 mg/g

ThexForte caplets OTC *vitamin supplement* [multiple B vitamins; vitamin C] ≛•500 mg

THF (thymic humoral factor) [q.v.]

thiabendazole (TBZ) USAN, USP *anthelmintic for strongyloidiasis (threadworm), larva migrans, and trichinosis* [also: tiabendazole]

thiabutazide [see: buthiazide]

thiacetarsamide sodium INN

thiacetazone BAN [also: thioacetazone]

thialbarbital INN [also: thialbarbitone]

thialbarbitone BAN [also: thialbarbital]

thialisobumal sodium [see: buthalital sodium]

thiamazole INN *thyroid inhibitor* [also: methimazole]

thiambutosine INN, BAN

Thiamilate enteric-coated tablets OTC *vitamin B_1 supplement* [thiamine HCl] 20 mg

thiamine (vitamin B_1) INN *water-soluble vitamin; enzyme cofactor* [also: thiamine HCl]

thiamine HCl (vitamin B_1) USP *water-soluble vitamin; enzyme cofactor* [also: thiamine] 50, 100, 250 mg oral; 100 mg/mL injection

thiamine mononitrate USP *vitamin B_1; enzyme cofactor*

thiamine propyl disulfide [see: prosultiamine]
thiaminogen *medicinal herb* [see: rice bran oil]
thiamiprine USAN *antineoplastic* [also: tiamiprine]
thiamphenicol USAN, INN, BAN *antibacterial*
thiamylal USP *barbiturate general anesthetic*
thiamylal sodium USP, JAN *barbiturate general anesthetic*
thiazesim HCl USAN *antidepressant* [also: tiazesim]
thiazides *a class of diuretic agents that increase urinary excretion of sodium and chloride in approximately equal amounts*
thiazinamium chloride USAN *antiallergic*
thiazinamium metilsulfate INN
4-thiazolidinecarboxylic acid [see: timonacic]
thiazolidinediones *a class of antidiabetic agents that increase insulin sensitivity and reduce plasma insulin levels*
thiazolsulfone [see: thiazosulfone]
thiazosulfone INN
thiazothielite [see: antienite]
thiazothienol [see: antazonite]
thienamycins *a class of antibiotics*
thienobenzodiazepines *a class of novel (atypical) antipsychotic agents*
thiethylperazine USAN, INN *antiemetic; antidopaminergic*
thiethylperazine malate USP *antiemetic; antipsychotic*
thiethylperazine maleate USAN, USP *antiemetic*
thihexinol methylbromide NF, INN
thimbleberry *medicinal herb* [see: blackberry]
thimerfonate sodium USAN *topical anti-infective* [also: sodium timerfonate]
thimerosal USP *topical anti-infective; preservative (49% mercury)* [also: thiomersal] 1:1000 topical
thioacetazone INN, DCF [also: thiacetazone]
thiocarbanidin (THC)
thiocarlide BAN [also: tiocarlide]
thiocolchicine glycoside [see: thiocolchicoside]
thiocolchicoside INN
thioctan; thioctacid; thioctic acid *natural antioxidant* [see: alpha lipoic acid]
thiocyanate sodium NF
thiodiglycol INN
thiodiphenylamine [see: phenothiazine]
thiofuradene INN
thioguanine (6-TG) USAN, USP *antimetabolite antineoplastic* [also: tioguanine] 40 mg oral
thiohexallymal [see: thialbarbital]
thiohexamide INN
Thiola sugar-coated tablets ℞ *prevention of cystine nephrolithiasis in homozygous cystinuria (orphan)* [tiopronin] 100 mg
thiomebumal sodium [see: thiopental sodium]
thiomersal INN, BAN *topical anti-infective; preservative* [also: thimerosal]
thiomesterone BAN [also: tiomesterone]
thiomicid [see: thioacetazone; thiacetazone]
thioparamizone [see: thioacetazone; thiacetazone]
thiopental sodium USP, INN, JAN *barbiturate general anesthetic; anticonvulsant* [also: thiopentone sodium] 2%, 2.5% (20, 25 mg/mL) injection
thiopentone sodium BAN *general anesthetic; anticonvulsant* [also: thiopental sodium]
thiophanate BAN
thiophosphoramide [see: thiotepa]
Thioplex powder for IV, intracavitary, or intravesical injection ℞ *alkylating antineoplastic for lymphomas and carcinoma of the breast, ovary, or bladder* [thiotepa] 15 mg
thiopropazate INN [also: thiopropazate HCl]
thiopropazate HCl NF [also: thiopropazate]
thioproperazine INN, BAN *phenothiazine antipsychotic* [also: thioproperazine mesylate]

thioproperazine mesylate *phenothiazine antipsychotic* [also: thioproperazine]
thioproperazine methanesulfonate [see: thioproperazine mesylate]
thioridazine USAN, USP, INN *phenothiazine antipsychotic; sedative*
thioridazine HCl USP *phenothiazine antipsychotic; sedative* 10, 15, 25, 50, 100, 150, 200 mg oral; 30, 100 mg/mL oral
thiosalan USAN *disinfectant* [also: tiosalan]
Thiosulfil Forte tablets (discontinued 2001) ℞ *broad-spectrum sulfonamide bacteriostatic* [sulfamethizole] 500 mg
thiosulfuric acid, disodium salt pentahydrate [see: sodium thiosulfate]
thiotepa USP, INN, BAN, JAN *alkylating antineoplastic for lymphomas and carcinoma of the breast, ovary, or bladder* 15 mg/vial injection
thiotetrabarbital INN
thiothixene USAN, USP, BAN *thioxanthene antipsychotic* [also: tiotixene] 1, 2, 5, 10, 20 mg oral
thiothixene HCl USAN, USP *thioxanthene antipsychotic* 5 mg/mL oral
thiouracil
thiourea *antioxidant*
thioxanthenes *a class of dopamine receptor antagonists with conventional (typical) antipsychotic activity*
thioxolone BAN [also: tioxolone]
thiphenamil HCl USAN *smooth muscle relaxant* [also: tifenamil]
thiphencillin potassium USAN *antibacterial* [also: tifencillin]
thiram USAN, INN *antifungal*
thistle, bitter; holy thistle; Saint Benedict thistle; spotted thistle *medicinal herb* [see: blessed thistle]
thistle, carline; ground thistle *medicinal herb* [see: carline thistle]
thonzonium bromide USAN, USP *detergent; surface-active agent* [also: tonzonium bromide]
thonzylamine HCl USAN, INN
Thorazine tablets, Spansules (capsules), IV or IM injection, syrup, suppositories, concentrate ℞ *conventional (typical) antipsychotic; antiemetic* [chlorpromazine] 10, 25, 50, 100, 200 mg; 30, 75, 150 mg; 25 mg/mL; 10 mg/5 mL; 25, 100 mg; 30, 100 mg/mL
thorium *element (Th)*
thorn, Egyptian *medicinal herb* [see: acacia]
thorn-apple *medicinal herb* [see: hawthorn; jimsonweed]
thousand-leaf; thousand seal *medicinal herb* [see: yarrow]
thozalinone USAN *antidepressant* [also: tozalinone]
THQ (tetrahydroxybenzoquinone) [see: tetroquinone]
THR (trishydroxyethyl rutin) [see: troxerutin]
Threamine DM syrup OTC *antitussive; decongestant; antihistamine* [dextromethorphan hydrobromide; phenylpropanolamine HCl; chlorpheniramine maleate] 10•12.5•2 mg/5 mL
Threamine Expectorant liquid OTC *decongestant; expectorant* [phenylpropanolamine HCl; guaifenesin; alcohol 5%] 12.5•100 mg/5 mL
3 in 1 Toothache Relief gum, liquid, lotion/gel OTC *topical oral anesthetic* [benzocaine]
357 HR Magnum tablets OTC *CNS stimulant; analeptic* [caffeine] 200 mg
three-leaved nightshade *medicinal herb* [see: birthroot]
3TC [now: lamivudine]
threonine (L-threonine) USAN, USP, INN *essential amino acid; symbols: Thr, T; investigational (orphan) for familial spastic paraparesis and amyotrophic lateral sclerosis* 500 mg oral
Threostat ℞ *investigational (orphan) for familial spastic paraparesis and amyotrophic lateral sclerosis* [L-threonine] 🔊 Triostat
Throat Discs lozenges OTC *analgesic; counterirritant* [capsicum; peppermint oil]
throatwort *medicinal herb* [see: figwort; foxglove]

Thrombate III powder for IV infusion ℞ *for thrombosis and pulmonary emboli of congenital AT-III deficiency (orphan)* [antithrombin III] 500, 1000 IU

thrombin USP, INN *topical local hemostatic*

Thrombinar powder ℞ *topical local hemostatic for surgery* [thrombin] 1000, 5000, 50 000 U

Thrombin-JMI powder ℞ *topical local hemostatic for surgery* [thrombin] 10 000, 20 000, 50 000 U

thrombinogen (prothrombin)

Thrombogen powder ℞ *topical local hemostatic for surgery* [thrombin] 1000, 5000, 10 000, 20 000 U

thrombolytics *a class of enzymes that dissolve blood clots, used emergently to treat stroke, pulmonary embolus, and myocardial infarct*

thromboplastin USP

thrombopoietin, recombinant human *investigational (orphan) adjunct to hematopoietic stem cell transplantation*

Thrombostat powder ℞ *topical local hemostatic for surgery* [thrombin] 5000, 10 000, 20 000 U

throw-wort *medicinal herb* [see: motherwort]

thulium *element (Tm)*

thunder god vine *(Tripterygium wilfordii)* plant *medicinal herb for abscesses, autoimmune diseases, boils, fever, inflammation, tumors, and viruses; also used as an insecticide to kill maggots or larvae and as a rat and bird poison* [also: triptolide]

thymalfasin USAN *vaccine enhancer for hepatitis C, cancer, and infectious diseases; investigational (Phase III, orphan) for chronic active hepatitis B; investigational (orphan) for DiGeorge syndrome with immune defects; investigational (orphan) for hepatocellular carcinoma*

thyme *(Thymus serpyllum; T. vulgaris)* plant *medicinal herb for acute bronchitis, colic, digestive disorders, gas, gout, headache, laryngitis, lung congestion, sciatica, and throat disorders*

thymic humoral factor, gamma 2 *investigational (Phase II) immunomodulator for HIV*

thymidylate synthase (TS) inhibitors *a class of folate-based antineoplastics*

Thymitaq ℞ *investigational (Phase III) antineoplastic* [nolatrexed dihydrochloride]

thymocartin INN

thymoctonan INN *investigational antiviral for HIV infection, genital herpes, and chronic viral hepatitis*

Thymoglobulin powder for IV infusion ℞ *immunosuppressant for acute renal transplant rejection* [antithymocyte globulin, rabbit] 25 mg

thymol NF *stabilizer; topical antiseptic*

thymol iodide NF

Thymone ℞ *investigational (orphan) for infant respiratory distress syndrome of prematurity* [protirelin]

thymopentin USAN, INN, BAN *immunoregulator; investigational (Phase III) for asymptomatic HIV infection*

thymopoietin 32-36 [now: thymopentin]

thymosin alpha-1 [now: thymalfasin]

thymostimulin INN *investigational (Phase III) immunomodulator for AIDS*

thymotrinan INN

thymoxamine BAN [also: moxisylyte]

Thymus serpyllum; T. vulgaris *medicinal herb* [see: thyme]

Thypinone IV injection ℞ *diagnostic aid for thyroid function* [protirelin] 500 µg/mL

Thyrar tablets (discontinued 1999) ℞ *natural thyroid replacement for hypothyroidism or thyroid cancer* [thyroid, desiccated bovine] 30, 60, 120 mg ⑨ Thyrolar

Thyrel-TRH IV injection ℞ *diagnostic aid for thyroid function* [protirelin] 500 µg/mL

Thyro-Block tablets ℞ *thyroid-blocking therapy* [potassium iodide] 130 mg

thyrocalcitonin [see: calcitonin]

Thyrogen IM injection ℞ *recombinant human thyroid-stimulating hormone (rhTSH); diagnostic aid for serum thyroglobulin (Tg) testing in thyroid cancer patients (orphan); investigational (NDA filed, orphan) treatment for thyroid cancer* [thyrotropin alfa] 1.1 mg/vial

thyroglobulin (TG) USAN, USP, INN *natural thyroid hormone*

thyroid USP *natural thyroid hormone* 15, 30, 60, 90, 120, 180, 240, 300 mg oral ⑨ euthroid

thyroid hormone (TH) [see: levothyroxine sodium]

Thyroid Strong tablets (discontinued 1999) ℞ *natural thyroid replacement for hypothyroidism or thyroid cancer* [thyroid, desiccated] 30, 60, 120, 180 mg

thyroid-stimulating hormone (TSH) [see: thyrotropin]

Thyrolar-0.25; -0.5; -1; -2; -3 tablets ℞ *synthetic thyroid hormone* [liotrix] 15 mg; 30 mg; 60 mg; 120 mg; 180 mg ⑨ Theolair; Thyrar

thyromedan HCl USAN *thyromimetic* [also: tyromedan]

thyropropic acid INN

thyrotrophic hormone [see: thyrotrophin]

thyrotrophin INN *thyroid-stimulating hormone* [also: thyrotropin]

thyrotropin *thyroid-stimulating hormone (TSH); in vivo diagnostic aid for thyroid function* [also: thyrotrophin]

thyrotropin alfa USAN *recombinant human thyroid-stimulating hormone (rhTSH); diagnostic aid for serum thyroglobulin (Tg) testing in thyroid cancer patients (orphan); investigational (NDA filed, orphan) treatment for thyroid cancer*

thyrotropin-releasing hormone (TRH) [see: protirelin]

thyroxine BAN *thyroid hormone* [also: levothyroxine sodium]

D-thyroxine [see: dextrothyroxine sodium]

L-thyroxine [see: levothyroxine sodium]

thyroxine I 125 USAN *radioactive agent*

thyroxine I 131 USAN *radioactive agent*

Thytropar powder for IM or subcu injection (discontinued 2001) ℞ *thyroid-stimulating hormone (TSH); in vivo diagnostic aid for thyroid function* [thyrotropin] 10 IU

tiabendazole INN *anthelmintic* [also: thiabendazole]

Tiabex (name changed to Gabitril upon marketing release in 1998)

tiacrilast USAN, INN *antiallergic*

tiacrilast sodium USAN *antiallergic*

tiadenol INN

tiafibrate INN

tiagabine INN *anticonvulsant adjunct for partial seizures*

tiagabine HCl USAN *anticonvulsant adjunct for partial seizures*

Tiamate extended-release film-coated tablets ℞ *antihypertensive; antianginal; antiarrhythmic; calcium channel blocker* [diltiazem maleate] 120, 180, 240 mg

tiamenidine USAN, INN *antihypertensive*

tiamenidine HCl USAN *antihypertensive*

tiametonium iodide INN

tiamiprine INN *antineoplastic* [also: thiamiprine]

tiamizide INN *diuretic; antihypertensive* [also: diapamide]

tiamulin USAN, INN *veterinary antibacterial*

tiamulin fumarate USAN *veterinary antibacterial*

tianafac INN

tianeptine INN

tiapamil INN, BAN *antagonist to calcium* [also: tiapamil HCl]

tiapamil HCl USAN *antagonist to calcium* [also: tiapamil]

tiapirinol INN

tiapride INN

tiaprofenic acid INN *nonsteroidal anti-inflammatory drug (NSAID)*

tiaprost INN

tiaramide INN, BAN *antiasthmatic* [also: tiaramide HCl]

tiaramide HCl USAN *antiasthmatic* [also: tiaramide]

Tiazac extended-release capsules ℞ *antihypertensive; antianginal; antiarrhythmic; calcium channel blocker* [diltiazem HCl] 120, 180, 240, 300, 360, 420 mg ⊠ Dyazide; thiazides

tiazesim INN *antidepressant* [also: thiazesim HCl]

tiazesim HCl [see: thiazesim HCl]

tiazofurin USAN *investigational (Phase II/III, orphan) antineoplastic for chronic myelogenous leukemia* [also: tiazofurine]

tiazofurine INN *antineoplastic for chronic myelogenous leukemia* [also: tiazofurin]

Tiazole ℞ *investigational (Phase II/III, orphan) antineoplastic for chronic myelogenous leukemia* [tiazofurin]

tiazuril USAN, INN *coccidiostat for poultry*

tibalosin INN

tibenelast sodium USAN *antiasthmatic; bronchodilator*

tibenzate INN

tibezonium iodide INN

tibolone USAN, INN, BAN *synthetic steroid; investigational (NDA filed) for osteoporosis and other postmenopausal symptoms*

tibric acid USAN, INN *antihyperlipoproteinemic*

tibrofan USAN, INN *disinfectant*

ticabesone INN *corticosteroid; anti-inflammatory* [also: ticabesone propionate]

ticabesone propionate USAN *corticosteroid; anti-inflammatory* [also: ticabesone]

Ticar powder for IV or IM injection ℞ *extended-spectrum penicillin antibiotic* [ticarcillin disodium] 1, 3, 6, 20, 30 g ⊠ Tigan

ticarbodine USAN, INN *anthelmintic*

ticarcillin INN *extended-spectrum penicillin antibiotic* [also: ticarcillin disodium]

ticarcillin cresyl sodium USAN *extended-spectrum penicillin antibiotic*

ticarcillin disodium USAN, USP *extended-spectrum penicillin antibiotic* [also: ticarcillin]

Tice BCG dermal puncture injection for TB, intravesical instillation for cancer ℞ *tuberculosis immunizing agent; antineoplastic for urinary bladder cancer* [BCG vaccine, Tice strain] 50 mg ($1-8 \times 10^8$ CFU)

tickweed *medicinal herb* [see: pennyroyal]

ticlatone USAN, INN *antibacterial; antifungal*

Ticlid film-coated tablets ℞ *platelet aggregation inhibitor for stroke* [ticlopidine HCl] 250 mg

ticlopidine INN, BAN *platelet aggregation inhibitor* [also: ticlopidine HCl]

ticlopidine HCl USAN *platelet aggregation inhibitor for stroke* [also: ticlopidine] 250 mg oral

ticolubant USAN *leukotriene B_4 receptor antagonist for psoriasis*

Ticon IM injection ℞ *antiemetic; anticholinergic* [trimethobenzamide HCl] 100 mg/mL

ticrynafen USAN *diuretic; uricosuric; antihypertensive* [also: tienilic acid]

tidembersat USAN *antimigraine*

tidiacic INN

tiemonium iodide INN, BAN

tienilic acid INN *diuretic; uricosuric; antihypertensive* [also: ticrynafen]

tienocarbine INN

tienopramine INN

tienoxolol INN

tifacogin USAN *anticoagulant; lipoprotein-associated coagulation inhibitor (LACI); investigational (Phase III) recombinant tissue factor pathway inhibitor*

tifemoxone INN

tifenamil INN *smooth muscle relaxant* [also: thiphenamil HCl]

tifenamil HCl [see: thiphenamil HCl]

tifencillin INN *antibacterial* [also: thiphencillin potassium]

tifencillin potassium [see: thiphencillin potassium]

tiflamizole INN

tiflorex INN

tifluadom INN

tiflucarbine INN

Tifolar ℞ *investigational antineoplastic* [pemetrexed disodium]

tiformin INN [also: tyformin]
tifurac INN *analgesic* [also: tifurac sodium]
tifurac sodium USAN *analgesic* [also: tifurac]
TIG (tetanus immune globulin) [q.v.]
Tigan capsules, IM injection ℞ *antiemetic; anticholinergic* [trimethobenzamide HCl] 100, 250 mg; 100 mg/mL ⓢ Ticar; Triban
Tigan suppositories, pediatric suppositories ℞ *antiemetic; anticholinergic* [trimethobenzamide HCl; benzocaine] 200 mg•2%; 100 mg•2% ⓢ Ticar; Triban
tigemonam INN *antimicrobial* [also: tigemonam dicholine]
tigemonam dicholine USAN *antimicrobial* [also: tigemonam]
tigestol USAN, INN *progestin*
tigloidine INN, BAN
tiglyl*pseudo*tropine [see: tigloidine]
tiglyltropeine [see: tropigline]
Tikosyn capsules ℞ *antiarrhythmic for atrial fibrillation/atrial flutter (AF/AFl); potassium channel blocker* [dofetilide] 125, 250, 500 µg
tilactase INN *digestive enzyme*
Tilad (Spanish name for U.S. product Tilade)
Tilade oral inhalation aerosol ℞ *respiratory anti-inflammatory; antiasthmatic; bronchoconstriction inhibitor* [nedocromil sodium] 1.75 mg/dose
tilbroquinol INN
tiletamine INN *anesthetic; anticonvulsant* [also: tiletamine HCl]
tiletamine HCl USAN *anesthetic; anticonvulsant* [also: tiletamine]
Tilia americana; T. cordata; T. europaea; T. platyphyllos *medicinal herb* [see: linden tree]
tilidate HCl BAN *analgesic* [also: tilidine HCl; tilidine]
tilidine INN *analgesic* [also: tilidine HCl; tilidate HCl]
tilidine HCl USAN *analgesic* [also: tilidine; tilidate HCl]
tiliquinol INN
tilisolol INN
tilmicosin USAN, INN, BAN *veterinary antibacterial*
tilmicosin phosphate USAN *veterinary antibacterial*
tilomisole USAN, INN *immunoregulator*
tilorone INN *antiviral* [also: tilorone HCl]
tilorone HCl USAN *antiviral* [also: tilorone]
tilozepine INN
tilsuprost INN
Tiltab (trademarked dosage form) *film-coated tablets*
tiludronate disodium USAN *bisphosphonate bone resorption inhibitor for Paget disease*
tiludronic acid INN
timcodar dimesylate USAN *antineoplastic adjunct to prevent emergence of multidrug-resistant tumors*
Timecap (trademarked dosage form) *sustained-release capsule*
Timecelle (trademarked dosage form) *timed-release capsule*
timefurone USAN, INN *antiatherosclerotic*
timegadine INN
Time-Hist sustained-release capsules ℞ *decongestant; antihistamine* [pseudoephedrine HCl; chlorpheniramine maleate] 120•8 mg
timelotem INN
Timentin powder or frozen premix for IV infusion ℞ *extended-spectrum penicillin antibiotic* [ticarcillin disodium; clavulanate potassium] 3•0.1 g
timepidium bromide INN
Timespan (trademarked dosage form) *timed-release tablets*
Timesules (dosage form) *sustained-release capsules*
timiperone INN
timobesone INN *topical adrenocortical steroid* [also: timobesone acetate]
timobesone acetate USAN *topical adrenocortical steroid* [also: timobesone]
Timodal (CAN) eye drops (discontinued 1998) ℞ *topical antiglaucoma agent (β-blocker)* [timolol maleate] 0.25%, 0.5%
timofibrate INN

Timolide 10-25 tablets ℞ *antihypertensive; β-blocker; diuretic* [timolol maleate; hydrochlorothiazide] 10•25 mg

timolol USAN, INN, BAN *topical antiglaucoma agent (β-blocker)* ⊠ atenolol

timolol hemihydrate *topical antiglaucoma agent (β-blocker)*

timolol maleate USAN, USP *antihypertensive; antiadrenergic (β-blocker); migraine prophylaxis; topical antiglaucoma agent* 5, 10, 20 mg oral; 0.25%, 0.5% eye drops

timonacic INN

timoprazole INN

Timoptic Ocumeter (eye drops), Ocudose (single-use eye drop dispenser) ℞ *topical antiglaucoma agent (β-blocker)* [timolol maleate] 0.25%, 0.5%

Timoptic-XE gel-forming Ocumeter (eye drops) ℞ *topical once-daily antiglaucoma agent (β-blocker)* [timolol maleate] 0.25%, 0.5%

Timunox ℞ *investigational (Phase III) immunomodulator for asymptomatic HIV infection* [thymopentin]

tin *element (Sn)*

tin chloride dihydrate [see: stannous chloride]

tin ethyl etiopurpurin (SnET2) [now: rostaporfin]

tin etiopurpurin dichloride *investigational (Phase I/II) photosensitizer for age-related macular degeneration (AMD)*

tin fluoride [see: stannous fluoride]

tinabinol USAN, INN *antihypertensive*

Tinactin cream, powder, spray powder, spray liquid, solution OTC *topical antifungal* [tolnaftate] 1% ⊠ Taractan

Tinactin for Jock Itch cream, spray powder OTC *topical antifungal* [tolnaftate] 1%

Tinactin Plus (CAN) powder, aerosol powder (discontinued 2000) OTC *topical antifungal* [tolnaftate] 1%

tinazoline INN

TinBen tincture OTC *skin protectant* [benzoin; alcohol 75–83%]

Tincture of Green Soap liquid OTC *antiseptic cleanser* [green soap; alcohol 28–32%]

Tine Test OT [see: Tuberculin Tine Test, Old]

Tine Test PPD single-use intradermal puncture test device *tuberculosis skin test* [tuberculin purified protein derivative] 5 U

Ting cream OTC *topical antifungal* [tolnaftate] 1%

Ting powder, spray liquid (discontinued 1998) OTC *topical antifungal* [tolnaftate] 1%

Ting spray powder OTC *topical antifungal* [miconazole nitrate] 2%

tinidazole USAN, INN *antiprotozoal*

tinisulpride INN

tinofedrine INN

tinoridine INN

Tinver lotion ℞ *topical antifungal; keratolytic; antipruritic; anesthetic* [sodium thiosulfate; salicylic acid; alcohol 10%] 25%•1%

tinzaparin sodium USAN, INN, BAN *a low molecular weight heparin–type anticoagulant and antithrombotic for the prevention of deep vein thrombosis (DVT)*

tiocarlide INN [also: thiocarlide]

tioclomarol INN

tioconazole USAN, USP, INN, BAN, JAN *topical antifungal*

tioctilate INN

tiodazosin USAN, INN *antihypertensive*

tiodonium chloride USAN, INN *antibacterial*

tiofacic [see: stepronin]

tioguanine INN *antineoplastic* [also: thioguanine]

tiomergine INN

tiomesterone INN [also: thiomesterone]

tioperidone INN *antipsychotic* [also: tioperidone HCl]

tioperidone HCl USAN *antipsychotic* [also: tioperidone]

tiopinac USAN, INN *anti-inflammatory; analgesic; antipyretic*

tiopronin INN *prevention of cystine nephrolithiasis in homozygous cystinuria (orphan)*

tiopropamine INN
tiosalan INN *disinfectant* [also: thiosalan]
tiosinamine [see: allylthiourea]
tiospirone INN *antipsychotic* [also: tiospirone HCl]
tiospirone HCl USAN *antipsychotic* [also: tiospirone]
tiotidine USAN, INN *antagonist to histamine H_2 receptors*
tiotixene INN *thioxanthene antipsychotic* [also: thiothixene]
tiotropium *investigational bronchodilator for chronic obstructive pulmonary disease (COPD)*
tioxacin INN
tioxamast INN
tioxaprofen INN
tioxidazole USAN, INN *anthelmintic*
tioxolone INN [also: thioxolone]
TIP (Taxol, isosfamide [with mesna rescue], Platinol) *chemotherapy protocol for head, neck, and esophageal cancers*
tipentosin INN, BAN *antihypertensive* [also: tipentosin HCl]
tipentosin HCl USAN *antihypertensive* [also: tipentosin]
tipepidine INN
tipetropium bromide INN
tipindole INN
tipranavir disodium USAN *antiviral protease inhibitor; investigational (Phase II) for HIV infection*
tipredane USAN, INN, BAN *topical adrenocortical steroid*
tiprenolol INN *antiadrenergic (β-receptor)* [also: tiprenolol HCl]
tiprenolol HCl USAN *antiadrenergic (β-receptor)* [also: tiprenolol]
tiprinast INN *antiallergic* [also: tiprinast meglumine]
tiprinast meglumine USAN *antiallergic* [also: tiprinast]
tipropidil INN *vasodilator* [also: tipropidil HCl]
tipropidil HCl USAN *vasodilator* [also: tipropidil]
tiprostanide INN, BAN
tiprotimod INN
tiqueside USAN, INN *antihyperlipidemic*
tiquinamide INN *gastric anticholinergic* [also: tiquinamide HCl]
tiquinamide HCl USAN *gastric anticholinergic* [also: tiquinamide]
tiquizium bromide INN
tirapazamine USAN, INN *antineoplastic*
tiratricol INN
tiratricol & levothyroxine sodium *investigational (orphan) to suppress thyroid-stimulating hormone (TSH) in thyroid cancer*
Tirend tablets (discontinued 1998) OTC *CNS stimulant; analeptic* [caffeine] 100 mg
tirilazad INN, BAN *lipid peroxidation inhibitor; 21-aminosteroid (lazaroid) antioxidant* [also: tirilizad mesylate]
tirilazad mesylate USAN *lipid peroxidation inhibitor; 21-aminosteroid (lazaroid) antioxidant; investigational (Phase I/II) protease inhibitor for HIV infection* [also: tirilizad]
tirofiban HCl USAN *glycoprotein (GP) IIb/IIIa receptor antagonist; platelet aggregation inhibitor for acute coronary syndrome, unstable angina, myocardial infarction, and cardiac surgery*
tiropramide INN
tisilfocon A USAN *hydrophobic contact lens material*
Tisit liquid, shampoo OTC *pediculicide for lice* [pyrethrins; piperonyl butoxide] 0.3%•2%; 0.3%•3%
Tisit Blue gel OTC *pediculicide for lice* [pyrethrins; piperonyl butoxide; petroleum distillate] 0.3%•3%•1.2%
tisocromide INN
TiSol solution OTC *anesthetic and antimicrobial throat irrigation* [benzyl alcohol; menthol] 1%•0.04%
tisopurine INN
tisoquone INN
tissue factor [see: thromboplastin]
tissue plasminogen activator (tPA; t-PA) [see: alteplase]
Tis-U-Sol solution ℞ *sterile irrigant* [physiological irrigating solution]
TIT (methotrexate, cytarabine, hydrocortisone) *chemotherapy protocol for CNS prophylaxis of pediatric*

acute lymphocytic leukemia; intrathecal (IT) administration

Titan solution OTC *cleaning solution for hard contact lenses*

titanium *element (Ti)*

titanium dioxide USP *topical protectant; astringent*

titanium oxide [see: titanium dioxide]

Titradose (trademarked dosage form) *scored tablet*

Titralac chewable tablets OTC *antacid* [calcium carbonate] 420, 750 mg

Titralac Plus chewable tablets, liquid OTC *antacid; antiflatulent* [calcium carbonate; simethicone] 420•21 mg; 500•20 mg/5 mL

tivanidazole INN

tivazine [see: piperazine citrate]

tixadil INN

tixanox USAN *antiallergic* [also: tixanoxum]

tixanoxum INN *antiallergic* [also: tixanox]

tixocortol INN *topical anti-inflammatory* [also: tixocortol pivalate]

tixocortol pivalate USAN *topical anti-inflammatory* [also: tixocortol]

Tixogel VP *investigational topical skin protectant for allergic contact dermatitis* [bentoquatam]

tizabrin INN

tizanidine INN, BAN *antispasmodic; central α_2 agonist* [also: tizanidine HCl]

tizanidine HCl USAN, JAN *antispasmodic for multiple sclerosis and spinal cord injury (orphan); central α_2 agonist* [also: tizanidine]

tizolemide INN

tizoprolic acid INN

T-Koff liquid ℞ *narcotic antitussive; decongestant; antihistamine* [codeine phosphate; phenylpropanolamine HCl; phenylephrine HCl; chlorpheniramine maleate] 10•20•20•5 mg/5 mL

^{201}Tl [see: thallous chloride Tl 201]

TLC C-53 *investigational cell adhesion antagonist for adult respiratory distress syndrome*

T-lymphotrophic virus antigens [see: human T-lymphotropic virus type III (HTLV-III) gp-160 antigens]

TMB (trimedoxime bromide) [q.v.]

TMP (trimethoprim) [q.v.]

TMP-SMZ (trimethoprim & sulfamethoxazole) [q.v.]

TNF (tumor necrosis factor) [q.v.]

TNKase powder for IV injection ℞ *thrombolytic/fibrinolytic for the treatment of acute myocardial infarction* [tenecteplase] 50 mg/vial

TNK-tPA *a genetically engineered mutation of tissue plasminogen activator (tPA); "TNK" refers to the three specific sites of genetic modification* [see: tenecteplase]

TNT (tumor necrosis therapy) [q.v.]

TOAP (thioguanine, Oncovin, [cytosine] arabinoside, prednisone) *chemotherapy protocol*

tobacco *dried leaves of the Nicotiana tabacum plant; narcotic sedative; emetic; diuretic; heart depressant; antispasmodic* [also see: nicotine]

tobacco, British *medicinal herb* [see: coltsfoot]

tobacco, Indian; wild tobacco *medicinal herb* [see: lobelia]

tobacco, sailor's *medicinal herb* [see: mugwort]

tobacco wood *medicinal herb* [see: witch hazel]

TOBI solution for inhalation ℞ *antibiotic for Pseudomonas aeruginosa lung infections in cystic fibrosis patients (orphan); investigational (Phase II) for bronchiectasis and pulmonary tuberculosis* [tobramycin] 300 mg/5 mL

toborinone USAN *cardiotonic*

TobraDex eye drop suspension ℞ *topical ophthalmic corticosteroidal anti-inflammatory; antibiotic* [dexamethasone; tobramycin] 0.1%•0.3% ⊠ Tobrex

TobraDex ophthalmic ointment ℞ *topical ophthalmic corticosteroidal anti-inflammatory; antibiotic* [dexamethasone; tobramycin; chlorobutanol] 0.1%•0.3%•0.5%

tobramycin USAN, USP, INN, BAN *aminoglycoside antibiotic; inhalant for Pseudomonas aeruginosa lung infections in cystic fibrosis patients (orphan)* 0.3% eye drops ⓢ Trobicin

tobramycin sulfate USP *aminoglycoside antibiotic* 10, 40 mg/mL injection

Tobrex Drop-Tainers (eye drops), ophthalmic ointment ℞ *topical ophthalmic antibiotic* [tobramycin] 0.3%; 3 mg/g ⓢ TobraDex

tobuterol INN

tocainide USAN, INN, BAN *antiarrhythmic*

tocainide HCl USP *antiarrhythmic*

tocamphyl USAN, INN *choleretic*

Tocicodendron diversilobum *medicinal herb* [see: poison oak]

tocladesine USAN *immunomodulator; antineoplastic*

tocofenoxate INN

tocofersolan INN *vitamin E supplement* [also: tocophersolan]

tocofibrate INN

tocolytics *a class of drugs used to inhibit uterine contractions*

tocopherol, *d*-alpha [see: vitamin E]

tocopherol, *dl*-alpha [see: vitamin E]

tocopherols, mixed [see: vitamin E]

tocopherols excipient NF *antioxidant*

tocophersolan USAN *vitamin E supplement* [also: tocofersolan]

tocopheryl acetate, *d*-alpha [see: vitamin E]

tocopheryl acetate, *dl*-alpha [see: vitamin E]

tocopheryl acid succinate, *d*-alpha [see: vitamin E]

tocopheryl acid succinate, *dl*-alpha [see: vitamin E]

tocopheryl polyethylene glycol succinate (TPGS) [see: tocophersolan]

todralazine INN, BAN

tofenacin INN *anticholinergic* [also: tofenacin HCl]

tofenacin HCl USAN *anticholinergic* [also: tofenacin]

tofesilate INN *combining name for radicals or groups*

tofetridine INN

tofisoline

tofisopam INN

Tofranil IM injection (discontinued 1999) ℞ *tricyclic antidepressant* [imipramine HCl] 25 mg/2 mL ⓢ Tepanil

Tofranil sugar-coated tablets ℞ *tricyclic antidepressant; treatment for childhood enuresis* [imipramine HCl] 10, 25, 50 mg ⓢ Tepanil

Tofranil-PM capsules ℞ *tricyclic antidepressant* [imipramine pamoate] 75, 100, 125, 150 mg

tolamolol USAN, INN *vasodilator; antiarrhythmic; antiadrenergic (β-receptor)*

tolazamide USAN, USP, INN, BAN *sulfonylurea antidiabetic* 100, 250, 500 mg oral

tolazoline INN *peripheral vasodilator* [also: tolazoline HCl]

tolazoline HCl USP *peripheral vasodilator for neonatal persistent pulmonary hypertension* [also: tolazoline]

tolboxane INN

tolbutamide USP, INN, BAN *sulfonylurea antidiabetic* 500 mg oral

tolbutamide sodium USP *diagnostic aid for pancreatic islet cell adenoma (insulinoma)*

tolcapone USAN, INN *antiparkinsonian; catechol-O-methyltransferase (COMT) inhibitor*

tolciclate USAN, INN *antifungal*

tolclotide [see: disulfamide]

toldimfos INN, BAN

Tolectin 200; Tolectin 600 tablets ℞ *antiarthritic; nonsteroidal anti-inflammatory drug (NSAID) for ankylosing spondylitis and acute bursitis/tendinitis* [tolmetin sodium] 200 mg; 600 mg

Tolectin DS capsules ℞ *antiarthritic; nonsteroidal anti-inflammatory drug (NSAID) for ankylosing spondylitis and acute bursitis/tendinitis* [tolmetin sodium] 400 mg

Tolerex powder OTC *enteral nutritional therapy* [lactose-free formula]

tolfamide USAN, INN *urease enzyme inhibitor*

tolfenamic acid INN, BAN

Tolfrinic film-coated tablets OTC *hematinic* [ferrous fumarate; cyanocobalamin; ascorbic acid] 200 mg•25 μg•100 mg

tolgabide USAN, INN, BAN *anticonvulsant*

tolhexamide [see: glycyclamide]

tolimidone USAN, INN *antiulcerative*

Tolinase tablets ℞ *sulfonylurea antidiabetic* [tolazamide] 100, 250, 500 mg ⓢ Orinase

tolindate USAN, INN *antifungal*

toliodium chloride USAN, INN *veterinary food additive*

toliprolol INN

tolmesoxide INN

tolmetin USAN, INN *antiarthritic; nonsteroidal anti-inflammatory drug (NSAID) for ankylosing spondylitis and acute bursitis/tendinitis*

tolmetin sodium USAN, USP *antiarthritic; nonsteroidal anti-inflammatory drug (NSAID) for ankylosing spondylitis and acute bursitis/tendinitis* 200, 400, 600 mg oral

tolnaftate USAN, USP, INN, BAN *antifungal* 1% topical

tolnapersine INN

tolnidamine INN

toloconium metilsulfate INN

tolofocon A USAN *hydrophobic contact lens material*

tolonidine INN

tolonium chloride INN *blue dye used in histology; diagnostic aid for oral cancer*

toloxatone INN

toloxichloral [see: toloxychlorinol]

toloxychlorinol INN

tolpadol INN

tolpentamide INN, BAN

tolperisone INN, BAN

tolpiprazole INN, BAN

tolpovidone I 131 USAN *hypoalbuminemia test; radioactive agent* [also: radiotolpovidone I 131]

tolpronine INN, BAN

tolpropamine INN, BAN

tolpyrramide USAN, INN *antidiabetic*

tolquinzole INN

tolrestat USAN, INN, BAN *aldose reductase inhibitor for diabetic neuropathy*

tolterodine USAN *muscarinic receptor antagonist for urinary incontinence*

tolterodine tartrate USAN *anticholinergic; muscarinic receptor antagonist for urinary frequency, urgency, and incontinence*

toltrazuril USAN, INN, BAN *veterinary coccidiostat*

tolu balsam USP *pharmaceutic aid*

***p*-toluenesulfone dichloramine** [see: dichloramine T]

tolufazepam INN

toluidine blue O [see: tolonium chloride]

toluidine blue O chloride [see: tolonium chloride]

Tolu-Sed DM syrup OTC *antitussive; expectorant* [dextromethorphan hydrobromide; guaifenesin; alcohol 10%] 10•100 mg/5 mL

tolycaine INN, BAN

tomelukast USAN, INN *antiasthmatic; leukotriene antagonist*

Tomocat concentrated oral suspension ℞ *radiopaque contrast medium for gastrointestinal imaging* [barium sulfate] 5%

tomoglumide INN

tomoxetine INN *antidepressant* [also: tomoxetine HCl]

tomoxetine HCl USAN *antidepressant* [also: tomoxetine]

tomoxiprole INN

Tomudex ℞ *antimetabolite antineoplastic; investigational (Phase III) thymidylate synthase inhibitor for colorectal cancer* [raltitrexed]

Tomycine (CAN) eye drops ℞ *topical antibiotic* [tobramycin] 0.3%

tonazocine INN *analgesic* [also: tonazocine mesylate]

tonazocine mesylate USAN *analgesic* [also: tonazocine]

tongue grass *medicinal herb* [see: chickweed]

tonics *a class of agents that restore normal tone to tissue and strengthen or invigorate organs (a term used in folk medicine)*

tonka bean *(Dipteryx odorata; D. oppositifolia)* fruit and seed *medicinal herb for cramps, nausea, and schistosomiasis*

Tonocard film-coated tablets ℞ *antiarrhythmic* [tocainide HCl] 400, 600 mg

Tonopaque powder for oral suspension ℞ *radiopaque contrast medium for gastrointestinal imaging* [barium sulfate] 95%

tonzonium bromide INN *detergent; surface-active agent* [also: thonzonium bromide]

tooth, lion's *medicinal herb* [see: dandelion]

Toothache gel OTC *topical oral anesthetic* [benzocaine]

toothache bush; toothache tree *medicinal herb* [see: prickly ash]

Topamax coated tablets, sprinkle caps ℞ *broad-spectrum sulfamate anticonvulsant for partial-onset and generalized tonic-clonic seizures; adjunctive treatment for Lennox-Gastaut syndrome (orphan)* [topiramate] 25, 100, 200 mg; 15, 25 mg

Topic gel OTC *topical analgesic; counterirritant* [benzyl alcohol; camphor; menthol; alcohol 30%] 5% • ? • ? 👂 Topicort

topical starch [see: starch, topical]

TopiCare (trademarked ingredient) *topical polyolprepolymer base for creams and gels*

Topicort ointment, cream, gel ℞ *topical corticosteroidal anti-inflammatory* [desoximetasone] 0.25%; 0.25%; 0.05% 👂 Topic

Topicort LP cream ℞ *topical corticosteroidal anti-inflammatory* [desoximetasone] 0.05%

Topicycline solution ℞ *topical antibiotic for acne* [tetracycline HCl] 2.2 mg/mL

Topiglan gel ℞ *investigational (Phase III) topical therapy for erectile dysfunction* [alprostadil]

topiramate USAN, INN, BAN *broad-spectrum sulfamate anticonvulsant for partial-onset and generalized tonic-clonic seizures; adjunctive treatment for Lennox-Gastaut syndrome (orphan)*

topo/CTX (topotecan, cyclophosphamide [with mesna rescue]) *chemotherapy protocol for pediatric bone and soft tissue sarcomas*

topoisomerase I inhibitors *a class of hormonal antineoplastics that prevent DNA replication of tumors by inhibiting the re-ligation of naturally occurring single-strand breaks*

Toposar IV injection ℞ *antineoplastic for testicular and small cell lung cancers* [etoposide; alcohol 30.5%] 20 mg/mL

topotecan INN, BAN *topoisomerase I inhibitor; antineoplastic for ovarian and small cell lung cancers* [also: topotecan HCl]

topotecan HCl USAN *topoisomerase I inhibitor; antineoplastic for ovarian and small cell lung cancers; investigational (Phase II) for AIDS-related progressive multifocal leukoencephalopathy (PML)* [also: topotecan]

toprilidine INN

Toprol-XL film-coated extended-release tablets ℞ *antihypertensive; long-term antianginal; antiadrenergic (β-blocker)* [metoprolol succinate] 25, 50, 100, 200 mg

topterone USAN, INN *antiandrogen*

TOPV (trivalent oral poliovirus vaccine) [see: poliovirus vaccine, live oral]

toquizine USAN, INN *anticholinergic*

Toradol film-coated tablets, Tubex (prefilled syringes) for IM or IV injection ℞ *nonsteroidal anti-inflammatory drug (NSAID); analgesic for acute, moderately severe, opioid-level pain* [ketorolac tromethamine] 10 mg; 15, 30 mg/mL

torasemide INN, BAN *antihypertensive; loop diuretic* [also: torsemide]

torbafylline INN

Torecan suppositories (discontinued 1997) ℞ *antiemetic* [thiethylperazine maleate] 10 mg

Torecan tablets, IM injection ℞ *antiemetic* [thiethylperazine maleate] 10 mg; 5 mg/mL

toremifene INN, BAN *antiestrogen antineoplastic* [also: toremifene citrate]

toremifene citrate USAN *antiestrogen antineoplastic for metastatic breast cancer (orphan); investigational (orphan) for desmoid tumors* [also: toremifene]

toripristone INN

tormentil *(Potentilla tormentilla; Tormentilla erecta)* root *medicinal herb used as an antiphlogistic, antiseptic, astringent, and hemostatic*

Tornalate oral inhalation aerosol, solution for inhalation ℞ *sympathomimetic bronchodilator* [bitolterol mesylate] 0.8%; 0.2%

torsemide USAN *antihypertensive; loop diuretic* [also: torasemide]

tosactide INN [also: octacosactrin]

tosifen USAN, INN *antianginal*

tosilate INN *combining name for radicals or groups* [also: tosylate]

tositumomab [see: iodine I 131 tositumomab]

Tostrex transdermal gel ℞ *investigational (Phase III) androgen replacement for male hypogonadism* [testosterone]

tosufloxacin USAN, INN *antibacterial*

tosulur INN

tosylate USAN, BAN *combining name for radicals or groups* [also: tosilate]

tosylchloramide sodium INN [also: chloramine-T]

Totacillin capsules, powder for oral suspension ℞ *aminopenicillin antibiotic* [ampicillin] 250, 500 mg; 125, 250 mg/5 mL

Totacillin-N powder for IV or IM injection (discontinued 1998) ℞ *aminopenicillin antibiotic* [ampicillin sodium] 0.25, 0.5, 1, 2, 10 g

Total solution OTC *cleaning/soaking/wetting solution for hard contact lenses*

Total Formula; Total Formula-2 tablets OTC *vitamin/mineral/iron supplement* [multiple vitamins & minerals; iron; folic acid; biotin] ≛•20•0.4•0.3 mg

Total Formula-3 without Iron tablets OTC *vitamin/mineral supplement* [multiple vitamins & minerals; folic acid; biotin] ≛•0.4•0.3 mg

touch-me-not; pale touch-me-not *medicinal herb* [see: celandine; jewelweed; Siberian ginseng]

toughened silver nitrate [see: silver nitrate, toughened]

Touro A & H; Touro Allergy timed-release capsules ℞ *decongestant; antihistamine* [pseudoephedrine HCl; brompheniramine maleate] 60•6 mg; 60•5.75 mg

Touro CC sustained-release tablets ℞ *antitussive; decongestant; expectorant* [dextromethorphan hydrobromide; pseudoephedrine HCl; guaifenesin] 30•60•575 mg

Touro DM extended-release tablets ℞ *antitussive; expectorant* [dextromethorphan hydrobromide; guaifenesin] 30•575 mg

Touro Ex sustained-release caplets ℞ *expectorant* [guaifenesin] 575 mg

Touro LA long-acting caplets ℞ *decongestant; expectorant* [pseudoephedrine HCl; guaifenesin] 120•500 mg

toxoids *a class of drugs used for active immunization that produce endogenous antibodies to toxins*

toywort *medicinal herb* [see: shepherd's purse]

tozalinone INN *antidepressant* [also: thozalinone]

TP-10 *investigational (Phase I/II) complement inhibitor for severe burns, adult respiratory distress syndrome; investigational (Phase I/II, orphan) for reperfusion injury* [also: sCR1]

TP-20 *investigational complement/selectin inhibitor for vascular inflammation*

tPA; t-PA (tissue plasminogen activator) [see: alteplase; anistreplase; lanoteplase; monteplase; reteplase; saruplase; tenecteplase]

TPCH (thioguanine, procarbazine, CCNU, hydroxyurea) *chemotherapy protocol*

TPDCV (thioguanine, procarbazine, DCD, CCNU, vincristine) *chemotherapy protocol*

TPGS (tocopheryl polyethylene glycol succinate) [see: tocophersolan]

T-Phyl timed-release tablets ℞ *antiasthmatic; bronchodilator* [theophylline] 200 mg

TPM Test kit for professional use *in vitro diagnostic aid for Toxoplasma gondii antibodies in serum* [indirect hemagglutination test]

TPN Electrolytes; TPN Electrolytes II; TPN Electrolytes III IV admixture ℞ *intravenous electrolyte therapy* [combined electrolyte solution]

traboxopine INN

Trac Tabs 2X tablets ℞ *urinary antibiotic; analgesic; antispasmodic; acidifier* [methenamine; phenyl salicylate; atropine sulfate; hyoscyamine sulfate; benzoic acid; methylene blue] 120•30•0.06•0.03•7.5•6 mg

tracazolate USAN, INN, BAN *sedative*

Trace Metals Additive in 0.9% NaCl IV injection ℞ *intravenous nutritional therapy* [multiple trace elements (metals)]

Tracelyte; Tracelyte II; Tracelyte with Double Electrolytes; Tracelyte II with Double Electrolytes IV admixture ℞ *intravenous nutritional therapy* [multiple trace elements (metals); electrolytes]

Tracleer oral doseform ℞ *investigational (NDA filed) endothelin receptor antagonist for pulmonary hypertension* [bosentan]

Tracrium IV infusion ℞ *nondepolarizing neuromuscular blocker; adjunct to anesthesia* [atracurium besylate] 10 mg/mL

trafermin USAN *investigational (Phase II/III) fibroblast growth factor for stroke and coronary artery disease*

tragacanth NF *suspending agent*

tralonide USAN, INN *corticosteroid; anti-inflammatory*

tramadol INN *central analgesic* [also: tramadol HCl]

tramadol HCl USAN *central analgesic* [also: tramadol]

tramazoline INN *adrenergic* [also: tramazoline HCl]

tramazoline HCl USAN *adrenergic* [also: tramazoline]

Trancopal caplets (discontinued 1998) ℞ *mild anxiolytic* [chlormezanone] 100, 200 mg

Trandate film-coated tablets, IV injection ℞ *antihypertensive; α- and β-blocker* [labetalol HCl] 100, 200, 300 mg; 5 mg/mL

trandolapril INN, BAN *antihypertensive; angiotensin converting enzyme (ACE) inhibitor*

trandolaprilat INN

tranexamic acid USAN, INN, BAN *systemic hemostatic; orphan status withdrawn 1996*

tranilast USAN, INN *antiasthmatic*

trans AMCHA (*trans*-aminomethyl cyclohexanecarboxylic acid) [see: tranexamic acid]

transcainide USAN, INN *antiarrhythmic*

transclomiphene [now: zuclomiphene]

Transderm Scōp transdermal patch ℞ *motion sickness preventative* [scopolamine hydrobromide] 1.5 mg (1 mg dose over 3 days)

Transderm-Nitro transdermal patch ℞ *antianginal; vasodilator* [nitroglycerin] 12.5, 25, 50, 75, 100 mg (0.1, 0.2, 0.4, 0.6, 0.8 mg/hr.)

transforming growth factor beta 2 *investigational (orphan) growth stimulator for full-thickness macular holes*

Transplatin ℞ *investigational (orphan) alkylating antineoplastic for ovarian and colorectal cancers* [oxaliplatin]

***trans*-π-oxocamphor** JAN *topical antipruritic; mild local anesthetic; counterirritant* [also: camphor]

***trans*-retinoic acid** [see: tretinoin]

Trans-Ver-Sal Adult-Patch; Trans-Ver-Sal Pedia-Patch; Trans-Ver-Sal Plantar-Patch transdermal patch OTC *topical keratolytic* [salicylic acid] 15%

trantelinium bromide INN

Tranxene T-Tabs ("T"-imprinted tablets) ℞ *benzodiazepine anxiolytic; minor tranquilizer; anticonvulsant adjunct; alcohol withdrawal aid* [clorazepate dipotassium] 3.75, 7.5, 15 mg

Tranxene-SD single-dose tablets ℞ *benzodiazepine anxiolytic; minor tranquilizer; anticonvulsant adjunct; alcohol withdrawal aid* [clorazepate dipotassium] 11.25, 22.5 mg

tranylcypromine INN, BAN *antidepressant; MAO inhibitor* [also: tranylcypromine sulfate]

tranylcypromine sulfate USP *antidepressant; MAO inhibitor* [also: tranylcypromine]

trapencaine INN

trapidil INN

trapymin [see: trapidil]

trastuzumab *antineoplastic monoclonal antibody to HER2 (human epidermal growth factor receptor 2) protein for metastatic breast cancer*

trastuzumab & paclitaxel *chemotherapy protocol for breast cancer*

Trasylol IV infusion ℞ *systemic hemostatic for coronary artery bypass graft (CABG) surgery (orphan)* [aprotinin] 10 000 KIU/mL (Kallikrein inhibitor units) ⊠ Travasol

TraumaCal ready-to-use liquid OTC *enteral nutritional therapy for moderate to severe stress or trauma* [multiple branched chain amino acids]

Travasol 2.75% in 5% (10%, 25%) Dextrose; Travasol 4.25% in 5% (10%, 25%) Dextrose IV infusion ℞ *total parenteral nutrition; peripheral parenteral nutrition* [multiple essential and nonessential amino acids; dextrose] ⊠ Trasylol

Travasol 3.5% (5.5%, 8.5%) with Electrolytes IV infusion ℞ *total parenteral nutrition (all except 3.5%); peripheral parenteral nutrition (all)* [multiple essential and nonessential amino acids; electrolytes]

Travasol 5.5% (8.5%, 10%) IV infusion ℞ *total parenteral nutrition; peripheral parenteral nutrition* [multiple essential and nonessential amino acids]

Travasorb HN; Travasorb MCT; Travasorb STD powder OTC *enteral nutritional therapy* [lactose-free formula]

Travasorb Renal Diet powder (discontinued 1998) OTC *enteral nutritional therapy for acute renal failure*

Travatan Drop-Tainers (eye drops) ℞ *prostaglandin* $F_{2\alpha}$ *analogue for glaucoma and ocular hypertension* [travoprost] 0.004%

traveler's joy *medicinal herb* [see: blue vervain; woodbine]

5% Travert and Electrolyte No. 2; 10% Travert and Electrolyte No. 2 IV infusion ℞ *intravenous nutritional/electrolyte therapy* [combined electrolyte solution; invert sugar (50% dextrose + 50% fructose)]

travoprost USAN *topical prostaglandin* $F_{2\alpha}$ *analogue for glaucoma and ocular hypertension*

traxanox INN

traxoprodil mesylate USAN *selective NMDA receptor antagonist for traumatic brain injury*

Traypak (trademarked packaging form) *multivial carton*

trazitiline INN

trazium esilate INN

trazodone INN *antidepressant used for panic disorders, aggressive behavior, alcoholism, and cocaine withdrawal; serotonin uptake inhibitor* [also: trazodone HCl]

trazodone HCl USAN *antidepressant used for panic disorders, aggressive behavior, alcoholism, and cocaine withdrawal; serotonin uptake inhibitor* [also: trazodone] 50, 100, 150, 300 mg oral

trazolopride INN

trebenzomine INN *antidepressant* [also: trebenzomine HCl]

trebenzomine HCl USAN *antidepressant* [also: trebenzomine]

trecadrine INN

Trecator-SC tablets ℞ *tuberculostatic* [ethionamide] 250 mg

trecetilide fumarate USAN *antiarrhythmic*

trecovirsen sodium USAN *antisense antiviral for HIV and AIDS*

trefentanil HCl USAN *analgesic*

trefoil, bean; bitter trefoil; marsh trefoil *medicinal herb* [see: buckbean]
treloxinate USAN, INN *antihyperlipoproteinemic*
Trelstar Depot IM injection (once monthly) ℞ *gonadotropin-releasing hormone (Gn-RH) agonist; antineoplastic for palliative treatment of advanced prostate cancer* [triptorelin pamoate] 3.75 mg
tremacamra USAN *antiviral; inhibits viral attachment to host cells*
trembling poplar; trembling tree *medicinal herb* [see: poplar]
trenbolone INN, BAN *veterinary anabolic steroid, also abused as a street drug* [also: trenbolone acetate]
trenbolone acetate USAN *veterinary anabolic steroid, also abused as a street drug* [also: trenbolone]
trenbolone hexahydrobenzylcarbonate *veterinary anabolic steroid, also abused as a street drug*
trengestone INN
trenizine INN
Trental film-coated controlled-release tablets ℞ *peripheral vasodilator to improve blood microcirculation in intermittent claudication* [pentoxifylline] 400 mg
treosulfan INN, BAN *investigational (orphan) for ovarian cancer*
trepibutone INN
trepipam INN *sedative* [also: trepipam maleate]
trepipam maleate USAN *sedative* [also: trepipam]
trepirium iodide INN
treprostinil sodium *investigational (NDA filed) prostacyclin analogue for pulmonary arterial hypertension (PAH) and peripheral vascular disease (PVD)*
treptilamine INN
trequinsin INN
trestolone INN *antineoplastic; androgen* [also: trestolone acetate]
trestolone acetate USAN *antineoplastic; androgen* [also: trestolone]
tretamine INN, BAN [also: triethylenemelamine]
trethinium tosilate INN
trethocanic acid INN
trethocanoic acid [see: trethocanic acid]
tretinoin USAN, USP, INN, BAN *keratolytic; treatment for acute promyelocytic leukemia (orphan); investigational (orphan) for other leukemias and ophthalmic squamous metaplasia; investigational (Phase II) for AIDS-related Kaposi sarcoma and non-Hodgkin lymphoma* 0.025%, 0.05%, 0.1% topical
tretoquinol INN
Trexall film-coated tablets ℞ *antimetabolite antineoplastic for leukemia; systemic antipsoriatic; antirheumatic* [methotrexate] 5, 7.5, 10, 15 mg
TRH (thyrotropin-releasing hormone) [see: protirelin]
Tri Vit with Fluoride drops ℞ *pediatric vitamin supplement and dental caries preventative* [vitamins A, C, and D; fluoride] 1500 IU•35 mg•400 IU•0.25 mg, 1500 IU•35 mg•400 IU•0.5 mg per mL
TRIAC (triiodothyroacetic acid) [q.v.]
Triacana ℞ *investigational (orphan) for suppression of thyroid-stimulating hormone (TSH) in thyroid cancer* [tiratricol; levothyroxine sodium]
Triacet cream ℞ *topical corticosteroidal anti-inflammatory* [triamcinolone acetonide] 0.1%
triacetin USP, INN *antifungal*
triacetyloleandomycin BAN *macrolide antibiotic* [also: troleandomycin]
Triacin-C Cough syrup ℞ *narcotic antitussive; decongestant; antihistamine* [codeine phosphate; pseudoephedrine HCl; triprolidine HCl; alcohol] 10•30•1.25 mg/5 mL
triaconazole [now: terconazole]
Triactin syrup OTC *decongestant; antihistamine* [phenylpropanolamine HCl; chlorpheniramine maleate] 6.25•1 mg/5 mL
Triad capsules ℞ *sedative; barbiturate analgesic* [acetaminophen; caffeine; butalbital] 325•40•50 mg

Triafed with Codeine syrup (discontinued 2000) ℞ *narcotic antitussive; decongestant; antihistamine* [codeine phosphate; pseudoephedrine HCl; triprolidine HCl] 10•30•1.25 mg/5 mL

triafungin USAN, INN *antifungal*

Triam Forte IM injection ℞ *corticosteroid; anti-inflammatory* [triamcinolone diacetate] 40 mg/mL

Triam-A IM, intra-articular, intrabursal, intradermal injection ℞ *corticosteroid; anti-inflammatory* [triamcinolone acetonide] 40 mg/mL

triamcinolone USP, INN, BAN, JAN *corticosteroid* 4 mg oral ⊡ Triaminicin

triamcinolone acetonide USP, JAN *corticosteroidal anti-inflammatory; treatment for chronic asthma and rhinitis* 0.025%, 0.1%, 0.5% topical; 10, 40 mg/mL injection

triamcinolone acetonide sodium phosphate USAN *corticosteroid*

triamcinolone benetonide INN *corticosteroid*

triamcinolone diacetate USP, JAN *corticosteroid* 40 mg/mL injection

triamcinolone furetonide INN *corticosteroid*

triamcinolone hexacetonide USAN, USP, INN, BAN *corticosteroid*

Triaminic chewable tablets, syrup OTC *pediatric decongestant and antihistamine* [phenylpropanolamine HCl; chlorpheniramine maleate] 6.25•0.5 mg; 6.25•1 mg/5 mL ⊡ Triaminicin; TriHemic

Triaminic oral infant drops (discontinued 2000) ℞ *pediatric decongestant and antihistamine* [phenylpropanolamine HCl; pyrilamine maleate; pheniramine maleate] 20•10•10 mg/mL

Triaminic Allergy; Triaminic Cold tablets OTC *decongestant; antihistamine* [phenylpropanolamine HCl; chlorpheniramine maleate] 25•4 mg; 12.5•2 mg

Triaminic AM Cough & Decongestant Formula liquid OTC *pediatric antitussive and decongestant* [dextromethorphan hydrobromide; pseudoephedrine HCl] 7.5•15 mg/5 mL

Triaminic AM Decongestant Formula syrup OTC *decongestant* [pseudoephedrine HCl] 15 mg/5 mL

Triaminic Cold & Allergy syrup OTC *decongestant; antihistamine* [phenylpropanolamine HCl; chlorpheniramine maleate] 6.25•1 mg/5 mL

Triaminic Cold & Cough soft chews OTC *pediatric antitussive, decongestant, and antihistamine* [dextromethorphan hydrobromide; pseudoephedrine HCl; chlorpheniramine maleate] 5•15•1 mg

Triaminic Cough soft chews OTC *pediatric antitussive* [dextromethorphan hydrobromide] 7.5 mg

Triaminic Decongestant oral infant drops OTC *pediatric decongestant* [pseudoephedrine HCl] 7.5 mg/0.8 mL

Triaminic DM syrup OTC *antitussive; decongestant* [dextromethorphan hydrobromide; phenylpropanolamine HCl] 5•6.25 mg/5 mL

Triaminic DM Day time (CAN) oral solution (discontinued 1998) OTC *pediatric antitussive, decongestant, and expectorant* [dextromethorphan hydrobromide; phenylpropanolamine HCl; guaifenesin] 1.5•1.75•7.5 mg/mL

Triaminic DM Night time for Children (CAN) liquid (discontinued 1998) OTC *pediatric antitussive, decongestant, and antihistamine* [dextromethorphan hydrobromide; pseudoephedrine HCl; chlorpheniramine maleate] 7.5•15•1 mg/5 mL

Triaminic Expectorant liquid OTC *decongestant; expectorant* [phenylpropanolamine HCl; guaifenesin] 6.25•50 mg/5 mL

Triaminic Expectorant DH liquid ℞ *narcotic antitussive; decongestant; antihistamine; expectorant* [hydrocodone bitartrate; phenylpropanolamine HCl; pyrilamine maleate; pheniramine maleate; guaifenesin; alcohol 5%] 1.67•12.5•6.25•6.25•100 mg/5 mL

Triaminic Expectorant with Codeine liquid ℞ *narcotic antitussive; decongestant; expectorant* [codeine phosphate; phenylpropanolamine HCl; guaifenesin; alcohol 5%] 10•12.5•100 mg/5 mL

Triaminic Nite Light liquid OTC *pediatric antitussive, decongestant, and antihistamine* [dextromethorphan hydrobromide; pseudoephedrine HCl; chlorpheniramine maleate] 7.5•15•1 mg/5 mL

Triaminic Severe Cold & Fever oral liquid OTC *antitussive; decongestant; antihistamine; analgesic; antipyretic* [dextromethorphan hydrobromide; pseudoephedrine HCl; chlorpheniramine maleate; acetaminophen] 7.5•15•1•160 mg/5 mL

Triaminic Softchews OTC *pediatric decongestant and antihistamine* [pseudoephedrine HCl; chlorpheniramine maleate] 15•1 mg

Triaminic Sore Throat Formula liquid OTC *pediatric antitussive, decongestant, and analgesic* [dextromethorphan hydrobromide; pseudoephedrine HCl; acetaminophen] 7.5•15•160 mg/5 mL

Triaminic Throat Pain & Cough soft chews OTC *pediatric antitussive, decongestant, and analgesic* [dextromethorphan hydrobromide; pseudoephedrine HCl; acetaminophen] 5•15•100 mg

Triaminic Vapor Patch OTC *counterirritant* [camphor; menthol] 4.7%•2.6%

Triaminic-12 sustained-release tablets OTC *decongestant; antihistamine* [phenylpropanolamine HCl; chlorpheniramine maleate] 75•12 mg

Triaminicin Cold, Allergy, Sinus tablets OTC *decongestant; antihistamine; analgesic* [phenylpropanolamine HCl; chlorpheniramine maleate; acetaminophen] 25•4•650 mg ⓢ triamcinolone; Triaminic

Triaminicol Multi-Symptom Cough and Cold tablets OTC *antitussive; decongestant; antihistamine* [dextromethorphan hydrobromide; phenylpropanolamine HCl; chlorpheniramine maleate] 10•12.5•2 mg

Triaminicol Multi-Symptom Relief liquid OTC *antitussive; decongestant; antihistamine* [dextromethorphan hydrobromide; phenylpropanolamine HCl; chlorpheniramine maleate] 10•12.5•2 mg/5 mL

Triaminicol Multi-Symptom Relief Colds with Cough liquid OTC *pediatric antitussive, decongestant, and antihistamine* [dextromethorphan hydrobromide; phenylpropanolamine HCl; chlorpheniramine maleate] 5•6.25•1 mg/5 mL

Triamolone 40 IM injection ℞ *corticosteroid; anti-inflammatory* [triamcinolone diacetate] 40 mg/mL

Triamonide 40 IM, intra-articular, intrabursal, intradermal injection ℞ *corticosteroid; anti-inflammatory* [triamcinolone acetonide] 40 mg/mL

triampyzine INN *anticholinergic* [also: triampyzine sulfate]

triampyzine sulfate USAN *anticholinergic* [also: triampyzine]

triamterene USAN, USP, INN, BAN, JAN *antihypertensive; potassium-sparing diuretic* ⓢ trimipramine

triamterene & hydrochlorothiazide *antihypertensive; potassium-sparing diuretic* 37.5•25 mg oral

trianisestrol [see: chlorotrianisene]

Triapine ℞ *investigational (Phase I) anticancer agent* ⓢ Triaprim

Triaprin capsules (discontinued 1998) ℞ *analgesic; sedative* [acetaminophen; butalbital] 325•50 mg ⓢ Triapine

Triavil tablets ℞ *conventional (typical) antipsychotic; antidepressant* [perphenazine; amitriptyline HCl] 2•10 mg; 2•25 mg; 4•10 mg; 4•25 mg

Triavil 4-50 tablets (discontinued 2000) ℞ *conventional (typical) antipsychotic; antidepressant* [perphenazine; amitriptyline HCl] 4•50 mg

Tri-A-Vite F drops ℞ *pediatric vitamin supplement and dental caries preventative*

[vitamins A, C, and D; fluoride] 1500 IU•35 mg•400 IU•0.5 mg per mL

Triaz gel, skin cleanser ℞ *topical keratolytic for acne* [benzoyl peroxide] 6%, 10%; 10%

triaziquone INN, BAN

triazolam USAN, USP, INN *benzodiazepine sedative; hypnotic* 0.125, 0.25 mg oral

Triban; Pediatric Triban suppositories ℞ *antiemetic; anticholinergic* [trimethobenzamide HCl; benzocaine] 200 mg•2%; 100 mg•2% ⑨ Tigan

tribasic calcium phosphate [see: calcium phosphate, tribasic]

tribavirin BAN *antiviral for severe lower respiratory tract infections* [also: ribavirin]

tribendilol INN

tribenoside USAN, INN *sclerosing agent*

Tribiotic Plus ointment OTC *topical antibiotic; anesthetic* [polymyxin B sulfate; bacitracin; neomycin sulfate; lidocaine] 5000 U•500 U•3.5 mg•40 mg per g

tribromoethanol NF

tribromomethane [see: bromoform]

tribromsalan USAN, INN *disinfectant*

tribuzone INN

tricalcium phosphate [see: calcium phosphate, tribasic]

tricarbocyanine dye [see: indocyanine green]

tricetamide USAN *sedative*

Trichinella extract USP

Tri-Chlor liquid ℞ *cauterant; keratolytic* [trichloroacetic acid] 80%

trichlorethoxyphosphamide [see: defosfamide]

trichlorfon USAN, USP *veterinary anthelmintic; investigational (NDA filed) acetylcholinesterase inhibitor for Alzheimer dementia* [also: metrifonate; metriphonate]

trichlorisobutylalcohol [see: chlorobutanol]

trichlormethiazide USP, INN *diuretic; antihypertensive* 4 mg oral

trichlormethine INN [also: trimustine]

trichloroacetic acid USP *strong keratolytic/cauterant*

trichlorocarbanilide (TCC) [see: triclocarban]

trichloroethylene NF, INN

trichlorofluoromethane [see: trichloromonofluoromethane]

trichlorofon [see: metrifonate]

trichloromonofluoromethane NF *aerosol propellant; topical anesthetic*

trichlorphon [see: metrifonate]

Tricholomopsis edodes *medicinal herb* [see: shiitake mushrooms]

Trichophyton extract *diagnosis and treatment of Trichophyton-induced skin infections*

trichorad [see: acinitrazole]

Trichosanthes kirilowii *medicinal herb* [see: Chinese cucumber]

trichosanthin *investigational (Phase II) antiviral for AIDS*

Trichotine Douche powder OTC *antiseptic/germicidal; vaginal cleanser and deodorizer; acidity modifier* [sodium perborate]

Trichotine Douche solution OTC *antiseptic/germicidal; vaginal cleanser and deodorizer; acidity modifier* [sodium borate]

triciribine INN *antineoplastic* [also: triciribine phosphate]

triciribine phosphate USAN *antineoplastic* [also: triciribine]

tricitrates (sodium citrate, potassium citrate, and citric acid) USP *systemic alkalizer; urinary alkalizer; antiurolithic*

triclabendazole INN

triclacetamol INN

triclazate INN

triclobisonium chloride NF, INN

triclocarban USAN, INN *disinfectant*

triclodazol INN

triclofenate INN *combining name for radicals or groups*

triclofenol piperazine USAN, INN *anthelmintic*

triclofos INN *hypnotic; sedative* [also: triclofos sodium]

triclofos sodium USAN *hypnotic; sedative* [also: triclofos]

triclofylline INN

triclonide USAN, INN *anti-inflammatory*
triclosan USAN, INN, BAN *disinfectant/antiseptic*
Tricodene Cough and Cold liquid ℞ *narcotic antitussive; antihistamine* [codeine phosphate; pyrilamine maleate] 8.2•12.5 mg/5 mL
Tricodene Forte; Tricodene NN liquid OTC *antitussive; decongestant; antihistamine* [dextromethorphan hydrobromide; phenylpropanolamine HCl; chlorpheniramine maleate] 10•12.5•2 mg/5 mL
Tricodene Pediatric Cough & Cold liquid OTC *pediatric antitussive and decongestant* [dextromethorphan hydrobromide; phenylpropanolamine HCl] 10•12.5 mg/5 mL
Tricodene Sugar Free liquid OTC *antitussive; antihistamine* [dextromethorphan hydrobromide; chlorpheniramine maleate] 10•2 mg/5 mL
Tricor capsules ℞ *antihyperlipidemic for primary hypercholesterolemia (types IIa and IIb hyperlipidemia), hypertriglyceridemia (types IV and V hyperlipidemia), and mixed dyslipidemia* [fenofibrate] 67, 134, 200 mg
tricosactide INN
Tricosal film-coated tablets ℞ *analgesic; antipyretic; antirheumatic* [choline magnesium trisalicylate] 500, 750, 1000 mg
tricyclamol chloride INN
Tri-Cyclen [see: Ortho Tri-Cyclen]
tricyclics *a class of antidepressants that inhibit reuptake of amines, norepinephrine, and serotonin*
Triderm cream ℞ *topical corticosteroidal anti-inflammatory* [triamcinolone acetonide] 0.1%
Tridesilon cream, ointment ℞ *topical corticosteroidal anti-inflammatory* [desonide] 0.05%
Tridesilon Otic [see: Otic Tridesilon]
Tri-Desogen (name changed to Mircette upon marketing release in 1998)
tridihexethyl chloride USP *peptic ulcer adjunct*
tridihexethyl iodide INN
Tridil IV infusion ℞ *antianginal; vasodilator; perioperative antihypertensive; for congestive heart failure with myocardial infarction* [nitroglycerin] 0.5, 5 mg/mL
Tridione capsules, Dulcets (chewable tablets) ℞ *anticonvulsant* [trimethadione] 300 mg; 150 mg
tridolgosir HCl USAN *chemoprotectant for solid tumor chemotherapy*
Tridrate Bowel Cleansing System oral solution + 3 tablets + 1 suppository OTC *pre-procedure bowel evacuant* [magnesium citrate (solution); bisacodyl (tablets and suppository)] 300 mL; 5 mg; 10 mg
trientine INN *chelating agent* [also: trientine HCl; trientine dihydrochloride]
trientine dihydrochloride BAN *chelating agent* [also: trientine HCl; trientine]
trientine HCl USAN, USP *copper chelating agent for Wilson disease (orphan)* [also: trientine; trientine dihydrochloride]
triest; triestrogen [see: estriol]
triethanolamine [now: trolamine]
triethyl citrate NF *plasticizer*
triethyleneiminobenzoquinone (TEIB) [see: triaziquone]
triethylenemelamine NF [also: tretamine]
triethylenethiophosphoramide (TSPA; TESPA) [see: thiotepa]
Trifed-C Cough syrup ℞ *narcotic antitussive; decongestant; antihistamine* [codeine phosphate; pseudoephedrine HCl; triprolidine HCl; alcohol 4.4%] 10•30•1.25 mg/5 mL
trifenagrel USAN, INN *antithrombotic*
trifezolac INN
triflocin USAN, INN *diuretic*
Tri-Flor-Vite with Fluoride drops ℞ *pediatric vitamin supplement and dental caries preventative* [vitamins A, C, and D; fluoride] 1500 IU•35 mg•400 IU•0.25 mg per mL
triflubazam USAN, INN *minor tranquilizer*
triflumidate USAN, INN *anti-inflammatory*
trifluomeprazine INN, BAN

trifluoperazine INN *phenothiazine antipsychotic; sedative* [also: trifluoperazine HCl]

trifluoperazine HCl USP *phenothiazine antipsychotic; sedative; anxiolytic* [also: trifluoperazine] 1, 2, 5, 10 mg oral; 10 mg/mL oral; 2 mg/mL injection

N-trifluoroacetyl adriamycin-14-valerate *investigational for carcinoma in situ of the urinary bladder; orphan status withdrawn 1998*

trifluorothymidine [see: trifluridine]

trifluperidol USAN, INN *antipsychotic*

triflupromazine USP, INN *phenothiazine antipsychotic; antiemetic*

triflupromazine HCl USP *phenothiazine antipsychotic; antiemetic*

trifluridine USAN, INN *ophthalmic antiviral* 1% eye drops

Triflusal ℞ *investigational agent for the prevention of stroke and dementia*

triflusal INN *investigational treatment for stroke and vascular dementia*

triflutate USAN, INN *combining name for radicals or groups*

Trifolium pratense *medicinal herb* [see: red clover]

trigevolol INN

α-triglycidyl isocyanurate (αTGI) [see: teroxirone]

Trigonella foenum-graecum *medicinal herb* [see: fenugreek]

TriHemic 600 film-coated tablets ℞ *hematinic* [ferrous fumarate; cyanocobalamin; ascorbic acid; vitamin E; intrinsic factor concentrate; docusate sodium; folic acid] 115 mg•25 μg•600 mg•30 IU•75 mg•50 mg•1 mg ⊠ Triaminic

Trihexy-2; Trihexy-5 tablets ℞ *anticholinergic; antiparkinsonian* [trihexyphenidyl HCl] 2 mg; 5 mg

trihexyphenidyl INN *anticholinergic; antiparkinsonian* [also: trihexyphenidyl HCl; benzhexol]

trihexyphenidyl HCl USP *anticholinergic; antiparkinsonian* [also: trihexyphenidyl; benzhexol] 2, 5 mg oral

TriHIBit IM injection ℞ *active immunizing agent for diphtheria, tetanus, pertussis, and Haemophilus influenzae type B* [diphtheria & tetanus toxoids & acellular pertussis (DTaP) vaccine; Hemophilus B conjugate vaccine] supplied as separate 0.5 mL vials of Tripedia (q.v.) and ActHib (q.v.)

Tri-Hydroserpine tablets ℞ *antihypertensive; vasodilator; diuretic* [hydrochlorothiazide; reserpine; hydralazine HCl] 15•0.1•25 mg

Tri-Immunol IM injection (discontinued 2001) ℞ *active immunizing agent for diphtheria, tetanus, and pertussis* [diphtheria & tetanus toxoids & whole-cell pertussis (DTwP) vaccine, adsorbed] 12.5 LfU•5 LfU•4 U/0.5 mL

triiodothyroacetic acid (TRIAC) *thyroid hormone analogue*

triiodothyronine sodium, levo [see: liothyronine sodium]

Tri-K liquid ℞ *potassium supplement* [potassium acetate; potassium bicarbonate; potassium citrate] 45 mEq/15 mL (K)

trikates USP *electrolyte replenisher*

Trikof-D sustained-release tablets OTC *antitussive; decongestant; expectorant* [dextromethorphan hydrobromide; phenylpropanolamine HCl; guaifenesin] 30•37.5•600 mg

Tri-Kort IM, intra-articular, intrabursal, or intradermal injection ℞ *corticosteroid; anti-inflammatory* [triamcinolone acetonide] 40 mg/mL

Trilafon coated tablets, oral concentrate, IV or IM injection ℞ *conventional (typical) antipsychotic; antiemetic* [perphenazine] 2, 4, 8, 16 mg; 16 mg/5 mL; 5 mg/mL

Trileptal film-coated tablets, oral suspension ℞ *anticonvulsant for partial seizures* [oxcarbazepine] 150, 300, 600 mg; 300 mg/5 mL

triletide INN

Tri-Levlen film-coated tablets (in Slidecases of 21 or 28) ℞ *triphasic oral contraceptive; emergency postcoital contraceptive* [levonorgestrel; ethinyl estradiol] Phase 1 (6 days): 50•30 μg;

Phase 2 (5 days): 75•40 µg;
Phase 3 (10 days): 125•30 µg

Trilisate tablets, liquid ℞ *analgesic; antipyretic; anti-inflammatory; antirheumatic* [choline salicylate; magnesium salicylate] 750, 1000 mg; 500 mg/5 mL

trilithium citrate tetrahydrate [see: lithium citrate]

Trillium erectum; T. grandiflorum; T. pendulum *medicinal herb* [see: birthroot]

Trilog IM, intra-articular, intrabursal, intradermal injection ℞ *corticosteroid; anti-inflammatory* [triamcinolone acetonide] 40 mg/mL

Trilone IM injection ℞ *corticosteroid; anti-inflammatory* [triamcinolone diacetate] 40 mg/mL

trilostane USAN, INN, BAN *adrenocortical suppressant; antisteroidal antineoplastic*

Trimazide capsules (discontinued 2000) ℞ *antiemetic; anticholinergic* [trimethobenzamide HCl] 100 mg

Trimazide suppositories, pediatric suppositories ℞ *antiemetic; anticholinergic* [trimethobenzamide HCl] 200 mg; 100 mg

trimazosin INN, BAN *antihypertensive* [also: trimazosin HCl]

trimazosin HCl USAN *antihypertensive* [also: trimazosin]

trimebutine INN *GI antispasmodic*

trimecaine INN

trimedoxime bromide INN

trimegestone USAN *progestin for postmenopausal hormone deficiency*

trimeperidine INN, BAN

trimeprazine BAN *phenothiazine antihistamine; antipruritic* [also: trimeprazine tartrate; alimemazine; alimemazine tartrate] ⑨ trimipramine

trimeprazine tartrate USP *phenothiazine antihistamine; antipruritic* [also: alimemazine; trimeprazine; alimemazine tartrate]

trimeproprimine [see: trimipramine]

trimetamide INN

trimetaphan camsilate INN *antihypertensive* [also: trimethaphan camsylate; trimetaphan camsylate]

trimetaphan camsylate BAN *antihypertensive* [also: trimethaphan camsylate; trimetaphan camsilate]

trimetazidine INN, BAN

trimethadione USP, INN *anticonvulsant* [also: troxidone]

trimethamide [see: trimetamide]

trimethaphan camphorsulfonate [see: trimethaphan camsylate] ⑨ trimethoprim

trimethaphan camsylate USP *emergency antihypertensive* [also: trimetaphan camsilate; trimetaphan camsylate]

trimethidinium methosulfate NF, INN

trimethobenzamide INN *antiemetic; anticholinergic* [also: trimethobenzamide HCl]

trimethobenzamide HCl USP *antiemetic; anticholinergic* [also: trimethobenzamide] 250 mg oral; 100, 200 mg suppositories; 100 mg/mL injection

trimethoprim (TMP) USAN, USP, INN, BAN *antibiotic* 100, 200 mg oral ⑨ trimethaphan

trimethoprim & dapsone *investigational for Pneumocystis carinii pneumonia; orphan status withdrawn 1998*

trimethoprim sulfate USAN *antibiotic*

trimethoprim sulfate & polymyxin B sulfate [CG] *topical ophthalmic antibiotic* 1 mg•10 000 U per mL

trimethoquinol [see: tretoquinol]

trimethylammonium chloride carbamate [see: bethanechol chloride]

3,3,5-trimethylcyclohexyl salicylate [see: homosalate]

trimethylene [see: cyclopropane]

trimethyltetradecylammonium bromide [see: tetradonium bromide]

trimetozine USAN, INN *sedative*

trimetrexate USAN, INN, BAN *antimetabolic antineoplastic; systemic antiprotozoal*

trimetrexate glucuronate USAN *antimetabolic antineoplastic; antiprotozoal for Pneumocystis carinii pneumonia of AIDS (orphan); investigational (orphan) for multiple cancers*

trimexiline INN

Triminol Cough syrup OTC *antitussive; decongestant; antihistamine* [dextromethorphan hydrobromide; phenylpropanolamine HCl; chlorpheniramine maleate] 10•12.5•2 mg/5 mL

trimipramine USAN, INN *tricyclic antidepressant* ⊡ imipramine; triamterene; trimeprazine

trimipramine maleate USAN *tricyclic antidepressant*

trimolide [see: trimetozine]

trimopam maleate [now: trepipam maleate]

trimoprostil USAN, INN *gastric antisecretory*

Trimo-San vaginal jelly OTC *antibacterial; astringent; antipruritic* [oxyquinoline sulfate; boric acid; sodium borate] 0.025%•1%•0.7%

Trimox capsules, powder for oral suspension, pediatric drops ℞ *aminopenicillin antibiotic* [amoxicillin] 250, 500 mg; 125, 250 mg/5 mL; 50 mg/mL

trimoxamine INN *antihypertensive* [also: trimoxamine HCl]

trimoxamine HCl USAN *antihypertensive* [also: trimoxamine]

Trimpex tablets ℞ *anti-infective; antibacterial* [trimethoprim] 100 mg

trimustine BAN [also: trichlormethine]

Trinalin Repetabs (repeat-action tablets) ℞ *decongestant; antihistamine* [pseudoephedrine sulfate; azatadine maleate] 120•1 mg

Trinam reservoir delivery device ℞ *investigational (Phase II, orphan) gene-based therapy for intimal hyperplasia* [vascular endothelial growth factor (VEGF)]

Tri-Nasal nasal spray ℞ *once-daily corticosteroidal anti-inflammatory for chronic allergic rhinitis* [triamcinolone acetonide] 50 μg/spray

trinecol (pullus) USAN *collagen derivative for treatment of rheumatoid arthritis*

Tri-Nefrin tablets OTC *decongestant; antihistamine* [phenylpropanolamine HCl; chlorpheniramine maleate] 25•4 mg

Trinipatch (CAN) transdermal patch ℞ *antianginal; vasodilator* [nitroglycerin] 22.4, 44.8, 67.2 mg (0.2, 0.4, 0.6 mg/hr.)

trinitrin [see: nitroglycerin]

trinitrophenol NF

Tri-Norinyl tablets (in Wallettes of 21 or 28) ℞ *triphasic oral contraceptive* [norethindrone; ethinyl estradiol]
Phase 1 (7 days): 0.5 mg•35 μg;
Phase 2 (9 days): 1 mg•35 μg;
Phase 3 (5 days): 0.5 mg•35 μg

Trinsicon capsules ℞ *hematinic* [ferrous fumarate; cyanocobalamin; ascorbic acid; intrinsic factor concentrate; folic acid] 110 mg•15 μg•75 mg•240 mg•0.5 mg

Triofed syrup OTC *decongestant; antihistamine* [pseudoephedrine HCl; triprolidine HCl] 30•1.25 mg/5 mL

triolein I 125 USAN *radioactive agent*

triolein I 131 USAN *radioactive agent*

trional [see: sulfonethylmethane]

Triostat IV injection ℞ *synthetic thyroid T_3 hormone; treatment for myxedema coma or precoma (orphan)* [liothyronine sodium] 10 μg/mL ⊡ Threostat

Triotann tablets ℞ *decongestant; antihistamine* [phenylephrine tannate; chlorpheniramine tannate; pyrilamine tannate] 25•8•25 mg

Tri-Otic ear drops ℞ *topical corticosteroidal anti-inflammatory; topical local anesthetic; antiseptic* [hydrocortisone; pramoxine HCl; chloroxylenol] 10•10•1 mg/mL

trioxifene INN *antiestrogen* [also: trioxifene mesylate]

trioxifene mesylate USAN *antiestrogen* [also: trioxifene]

trioxsalen USAN, USP *systemic psoralens for repigmentation of idiopathic vitiligo; also used to enhance pigmentation and increase tolerance to sunlight* [also: trioxysalen]

trioxyethylrutin [see: troxerutin]

trioxymethylene [see: paraformaldehyde]

trioxysalen INN *systemic psoralens for repigmentation of idiopathic vitiligo;*

also used to enhance pigmentation and increase tolerance to sunlight [also: trioxsalen]

Tri-P oral infant drops ℞ *decongestant; antihistamine* [phenylpropanolamine HCl; pyrilamine maleate; pheniramine maleate] 20•10•10 mg/mL

tripamide USAN, INN *antihypertensive; diuretic*

triparanol INN *(withdrawn from market)*

Tripedia IM injection ℞ *active immunizing agent for diphtheria, tetanus, and pertussis* [diphtheria & tetanus toxoids & acellular pertussis (DTaP) vaccine, adsorbed] 6.7 LfU•5 LfU•46.8 μg per 0.5 mL

tripelennamine INN *ethylenediamine antihistamine* [also: tripelennamine citrate]

tripelennamine citrate USP *ethylenediamine antihistamine* [also: tripelennamine]

tripelennamine HCl USP *ethylenediamine antihistamine*

Triphasil tablets (in packs of 21 or 28) ℞ *triphasic oral contraceptive; emergency postcoital contraceptive* [levonorgestrel; ethinyl estradiol]
Phase 1 (6 days): 50•30 μg;
Phase 2 (5 days): 75•40 μg;
Phase 3 (10 days): 125•30 μg

Tri-Phen-Chlor syrup, pediatric syrup, pediatric drops ℞ *decongestant; antihistamine* [phenylpropanolamine HCl; phenylephrine HCl; chlorpheniramine maleate; phenyltoloxamine citrate] 20•5•2.5•7.5 mg/5 mL; 5•1.25•0.5•2 mg/5 mL; 5•1.25•0.5•2 mg/mL

Tri-Phen-Chlor T.R. timed-release tablets ℞ *decongestant; antihistamine* [phenylpropanolamine HCl; phenylephrine HCl; chlorpheniramine maleate; phenyltoloxamine citrate] 40•10•5•15 mg

Tri-Phen-Mine syrup, drops ℞ *pediatric decongestant and antihistamine* [phenylpropanolamine HCl; phenylephrine HCl; chlorpheniramine maleate; phenyltoloxamine citrate] 5•1.25•0.5•2 mg/5 mL; 5•1.25•0.5•2 mg/mL

Tri-Phen-Mine S.R. timed-release tablets ℞ *decongestant; antihistamine* [phenylpropanolamine HCl; phenylephrine HCl; chlorpheniramine maleate; phenyltoloxamine citrate] 40•10•5•15 mg

Triphenyl syrup OTC *decongestant; antihistamine* [phenylpropanolamine HCl; chlorpheniramine maleate] 6.25•1 mg/5 mL

Triphenyl Expectorant liquid OTC *decongestant; expectorant* [phenylpropanolamine HCl; guaifenesin; alcohol 5%] 12.5•100 mg/5 mL

Triple Antibiotic ointment OTC *topical antibiotic* [polymyxin B sulfate; neomycin sulfate; bacitracin] 5000 U•3.5 mg•400 U per g

Triple Antibiotic ophthalmic ointment (discontinued 2000) ℞ *topical ophthalmic antibiotic* [polymyxin B sulfate; neomycin sulfate; bacitracin zinc] 5000 U•3.5 mg•400 U per g

Triple Sulfa vaginal cream ℞ *broad-spectrum bacteriostatic* [sulfathiazole; sulfacetamide; sulfabenzamide] 3.42%•2.86%•3.7%

triple sulfa (sulfathiazole, sulfacetamide, and sulfabenzamide) [q.v.]

Triple Vitamin ADC with Fluoride drops ℞ *pediatric vitamin supplement and dental caries preventative* [vitamins A, C, and D; fluoride] 1500 IU•35 mg•400 IU•0.5 mg per mL

Triple X Kit liquid + shampoo OTC *pediculicide for lice* [pyrethrins; piperonyl butoxide; petroleum distillate] 0.3%•3%•?

Triposed tablets, syrup OTC *decongestant; antihistamine* [pseudoephedrine HCl; triprolidine HCl] 60•2.5 mg; 30•1.25 mg/5 mL

tripotassium citrate monohydrate [see: potassium citrate]

triproamylin [see: pramlintide]

triprolidine INN *antihistamine* [also: triprolidine HCl]

triprolidine HCl USP *antihistamine* [also: triprolidine]

Tripterygium wilfordii *medicinal herb* [see: thunder god vine]

triptolide *investigational immunosuppressive and antineoplastic*

Triptone long-acting caplets OTC *antinauseant; antiemetic; antivertigo; motion sickness preventative* [dimenhydrinate] 50 mg

triptorelin USAN, INN *gonadotropin-releasing hormone (Gn-RH) antineoplastic*

triptorelin pamoate USAN *gonadotropin-releasing hormone (Gn-RH) agonist; antineoplastic for palliative treatment of advanced prostate cancer*

trisaccharides A & B *investigational (orphan) for newborn hemolytic disease and ABO blood incompatibility of organ or bone marrow transplants*

Trisan (CAN) foaming gel OTC *medicated cleanser for acne* [triclosan] 0,25%

Trisenox injection ℞ *antineoplastic for acute promyelocytic leukemia (APL)* [arsenic trioxide] 10 mg/10 mL

trisodium citrate [see: sodium citrate]

trisodium citrate dihydrate [see: sodium citrate]

trisodium hydrogen ethylenediaminetetraacetate [see: edetate trisodium]

Trisoralen tablets ℞ *systemic psoralens for repigmentation of idiopathic vitiligo; also used to enhance pigmentation and increase tolerance to sunlight* [trioxsalen] 5 mg

Tri-Statin II cream ℞ *topical corticosteroidal anti-inflammatory; antifungal* [triamcinolone acetonide; nystatin] 0.1%•100 000 U per g

Tristoject IM injection ℞ *corticosteroid; anti-inflammatory* [triamcinolone diacetate] 40 mg/mL

trisulfapyrimidines USP (a mixture of sulfadiazine, sulfamerazine, and sulfamethazine) *broad-spectrum bacteriostatic*

Tri-Super Flavons 1000 tablets OTC *dietary supplement* [mixed bioflavonoids] 1000 mg

Tritan tablets ℞ *decongestant; antihistamine* [phenylephrine tannate; chlorpheniramine tannate; pyrilamine tannate] 25•8•25 mg

Tri-Tannate tablets, pediatric oral suspension ℞ *decongestant; antihistamine* [phenylephrine tannate; chlorpheniramine tannate; pyrilamine tannate] 25•8•25 mg; 5•2•12.5 mg/5 mL

Tri-Tannate Plus Pediatric oral suspension ℞ *pediatric antitussive, decongestant, and antihistamine* [carbetapentane tannate; phenylephrine tannate; ephedrine tannate; chlorpheniramine tannate] 30•5•5•4 mg/5 mL

Tritec film-coated tablets ℞ *histamine H_2 antagonist for duodenal ulcers with H. pylori infection* [ranitidine bismuth citrate] 400 mg

tritheon [see: acinitrazole]

tritiated water USAN *radioactive agent*

Triticum repens *medicinal herb* [see: couch grass]

tritiozine INN

tritoqualine INN

Triva Douche powder OTC *antiseptic/germicidal; vaginal cleanser and deodorizer* [oxyquinoline sulfate] 2%

Trivagizole 3 vaginal cream OTC *topical antifungal for yeast infections* [clotrimazole] 2%

trivalent oral poliovirus vaccine (TOPV) [see: poliovirus vaccine, live oral]

Tri-Vi-Flor chewable tablets, drops ℞ *pediatric vitamin supplement and dental caries preventative* [vitamins A, C, and D; sodium fluoride] 2500 IU•60 mg•400 IU•1 mg; 1500 IU•35 mg•400 IU•0.25 mg, 1500 IU•35 mg•400 IU•0.5 mg per mL

Tri-Vi-Flor with Iron drops ℞ *pediatric vitamin/iron supplement and dental caries preventative* [vitamins A, C, and D; iron; sodium fluoride] 1500 IU•35 mg•400 IU•0.25 mg per mL

Tri-Vi-Sol drops OTC *pediatric vitamin supplement* [vitamins A, C, and D] 1500 IU•35 mg•400 IU per mL

Tri-Vi-Sol with Iron drops OTC *vitamin/iron supplement* [vitamins A, C, and D; ferrous sulfate] 1500 IU•35 mg•400 IU•10 mg per mL

Trivitamin Fluoride chewable tablets, drops ℞ *pediatric vitamin supplement and dental caries preventative* [vitamins A, C, and D; fluoride] 2500 IU•60 mg•400 IU•1 mg; 1500 IU•35 mg•400 IU•0.25 mg, 1500 IU•35 mg•400 IU•0.5 mg per mL

Tri-Vitamin Infants' Drops OTC *vitamin supplement* [vitamins A, C, and D] 1500 IU•35 mg•400 IU per mL

Tri-Vitamin with Fluoride drops ℞ *pediatric vitamin supplement and dental caries preventative* [vitamins A, C, and D; fluoride] 1500 IU•35 mg•400 IU•0.5 mg per mL

Trivora-28 tablets (in packs of 28) ℞ *triphasic oral contraceptive; emergency postcoital contraceptive* [levonorgestrel; ethinyl estradiol]
Phase 1 (6 days): 0.05 mg•30 μg;
Phase 2 (5 days): 0.075 mg•40 μg;
Phase 3 (10 days): 0.125 mg•30 μg

trixolane INN

Trizivir film-coated caplets ℞ *antiretroviral nucleoside reverse transcriptase inhibitor (NRTI) for HIV infection* [abacavir sulfate; zidovudine; lamivudine] 300•300•150 mg

trizoxime INN

Trizyme (ingredient) OTC *digestive enzymes* [amylolytic, proteolytic and cellulolytic enzymes (amylase; protease; cellulase)]

Trobicin powder for IM injection ℞ *antibiotic* [spectinomycin HCl] 400 mg/mL ⑨ tobramycin

Trocade ℞ *matrix metalloproteinase inhibitor; investigational cartilage protective agent for rheumatoid arthritis* [cipemastat]

Trocaine lozenges OTC *topical oral anesthetic* [benzocaine] 10 mg

Trocal lozenges OTC *antitussive* [dextromethorphan hydrobromide] 7.5 mg

trocimine INN

troclosene potassium USAN, INN *topical anti-infective*

trofosfamide INN

troglitazone USAN, INN *thiazolidinedione antidiabetic; increases cellular response to insulin without increasing insulin secretion*

trolamine USAN, NF *alkalizing agent; analgesic*

trolamine polypeptide oleate-condensate *cerumenolytic to emulsify and disperse ear wax*

troleandomycin USAN, USP *macrolide antibiotic; investigational (orphan) for severe asthma* [also: triacetyloleandomycin]

trolnitrate INN

trolnitrate phosphate [see: trolnitrate]

tromantadine INN

trometamol INN, BAN *alkalizer for cardiac bypass surgery* [also: tromethamine]

tromethamine USAN, USP *alkalizer for cardiac bypass surgery* [also: trometamol]

Tronolane anorectal cream OTC *topical local anesthetic* [pramoxine HCl] 1% ⑨ Tronothane

Tronolane rectal suppositories OTC *astringent; emollient* [zinc oxide] 11%

Tronothane HCl cream OTC *topical local anesthetic* [pramoxine HCl] 1% ⑨ Tronolane

tropabazate INN

Tropaeolum majus *medicinal herb* [see: Indian cress]

tropanserin INN, BAN *migraine-specific serotonin receptor antagonist* [also: tropanserin HCl]

tropanserin HCl USAN *migraine-specific serotonin receptor antagonist* [also: tropanserin]

tropapride INN

tropatepine INN

tropenziline bromide INN

TrophAmine 6%; TrophAmine 10% IV infusion ℞ *total parenteral* *nutrition; peripheral parenteral nutrition* [multiple essential and nonessential amino acids]

Trophite + Iron liquid OTC *hematinic* [ferric pyrophosphate; vitamins B_1 and B_{12}] 60 mg•30 mg•75 µg per 15 mL

trophosphamide [see: trofosfamide]

Tropicacyl eye drops ℞ *cycloplegic; mydriatic* [tropicamide] 0.5%, 1%

tropicamide USAN, USP, INN *ophthalmic anticholinergic; cycloplegic; short-acting mydriatic*

tropigline INN, BAN

tropirine INN

tropisetron INN, BAN *investigational treatment for nausea and vomiting related to chemotherapy*

Tropi-Storz eye drops ℞ *cycloplegic; mydriatic* [tropicamide] 0.5%, 1%

tropodifene INN

troquidazole INN

trospectomycin INN, BAN *broad-spectrum aminocyclitol antibiotic* [also: trospectomycin sulfate]

trospectomycin sulfate USAN *broad-spectrum aminocyclitol antibiotic* [also: trospectomycin]

trospium chloride INN

trovafloxacin mesylate USAN *broad-spectrum fluoroquinolone antibiotic*

Trovan film-coated tablets ℞ *broad-spectrum fluoroquinolone antibiotic* [trovafloxacin mesylate] 100, 200 mg

Trovan IV infusion ℞ *broad-spectrum fluoroquinolone antibiotic* [alatrofloxacin mesylate] 5 mg/mL ⑨ Atrovent

Trovan/Zithromax Compliance Pak ℞ *single-dose antibiotic treatment for sexually transmitted diseases* [Trovan (trovafloxacin mesylate); Zithromax (azithromycin)] 100 mg tablet; 1 g packet for oral suspension

Trovert ℞ *investigational (Phase II, orphan) growth hormone antagonist for acromegaly* [B2036-PEG (code name —generic name not yet assigned)] ⑨ Provir; Provera

troxacitabine USAN *antineoplastic for various leukemias and solid tumors*

troxerutin INN, BAN *vitamin* P_4

troxidone BAN *anticonvulsant* [also: trimethadione]

troxipide INN

troxolamide INN

troxonium tosilate INN [also: troxonium tosylate]

troxonium tosylate BAN [also: troxonium tosilate]

troxundate INN *combining name for radicals or groups*

troxypyrrolium tosilate INN [also: troxypyrrolium tosylate]

troxypyrrolium tosylate BAN [also: troxypyrrolium tosilate]

true ivy *medicinal herb* [see: English ivy]

T.R.U.E. Test patch *diagnostic aid for contact dermatitis* [skin test antigens (23 different) plus 1 negative control]

Truphylline suppositories ℞ *antiasthmatic; bronchodilator* [aminophylline] 250, 500 mg

Trusopt eye drops ℞ *topical carbonic anhydrase inhibitor for glaucoma* [dorzolamide HCl] 2%

truxicurium iodide INN

truxipicurium iodide INN

trypaflavine [see: acriflavine HCl]

tryparsamide USP, INN

trypsin, crystallized USP *topical proteolytic enzyme; necrotic tissue debridement*

tryptizol [see: amitriptyline]

tryptizol HCl [see: amitriptyline HCl]

tryptophan (L-tryptophan) USAN, USP, INN *essential amino acid; serotonin precursor (The FDA has recalled all OTC tryptophan supplements.)*

Trysul vaginal cream (discontinued 2001) ℞ *broad-spectrum bacteriostatic* [sulfathiazole; sulfacetamide; sulfabenzamide] 3.42%•2.86%•3.7%

TSC (technetium sulfur colloid) [see: technetium Tc 99m sulfur colloid]

T/Scalp liquid OTC *topical corticosteroidal anti-inflammatory* [hydrocortisone] 1%

TSH (thyroid-stimulating hormone) [see: thyrotropin]

TSPA (triethylenethiophosphoramide) [see: thiotepa]

TST (tuberculin skin test) [see: tuberculin]

T-Stat topical solution, medicated pads ℞ *topical antibiotic for acne* [erythromycin] 2%

Tsuga canadensis *medicinal herb* [see: hemlock]

T-Tabs (trademarked form) *tablets with a "T" imprint*

tuaminoheptane USP, INN *adrenergic; vasoconstrictor*

tuaminoheptane sulfate USP

tuberculin USP *dermal tuberculosis test*

tuberculin, crude [see: tuberculin]

tuberculin, old (OT) [see: tuberculin]

tuberculin purified protein derivative (PPD) [see: tuberculin]

Tuberculin Tine Test, Old single-use intradermal puncture test device *tuberculosis skin test* [old tuberculin] 5 U

tuberculosis vaccine [see: BCG vaccine]

Tubersol intradermal injection ℞ *tuberculosis skin test* [tuberculin purified protein derivative] 1, 5, 250 U/0.1 mL

Tubex (trademarked delivery system) *cartridge-needle unit*

tubocurarine chloride USP, INN, BAN *neuromuscular blocker; muscle relaxant* 3 mg (20 U)/mL injection

tubocurarine chloride HCl pentahydrate [see: tubocurarine chloride]

tubulozole INN *antineoplastic; microtubule inhibitor* [also: tubulozole HCl]

tubulozole HCl USAN, INN *antineoplastic; microtubule inhibitor* [also: tubulozole]

tucaresol INN, BAN *investigational (Phase II) immunopotentiator for HIV infection*

Tucks; Tucks Take-Alongs cleansing pads OTC *moisturizer and cleanser for the perineal area; astringent* [witch hazel; glycerin] 50%•10%

Tucks Clear gel OTC *astringent* [hamamelis water; glycerin] 50%•10%

tuclazepam INN

Tuinal Pulvules (capsules) ℞ *sedative; hypnotic; also abused as a street drug* [amobarbital sodium; secobarbital sodium] 50•50, 100•100 mg ⓓ Luminal; Tylenol

tulobuterol INN, BAN, JAN [also: tulobuterol HCl]

tulobuterol HCl JAN [also: tulobuterol]

tulopafant INN

tumeric root *medicinal herb* [see: goldenseal]

tumor necrosis factor (TNF) *investigational (Phase I) antiviral for HIV infection* [also see: anti-TNF MAb]

tumor necrosis factor-binding protein I and II *investigational (orphan) for symptomatic AIDS patients*

tumor necrosis therapy (TNT) *investigational (orphan) radioactive chimeric monoclonal antibody for malignant glioma and astrocytoma*

Tums; Tums E-X; Tums Ultra; Tums Calcium for Life PMS; Tums Calcium for Life Bone Health chewable tablets OTC *antacid; calcium supplement* [calcium carbonate] 500 mg; 750 mg; 1 g; 750 mg; 1250 mg

Tums 500 chewable tablets (discontinued 2000) OTC *antacid; calcium supplement* [calcium carbonate] 1.25 g

tung seed *(Aleurites cordata; A. moluccana)* seed and oil *medicinal herb for asthma, bowel evacuation, and tumors; not generally regarded as safe, as it is highly toxic*

tungsten *element (W)*

Turbinaire (trademarked delivery system) *nasal inhalation aerosol*

Turbuhaler (trademarked delivery system) *dry powder in a metered-dose inhaler*

turkey corn *(Corydalis formosa)* root *medicinal herb used as an antisyphilitic, bitter tonic, and diuretic*

turkey pea; wild turkey pea *medicinal herb* [see: turkey corn]

turmeric *(Curcuma domestica; C. longa)* rhizomes *medicinal herb for flatulence, hemorrhage, hepatitis and jaundice, topical analgesia, and ringworm*

Turnera aphrodisiaca; T. diffusa; T. microphylla *medicinal herb* [see: damiana]

turosteride INN

turpentine *(Pinus palustris)* gum *natural treatment for colds, cough, and toothache; also used topically as a counterirritant for muscle pain and rheumatic disorders*

turtlebloom *(Chelone glabra)* leaves *medicinal herb used as an anthelmintic, aperient, cholagogue, and detergent*

Tusibron syrup OTC *expectorant* [guaifenesin; alcohol 3.5%] 100 mg/5 mL ⊡ Tussigon

Tusibron-DM syrup OTC *antitussive; expectorant* [dextromethorphan hydrobromide; guaifenesin] 15•100 mg/5 mL

Tusquelin syrup ℞ *antitussive; decongestant; antihistamine; analgesic* [dextromethorphan hydrobromide; phenylpropanolamine HCl; phenylephrine HCl; chlorpheniramine maleate; alcohol 5%] 15•5•5•2 mg/5 mL

Tussafed syrup, pediatric drops ℞ *antitussive; decongestant; antihistamine* [dextromethorphan hydrobromide; pseudoephedrine HCl; carbinoxamine maleate; menthol] 15•60•4 mg/5 mL; 4•25•2 mg/mL ⊡ Tussafin

Tussafed HC syrup ℞ *narcotic antitussive; decongestant; expectorant* [hydrocodone bitartrate; phenylephrine HCl; guaifenesin] 2.5•7.5•50 mg/5 mL

Tussafed-LA sustained-release tablets ℞ *antitussive; decongestant; expectorant* [dextromethorphan hydrobromide; pseudoephedrine HCl; guaifenesin] 30•60•600 mg

Tussafin Expectorant liquid ℞ *narcotic antitussive; decongestant; expectorant* [hydrocodone bitartrate; pseudoephedrine HCl; guaifenesin; alcohol 12.5%] 5•60•200 mg/5 mL ⊡ Tussafed

Tuss-Allergine Modified T.D. capsules ℞ *antitussive; decongestant* [caramiphen edisylate; phenylpropanolamine HCl] 40•75 mg

Tussanil DH syrup ℞ *narcotic antitussive; decongestant; antihistamine* [hydrocodone bitartrate; phenylephrine HCl; chlorpheniramine maleate; alcohol 5%] 2.5•10•4 mg/5 mL

Tussanil DH tablets ℞ *narcotic antitussive; decongestant; expectorant; analgesic* [hydrocodone bitartrate; phenylpropanolamine HCl; guaifenesin; salicylamide] 1.66•25•100•300 mg

Tussar DM syrup OTC *antitussive; decongestant; antihistamine* [dextromethorphan hydrobromide; pseudoephedrine HCl; chlorpheniramine maleate] 15•30•2 mg/5 mL

Tussar SF; Tussar-2 liquid ℞ *narcotic antitussive; antihistamine; expectorant* [codeine phosphate; pseudoephedrine HCl; guaifenesin; alcohol 2.5%] 10•30•100 mg/5 mL

Tuss-DM tablets OTC *antitussive; expectorant* [dextromethorphan hydrobromide; guaifenesin] 10•200 mg

Tussend syrup ℞ *narcotic antitussive; decongestant; antihistamine* [hydrocodone bitartrate; pseudoephedrine HCl; chlorpheniramine maleate; alcohol 5%] 2.5•30•2 mg/5 mL

Tussex Cough syrup OTC *antitussive; decongestant; expectorant* [dextromethorphan hydrobromide; phenylephrine HCl; guaifenesin] 10•5•100 mg/5 mL ⊡ Tussionex; Tussirex

Tussi-12 tablets, oral suspension ℞ *pediatric antitussive, decongestant, and antihistamine* [carbetapentane tannate; phenylephrine tannate; chlorpheniramine tannate] 60•10•5 mg; 30•5•4 mg/5 mL

Tussigon tablets ℞ *narcotic antitussive; anticholinergic* [hydrocodone bitartrate; homatropine methylbromide] 5•1.5 mg ⊡ Tusibron

Tussilago farfara *medicinal herb* [see: coltsfoot]

Tussionex Pennkinetic extended-release suspension ℞ *narcotic antitussive; antihistamine* [hydrocodone polistirex; chlorpheniramine polistirex] 10•8 mg/5 mL ⊡ Tussex; Tussirex

Tussi-Organidin DM NR; Tussi-Organidin DM-S NR liquid (S includes a 10 mL oral syringe) ℞ *antitussive; expectorant* [dextromethorphan hydrobromide; guaifenesin] 10•100 mg/5 mL

Tussi-Organidin NR; Tussi-Organidin-S NR liquid (S includes a 10 mL oral syringe) ℞ *narcotic antitussive; expectorant* [codeine phosphate; guaifenesin] 10•100 mg/5 mL

Tussirex syrup, sugar-free liquid ℞ *narcotic antitussive; decongestant; antihistamine; expectorant; analgesic* [codeine phosphate; phenylephrine HCl; pheniramine maleate; sodium citrate; sodium salicylate; caffeine citrate] 10•4.17•13.33•83.3•83.33•25 mg/5 mL ⓢ Tussex; Tussionex

Tuss-LA sustained-release tablets ℞ *decongestant; expectorant* [pseudoephedrine HCl; guaifenesin] 120•500 mg

Tusso-DM liquid ℞ *antitussive; expectorant* [dextromethorphan hydrobromide; iodinated glycerol] 10•30 mg/5 mL

Tussogest extended-release capsules ℞ *antitussive; decongestant* [caramiphen edisylate; phenylpropanolamine HCl] 40•75 mg

Tuss-Ornade Spansules (sustained-release capsules), liquid (discontinued 1997) ℞ *antitussive; decongestant* [caramiphen edisylate; phenylpropanolamine HCl] 40•75 mg; 6.7•12.5 mg/5 mL

Tuss-Tan tablets, pediatric oral suspension ℞ *antitussive; decongestant; antihistamine* [carbetapentane tannate; phenylephrine tannate; ephedrine tannate; chlorpheniramine tannate] 60•10•10•5 mg; 30•5•5•4 mg/5 mL

Tusstat syrup ℞ *antihistamine; antitussive* [diphenhydramine HCl; alcohol 5%] 12.5 mg/5 mL

tuvatidine INN

tuvirumab USAN, INN *investigational (Phase II) antiviral monoclonal antibody for hepatitis B*

TVC-2 Dandruff Shampoo (discontinued 1998) OTC *antiseborrheic; antibacterial; antifungal* [pyrithione zinc] 2%

T-Vites tablets OTC *vitamin/mineral supplement* [multiple vitamins & minerals; biotin] ≛•30 μg

12 Hour nasal spray OTC *nasal decongestant* [oxymetazoline HCl] 0.05%

12 Hour Cold sustained-release tablets OTC *decongestant; antihistamine* [pseudoephedrine sulfate; dexbrompheniramine maleate] 120•6 mg

20-20 tablets OTC *CNS stimulant; analeptic* [caffeine] 200 mg

Twice-A-Day nasal spray OTC *nasal decongestant* [oxymetazoline HCl] 0.05%

Twilite caplets OTC *antihistaminic sleep aid* [diphenhydramine HCl] 50 mg

twin leaf *(Jeffersonia diphylla)* root *medicinal herb used as an antirheumatic, antispasmodic, antisyphilitic, diuretic, emetic, and expectorant*

Twin-K liquid ℞ *potassium supplement* [potassium gluconate; potassium citrate] 20 mEq/15 mL (K)

Twinrix IM injection ℞ *immunizing agent for hepatitis A, B, and D in adults* [hepatitis A vaccine, inactivated; hepatitis B virus vaccine, recombinant] 720 EL.U.•20 μg per mL

TwoCal HN ready-to-use liquid OTC *enteral nutritional therapy* [lactose-free formula]

Two-Dyne capsules (discontinued 1998) ℞ *analgesic; sedative* [acetaminophen; caffeine; butalbital] 325•40•50 mg

tybamate USAN, NF, INN, BAN *minor tranquilizer*

tyformin BAN [also: tiformin]

tylcalsin [see: calcium acetylsalicylate]

tylemalum [see: carbubarb]

Tylenol tablets, caplets, gelcaps, liquid OTC *analgesic; antipyretic* [acetaminophen] 325, 500 mg; 325, 650 mg; 500 mg; 500 mg/15 mL ℞ Tuinal

Tylenol, Children's chewable tablets, oral liquid OTC *analgesic; antipyretic* [acetaminophen] 80 mg; 160 mg/5 mL

Tylenol Allergy Sinus caplets, gelcaps OTC *decongestant; antihistamine; analgesic* [pseudoephedrine HCl; chlorpheniramine maleate; acetaminophen] 30•2•500 mg

Tylenol Allergy Sinus NightTime caplets OTC *decongestant; antihistamine; analgesic* [pseudoephedrine HCl; diphenhydramine HCl; acetaminophen] 30•25•500 mg

Tylenol Arthritis Extended Relief extended-release caplets OTC *analgesic; antipyretic* [acetaminophen] 650 mg

Tylenol Cold, Children's chewable tablets, liquid OTC *pediatric decongestant, antihistamine and analgesic* [pseudoephedrine HCl; chlorpheniramine maleate; acetaminophen] 7.5•0.5•80 mg; 15•1•160 mg/5 mL

Tylenol Cold, Multi-Symptom caplets, tablets OTC *antitussive; decongestant; antihistamine; analgesic* [dextromethorphan hydrobromide; pseudoephedrine HCl; chlorpheniramine maleate; acetaminophen] 10•30•2•325 mg

Tylenol Cold Multi Symptom Plus Cough, Children's liquid OTC *pediatric antitussive, decongestant, antihistamine, and analgesic* [dextromethorphan hydrobromide; pseudoephedrine HCl; chlorpheniramine maleate; acetaminophen] 5•15•1•160 mg/5 mL

Tylenol Cold No Drowsiness caplets, gelcaps OTC *antitussive; decongestant; analgesic* [dextromethorphan hydrobromide; pseudoephedrine HCl; acetaminophen] 15•30•325 mg

Tylenol Cold Plus Cough, Children's chewable tablets OTC *antitussive; decongestant; antihistamine; analgesic* [dextromethorphan hydrobromide; pseudoephedrine HCl; chlorpheniramine maleate; acetaminophen] 2.5•7.5•0.5•80 mg

Tylenol Cough, Multi-Symptom liquid OTC *antitussive; analgesic* [dextromethorphan hydrobromide; acetaminophen; alcohol 5%] 10•216.7 mg/5 mL

Tylenol Cough with Decongestant, Multi-Symptom liquid OTC *antitussive; decongestant; analgesic* [dextromethorphan hydrobromide; pseudoephedrine HCl; acetaminophen; alcohol 5%] 10•20•200 mg/5 mL

Tylenol Extended Relief (name changed to Tylenol Arthritis Extended Relief in 1998)

Tylenol Flu gelcaps OTC *antitussive; decongestant; analgesic* [dextromethorphan hydrobromide; pseudoephedrine HCl; acetaminophen] 15•30•500 mg

Tylenol Flu NightTime gelcaps, powder OTC *decongestant; antihistamine; analgesic* [pseudoephedrine HCl; diphenhydramine HCl; acetaminophen] 30•25•500 mg; 60•50•1000 mg/packet

Tylenol Headache Plus caplets (discontinued 2000) OTC *analgesic; antipyretic; antacid* [acetaminophen; calcium carbonate] 500•250 mg

Tylenol Infants' Drops solution OTC *analgesic; antipyretic* [acetaminophen] 100 mg/mL

Tylenol Junior Strength chewable tablets OTC *analgesic; antipyretic* [acetaminophen] 160 mg

Tylenol Menstrual (CAN) tablets OTC *analgesic; diuretic; antihistamine* [acetaminophen; pamabrom; pyrilamine maleate] 500•25•15 mg

Tylenol Multi-Symptom Hot Medication powder for oral solution OTC *antitussive; decongestant; antihistamine; analgesic* [dextromethorphan hydrobromide; pseudoephedrine HCl; chlorpheniramine maleate; acetaminophen] 30•60•4•650 mg/packet

Tylenol Multi-Symptom Menstrual Relief, Women's caplets OTC *anal-*

gesic; diuretic [acetaminophen; pamabrom] 500•25 mg

Tylenol No. 2, No. 3, and No. 4 [see: Tylenol with Codeine]

Tylenol PM tablets, caplets, gelcaps OTC *antihistaminic sleep aid; analgesic* [diphenhydramine HCl; acetaminophen] 25•500 mg

Tylenol Severe Allergy caplets OTC *antihistamine; analgesic* [diphenhydramine HCl; acetaminophen] 12.5•500 mg

Tylenol Sinus tablets, caplets, geltabs, gelcaps OTC *decongestant; analgesic; antipyretic* [pseudoephedrine HCl; acetaminophen] 30•500 mg

Tylenol Sore Throat oral liquid OTC *analgesic; antipyretic* [acetaminophen] 1000 mg/30 mL

Tylenol with Codeine elixir ℞ *narcotic analgesic* [codeine phosphate; acetaminophen] 12•120 mg/5 mL

Tylenol with Codeine No. 2, No. 3, and No. 4 tablets ℞ *narcotic analgesic; sometimes abused as a street drug* [codeine phosphate; acetaminophen] 15•300 mg; 30•300 mg; 60•300 mg

tylosin INN, BAN

Tylox capsules ℞ *narcotic analgesic* [oxycodone HCl; acetaminophen] 5•500 mg

tyloxapol USAN, USP, INN, BAN *detergent; wetting agent; cleaner/lubricant for artificial eyes; investigational (orphan) for cystic fibrosis*

Tympagesic ear drops ℞ *topical local anesthetic; analgesic; decongestant* [benzocaine; antipyrine; phenylephrine HCl] 5%•5%•0.25%

Typherex (commercially available in England) ℞ *investigational vaccine for typhoid fever*

Typherix (CAN) IM injection in prefilled syringe ℞ *typhoid vaccine for adults and children over 2 years* [typhoid vaccine (Ty-2), Vi polysaccharide] 25 µg/0.5 mL

Typhim Vi IM injection ℞ *typhoid vaccine for adults and children over 2 years* [typhoid vaccine (Ty-2), Vi polysaccharide] 25µg/0.5 mL

typhoid vaccine USP *active bacterin for typhoid fever (Salmonella typhi Ty21a, attenuated)*

Typhoid Vaccine (AKD) subcu injection by jet injectors only ℞ *typhoid vaccine for military use only* [typhoid vaccine (Ty-2), acetone-killed and dried] 8 U/mL

Typhoid Vaccine (H-P) subcu injection (incompatible with jet injectors) ℞ *typhoid vaccine for adults and children* [typhoid vaccine (Ty-2), heat- and phenol-inactivated] 8 U/mL

typhoid Vi capsular polysaccharide vaccine *active bacterin for typhoid fever (Salmonella typhi Ty-2, inactivated)*

typhus vaccine USP

"typical" antipsychotics [see: conventional antipsychotics]

Tyrex-2 powder OTC *enteral nutritional therapy for tyrosinemia type II*

Tyrodone liquid ℞ *antitussive; decongestant* [hydrodocone bitartrate; pseudoephedrine HCl; alcohol 5%] 5•60 mg/5 mL

tyromedan INN *thyromimetic* [also: thyromedan HCl]

tyromedan HCl [see: thyromedan HCl]

Tyromex-1 powder OTC *formula for infants with tyrosinemia type I*

tyropanoate sodium USAN, USP *oral radiopaque contrast medium for cholecystography (57.4% iodine)* [also: sodium tyropanoate]

tyrosine (L-tyrosine) USAN, USP, INN *nonessential amino acid; symbols: Tyr, Y*

Tyrosum Cleanser liquid, packets OTC *topical cleanser for acne* [isopropanol; acetone] 50%•10%

tyrothricin USP, INN *antibacterial*

Tyzine nasal spray, nose drops, pediatric drops ℞ *nasal decongestant* [tetrahydrozoline HCl] 0.1%; 0.1%; 0.05%

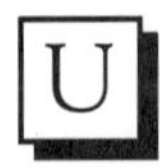

UAA sugar-coated tablets ℞ *urinary antibiotic; analgesic; antispasmodic; acidifier* [methenamine; phenyl salicylate; atropine sulfate; methylene blue; hyoscyamine sulfate; benzoic acid] 40.8•18.1•0.03•5.4•0.03•4.5 mg

UAD Otic ear drop suspension ℞ *topical corticosteroidal anti-inflammatory; antibiotic* [hydrocortisone; neomycin sulfate; polymyxin B sulfate] 1%•5 mg•10 000 U per mL

ubenimex INN

ubidecarenone INN

ubiquinone [see: coenzyme Q10]

ubisindine INN

UBT Breath Test for H. pylori test for professional use *diagnostic aid for the detection of ulcers*

Ucephan oral solution ℞ *to prevent and treat hyperammonemia of urea cycle enzymopathy (orphan)* [sodium benzoate; sodium phenylacetate] 10•10 g/100 mL

UCG Beta Slide Monoclonal II slide tests for professional use *in vitro diagnostic aid; urine pregnancy test*

UCG Slide tests for professional use *in vitro diagnostic aid; urine pregnancy test* [latex agglutination test]

U-Cort cream (discontinued 1997) ℞ *topical corticosteroidal anti-inflammatory* [hydrocortisone acetate] 1%

UDIP (trademarked packaging form) *unit-dose identification package*

Uendex ℞ *investigational (Phase II) antiviral for HIV and AIDS; investigational (orphan) for cystic fibrosis* [dextran sulfate]

ufenamate INN

ufiprazole INN

UFT capsules ℞ *antimetabolite antineoplastic; investigational (NDA filed) adjunct to leucovorin calcium for advanced colorectal cancer* [uracil; tegafur] 1:4

U-Ject (trademarked delivery system) *prefilled disposable syringe*

Ulcerease mouth rinse OTC *topical antipruritic/counterirritant; mild local anesthetic* [phenol] 0.6%

uldazepam USAN, INN *sedative*

ulinastatin INN

Ulmus fulva; U. rubra *medicinal herb* [see: slippery elm]

ulobetasol INN *topical corticosteroidal anti-inflammatory* [also: halobetasol propionate]

ULR-LA long-acting tablets ℞ *decongestant; expectorant* [phenylpropanolamine HCl; guaifenesin] 75•400 mg

Ultane liquid for vaporization ℞ *inhalation general anesthetic* [sevoflurane]

Ultiva powder for IV infusion ℞ *short-acting narcotic analgesic for general anesthesia* [remifentanil HCl] 1 mg/mL

Ultra Derm lotion, bath oil OTC *moisturizer; emollient*

Ultra KLB6 tablets OTC *dietary supplement* [vitamin B_6; multiple food supplements] 16.7•≛ mg

Ultra Mide 25 lotion OTC *moisturizer; emollient; keratolytic* [urea] 25%

Ultra Tears eye drops OTC *ophthalmic moisturizer/lubricant* [hydroxypropyl methylcellulose] 1%

Ultra Vent (trademarked delivery system) *jet nebulizer*

Ultra Vita Time tablets OTC *dietary supplement* [multiple vitamins & minerals; multiple food products; iron; folic acid; biotin] ≛•6•0.4•1 mg

UltraBrom sustained-release capsules ℞ *decongestant; antihistamine* [pseudoephedrine HCl; brompheniramine maleate] 120•12 mg

UltraBrom PD timed-release capsules ℞ *pediatric decongestant and antihistamine* [pseudoephedrine HCl; brompheniramine maleate] 60•6 mg

Ultracal liquid OTC *enteral nutritional therapy* [lactose-free formula]

Ultra-Care solution + tablets OTC *two-step chemical disinfecting system for soft contact lenses* [hydrogen peroxide-based] 3%

Ultracet tablets ℞ *central analgesic for acute pain* [tramadol HCl; acetaminophen] 37.5•325 mg

Ultra-Freeda; Ultra Freeda, Iron Free tablets OTC *geriatric vitamin/mineral supplement* [multiple vitamins & minerals; folic acid; biotin] ≛•270•100 μg

UltraJect prefilled syringe ℞ *narcotic analgesic* [morphine sulfate]

Ultralan liquid OTC *enteral nutritional therapy* [lactose-free formula]

Ultram film-coated tablets ℞ *central analgesic* [tramadol HCl] 50 mg

Ultram XL ℞ *investigational (Phase III) extended-release formulation* [tramadol HCl]

UltraMide 25 (CAN) lotion OTC *moisturizer; emollient* [urea] 25%

Ultra-Natal tablets ℞ *vitamin/mineral/iron supplement for pregnancy and lactation* [multiple vitamins & minerals; carbonyl iron; folic acid] ≛•90 mg iron•1 mg

Ultrase; Ultrase MT 12; Ultrase MT 18; Ultrase MT 20 capsules ℞ *digestive enzymes* [lipase; protease; amylase] 4500•25 000•20 000 U; 12 000•39 000•39 000 U; 18 000•58 500•58 500 U; 20 000•65 000•65 000 U

Ultravate ointment, cream ℞ *topical corticosteroidal anti-inflammatory* [halobetasol propionate] 0.05%

Ultravist IV injection ℞ *radiopaque contrast medium for imaging of the head, heart, peripheral vascular system, and genitourinary tract* [iopromide (39% iodine)] 311.7, 498.72, 623.4, 768.86 mg/mL (150, 240, 300, 370 mg/mL)

Ultrazyme Enzymatic Cleaner effervescent tablets OTC *enzymatic cleaner for soft contact lenses* [subtilisin A]

Umatrope ℞ *investigational treatment for short bowel syndrome (SBS) in children* [somatropin]

umespirone INN

uña de gato *medicinal herb* [see: cat's claw]

Unasyn powder for IV or IM injection ℞ *aminopenicillin antibiotic plus synergist* [ampicillin sodium; sulbactam sodium] 1•0.5, 2•1, 10•5 g 🔊 Anacin; Unisom

Uncaria guianensis; U. tomentosa *medicinal herb* [see: cat's claw]

10-undecenoic acid [see: undecylenic acid]

10-undecenoic acid, calcium salt [see: calcium undecylenate]

undecoylium chloride-iodine

undecylenic acid USP *antifungal*

Unguentine ointment OTC *minor burn treatment* [phenol; zinc oxide; eucalyptus oil] 1%•?•?

Unguentine Plus cream OTC *topical local anesthetic* [lidocaine HCl; phenol] 2%•0.5%

Unguentum Bossi cream ℞ *topical antipsoriatic; anti-infective; bactericidal* [ammoniated mercury; methenamine sulfosalicylate; coal tar] 5%•2%•2%

Uni-Ace drops OTC *analgesic; antipyretic* [acetaminophen] 100 mg/mL

Uni-Amp (trademarked packaging form) *single-dose ampule*

Unibase OTC *ointment base*

Uni-Bent Cough syrup OTC *antihistamine; antitussive* [diphenhydramine HCl; alcohol 5%] 12.5 mg/5 mL

Unicap capsules, tablets OTC *vitamin supplement* [multiple vitamins; folic acid] ≛•0.4 mg

Unicap Jr. chewable tablets OTC *vitamin supplement* [multiple vitamins; folic acid] ≛•0.4 mg

Unicap M; Unicap T tablets OTC *vitamin/mineral/iron supplement* [multiple vitamins & minerals; iron; folic acid] ≛•18•0.4 mg

Unicap Plus Iron tablets OTC *vitamin/iron supplement* [multiple vitamins; iron; folic acid] ≛•22.5•0.4 mg

Unicap Sr. tablets OTC *vitamin/mineral/iron supplement* [multiple vitamins & minerals; iron; folic acid] ≛•10•0.4 mg

Unicomplex T & M tablets OTC *vitamin/mineral/iron supplement* [multiple vitamins & minerals; iron; folic acid] ≛•18•0.4 mg

Uni-Decon sustained-release tablets ℞ *decongestant; antihistamine* [phenylpropanolamine HCl; phenylephrine HCl; chlorpheniramine maleate; phenyltoloxamine citrate] 40•10•5•15 mg

Uni-Dur extended-release tablets ℞ *once-daily antiasthmatic/bronchodilator* [theophylline] 400, 600 mg

Unifiber powder OTC *bulk laxative* [cellulose powder]

unifocon A USAN *hydrophobic contact lens material*

Unilax capsules (discontinued 1998) OTC *stimulant laxative; stool softener* [phenolphthalein; docusate sodium] 130•230 mg

Unimatic (trademarked delivery system) *prefilled disposable syringe*

Uni-nest (trademarked packaging form) *ampule*

Unipak (packaging form) *dispensing pack*

Unipen capsules ℞ *penicillinase-resistant penicillin antibiotic* [nafcillin sodium] 250 mg ⊡ Omnipen

Unipen film-coated tablets, powder for IV or IM injection (discontinued 1998) ℞ *penicillinase-resistant penicillin antibiotic* [nafcillin sodium] 500 mg; 0.5, 1, 2, 10 g ⊡ Omnipen

Uniphyl timed-release tablets ℞ *antiasthmatic; bronchodilator* [theophylline] 400, 600 mg

Uniprost (name changed to Remodulin for NDA 2001)

Uniquin (foreign name for U.S. product Maxaquin)

Uniretic tablets ℞ *antihypertensive; angiotensin-converting enzyme (ACE) inhibitor; diuretic* [moexipril HCl; hydrochlorothiazide] 7.5•12.5, 15•25 mg

Uni-Rx (trademarked packaging form) *unit-dose containers and packages*

Unisert (trademarked dosage form) *suppository*

Unisol; Unisol 4 solution OTC *rinsing/storage solution for soft contact lenses* [sodium chloride (saline solution)]

Unisol Plus aerosol solution OTC *rinsing/storage solution for soft contact lenses* [sodium chloride (saline solution)]

Unisom Natural Source (CAN) gel capsules OTC *herbal sleep aid* [valerian extract (from valerian root)] 100 mg (400 mg)

Unisom Nighttime Sleep-Aid tablets OTC *antihistaminic sleep aid* [doxylamine succinate] 25 mg ⊡ Anacin; Unasyn

Unisom SleepGels (capsules) OTC *antihistaminic sleep aid* [diphenhydramine HCl] 50 mg ⊡ Anacin; Unasyn

Unisom with Pain Relief tablets OTC *antihistaminic sleep aid; analgesic* [diphenhydramine citrate; acetaminophen] 50•650 mg ⊡ Anacin; Unasyn

Unistep hCG test kit for professional use *in vitro diagnostic aid; urine pregnancy test*

Unithroid tablets ℞ *synthetic thyroid T_4 hormone* [levothyroxine sodium] 25, 50, 75, 88, 100, 112, 125, 150, 175, 200, 300 µg

Unitrol timed-release capsules OTC *diet aid* [phenylpropanolamine HCl] 75 mg

Unituss HC syrup ℞ *narcotic antitussive; decongestant; antihistamine* [hydrocodone bitartrate; phenylephrine HCl; chlorpheniramine maleate] 2.5•5•2 mg/5 mL

Uni-Tussin syrup OTC *expectorant* [guaifenesin; alcohol 3.5%] 100 mg/5 mL

Uni-Tussin DM syrup OTC *antitussive; expectorant* [dextromethorphan hydrobromide; guaifenesin] 10•100 mg/5 mL

Univasc film-coated tablets ℞ *antihypertensive; angiotensin-converting enzyme (ACE) inhibitor* [moexipril HCl] 7.5, 15 mg

Univial (trademarked form) *single-dose vials*

Unna's boot [see: Dome-Paste bandage]

unoprostone isopropyl *topical prostaglandin $F_{2\alpha}$ analogue for glaucoma and ocular hypertension*

Uprima sublingual tablets ℞ *investigational (NDA filed) dopamine receptor agonist for erectile dysfunction* [apomorphine HCl] 2, 3, 4 mg
Uracid capsules ℞ *urinary acidifier to control ammonia production* [racemethionine] 200 mg ⓢ uracil; Urised; Urocit
uracil USAN *antineoplastic potentiator for tegafur (not available separately; combined with tegafur in a 1:4 ratio)*
uracil mustard USAN, USP *nitrogen mustard-type alkylating antineoplastic* [also: uramustine] ⓢ Uracel; Uracid
Uracyst-S; Uracyst-S Concentrate (CAN) liquid for bladder instillation ℞ *glycosaminoglycan temporary replacement* [chondroitan sulfate sodium] 2 mg/mL; 20 mg/mL
uradal [see: carbromal]
uralenic acid [see: enoxolone]
uramustine INN, BAN *nitrogen mustard-type alkylating antineoplastic* [also: uracil mustard]
uranin [see: fluorescein sodium]
uranium *element (U)*
urapidil INN, BAN
urea USP *osmotic diuretic; keratolytic; emollient*
urea peroxide [see: carbamide peroxide]
Ureacin-10 lotion OTC *moisturizer; emollient; keratolytic* [urea] 10%
Ureacin-20 cream OTC *moisturizer; emollient; keratolytic* [urea] 20%
Ureaphil IV infusion ℞ *osmotic diuretic* [urea] 40 g/150 mL
Urecholine tablets, subcu injection (discontinued 2001) ℞ *cholinergic urinary stimulant for postsurgical and postpartum urinary retention* [bethanechol chloride] 5, 10, 25, 50 mg; 5 mg/mL
uredepa USAN, INN *antineoplastic*
uredofos USAN, INN *veterinary anthelmintic*
urefibrate INN
***p*-ureidobenzenearsonic acid** [see: carbarsone]
urethan NF [also: urethane]
urethane INN, BAN [also: urethan]
urethane polymers [see: polyurethane foam]
Urex tablets ℞ *urinary antibiotic* [methenamine hippurate] 1 g ⓢ Eurax; Serax
Urginea indica; U. maritima; U. scilla *medicinal herb* [see: squill]
Uricult culture paddles for professional use *in vitro diagnostic aid for nitrate, uropathogens, or bacteria in the urine*
uridine 5′-triphosphate *investigational (Phase I/II, orphan) for cystic fibrosis and primary ciliary dyskinesia*
Uridon Modified sugar-coated tablets ℞ *urinary antibiotic; analgesic; antispasmodic; acidifier* [methenamine; phenyl salicylate; atropine sulfate; methylene blue; hyoscyamine sulfate; benzoic acid] 40.8•18.1•0.03•5.4•0.03•4.5 mg
Urimar-T tablets ℞ *urinary antibiotic; antiseptic; analgesic; antispasmodic* [methenamine; sodium biphosphate; phenyl salicylate; methylene blue; hyoscyamine sulfate] 81.6•40.8•36.2•10.8•0.12 mg
Urimax film-coated tablets ℞ *urinary antibiotic; analgesic; antispasmodic; acidifier* [methenamine; phenyl salicylate; methylene blue; hyoscyamine sulfate; sodium biphosphate] 81.6•36.2•10.8•0.12•40.8 mg
Urinary Antiseptic No. 2 tablets ℞ *urinary antibiotic; analgesic; antispasmodic; acidifier* [methenamine; phenyl salicylate; atropine sulfate; methylene blue; hyoscyamine sulfate; benzoic acid] 40.8•18.1•0.03•5.4•0.03•4.5 mg
Urised sugar-coated tablets ℞ *urinary antibiotic; analgesic; antispasmodic; acidifier* [methenamine; phenyl salicylate; atropine sulfate; methylene blue; hyoscyamine sulfate; benzoic acid] 40.8•18.1•0.03•5.4•0.03•4.5 mg ⓢ Uracel; Uracid; Urispas
Urisedamine tablets ℞ *urinary antibiotic; antispasmodic* [methenamine mandelate; hyoscyamine] 500•0.15 mg

Urispas film-coated tablets ℞ *urinary antispasmodic* [flavoxate HCl] 100 mg (200 mg available in Canada) ⊡ Urised

Uristat tablets ℞ *urinary analgesic* [phenazopyridine HCl] 95 mg

Uristix; Uristix 4 reagent strips *in vitro diagnostic aid for multiple urine products*

Uri-Tet capsules (discontinued 1997) ℞ *broad-spectrum tetracycline antibiotic* [oxytetracycline HCl] 250 mg

Uritin tablets ℞ *urinary antibiotic; analgesic; antispasmodic; acidifier* [methenamine; phenyl salicylate; atropine sulfate; methylene blue; hyoscyamine sulfate; benzoic acid] 40.8•18.1•0.03•5.4•0.03•4.5 mg

Urobak tablets ℞ *broad-spectrum bacteriostatic* [sulfamethoxazole] 500 mg

Urobiotic-250 capsules (discontinued 1997) ℞ *urinary anti-infective; urinary analgesic* [oxytetracycline HCl; sulfamethizole; phenazopyridine HCl] 250•250•50 mg ⊡ Otobiotic

Urocit-K tablets ℞ *urinary alkalizer for nephrolithiasis and hypocitruria prevention (orphan)* [potassium citrate] 5, 10 mEq ⊡ Uracid

Urodine tablets (discontinued 1997) ℞ *urinary analgesic* [phenazopyridine HCl] 100, 200 mg

urofollitrophin BAN *follicle-stimulating hormone (FSH)* [also: urofollitropin]

urofollitropin USAN, INN *follicle-stimulating hormone (FSH); ovulation stimulant for polycystic ovarian disease (orphan) and assisted reproductive techniques (ARTs); investigational (orphan) for spermatogenesis in hormone-deficient males* [also: urofollitrophin]

urogastrone *investigational (orphan) for recovery from corneal transplant surgery*

Urogesic tablets ℞ *urinary analgesic* [phenazopyridine HCl] 100 mg

Urogesic Blue sugar-coated tablets ℞ *urinary antibiotic; antiseptic; analgesic; antispasmodic* [methenamine; sodium biphosphate; phenyl salicylate; methylene blue; hyoscyamine sulfate] 81.6•40.8•36.2•10.8•0.12 mg

urokinase USAN, INN, BAN, JAN *plasminogen activator; thrombolytic enzyme*

urokinase alfa USAN *plasminogen activator; thrombolytic enzyme*

Uro-KP-Neutral film-coated tablets ℞ *urinary acidifier; phosphorus supplement* [sodium phosphate; potassium phosphate; monobasic sodium phosphate] 250 mg (P)

Urolene Blue tablets ℞ *urinary anti-infective and antiseptic; antidote to cyanide poisoning* [methylene blue] 65 mg

Uro-Mag capsules OTC *antacid; magnesium supplement* [magnesium oxide] 140 mg

uronal [see: barbital]

Uro-Phosphate film-coated tablets ℞ *urinary antibiotic; acidifier* [methenamine; sodium biphosphate] 300•434.78 mg

Uroqid-Acid No. 2 film-coated tablets ℞ *urinary antibiotic; acidifier* [methenamine mandelate; sodium acid phosphate] 500•500 mg

Urovist Cysto intracavitary instillation (discontinued 1999) ℞ *radiopaque contrast medium for cystourethrography* [diatrizoate meglumine (46.67% iodine)] 30% (14.1%)

Urovist Meglumine DIU/CT injection (discontinued 1999) ℞ *radiopaque contrast medium* [diatrizoate meglumine (46.67% iodine)] 30%

Urovist Sodium 300 injection (discontinued 1999) ℞ *radiopaque contrast medium* [diatrizoate sodium (59.87% iodine)] 50%

Ursinus Inlay-Tabs (tablets) OTC *decongestant; analgesic; antipyretic* [pseudoephedrine HCl; aspirin] 30•325 mg

Urso tablets ℞ *bile acid for primary biliary cirrhosis (orphan); investigational for hypercholesterolemia, type IIa and IIb* [ursodiol] 250 mg

ursodeoxycholic acid INN, BAN *naturally occurring bile acid; anticholelithogenic* [also: ursodiol]

ursodiol USAN *naturally occurring bile acid for primary biliary cirrhosis (orphan); investigational for hypercholesterolemia, type IIa and IIb* [also: ursodeoxycholic acid]

ursulcholic acid INN

Urtica dioica; U. urens *medicinal herb* [see: nettle]

uva ursi *(Arbutus uva ursi; Arctostaphylos uva ursi)* leaves *medicinal herb for bladder and kidney infections, Bright disease, constipation, diabetes, gonorrhea, nephritis, spleen disorders, urethritis, and uterine ulcerations*

Uvadex extracorporeal solution (leukocytes are collected, photoactivated with the UVAR Photopheresis System, then reinfused) ℞ *palliative treatment for cutaneous T-cell lymphoma (CTCL); investigational (orphan) treatment of diffuse systemic sclerosis and to prevent rejection of cardiac allografts* [methoxsalen] 20 µg/mL

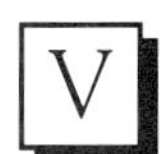

VA (vincristine, actinomycin D) *chemotherapy protocol*

VA-10367 *investigational neurophilic compound that accelerates functional recovery and nerve regeneration in spinal cord and peripheral nerve injury*

VAAP (vincristine, asparaginase, Adriamycin, prednisone) *chemotherapy protocol*

VAB; VAB-I (vinblastine, actinomycin D, bleomycin) *chemotherapy protocol*

VAB-II (vinblastine, actinomycin D, bleomycin, cisplatin) *chemotherapy protocol*

VAB-III (vinblastine, actinomycin D, bleomycin, cisplatin, chlorambucil, cyclophosphamide) *chemotherapy protocol*

VAB-V (vinblastine, actinomycin D, bleomycin, cyclophosphamide, cisplatin) *chemotherapy protocol*

VAB-6 (vinblastine, actinomycin D, bleomycin, cyclophosphamide, cisplatin) *chemotherapy protocol for testicular cancer*

VABCD (vinblastine, Adriamycin, bleomycin, CCNU, DTIC) *chemotherapy protocol*

VAC (vincristine, Adriamycin, cisplatin) *chemotherapy protocol*

VAC (vincristine, Adriamycin, cyclophosphamide) *chemotherapy protocol for small cell lung cancer* [also: CAV]

VAC pulse; VAC standard (vincristine, actinomycin D, cyclophosphamide) *chemotherapy protocol for sarcomas*

VACA (vincristine, actinomycin D, cyclophosphamide, Adriamycin) *chemotherapy protocol*

VACAD (vincristine, actinomycin D, cyclophosphamide, Adriamycin, dacarbazine) *chemotherapy protocol*

VACAdr (vincristine, actinomycin D, cyclophosphamide, Adriamycin) *chemotherapy protocol for pediatric bone and soft tissue sarcomas*

VACAdr-IfoVP (vincristine, actinomycin D, cyclophosphamide, Adriamycin, ifosfamide, VePesid) *chemotherapy protocol*

vaccines *a class of drugs used for active immunization that consist of antigens which induce endogenous production of antibodies*

vaccinia immune globulin (VIG) USP *passive immunizing agent*

vaccinia immune human globulin [now: vaccinia immune globulin]

vaccinia virus vaccine for human papillomavirus (HPV), recombinant *investigational (orphan) for cervical cancer*

Vaccinium edule; V. erythrocarpum; V. macrocarpon; V. oxycoccos; V. vitis *medicinal herb* [see: cranberry]

Vaccinium myrtillus *medicinal herb* [see: bilberry]

VACP (VePesid, Adriamycin, cyclophosphamide, Platinol) *chemotherapy protocol*

VAD (vincristine, Adriamycin, dactinomycin) *chemotherapy protocol for pediatric Wilms tumor*

VAD (vincristine, Adriamycin, dexamethasone) *chemotherapy protocol for multiple myeloma and acute lymphocytic leukemia (ALL)*

Vademin-Z capsules OTC *vitamin/mineral supplement* [multiple vitamins & minerals]

vadocaine INN

VAdrC (vincristine, Adriamycin, cyclophosphamide) *chemotherapy protocol*

VAD/V (vincristine, Adriamycin, dexamethasone, verapamil) *chemotherapy protocol*

VAFAC (vincristine, amethopterin, fluorouracil, Adriamycin, cyclophosphamide) *chemotherapy protocol*

Vagifem film-coated vaginal tablets ℞ *estrogen replacement for postmenopausal atrophic vaginitis* [estradiol hemihydrate] 25 µg

Vagi-Gard; Vagi-Gard Advanced Sensitive Formula vaginal cream OTC *topical local anesthetic; keratolytic; antifungal* [benzocaine; resorcinol] 20%•3%; 5%•2%

Vaginex vaginal cream OTC *topical antihistamine* [tripelennamine HCl]

Vagisec Douche solution ℞ *vaginal cleanser and deodorizer*

Vagisec Plus vaginal suppositories ℞ *antibacterial* [aminacrine HCl] 6 mg

Vagisil cream OTC *topical local anesthetic; antipruritic; antifungal* [benzocaine; resorcinol] 5%•2%

Vagisil powder OTC *absorbs vaginal moisture* [cornstarch; aloe]

Vagistat-1 vaginal ointment in prefilled applicator OTC *antifungal* [tioconazole] 6.5%

VAI (vincristine, actinomycin D, ifosfamide) *chemotherapy protocol*

valaciclovir INN *antiviral for herpes zoster and herpes simplex* [also: valacyclovir HCl]

valacyclovir HCl USAN *antiviral for herpes zoster and herpes simplex* [also: valaciclovir]

valconazole INN

Valcyte tablets ℞ *nucleoside analogue antiviral for AIDS-related cytomegalovirus retinitis* [valganciclovir HCl] 450 mg

valdecoxib USAN *COX-2 inhibitor; investigational (Phase III) anti-inflammatory and analgesic for osteoarthritis*

valdetamide INN

valdipromide INN

Valentine tablets OTC *CNS stimulant; analeptic* [caffeine] 200 mg

valepotriate [see: valtrate]

Valergen 20; Valergen 40 IM injection ℞ *estrogen replacement therapy for postmenopausal symptoms; antineoplastic for prostatic cancer* [estradiol valerate in oil] 20 mg/mL; 40 mg/mL

valerian *(Valeriana officinalis)* root *medicinal herb for convulsions, hypertension, hysteria, hypochondria, nervousness, pain, and sedation* [500 mg oral (CAN)]

valerian, false *medicinal herb* [see: life root]

Valertest No. 1 IM injection ℞ *hormone replacement therapy for postmenopausal symptoms* [estradiol valerate; testosterone enanthate] 4•90 mg/mL

valethamate bromide NF

valganciclovir HCl USAN *nucleoside analogue antiviral for AIDS-related cytomegalovirus retinitis; oral prodrug of ganciclovir*

valine (L-valine) USAN, USP, INN, JAN *essential amino acid; symbols: Val, V*

valine & isoleucine & leucine *investigational (orphan) for hyperphenylalaninemia*

Valisone ointment, cream, lotion ℞ *topical corticosteroidal anti-inflammatory* [betamethasone valerate] 0.1%

Valisone Reduced Strength cream ℞ *topical corticosteroidal anti-inflammatory* [betamethasone valerate] 0.01%

Valium tablets, IV or IM injection, Tel-E-Ject syringes ℞ *benzodiazepine sedative; anxiolytic; anticonvulsant; skeletal muscle relaxant; also abused as a street drug* [diazepam] 2, 5, 10 mg; 5 mg/mL; 10 mg ⑨ thallium; Valpin

Valium Roche Oral (CAN) tablets ℞ *benzodiazepine sedative; anxiolytic; anticonvulsant; skeletal muscle relaxant; also abused as a street drug* [diazepam] 5, 10 mg

valnoctamide USAN, INN *tranquilizer*

valofane INN

valomaciclovir stearate USAN *DNA polymerase inhibitor antiviral for herpes zoster infections*

valperinol INN

valproate pivoxil INN

valproate semisodium INN *anticonvulsant; antipsychotic for manic episodes; migraine prophylaxis* [also: divalproex sodium; semisodium valproate]

valproate sodium USAN *anticonvulsant; investigational for migraine relief* 250 mg/5 mL oral

valproic acid USAN, USP, INN, BAN *anticonvulsant* 250 mg oral

valpromide INN

valrubicin USAN *anthracycline antibiotic antineoplastic for bladder cancer (orphan)*

valsartan USAN, INN *antihypertensive; angiotensin II receptor antagonist*

valspodar USAN *investigational (Phase III) cyclosporine-derived P-glycoprotein (P-gp) inhibitor for multi-drug–resistant (MDR) cancers, including acute myelogenous leukemia (AML), multiple myeloma, and ovarian cancer*

Valstar intravesical solution ℞ *anthracycline antibiotic antineoplastic for bladder cancer (orphan)* [valrubicin] 40 mg/mL

Valtaxin (CAN) intravesical solution ℞ *anthracycline antibiotic antineoplastic for bladder cancer (orphan)* [valrubicin] 40 mg/mL

valtrate INN

Valtrex film-coated caplets ℞ *antiviral for herpes zoster, herpes simplex, and genital herpes* [valacyclovir HCl] 500, 1000 mg

VAM (vinblastine, Adriamycin, mitomycin) *chemotherapy protocol*

VAM (VP-16-213, Adriamycin, methotrexate) *chemotherapy protocol*

VAMP (vincristine, actinomycin, methotrexate, prednisone) *chemotherapy protocol*

VAMP (vincristine, Adriamycin, methylprednisolone) *chemotherapy protocol*

VAMP (vincristine, amethopterin, mercaptopurine, prednisone) *chemotherapy protocol*

vanadium *element (V)*

Vancenase Pockethaler (nasal inhalation aerosol) ℞ *corticosteroidal anti-inflammatory for seasonal or perennial rhinitis* [beclomethasone dipropionate] 42 μg/dose

Vancenase AQ nasal spray ℞ *corticosteroidal anti-inflammatory for seasonal or perennial rhinitis* [beclomethasone dipropionate] 0.084%

Vanceril; Vanceril Double Strength oral inhalation aerosol ℞ *corticosteroidal anti-inflammatory for chronic asthma* [beclomethasone dipropionate] 42 μg/dose; 84 μg/dose

Vancocin Pulvules (capsules), powder for oral solution, powder for IV or IM injection ℞ *tricyclic glycopeptide antibiotic* [vancomycin HCl] 125, 250 mg; 1, 10 g; 0.5, 1, 10 g

Vancoled powder for IV or IM injection ℞ *tricyclic glycopeptide antibiotic* [vancomycin HCl] 0.5, 1, 5 g

vancomycin INN, BAN *tricyclic glycopeptide antibiotic* [also: vancomycin HCl]

vancomycin HCl USP *tricyclic glycopeptide antibiotic* [also: vancomycin] 1 g oral; 0.5, 1, 5, 10 g/vial injection

vaneprim INN

Vanex Expectorant liquid ℞ *narcotic antitussive; decongestant; expectorant* [hydrocodone bitartrate; pseudoephedrine HCl; guaifenesin; alcohol 5%] 2.5•30•100 mg/5 mL

Vanex Forte sustained-release caplets ℞ *decongestant; antihistamine* [phenylpropanolamine HCl; phenylephrine HCl; chlorpheniramine maleate; pyrilamine maleate] 50•10•4•25 mg

Vanex Forte-R sustained-release capsules ℞ *decongestant; antihistamine* [phenylpropanolamine HCl; chlorpheniramine maleate] 75•12 mg

Vanex-HD liquid ℞ *narcotic antitussive; decongestant; antihistamine* [hydrocodone bitartrate; phenylephrine HCl; chlorpheniramine maleate] 1.67•5•2 mg/5 mL

Vanicream OTC *cream base*

vanilla NF *flavoring agent*

vanilla *(Vanilla fragrans; V. planifolia; V. tahitensis)* bean *medicinal herb for CNS stimulation, fever, and flatulence; also used as an aphrodisiac*

vanillin NF *flavoring agent*

N-vanillylnonamide [see: nonivamide]

N-vanillyloleamide [see: olvanil]

Vaniqa cream ℞ *hair growth inhibitor for unwanted facial hair on women* [eflornithine HCl] 13.9%

vanitiolide INN

Vanlev ℞ *vasopeptidase inhibitor (VPI); investigational (NDA filed) endopeptidase and angiotensin-converting enzyme (ACE) inhibitor for hypertension and congestive heart failure* [omapatrilat]

Vanocin lotion ℞ *topical acne treatment* [sulfacetamide sodium; sulfur] 10%•5%

Vanoxide lotion OTC *topical keratolytic for acne* [benzoyl peroxide] 5%

Vanoxide-HC lotion ℞ *topical corticosteroidal anti-inflammatory and keratolytic for acne* [benzoyl peroxide; hydrocortisone] 5%•0.5%

Vanquish caplets OTC *analgesic; antipyretic; anti-inflammatory* [acetaminophen; aspirin (buffered with magnesium hydroxide and aluminum hydroxide); caffeine] 194•227•(50•25)•33 mg

Vansil capsules ℞ *anthelmintic for schistosomiasis (flukes)* [oxamniquine] 250 mg

Vanticon (German name for U.S. product Accolate)

Vantin film-coated tablets, granules for suspension ℞ *broad-spectrum cephalosporin antibiotic* [cefpodoxime proxetil] 100, 200 mg; 50, 100 mg/5 mL ⑨ Banthine; Bantron

vanyldisulfamide INN

VAP (vinblastine, actinomycin D, Platinol) *chemotherapy protocol*

VAP (vincristine, Adriamycin, prednisone) *chemotherapy protocol*

VAP (vincristine, Adriamycin, procarbazine) *chemotherapy protocol*

VAP (vincristine, asparaginase, prednisone) *chemotherapy protocol*

vapiprost INN, BAN *antagonist to thromboxane A_2* [also: vapiprost HCl]

vapiprost HCl USAN *antagonist to thromboxane A_2* [also: vapiprost]

Vaponefrin solution for inhalation (discontinued 1999) OTC *sympathomimetic bronchodilator* [racepinephrine] 2%

Vaporole (trademarked dosage form) *crushable ampule for inhalation*

vapreotide USAN *antineoplastic*

Vaqta IM injection ℞ *immunization against hepatitis A virus (HAV)* [hepatitis A vaccine, inactivated] 25 U/0.5 mL (pediatric), 50 U/mL (adult)

vardenafil *phosphodiesterase-5 (PDE-5) inhibitor; investigational (Phase III) for erectile dysfunction*

varicella virus vaccine *live, attenuated vaccine for chickenpox*

varicella-zoster immune globulin (VZIG) USP *passive immunizing agent for children or immunocompromised adults exposed to chickenpox or zoster* 125 U/2.5 mL

Varivax powder for subcu injection ℞ *vaccine for chickenpox* [varicella virus vaccine, live attenuated] 1350 PFU/0.5 mL dose

Varoniscastrum virgincum *medicinal herb* [see: Culver root]

VAS-972 *investigational immune modulation therapy for contact hypersensitivity*

Vascor film-coated tablets ℞ *antianginal* [bepridil HCl] 200, 300, 400 mg

Vascoray injection ℞ *radiopaque contrast medium* [iothalamate meglumine; iothalamate sodium (51.3% total iodine)] 520•260 mg/mL (400 mg/mL)

vascular endothelial growth factor (VEGF) *investigational (Phase II, orphan) gene therapy for peripheral vascular disease and coronary artery disease*

vascular serotonin $5\text{-}HT_1$ receptor agonists *a class of antimigraine agents that constrict cranial blood vessels and inhibit the release of inflammatory neuropeptides*

Vaseretic 5-12.5; Vaseretic 10-25 tablets ℞ *antihypertensive; angiotensin-converting enzyme (ACE) inhibitor; diuretic* [enalapril maleate; hydrochlorothiazide] 5•12.5 mg; 10•25 mg

vasoactive intestinal polypeptide (VIP) *investigational (NDA filed) treatment for male sexual dysfunction; investigational (orphan) for acute esophageal food impaction*

VasoCare ℞ *investigational agent that reduces stress* ▣ VasoClear

Vasocidin eye drops ℞ *topical ophthalmic corticosteroidal anti-inflammatory; antibiotic* [prednisolone sodium phosphate; sulfacetamide sodium] 0.25%•10% ▣ Vasodilan

Vasocidin ophthalmic ointment ℞ *topical ophthalmic corticosteroidal anti-inflammatory; antibiotic* [prednisolone acetate; sulfacetamide sodium] 0.5%•10%

Vasocine ophthalmic ointment ℞ *topical ophthalmic corticosteroidal anti-inflammatory; antibiotic* [prednisolone acetate; sulfacetamide sodium] 0.5%•10% ▣ Vaseline

VasoClear eye drops OTC *topical ophthalmic decongestant* [naphazoline HCl] 0.02% ▣ VasoCare

VasoClear A eye drops OTC *topical ophthalmic decongestant and astringent* [naphazoline HCl; zinc sulfate] 0.02%•0.25%

Vasocon Regular eye drops ℞ *topical ophthalmic decongestant and vasoconstrictor* [naphazoline HCl] 0.1%

Vasocon-A eye drops ℞ *topical ophthalmic decongestant and antihistamine* [naphazoline HCl; antazoline phosphate] 0.05%•0.5%

vasoconstrictors *a class of cardiovascular drugs that narrow the blood vessels*

Vasodilan tablets ℞ *peripheral vasodilator* [isoxsuprine HCl] 10, 20 mg ▣ Vasocidin

vasodilators *a class of cardiovascular drugs that dilate the blood vessels*

Vasofem ℞ *investigational (NDA filed) oral treatment for female sexual arousal disorder* [phentolamine mesylate]

Vasoflux ℞ *investigational (Phase II) anticoagulant for use in acute myocardial infarction patients* ▣ Vasoprost; Vasosulf

Vasomax ℞ *investigational (NDA filed) oral treatment for erectile dysfunction* [phentolamine mesylate]

vasopressin (VP) USP, INN *posterior pituitary hormone; antidiuretic for diabetes insipidus or prevention of abdominal distention* 20 U/mL injection

vasopressin tannate USP *posterior pituitary hormone; antidiuretic*

vasopressors *a class of posterior pituitary hormones that raise blood pressure by causing contraction of capillaries and arterioles; a class of sympathomimetic agents that raise blood pressure by increasing myocardial contractility* [also called: vasopressins]

Vasoprost ℞ *investigational (orphan) prostaglandin for severe peripheral arterial occlusive disease* [alprostadil] ▣ Vasoflux

Vasosulf eye drops ℞ *topical ophthalmic antibiotic and decongestant* [sulfacetamide sodium; phenylephrine HCl] 15%•0.125% ⊠ Velosef; Vasoflux

Vasotate HC ear drops ℞ *topical corticosteroidal anti-inflammatory; antibacterial; antifungal* [hydrocortisone; acetic acid] 1%•2%

Vasotec tablets ℞ *antihypertensive; angiotensin-converting enzyme (ACE) inhibitor* [enalapril maleate] 2.5, 5, 10, 20 mg

Vasotec I.V. injection ℞ *antihypertensive; angiotensin-converting enzyme (ACE) inhibitor* [enalaprilat] 1.25 mg/mL

Vasoxyl IV or IM injection ℞ *vasopressor for hypotensive shock during surgery* [methoxamine HCl] 20 mg/mL

VAT (vinblastine, Adriamycin, thiotepa) *chemotherapy protocol*

VATD; VAT-D (vincristine, ara-C, thioguanine, daunorubicin) *chemotherapy protocol*

VATH (vinblastine, Adriamycin, thiotepa, Halotestin) *chemotherapy protocol for breast cancer*

Vatronol [see: Vicks Vatronol]

VAV (VP-16-213, Adriamycin, vincristine) *chemotherapy protocol*

Vaxigrip (CAN) IM injection ℞ *flu vaccine* [influenza split-virus vaccine] 0.5 mL/dose

VaxSyn HIV-1 ℞ *investigational (orphan) antiviral (therapeutic, Phase II) and vaccine (preventative, Phase I) for HIV and AIDS* [gp160 antigens]

VB (vinblastine, bleomycin) *chemotherapy protocol*

VBA (vincristine, BCNU, Adriamycin) *chemotherapy protocol*

VBAP (vincristine, BCNU, Adriamycin, prednisone) *chemotherapy protocol for multiple myeloma*

VBC (VePesid, BCNU, cyclophosphamide) *chemotherapy protocol*

VBC (vinblastine, bleomycin, cisplatin) *chemotherapy protocol*

VBCMP (vincristine, BCNU, cyclophosphamide, melphalan, prednisone) *chemotherapy protocol for multiple myeloma*

VBD (vinblastine, bleomycin, DDP) *chemotherapy protocol*

VBM (vincristine, bleomycin, methotrexate) *chemotherapy protocol*

VBMCP (vincristine, BCNU, melphalan, cyclophosphamide, prednisone) *chemotherapy protocol*

VBMF (vincristine, bleomycin, methotrexate, fluorouracil) *chemotherapy protocol*

VBP (vinblastine, bleomycin, Platinol) *chemotherapy protocol*

VC (VePesid, carboplatin) *chemotherapy protocol*

VC (vincristine) [q.v.]

VC (vinorelbine, cisplatin) *chemotherapy protocol for non–small cell lung cancer (NSCLC)*

VCAP (vincristine, cyclophosphamide, Adriamycin, prednisone) *chemotherapy protocol for multiple myeloma*

V-CAP III (VP-16-213, cyclophosphamide, Adriamycin, Platinol) *chemotherapy protocol*

VCF (vaginal contraceptive film) OTC *spermicidal contraceptive* [nonoxynol 9] 28%

VCF (vincristine, cyclophosphamide, fluorouracil) *chemotherapy protocol*

V-Cillin K powder for oral solution (discontinued 1997) ℞ *natural penicillin antibiotic* [penicillin V potassium] 125, 250 mg/5 mL ⊠ Bicillin; Wycillin

V-Cillin K tablets (discontinued 1998) ℞ *natural penicillin antibiotic* [penicillin V potassium] 125, 250, 500 mg ⊠ Bicillin; Wycillin

VCMP (vincristine, cyclophosphamide, melphalan, prednisone) *chemotherapy protocol for multiple myeloma* [also: VMCP]

VCP (vincristine, cyclophosphamide, prednisone) *chemotherapy protocol*

VCP 205 *investigational (Phase II) vaccine for HIV* [also: ALVAC-120TMG]
VCR (vincristine) [q.v.]
VD (vinorelbine, doxorubicin) *chemotherapy protocol for breast cancer*
VDA (vincristine, daunorubicin, asparaginase) *chemotherapy protocol*
V-Dec-M sustained-release tablets ℞ *decongestant; expectorant* [pseudoephedrine HCl; guaifenesin] 120•500 mg
VDP (vinblastine, dacarbazine, Platinol) *chemotherapy protocol*
VDP (vincristine, daunorubicin, prednisone) *chemotherapy protocol*
Vectrin capsules ℞ *tetracycline antibiotic* [minocycline HCl] 50, 100 mg
vecuronium bromide USAN, INN, BAN *nondepolarizing neuromuscular blocker; muscle relaxant; adjunct to anesthesia* 10, 20 mg injection
Veetids film-coated tablets ℞ *natural penicillin antibiotic* [penicillin V potassium] 250, 500 mg
Veetids '125'; Veetids '250' powder for oral solution ℞ *natural penicillin antibiotic* [penicillin V potassium] 125 mg/5 mL; 250 mg/5 mL
vegetable oil, hydrogenated NF *tablet and capsule lubricant*
vegetable tallow; vegetable wax *medicinal herb* [see: bayberry]
VEGF (vascular endothelial growth factor) [q.v.]
Vehicle/N; Vehicle/N Mild OTC *lotion base*
VeIP (Velban, ifosfamide [with mesna rescue], Platinol) *chemotherapy protocol for genitourinary and testicular cancer*
Velban powder for IV injection ℞ *antineoplastic for lung, breast and testicular cancers, lymphomas, sarcomas, and neuroblastoma* [vinblastine sulfate] 10 mg/vial ⓢ Valpin
Veldona low-dose oral lozenge ℞ *investigational (Phase II) treatment for AIDS-related xerostomia; investigational (Phase I) cytokine for AIDS and hepatitis B; investigational (orphan) oral papillomavirus warts in HIV-infected patients* [interferon alfa]
velnacrine INN, BAN *cholinesterase inhibitor* [also: velnacrine maleate]
velnacrine maleate USAN *cholinesterase inhibitor for Alzheimer disease* [also: velnacrine]
Velosef capsules, oral suspension, powder for IV or IM injection ℞ *cephalosporin antibiotic* [cephradine] 250, 500 mg; 125, 250 mg/5 mL; 250, 500, 1000, 2000 mg ⓢ Vasosulf
Velosulin BR subcu injection OTC *antidiabetic* [human insulin (rDNA)] 100 U/mL
Veltane tablets (discontinued 1997) ℞ *antihistamine* [brompheniramine maleate] 4 mg
Velvachol OTC *cream base*
Vendona ℞ *investigational cytokine for AIDS*
Venice turpentine *medicinal herb* [see: larch]
venlafaxine INN, BAN *antidepressant; anxiolytic; serotonin and norepinephrine reuptake inhibitor* [also: venlafaxine HCl]
venlafaxine HCl USAN *antidepressant; anxiolytic; serotonin and norepinephrine reuptake inhibitor* [also: venlafaxine]
Venofer IV injection ℞ *hematinic for iron deficiency anemia in patients undergoing chronic dialysis* [iron sucrose] 20 mg/mL
Venoglobulin-I powder for IV infusion (discontinued 2001; replaced by Venoglobulin-S) ℞ *passive immunizing agent for HIV and idiopathic thrombocytopenic purpura (ITP)* [immune globulin] 50 mg/mL
Venoglobulin-S powder for IV infusion ℞ *passive immunizing agent for HIV and idiopathic thrombocytopenic purpura (ITP)* [immune globulin, solvent/detergent treated] 5%, 10%
Venomil subcu or IM injection ℞ *venom sensitivity testing (subcu); venom desensitization therapy (IM)* [extracts of honeybee, yellow jacket,

yellow hornet, white-faced hornet, mixed vespid, and wasp venom]

Ventolin (CAN) Diskus (inhalation powder device) ℞ *sympathomimetic bronchodilator* [albuterol sulfate] 200 µg/dose

Ventolin inhalation aerosol ℞ *sympathomimetic bronchodilator* [albuterol] 90 µg/dose ⓢ phentolamine

Ventolin Rotacaps (encapsulated powder for inhalation), tablets, solution for inhalation, Nebules (unit-dose solution for inhalation), syrup ℞ *sympathomimetic bronchodilator* [albuterol sulfate] 200 µg/dose; 2, 4 mg; 0.05%; 0.083%; 2 mg/5 mL

Ventolin HFA CFC-free inhalation aerosol ℞ *sympathomimetic bronchodilator* [albuterol] 90 µg/dose

VePesid IV injection, capsules ℞ *antineoplastic for testicular and small cell lung cancers* [etoposide] 20 mg/mL; 50 mg

Veracolate tablets (discontinued 1998) OTC *stimulant laxative* [phenolphthalein; cascara sagrada extract; capsicum oleoresin] 32.4•75•0.05 mg

veradoline INN *analgesic* [also: veradoline HCl]

veradoline HCl USAN *analgesic* [also: veradoline]

veralipride INN

verapamil USAN, INN, BAN *coronary vasodilator; calcium channel blocker*

verapamil HCl USAN, USP *antianginal; antiarrhythmic; antihypertensive; calcium channel blocker* 40, 80, 120, 180, 240, 360 mg oral; 5 mg/2 mL injection

***Veratrum* species** *medicinal herb* [see: hellebore]

veratrylidene-isoniazid [see: verazide]

verazide INN, BAN

Verazinc capsules OTC *zinc supplement* [zinc sulfate] 220 mg

Verbascum nigrum; V. phlomoides; V. thapsiforme; V. thapsus *medicinal herb* [see: mullein]

Verbena hastata *medicinal herb* [see: blue vervain]

Verdia ℞ *investigational angiotensin II receptor antagonist for hypertension (NDA withdrawn 1998)* [tasosartan]

Verelan sustained-release capsules ℞ *antihypertensive; antianginal; antiarrhythmic; calcium channel blocker* [verapamil HCl] 120, 180, 240, 360 mg

Verelan PM delayed-onset, extended-release capsules ℞ *antihypertensive; calcium channel blocker* [verapamil HCl] 100, 200, 300 mg

Vergon capsules OTC *anticholinergic; antihistamine; antivertigo agent; motion sickness preventative* [meclizine HCl] 30 mg

verilopam INN *analgesic* [also: verilopam HCl]

verilopam HCl USAN *analgesic* [also: verilopam]

verlukast USAN, INN *bronchodilator; antiasthmatic*

Verluma technetium Tc 99 prep kit ℞ *monoclonal antibody imaging agent for small cell lung cancer* [nofetumomab merpentan]

vermicides; vermifuges *a class of drugs effective against parasitic infections* [also called: anthelmintics]

Vermox chewable tablets ℞ *anthelmintic for trichuriasis, enterobiasis, ascariasis, and uncinariasis* [mebendazole] 100 mg

verofylline USAN, INN *bronchodilator; antiasthmatic*

veronal [see: barbital]

veronal sodium [see: barbital sodium]

veronica, tall *medicinal herb* [see: Culver root]

Veronica beccabunga *medicinal herb* [see: brooklime]

Veronica officinalis *medicinal herb* [see: speedwell]

Verr-Canth liquid (discontinued 1997) ℞ *topical keratolytic* [cantharidin] 0.7%

Verrex liquid (discontinued 1997) ℞ *topical keratolytic* [salicylic acid; podophyllum] 30%•10%

Versacaps prolonged-action capsules ℞ *decongestant; expectorant* [pseudoephedrine HCl; guaifenesin] 60•300 mg

Versed IV or IM injection, Tel-E-Ject syringes, pediatric syrup ℞ *short-acting benzodiazepine general anesthetic adjunct for preoperative sedation* [midazolam HCl] 1, 5 mg/mL; 2 mg/mL

versetamide USAN *stabilizer; carrier agent for gadoversetamide*

Versiclear lotion ℞ *topical antifungal; keratolytic; antipruritic; anesthetic* [sodium thiosulfate; salicylic acid; alcohol 10%] 25%•1%

verteporfin USAN *antineoplastic and treatment for wet age-related macular degeneration (used with phototherapy)*

vervain *medicinal herb* [see: blue vervain]

Vesanoid capsules ℞ *antineoplastic for acute promyelocytic leukemia (orphan); investigational (orphan) for other leukemias and ophthalmic squamous metaplasia* [tretinoin] 10 mg

vesicants *a class of agents that cause blisters*

vesnarinone USAN, INN *cardiotonic; investigational inotropic for congestive heart failure (clinical trials discontinued 1996)*

vesperal [see: barbital]

Vesprin IV or IM injection ℞ *conventional (typical) antipsychotic; antiemetic* [triflupromazine HCl] 10, 20 mg/mL

Vestra tablets ℞ *investigational (NDA filed) fast-acting selective norepinephrine reuptake inhibitor for depression* [reboxetine mesylate]

vetrabutine INN, BAN

Vetuss HC syrup ℞ *narcotic antitussive; decongestant; antihistamine* [hydrocodone bitartrate; phenylpropanolamine HCl; phenylephrine HCl; pyrilamine maleate; pheniramine maleate; alcohol 5%] 1.7•3.3•5•3.3•3.3 mg/5 mL

Vexol eye drop suspension ℞ *topical ophthalmic corticosteroidal anti-inflammatory* [rimexolone] 1%

Viactiv chewable tablets OTC *calcium supplement* [calcium carbonate; vitamin D; vitamin K] 1.25 g•100 IU•40 µg

Viadur DUROS (once-yearly subcu implant) ℞ *antihormonal antineoplastic for the palliative treatment of advanced prostate cancer* [leuprolide acetate] 120 µg/day

Viaflex (trademarked form) *ready-to-use IV*

ViaFoam ℞ *investigational (Phase III) corticosteroid foam for psoriasis of the scalp* [clobetasol propionate]

Viagra film-coated tablets ℞ *selective vasodilator for erectile dysfunction* [sildenafil citrate] 25, 50, 100 mg

Vianain ℞ *investigational (orphan) proteolytic enzymes for debridement of severe burns* [ananain; comosain; bromelains]

vibesate

Vibramycin capsules, powder for IV injection ℞ *tetracycline antibiotic* [doxycycline hyclate] 50, 100 mg; 100, 200 mg

Vibramycin powder for oral suspension ℞ *tetracycline antibiotic* [doxycycline] 25 mg/5 mL

Vibramycin syrup ℞ *tetracycline antibiotic* [doxycycline calcium] 50 mg/5 mL

Vibra-Tabs tablets ℞ *tetracycline antibiotic* [doxycycline hyclate] 100 mg

Viburnum opulus *medicinal herb* [see: cramp bark]

VIC (VePesid, ifosfamide [with mesna rescue], carboplatin) *chemotherapy protocol for non–small cell lung cancer (NSCLC)* [also: CVI]

VIC (vinblastine, ifosfamide, CCNU) *chemotherapy protocol*

Vicam injection ℞ *parenteral vitamin therapy* [multiple B vitamins; vitamin C] ≛•50 mg/mL

Vicks 44 Non-Drowsy Cold & Cough LiquiCaps (capsules) OTC *antitussive; decongestant* [dextromethorphan hydrobromide; pseudoephedrine HCl] 30•60 mg

Vicks 44D Cough & Head Congestion; Vicks Formula 44D Cough & Decongestant; Vicks Pediatric

Formula 44d Cough & Decongestant liquid OTC *antitussive; decongestant* [dextromethorphan hydrobromide; pseudoephedrine HCl] 10•20 mg/5 mL; 10•20 mg/5 mL; 5•10 mg/5 mL

Vicks 44E liquid OTC *antitussive; expectorant* [dextromethorphan hydrobromide; guaifenesin] 6.7•66.7 mg/5 mL

Vicks 44M Cold, Flu & Cough LiquiCaps (capsules) OTC *antitussive; decongestant; antihistamine; analgesic* [dextromethorphan hydrobromide; pseudoephedrine HCl; chlorpheniramine maleate; acetaminophen] 10•30•2•250 mg

Vicks Cough Drops; Vicks Menthol Cough Drops OTC *topical analgesic; counterirritant; mild local anesthetic* [menthol] 10 mg; 8.4 mg

Vicks Cough Silencers lozenges OTC *antitussive; topical oral anesthetic* [dextromethorphan hydrobromide; benzocaine] 2.5•1 mg

Vicks Dry Hacking Cough syrup OTC *antitussive* [dextromethorphan hydrobromide; alcohol 10%] 15 mg/5 mL

Vicks Inhaler OTC *nasal decongestant* [*l*-desoxyephedrine] 50 mg

Vicks NyQuil products [see: NyQuil]

Vicks Pediatric 44d Dry Hacking Cough and Head Congestion syrup OTC *antitussive* [dextromethorphan hydrobromide] 15 mg/15 mL

Vicks Pediatric Formula 44e liquid OTC *antitussive; expectorant* [dextromethorphan hydrobromide; guaifenesin] 3.3•33.3 mg/5 mL

Vicks Pediatric Formula 44m Multi-Symptom Cough & Cold liquid OTC *pediatric antitussive, decongestant, and antihistamine* [dextromethorphan hydrobromide; pseudoephedrine HCl; chlorpheniramine maleate] 5•10•0.67 mg/5 mL

Vicks Sinex products [see: Sinex]

Vicks VapoRub vaporizing ointment, cream OTC *counterirritant* [camphor; menthol; eucalyptus oil] 4.7%•2.6%•1.2%

Vicks Vitamin C Drops (lozenges) OTC *vitamin C supplement* [ascorbic acid and sodium ascorbate] 25 mg

Vicodin; Vicodin ES; Vicodin HP tablets ℞ *narcotic analgesic* [hydrocodone bitartrate; acetaminophen] 5•500 mg; 7.5•750 mg; 10•660 mg

Vicodin Tuss syrup ℞ *narcotic antitussive; expectorant* [hydrocodone bitartrate; guaifenesin] 5•100 mg/5 mL ⑨ Hycodan; Hycomine

Vicon Forte capsules ℞ *vitamin/mineral supplement* [multiple vitamins & minerals; folic acid] ≛•1 mg

Vicon Plus capsules OTC *vitamin/mineral supplement* [multiple vitamins & minerals] ≛

Vicon-C capsules OTC *vitamin/mineral supplement* [multiple B vitamins & minerals; vitamin C] ≛•300 mg

Vicoprofen film-coated tablets ℞ *narcotic analgesic* [hydrocodone bitartrate; ibuprofen] 7.5•200 mg

vicotrope [see: cosyntropin]

vidarabine USAN, USP, INN, BAN *antiviral* ⑨ cytarabine

vidarabine monohydrate [see: vidarabine]

vidarabine phosphate USAN *antiviral*

vidarabine sodium phosphate USAN *antiviral*

Vi-Daylin chewable tablets OTC *vitamin supplement* [multiple vitamins; folic acid] ≛•0.3 mg

Vi-Daylin ADC drops OTC *vitamin supplement* [vitamins A, C, and D] 1500 IU•35 mg•400 IU per mL

Vi-Daylin ADC Vitamins + Iron drops OTC *vitamin/iron supplement* [vitamins A, C, and D; ferrous gluconate] 1500 IU•35 mg•400 IU•10 mg per mL

Vi-Daylin Multivitamin liquid, drops OTC *vitamin supplement* [multiple vitamins]

Vi-Daylin Multivitamin + Iron chewable tablets OTC *vitamin/iron supplement* [multiple vitamins; iron; folic acid] ≛•12•0.3 mg

Vi-Daylin Multivitamin + Iron liquid, drops OTC *vitamin/iron supplement* [multiple vitamins; ferrous gluconate] ≛•10 mg/5 mL; ≛•10 mg/mL

Vi-Daylin/F ADC drops ℞ *pediatric vitamin supplement and dental caries preventative* [vitamins A, C, and D; sodium fluoride] 1500 IU•35 mg•400 IU•0.25 mg per mL

Vi-Daylin/F ADC + Iron drops ℞ *pediatric vitamin/iron supplement and dental caries preventative* [vitamins A, C, and D; sodium fluoride; ferrous sulfate] 1500 IU•35 mg•400 IU•0.25 mg•10 mg per mL

Vi-Daylin/F Multivitamin chewable tablets ℞ *pediatric vitamin supplement and dental caries preventative* [multiple vitamins; sodium fluoride; folic acid] ≛•1•0.3 mg

Vi-Daylin/F Multivitamin drops ℞ *pediatric vitamin supplement and dental caries preventative* [multiple vitamins; sodium fluoride] ≛•0.25 mg/mL

Vi-Daylin/F Multivitamin + Iron chewable tablets ℞ *pediatric vitamin/iron supplement and dental caries preventative* [multiple vitamins; sodium fluoride; ferrous sulfate; folic acid] ≛•1•12•0.3 mg

Vi-Daylin/F Multivitamin + Iron drops ℞ *pediatric vitamin/iron supplement and dental caries preventative* [multiple vitamins; sodium fluoride; ferrous sulfate] ≛•0.25•10 mg/mL

Videx chewable/dispersible tablets, powder for oral solution, powder for pediatric oral solution ℞ *antiviral for advanced HIV infection* [didanosine] 25, 50, 100, 150, 200 mg; 100, 167, 250 mg/packet; 2, 4 g/bottle

Videx EC delayed-release capsules with enteric-coated beads ℞ *antiviral for advanced HIV infection* [didanosine] 125, 200, 250, 400 mg

VIE (vincristine, ifosfamide, etoposide) *chemotherapy protocol*

vifilcon A USAN *hydrophilic contact lens material*

vifilcon B USAN *hydrophilic contact lens material*

Vi-Flor [see: Poly-Vi-Flor; Tri-Vi-Flor]

VIG (vaccinia immune globulin) [q.v.]

vigabatrin USAN, INN, BAN *anticonvulsant for tardive dyskinesia*

Vigomar Forte tablets OTC *vitamin/mineral/iron supplement* [multiple vitamins & minerals; iron] ≛•12 mg

Vigortol liquid OTC *geriatric vitamin/mineral supplement* [multiple B vitamins & minerals; alcohol 18%] ≛

VIL ℞ *investigational (orphan) for hyperphenylalaninemia* [valine; isoleucine; leucine]

viloxazine INN, BAN *bicyclic antidepressant* [also: viloxazine HCl]

viloxazine HCl USAN *bicyclic antidepressant* [also: viloxazine]

Viminate liquid OTC *geriatric vitamin/mineral supplement* [multiple B vitamins & minerals] ≛

viminol INN

VIMRxyn ℞ *investigational (Phase I) antiviral for HIV and AIDS* [hypericin (synthetic)]

vinafocon A USAN *hydrophobic contact lens material*

vinbarbital NF, INN [also: vinbarbitone]

vinbarbital sodium NF

vinbarbitone BAN [also: vinbarbital]

vinblastine INN *vinca alkaloid antineoplastic* [also: vinblastine sulfate]

vinblastine sulfate USAN, USP *vinca alkaloid antineoplastic* [also: vinblastine] 10 mg/vial, 1 mg/mL injection

vinblastine sulfate & estramustine *chemotherapy protocol for prostate cancer*

vinburnine INN

vinca alkaloids *a class of natural antineoplastics*

Vinca major; V. minor *medicinal herb* [see: periwinkle]

vincaleukoblastine sulfate [see: vinblastine sulfate]

vincamine INN, BAN

vincanol INN

vincantenate [see: vinconate]

vincantril INN

Vincasar PFS IV injection ℞ *antineoplastic* [vincristine sulfate] 1 mg/mL
vincofos USAN, INN *anthelmintic*
vinconate INN
vincristine (VC; VCR) INN *antineoplastic* [also: vincristine sulfate]
vincristine sulfate USAN, USP *antineoplastic* [also: vincristine] 1 mg/mL injection
vindeburnol INN
vindesine USAN, INN, BAN *synthetic vinca alkaloid antineoplastic*
vindesine sulfate USAN, JAN *investigational (NDA filed) synthetic vinca alkaloid antineoplastic*
vinegar [see: acetic acid]
vinepidine INN *antineoplastic* [also: vinepidine sulfate]
vinepidine sulfate USAN *antineoplastic* [also: vinepidine]
vinformide INN
vinglycinate INN *antineoplastic* [also: vinglycinate sulfate]
vinglycinate sulfate USAN *antineoplastic* [also: vinglycinate]
vinleurosine INN *antineoplastic* [also: vinleurosine sulfate]
vinleurosine sulfate USAN *antineoplastic* [also: vinleurosine]
vinmegallate INN
vinorelbine INN *antineoplastic* [also: vinorelbine tartrate]
vinorelbine tartrate USAN *antineoplastic for non–small cell lung cancer (NSCLC)* [also: vinorelbine]
vinorelbine tartrate & cisplatin *chemotherapy protocol for cervical cancer*
vinorelbine tartrate & paclitaxel *chemotherapy protocol for breast cancer*
vinpocetine USAN, INN
vinpoline INN
vinrosidine INN *antineoplastic* [also: vinrosidine sulfate]
vinrosidine sulfate USAN *antineoplastic* [also: vinrosidine]
vintiamol INN
vintoperol INN
vintriptol INN
vinyl alcohol polymer [see: polyvinyl alcohol]
vinyl ether USP
vinyl gamma-aminobutyric acid [see: vigabatrin]
vinylbital INN [also: vinylbitone]
vinylbitone BAN [also: vinylbital]
vinylestrenolone [see: norgesterone]
vinymal [see: vinylbital]
vinyzene [see: bromchlorenone]
vinzolidine INN *antineoplastic* [also: vinzolidine sulfate]
vinzolidine sulfate USAN *antineoplastic* [also: vinzolidine]
Vioform cream, ointment (discontinued 2000) OTC *topical antifungal; antibacterial* [clioquinol] 3%
Viogen-C capsules OTC *vitamin/mineral supplement* [multiple B vitamins & minerals; vitamin C] ≛ • 300 mg
Viokase tablets, powder ℞ *digestive enzymes* [lipase; protease; amylase] 8000 • 30 000 • 30 000 U; 16 800 • 70 000 • 70 000 U/0.7 g
Viola odorata *medicinal herb* [see: violet]
Viola tricolor *medicinal herb* [see: pansy]
violet (*Viola odorata*) flowers and leaves *medicinal herb for asthma, bronchitis, cancer, colds, cough, sinus congestion, tumors, and ulcers*
violet, garden *medicinal herb* [see: pansy]
violetbloom *medicinal herb* [see: bittersweet nightshade]
viomycin INN [also: viomycin sulfate]
viomycin sulfate USP [also: viomycin]
viosterol in oil [see: ergocalciferol]
Vioxx tablets, oral suspension ℞ *analgesic; antiarthritic; antipyretic; COX-2 inhibitor; nonsteroidal anti-inflammatory drug (NSAID)* [rofecoxib] 12.5, 25, 50 mg; 12.5, 25 mg/5 mL
VIP (vasoactive intestinal polypeptide) [q.v.]
VIP; VIP-1; VIP-2 (VePesid, ifosfamide [with mesna rescue], Platinol) *chemotherapy protocol for genitourinary, testicular, and small cell and non–small cell lung cancer (NSCLC)*
VIP (vinblastine, ifosfamide [with mesna rescue], Platinol) *chemotherapy protocol*

VIP-B (VP-16, ifosfamide, Platinol, bleomycin) *chemotherapy protocol*

Viprinex (CAN) subcu injection, IV infusion ℞ *anticoagulant for deep vein thrombosis (DVT) and severe chronic peripheral circulatory disorders* [ancrod] 70 IU/mL

viprostol USAN, INN, BAN *hypotensive; vasodilator*

viprynium embonate BAN *anthelmintic* [also: pyrvinium pamoate]

viqualine INN

viquidil INN

Viquin Forte cream ℞ *hyperpigmentation bleaching agent; sunscreen* [hydroquinone; padimate O; dioxybenzone; oxybenzone] 4%•8%•3%•2%

Vira-A ophthalmic ointment ℞ *topical antiviral for acute keratoconjunctivitis and recurrent epithelial keratitis due to herpes simplex virus infection* [vidarabine] 3%

Viracept film-coated tablets, powder for oral solution ℞ *antiretroviral HIV-1 protease inhibitor* [nelfinavir mesylate] 250 mg; 50 mg/g

Viractin cream, gel (name changed to Cēpacol Viractin in 2001)

Viramune tablets, oral suspension ℞ *antiviral non-nucleoside reverse transcriptase inhibitor (NNRTI) for HIV-1* [nevirapine] 200 mg; 50 mg/5 mL

Virazole powder for inhalation aerosol ℞ *antiviral for severe lower respiratory tract infections; investigational (Phase II/III) for HIV; investigational (orphan) for hemorrhagic fever with renal syndrome* [ribavirin] 6 g/100 mL vial (20 mg/mL reconstituted)

Viread ℞ *investigational (NDA filed) oral antiviral nucleoside reverse transcriptase inhibitor (NRTI) for HIV infection* [tenofovir disoproxil fumarate]

Virend ℞ *investigational (Phase II) antiviral for AIDS-related genital herpes* [crofelemer]

Virginia mountain mint; Virginia thyme *medicinal herb* [see: wild hyssop]

Virginia silk *medicinal herb* [see: milkweed]

virginiamycin USAN, INN *antibacterial; veterinary food additive*

virginiamycin factor M_1 [see: virginiamycin]

virginiamycin factor S [see: virginiamycin]

virgin's bower *medicinal herb* [see: woodbine]

viridofulvin USAN, INN *antifungal*

Virilon capsules, IM injection ℞ *androgen replacement for hypogonadism or testosterone deficiency in men, delayed puberty in boys, and metastatic breast cancer in women; also abused as a street drug* [methyltestosterone] 10 mg; 200 mg/mL

Virogen Herpes slide test for professional use *in vitro diagnostic aid for herpes simplex virus antigen in lesions or cell cultures* [latex agglutination test]

Virogen Rotatest slide test for professional use *in vitro diagnostic aid for fecal rotavirus* [latex agglutination test]

Viroptic Drop-Dose (eye drops) ℞ *ophthalmic antiviral for keratoconjunctivitis and epithelial keratitis due to herpes simplex virus infection* [trifluridine] 1%

viroxime USAN, INN *antiviral*

viroxime component A [see: zinviroxime]

viroxime component B [see: enviroxime]

Virulizin *investigational (orphan) immunostimulant for malignant melanoma and pancreatic cancer; investigational (Phase I/II) macrophage activator for AIDS-related lymphomas and Kaposi sarcoma*

Viscoat prefilled syringes ℞ *viscoelastic agent for ophthalmic surgery* [hyaluronate sodium; chondroitin sulfate sodium] 30•40 mg/mL

Viscum album *medicinal herb* [see: mistletoe]

Visicol tablets ℞ *saline laxative; pre-procedure bowel evacuant* [sodium phosphate (monobasic and dibasic)] 1.5 g (1.102•0.398 g)

visilizumab USAN *anti-CD3 monoclonal antibody for organ transplants, autoimmune diseases, and other T-lymphocyte disorders*

visiluzumab [now: visilizumab]

Visine Allergy Relief eye drops OTC *topical ophthalmic decongestant and astringent* [tetrahydrozoline HCl; zinc sulfate] 0.05%•0.25%

Visine L.R. eye drops OTC *topical ophthalmic decongestant and vasoconstrictor* [oxymetazoline HCl] 0.025%

Visine Moisturizing eye drops OTC *topical ophthalmic decongestant, vasoconstrictor, and lubricant* [tetrahydrozoline HCl; polyethylene glycol 400] 0.05%•1%

Vision (trademarked device) OTC *needle-free insulin injection system*

Vision Care Enzymatic Cleaner tablets OTC *enzymatic cleaner for soft contact lenses* [pork pancreatin]

Visipak (trademarked packaging form) *reverse-numbered package*

Visipaque intra-arterial or IV injection ℞ *radiopaque contrast medium for CT, x-ray and visceral digital subtraction angiography* [iodixanol (49.1% iodine)] 550, 653 mg/mL (270, 320 mg/mL)

Visken tablets ℞ *antihypertensive; antiadrenergic (β-blocker)* [pindolol] 5, 10 mg

visnadine INN, BAN

visnafylline INN

Vi-Sol [see: Ce-Vi-Sol; Poly-Vi-Sol; Tri-Vi-Sol]

Vistacon IM injection (discontinued 1998) ℞ *anxiolytic; antiemetic* [hydroxyzine HCl] 50 mg/mL

Vistaquel 50 IM injection (discontinued 1997) ℞ *anxiolytic* [hydroxyzine HCl] 50 mg/mL

Vistaril capsules, oral suspension ℞ *anxiolytic; minor tranquilizer; antihistamine for allergic pruritus* [hydroxyzine pamoate] 25, 50, 100 mg; 25 mg/5 mL ⑨ Restoril

Vistaril deep IM injection ℞ *anxiolytic; antiemetic; antihistamine for allergic pruritus; adjunct to preoperative or prepartum analgesia* [hydroxyzine HCl] 25, 50 mg/mL ⑨ Restoril; Zestril

vistatolon INN *antiviral* [also: statolon]

Vistazine 50 IM injection ℞ *anxiolytic; antiemetic; antihistamine for allergic pruritus* [hydroxyzine HCl] 50 mg/mL

Vistide IV infusion ℞ *nucleoside antiviral for AIDS-related cytomegalovirus retinitis* [cidofovir] 75 mg/mL

Visual-Eyes ophthalmic solution OTC *extraocular irrigating solution* [sterile isotonic solution]

Visudyne IV injection ℞ *treatment for wet age-related macular degeneration (AMD), for use with the Opal Photoactivator laser* [verteporfin] 2 mg/mL (15 mg/vial)

Vita-bee with C Captabs (capsule-shaped tablets) OTC *vitamin supplement* [multiple B vitamins; vitamin C] ≛•300 mg

Vita-Bob softgel capsules OTC *vitamin supplement* [multiple vitamins; folic acid] ≛•0.4 mg

Vita-C crystals OTC *vitamin C supplement* [ascorbic acid] 4 g/tsp.

VitaCarn oral solution ℞ *dietary amino acid for primary and secondary genetic carnitine deficiency (orphan) and end-stage renal disease (orphan); investigational (orphan) for pediatric cardiomyopathy* [levocarnitine]

Vita-Feron tablets (discontinued 1998) OTC *hematinic* [iron; folic acid; vitamin B_{12}] 150•0.8•0.006 mg

Vitafōl syrup ℞ *hematinic* [ferric pyrophosphate; multiple B vitamins; folic acid] 90•≛•0.75 mg/15 mL

Vitafōl; Vitafōl-PN film-coated caplets ℞ *hematinic; vitamin supplement* [ferrous fumarate; multiple vitamins; folic acid] 65 mg•≛•1 mg

Vita-Kid chewable wafers OTC *vitamin supplement* [multiple vitamins; folic acid] ≛•0.3 mg

Vital B-50 timed-release tablets OTC *vitamin supplement* [multiple B vitamins; folic acid; biotin] ≛•100•50 µg

Vital High Nitrogen powder OTC *enteral nutritional therapy* [lactose-free formula] 79 g
Vitalets chewable tablets OTC *vitamin/mineral/iron supplement* [multiple vitamins & minerals; iron; biotin] ≛ •10 mg•25 μg
Vitalize SF liquid OTC *hematinic* [ferric pyrophosphate; multiple B vitamins; lysine] 66•≛•300 mg/15 mL
Vitalux (CAN) time-release tablet OTC *vitamin/antioxidant supplement* [multiple vitamins; multiple minerals]
vitamin A USP *fat-soluble vitamin; antixerophthalmic; topical emollient; essential for vision, dental development, growth, cortisone synthesis, epithelial tissue differentiation, embryonic development, reproduction, and mucous membrane maintenance* 10 000, 15 000, 25 000 IU oral
vitamin A acid [see: tretinoin]
vitamin A palmitate
vitamin A_1 [see: retinol]
Vitamin B Complex 100 injection ℞ *parenteral vitamin therapy* [multiple B vitamins] ≛
vitamin B_1 [see: thiamine HCl]
vitamin B_1 mononitrate [see: thiamine mononitrate]
vitamin B_2 [see: riboflavin]
vitamin B_3 [see: niacin; niacinamide]
vitamin B_5 [see: calcium pantothenate]
vitamin B_6 [see: pyridoxine HCl]
vitamin B_8 [see: adenosine phosphate]
vitamin B_{12} [now: cyanocobalamin; hydroxocobalamin]
vitamin B_c [see: folic acid]
vitamin B_t [see: carnitine]
vitamin C [see: ascorbic acid; calcium ascorbate; sodium ascorbate]
vitamin D *a family of fat-soluble vitamins consisting of ergocalciferol (vitamin D_2) and cholecalciferol (vitamin D_3), which is converted to calcitriol (the active form) in the body; considered a non-endogenous hormone* [see also: alfacalcidol; calcifediol; dihydrotachysterol; doxercalciferol; paricalcitol] 400, 1000 IU oral (CAN)
Vitamin D Oral Drops (discontinued 1999) OTC *vitamin supplement* [ergocalciferol (vitamin D_2)] 8000 IU/mL
vitamin D_1 [see: dihydrotachysterol]
vitamin D_2 [see: ergocalciferol]
vitamin D_3 [see: cholecalciferol]
vitamin E USP *fat-soluble vitamin; antioxidant; platelet aggregation inhibitor; topical emollient* [note relative potencies at alpha tocopherol, et seq.] 100, 200, 400, 500, 800, 1000 IU oral; 15 IU/30 mL oral
Vitamin E with Mixed Tocopherols tablets OTC *vitamin supplement* [vitamin E] 100, 200, 400 IU
vitamin E-TPGS (tocopheryl polyethylene glycol succinate) [see: tocophersolan]
vitamin G [see: riboflavin]
vitamin H [see: biotin]
vitamin K_1 [see: phytonadione]
vitamin K_2 [see: menaquinone]
vitamin K_3 [see: menadione]
vitamin K_4 [see: menadiol sodium diphosphate]
vitamin M [see: folic acid]
vitamin P [see: bioflavonoids]
vitamin P_4 [see: troxerutin]
Vitamin-Mineral Supplement liquid OTC *vitamin/mineral supplement* [multiple B vitamins & minerals; alcohol 18%]
Vitaneed liquid OTC *enteral nutritional therapy* [lactose-free formula]
Vita-Plus E softgels OTC *vitamin supplement* [vitamin E (as *d*-alpha tocopheryl acetate)] 400 IU
Vita-Plus G softgel capsules OTC *geriatric vitamin/mineral supplement* [multiple vitamins & minerals]
Vita-Plus H softgel capsules OTC *vitamin/mineral/iron supplement* [multiple vitamins & minerals; iron] ≛•13.4 mg
Vita-PMS; Vita-PMS Plus tablets OTC *vitamin/mineral supplement; digestive enzymes* [multiple vitamins & minerals; folic acid; biotin; amylase; protease; lipase; betaine acid HCl]

≛•0.33 mg•10.4 μg•2500 U•2500 U•200 U•16.7 mg

Vitarex tablets OTC *vitamin/mineral/iron supplement* [multiple vitamins & minerals; iron] ≛•15 mg

Vitaxin ℞ *investigational (Phase II) angiogenesis inhibitor for leiomyosarcoma*

Vite E cream OTC *emollient* [vitamin E] 50 mg/g

Vitec cream OTC *emollient* [vitamin E]

Vitelle Irospan timed-release tablets, timed-release capsules OTC *hematinic; iron supplement* [iron (from ferrous sulfate, dried); ascorbic acid] 65•150 mg

Vitelle Lurline PMS tablets OTC *analgesic; antipyretic; diuretic; vitamin B_6* [acetaminophen; pamabrom; pyridoxine HCl] 500•25•50 mg

Vitelle Nesentials tablets OTC *vitamin/mineral supplement* [multiple vitamins & minerals]

Vitelle Nestabs OTC tablets OTC *prenatal vitamin/calcium/iron supplement* [multiple vitamins; calcium; iron; folic acid] ≛•200•29•0.8 mg

Vitelle Nestrex tablets OTC *vitamin B_6 supplement* [pyridoxine HCl] 25 mg

vitellin *natural remedy* [see: lecithin]

Vitex agnus-castus *medicinal herb* [see: chaste tree]

Vitinoin (CAN) cream, gel (discontinued 2001) ℞ *topical keratolytic for acne* [tretinoin] 0.025%, 0.05%, 0.1%; 0.025%

Vitis coigetiae; V. vinifera *medicinal herb* [see: grape seed]

Vitrase ℞ *investigational (Phase III) agent to clear vitreous hemorrhage*

Vitrasert intraocular implant (5–8 months' duration) ℞ *antiviral for AIDS-related CMV retinitis (orphan)* [ganciclovir] 4.5 mg

Vitravene intravitreal injection ℞ *ophthalmic antiviral for AIDS-related CMV retinitis* [fomivirsen sodium] 6.6 mg/mL

Vitron-C chewable tablets OTC *hematinic* [iron (from ferrous fumarate); ascorbic acid] 66•125 mg ⑨ Vytone

Vitron-C-Plus tablets (discontinued 1998) OTC *hematinic* [iron (from ferrous fumarate); ascorbic acid] 132•250 mg

Vivactil film-coated tablets ℞ *tricyclic antidepressant* [protriptyline HCl] 5, 10 mg

Viva-Drops eye drops OTC *ocular moisturizer/lubricant*

Vivarin tablets OTC *CNS stimulant; analeptic* [caffeine] 200 mg

Vivelle; Vivelle-Dot transdermal patch ℞ *estrogen replacement therapy for postmenopausal symptoms* [estradiol] 25, 37.5, 50, 75, 100 μg/day

Vivonex T.E.N. powder OTC *enteral nutritional therapy* [lactose-free formula]

Vivotif Berna enteric-coated capsules ℞ *typhoid fever vaccine* [typhoid vaccine (Ty21a), live attenuated] $2–6 \times 10^9$ viable CFU + $5–50 \times 10^9$ nonviable cells

Vi-Zac capsules OTC *vitamin/zinc supplement* [vitamins A, C, and E; zinc] 5000 IU•500 mg•50 mg•18 mg

V-Lax powder (discontinued 1999) OTC *bulk laxative* [psyllium hydrophilic mucilloid] 50%

VLP (vincristine, L-asparaginase, prednisone) *chemotherapy protocol*

VM (vinblastine, mitomycin) *chemotherapy protocol for breast cancer*

VM-26 [see: teniposide]

VM-26PP (teniposide, procarbazine, prednisone) *chemotherapy protocol*

VMAD (vincristine, methotrexate, Adriamycin, actinomycin D) *chemotherapy protocol*

VMCP (vincristine, melphalan, cyclophosphamide, prednisone) *chemotherapy protocol for multiple myeloma* [also: VCMP]

VML-262 *investigational (Phase II) topical treatment for psoriasis*

VMP (VePesid, mitoxantrone, prednimustine) *chemotherapy protocol*

VOCAP (VP-16-213, Oncovin, cyclophosphamide, Adriamycin, Platinol) *chemotherapy protocol*

Vofenal (CAN) eye drops (discontinued 2001) ℞ *topical nonsteroidal anti-inflammatory drug (NSAID)* [diclofenac sodium] 0.1%

vofopitant dihydrochloride USAN *tachykinin NK_1 receptor antagonist; antiemetic*

voglibose USAN *investigational α-glucosidase inhibitor; antidiabetic*

volatile nitrites *amyl nitrite, butyl nitrite, and isobutyl nitrite vapors that produce coronary stimulant effects, abused as street drugs* [see also: nitrous oxide; petroleum distillate inhalants]

volazocine USAN, INN *analgesic*

Volmax extended-release tablets ℞ *sympathomimetic bronchodilator* [albuterol sulfate] 4, 8 mg

Voltaren delayed-release tablets ℞ *analgesic; antiarthritic; nonsteroidal anti-inflammatory drug (NSAID) for ankylosing spondylitis* [diclofenac sodium] 25, 50, 75 mg

Voltaren (CAN) suppositories ℞ *analgesic; antiarthritic; nonsteroidal anti-inflammatory drug (NSAID)* [diclofenac sodium] 50, 100 mg

Voltaren Ophtha (CAN) eye drops ℞ *ocular nonsteroidal anti-inflammatory drug (NSAID) for postoperative treatment following cataract extraction* [diclofenac sodium] 0.1%

Voltaren Ophthalmic eye drops ℞ *ocular nonsteroidal anti-inflammatory drug (NSAID) for postoperative treatment following cataract extraction* [diclofenac sodium] 0.1%

Voltaren Rapide (CAN) tablets ℞ *analgesic; antiarthritic; nonsteroidal anti-inflammatory drug (NSAID)* [diclofenac potassium] 50 mg

Voltaren SR (CAN) slow-release tablets ℞ *once-daily antiarthritic; nonsteroidal anti-inflammatory drug (NSAID)* [diclofenac sodium] 75, 100 mg

Voltaren XR extended-release tablets ℞ *once-daily antiarthritic; nonsteroidal anti-inflammatory drug (NSAID)* [diclofenac sodium] 100 mg

von Willebrand factor [see: antihemophilic factor]

Vontrol tablets (discontinued 1998) ℞ *antiemetic; antivertigo agent* [diphenidol HCl] 25 mg ⊡ Bontril

vorozole USAN, INN, BAN *antineoplastic; aromatase inhibitor*

vortel [see: clorprenaline HCl]

VōSol HC Otic ear drops ℞ *topical corticosteroidal anti-inflammatory; antibacterial; antifungal* [hydrocortisone; acetic acid] 1%•2%

VōSol Otic ear drops ℞ *antibacterial; antifungal* [acetic acid] 2%

votumumab USAN *monoclonal antibody for cancer imaging and therapy*

voxergolide INN

Voxsuprine tablets ℞ *peripheral vasodilator* [isoxsuprine HCl] 10, 20 mg

VP (vasopressin) [q.v.]

VP (VePesid, Platinol) *chemotherapy protocol for small cell lung cancer*

VP (vincristine, prednisone) *chemotherapy protocol*

VP + A (vincristine, prednisone, asparaginase) *chemotherapy protocol*

VP-16 [see: etoposide]

VPB (vinblastine, Platinol, bleomycin) *chemotherapy protocol*

VPBCPr (vincristine, prednisone, vinblastine, chlorambucil, procarbazine) *chemotherapy protocol*

VPCA (vincristine, prednisone, cyclophosphamide, ara-C) *chemotherapy protocol*

VPCMF (vincristine, prednisone, cyclophosphamide, methotrexate, fluorouracil) *chemotherapy protocol*

VP-L-asparaginase (vincristine, prednisone, L-asparaginase) *chemotherapy protocol*

VPP (VePesid, Platinol) *chemotherapy protocol*

VT-1 *investigational stem cell transplant adjunct for multiple myeloma and other blood-related cancers*

V-TAD (VePesid, thioguanine, ara-C, daunorubicin) *chemotherapy protocol for acute myelocytic leukemia (AML)*

vulneraries *a class of agents that promote wound healing*

Vumon IV infusion ℞ *antineoplastic for acute lymphocytic leukemia (orphan) and bladder cancer* [teniposide] 50 mg (10 mg/mL)

V.V.S. vaginal cream (discontinued 2001) ℞ *broad-spectrum bacteriostatic* [sulfathiazole; sulfacetamide; sulfabenzamide] 3.42%•2.86%•3.7%

VX-497 *investigational (Phase II) inosine monophosphate dehydrogenase (IMPDH) inhibitor for the oral treatment of hepatitis C and autoimmune diseases*

VX-740 *investigational anti-inflammatory agent*

Vytone cream ℞ *topical corticosteroidal anti-inflammatory; antifungal; antibacterial* [hydrocortisone; iodoquinol] 1%•1% ⓓ Hytone; Vitron

VZIG (varicella-zoster immune globulin) [q.v.]

wahoo ***(Euonymus atropurpureus)*** bark *medicinal herb used as a diuretic, expectorant, and laxative*

wakerobin *medicinal herb* [see: birthroot]

wallflower; western wallflower *medicinal herb* [see: dogbane]

walnut (*Juglans* spp.) *medicinal herb* [see: black walnut; butternut; English walnut]

walnut, lemon; white walnut *medicinal herb* [see: butternut]

Walpole tea *medicinal herb* [see: New Jersey tea]

wandering milkweed *medicinal herb* [see: dogbane]

warfarin INN, BAN *coumarin-derivative anticoagulant* [also: warfarin potassium]

warfarin potassium USP *coumarin-derivative anticoagulant* [also: warfarin]

warfarin sodium USP *coumarin-derivative anticoagulant* 1, 2, 2.5, 4, 5, 7.5, 10 mg oral

Wart Remover liquid OTC *topical keratolytic* [salicylic acid in flexible collodion] 17%

Wartec ⓒⓐⓝ solution ℞ *topical antimitotic for external genital warts* [podofilox] 0.5%

Wart-Off liquid OTC *topical keratolytic* [salicylic acid in flexible collodion] 17%

water, purified USP *solvent*

water, tritiated [see: tritiated water]

water cabbage *medicinal herb* [see: white pond lily]

water dock ***(Rumex aquaticus)*** *medicinal herb* [see: yellow dock]

water eryngo ***(Eryngium aquaticum)*** root *medicinal herb used as a diaphoretic, diuretic, emetic, expectorant, and stimulant*

water fern *medicinal herb* [see: buckhorn brake]

water flag *medicinal herb* [see: blue flag]

water hemlock; water parsley *medicinal herb* [see: poison hemlock]

water lily *medicinal herb* [see: blue flag; white pond lily]

water lily, sweet; sweet-scented water lily; white water lily *medicinal herb* [see: white pond lily]

water moccasin snake antivenin [see: antivenin (Crotalidae) polyvalent]

water O 15 USAN *radioactive diagnostic aid for vascular disorders*

water pepper *medicinal herb* [see: knotweed]

water pimpernel; water purslain *medicinal herb* [see: brooklime]

water shamrock *medicinal herb* [see: buckbean]

water smartweed *medicinal herb* [see: knotweed]

[^{15}O]water [see: water O 15]

watercress *(Nasturtium officinale)* plant *medicinal herb for anemia, cramps, kidney and liver disorders, nervousness, and rheumatism*

water-d$_2$ [see: deuterium oxide]

wax, carnauba NF *tablet-coating agent*

wax, emulsifying NF *emulsifying and stiffening agent*

wax, microcrystalline NF *stiffening and tablet-coating agent*

wax, white NF *stiffening agent* [also: beeswax, white]

wax, yellow NF *stiffening agent* [also: beeswax, yellow]

wax cluster *medicinal herb* [see: wintergreen]

wax myrtle *medicinal herb* [see: bayberry]

weeping spruce *medicinal herb* [see: hemlock]

Welchol tablets ℞ *nonabsorbed cholesterol-lowering polymer for hyperlipidemia* [colesevelam HCl] 625 mg

Wellbutrin tablets ℞ *aminoketone antidepressant* [bupropion HCl] 75, 100 mg

Wellbutrin SR sustained-release film-coated tablets ℞ *aminoketone antidepressant* [bupropion HCl] 100, 150 mg

Wellcovorin powder for IV infusion ℞ *chemotherapy "rescue" agent (orphan)* [leucovorin calcium] 100 mg/vial

Wellcovorin tablets ℞ *chemotherapy "rescue" agent (orphan); antidote to folic acid antagonist overdose* [leucovorin calcium] 5, 25 mg

Wellferon subcu or IM injection (discontinued 2000) ℞ *biological response modifier for chronic hepatitis C (orphan); investigational (Phase III) for HIV* [interferon alfa-n1] 3 MU/mL

Wellferon (CAN) subcu or IM injection (discontinued 2001) ℞ *biological response modifier for hairy cell leukemia, laryngeal papillomatosis, condylomata acuminata, and chronic hepatitis B and C* [interferon alfa-n1] 3, 5, 10 MU/mL

Westcort ointment, cream ℞ *topical corticosteroidal anti-inflammatory* [hydrocortisone valerate] 0.2%

western wallflower *medicinal herb* [see: dogbane]

Wet-N-Soak solution OTC *rewetting solution for rigid gas permeable contact lenses*

Wet-N-Soak Plus solution OTC *disinfecting/wetting/soaking solution for rigid gas permeable contact lenses* [note: RGP contact indication different from hard contact indication for same product]

Wet-N-Soak Plus solution OTC *wetting/soaking solution for hard contact lenses* [note: hard contact indication different from RGP contact indication for same product]

Wetting solution OTC *wetting solution for hard contact lenses*

Wetting & Soaking solution OTC *disinfecting/wetting/soaking solution for rigid gas permeable contact lenses* [note: one of two different products with the same name]

Wetting & Soaking solution OTC *wetting/soaking solution for hard contact lenses* [note: one of two different products with the same name]

wheat germ oil (octacosanol) *natural supplement for increasing muscle endurance*

WHF Lubricating Gel OTC *vaginal antimicrobial and lubricant* [chlorhexidine gluconate; glycerin]

white bay *medicinal herb* [see: magnolia]

white beeswax [see: beeswax, white]

White Cloverine Salve ointment OTC *skin protectant* [white petrolatum] 97%

White Cod Liver Oil Concentrate capsules, chewable tablets OTC *vitamin supplement* [vitamins A, D, and E] 10 000•400•$\stackrel{?}{=}$ IU; 4000•200•$\stackrel{?}{=}$ IU

White Cod Liver Oil Concentrate with Vitamin C chewable tablets OTC *vitamin supplement* [vitamins A, C, and D] 4000 IU•50 mg•200 IU

white cohosh *(Actaea alba; A. pachypoda; A. rubra)* plant and root *medicinal herb for arthritis, bowel evacuation, colds, cough, itching, promoting labor, reviving those near death,* *rheumatism, stimulating menses, stomach disorders, and urogenital disorders*

white endive *medicinal herb* [see: dandelion]

white fringe *medicinal herb* [see: fringe tree]

white hellebore *(Veratrum album)* [see: hellebore]

white horehound *medicinal herb* [see: horehound]

white lotion USP *astringent; topical protectant*

white mineral oil [see: petrolatum, white]

white mustard; white mustard seed *medicinal herb* [see: mustard]

white nettle *medicinal herb* [see: blind nettle]

white oak *(Quercus alba)* bark *medicinal herb for internal and external bleeding, menstrual disorders, mouth sores, skin irritation, toothache, strep throat, ulcers, and urinary bleeding*

white ointment [see: ointment, white]

white petrolatum [see: petrolatum, white]

white phenolphthalein [see: phenolphthalein]

white pine *(Pinus strobus)* bark *medicinal herb for bronchitis, dysentery, laryngitis, and mucous build-up*

white pond lily *(Nymphaea odorata)* root *medicinal herb used as an antiseptic, astringent, demulcent, discutient, and vulnerary*

white root *medicinal herb* [see: pleurisy root]

white sorrel *medicinal herb* [see: wood sorrel]

white walnut *medicinal herb* [see: butternut]

white water lily *medicinal herb* [see: white pond lily]

white wax [see: wax, white]

white willow *(Salix alba)* *medicinal herb* [see: willow]

whitethorn *medicinal herb* [see: hawthorn]

Whitfield's ointment [see: benzoic & salicylic acids]

Whitfield's Ointment OTC *topical antifungal; keratolytic* [benzoic acid; salicylic acid] 6%•3%

whole blood [see: blood, whole]

whole root rauwolfia [see: rauwolfia serpentina]

whole-cell pertussis vaccine [see: diphtheria & tetanus toxoids & whole-cell pertussis (DTwP) vaccine, adsorbed]

whorlywort *medicinal herb* [see: Culver root]

Wibi lotion OTC *moisturizer; emollient*

widow spider species antivenin [now: antivenin (Latrodectus mactans)]

Wigraine suppositories ℞ *migraine-specific vasoconstrictor* [ergotamine tartrate; caffeine; tartaric acid] 2•100•21.5 mg

Wigraine tablets ℞ *migraine-specific vasoconstrictor* [ergotamine tartrate; caffeine] 1•100 mg

wild bergamot *(Monarda fistulosa)* leaves *medicinal herb used as a carminative and stimulant*

wild black cherry *(Prunus serotina)* bark *medicinal herb used as an astringent, pectoral, sedative, and stimulant*

wild carrot *medicinal herb* [see: carrot]

wild cherry *(Prunus virginiana)* bark *medicinal herb for asthma, bronchitis, cough, fever, hypertension, and mucosal inflammation with discharge; also used as an expectorant*

wild cherry syrup USP

wild chicory *medicinal herb* [see: chicory]

wild clover *medicinal herb* [see: red clover]

wild cranesbill *medicinal herb* [see: alum root]

wild daisy *(Bellis perennis)* flowers and leaves *medicinal herb used as an analgesic, antispasmodic, demulcent, digestive, expectorant, laxative, and purgative*

wild endive *medicinal herb* [see: dandelion]

wild fennel *medicinal herb* [see: fennel]

wild geranium *medicinal herb* [see: alum root]

wild ginger *(Asarum canadense)* root *medicinal herb used as a carminative, diaphoretic, expectorant, and irritant; sometimes used as a substitute for ginger (Zingiber)*

wild hydrangea *medicinal herb* [see: hydrangea]

wild hyssop *medicinal herb* [see: blue vervain]

wild hyssop *(Pycnanthemum virginianum)* plant *medicinal herb used as an antispasmodic, carminative, diaphoretic, and stimulant*

wild indigo *(Baptisia tinctoria)* plant *medicinal herb used as an antiseptic, astringent, emetic, purgative, and stimulant*

wild jalap *(Ipomoea pandurata)* root *medicinal herb used as a strong cathartic*

wild lemon *medicinal herb* [see: mandrake]

wild lettuce *(Lactuca virosa)* leaves, flowers, and seeds *medicinal herb for asthma, bronchitis, chronic pain, circulatory disorders, cramps, laryngitis, nervous disorders, stimulating lactation, swollen genitals, and urinary tract infections*

wild marjoram *medicinal herb* [see: marjoram]

wild Oregon grape *medicinal herb* [see: Oregon grape]

wild pepper *medicinal herb* [see: mezereon; Siberian ginseng]

wild potato; wild scammony; wild sweet potato vine *medicinal herb* [see: wild jalap]

wild red raspberry *medicinal herb* [see: red raspberry]

wild senna *medicinal herb* [see: senna]

wild snowball *medicinal herb* [see: New Jersey tea]

wild strawberry *medicinal herb* [see: strawberry]

wild tobacco *medicinal herb* [see: lobelia]

wild turkey pea *medicinal herb* [see: turkey corn]

wild valerian, great *medicinal herb* [see: valerian]

wild woodbine *medicinal herb* [see: American ivy]

wild yam *(Dioscorea villosa)* root *medicinal herb for arthritis, bilious colic, bowel spasms, gas, menstrual cramps, morning sickness, and spasmodic asthma*

Willard water *natural remedy for acne, alopecia, anxiety, arthritis, hypertension, and stomach ulcers*

willow *(Salix alba; S. caprea; S. nigra; S. purpurea)* bark and buds *medicinal herb for analgesia, diuresis, eczema, fever, inducing diaphoresis, headache, nervousness, rheumatism, and ulcerations; also used as an anaphrodisiac, antiseptic, and astringent*

wind root *medicinal herb* [see: pleurisy root]

wineberry *medicinal herb* [see: currant]

winged elm *medicinal herb* [see: slippery elm]

WinRho SD IV or IM injection (discontinued 2000; replaced by WinRho SDF) ℞ *obstetric Rh factor immunity suppressant; treatment for immune thrombocytopenic purpura (orphan)* [Rh_0(D) immune globulin, solvent/detergent treated] 600, 1500, 5000 IU (120, 300, 1000 μg)

WinRho SDF freeze-dried powder for IV or IM injection ℞ *obstetric Rh factor immunity suppressant; treatment for immune thrombocytopenic purpura (orphan)* [Rh_0(D) immune globulin, solvent/detergent treated] 600, 1500, 5000 IU (120, 300, 1000 μg)

Winstrol tablets ℞ *anabolic steroid for hereditary angioedema* [stanozolol] 2 mg

winter bloom *medicinal herb* [see: witch hazel]

winter clover *medicinal herb* [see: squaw vine]

winter marjoram; winter sweet *medicinal herb* [see: marjoram]

winter savory *(Calamintha montana; Satureja montana; S. obovata)* leaves and stems *medicinal herb for* *diarrhea, nausea, promoting expectoration, relieving gas and flatulence, and stimulation of menstruation; also used as an aphrodisiac*

winterberry *(Ilex verticillata)* bark and fruit *medicinal herb used as an astringent, bitter tonic, and febrifuge*

wintergreen *(Gaultheria procumbens)* leaves and oil *medicinal herb for aches and pains, colds, gout, lumbago, and migraine headache; also used topically as an astringent and rubefacient*

wintergreen, bitter; false wintergreen *medicinal herb* [see: pipsissewa]

wintergreen oil [see: methyl salicylate]

winterlein *medicinal herb* [see: flaxseed]

Wintersteiner's compound F [see: hydrocortisone]

winterweed *medicinal herb* [see: chickweed]

witch hazel *(Hamamelis virginiana)* bark *medicinal herb for bruises, burns, colds, colitis, diarrhea, dysentery, eye irritations, hemorrhoids, internal and external bleeding, mucous membrane inflammation of mouth, gums, and throat, tuberculosis, and varicose veins*

withania *(Withania somnifera)* fruit and roots *medicinal herb for diuresis, inducing emesis, liver disorders, inflammation, sedation, tuberculosis, and tumors*

withe; withy *medicinal herb* [see: willow]

wobe-mugos *investigational (orphan) enzyme combination adjunct to chemotherapy for multiple myeloma*

wolf claw *medicinal herb* [see: club moss]

Women's Daily Formula capsules OTC *vitamin/calcium/iron supplement* [multiple vitamins; calcium; iron; folic acid] ≛ •450•25•0.4 mg

Women's Gentle Laxative enteric-coated tablets OTC *stimulant laxative* [bisacodyl] 5 mg

Wonder Ice gel OTC *topical analgesic; counterirritant* [menthol] 5.25%

Wonderful Dream salve (discontinued 1998) OTC *topical antiseptic and antimicrobial* [phenylmercuric nitrate] 1:5000

Wondra lotion OTC *moisturizer; emollient* [lanolin]

wood betony *medicinal herb* [see: betony]

wood creosote [see: creosote carbonate]

wood sanicle *medicinal herb* [see: sanicle]

wood sorrel *(Oxalis acetosella)* plant *medicinal herb used as an anodyne, diuretic, emmenagogue, irritant, and stomachic*

wood strawberry *medicinal herb* [see: strawberry]

woodbine *(Clematis virginiana)* leaves *medicinal herb for bowel evacuation, cancer, edema, fever, hypertension, inflammation, insomnia, itching, kidney disorders, skin cuts and sores, tuberculous cervical lymphadenitis, tumors, and venereal eruptions; not generally regarded as safe and effective*

woodbine; American woodbine; wild woodbine *medicinal herb* [see: American ivy]

woodruff *medicinal herb* [see: sweet woodruff]

woody nightshade *medicinal herb* [see: bittersweet nightshade]

Woolley's antiserotonin [see: benanserin HCl]

wooly parsnip *medicinal herb* [see: masterwort]

wormwood *(Artemisia absinthium)* plant and leaves *medicinal herb for aiding digestion, constipation, debility, fever, intestinal worms, jaundice, labor pains, menstrual cramps, and stomach and liver disorders; not generally regarded as safe and effective*

wound weed *medicinal herb* [see: goldenrod]

woundwort *(Prunella vulgaris)* plant *medicinal herb used as an antispasmodic, astringent, bitter tonic, diuretic, hemostatic, vermifuge, and vulnerary*

woundwort, soldier's *medicinal herb* [see: yarrow]

WOWtabs (trademarked dosage form) *quickly dissolving "without water" tablets*

WX-G250RIT *investigational (orphan) antineoplastic for renal cell carcinoma*
Wyamine Sulfate IV or IM injection ℞ *vasopressor for hypotensive shock* [mephentermine sulfate] 15, 30 mg/mL
Wyanoids Relief Factor rectal suppositories OTC *emollient* [cocoa butter; shark liver oil] 79%•3%
Wycillin IM, IV, intrapleural, or intrathecal injection, Tubex (cartridge-needle units) ℞ *natural penicillin antibiotic* [penicillin G procaine] 600 000, 1 200 000, 2 400 000 U ⑨ Bicillin; V-Cillin
Wydase IV or subcu injection, powder for injection (discontinued 2001) ℞ *adjuvant to increase absorption and dispersion of injected drugs* [hyaluronidase] 150 U/mL; 150, 1500 U/vial ⑨ Lidex
Wygesic tablets ℞ *narcotic analgesic* [propoxyphene HCl; acetaminophen] 65•650 mg
wymote *medicinal herb* [see: marsh mallow]
Wymox capsules, powder for oral suspension ℞ *aminopenicillin antibiotic* [amoxicillin] 250, 500 mg; 125, 250 mg/5 mL
Wyseal (trademarked dosage form) *film-coated tablet*
Wytensin tablets ℞ *antihypertensive* [guanabenz acetate] 4, 8 mg

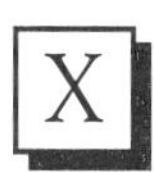

Xalatan eye drops ℞ *prostaglandin agonist for glaucoma and ocular hypertension* [latanoprost] 0.005% (50 µg/mL) ⑨ Dilantin
Xalcom ℞ *investigational (NDA filed) combination agent for glaucoma and ocular hypertension* [latanoprost; timolol]
xaliprodene *investigational (Phase III) nerve growth factor–like agent for amyotrophic lateral sclerosis; investigational (Phase II) for Alzheimer disease*
xamoterol USAN, INN, BAN *cardiac stimulant*
xamoterol fumarate USAN *cardiac stimulant*
Xanax tablets ℞ *benzodiazepine anxiolytic* [alprazolam] 0.25, 0.5, 1, 2 mg ⑨ Tenex; Zantac
xanomeline USAN *cholinergic agonist for Alzheimer disease*
xanomeline tartrate USAN *cholinergic agonist for Alzheimer disease*
xanoxate sodium USAN *bronchodilator*
xanoxic acid INN
xanthan gum NF *suspending agent*
xanthines, xanthine derivatives *a class of bronchodilators*
xanthinol niacinate USAN *peripheral vasodilator* [also: xantinol nicotinate]
xanthiol INN
xanthiol HCl [see: xanthiol]
xanthocillin BAN [also: xantocillin]
Xanthorhiza simplicissima *medicinal herb* [see: yellow root]
xanthotoxin [see: methoxsalen]
Xanthoxylum americanum; X. fraxineum *medicinal herb* [see: prickly ash]
xantifibrate INN
xantinol nicotinate INN *peripheral vasodilator* [also: xanthinol niacinate]
xantocillin INN [also: xanthocillin]
xantofyl palmitate INN
Xcytrin injection ℞ *investigational (Phase III) radiosensitizer for brain metastases* [motexafin gadolinium]
^{127}**Xe** [see: xenon Xe 127]
^{133}**Xe** [see: xenon Xe 133]
Xeloda film-coated tablets ℞ *antineoplastic for metastatic breast and colorectal cancer* [capecitabine] 150, 500 mg
xemilofiban HCl USAN *antianginal; investigational (Phase II) antithrombotic to prevent reocclusion of coronary*

arteries after PTCA (clinical trials discontinued 1999)
xenalamine [see: xenazoic acid]
xenaldial [see: xenygloxal]
xenalipin USAN, INN *hypolipidemic*
xenazoic acid INN
xenbucin USAN, INN *antihypercholesterolemic*
xenbuficin [see: xenbucin]
Xenical capsules ℞ *lipase inhibitor for weight loss* [orlistat] 120 mg
xenipentone INN
xenon *element (Xe)*
xenon (^{133}Xe) INN *radioactive agent* [also: xenon Xe 133]
xenon Xe 127 USP *diagnostic aid; medicinal gas; radioactive agent*
xenon Xe 133 USAN, USP *radioactive agent* [also: xenon (^{133}Xe)]
xenthiorate INN
xenygloxal INN
xenyhexenic acid INN
xenysalate INN, BAN *topical anesthetic; antibacterial; antifungal* [also: biphenamine HCl]
xenysalate HCl [see: biphenamine HCl]
xenytropium bromide INN
Xerac AC liquid ℞ *topical cleanser for acne* [aluminum chloride; alcohol] 6.25%•96%
Xerecept *investigational (Phase I/II, orphan) agent for peritumoral brain edema* [corticotropin-releasing factor]
Xeroderm lotion (discontinued 1998) OTC *moisturizer; emollient*
xibenolol INN
xibornol INN, BAN
Xigris IV injection ℞ *investigational (NDA filed) recombinant human activated protein C (rhAPC) for severe sepsis* [drotrecogin alfa]
xilobam USAN, INN *muscle relaxant*
ximoprofen INN
xinafoate USAN, INN, BAN *combining name for radicals or groups*
xinidamine INN
xinomiline INN
xipamide USAN, INN *antihypertensive; diuretic*
xipranolol INN
Xiral sustained-release tablets ℞ *decongestant; antihistamine; anticholinergic* [pseudoephedrine HCl; chlorpheniramine maleate; methscopolamine nitrate] 120•8•2.5 mg
Xolair IV and subcu injection ℞ *investigational (NDA filed) anti-IgE monoclonal antibody for asthma and allergic rhinitis* [omalizumab]
XomaZyme-H65 *orphan status withdrawn 1997* [CD5-T lymphocyte immunotoxin]
Xopenex inhalation solution ℞ *sympathomimetic bronchodilator* [levalbuterol HCl] 0.63, 1.25 mg/3 mL dose
xorphanol INN *analgesic* [also: xorphanol mesylate]
xorphanol mesylate USAN *analgesic* [also: xorphanol]
X-Prep liquid OTC *pre-procedure bowel evacuant* [senna extract] 74 mL
X-Prep Bowel Evacuant Kit-1 oral liquid + 2 tablets + 1 suppository OTC *pre-procedure bowel evacuant* [X-Prep liquid (q.v.); Senokot-S tablets (q.v.); Rectolax suppository (q.v.)]
X-Prep Bowel Evacuant Kit-2 oral liquid + granules + 1 suppository OTC *pre-procedure bowel evacuant* [X-Prep liquid (q.v.); Citralax granules (q.v.); Rectolax suppository (q.v.)]
XR-9576 *investigational (Phase III) antineoplastic*
XRT (x-ray therapy) *adjunct to chemotherapy* [not a pharmaceutical agent]
X-Seb shampoo OTC *antiseborrheic; keratolytic* [salicylic acid] 4%
X-Seb Plus shampoo OTC *antiseborrheic; keratolytic; antibacterial; antifungal* [salicylic acid; pyrithione zinc] 2%•1%
X-Seb T shampoo OTC *antiseborrheic; antipsoriatic; keratolytic* [coal tar; salicylic acid] 10%•4%
X-Seb T Plus shampoo OTC *antiseborrheic; antipsoriatic; keratolytic* [coal tar; salicylic acid; menthol] 10%•3%•1%
xylamidine tosilate INN *serotonin inhibitor* [also: xylamidine tosylate]

xylamidine tosylate USAN *serotonin inhibitor* [also: xylamidine tosilate]
xylazine INN *analgesic; veterinary muscle relaxant* [also: xylazine HCl]
xylazine HCl USAN *analgesic; veterinary muscle relaxant* [also: xylazine]
xylitol NF *sweetened vehicle*
Xylocaine injection ℞ *injectable local anesthetic* [lidocaine HCl] 0.5%, 1%, 2%
Xylocaine liquid, solution, ointment, jelly ℞ *mucous membrane anesthetic* [lidocaine HCl] 5%; 4%; 5%; 2%
Xylocaine ointment OTC *topical local anesthetic* [lidocaine] 2.5%
Xylocaine 10% Oral spray ℞ *mucous membrane anesthetic* [lidocaine HCl] 10%
Xylocaine HCl injection ℞ *injectable local anesthetic* [lidocaine HCl; dextrose] 1.5%•7.5%
Xylocaine HCl injection ℞ *injectable local anesthetic* [lidocaine HCl; epinephrine] 0.5%•1:200 000, 1%•1:100 000, 1%•1:200 000, 2%•1:50 000, 2%•1:100 000, 2%•1:200 000
Xylocaine HCl IV for Cardiac Arrhythmias IV injection, IV admixture ℞ *antiarrhythmic* [lidocaine HCl] 1%, 2%, 4%, 20%
Xylocaine MPF injection ℞ *injectable local anesthetic* [lidocaine HCl] 0.5%, 1%, 1.5%, 2%, 4%
Xylocaine MPF injection ℞ *injectable local anesthetic* [lidocaine HCl; epinephrine] 1%•1:200 000, 1.5%•1:200 000, 2%•1:200 000
Xylocaine MPF injection ℞ *injectable local anesthetic* [lidocaine HCl; glucose] 5%•7.5%
Xylocaine Viscous solution ℞ *mucous membrane anesthetic* [lidocaine HCl] 2%
xylocoumarol INN
xylofilcon A USAN *hydrophilic contact lens material*
xylometazoline INN, BAN *vasoconstrictor; nasal decongestant* [also: xylometazoline HCl]
xylometazoline HCl USP *vasoconstrictor; nasal decongestant* [also: xylometazoline]
Xylo-Pfan tablets OTC *diagnostic aid for intestinal function* [xylose] 25 g
xylose (D-xylose) USP *diagnostic aid for intestinal function*
xyloxemine INN
Xyrem oral solution ℞ *investigational (NDA filed, orphan) treatment for cataplexy* [sodium oxybate]
Xyvion ℞ *investigational (NDA filed) synthetic steroid for osteoporosis and other postmenopausal symptoms* [tibolone]

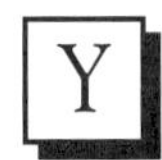

yam *medicinal herb* [see: wild yam]
yarrow *(Achillea millefolium)* flower *medicinal herb for bowel hemorrhage, colds, fever, flu, hypertension, inducing sweating, measles, mucosal inflammation with discharge, nosebleed, reducing heavy menstrual bleeding and pain, thrombosis, and topical hemostasis*
Yasmin tablets (in packs of 28) ℞ *monophasic oral contraceptive* [drospirenone; ethinyl estradiol] 3 mg•30 µg
yatren [see: chiniofon]
^{169}Yb [see: pentetate calcium trisodium Yb 169]
^{169}Yb [see: ytterbium Yb 169 pentetate]
yeast, dried NF
yeast cell derivative *claimed to promote wound healing*

Yeast-Gard vaginal suppositories OTC *for vaginal irritations, itching, and burning* [pulsatilla 28x; *Candida albicans* 28x]

Yeast-Gard; Yeast-Gard Sensitive Formula vaginal cream (name changed to Vagi-Gard in 1998)

Yeast-Gard Medicated Disposable Douche Premix solution OTC *antifungal; vaginal cleanser and deodorizer; acidity modifier* [sodium benzoate; lactic acid]

Yeast-Gard Medicated Douche; Yeast-Gard Medicated Disposable Douche solution OTC *antiseptic/germicidal; vaginal cleanser and deodorizer* [povidone-iodine] 10%; 0.3%

Yeast-X powder (discontinued 1998) OTC *absorbs vaginal moisture; astringent* [cornstarch; zinc oxide]

Yeast-X vaginal suppositories OTC *for vaginal irritations, itching, and burning* [pulsatilla 28x]

Yelets tablets OTC *vitamin/mineral/iron supplement* [multiple vitamins & minerals; ferrous fumarate; folic acid] ≛•20•0.1 mg

yellow bedstraw; yellow cleavers *medicinal herb* [see: bedstraw]

yellow beeswax [see: beeswax, yellow]

yellow dock *(Rumex crispus)* root *medicinal herb for anemia, blood cleansing, constipation, itching, liver congestion, rheumatism, skin problems, and eyelid ulcerations; also used as a dentifrice*

yellow ferric oxide [see: ferric oxide, yellow]

yellow fever vaccine USP *active immunizing agent for yellow fever*

yellow gentian *medicinal herb* [see: gentian]

yellow ginseng *medicinal herb* [see: blue cohosh]

yellow Indian paint *medicinal herb* [see: goldenseal]

yellow jessamine *medicinal herb* [see: gelsemium]

yellow mercuric oxide [see: mercuric oxide, yellow]

yellow ointment [see: ointment, yellow]

yellow paint root; yellow root *medicinal herb* [see: goldenseal]

yellow petrolatum JAN *ointment base; emollient/protectant* [also: petrolatum]

yellow phenolphthalein [see: phenolphthalein, yellow]

yellow precipitate [see: mercuric oxide, yellow]

yellow puccoon *medicinal herb* [see: goldenseal]

yellow root *(Xanthorhiza simplicissima)* *medicinal herb used for diabetes and hypertension*

yellow root; yellow paint root *medicinal herb* [see: goldenseal]

yellow wax [see: wax, yellow]

yellow wood; yellow wood berries *medicinal herb* [see: prickly ash]

yerba maté *(Ilex paraguariensis)* leaves *medicinal herb used as a* CNS *stimulant, diuretic, and purifier*

yerba santa *(Eriodictyon californicum)* leaves *medicinal herb for asthma, bronchial congestion, colds, hay fever, inducing expectoration, inflammation, rheumatic pain, and tuberculosis*

yew (*Taxus bacatta* and other species) leaves *medicinal herb for liver disorders, rheumatism, and urinary tract disorders*

YF-Vax subcu injection ℞ *yellow fever vaccine* [yellow fever vaccine] 0.5 mL

YKP-10A *investigational (Phase II) antidepressant*

Yocon tablets ℞ *no FDA-approved uses; sympatholytic; mydriatic; aphrodisiac* [yohimbine HCl] 5.4 mg

Yodoxin tablets, powder ℞ *amebicide* [iodoquinol] 210, 650 mg; 25 g

yohimbe *(Corynanthe johimbe; Pausinystalia johimbe)* bark *medicinal herb for angina, hypertension, and impotence and other sexual dysfunction; also used as an aphrodisiac*

yohimbic acid INN

yohimbine HCl *alpha$_2$-adrenergic blocker; claimed to be an aphrodisiac; no FDA-sanctioned uses* 5.4 mg oral

Yohimex tablets ℞ *no FDA-approved uses; sympatholytic; mydriatic; aphrodisiac* [yohimbine HCl] 5.4 mg

Your Choice Non-Preserved Saline solution OTC *rinsing/storage solution for soft contact lenses* [sodium chloride (saline solution)]

Your Choice Sterile Preserved Saline solution OTC *rinsing/storage solution for soft contact lenses* [sodium chloride (preserved saline solution)]

youthwort *medicinal herb* [see: masterwort]

ytterbium *element (Yb)*

ytterbium Yb 169 pentetate USP *radioactive agent*

yttrium *element (Y)*

yttrium Y 90 murine MAb (2B8-MXDTPA) & indium In 111 murine MAb (2B8-MXDTPA) *investigational (orphan) for non-Hodgkin B-cell lymphoma*

yucca *(Yucca glauca)* root *medicinal herb for arthritis, colitis, hypertension, migraine headache, and rheumatism*

yuma *medicinal herb* [see: wild yam]

Yurelax (Spanish name for U.S. product Flexeril)

Yutopar IV infusion ℞ *uterine relaxant to arrest preterm labor* [ritodrine HCl] 10, 15 mg/mL

Z

zabicipril INN

zacopride INN *antiemetic; peristaltic stimulant* [also: zacopride HCl]

zacopride HCl USAN, INN *antiemetic; peristaltic stimulant* [also: zacopride]

Zacutex IV injection ℞ *investigational (Phase III) platelet activating factor (PAF) antagonist for acute pancreatitis* [lexipafant]

Zadaxin (commercially available in several countries) ℞ *investigational (Phase III) influenza vaccine and vaccine enhancer for lung cancer; investigational (Phase III, orphan) for chronic hepatitis B; investigational (orphan) for DiGeorge syndrome with immune defects; investigational (orphan) for hepatocellular carcinoma* [thymalfasin]

Zaditen Ophthalmic (foreign name for U.S. product Zaditor)

Zaditor eye drops ℞ *topical ophthalmic antihistamine and mast cell stabilizer for allergic conjunctivitis* [ketotifen fumarate] 0.025%

zafirlukast USAN, INN, BAN *antiasthmatic; leukotriene receptor antagonist (LTRA)*

zafuleptine INN

Zagam film-coated tablets ℞ *once-daily broad-spectrum fluoroquinolone antibiotic for community-acquired respiratory infections* [sparfloxacin] 200 mg

zalcitabine USAN *nucleoside reverse transcriptase inhibitor (NRTI) antiviral for HIV infection (orphan)*

zaleplon USAN *pyrazolopyrimidine hypnotic for the short-term treatment of insomnia*

zalospirone INN *anxiolytic* [also: zalospirone HCl]

zalospirone HCl USAN *anxiolytic* [also: zalospirone]

zaltidine INN, BAN *antagonist to histamine H_2 receptors* [also: zaltidine HCl]

zaltidine HCl USAN *antagonist to histamine H_2 receptors* [also: zaltidine]

zamifenacin INN, BAN *investigational treatment for irritable bowel syndrome*

Zanaflex tablets ℞ *antispasmodic for multiple sclerosis and spinal cord injury (orphan)* [tizanidine HCl] 4 mg

zanamivir USAN *antiviral; neuraminidase inhibitor for the treatment of acute influenza A and B infections*

Zanfel cream OTC *topical poison ivy treatment*

zankiren HCl USAN *antihypertensive*

Zanosar powder for IV injection ℞ *nitrosourea-type alkylating antineoplastic for metastatic islet cell carcinoma of pancreas* [streptozocin] 1 g (100 mg/mL)

zanoterone USAN *antiandrogen*

Zantac film-coated tablets, syrup, IV or IM injection ℞ *histamine H_2 antagonist for gastric and duodenal ulcers* [ranitidine HCl] 150, 300 mg; 15 mg/mL; 0.5, 25 mg/mL ⑨ Xanax

Zantac 75 tablets OTC *histamine H_2 antagonist for episodic heartburn* [ranitidine HCl] 75 mg

Zantac EFFERdose effervescent tablets, effervescent granules ℞ *histamine H_2 antagonist for gastric and duodenal ulcers* [ranitidine HCl] 150 mg; 150 mg/packet

Zantac GELdose capsules ℞ *histamine H_2 antagonist for gastric and duodenal ulcers* [ranitidine HCl] 150, 300 mg

Zanthorhiza apiifolia *medicinal herb* [see: yellow root]

Zantryl capsules ℞ *anorexiant; CNS stimulant* [phentermine HCl] 30 mg

Zanzibar aloe *medicinal herb* [see: aloe]

zapizolam INN

zaprinast INN, BAN

zardaverine INN

Zarontin capsules, syrup ℞ *anticonvulsant* [ethosuximide] 250 mg; 250 mg/5 mL ⑨ Zaroxolyn

Zaroxolyn tablets ℞ *antihypertensive; diuretic* [metolazone] 2.5, 5, 10 mg ⑨ Zarontin; Zeroxin

zatosetron INN, BAN *antimigraine* [also: zatosetron maleate]

zatosetron maleate USAN *antimigraine* [also: zatosetron]

Zavedos (European name for U.S. product Idamycin)

Z-Bec tablets OTC *vitamin/zinc supplement* [multiple vitamins; zinc sulfate] ≛•22.5 mg

ZBT Baby powder OTC *topical diaper rash treatment* [talc]

ZDV (zidovudine) [q.v.]

ZE Caps soft capsules OTC *dietary supplement* [vitamin E; zinc gluconate] 200•9.6 mg

Zea mays *medicinal herb* [see: Indian corn]

ZeaSorb (CAN) powder OTC *absorbent; antibacterial; antifungal* [microporous cellulose; chloroxylenol] 45%•0.5%

ZeaSorb AF (CAN) powder OTC *topical antifungal* [tolnaftate] 1%

Zeasorb-AF powder OTC *topical antifungal* [miconazole nitrate] 2%

zeaxanthin *natural carotenoid used to prevent and treat age-related macular degeneration (AMD), retinitis pigmentosa (RP), and other retinal dysfunction*

Zebeta film-coated tablets ℞ *antihypertensive; antiadrenergic (β-blocker)* [bisoprolol fumarate] 5, 10 mg

Zecnil (discontinued 1997) ℞ *investigational (orphan) for secreting cutaneous gastrointestinal fistulas and bleeding esophageal varices* [somatostatin]

Zefazone powder or frozen premix for IV injection ℞ *cephalosporin antibiotic* [cefmetazole sodium] 1, 2 g ⑨ cefazolin

Zeffix ℞ *investigational oral treatment for hepatitis B* [lamivudine]

zein NF *coating agent*

Zeldox European name for U.S. product Geodon

Zelmac tablets ℞ *investigational (NDA filed) selective serotonin 5-HT_4 receptor antagonist for irritable bowel syndrome* [tegaserod]

Zemaphyte ℞ *investigational (Phase III) treatment for eczema*

Zemplar parenteral injection during dialysis ℞ *synthetic vitamin D analogue for osteodystrophy and hyperparathyroidism secondary to chronic renal failure* [paricalcitol] 5 µg/mL

Zemuron IV injection ℞ *neuromuscular blocking agent for anesthesia* [rocuronium bromide] 10 mg/mL

Zenapax injection ℞ *preventative for acute renal allograft rejection and acute graft vs. host disease following organ or bone marrow transplant (orphan);*

investigational (Phase I/II) for uveitis [daclizumab] 25 mg/5 mL

zenarestat USAN *investigational (Phase III) aldose reductase inhibitor for diabetic neuropathy*

Zenate, Advanced Formula film-coated tablets ℞ *vitamin/iron supplement* [multiple vitamins; iron; folic acid] ≛•65•1 mg

zenazocine mesylate USAN *analgesic*

zepastine INN

Zephiran Chloride tincture, tincture spray, aqueous solution, towelettes, disinfectant concentrate OTC *topical antiseptic* [benzalkonium chloride] 1:750; 1:750; 1:750; 1:750; 17%

zephirol [see: benzalkonium chloride]

Zephrex film-coated tablets ℞ *decongestant; expectorant* [pseudoephedrine HCl; guaifenesin] 60•400 mg

Zephrex LA timed-release tablets ℞ *decongestant; expectorant* [pseudoephedrine HCl; guaifenesin] 120•600 mg

zeranol USAN, INN *anabolic*

Zerit capsules, powder for oral solution ℞ *nucleoside reverse transcriptase inhibitor (NRTI) antiviral for HIV-1 infection* [stavudine] 15, 20, 30, 40 mg; 1 mg/mL

Zestoretic tablets ℞ *antihypertensive; angiotensin-converting enzyme (ACE) inhibitor; diuretic* [hydrochlorothiazide; lisinopril] 12.5•10, 25•20 mg

Zestril tablets ℞ *antihypertensive; angiotensin-converting enzyme (ACE) inhibitor* [lisinopril] 2.5, 5, 10, 20, 30, 40 mg ⊡ Restoril; Vistaril

Zetar shampoo OTC *antiseborrheic; antipsoriatic; antipruritic; antibacterial* [coal tar] 1%

Zetar Emulsion bath oil ℞ *antipsoriatic; antiseborrheic; antipruritic; emollient* [coal tar] 30%

zetidoline INN, BAN

Zevalin ℞ *investigational (orphan) radioimmunotherapy for non-Hodgkin B-cell lymphoma* [ibritumomab tiuxetan]

Z-gen tablets OTC *vitamin/zinc supplement* [multiple vitamins; zinc] ≛•22.5 mg

Zhuzishen *(Panax pseudoginseng)* *medicinal herb* [see: ginseng]

Ziac tablets ℞ *antihypertensive; β-blocker; diuretic* [hydrochlorothiazide; bisoprolol fumarate] 6.25•2.5, 6.25•5, 6.25•10 mg

Ziagen film-coated caplets, oral solution ℞ *antiviral nucleoside reverse transcriptase inhibitor for HIV infection* [abacavir sulfate] 300 mg; 20 mg/mL

ziconotide USAN *investigational (NDA filed) intrathecal calcium channel blocker for chronic malignant pain of cancer or AIDS; investigational (Phase II) for acute postsurgical pain*

zidapamide INN

zidometacin USAN, INN *anti-inflammatory*

zidovudine (ZDV) USAN, INN, BAN *nucleoside reverse transcriptase inhibitor (NRTI) antiviral for HIV, AIDS, and AIDS-related complex (orphan)*

zidovudine & amprenavir & lamivudine *investigational (Phase III) second-generation protease inhibitor combination for AIDS*

zidovudine & didanosine *investigational (Phase II) heterodimer antiviral combination for AIDS*

zidovudine & didanosine & nevirapine *investigational (Phase III) antiviral combination for HIV infection*

zidovudine & efavirenz & lamivudine *investigational (Phase III) antiviral combination for HIV and AIDS*

zidovudine & saquinavir mesylate & ritonavir *investigational (Phase II) protease inhibitor combination for HIV infection*

zifrosilone USAN *acetylcholinesterase inhibitor for Alzheimer disease*

Ziks cream OTC *topical analgesic; counterirritant* [methyl salicylate; menthol; capsaicin] 12%•1%•0.025% ⊡ Vicks

Zilactin Medicated gel OTC *astringent for oral canker and herpes lesions* [tannic acid; alcohol 80%] 7%

Zilactin-B Medicated gel OTC *topical oral anesthetic* [benzocaine; alcohol 76%] 10%

Zilactin-L liquid OTC *topical local anesthetic* [lidocaine] 2.5%
zilantel USAN, INN *anthelmintic*
zileuton USAN, INN, BAN *5-lipoxygenase inhibitor; leukotriene receptor inhibitor; for prophylaxis and chronic treatment of asthma*
zilpaterol INN
zimeldine INN, BAN *antidepressant* [also: zimeldine HCl]
zimeldine HCl USAN *antidepressant* [also: zimeldine]
zimelidine HCl [now: zimeldine HCl]
zimidoben INN
Zinacef powder or frozen premix for IV or IM injection ℞ *cephalosporin antibiotic* [cefuroxime sodium] 0.75, 1.5, 7.5 g
zinc *element (Zn)*
Zinc 15 tablets OTC *zinc supplement* [zinc sulfate] 66 mg
zinc acetate USP *copper blocking/complexing agent for Wilson disease (orphan)*
zinc acetate, basic INN
zinc acetate dihydrate [see: zinc acetate]
zinc bacitracin [see: bacitracin zinc]
zinc caprylate *antifungal*
zinc carbonate USAN *zinc supplement*
zinc chloride USP *astringent; dentin desensitizer; dietary zinc supplement*
zinc chloride Zn 65 USAN *radioactive agent*
zinc complex bacitracins [see: bacitracin zinc]
zinc gelatin USP
zinc gluconate USP *dietary zinc supplement* 10, 15, 50, 78 mg oral
Zinc Lozenges OTC *topical anti-infective to relieve sore throat* [zinc citrate and zinc gluconate] 23 mg
zinc mesoporphyrin & hemin *investigational (orphan) for acute porphyric syndromes*
zinc oleate NF
zinc oxide USP, JAN *astringent; topical protectant; emollient; antiseptic* 20% topical
zinc peroxide, medicinal USP
zinc phenolsulfonate NF *not generally regarded as safe and effective as an antidiarrheal*
zinc propionate *antifungal*
zinc pyrithione [see: pyrithione zinc]
zinc stearate USP *dusting powder; tablet and capsule lubricant; antifungal*
zinc sulfate USP, JAN *ophthalmic astringent; dietary zinc supplement* 200, 220, 250 mg oral; 1, 5 mg/mL injection
zinc sulfate heptahydrate [see: zinc sulfate]
zinc sulfate monohydrate [see: zinc sulfate]
zinc sulfocarbolate [see: zinc phenolsulfonate]
zinc undecylenate USP *antifungal*
zinc valerate USP
Zinc-220 capsules OTC *zinc supplement* [zinc sulfate] 220 mg
Zinca-Pak IV injection ℞ *intravenous nutritional therapy* [zinc sulfate] 1, 5 mg/mL
Zincate capsules ℞ *zinc supplement* [zinc sulfate] 220 mg
zinc-eugenol USP
Zincfrin Drop-Tainers (eye drops) OTC *topical ocular decongestant and astringent* [phenylephrine HCl; zinc sulfate] 0.12%•0.25%
Zincon shampoo OTC *antiseborrheic; antibacterial; antifungal* [pyrithione zinc] 1%
Zincvit capsules ℞ *vitamin/mineral supplement* [multiple vitamins & minerals; folic acid] ≛•1 mg
zindotrine USAN, INN *bronchodilator*
zindoxifene INN
Zinecard powder for IV drip or push ℞ *cardioprotectant for doxorubicin-induced cardiomyopathy (orphan)* [dexrazoxane] 250, 500 mg/vial
Zingiber officinale *medicinal herb* [see: ginger]
zinoconazole INN *antifungal* [also: zinoconazole HCl]
zinoconazole HCl USAN *antifungal* [also: zinoconazole]
zinostatin USAN, INN *antineoplastic* ⊡ Sandostatin; simvastatin

zinterol INN *bronchodilator* [also: zinterol HCl]
zinterol HCl USAN *bronchodilator* [also: zinterol]
Zintevir ℞ *investigational (Phase I/II) integrase inhibitor for HIV infection* [AR-177 (code name—generic name not yet assigned)]
zinviroxime USAN, INN *antiviral*
zipeprol INN
ziprasidone *benzisoxazole-type atypical antipsychotic for schizophrenia*
ziprasidone HCl *serotonin 5-HT_2 and dopamine D_2 antagonist; benzisoxazole-type atypical antipsychotic for schizophrenia*
ziprasidone mesylate USAN *serotonin 5-HT_2 and dopamine D_2 antagonist; benzisoxazole-type atypical antipsychotic for schizophrenia*
Ziracin ℞ *investigational antibiotic* [evernimicin]
Ziradryl lotion OTC *topical antihistamine; astringent; antiseptic* [diphenhydramine HCl; zinc oxide; alcohol 2%] 1%•2%
zirconium *element (Zr)*
zirconium oxide *astringent*
Zithromax tablets, powder for oral suspension, powder for IV or IM injection ℞ *macrolide antibiotic* [azithromycin] 250, 600 mg; 100, 200 mg/5 mL, 1 g packet; 500 mg/vial
Zixoryn ℞ *investigational (orphan) for neonatal hyperbilirubinemia* [flumecinol]
Z-Max (Mexican name for U.S. product Vasomax)
^{65}Zn [see: zinc chloride Zn 65]
ZNP cleansing bar OTC *antiseborrheic; antibacterial; antifungal* [pyrithione zinc] 2%
zocainone INN
Zocor film-coated tablets ℞ *HMG-CoA reductase inhibitor for hyperlipidemia, hypertriglyceridemia, and coronary heart disease* [simvastatin] 5, 10, 20, 40, 80 mg
Zodeac-100 tablets ℞ *hematinic; vitamin/mineral supplement* [ferrous fumarate; multiple vitamins & minerals; folic acid; biotin] 60 mg•≛•1 mg•300 µg
zofenopril INN, BAN *angiotensin-converting enzyme (ACE) inhibitor* [also: zofenopril calcium]
zofenopril calcium USAN *angiotensin-converting enzyme (ACE) inhibitor* [also: zofenopril]
zofenoprilat INN *antihypertensive* [also: zofenoprilat arginine]
zofenoprilat arginine USAN *antihypertensive* [also: zofenoprilat]
zoficonazole INN
Zofran film-coated tablets, oral solution, IV infusion, IM injection ℞ *serotonin 5-HT_3 antagonist; antiemetic for nausea following chemotherapy, radiation, or surgery* [ondansetron HCl] 4, 8, 24 mg; 4 mg/5 mL; 32 mg/50 mL; 2 mg/mL
Zofran ODT (orally disintegrating tablets) ℞ *serotonin 5-HT_3 receptor antagonist; antiemetic for nausea following chemotherapy, radiation, or surgery* [ondansetron HCl] 4, 8 mg
Zoladex subcu implant in preloaded syringe ℞ *hormonal antineoplastic for palliative treatment of prostatic carcinoma and breast cancer; LH-RH agonist for endometriosis and endometrial thinning* [goserelin acetate] 3.6 mg (1-month implant), 10.8 mg (3-month implant) ⓢ sulindac
Zoladex LA (CAN) subcu implant in preloaded syringe ℞ *hormonal antineoplastic for palliative treatment of prostatic carcinoma; LH-RH agonist for endometriosis* [goserelin acetate] 10.8 mg (3-month implant)
zolamine INN *antihistamine; topical anesthetic* [also: zolamine HCl]
zolamine HCl USAN *antihistamine; topical anesthetic* [also: zolamine]
zolazepam INN, BAN *sedative* [also: zolazepam HCl]
zolazepam HCl USAN *sedative* [also: zolazepam]
zoledronate disodium USAN *bone resorption inhibitor for osteoporosis*

zoledronate trisodium USAN *bone resorption inhibitor for osteoporosis*

zoledronic acid USAN *bisphosphonate bone resorption inhibitor for hypercalcemia of malignancy and metabolic bone disorders such as Paget disease*

zolenzepine INN

zolertine INN *antiadrenergic; vasodilator* [also: zolertine HCl]

zolertine HCl USAN *antiadrenergic; vasodilator* [also: zolertine]

Zolicef powder for IV or IM injection ℞ *cephalosporin antibiotic* [cefazolin sodium] 0.5, 1 g

zolimidine INN

zolimomab aritox USAN *anti-T lymphocyte monoclonal antibody*

zoliprofen INN

zoliridine [see: zolimidine]

zolmitriptan USAN *vascular serotonin 5-HT$_1$ receptor agonist for migraine headache*

Zoloft (CAN) capsules ℞ *selective serotonin reuptake inhibitor (SSRI) for depression, obsessive-compulsive disorder (OCD), and panic disorder* [sertraline HCl] 25, 50, 100 mg

Zoloft film-coated tablets, oral drops ℞ *selective serotonin reuptake inhibitor (SSRI) for depression, obsessive-compulsive disorder (OCD), panic disorder, and post-traumatic stress disorder (PTSD)* [sertraline HCl] 25, 50, 100 mg; 20 mg/mL

zoloperone INN

zolpidem INN, BAN *imidazopyridine sedative and hypnotic* [also: zolpidem tartrate]

zolpidem tartrate USAN *imidazopyridine sedative and hypnotic* [also: zolpidem]

Zomaril ℞ *investigational (Phase III) antipsychotic for schizophrenia* [iloperidone]

zomebazam INN

zomepirac INN, BAN *analgesic; anti-inflammatory* [also: zomepirac sodium]

zomepirac sodium USAN, USP *analgesic; anti-inflammatory* [also: zomepirac]

Zometa powder for IV infusion ℞ *bone resorption inhibitor for hypercalcemia of malignancy and metabolic bone disorders such as Paget disease* [zoledronic acid] 4 mg/vial

zometapine USAN *antidepressant*

Zomig film-coated tablets ℞ *vascular serotonin 5-HT$_1$ receptor agonist for migraine headache* [zolmitriptan] 2.5, 5 mg ⊡ Flomax; Slow-Mag

Zomig (CAN) Rapimelt (orally disintegrating tablets) ℞ *vascular serotonin 5-HT$_1$ receptor agonist for migraine headache* [zolmitriptan] 2.5 mg

Zomig-ZMT orally disintegrating tablets ℞ *vascular serotonin 5-HT$_1$ receptor agonist for migraine headache* [zolmitriptan] 2.5, 5 mg ⊡ Flomax; Slow-Mag

Zonalon cream ℞ *topical antihistamine and antipruritic* [doxepin HCl] 5%

Zone-A Forte lotion ℞ *topical corticosteroidal anti-inflammatory; local anesthetic* [hydrocortisone acetate; pramoxine] 2.5%•1%

Zonegran capsules ℞ *sulfonamide anticonvulsant for partial seizures* [zonisamide] 100 mg

zoniclezole INN *anticonvulsant* [also: zoniclezole HCl]

zoniclezole HCl USAN *anticonvulsant* [also: zoniclezole]

zonisamide USAN, INN, BAN *sulfonamide anticonvulsant*

Zonite Douche solution concentrate OTC *antiseptic; antipruritic/counterirritant; vaginal cleanser and deodorizer* [benzalkonium chloride; menthol; thymol]

Zophren (European name for U.S. product Zofran)

zopiclone INN, BAN, JAN *sedative; hypnotic*

(S)-zopiclone [see: esopiclone]

zopolrestat USAN *antidiabetic; aldose reductase inhibitor*

zorbamycin USAN *antibacterial*

ZORprin Zero Order Release tablets ℞ *analgesic; antipyretic; anti-inflammatory; antirheumatic* [aspirin] 800 mg

zorubicin INN *antineoplastic* [also: zorubicin HCl]

zorubicin HCl USAN *antineoplastic* [also: zorubicin]

Zostrix; Zostrix-HP cream OTC *topical analgesic* [capsaicin] 0.025%; 0.075%

Zosyn powder or frozen premix for IV injection ℞ *extended-spectrum penicillin antibiotic* [piperacillin sodium; tazobactam sodium] 2•0.25, 3•0.375, 4•0.5, 36•4.5 g

zotepine INN, JAN *investigational antipsychotic*

Zoto-HC ear drops ℞ *topical corticosteroidal anti-inflammatory; antibacterial; local anesthetic* [hydrocortisone; chloroxylenol; pramoxine HCl] 10%•1%•10%

Zovant ℞ *investigational (Phase III) recombinant human activated protein C for severe sepsis*

Zovia 1/35E; Zovia 1/50E tablets (in packs of 21 or 28) ℞ *monophasic oral contraceptive* [ethynodiol diacetate; ethinyl estradiol] 1 mg•35 µg; 1 mg•50 µg

Zovirax powder for IV infusion ℞ *antiviral for herpes infections* [acyclovir sodium] 500, 1000 mg

Zovirax tablets, capsules, oral suspension, ointment ℞ *antiviral for herpes simplex, herpes zoster, and adult-onset chickenpox* [acyclovir] 400, 800 mg; 200 mg; 200 mg/5 mL; 5%

zoxazolamine NF, INN

zucapsaicin USAN *topical analgesic*

zuclomifene INN

zuclomiphene USAN

zuclopenthixol INN, BAN *thioxanthene antipsychotic*

Zyban sustained-release film-coated tablets ℞ *non-nicotine aid to smoking cessation* [bupropion HCl] 150 mg

Zydis (trademarked dosage form) *orally disintegrating tablets*

Zydis ℞ *investigational (orphan) treatment for late-stage Parkinson disease* [apomorphine HCl]

Zydone tablets, capsules ℞ *narcotic analgesic* [hydrocodone bitartrate; acetaminophen] 5•400, 7.5•400, 10•400 mg; 5•500 mg

Zyflo film-coated tablets ℞ *5-lipoxygenase inhibitor; leukotriene receptor inhibitor; prophylaxis and treatment for chronic asthma* [zileuton] 600 mg

zylofuramine INN

Zyloprim tablets ℞ *xanthine oxidase inhibitor for gout and hyperuricemia; antineoplastic adjunct for reducing uric acid levels following chemotherapy for leukemia, lymphoma, and solid tumor malignancies (orphan)* [allopurinol] 100, 300 mg

Zymacap capsules OTC *vitamin supplement* [multiple vitamins; folic acid] ≛•0.4 mg

Zymase capsules containing enteric-coated spheres ℞ *digestive enzymes* [lipase; protease; amylase] 12 000•24 000•24 000 U

Zyprexa film-coated tablets, Zydis (orally disintegrating tablets) ℞ *novel (atypical) antipsychotic for manic episodes of a bipolar disorder* [olanzapine] 2.5, 5, 7.5, 10, 15, 20 mg; 5, 10 mg

Zyprexa IntraMuscular IM injection ℞ *investigational doseform* [olanzapine]

Zyrkamine *investigational (orphan) for non-Hodgkin lymphoma* [mitoguazone]

Zyrtec film-coated tablets, syrup ℞ *nonsedating antihistamine for allergic rhinitis and chronic idiopathic urticaria* [cetirizine HCl] 5, 10 mg; 5 mg/5 mL

Zyrtec-D extended-release tablets ℞ *nonsedating antihistamine and decongestant for allergic rhinitis* [cetirizine HCl; pseudoephedrine HCl] 5•120 mg

Zyvox tablets, powder for oral suspension, IV infusion ℞ *oxazolidinone antibiotic for gram-positive bacterial infections* [linezolid] 400, 600 mg; 100 mg/5 mL; 2 mg/mL

Zyvoxam (CAN) tablets, IV infusion ℞ *oxazolidinone antibiotic for gram-positive bacterial infections* [linezolid] 600 mg; 2 mg/mL

APPENDIX **A**

Sound-Alikes

Listed below are 706 drug names that may be confused in transcription, followed by one or more possible "sound-alike" names. The list is not all-inclusive, and we would appreciate hearing of any additions the reader might suggest. These sound-alikes have also been included in the main section of the book. Look for the "ear" icon (𝟗).

Accurbron	Accutane
Accutane	Accurbron
Aciphex	AcuTect
Actifed	Actidil
actinomycin	Achromycin; Aureomycin
AcuTect	Aciphex
adrenaline	adrenalone
adrenalone	adrenaline
Advil	Avail
Afrin	aspirin
Agoral	Argyrol
Akne-mycin	Ak-Mycin
Alamag	Alma-Mag
Alco-Gel	aloe gel
Aldactazide	Aldactone
Aldactone	Aldactazide
Aldoril	Elavil; Eldepryl; Enovil; Equanil; Mellaril
Allergan	allergen; Auralgan
aloe	Alco-Gel
ALOMAD	Alomide
Alomide	ALOMAD
Alustra	Lustra
Ambenyl	Aventyl
Amicar	Amikin
Amikin	Amicar
amitriptyline	nortriptyline
amoxapine	amoxicillin; Amoxil
amoxicillin	amoxapine
Amoxil	amoxapine
Amphojel	Amphocil
Anacin	Unisom; Unasyn
Anafranil	enalapril
Analpram	Analbalm
Ancobon	Oncovin
Ansaid	NSAID
Anturane	Artane

Anusol	Aplisol
Aplisol	Anusol; Apresoline
Appedrine	aprindine; ephedrine
aprindine	Appedrine; ephedrine
ara-C	ERYC
Aralen	Arlidin
Aricept	Erycette
Artane	Anturane
aspirin	Afrin
Atacand	Ativan
Atarax	Marax
atenolol	timolol
Ativan	Atacand; Adapin; Avitene
Atrovent	Trovan
Auralgan	Allergan; allergen
Avail	Advil
Aventyl	Ambenyl; Bentyl
Avita	Evista
Avitene	Ativan
Axid	Biaxin
azolimine	Azulfidine
Azulfidine	Silvadene
Bacid	Banacid
bacitracin	Bacitrin; Bactrim
Bactocill	Pathocil
Bactrim	bacitracin
BAL in Oil	Balneol
Balneol	BAL in Oil
Banophen	Barophen
Banthīne	Brethine; Vantin
Bantron	Vantin
Beminal	Benemid
Benadryl	Bentyl; Benylin; Caladryl
Benadryl	Bentyl; Benylin; Caladryl
Benemid	Beminal
Benoxyl	PanOxyl
Bentyl	Aventyl; Benadryl; Bontril
Benylin	Benadryl
Betagan	Betagen
Betagen	Betagan
Betapen	Adapin; Phenaphen
Biaxin	Axid
Bichloracetic Acid	dichloroacetic acid
Bicillin	V-Cillin; Wycillin
bleomycin	Cleocin
Bonamine	Bonine
Bonine	Bonamine
Bontril	Bentyl; Vontrol
Boyol	boil
Brethine	Banthine

Bretylol	Brevital
Brevital	Bretylol
Bromfed	Bromphen
Bromophen	Bromfed; Bromphen
Bromphen	Bromfed; Bromophen
Broncholate	Brondelate
Brondelate	Broncholate
butabarbital	butalbital
butalbital	butabarbital; Butibel
Butibel	butalbital
Byclomine	Hycomine
Bydramine	Hydramine
Caladryl	Benadryl
Calamox	Camalox
Calan	kaolin; Kaon
calcitonin	calcitriol
calcitriol	calcitonin
Capastat	Cepastat
Capitrol	captopril
captopril	Capitrol
Cardene	Cardizem
Cardizem	Cardene
Catapres	Catarase; Combipres; Ser-Ap-Es
Catarase	Catapres
Cefadyl	Cefzil
cefazolin	cephalothin; Zefazone
cefotaxime	cefoxitin
cefoxitin	cefotaxime
ceftizoxime	cefuroxime
cefuroxime	ceftizoxime
Cefzil	Cefadyl; Kefzol
Celebrex	Cerebyx
Cēpastat	Capastat
cephalexin	cefazolin; cephalothin
cephalothin	cefazolin
cephapirin	cephradine
cephradine	cephapirin
Cerebyx	Celebrex
chlorpheniramine	chlorphentermine
chlorphentermine	chlorpheniramine
cimetidine	dimethicone
Cipro	Septa; Septra
Citracal	Citrucel
Citrucel	Citracal
clara cell	Clearasil
claretin	Claritin; Clarityne
clarithromycin	dirithromycin; erythromycin
Claritin	claretin; Clarityne
Clarityne	claretin; Claritin
Clearasil	clara cell

Cleocin	bleomycin; Lincocin
clioxanide	Clinoxide
clomiphene	clonidine
clonidine	clomiphene; Klonopin; quinidine
clotrimazole	co-trimoxazole
Codegest	Codehist
Codehist	Codegest
codeine	Kaodene
Colestid	colistin
colestipol	colistin
colistin	Colestid; colestipol
Combipres	Catapres
Cort-Dome	Cortone
Cortenema	quart enema
cortisone	Cortizone
Cortizone	cortisone
Cortone	Cort-Dome
Cotrim	Cortin
co-trimoxazole	clotrimazole
Coumadin	Kemadrin
Covera	Provera
cytarabine	vidarabine
dacarbazine	Dicarbosil; procarbazine
Dalmane	Dialume
danthron	Dantrium
Dantrium	danthron
Daranide	Daraprim
Daraprim	Daranide
Daricon	Darvon
Darvocet-N	Darvon-N
Darvon	Daricon
daunorubicin	doxorubicin
Decadron	Decaderm; Percodan
Deconsal	Deconal
Delcort	Dilacor
Demulen	Demerol; Demolin
Dermacort	DermiCort
deserpidine	desipramine
Desferal	Disophrol
desipramine	deserpidine
desoximetasone	dexamethasone
Desoxyn	digitoxin; digoxin
dexamethasone	desoximetasone
Dexedrine	dextran
dextran	Dexedrine; dextrin
dextrin	dextran
Dialume	Dalmane
Dicarbosil	dacarbazine
dichloroacetic acid	Bichloracetic acid
dicumarol	Demerol

digitoxin	Desoxyn; digoxin
digoxin	Desoxyn; digitoxin
Dilacor	Delcort
Dilantin	Milontin; Mylanta; Xalatan
Dimacol	dimercaprol
dimenhydrinate	diphenhydramine
dimercaprol	Dimacol
Dimetabs	Dimetane; Dimetapp
Dimetane	Dimetabs
Dimetapp	Dimetabs
dimethicone	cimetidine
diphenhydramine	dimenhydrinate
Diphenylan	Diphenylin
dirithromycin	clarithromycin; erythromycin
Disophrol	Desferal; disoprofol; Stilphostrol
disoprofol	Disophrol
Ditropan	Intropin
Diutensen	Salutensin
dobutamine	dopamine
Donnagel	Donnatal
Donnatal	Donnagel
Donnazyme	Entozyme
dopamine	dobutamine; Dopram
Dopar	Dopram
Dopram	dopamine; Dopar
doxepin	Doxidan; Loxitane
Doxidan	doxepin
doxorubicin	daunorubicin
Dramanate	Dommanate
Duranest	Duratest
Duratest	Duranest; Duratuss
Duratuss	Duratest
Dyazide	thiazides; Tiazac
Dymelor	Demerol; Pamelor
Dyrenium	Pyridium
Ecotrin	Edecrin
Edecrin	Ecotrin; Ethaquin
Elavil	Aldoril; Eldepryl; Enovil; Equanil; Mellaril
Eldepryl	Aldoril; Elavil; Enovil; Equanil; Mellaril
emetine	Emetrol
Emetrol	emetine
Enbrel	Incel
Endal	Intal
Enduron	Imuran; Inderal
Enduronyl	Inderal
ephedrine	Appedrine; aprindine
Epifrin	epinephrine; EpiPen
Epinal	Epitol
epinephrine	Epifrin
EpiPen	Epifrin

Epitol	Epinal
Epogen	"amp and gent" (ampicillin & gentamicin)
Equanil	Aldoril; Elavil; Eldepryl; Enovil; Mellaril
ERYC	ara-C
Erycette	Aricept
erythromycin	clarithromycin; dirithromycin
Esidrix	Lasix
Esimil	Estinyl; Isomil
Estinyl	Esimil
Estraderm	Estradurin
Estratab	Ethatab
ethacridine	ethacrynic
ethacrynic acid	ethacridine
ethinamate	ethionamide
Ethiodol	ethynodiol
ethionamide	ethinamate
ethynodiol	Ethiodol
Eurax	Serax; Urex
Evac-Q-Kit	Evac-Q-Kwik
Evac-Q-Kwik	Evac-Q-Kit
Evista	Avita
Femiron	Remeron
fentanyl	Sentinel
Feosol	Feostat; Fer-In-Sol; Festal
Feostat	Feosol
Fer-In-Sol	Feosol
Feverall	Fiberall
Fiberall	Feverall
Fioricet	Lorcet
Fiorinal	Florinef
Flexeril	Flaxedil
Flomax	Slow-Mag; Zomig
Florinef	Fiorinal
folacin	Fulvicin
Fostex	pHisoHex
Fulvicin	folacin; Furacin
Furacin	Fulvicin
Gabitril	Carbatrol
Garamycin	Gamastan; kanamycin; Terramycin; Theramycin
Gelfoam	Ger-O-Foam
Genatap	Genapap
Generet	Gentap
gentamicin	Jenamicin; kanamycin
glucose	Glutose
Glutose	glucose
Glycotuss	Glytuss
Glytuss	Glycotuss
Gonak	Gonic
Gonic	Gonak
guaifenesin	guanfacine

guanethidine	guanidine
guanfacine	guaifenesin
guanidine	guanethidine
Guiatuss	Guiatussin
Guiatussin	Guiatuss
Haldol	Halenol; Halog
Halog	Haldol
Halotestin	Halotex; Halotussin
Halotex	Halotestin
Halotussin	Halotestin
Hespan	Histatan
Hexadrol	Hexalol
Hexalen	Hexalol
Hycodan	Hycomine; Vicodin
Hycomine	Byclomine; Hycodan; Vicodin
Hydergine	Hydramine
Hydramyn	Hydramine; Hytramyn
Hygroton	Regroton
HyperHep	Hyper-Tet; Hyperstat
Hyperstat	Hyper-Tet; HyperHep; Nitrostat
Hyper-Tet	HyperHep; Hyperstat
Hytone	Vytone
Ilosone	inosine
imipramine	Imferon; Norpramin; trimipramine
Imuran	Enduron; Imferon
Incel	Enbrel
Inderal	Enduron; Enduronyl; Inderide
Inderide	Inderal
Indocin	Lincocin; Minocin
InFeD	NSAID
inosine	Ilosone
insulin	inulin
Intal	Endal
Intropin	Ditropan; Isoptin
inulin	insulin
Ismelin	Ritalin
Isomil	Esimil
Isoptin	Intropin
Isopto Carpine	Isopto Eserine
Isordil	Isuprel
Isuprel	Isordil
kanamycin	Garamycin; gentamicin
Kaochlor	K-Lor
Kaodene	codeine
kaolin	Calan; Kaon
Kaon	Calan; kaolin
Kaon-Cl	Calan; kaolin
Kaopectate	Kapectalin
Kapectolin	Kaopectate
Kay Ciel	KCl

KCl	Kay Ciel
Keflex	Keflet; Keflin
Kefzol	Cefzil
Kemadrin	Coumadin
Kenalog	Ketalar
Ketalar	Kenalog
Klonopin	clonidine
K-Lor	Kaochlor
Klotrix	Liotrix
Koromex	Komex
lanolin	Lanoline
Lasix	Esidrix; Lidex
levallorphan	levorphanol
levodopa	methyldopa
levorphanol	levallorphan
levothyroxine	liothyronine
Lidex	Lasix; Lidox; Wydase
Lincocin	Cleocin; Indocin
liothyronine	levothyroxine
liotrix	Klotrix
Loniten	clonidine
Lonox	Lovenox
Lorcet	Fioricet
Lotrimin	Otrivin
Lovenox	Lonox
Loxitane	doxepin
Luminal	Tuinal
Lupron	Mepron; Napron
Lustra	Alustra
Maalox	Marax
Mandol	nadolol
Marax	Atarax; Maalox
Marcaine	Narcan
Maxzide	Microzide
mazindol	mebendazole
Mebaral	Medrol
mebendazole	mazindol
Meclan	Meclomen; Mezlin
meclizine	mescaline
meclozine	mescaline
Medrol	Mebaral
Mellaril	Aldoril; Elavil; Eldepryl; Enovil; Equanil; Moderil
meperidine	meprobamate
mephenytoin	Mephyton; Mesantoin
Mephyton	mephenytoin; methadone
meprobamate	meperidine
Mepron	Lupron; Napron
Meprospan	Naprosyn
Mesantoin	mephenytoin; Mestinon; Metatensin
mescaline	meclizine

Mestinon	Mesantoin; Metatensin
Metahydrin	Metandren
metaproterenol	metoprolol
Metatensin	Mesantoin; Mestinon
metaxalone	metolazone
metesind	medicine
methadone	Mephyton
methenamine	methionine
methionine	methenamine
methixene	methoxsalen
methoxsalen	methixene
methyldopa	levodopa
metolazone	metaxalone
Metopirone	metyrapone
metoprolol	metaproterenol
metyrapone	Metopirone; metyrosine
metyrosine	metyrapone
Mezlin	Meclan
MICRhoGAM	microgram
Microzide	Maxzide
Midrin	Mydfrin
Milontin	Dilantin; Miltown; Mylanta
Miltown	Milontin
Minocin	Indocin; Mithracin; niacin
Mithracin	Minocin
mithramycin	mitomycin
mitomycin	mithramycin; Mutamycin
Moban	Mobidin; Modane
Mobidin	Moban
Modane	Moban; Mudrane
Modicon	Mylicon
Moi-Stir	moisture
Monocaps	Monoclate; Monoket
Monocid	Monocete
Monoclate	Monocaps; Monoket
Monoket	Monocete
Mudrane	Modane
Mutamycin	mitomycin
Myambutol	Nembutal
Mydfrin	Midrin; Myfedrine
Mylanta	Dilantin; Milontin
Myleran	Mylicon
Mylicon	Modicon; Myleran
nadolol	Nandol
Naldecon	Nalfon
Nalfon	Naldecon
Napron	Lupron; Mepron
Naprosyn	Meprospan; Natacyn
Narcan	Marcaine
Nardil	Norinyl

Natacyn	Naprosyn
Nembutal	Myambutal
Neomixin	neomycin
neomycin	Neomixin
Neovastat	Novastan
niacin	Minocin
Nicobid	Nitro-Bid
Nilstat	Nitrostat; nystatin
Nitro-Bid	Nicobid
nitroglycerin	Nitroglyn
Nitroglyn	nitroglycerin
Norinyl	Nardil
Norpramin	imipramine
nortriptyline	amitriptyline
Novastan	Neovastat; Ovastat
NSAID	InFeD
nystatin	Nilstat; Nitrostat
Omnipen	Unipen
Oncovin	Ancobon
Orabase	Orinase
orarsan	Oracin; Orasone
Orasone	Oracin; orarsan
Oretic	Oreton
Oreton	Oretic
Orinase	Orabase; Ornade; Ornex; Tolinase
Ornade	Orinase; Ornex
Ornex	Orex; Orinase; Ornade
Orthoclone	Ortho-Creme
Otobiotic	Urobiotic
Otrivin	Lotrimin
OvaRex	O-Vax
Ovastat	Novastan
O-Vax	Ovarex
oxymetazoline	oxymetholone
oxymetholone	oxymetazoline; oxymorphone
oxymorphone	oxymetholone
Pamelor	Dymelor; Panlor
Panasol	Panscol
Panlor	Pamelor
Panorex	Panarex
Panoxyl	Benoxyl
Panscol	Panasol
Parafon	Pantopon
paramethadione	paramethasone
paramethasone	paramethadione
Pathilon	Pathocil
Pathocil	Bactocill; Pathilon; Placidyl
Pavabid	Pavased
Pavatine	Pavatym
Paverolan	Pavulon

Pavulon	Paverolan
penicillamine	penicillin
penicillin	penicillamine; Polycillin
Pentazine	Phenazine
pentobarbital	phenobarbital
Pentothal	pentrinitrol
Pentothal	pentrinitrol;
pentrinitrol	Pentothal
Percodan	Decadron
Perdiem	Pyridium
Periactin	Taractan
Persantine	Pertofrane
Phazyme	Pherazine
phenacetin	phenazocine
Phenazine	Pentazine; phenelzine; Phenoxine; Pherazine
phenazocine	phenacetin
phenelzine	Phenazine; Phenylzin
Phenergan	Phenaphen; Theragran
phenobarbital	pentobarbital
Phenoxine	Phenazine
phentermine	phentolamine
phentolamine	phentermine; Ventolin
pHisoHex	Fostex
physostigmine	pyridostigmine; Prostigmin
piperacetazine	piperazine
piperazine	piperacetazine
piracetam	piroxicam
piroxicam	piracetam
Pitocin	Pitressin
Pitressin	Pitocin
Placidyl	Pathocil
Plendil	Prinivil
Podofin	podophyllin
podophyllin	Podofin
Polycillin	penicillin
Ponstel	Pronestyl
Posicor	Proscar
pralidoxime	pyridoxine; pramoxine
Pramosone	pramoxine
pramoxine	pralidoxime; Pramosone
Pravachol	Primacor
prazepam	prazepine; prazosin
prazepine	prazepam
prazosin	prazepam
prednisolone	prednisone
prednisone	prednisolone
Preven	Preveon
Preveon	Preven
Prilosec	Prozac
Primacor	Pravachol

Prinivil	Plendil
Priscoline	Apresoline
procaine	Procan
procarbazine	dacarbazine
proline	Prolene
promazine	Promethazine
Pronestyl	Ponstel
Proscar	Posicor
Prostigmin	physostigmine
Protopam	Protamine
Provera	Covera; Provir; Trovert
Provir	Provera; Trovert
Prozac	Prilosec
Pyridium	Dyrenium; pyridoxine; pyrithione; pyritidium
pyridostigmine	physostigmine
pyridoxine	pralidoxime; Pyridium
pyrithione	Pyridium
Quarzan	Questran
quinacrine	quinidine
quinidine	clonidine; quinacrine; Quinatime; quinine
quinine	quinidine
Rēgain	Rogaine
Reglan	Regonol
Regonol	Reglan
Regroton	Hygroton
Remeron	Femiron
Repan	Riopan
Restoril	Risperdal; Vistaril; Zestril
Rheumatex	Rheumatrex
Rheumatrex	Rheumatex
Rifadin	Ritalin
Risperdal	Restoril
Ritalin	Ismelin; Rifadin
Robaxisal	Robaxacet
Rogaine	Rēgain
Salutensin	Diutensen
Sandostatin	simvastatin; zinostatin
Sentinel	fentanyl
Septa	Cipro; Septra
Septra	Cipro; Septa
Ser-Ap-Es	Catapres
Serax	Eurax; Urex; Xerac
Serentil	Surital
Silvadene	Azulfidine
Simplet	Singlet
simvastatin	Sandostatin; zinostatin
Singlet	Simplet
Slow-Mag	Flomax; Zomig
stilbestrol	Stilphostrol
Stilphostrol	Disophrol; stilbestrol

Streptase	Streptonase
streptokinase	Streptonase
Streptonase	Streptase; streptokinase
sucrase	sucrose
sucrose	sucrase
Sulf-10	Sulten-10
sulfamethizole	sulfamethoxazole
sulfamethoxazole	sulfamethizole
sulfathiazole	sulfisoxazole
sulfisoxazole	sulfathiazole
sulindac	Zoladex
Synthroid	Euthroid
Tagamet	Tegopen
Targretin	Tegopen; Tegrin
Tegopen	Tagamet; Tegrin; Targretin
Tegretol	Tegrin
Tegrin	Tegopen; Tegretol; Targretin
Teldrin	Tedral
Tenex	Xanax
Terramycin	Garamycin; Theramycin
testolactone	testosterone
testosterone	testolactone
thallium	Valium
Theoclear	Theolair
Theolair	Theoclear; Thyrolar
TheraFlu	Thera-Flur
Thera-Flur	TheraFlu
Theragran	Theragyn; Phenergan
Theragyn	Theragran
Theramycin	Garamycin; Terramycin
Theravite	Therevac
Therevac	Theravite
Threostat	Triostat
Thyrar	Thyrolar
thyroid	euthroid
Thyrolar	Theolair; Thyrar
Tiazac	Dyazide; thiazides
Ticar	Tigan
Tigan	Ticar; Triban
timolol	atenolol
Tinactin	Taractan
TobraDex	Tobrex
tobramycin	Trobicin
Tobrex	TobraDex
Tofranil	Tepanil
Tolinase	Orinase
Topic	Topicort
Topicort	Topic
Trasylol	Travasol
Travasol	Trasylol

triamcinolone	Triaminicin
Triaminic	Triaminicin; TriHemic
Triaminicin	triamcinolone; Triaminic
triamterene	trimipramine
Triapine	Triaprim
Triaprin	Triapine
Triban	Tigan
TriHemic	Triaminic
trimeprazine	trimipramine
trimethaphan	trimethoprim
trimethoprim	trimethaphan
trimipramine	imipramine; triamterene; trimeprazine
Triostat	Threostat
Trobicin	tobramycin
Tronolane	Tronothane
Tronothane	Tronolane
Trovan	Atrovent
Trovert	Provir; Provera
Tuinal	Luminal; Tylenol
Tusibron	Tussigon
Tussafed	Tussafin
Tussafin	Tussafed
Tussex	Tussionex; Tussirex
Tussigon	Tusibron
Tussionex	Tussex; Tussirex
Tussirex	Tussex; Tussionex
Tylenol	Tuinal
Unasyn	Anacin; Unisom
Unipen	Omnipen
Unisom	Anacin; Unasyn
Uracid	uracil; Urised; Urocit
uracil	Uracel; Uracid
Urex	Eurax; Serax
Urised	Uracel; Uracid; Urispas
Urispas	Urised
Urobiotic	Otobiotic
Urocit	Uracid
Valium	thallium; Valpin
Vantin	Banthine; Bantron
VasoCare	VasoClear
Vasocidin	Vasodilan
Vasocine	Vaseline
VasoClear	VasoCare
Vasodilan	Vasocidin
Vasoflux	Vasoprost; Vasosulf
Vasoprost	Vasoflux
Vasosulf	Velosef; Vasoflux
V-Cillin	Bicillin; Wycillin
Velban	Valpin
Velosef	Vasosulf

Ventolin	phentolamine
Vicodin	Hycodan; Hycomine
vidarabine	cytarabine
Vistaril	Restoril; Zestril
Vitron	Vytone
Vontrol	Bontril
Vytone	Hytone; Vitron
Wycillin	Bicillin; V-Cillin
Wydase	Lidex
Xalatan	Dilantin
Xanax	Tenex; Zantac
Zantac	Xanax
Zarontin	Zaroxolyn
Zaroxolyn	Zarontin; Zeroxin
Zefazone	cefazolin
Zestril	Restoril; Vistaril
Ziks	Vicks
zinostatin	Sandostatin; simvastatin
Zoladex	sulindac
Zomig	Flomax; Slow-Mag

APPENDIX **B**

Abbreviations Used with Medications and Dosages

Abbreviation/Term	*Literally*	*Meaning*
a.c.	ante cibum	before meals or food
ad	ad	to, up to
A.D., AD	auris dextra	right ear
ad lib.	ad libitum	at pleasure
A.L.	auris laeva	left ear
a.m., A.M.	ante meridiem	morning
Aq.	aqua	water
A.S., AS	auris sinistra	left ear
A.U., AU*	auris uterque	each ear
b.i.d.	bis in die	twice daily
b.m.	bowel movement	
cc, cm^3	cubic centimeter	
CFU	colony-forming unit(s)	
d.	die	day
EL.U.	ELISA unit(s)	
et	et	and
g	gram(s)	
gt. (plural gtt.)	gutta (plural guttae)	a drop (drops)
h.	hora	hour
HAU	hemagglutinating unit(s)	
h.s.	hora somni	at bedtime
IM†	intramuscular	
IU	international unit(s)	
IV†	intravenous	
LfU	limes flocculating unit(s) limit of flocculation unit(s)	
mcg, μg	microgram(s)	
mg	milligram(s)	
mEq	milliequivalent(s)	
mkat	millikatal unit(s)	
mL, ml	milliliter(s)	
mU, mIU	milliunit(s)	
MU, MIU	megaunit(s)	one million (10^6) IU
nkat	nanokatal unit(s)	
O.D.	oculus dexter	right eye
O.L.	oculus laevus	left eye
O.S.	oculus sinister	left eye
O.U.§	oculus uterque	each eye
p.c.	post cibum	after meals

Abbreviation/Term	Literally	Meaning
p.m., P.M.	post meridiem	afternoon or evening
p.o.	per os	by mouth
p.r.n.	pro re nata	as needed
q.d.	quaque die	every day
q.h.	quaque hora	every hour
q.i.d.	quater in die	four times a day
q.o.d.		every other day
q.s.	quantum satis	sufficient quantity
q.s. ad	quantum satis ad	a sufficient quantity to make
℞, Rx	recipe	take; a recipe
Sig.	signetur	label
s.o.s.	si opus sit	if there is need
stat	statim	at once, immediately
subcu, subq, SQ	subcutaneous	beneath the skin
t.i.d.	ter in die	three times a day
tsp.	teaspoonful	
μg, mcg	microgram(s)	

[*] Although some references have aures unitas (Latin, both ears), this cannot be justified by classical Latin.

[†] Some references suggest that IM and IV be typed with periods to distinguish from Roman numerals, but we believe context is sufficient to make this distinction.

[§] Although some references have oculi unitas (Latin, both eyes), this cannot be justified by classical Latin.

APPENDIX C

Therapeutic Drug Levels

Drug	*Class*	*Serum Levels* metric units (SI units)
amantadine	antiviral	300 ng/mL
amikacin	aminoglycoside	16–32 μg/mL
amiodarone	antiarrhythmic	0.5–2.5 μg/mL
amitriptyline	antidepressant	110–250 ng/mL
amoxapine	antidepressant	200–500 ng/mL
amrinone	cardiotonic	3.7 μg/mL
bretylium	antiarrhythmic	0.5–1.5 μg/mL
bupropion	antidepressant	25–100 ng/mL
carbamazepine	anticonvulsant	4–12 μg/mL (17–51 μmol/L)
chloramphenicol	antibiotic	10–20 μg/mL (31–62 μmol/L)
chlorpromazine	antipsychotic	30–500 ng/mL
clomipramine	antidepressant	80–100 ng/mL
cyclosporine	immunosuppressive	250–800 ng/mL (whole blood, RIA*)
trough values:		50–300 ng/mL (plasma,RIA*)
desipramine	antidepressant	125–300 ng/mL
digitoxin	antiarrhythmic	9–25 μg/L (11.8–32.8 nmol/L)
digoxin	antiarrhythmic	0.5–2.2 ng/mL (0.6–2.8 nmol/L)
disopyramide	antiarrhythmic	2–8 μg/mL (6–18 μmol/L)
doxepin	antidepressant	100–200 ng/mL
flecainide	antiarrhythmic	0.2–1 μg/mL
fluphenazine	antipsychotic	0.13–2.8 ng/mL
gentamicin	aminoglycoside	4–8 μg/mL
haloperidol	antipsychotic	5–20 ng/mL
hydralazine	antihypertensive	100 ng/mL
imipramine	antidepressant	200–350 ng/mL
kanamycin	aminoglycoside	15–40 μg/mL
lidocaine	antiarrhythmic	1.5–6 μg/mL (4.5–21.5 μmol/L)
lithium	antipsychotic	0.5–1.5 mEq/L (0.5–1.5 mmol/L)
maprotiline	antidepressant	200–300 ng/mL
mexiletine	antiarrhythmic	0.5–2 μg/mL
netilmicin	aminoglycoside	6–10 μg/mL

Drug	*Class*	***Serum Levels*** *metric units (SI units)*
nortriptyline	antidepressant	50–150 ng/mL
perphenazine	antipsychotic	0.8–1.2 ng/mL
phenobarbital	anticonvulsant	15–40 μg/mL (65–172 μmol/L)
phenytoin	anticonvulsant	10–20 μg/mL (40–80 μmol/L)
primidone	anticonvulsant	5–12 μg/mL (25–46 μmol/L)
procainamide	antiarrhythmic	4–8 μg/mL (17–34 μmol/L)
propranolol	antiarrhythmic	50–200 ng/mL (190–770 nmol/L)
protriptyline	antidepressant	100–200 ng/mL
quinidine	antiarrhythmic	2–6 μg/mL (4.6–9.2 μmol/L)
salicylate	analgesic	100–200 mg/L (725–1448 μmol/L)
streptomycin	aminoglycoside	20–30 μg/mL
sulfonamide	antibiotic	5–15 mg/dL
terbutaline	bronchodilator	0.5–4.1 ng/mL
theophylline	bronchodilator	10–20 μg/mL (55–110 μmol/L)
thiothixene	antipsychotic	2–57 ng/mL
tobramycin	aminoglycoside	4–8 μg/mL
tocainide	antiarrhythmic	4–10 μg/mL
trazodone	antidepressant	800–1600 ng/mL
valproic acid	anticonvulsant	50–100 μg/mL (350–700 μmol/L)
vancomycin	antibiotic	30–40 ng/mL (peak)
verapamil	antiarrhythmic	0.08–0.3 μg/mL

* radioimmunoassay

APPENDIX **D**

The Most Prescribed Drugs

Drug	*Class/Indication(s)*
Accupril (quinapril HCl)	antihypertensive, ACE inhibitor
Accutane (isotretinoin)	oral keratolytic for severe cystic acne
acetaminophen with codeine	analgesic, anti-inflammatory
Aciphex (rabeprazole sodium)	proton pump inhibitor for GERD
Actos (pioglitazone HCl)	antidiabetic; decreases insulin resistance
acyclovir	antibiotic
Adalat CC (nifedipine)	antianginal, antihypertensive
Adalat XL CAN (nifedipine)	antianginal, antihypertensive
Adderall (mixed amphetamines)	CNS stimulant for ADHD
albuterol sulfate	bronchodilator
Alesse (levonorgestrel, ethinyl estradiol)	monophasic oral contraceptive
Allegra (fexofenadine HCl)	nonsedating antihistamine
Allegra-D (fexofenadine HCl, pseudoephedrine HCl)	antihistamine, decongestant
allopurinol	treatment for gout and hyperuricemia
alprazolam	anxiolytic, sedative
Altace (ramipril)	antihypertensive, ACE inhibitor
Alti-MPA CAN (medroxyprogesterone acetate)	oral progestin
Amaryl (glimepiride)	oral sulfonylurea antidiabetic
Ambien (zolpidem tartrate)	sedative, hypnotic
amitriptyline HCl	tricyclic antidepressant
amoxicillin trihydrate	antibiotic
Amoxil (amoxicillin trihydrate)	antibiotic
Apo-Amitriptyline CAN (amitriptyline HCl)	tricyclic antidepressant
Apo-Amoxi CAN (amoxicillin trihydrate)	antibiotic
Apo-Atenol CAN (atenolol)	antihypertensive, antianginal
Apo-Clonazepam CAN (clonazepam)	anticonvulsant
Apo-Diazepam CAN (diazepam)	anxiolytic, skeletal muscle relaxant
Apo-Diltiaz CD CAN (diltiazem HCl)	antihypertensive, antianginal
Apo-Furosemide CAN (furosemide)	diuretic, antihypertensive
Apo-Glyburide CAN (glyburide)	antidiabetic
Apo-Hydro CAN (hydrochlorothiazide)	diuretic, antihypertensive
Apo-Lorazepam CAN (lorazepam)	anxiolytic, tranquilizer
Apo-Metoprolol L CAN (metoprolol tartrate)	antianginal, antihypertensive
Apo-Naproxen CAN (naproxen)	antiarthritic, analgesic, NSAID
Apo-Oxazepam CAN (oxazepam)	anxiolytic
Apo-Pen VK CAN (penicillin V potassium)	natural antibiotic
Apo-Prednisone CAN (prednisone)	corticosteroidal anti-inflammatory

Drug	*Class/Indication(s)*
Apo-Salvent CAN (salbutamol)	bronchodilator
Apo-Temazepam CAN (temazepam)	tranquilizer, hypnotic
Arthrotec CAN (diclofenac sodium, misoprostol)	antiarthritic, NSAID
atenolol	antihypertensive, antianginal
Ativan CAN (lorazepam)	anxiolytic, tranquilizer
Atrovent (ipratropium bromide)	bronchodilator
Augmentin (amoxicillin trihydrate, clavulanate potassium)	antibiotic
Avandia (rosiglitazone maleate)	antidiabetic; decreases insulin resistance
Avapro (irbesartan)	antihypertensive
Azmacort (triamcinolone acetonide)	corticosteroid for asthma
Bactroban (mupirocin)	topical antibiotic
Benzamycin (erythromycin, benzoyl peroxide)	topical antibiotic and keratolytic for acne
benzonatate	antitussive
Biaxin (clarithromycin)	antibiotic
BuSpar (buspirone HCl)	anxiolytic
butalbital/acetaminophen/caffeine	analgesic, sedative
captopril	antihypertensive, ACE inhibitor
Cardizem CD (diltiazem HCl)	antihypertensive, antianginal
Cardura (doxazosin mesylate)	antihypertensive, antiadrenergic
carisoprodol	skeletal muscle relaxant
Cartia XT (diltiazem HCl)	antihypertensive, antianginal
Ceftin (cefuroxime axetil)	antibiotic
Cefzil (cefprozil)	antibiotic
Celebrex (celecoxib)	antiarthritic, NSAID, COX-2 inhibitor
Celestoderm-V CAN (betamethasone valerate)	topical steroidal anti-inflammatory
Celexa (citalopram hydrobromide)	antidepressant, SSRI
C.E.S. CAN (conjugated estrogens)	oral estrogens for postmenopausal HRT
cephalexin	antibiotic
Ciloxan (ciprofloxacin HCl)	ophthalmic antibiotic
cimetidine	histamine antagonist for gastric ulcers
Cipro (ciprofloxacin)	antibiotic
Claritin (loratadine)	antihistamine
Claritin-D (loratadine, pseudoephedrine sulfate)	antihistamine, decongestant
clindamycin HCl	antibiotic
clonazepam	anticonvulsant
clonidine	antihypertensive
Combivent (ipratropium bromide, albuterol sulfate)	bronchodilator for COPD
Contuss (phenylpropanolamine HCl, phenylephrine HCl, guaifenesin)	decongestant, expectorant
Cortate CAN (hydrocortisone)	topical steroidal anti-inflammatory
Coumadin (warfarin sodium)	anticoagulant
Cozaar (losartan potassium)	antihypertensive

Drug	*Class/Indication(s)*
cyclobenzaprine HCl	skeletal muscle relaxant
Depakote (divalproex sodium)	anticonvulsant
Detrol (tolterodine tartrate)	for urinary frequency and incontinence
diazepam	anxiolytic, skeletal muscle relaxant
diclofenac sodium	antiarthritic, analgesic, NSAID
Didrocal CAN (etidronate disodium, calcium carbonate)	bone resorption inhibitor
Diflucan (fluconazole)	systemic antifungal
digoxin	antiarrhythmic
Dilantin (phenytoin sodium)	anticonvulsant
Diovan (valsartan)	antihypertensive, angiotensin II blocker
Diovan HCT (valsartan, hydrochlorothiazide)	antihypertensive, angiotensin II blocker, diuretic
doxepin HCl	tricyclic antidepressant, anxiolytic
doxycycline hyclate	antibiotic
Duragesic (fentanyl)	transdermal narcotic analgesic
Effexor XR (venlafaxine)	antidepressant, anxiolytic
Elocom CAN (mometasone furoate)	topical steroidal anti-inflammatory
Elocon (mometasone furoate)	topical steroidal anti-inflammatory
Eltroxin CAN (levothyroxine sodium)	thyroid hormone
Endocet (oxycodone HCl, acetaminophen)	narcotic analgesic
Ery-Tab (erythromycin)	antibiotic
estradiol	oral estrogen for postmenopausal HRT
Evista (raloxifene HCl)	postmenopausal osteoporosis treatment
Flomax (tamsulosin HCl)	benign prostatic hypertrophy treatment
Flonase (fluticasone propionate)	steroidal anti-inflammatory
Flovent (fluticasone propionate)	steroidal anti-inflammatory
folic acid	hematopoietic, prevents birth defects
Fosamax (alendronate sodium)	postmenopausal osteoporosis treatment
Fucidin CAN (fusidic acid/fusidate sodium)	topical antibiotic
furosemide	diuretic, antihypertensive
gemfibrozil	antihyperlipidemic
Gen-Glybe CAN (gluburide)	antidiabetic
Gen-Metformin CAN (metformin HCl)	antidiabetic
Gen-Ranitidine CAN (ranitidine HCl)	histamine antagonist for gastric ulcers
glipizide	antidiabetic
Glucophage (metformin HCl)	antidiabetic
Glucotrol XL (glipizide)	antidiabetic
glyburide	antidiabetic
Humulin N; Humulin 70/30 (insulin)	antidiabetic
hydrochlorothiazide	diuretic, antihypertensive
hydrocodone/acetaminophen	antitussive, analgesic
hydroxyzine HCl	anxiolytic, minor tranquilizer
hyoscyamine sulfate	gastrointestinal/urinary antispasmodic
Hyzaar (losartan potassium, hydrochlorothiazide)	antihypertensive, angiotensin II blocker, diuretic
ibuprofen	antiarthritic, analgesic, NSAID

Drug	*Class/Indication(s)*
Imitrex (sumatriptan succinate)	antimigraine
isosorbide mononitrate	coronary vasodilator, antianginal
K-Dur (potassium chloride)	potassium supplement
Klor-Con (potassium chloride)	potassium supplement
Lanoxin (digoxin)	antiarrhythmic
Lescol (fluvastatin sodium)	antihyperlipidemic
Levaquin (levofloxacin)	fluoroquinolone antibiotic
Levothroid (levothyroxine sodium)	thyroid hormone
Levoxyl (levothyroxine sodium)	thyroid hormone
Lipitor (atorvastatin calcium)	antihyperlipidemic
Lo/Ovral (ethinyl estradiol, norgestrel)	monophasic oral contraceptive
Loestrin Fe (norethindrone acetate, ethinyl estradiol, ferrous fumarate)	monophasic oral contraceptive, iron supplement
lorazepam	anxiolytic, tranquilizer
Losec (CAN) (omeprazole magnesium)	proton pump inhibitor for GERD
Lotensin (benazepril HCl)	antihypertensive, ACE inhibitor
Lotrel (amlodipine besylate, benazepril HCl)	antihypertensive, ACE inhibitor, calcium channel blocker
Lotrisone (betamethasone dipropionate, clotrimazole)	topical corticosteroid, antifungal
Macrobid (nitrofurantoin macrocrystals, nitrofurantoin monohydrate)	urinary antibacterial
Marvelon (CAN) (desogestrel, ethinyl estradiol)	monophasic oral contraceptive
meclizine HCl	antiemetic for motion sickness, vertigo
medroxyprogesterone	progestin
methocarbamol	skeletal muscle relaxant
methylphenidate HCl	CNS stimulant for ADHD
methylprednisolone	corticosteroidal anti-inflammatory
metoclopramide HCl	antiemetic for chemotherapy
metoprolol tartrate	antianginal, antihypertensive
Metrogel Vaginal (metronidazole)	antibacterial for bacterial vaginosis
metronidazole	oral antibiotic
Miacalcin (calcitonin salmon)	calcium regulator for osteoporosis
minocycline HCl	broad-spectrum antibiotic
Mircette (desogestrel, ethinyl estradiol)	biphasic oral contraceptive
Monopril (fosinopril sodium)	antihypertensive, ACE inhibitor
naproxen sodium	antiarthritic, analgesic, NSAID
Nasonex (mometasone furoate)	nasal steroid for allergic rhinitis
Necon (norethindrone, ethinyl estradiol)	monophasic oral contraceptive
neomycin/polymyxin/hydrocortisone	antibiotic, steroidal anti-inflammatory
Neurontin (gabapentin)	anticonvulsant
nitroglycerin	antianginal, coronary vasodilator
NitroQuick (nitroglycerin)	antianginal, coronary vasodilator
nortriptyline HCl	tricyclic antidepressant
Norvasc (amlodipine)	antianginal, antihypertensive
Novamoxin (CAN) (amoxicillin trihydrate)	antibiotic
Novo-Glyburide (CAN) (glyburide)	antidiabetic

Drug	*Class/Indication(s)*
Novo-Hydrazide (CAN) (hydrochlorothiazide)	diuretic, antihypertensive
Novo-Lorazem (CAN) (lorazepam)	anxiolytic, tranquilizer
Novo-Medrone (CAN) (medroxyprogesterone acetate)	oral progestin
Novo-Metformin (CAN) (metformin HCl)	antidiabetic
Novo-Metoprol (CAN) (metoprolol tartrate)	antianginal, antihypertensive
Novo-Ranidine (CAN) (ranitidine HCl)	histamine antagonist for gastric ulcers
Novo-Salmol (CAN) (salbutamol)	bronchodilator
Novo-Semide (CAN) (furosemide)	diuretic, antihypertensive
Novo-Triptyn (CAN) (amitriptyline HCl)	tricyclic antidepressant
Novoxapam (CAN) (oxazepam)	anxiolytic
Ortho-Cyclen (norgestimate, ethinyl estradiol)	monophasic oral contraceptive
Ortho-Novum 7/7/7 (norethindrone, ethinyl estradiol)	triphasic oral contraceptive
Ortho Tri-Cyclen (norgestimate, ethinyl estradiol)	triphasic oral contraceptive
oxycodone HCl/acetaminophen	narcotic analgesic, NSAID
OxyContin (oxycodone HCl)	narcotic analgesic
Oxycoset (CAN) (oxycodone HCl, acetaminophen)	narcotic analgesic
Pantoloc (CAN) (pantoprazole sodium)	proton pump inhibitor for GERD
Patanol (olopatadine HCl)	ophthalmic antihistamine for allergy
Paxil (paroxetine HCl)	antidepressant
penicillin VK (penicillin V potassium)	natural antibiotic
Pepcid (famotidine)	histamine antagonist for gastric ulcers
Percocet (oxycodone HCl, acetaminophen)	narcotic analgesic
phenazopyridine HCl	urinary tract analgesic
Phenergan (promethazine HCl)	antihistamine, antiemetic, sedative
phenobarbital; phenobarbital sodium	anticonvulsant, hypnotic, sedative
phenylpropanolamine HCl/guaifenesin	decongestant, expectorant
Plavix (clopidogrel bisulfate)	platelet aggregation inhibitor
Plendil (felodipine)	antihypertensive
potassium chloride	potassium supplement
Pravachol (pravastatin sodium)	antihyperlipidemic
prednisone	corticosteroidal anti-inflammatory
Premarin (conjugated estrogens)	estrogen replacement
Prempro (conjugated estrogens, medroxyprogesterone acetate)	hormone replacement therapy
Prepulsid (CAN) (cisapride)	treatment for nocturnal GERD
Prevacid (lansoprazole)	antisecretory, antiulcer
Prilosec (omeprazole)	proton pump inhibitor for GERD
Prinivil (lisinopril)	antihypertensive, ACE inhibitor
Procardia XL (nifedipine)	antianginal, antihypertensive
promethazine HCl	antihistamine, antiemetic
promethazine with codeine	narcotic antitussive, antihistamine

Drug	*Class/Indication(s)*
Prometrium [CAN] (progesterone)	oral progestin
propoxyphene napsylate/acetaminophen	narcotic analgesic, NSAID
propranolol HCl	antihypertensive, antiarrhythmic
Proventil HFA (albuterol)	bronchodilator
Provera [CAN] (medroxyprogesterone acetate)	oral progestin
Prozac (fluoxetine HCl)	antidepressant
Pulmicort [CAN] (budesonide)	steroidal anti-inflammatory for asthma
ranitidine	histamine antagonist for gastric ulcers
Relafen (nabumetone)	antiarthritic, NSAID
Remeron (mirtazapine)	tetracyclic antidepressant
Risperdal (risperidone)	antipsychotic
Ritalin (methylphenidate HCl)	CNS stimulant for ADHD
Roxicet (oxycodone HCl, acetaminophen)	narcotic analgesic, NSAID
salbutamol sulfate	bronchodilator
Serevent (salmeterol xinafoate)	antiasthmatic, bronchodilator
Serzone (nefazodone HCl)	antidepressant
Singulair (montelukast sodium)	antiasthmatic
Skelaxin (metaxalone)	skeletal muscle relaxant
spironolactone	antihypertensive, diuretic
Synthroid (levothyroxine sodium)	thyroid replacement
tamoxifen citrate	antineoplastic for breast cancer
temazepam	tranquilizer, hypnotic
Tequin (gatifloxacin)	broad-spectrum antibiotic
Terazol 7 (terconazole)	vaginal antifungal
terazosin HCl	α-blocker for hypertension and BPH
theophylline (sustained-release form)	bronchodilator
Tiazac (diltiazem HCl)	antihypertensive, antianginal
Tobradex (tobramycin, dexamethasone)	ophthalmic antibiotic and steroid
Toprol XL (metoprolol succinate)	antihypertensive, antianginal
trazodone HCl	tetracyclic antidepressant
triamcinolone acetonide	topical steroidal anti-inflammatory
triamterene/hydrochlorothiazide	diuretic, antihypertensive
trimethoprim/sulfamethoxazole	anti-infective, antibacterial
Trimox (amoxicillin trihydrate)	antibiotic
Triphasil (levonorgestrel, ethinyl estradiol)	triphasic oral contraceptive
Tussionex Pennkinetic (hydrocodone polistirex, chlorpheniramine polistirex)	narcotic antitussive, antihistamine
Tylenol with Codeine #2, #3 (acetaminophen, codeine phosphate)	analgesic, anti-inflammatory
Ultram (tramadol HCl)	analgesic
Valtrex (valacyclovir HCl)	oral antiviral
Vasotec (enalaprilat maleate)	antihypertensive, ACE inhibitor
Veetids (penicillin V potassium)	antibiotic
verapamil HCl (sustained-release form)	antianginal, antiarrhythmic, calcium channel blocker

Drug	*Class/Indication(s)*
Viagra (sildenafil citrate)	vasodilator for erectile dysfunction
Vicoprofen (hydrocodone bitartrate, ibuprofen)	narcotic analgesic
Vioxx (rofecoxib)	antiarthritic, NSAID, COX-2 inhibitor
warfarin sodium	anticoagulant
Wellbutrin SR (bupropion HCl)	antidepressant
Xalatan (latanoprost)	antiglaucoma
Zestoretic (hydrochlorothiazide, lisinopril)	antihypertensive, ACE inhibitor, diuretic
Zestril (lisinopril)	antihypertensive
Ziac (hydrochlorothiazide, bisoprolol fumarate)	antihypertensive
Zithromax (azithromycin dihydrate)	antibiotic
Zocor (simvastatin)	antihyperlipidemic
Zoloft (sertraline)	antidepressant
Zyban (CAN) (bupropion HCl)	smoking cessation aid
Zyprexa (olanzapine)	antipsychotic, antimanic
Zyrtec (cetirizine HCl)	antihistamine

Dropped from the previous year's list:

Alphagan (brimonidine tartrate)	antiglaucoma, ocular antihypertensive
Aricept (donepezil HCl)	cognition enhancer
Arthrotec (diclofenac sodium, misoprostol)	antiarthritic, NSAID
Axid (nizatidine)	histamine antagonist for gastric ulcers
Climara (estradiol)	transdermal estrogen for menopause
Cycrin (medroxyprogesterone acetate)	progestin
Daypro (oxaprozin)	NSAID
Desogen (ethinyl estradiol, desogestrel)	monophasic oral contraceptive
Estrace (estradiol)	topical estrogen
Hytrin (terazosin HCl)	antihypertensive
Imdur (isosorbide mononitrate)	antianginal
Lamisil (terbinafine HCl)	systemic antifungal
Mevacor (lovastatin)	antihyperlipidemic
Nitrostat (nitroglycerin)	antianginal, coronary vasodilator
Propulsid (cisapride)	gastroesophageal reflux treatment
Rezulin (troglitazone)	oral antidiabetic agent
Vancenase AQ, DS (beclomethasone dipropionate)	steroidal anti-inflammatory